Oski's
ESSENTIAL
PEDIATRICS

OSKI'S
ESSENTIAL
PEDIATRICS

Editors

KEVIN B. JOHNSON, M.D., M.S.
Assistant Professor of Pediatrics
The Johns Hopkins University School of Medicine
Department of Pediatrics
The Johns Hopkins Hospital
Baltimore, Maryland

FRANK A. OSKI, M.D.
Distinguished Service Professor
The Johns Hopkins University School of Medicine
Department of Pediatrics
The Johns Hopkins Hospital
Baltimore, Maryland

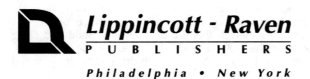

Lippincott - Raven
PUBLISHERS

Philadelphia • New York

Acquisitions Editor: Paula Callaghan
Assistant Editor: Julia Benson
Project Editor: Erika Kors
Production Manager: Helen Ewan
Production Coordinator: Patricia McCloskey
Design Coordinator: Kathy Kelley-Luedtke

9 8 7 6 5 4 3 2 1

Library of Congress Cataloging-in-Publications Data

Oski's essential pediatrics / editors, Kevin B. Johnson, Frank A. Oski.
    p. cm.
    Includes index.
    Consolidated version of: Principles and practice of pediatrics /
editor-in-chief, Frank A. Oski. 2nd ed. c 1994.
    ISBN 0-397-51514-6
    1. Pediatrics.   I. Johnson, Kevin B., M.D.   II. Oski, Frank A.
III. Principles and practice of pediatrics.
    [DNLM: 1. Pediatrics.   WS 200 082 1997]
    RJ45.085   1997
    618.92 - - dc20
    DNLM/DLC
    for Library of Congress   96-38508
                                                     CIP

Care has been taken to confirm the accuracy of the information presented and to
describe generally accepted practices. However, the authors, editors, and publisher are not
responsible for errors or omissions or for any consequences from application of the information in this book and make no warranty, express or implied, with respect to the contents
of the publication.

The authors, editors and publisher have exerted every effort to ensure that drug selection and dosage set forth in this text are in accordance with current recommendations and
practice at the time of publication. However, in view of ongoing research, changes in government regulations, and the constant flow of information relating to drug therapy and
drug reactions, the reader is urged to check the package insert for each drug for any change
in indications and dosage and for added warnings and precautions. This is particularly
important when the recommended agent is a new or infrequently employed drug.

Some drugs and medical devices presented in this publication have Food and Drug
Administration (FDA) clearance for use in restricted research settings. It is the responsibility of the health care provider to ascertain the FDA status of each drug or device planned
for use in their clinical practice.

Contributors

Hoover Adger

Donald C. Anderson

Carol J. Baker

William F. Balistreri

Gerald Barber

Lewis A. Barness

Nancy M. Bauman

William M. Belknap

Phillip L. Berry

Marc L. Boom

Kenneth M. Boyer

Ira K. Brandt

Eileen D. Brewer

David A. Bross

Marilyn R. Brown

Iley Browning

Rebecca L. Byers

John L. Carroll

Thomas B. Casale

James F. Casella

William J. Cashore

James T. Cassidy

Frank Cecchin

John P. Cheatham

James D. Cherry

Myra Chiang

William D. Cochran

Mary E. D'Alton

Gail J. Demmler

Darryl C. DeVivo

Elliot C. Dick

Harry C. Dietz

Salvatore DiMauro

Patricia A. Donohoue

ZoAnn E. Dreyer

David J. Driscoll

Christopher Duggan

Lisa M. Dunkle

Peyton A. Eggleston

Lamia Elerian

Galal M. El-Said

B. Keith English

Jose A. Ettedgui

Ralph D. Feigin

Donald J. Fernbach

Marvin A. Fishman

David E. Fixler

J.D. Fortenberry

Robert W. Frenck, Jr.

Lisa M. Frenkel

Richard A. Friedman

Glenn T. Furuta

Daniel G. Glaze

W. Paul Glezen

William J. Glish

Julius G. Goepp

Edmond T. Gonzales, Jr.

Robert J. Gorlin

Richard J. Grand

Charles Grose

Ian Gross

Carl H. Gumbiner

Margaret R. Hammerschlag

Paul E. Hammerschlag

Brian D. Hanna

I. Celine Hanson

William R. Hayden

Robert Herzlinger

Peter W. Hiatt

L. Leighton Hill

Richard Hong

Richard L. Hurwitz

Nancy Hutton

W. Daniel Jackson

Joseph Jankovic

Victoria E. Judd

Sheldon L. Kaplan

Kathleen A. Kennedy

Bradley Howard Kessler

John L. Kirkland

Rebecca T. Kirkland

Mark W. Kline

William J. Klish

Edward C. Kohaut

Steve Kohl

Andrew J. Kornberg

Seth Paul Kravitz

Gregory L. Landry

Claire Langston

Marc H. Lebel

Howard M. Lederman

Carlton K. K. Lee

Carlos H. Lifschitz

Sarah S. Long

Martin I. Lorin

Gerald M. Loughlin

Penelope Terhune Louis

Donald H. Mahoney, Jr.

Carole L. Marcus

M. Michele Mariscalco

Paul L. Martin

Steven R. Martin

John J. Mathewson

David O. Matson

Irene H. Maumenee

Steven R. Mayfield

Edward R. B. McCabe

Kenneth L. McClain

Colston McEvoy

Julia McMillan

Dan G. McNamara

Patricia Mena

Laura R. Ment

John F. Modlin

Mary J. H. Morriss

Immanuela R. Moss

Kathleen J. Motil

Charles E. Mullins

William H. Neches

Donald A. Novak

Frank A. Oski

Marc Paquet

Sang C. Park

Julia Thorne Parke

Wade P. Parks

Lori E.R. Patterson

Howard A. Pearson

Alan K. Percy

Larry K. Pickering

Leslie P. Plotnick

William J. Pokorny

David R. Powell

Arthur L. Prensky

Guy Randolph

Vincent M. Riccardi

Beryl J. Rosenstein

N. Paul Rosman

David R. Roth

Peter C. Rowe

G.M. Ruiz-Palacios

Hugh A. Sampson

Pablo J. Sánchez

Mathuram Santosham

Kenneth C. Schuberth

Paula J. Schweich

Gwendolyn B. Scott

Larry J. Shapiro

Bennett A. Shaywitz

William T. Shearer

Jane D. Siegel

Richard H. Sills

F. Estelle R. Simons

C. Wayne Smith

Richard J. H. Smith

Paul D. Sponseller

Jeffery R. Starke

C. Philip Steuber

Frederick J. Suchy

Ciro V. Sumaya

Larry H. Taber

Norman S. Talner

Jack L. Titus

Elias I. Traboulsi

Walter W. Tunnessen, Jr.

Ricardo Uauy

Jon A. Vanderhoof

G. Wesley Vick III

Ellen R. Wald

W. Allan Walker

Rebecca S. Wappner

Kent E. Ward

Joseph B. Warshaw

Steven L. Werlin

Michele Diane Wilson

Modena Hoover Wilson

Jerry A. Winkelstein

Preface

The field of Pediatrics can be daunting to the uninitiated. The incessant crying of young infants, the apparent frailty of the newborn or chronically ill child, and the breadth of diseases known by acronyms or proper names can be overwhelming to the new student of this field. Add to this the sheer bulk of a standard textbook of Pediatrics, and you have a fairly intimidating clinical clerkship.

An old adage, often used to compare pediatrics to internal medicine, is appropriate here: *Essential Pediatrics* is not just a little *Principles and Practice of Pediatrics*. Like the "big book," *Essential Pediatrics* has content formatted for most situations students encounter. Problem-focused learning is addressed both in the initial chapters, "The Pediatric History and Physical Examination," and "Diagnostic Process," as well as in the section "Pediatrician's Companion." The Companion, along with information on laboratory evaluations and values, contains artists' renditions of syndromes with dysmorphic features. The student faced with a patient with a particular diagnosis will be pleased to find the clinically comprehensive sections for common specialty diagnoses. Finally, in this era of managed care, the student assigned to an ambulatory experience will be able to make use of the entire book, but will especially benefit from the section devoted to Ambulatory Pediatrics, with its up-to-date immunizations information and very comprehensive coverage of injury prevention and emergency situations.

The comparison between *Essential Pediatrics* and the "big book" stops here. The aim of this book is to consolidate and to summarize the core elements of Pediatrics in a manner suitable to both the student new to Pediatrics and for the student reviewing the basics of the field. We have made every effort to include only information that will be of use in a "just-in-time" learning mode. The student will, for example, encounter information about the pathophysiology of a particular disease only when that discussion is relevant to immediate decision making. We have tried to add tables and figures that are easy to both read and remember. Conversely, we have carefully removed text and tables that were not vital to an overview about any topic. The student preparing a thorough discussion about a subject is encouraged to conduct a literature search, or to review the "big book" for more salient detail.

We hope that this book serves its intended purpose, and that students using it will feel a little more comfortable during their rotation as a result. We are confident that our efforts for the past two years have resulted in at least one thing: your weighty fund of knowledge and light book bag will be the envy of your colleagues!

Kevin B. Johnson, MD
Frank A. Oski, MD

Contents

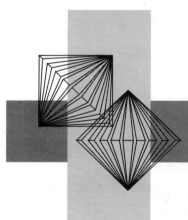

PART I

General Considerations

Oski's Essential Pediatrics,
edited by Kevin B. Johnson and Frank A. Oski.
Lippincott–Raven Publishers,
Philadelphia © 1997

1

The Pediatric History and Physical Examination

■ HISTORY

Obtaining a complete history on a pediatric patient not only is necessary but also leads to the correct diagnosis in the vast majority of children. The history usually is learned from the parent, the older child, or the caretaker of a sick child. After learning the fundamentals of obtaining and recording historic data, the nuances associated with the giving of information must be interpreted.

For the acutely ill child, a short, rapidly obtained report of the events of the immediate past may suffice temporarily, but as soon as the crisis is controlled, a more complete history is necessary. A convenient method of learning to obtain a meaningful history is to ask systematically and directly all of the questions outlined below. After confidence is gained with experience, questions can be problem-directed and asked in an order designed to elicit more specific information about a suspected disease state or diagnosis. Some psychosocial implications will be obvious. More subtle details often are obtained by asking open-ended questions. Those with organic illness usually have short histories; those with psychosomatic illness have a longer list of symptoms and complaints.

During the interview, it is important to convey to the parent interest in the child as well as the illness. The parent is allowed to talk freely at first and to express concerns in his or her own words. The interviewer should look directly either at the parent or the child intermittently and not only at the writing instruments. A sympathetic listener who addresses the parent and child by name frequently obtains more accurate information than does a harried, distracted interviewer. Careful observation during the interview frequently uncovers stresses and concerns that otherwise are not apparent.

The written record is not only helpful in determining a diagnosis and making decisions but also is necessary for observing the growth and development of the child. A well-organized record facilitates the retrieval of information and obviates problems if it is required for legal review.

The following guidelines indicate the information needed. If preferred, a number of printed forms are available, which contain similar material, or forms may be modified as long as consistency is maintained.

General Information

Identifying data include the date, name, age and birth date, sex, race, referral source if pertinent, relationship of the child and informant, and some indication of the mental state

or reliability of the informant. It frequently is helpful to include the ethnic or racial background, address, and telephone numbers of the informants.

Chief Complaint

After the identifying data, the chief complaint should be recorded. Given in the informant's or patient's own words, the chief complaint is a brief statement of the reason why the patient was brought to be seen. It is not unusual that the stated complaint is not the true reason the child was brought for attention. Expanding the question of "Why did you bring him?" to "What concerns you?" allows the informant to focus on the complaint more accurately. Carefully phrased questions can elicit information without prying.

History of Present Illness

Next, the details of the present illness are recorded in chronologic order. For the sick child, it is helpful to begin: "The child was well until _____ days before this visit." This is followed by a daily documentation of events leading up to the present time, including signs, symptoms, and treatment, if any. Statements should be recorded in number of days before the visit or dates, but not in days of the week, because chronology will be difficult to retrieve even a short time later if days of the week are used. If the child is taking medicine, the amount being taken, the name of the medicine, the frequency of administration, and how well and how long it has been or is being taken are needed.

For the well child, a simple statement such as "No complaints" or "No illness" suffices. A question about school attendance may be pertinent. If the past medical history is significant to the current illness, a brief summary is included. If information is obtained from old records, it should be noted here or may be recorded in the past medical history.

Past Medical History

Obtaining the past medical history serves not only to provide a record of data that may be significant either now or later to the well-being of the child but also to provide evidence of children who are at risk for health or psychosocial problems.

Prenatal History

If a prenatal interview has been held (see below), this information already may be available. Questions to be answered include those regarding the health of the mother during this pregnancy, especially in regard to any infections, other illnesses, vaginal bleeding, toxemia, or care of animals, such as cats, which may induce toxoplasmosis or other animal-borne diseases, all of which can have permanent effects on the embryo and child. The time and type of movements the fetus made in utero should be determined. The number of previous pregnancies and their results, radiographs or medications taken during the pregnancy, results of serology and blood typing of the mother and baby, and results of other tests such as amniocentesis should be recorded. If the mother's weight gain has been excessive or insufficient, this also should be noted.

Birth History

The duration of pregnancy, the ease or difficulty of labor, and the duration of labor may be important, especially if there is a question of developmental delay. The type of delivery (spontaneous, forceps-assisted, or cesarean section), type of anesthesia or analgesia used during delivery, attendance by other family members at delivery, and presenting part (if known) are recorded. The child's birth order (if there have been multiple births) and birth weight should also be noted.

Neonatal History

Many informants are aware of Apgar scores at birth and at 5 minutes, any unusual appearance of the child such as cyanosis or respiratory distress, and any resuscitative efforts that took place and their duration. If the mother was delayed in seeing the infant after birth, reasons should be sought. Jaundice, anemia, convulsions, dysmorphic states, and congenital anomalies or infections in the mother or infant are some of the reasons that viewing or handling of the newborn by the mother may be delayed. The time of onset of any of these abnormal states may be significant.

Feeding History

Note whether the baby was breast- or bottle-fed and how well the baby took the first feeding. Poor sucking at the first feeding may be the result of sleepiness of the baby but also is a warning sign of neurologic abnormality, which may not become manifest until much later in life. By the second or third feeding, even brain-damaged children usually nurse well.

If the infant has been bottle-fed, inquire about the type of formula used and the amount taken during a 24-hour period. At the same time, ask about the mother's initial reaction to her baby, the nature of bonding and eye-to-eye contact, and the patterns of crying, sleeping, urinating, and defecating. Requirements for supplemental feeding, vomiting, regurgitation, colic, diarrhea, or other gastrointestinal or feeding problems should be noted.

Determine the ages at which solid foods were introduced and supplementation with vitamins or fluoride took place, as well as the age at which weaning occurred and the method used to wean. In addition, note the age at which baby foods, toddlers' foods, and table food were introduced, the response to these, and any evidence of food intolerance or vomiting. If feeding difficulties are present, determine the onset of the problem, methods of feeding, reasons for changes, interval between feedings, amount taken at each feeding, vomiting, crying, and weight changes. With any feeding problem, evaluate the effect on the family by asking, "How did you manage the problem?"

For an older child, ask the informant to supply some breakfast, lunch, and dinner (supper) menus, likes and dislikes, and response of the family to eating problems.

Developmental History

Estimation of physical growth rate is important. Attempt to ascertain the birth weight and the weights at 6 months, 1 year, 2 years, 5 years, and 10 years. Lengths at similar ages are desirable. These data are plotted on physical growth charts. Any sudden gain or loss in physical growth should be noted particularly because its onset may correspond to the onset of organic or psychosocial illness. It may be helpful to compare the child's growth with the rate of growth of siblings or parents.

Ages at which major developmental milestones were met aid in indicating deviations from normal. Some such milestones include following a person with the eyes, holding the head erect, smiling responsively, reaching for objects, transferring objects, sitting alone, walking with support and alone, speaking the first words and sentences, and experiencing tooth eruption. Ages of dressing self, tying own shoes, hopping, skipping, and riding a tricycle and bicycle should be noted, as well as grade in school and school performance.

In addition, note should be made of the age at which bowel and bladder control were achieved. If problems exist, the ages at which toilet teaching began also may indicate reasons for problems.

Behavior History

Amount of sleep and sleep problems, and habits such as pica, smoking, and use of alcohol or drugs should be questioned. The informant should state whether the child is happy or difficult to manage, and should indicate the child's response to new situations, strangers, and school. Temper tantrums, excessive or unprovoked crying, nail biting, and nightmares and night terrors should be recorded. Question the child regarding masturbation, dating, dealing with the opposite sex, and parents' responses to menstruation and sexual development.

Immunization History

The types of immunizations received, with the number, dates, sites given, and reactions should be recorded as part of the history. In addition, it is helpful to record these immunizations on the front of the chart or in a conveniently obvious place with a lot number for future reference when completing school physical examinations or when determining need for booster immunizations or possible reactions.

History of Past Illnesses

A general statement should be made about the child's general health before the present encounter, such as weight change, fever, weakness, or mood alterations. Specific inquiry is helpful regarding the results of any screening tests and regarding any history of roseola, rubeola, rubella, pertussis, mumps, varicella, scarlet fever, tuberculosis, anemia, recurrent tonsillitis, otitis media, pneumonia, meningitis, encephalitis or other nervous system disease, gastrointestinal tract disease, or any other illness, as well as specific treatment, results, and residua. The history of each past illness should include dates of onset, course, and termination. If hospitalization or surgery was necessary, the diagnoses, dates, and name of the hospital should be included. Questions concerning allergies include the occurrence and type of any drug reactions, food allergies, hay fever, and asthma. Accidents, injuries, and poisonings should be noted.

Review of Systems

The review of systems serves as a checklist for pertinent information that might have been omitted. If information has been obtained previously, simply state, "See history of present illness" or "See history of past illnesses." Questions concerning each system may be introduced with a question such as: "Are there any symptoms related to ...?"

Head (*eg*, injuries, headache)

Eyes (*eg*, visual changes, crossed or tendency to cross, discharge, redness, puffiness, injuries, glasses)

Ears (*eg*, difficulty with hearing, pain, discharge, ear infections, myringotomy, ventilation tubes)

Nose (*eg*, discharge, watery or purulent, difficulty in breathing through nose, epistaxis)

Mouth and throat (*eg*, sore throat or tongue, difficulty in swallowing, dental defects)

Neck (*eg*, swollen glands, masses, stiffness, symmetry)

Breasts (*eg*, lumps, pain, asymmetry, nipple discharge)

Lungs (*eg*, shortness of breath, ability to keep up with peers, cough with time of cough and character, hoarseness, wheezing, hemoptysis, pain in chest)

Heart (*eg*, cyanosis, edema, heart murmurs or "heart trouble," pain over heart)

Gastrointestinal (*eg*, appetite, nausea, vomiting with relation to feeding, amount, color, blood- or bile-stained, or projectile, bowel movements with number and character, abdominal pain or distention, jaundice)

Genitourinary (*eg*, dysuria, hematuria, frequency, oliguria, character of urinary stream, enuresis, urethral or vaginal discharge, menstrual history, attitude toward menses and opposite sex, sores, pain, intercourse, venereal disease, abortions, birth control method)

Extremities (*eg*, weakness, deformities, difficulty in moving extremities or in walking, joint pains and swelling, muscle pains or cramps)

Neurologic (*eg*, headaches, fainting, dizziness, incoordination, seizures, numbness, tremors)

Skin (*eg*, rashes, hives, itching, color change, hair and nail growth, color and distribution, easy bruising or bleeding)

Psychiatric (*eg*, usual mood, nervousness, tension, drug use or abuse)

Family History

The family history provides evidence for considering familial diseases as well as infections or contagious illnesses.

A genetic type chart is easy to read and very helpful. It should include parents, siblings, and grandparents, with their ages, health, or cause of death. If problems with genetic implications exist, all known relatives should be inquired about. If a genetic type chart is used, pregnancies should be listed in a series and should include the health of the siblings (Figure 1–1).

Family diseases, such as allergy; blood, heart, lung, venereal, or kidney disease; tuberculosis; diabetes; rheumatic fever; convulsions; skin, gastrointestinal, behavioral, or mental disorders; cancer; or other disease the informant mentions, should be included. These diseases may have a heritable or contagious effect. Pertinent negatives should be included also.

Social History

Details of the family unit include the number of people in the habitat and its size, the presence of grandparents, the marital status of the parents, the significant caretaker, the

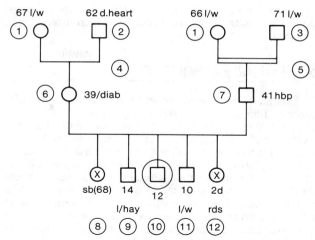

Figure 1-1. Genetic type chart. (*Circle*, female, *square*, male.) *1*, maternal grandmother, 67 years old, living and well; paternal grandmother, 66, living and well. *2*, Maternal grandfather, died at 62 of heart disease. *3*, Paternal grandfather, 71, living and well. *4, Single horizontal line*, married. *5, Double horizontal line*, consanguineous marriage. *6*, Mother, 39 years old, living, diabetic. *7*, Father, 41 years old, living, hypertensive. *8*, Stillbirth, 1968 (x, died). *9*, Male sibling, 14 years old, living, hay fever. *10*, Patient, 12 years old (note *light circle*). *11*, Brother, 10 years old, living and well. *12*, Female, died at 2 days old of respiratory distress (year can be included).

total family income and its source, and whether the mother and father work outside the home. If it is pertinent to the current problems of the child, inquire about the family's attitude toward the child and toward each other, the type of discipline used, and the major disciplinarian. If the problem is psychosocial and only one parent is the informant, it may be necessary to interview the other parent, and to outline a typical day in the life of the child.

Prenatal History

It is desirable, if feasible, to interview the mother and father before the child is born. Not only can some necessary data be obtained, but also the parents can become acquainted with the doctor who will be seeing them shortly after the arrival of their newborn. The health of the mother, whether she will nurse or bottle-feed the baby and whether the husband supports her choice, the preparation for the baby on arrival home, and whether help will be available can be ascertained. Because the father may feel bypassed by the pregnancy except for the initial event, it is important to direct some questions to him, such as, "Do you want your son circumcised?," and to get the family history of diseases first from him.

History From the Child

Even young children should be asked about their symptoms and their understanding of their problem. This also provides an opportunity to determine the interaction of the child with the parent. For most adolescents, it is important to take part of the history from the adolescent alone after asking for his or her approval. Regardless of your own opinion, obtain the history objectively without any moral implications, starting with open-ended questions related to the initial complaint and then directing the questions.

■ PHYSICAL EXAMINATION

Examination of the infant and young child begins with observing him or her and establishing rapport. The order of the examination should fit the child and the circumstances. It is wise to make no sudden movements and to complete first those parts of the examination that require the child's cooperation. Painful or disagreeable procedures should be deferred to the end of the examination, and these should be explained to the child before proceeding. For the older child and adolescent, examination can begin with the head and conclude with the extremities. The approach is gentle, but expeditious and complete. For the young, apprehensive child, chatter, reassurance, or other communication frequently permits an orderly examination. Some children are best held by the parent during the examination. For others, part of the examination may require restraint by the parent or assistant.

When the complaint includes a report of pain in a certain area, this area should be examined last. If the child has obvious deformities, that area should be examined in a routine fashion without undue emphasis, because extra attention may increase embarrassment or guilt.

Because the entire child is to be examined, at some time all of the clothing must be removed. This does not necessarily mean that it must be removed at the same time. Only the part that is being examined needs to be uncovered and then it can be reclothed. Except during infancy, modesty should be respected and the child should be kept as comfortable as possible.

With practice, the examination of the child can be completed quickly even in most critical emergency states. Only in those with apnea, shock, absence of pulse, or, occasionally, seizures is the complete examination delayed. Although the method of procedure may vary, the record of examination should be in the same format for all children. This provides easy access to needed information later. The description that follows is the usual way of recording the examination and not necessarily its required order. When diseases are given with a sign, these are examples and not a complete differential for that sign. The significance of a previous examination cannot be overstressed. A murmur that was not heard a year ago but now is easily audible has far different significance than does a similar murmur heard many years before.

Completion of the history can be accomplished during the physical examination. Talking to the parent frequently reassures the child. Praising the young child, explaining the parts of the examination to the older child, and reassuring the adolescent of normal findings facilitates the examination. Usually, if the examiner enjoys the spontaneity and responsiveness of children, the examination will be easier and more thorough.

Measurements (Vital Signs)

Temperature is taken in the axilla or rectum in the young child and by mouth after 5 or 6 years of age, when the child can understand how to hold the thermometer. Electronic thermometer probes inserted as usual or in the ear canal give rapid, accurate determinations. Elevated temperature occurs with infection, excitement, anxiety, exercise, hyperthyroidism, collagen-vascular disease, or tumor.

Decreased temperature occurs with chilling, shock, hypothyroidism, or inactivity. Temperature may be decreased after taking certain drugs, with hypocortisolism, or with overwhelming infection.

The pulse rate can be obtained at any peripheral pulse (femoral, radial, or carotid) or by palpation over the heart. The normal rate varies from 70 to 170 beats per minute at birth to 120 to 140 shortly after birth, and ranges from 80 to 140 at 1 to 2 years, from 80 to 120 at 3 years, and from 70 to 115 after 3 years. The sleeping pulse after the age of 2 years normally is about 20 beats per minute less than the awake pulse, but does not decrease with rheumatic fever or thyrotoxicosis. For each degree of temperature rise, the pulse rate increases about 10 beats per minute. The pulse rate is elevated with excitement, exercise, or hypermetabolic states, and is decreased with hypometabolic states, hypertension, or increased intracranial pressure. Irregularity may be caused by sinus arrhythmia, but can indicate underlying heart disease. Absence of the femoral pulse is a cardinal sign of postductal coarctation of the aorta.

Respiratory Rate

The respiratory rate should be determined by observing the movement of the chest or abdomen or by auscultating the chest. The normal newborn rate is 30 to 80 breaths per minute; the rate decreases to 20 to 40 in early infancy and childhood and then to 15 to 25 in late childhood and adolescence. Exercise, anxiety, infection, and hypermetabolic states increase the rate; central nervous system lesions, metabolic abnormalities, alkalosis, depressants, and other poisons decrease the rate.

Blood Pressure

The blood pressure should be measured with a cuff, with the bladder completely encircling the extremity and the width covering one half to two thirds of the length of the upper arm or upper leg. The pressure should be recorded and compared with normal readings (Figure 1–2). High systolic pressure occurs with excitement, anxiety, and hypermetabolic states. High systolic and diastolic pressures occur with renal diseases, pheochromocytoma, adrenal disease, arteritis, or coarctation of the aorta.

Height, Weight, Head Circumference

To obtain height and weight recordings, measure the infant supine up to the age of 2 years, and standing thereafter. Measure head circumference in all infants less than 2 years of age and in those with misshapen heads. Record height, weight, and head circumference measurements with percentiles on a chart (Figures 1–3 through 1–10).

Shortness may be caused by malabsorption, chronic illness, psychosocial deprivation, hormonal disorders, familial patterns, or syndromes with dwarfism. Gigantism may be the result of pituitary abnormalities. Compare sitting height and total height in dwarfs to standard measurements to determine the type of syndrome present.

Decreased weight can be caused by conditions similar to those that cause decreased height. In states of malnutrition, weight percentile is less than height percentile; head circumference remains normal unless the condition is severe and persists. Overweight usually is exogenous and associated with increased height until epiphyseal closure. Overweight

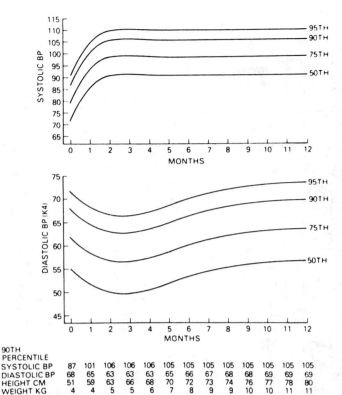

Figure 1-2. Age-specific percentiles of blood pressure (*BP*) measurements in boys—birth to 12 months of age; Korotkoff phase IV (*K4*) used for diastolic BP. (American Academy of Pediatrics. Task Force on Blood Pressure. *Pediatrics* 1987;79:1.)

90TH PERCENTILE													
SYSTOLIC BP	87	101	106	106	106	105	105	105	105	105	105	105	105
DIASTOLIC BP	68	65	63	63	63	65	66	67	68	68	69	69	69
HEIGHT CM	51	59	63	66	68	70	72	73	74	76	77	78	80
WEIGHT KG	4	4	5	5	6	7	8	9	9	10	10	11	11

resulting from endocrine disorders is associated with decreased linear growth.

General Appearance

A statement should be recorded about the alertness, distress, general development, and nutrition of the child. Mental status, activity, unusual positions, or apprehension or cooperativeness may direct one to consider an acute or chronic illness or no illness at all. The child who lies quietly, staring into space, may be gravely ill. The child who lies quietly but becomes irritable when held by his mother (paradoxic irritability) may have meningitis or pain in motion. Note any unusual odor, which may suggest the presence of a foreign body in one of the orifices or certain metabolic diseases or toxins.

Skin

In examining the skin, record its color and turgor, the type of any lesions, and the condition of body and scalp hair and nails.

Normal color of the skin is the result of the presence of melanin; depigmented areas are vitiligo; absence of pigment occurs in albinism. Cyanosis is caused by unsaturation of or abnormal forms of hemoglobin; jaundice is caused by excessive bilirubin deposited in the adipose tissue. Note the size and borders of nevi, which usually are darkly pigmented areas, and café au lait spots, which are brownish areas that may signal neurofibromatosis. White spots shaped like a leaf

suggest tuberous sclerosis. Ecchymoses or petechiae and scars may indicate abuse.

Swelling may be caused by edema. Lack of turgor occurs with dehydration or recent weight loss. Describe any rashes, many of which are characteristic of viral or bacterial infection.

Head and Face

Record the shape, symmetry, and any defects of the head; the distribution of hair; and the size and tension of fontanelles. A large head may be an early sign of hydrocephalus or an intracranial mass. A small head may be a result of early closure of sutures or lack of brain development. For any deviation from normal head size, frequent measurements are necessary. The fontanelles normally are flat. The posterior fontanelle closes by 2 months of age, and the anterior fontanelle closes by 12 to 18 months of age. Unusual hair whorls are associated with severe intracranial abnormalities.

The face may appear distinctive for a number of syndromes. For example, unilateral facial paralysis may be associated with congenital heart disease. Coarse facies occur with storage diseases. Epicanthal folds occur in a number of syndromes, including Down and trisomy 21.

Eyes

Test vision grossly in the young child with brightly colored objects. In the older child, test with Snellen's E chart. Evaluate for strabismus by noting the position of the reflection of light on the cornea from a distant source. Evaluate the range of eye movements and the presence of nystagmus. Both eyelids should open equally. Failure to open is ptosis and may be caused by neurologic or systemic diseases. Upward slanting of the palpebral fissures with covering of the inner canthus (epicanthal folds) is a sign of Down syndrome. The conjunctivae should be pink, but not inflamed; the sclerae should be white. Examine the cornea for haziness (a sign of glaucoma) or opacities. Record the size and shape of the pupils, the color of the iris, and the response of the iris to light and accommodation. In the fundoscopic examination, use a zero lens and note the presence of a red reflex, or hemorrhages or pigmented areas, and the size of the veins compared to the arteries. Any obstruction, such as corneal or lenticular cataract, will obliterate part or all of the red reflex. The disc borders should be sharp. They are blurred with increased intracranial pressure. The macula may not be clear, which is a sign of degenerative diseases. Obtain the corneal reflex by lightly touching the cornea with a piece of cotton. Failure to blink indicates trigeminal or facial nerve injury.

Ears

Note the position of the ears and abnormalities of the external ear, the pinna. Low-set ears may suggest the presence of renal agenesis. Tags and deformities frequently are associated with other minor or major anomalies. Grossly evaluate hearing, then proceed with examination of the inner ear. Pull the earlobe up and anteriorly. Grasp an otoscope equipped with a bright light so that the holding hand rests on the child's head and moves with any movement of the head, and use the largest speculum that will fit into the canal. The canal should be clear, and the drum should be pearly gray in color and concave. A cone of light, the malleus, and sometimes the incus will be identified. If the bones are not visualized, the drum is not gray in color or is

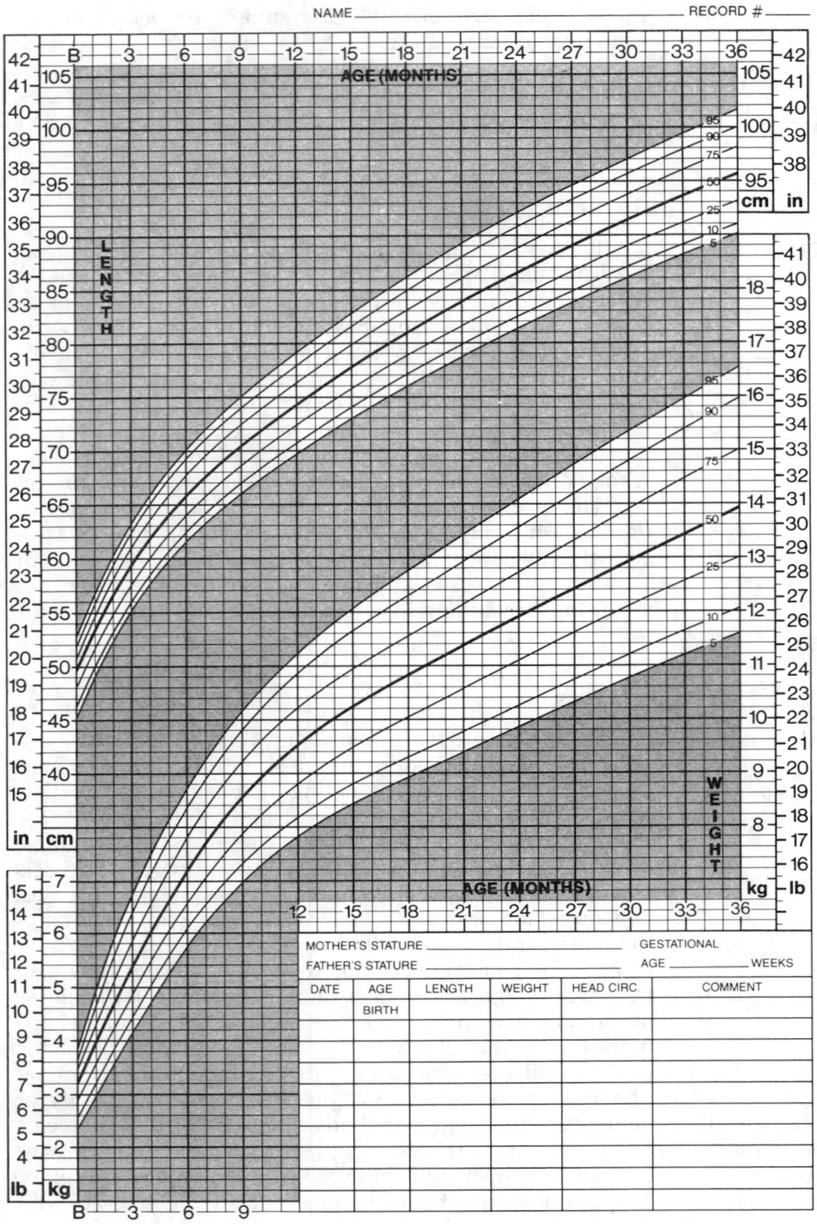

Figure 1-3. NCHS percentiles of physical growth in girls—birth to 36 months of age. (©1982 Ross Laboratories, Columbus OH 43216. Adapted from Hamill PVV, Drizd TA, Johnson CL, et al. Physical growth: National Center for Health Statistics percentiles. *Am J Clin Nutr.* 1979;32:607. Data from the Fels Research Institute, Wright State University School of Medicine, Yellow Springs, OH.)

infected, or the drum is not concave, fluid may be in the inner ear, which is diagnostic of otitis media.

Nose

Raise the tip of the nose and look up the nose with a bright light. Deformities of the septum, bleeding, or discharges should be recorded. The normal nasal mucosa is light pink in color. Tap on the maxillary and frontal sinuses for tenderness. Feel for air egress from both nares.

Mouth and Throat

Examination of the mouth and throat usually is the most resistant part of the examination and should be performed near the end of the examination. The child should be sitting so that the tongue is less likely to obstruct the pharynx. Deformi-

ties or infections around the lips are recorded. Count the number and note the condition of the teeth. Similarly, note the condition and color of the tongue, buccal mucosa, palate, tonsils, and posterior pharynx. Normally, these are pink in color. Exudate indicates infection by bacteria, viruses, or fungi, but etiology usually cannot be determined by physical examination alone. Note also the presence of the gag reflex and the voice or cry. If the child seems hoarse, question the parent concerning the normal voice. Laryngitis can lead to airway obstruction. After the age of 2 years, children should not drool. Chronic drooling may suggest mental deficiency, but acute onset of drooling is a grave sign of epiglottitis or poison ingestion.

Neck

Feel in the neck for lymph nodes, which normally are nontender and up to 1 cm in diameter in both the anterior and posterior cervical triangles. Larger or tender nodes occur with

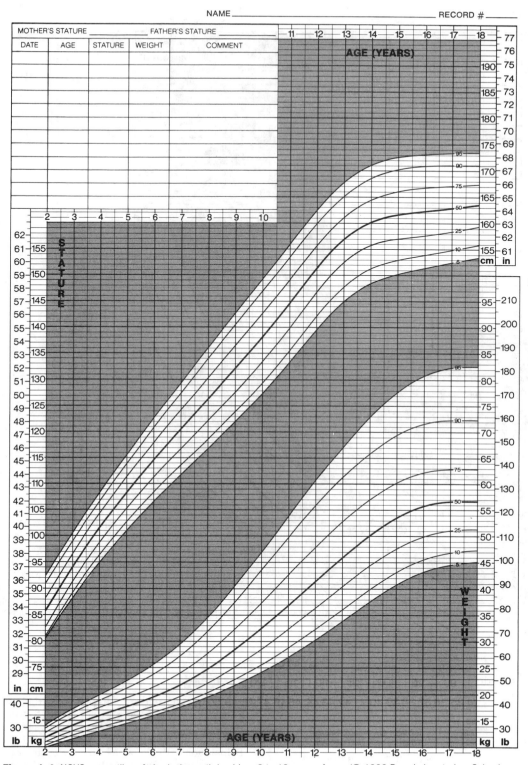

Figure 1-4. NCHS percentiles of physical growth in girls—2 to 18 years of age. (© 1982 Ross Laboratories, Columbus OH 43216. Adapted from Hamill PVV, Drizd TA, Johnson CL, et al. Physical growth: National Center for Health Statistics percentiles. *Am J Clin Nutr*. 1979;32:607. Data from the National Center for Health Statistics (NCHS), Hyattsville, MD.)

local or systemic infection or malignancies. Feel the trachea in the midline. The thyroid may not be palpable. Other masses may be present and are always abnormal. Flex the neck. Resistance to flexion is a cardinal sign of meningitis, but this also occurs with severe infections around the neck or dislocation of the cervical vertebrae.

Lymph Nodes

In addition to the lymph nodes in the neck, palpate inguinal, epitrochlear, supraclavicular, axillary, and posterior occipital nodes. Normally, inguinal nodes may be up to 1 cm in diameter; the others are nonpalpable or less than 5

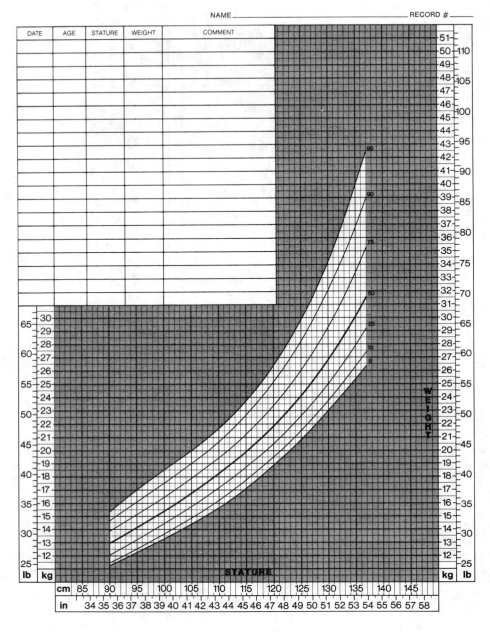

Figure 1-5. NCHS percentiles of prepubescent physical growth in girls. (©1982 Ross Laboratories, Columbus OH 43216. Adapted from Hamill PVV, Drizd TA, Johnson CL, et al. Physical growth: National Center for Health Statistics percentiles. *Am J Clin Nutr.* 1979;32:607. Data from the National Center for Health Statistics (NCHS), Hyattsville, MD.)

mm. Larger or tender nodes hold significance similar to that described for abnormal cervical glands.

Chest

Observe the chest for shape and symmetry. The chest wall is almost round in infancy and in children with obstructive lung disease. Respirations are predominantly abdominal until about 6 years of age, when they become thoracic. Note suprasternal, intercostal, and subcostal retractions, which are signs of increased respiratory work. Swelling at the costochondral junctions is an indication of rickets. Edema of the chest wall occurs in children with superior vena cava obstruction. Asymmetry of expansion occurs with diaphragmatic paralysis, pneumothorax, or other intrathoracic abnormalities.

Breasts

Breasts normally are hypertrophied at birth; they regress within 6 months and develop with the onset of puberty. Development during adolescence is staged. Breast development in both boys and girls usually begins asymmetrically. Palpate for nodules, which may be cysts or tumors. Redness, heat, and tenderness usually indicate infection.

Lungs

Examination of the lungs includes observation, palpation, percussion, auscultation, and, if indicated, transillumination.

Observation

Note the type and rate of the child's breathing. The rate of respiration varies, as described previously. Rapid rates,

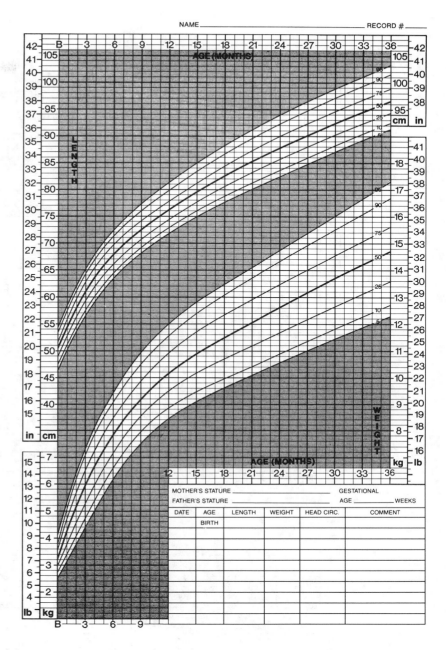

Figure 1-6. NCHS percentiles of physical growth in boys—birth to 36 months of age. (©1982 Ross Laboratories, Columbus OH 43216. Adapted from Hamill PVV, Drizd TA, Johnson CL, et al. Physical growth: National Center for Health Statistics percentiles. *Am J Clin Nutr.* 1979; 32:607. Data from the Fels Research Institute, Wright State University School of Medicine, Yellow Springs, OH.)

known as tachypnea, are associated with infection, fever, excitement, exercise, heart failure, or intoxicants. Slower rates are characteristic of intracranial lesions, depression caused by sedative drugs, heart block, or alkalosis. Cheyne-Stokes breathing, which is characterized by periods of deep, rapid respirations followed by slow, shallow respirations, is common in premature and newborn infants, and in those with intracranial or metabolic abnormalities. Dyspnea, or distress during breathing, is associated with flaring of the intercostal spaces and nares. Inspiratory dyspnea is more common with obstruction high in the respiratory system and expiratory dyspnea is more common with lower respiratory diseases.

Palpation

Feel the entire chest with the palms and fingertips. Note masses or areas of tenderness. Tactile fremitus, a vibratory sensation during crying or speaking, normally is felt over the entire chest. Fremitus is absent if the airway is obstructed.

Percussion

Either direct percussion (tapping the chest wall directly with either the index or middle fingers) or indirect percussion (placing a finger of one hand *firmly* on the chest wall and tapping that finger with the index or middle finger of the opposite hand) may be used in children. The entire chest wall is percussed anteriorly, posteriorly, and along the midaxillary line. A resonant sound will be obtained over most of the chest except over the scapulae, diaphragm, liver, and heart, where dullness is elicited. Dullness detects consolidation in the lungs, as well as the size and position of the liver and heart. Scratch percussion, which involves tapping the chest wall with a finger while listening with a bell stethoscope over the heart and liver, is especially useful in determining heart and liver size. Increased resonance is found with increased trapped air, emphysema, or air in the pleural space (pneumothorax).

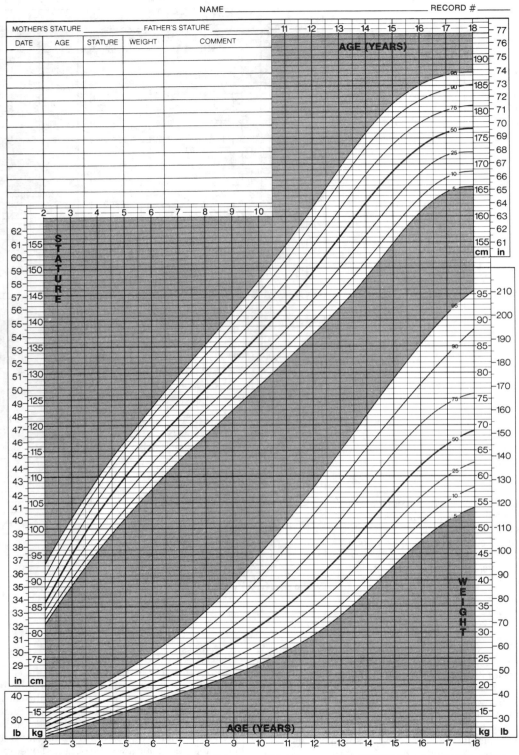

Figure 1-7. NCHS percentiles of physical growth in boys—2 to 18 years of age.(©1982 Ross Laboratories, Columbus OH 43216. Adapted from Hamill PVV, Drizd TA, Johnson CL, et al. Physical growth: National Center for Health Statistics percentiles. *Am J Clin Nutr.* 1979;32:607. Data from the National Center for Health Statistics (NCHS), Hyattsville, MD.)

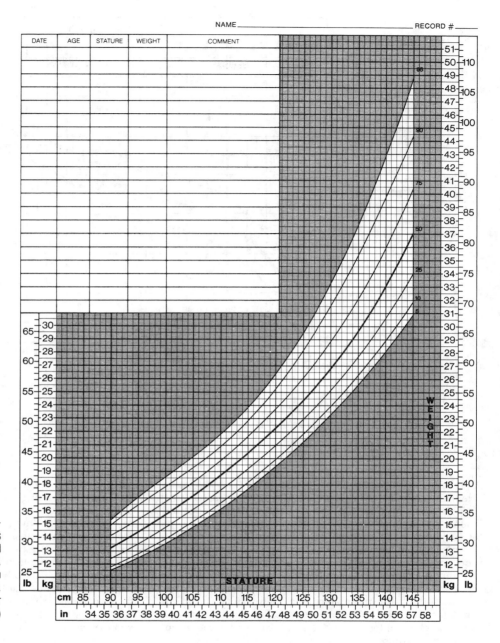

Figure 1-8. NCHS percentiles of prepubescent physical growth in boys. (©1982 Ross Laboratories, Columbus OH 43216. Adapted from Hamill PVV, Drizd TA, Johnson CL, et al. Physical growth: National Center for Health Statistics percentiles. *Am J Clin Nutr.* 1979;32:607. Data from the National Center for Health Statistics (NCHS), Hyattsville, MD.)

Auscultation

To auscultate the lungs in children, listen with a small bell in small children and with the diaphragm in older children. Normal breath sounds are bronchovesicular and inspiration is twice as long as expiration in young children; breath sounds are vesicular and inspiration is three times as long as expiration in older children. Breath sounds are decreased with consolidation or pleural fluid in the young child and increased with pneumonia in the older child. Fine crackles either in inspiration or expiration (rales) indicate foreign substances, usually fluid, in the alveoli or smaller bronchi, as occurs in bronchitis, pneumonia, or heart failure. Coarse extraneous sounds (rhonchi) are the result of foreign substances in the larger airways, as in crying or upper respiratory infection. Musical extraneous sounds (wheezes) are caused by airflow through compromised larger airways, as in asthma.

Transillumination

If pneumothorax is present, the chest will transilluminate. This is especially useful in the newborn.

Heart

In addition to the heart's rate (pulse) and rhythm, and the blood pressure, note the size, shape, sound quality, and presence of murmurs when examining the heart.

Precordial bulging is a sign of right-sided enlargement. A cardiac impulse may not be noted in a young child, but in a thin, active child, it may suggest the size and position of the heart. An apex beat outside the midclavicular line in the fifth interspace indicates cardiomegaly, which is a significant sign of heart disease or heart failure. Palpation and percussion are described above. Auscultate both in the sitting and the supine position. Determine the heart rate and rhythm if this was not

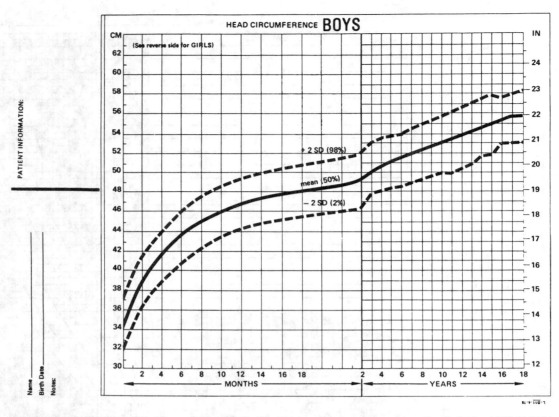

Figure 1-9. Head circumference, boys. (Nellhaus G. Composite international and interracial graphs. *Pediatrics.* 1968;41:106.)

done previously. Auscultate initially over the apex (mitral area), then over the lower right sternal border (tricuspid area), the second left intercostal space at the sternal edge (pulmonary area), and the second right intercostal space at the sternal edge (aortic area). Next, proceed to the remainder of the precordium, the axillae, back, and neck. Note heart sounds and any arrhythmia. A loud first sound at the apex occurs with mitral stenosis, a loud second sound at the pulmonary area occurs with pulmonary hypertension, and a fixed split-second sound in the pulmonary area occurs with an atrial septal defect. Innocent murmurs are systolic, musical, or vibratory and of low intensity, and usually are heard at the second left interspace, just inside the apex, or beneath either clavicle. The latter is a venous hum that may be continuous and that disappears when the patient is supine. Diastolic murmurs are almost always significant. Significant systolic murmurs may be stenotic and are loudest in midsystole over the aortic or pulmonary areas. Regurgitant murmurs begin immediately after the first sound. Over the mitral or tricuspid area, they indicate valvular insufficiency. A continuous or uneven systolic murmur along the upper left sternal border indicates patent ductus arteriosus.

Abdomen

Observe the shape of the abdomen. A flat abdomen may indicate diaphragmatic hernia; a distended abdomen may indicate intestinal obstruction or ascites. Auscultate before percussing or palpating. Normally, peristaltic sounds are heard every 10 to 30 seconds. High-pitched frequent sounds occur with obstruction or peritonitis; absent sounds indicate

ileus. Next, palpate gently, beginning in the left lower quadrant and proceeding to the left upper, right upper, right lower, and midline areas. Then palpate more deeply in the same areas and follow with palpation in the same areas with the unused hand, pushing toward the front hand from the child's back. Feel especially for the liver in the right upper quadrant and the spleen in the left upper quadrant, and estimate their size. Any other masses are abnormal. Determine tenderness and attempt to locate the maximum point of any tenderness, which may indicate intra-abdominal infection such as peritonitis, cystitis, or appendicitis, or rapid enlargement of organs, as occurs with enlargement of the liver in heart failure. Percuss to verify findings. Feel in the costovertebral angles to determine kidney size. Tenderness usually indicates pyelonephritis.

Genitalia

A child's stage of pubertal development is estimated from the presence of pubic hair. Average adolescent development in girls proceeds as follows: breast development after 8 years of age, pubic hair after 12 years of age, increase in height velocity after 12 years of age, and menarche and axillary hair after 13 years of age. Average development in boys proceeds as follows: testicular enlargement at 11.5 years of age, pubic hair at 12.5 years of age, increase in height velocity at 14 years of age, and facial and axillary hair at 14.5 years of age. Variations in order of development suggest hormonal abnormalities. Modesty of the child should be respected during the examination, especially of the genitalia.

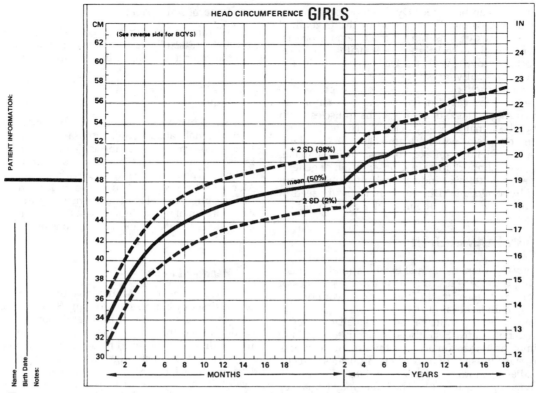

Figure 1-10. Head circumference, girls. (Nellhaus G. Composite international and interracial graphs. *Pediatrics*. 1968;41:106.)

Inspect the genitalia for urethral discharges, which are always pathologic and indicate infection anywhere in the genitourinary systems.

In a girl, vaginal bleeding after the newborn period and before puberty may be the result of injury or foreign body. Fused labia minora usually part with hygiene. Imperforate hymen causes hydrocolpos before puberty and hematocolpos after menarche. Vaginal discharge may be the result of injury or foreign body in a young girl, usually is normal at the start of puberty, and suggests infection in an older girl. Adolescents with vaginal discharge, dysuria, lower abdominal pain, irregular bleeding, or sexual activity require a complete vaginal examination. The uterus in a younger child is palpated for size, shape, and tenderness with one hand over the lower abdomen and a finger of the other hand in the rectum. For an older child, the cervix is visualized with a vaginoscope or small speculum, and cultures are obtained.

In boys, testes should be in the scrotum after birth, although active cremasteric reflexes may empty the scrotum temporarily. The meatal opening should be slitlike and the urinary stream should be strong. Hydroceles, which do not reduce and do transilluminate, and hernias, which reduce but do not transilluminate, enlarge the scrotum. Testicular tenderness suggests torsion of the testis or epididymitis.

Rectum

Inspect the anus for fissures, inflammation, or lack of tone. The latter may indicate child abuse. The rectum is not examined routinely, but is examined in all children with abdominal or gastrointestinal complaints, including diarrhea, constipation, or bleeding from the rectum.

Extremities and Back

Asymmetry, anomalies, unusual size, pain, tenderness, heat, and swelling deformities of the extremities and back must be distinguished from congenital malformations, osteomyelitis, cellulitis, myositis, or, rarely, rickets and scurvy. Joint heat, tenderness, swelling, effusion, redness, and limitation or pain on motion may indicate arthritis, arthralgia, synovitis or injury, or septic arthritis (which is a medical emergency). Observe as the child walks for the presence of a limp. Clubbing of the fingers is a sign of chronic hypoxemia, as in congenital heart or chronic pulmonary diseases.

The spine should be straight with mild lumbar lordosis. Kyphosis, scoliosis, masses, tenderness, limitation of motion, spina bifida, pilonidal dimples, or cysts may be caused by injury, malformation, infections, or tumors.

Weakness, tenderness, or paresis of the muscles suggests inflammatory muscle disease, congenital or metabolic neuromuscular diseases, or central nervous system abnormalities.

Neurologic Examination

Mental status and orientation help determine the acuteness of a child's illness, depending on the environmental conditions. Position at rest and abnormal movements such as tremors, twitchings, choreiform movements, and athetosis are characteristic of hyperirritability of the central nervous system. Incoordination of gait usually indicates cerebellar dysfunction. Kernig's sign (inability to extend the leg with the hip flexed) and Brudzinski's sign (flexing the neck with resultant flexion of the hip or knee) are indications of meningeal irritation.

Cranial nerves can be tested. Dysfunction of olfactory nerve I results in anosmia. Dysfunction of the trigeminal nerve V results in lack of sensation of the face and tongue. With peripheral facial nerve VII paralysis, neither the forehead nor the face moves. With nuclear VII paralysis, the forehead moves. Difficulty in swallowing and loss of pharygeal reflexes are caused by dysfunction of the glossopharyngeal nerve IX or the vagus nerve X. Patients cannot contract the sternocleidomastoid or trapezius muscles with involvement of the spinal accessory nerve XI. The tongue protrudes to the involved side with hypoglossal nerve XII lesions.

Examination of tendon reflexes (biceps, triceps, patellar, and Achilles) is less important than is observation of general activity. Hyperactive reflexes indicate an upper motor neuron lesion or hypocalcemia. Decreased reflexes are seen in lower motor neuron lesions or the muscular dystrophies.

■ NEWBORN EXAMINATION

In the delivery room, a minimal examination is needed. The general appearance is noted and, at 1 and 5 minutes of age, an Apgar score is assigned (Table 1–1). A score of 7 or less indicates that an infant is at risk.

The infant is placed in a warmer. A small catheter is passed through both nares. Secretions are aspirated, and the tube is continued into the stomach and the stomach contents are aspirated. Easy passage of the catheter indicates patency of both nares. Passage into the stomach obviates blind pouch types of tracheoesophageal fistula. The infant may urinate or defecate, indicating patency of these orifices. The mouth is inspected for cleft palate. Gestational age is assessed based on neurodevelopmental signs. Newborn care then is given, and further examination is deferred to the nursery.

Preferably within the first few hours of birth, an admission newborn examination is performed in the presence of the parents. The examiner should develop a routine for the newborn examination so that critical areas are never omitted. In the first few hours of life, the newborn usually is awake, but after 4 hours, he or she may be sleepy. The pressing question to be answered in the first examination is: "Is my child normal?" Although the order of the examination may vary, as with the history, a stereotyped order of recording should be initiated for easy retrieval of information if it is needed later.

Vital Signs

Vital signs include temperature, heart rate, respiratory rate, blood pressure (using an apparatus for newborns) in an upper and a lower extremity, weight, length, and head, chest, and abdominal circumferences. In addition to recording these, it is essential that they also be plotted on a chart (see Figures 1–3 and 1–6).

General Appearance

Within a few moments, observe the movement of the four extremities, the appearance of the head and neck, body symmetry, and any gross abnormalities.

Skin

The skin may be covered by a white, greasy, easily removable material called vernix caseosa. Note skin color, consistency, and hydration. Cyanosis, jaundice, eruptions, edema, bruises, petechiae, and pallor are significant abnormalities. Note also hemangiomas and nevi, their size and location. Mongolian (brown) spots over the back are not suggestive of disease, but café au lait spots, if they are numerous, may be a cardinal sign of neurofibromatosis. Papules and pustules must be identified as either normal eruptions or infections.

Head and Neck

The fontanelle size and head circumference are variable on the first day because of molding. Scalp edema (caput succedaneum) crosses the midline and may be present; this is distinguished from cephalhematoma, which does not cross the midline and is caused by subperiosteal bleeding.

Unusual facies suggests dysmorphic syndromes. Peripheral facial nerve palsies are common. Edema of the eyelids is a result of birth processes or reaction to silver nitrate prophylaxis. Subconjunctival and retinal hemorrhages are found frequently. Red reflex from the fundus, if not visible, indicates some obstruction in the preretinal chambers. Malformation of the pinnae of the ears often is accompanied by severe congenital malformations. If the nose was not found to be patent in the first examination, it should be examined at this time by passing a catheter through both nares. The mouth should be reexamined for cleft palate. The neck should be examined for shortening (as in Klippel-Feil syndrome), redundant skin folds (as in gonadal dysgenesis), vertebral anomalies, cysts, sinuses, and limitation of motion (torticollis).

Chest

The chest normally is barrel-shaped and smooth at birth, and expands symmetrically with no retractions. Unequal expansion or asymmetry suggests intrathoracic pathology such as cardiac enlargement, pneumothorax, or diaphragmatic hernia. The respiratory rate normally is less than 60 breaths per minute. Occasional irregularities with apnea up to 10 seconds can be normal. Auscultation may reveal adventitious sounds for the first 4 to 6 hours. Per-

TABLE 1-1. Apgar Score

Rating	0	1	2
Appearance	Pale or blue	Body pink, extremities blue	Pink all over
Pulse	Absent	100	100
Grimace	None	Weak	Strong
Activity (tone)	Limp	Some flexion	Spontaneous movement
Respiratory effort	Absent	Hypoventilation, gasping	Coordinated, vigorous cry

cussion is resonant throughout. Maximal cardiac impulse is felt in the fourth interspace close to the sternum. Thrills, if they are present, usually indicate cardiac abnormalities. Murmurs are present in 60% of normal newborns, but the lack of a murmur does not eliminate a diagnosis of congenital heart disease. Brachial and femoral pulses, if they are not of equal intensity, suggest vascular anomalies such as coarctation of the aorta. If chest expansion is unequal, transilluminate the chest. Transillumination occurs with pneumothorax and occasionally with diaphragmatic hernia.

Abdomen

Distention of the abdomen occurs with sepsis, intestinal or urinary system obstruction, ascites, tumors, or pneumoperitoneum. Scaphoid abdomen suggests a diaphragmatic hernia. Palpate gently. The liver's edge usually is felt 1 to 2 cm below the costal margin and the spleen tip is barely palpable. The bladder, if it is palpable, should be reexamined after voiding. Palpation of the costovertebral angle with ballottement helps to determine the size of the kidneys. The umbilical cord contains two arteries, which are small and thick-walled, and one vein, which is larger and thin-walled. A single umbilical artery is associated with an increased incidence of congenital anomalies. Erythema at the base of the cord suggests omphalitis. Note the patency of the urethral meatus by observing voiding and the patency of the anus either by observing the passage of meconium or by inserting a small rubber catheter.

Extremities

Asymmetric posturing requires careful palpation of the clavicles, shoulders, and extremities for fractures or brachial plexus injuries. Anomalies of the hands and feet such as webbing, polydactyly, and clubfoot are noted. Abduct both legs to determine any limitation of movement or instability of the hips, which is characteristic of dislocated hips.

Genitalia

Testes normally are in the scrotum of term infants. Determine the position and size of the urethral meatus. The newborn's penis is greater than 2 cm in length. An enlarged clitoris can be confused with a small penis and requires evaluation for chromosomal sex and other abnormalities of the genitourinary system. The vaginal opening is inspected, and mucosal tags, imperforate hymen, and ambiguous genitalia are sought.

Neurologic Examination

Assess muscle tone and strength. Extremities normally recoil spontaneously when they are extended from a flexed position and thrash about when irritated. Moro's reflex, which is obtained by loud noise or sudden motion, involves abduction of the upper arms and legs, and extension at the elbows and knees, followed by flexion. Absence of this reflex indicates central nervous system depression. Asymmetry suggests extremity fracture or peripheral nerve injury.

(Abridged from Lewis A. Barness, The Pediatric History and Physical Examination, in Oski, DeAngelis, Feigin, McMillan, Warshaw: *Principles and Practice of Pediatrics, Second Edition*, J.B. Lippincott, 1994.)

Oski's Essential Pediatrics, edited by Kevin B. Johnson and Frank A. Oski. Lippincott–Raven Publishers, Philadelphia © 1997

2

The Diagnostic Process

Diagnosis is one of the most important tasks of the clinician. Problem solving in medicine has been described, somewhat cynically, as "the process of making adequate decisions with inadequate information."

If the diagnosis is correct and treatment is available, proper care usually follows. If no specific treatment is available, correct diagnosis is still important because it provides a basis for prognosis and advice to patients or parents.

The need for a logical approach to medical diagnosis is vitally important to the economy of the United States, where health costs account for about 10% of the gross national product. Former US Secretary of Health, Education and Welfare (HEW) Joseph A. Califano observed that "the physician is the central decision maker for more than 70% of health care services." These decisions include those for hospitalization, duration of hospitalization, medications employed, and diagnostic tests used.

The cognitive processes used in making a diagnosis are not fully understood. Perhaps nowhere else in medicine do the art and the science of medicine blend as imperceptibly as they do in the process of making a diagnosis.

Physicians use four basic approaches to reach a diagnosis: pattern recognition, sampling the universe, clinical algorithms, and hypothesis generation.

Pattern recognition is the process by which a diagnosis is made based on physical clues or linkage identification. For example, a diagnosis of Down's syndrome can be made by recognizing the physical findings that make up this genetic abnormality. Similarly, the diagnosis of Henoch-Schönlein purpura is immediately apparent if the rash has a characteristic pattern and distribution. Diagnosis by pattern identification requires familiarity with diseases through experience or study. The expression "the more you see, the more you know, and the more you know, the more you see" describes how pattern recognition develops. Linkage identification is a form of pattern recognition. A diagnosis is based on history and physical or laboratory findings. For example, the finding of a micropenis and hypoglycemia in a neonate would result in a prompt diagnosis of congenital hypopituitarism. A history of bloody diarrhea in association with a white blood cell count demonstrating more band forms than mature polymorphonuclear leukocytes would result in an immediate diagnosis of *Shigella* gastroenteritis. Skill in linkage identification, like pattern recognition, is gained by observation and study. The seemingly intuitive diagnosis, often the hallmark of the older physician, is usually a result of linkage identification.

Sampling the universe refers to the mindless ordering of laboratory studies in hopes that an abnormality will appear that will result in a diagnosis. This is a diagnostic process to be decried. In the United States, about $27 billion per year are spent on laboratory tests, and another $2 billion per year are spent on chest roentgenograms. An estimated 20% to 60% of these tests are unnecessary. If the estimates are accurate, then $6 to $12 billion per year are spent on procedures that do not aid in the diagnosis or treatment of illness. The amount spent specifically on pediatric patients is unknown.

Laboratory tests should be obtained only to support a hypothesis. If the history and physical diagnosis do not suggest an underlying organic disorder, there is no rationale for ordering a battery of laboratory tests in an attempt to uncover an occult disease. The evaluation of infants and children with failure to thrive is an example of this form of behavior. In a 1978 review of 2607 laboratory studies performed on 185 patients with failure to thrive, Sills found that only 1.4% of the tests were of any positive diagnostic assistance, and all of them were specifically indicated by the history or physical examination.

A *clinical algorithm* is a protocol, presented as a flow chart, that contains branch points that require decisions. The clinical algorithm enables the user to reach a diagnosis. The clinical algorithm is a by-product of computer science and is based on the belief that the medical diagnostic process can be automated. A number of clinical situations have been adapted successfully to algorithms, but the majority have not. An example of a clinical algorithm is depicted in Figure 2–1.

Early algorithms were comprehensive and required many laboratory tests and physical findings. Many of these procedures were found to be unnecessary, and algorithms were simplified. An algorithm is not merely a list of symptoms or diagnostic procedures, but a logical flow chart or decision table that helps clinicians make decisions. They often require a precise yes or no answer; not all clinical questions can be answered so crisply. "Maybe" or any other vague answer blocks the progression in the typical algorithm. Algorithms have not been developed for every clinical situation or patient complaint. Algorithms are not yet a substitute for decision analysis or hypothesis generation in the establishment of a diagnosis.

Hypothesis generation, the development of explanations for the patient's problem, is the most common and intellectually satisfying technique for arriving at a diagnosis. The development of hypotheses distinguishes the problem-solving process from mere data collection. The stockpiling of facts, without a hypothesis, has been likened to baseball statisticians with a great number of facts available to them but no way of determining what they really mean.

Hypotheses, or potential diagnoses, are generated early in patient encounters. Studies demonstrate that the competent physician begins to generate hypotheses the moment the chief complaint is heard. The generation of hypotheses continues as the remainder of the history unfolds. These hypotheses guide further inquiry. This immediate hypothesis generation directly contrasts the conventional strategy taught to medical students to defer all hypotheses until history taking and physical examination are completed.

Many physicians employ a common strategy to analyze presenting complaints. Initially, they interpret complaints anatomically; next, they interpret complaints physiologically; and, finally, they interpret major symptoms pathophysiologically.

Fulginiti (1981) lists seven principles used to establish a clinical hypothesis:

1. Common diseases and conditions occur commonly.
2. A single process should be invoked to explain most of the data, if not all of it.
3. Simple problems usually have simple explanations.
4. Hypotheses should derive from the data and not be imposed on them.
5. The hypothesis should be consistent with known pathophysiologic mechanisms.
6. Serious consideration of an individual hypothesis should be based on its probability.
7. Hypotheses may be formulated, accepted, rejected, or modified at any point in the course of problem solving.

As mentioned, research reveals that competent physicians tend to generate hypotheses the moment the chief com-

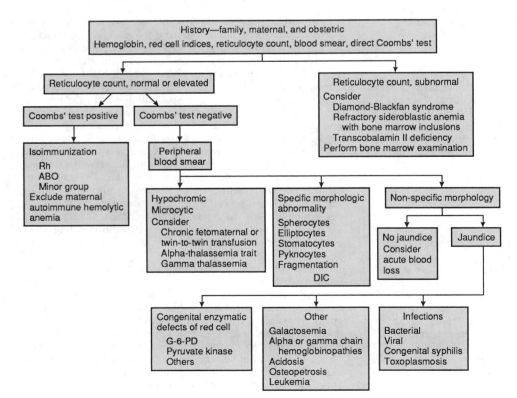

Figure 2-1. An approach to the differential diagnosis of anemia in the newborn (Oski FA, Naima JL. *Hematologic problems of the newborn.* Philadelphia: WB Saunders; 1982:72.)

plaint is heard. The same research demonstrates that a limited number of hypotheses are entertained simultaneously. It is uncommon for more than five hypotheses to be actively retained, and never are more than seven considered. Investigation often is limited to the hypotheses that survive revisions that occur while the history and physical examination are performed. Several things can go wrong. The physician may retain hypotheses that are too general and often not easily tested. Facts and findings may be ignored because they are inconsistent with a hypothesis. Physicians appear loath to generate new hypotheses after the initial list is formulated, and equally loath to discard an existing one.

The human mind needs to perceive problems as having limited degrees of complexity. We oversimplify by assigning new information to existing hypotheses rather than forming new hypotheses, even when the information does not fit. The labeling of a condition as atypical or as a "form fruste" is an example of the parsimony of the human mind and is responsible for the slow recognition of new diseases.

■ SUGGESTED GUIDELINES FOR ESTABLISHING A DIAGNOSIS

1. Always think of a number of diagnostic possibilities that are compatible with the chief complaint or the initial physical findings. Always consider the most common diagnosis first, but always include among your diagnoses those conditions, no matter how rare, for which treatment is available and which, if missed and untreated, would produce irreparable harm or even death to your patient.

2. Form a reasoned plan for testing your hypothesis. Sequence laboratory tests to establish, or rule out, the most common diseases first as well as the diseases requiring urgent treatment.

3. Don't rush to make a diagnosis for which no treatment is available.

4. Never perform a diagnostic procedure that is not related to any of your diagnostic possibilities (eg, a urinalysis in a patient being evaluated for inspiratory stridor).

5. Do not pursue a differential among diagnoses that will not alter your course of action.

6. Always consider the harm that tests might do as well as their costs. Balance the harm and the costs against the information that may be gained.

7. Be constantly aware of the natural tendency to discount, or even disregard, evidence likely to eliminate your favored diagnosis.

8. Never dismiss the possibility that a patient with multiple complaints or problems may have more than one disease. The chances of having two common diseases simultaneously is greater than the chance of having one rare disease.

9. If you cannot rule out the possibility of the presence of a disease that would result in serious harm to the patient if left untreated, then treat the patient as if the disease was present.

Probability and utility should always guide your actions.

(Abridged from Frank A. Oski, The Diagnostic Process, in Oski, DeAngelis, Feigin, McMillan, Warshaw: *Principles and Practice of Pediatrics, Second Edition,* J.B. Lippincott, 1994.)

Oski's Essential Pediatrics,
edited by Kevin B. Johnson and Frank A. Oski.
Lippincott–Raven Publishers,
Philadelphia © 1997

3

The Newborn

Two hundred years from now, if we were asked what is clinically most the same now as 200 years before, we would probably be safe to answer, a newborn infant. Even so, newborns are, in reality, extremely complex genetically engineered organisms waiting to act and react with their environment. However, they are pretty consistently the same model, year after year. This chapter deals with the usual medical care and evaluation of normal newborns and those with common variations.

■ THE BIRTH AND NEWBORN ENVIRONMENT

Efforts are now made to create a natural and comfortable environment for childbirth in hospitals. A combination labor, delivery, and recovery room (occasionally even a postpartum room as well) has been incorporated into the construction of almost all new hospitals, and fathers and others close to the mother now can be present during the birthing process. Mothers should be encouraged to hold the infant as soon after delivery as possible. This provides assurance of normalcy, and maternal attachment may also be enhanced during the hyperalert state that characterizes the newborn in the early minutes after delivery.

Because newborns are warmer than their mothers by about 0.5°C, they are born vasodilated and tend to lose heat rapidly. Also contributing to their heat loss is evaporative heat loss in the often too-cold environment. It is important to dry and wrap the newborn. A stocking cap placed immediately over the head while the rest of the infant is being dried helps to blunt this initial heat loss. Marked heat loss and consequent lowering of the infant's core temperature can cause an otherwise well infant to exhibit grunting respiration and cyanosis and to develop a measurable metabolic acidosis.

Apgar scores should be assigned (see Chapter 1), and a brief but essential examination of the baby should be done in the delivery room. This will determine whether the infant goes to the regular nursery or to a more acute care nursery. Major anomalies, labor- or drug-induced asphyxia or depression, and expected or unexpected prematurity should be recognized in the delivery room. It is also important for babies with malformations to be seen by the mother and father, with appropriate support and explanation.

■ INITIAL PHYSICAL EXAMINATION

A thorough examination should be done within 24 hours of birth. Many pediatricians use warming lights during this examination, to keep the infant warm and, hence, less fussy. It is important to have an appropriate prenatal and delivery history available, as well as information provided by nurses concerning infant behavior and feeding patterns. Evaluations by nursery nurses are done at least every 8 hours and usually much more frequently close to admission or when deviations from normal such as hypothermia, grunting and retracting, questionable cyanosis, or hypotonia or jitteriness are noted. Febrile infants with rectal temperatures of 100°F or higher need especially careful observation and evaluation.

Three percent of all newborns have a major malformation, so unexpected anomalies such as those of the central nervous system (CNS), heart, skeleton, or gastrointestinal tract may be found. There may also be evidence of physical or hypoxic stress caused by the labor or the delivery process. The examiner should also be aware of risk factors for infection or hemolytic disease. The experienced examiner is alert for subtle signs related to newborn tone or level of arousal. An infant who becomes "alert" and stops moving or fretting in the presence of conversation can probably hear. Bright lights or a flashlight beam will almost always cause a blink, initially providing assurance of at least grossly intact vision.

Experienced examiners evaluate the neurologic system throughout the examination, using the infant's response to the general examination as an indicator of neurologic status. Painful components of the examination usually elicit an aversion response, the absence of which might indicate CNS pathology. Redressing or briefly holding and cuddling an infant will usually quiet a crying infant, although using a pacifier is often the most effective method. The infant's general patterns of response may provide clues to underlying pathology.

Heart and Lungs

The heart and lungs are commonly examined first, while the infant is still quiet and unchilled. This part of the examination can be done with just the shirt pulled up and the diapers on, thus causing the least disturbance to and chilling of the baby. The infant should be examined for the presence of central cyanosis. *Acrocyanosis*—blue hands, blue feet, and occasionally even blue lips (but a pink tongue)—is normal, especially if the baby is cold. All the rest of the skin should be pink. Heart sounds loudest on the right suggest dextrocardia or possibly a left pneumothorax. Rate and rhythm should be noted; a rate between 90 and 160 is in the normal range. Some irregularity of rhythm, usually from premature ventricular contractions, is common, and, if it is an isolated finding, this is usually benign and transient. Systolic murmurs are common on the first day and usually reflect the closing ductus arteriosus or are simple flow murmurs. Persistent murmurs or murmurs accompanied by an overactive heart or in the presence of a fixed rate or tachycardia need careful evaluation. Femoral pulses may be difficult to palpate but should be sought in the presence of systolic murmurs to rule out coarctation of the aorta.

A pink, apparently well-oxygenated infant who is breathing quietly without retractions and grunting is immediately reassuring to the examiner. Most infants breathe rather irregularly in the first day or two of life, and the depth of each breath varies as well. Their abdomens often rise and fall because they use their diaphragms more than their intercostal muscles. Asymmetry, intercostal retractions, and tachypnea (a respiratory rate over 60) are worrisome if they are more than transient findings.

Abdomen

Examination of the abdomen should be done with the infant naked. Again, observation is important. In the first day, the newborn abdomen is full and rounded, not asymmetric or scaphoid. *Diastasis recti*, nonunion of the two rectus muscles from the umbilicus to the xiphoid, often causes a mild hernia-

tion in the midline. Asymmetry, unless it is due to a big stomach bubble (often just after eating or crying), may be a clue to an abnormal abdominal mass. A scaphoid abdomen, usually with accompanying respiratory symptoms, might indicate a diaphragmatic hernia with some of the abdominal contents up in the chest. The veins in the skin over the upper abdomen often appear dilated. The cord and its three vessels will have been evaluated at delivery but can be rechecked quickly. A two-vessel cord is accompanied by another major anomaly at least 10% of the time, so this should alert the examiner. The spleen is usually not palpable.

In the newborn, the liver edge can best be evaluated by approaching it from below with the thumb, held flattened on the abdomen and placed between the midline and axillary line, beginning the palpation at the level of the umbilicus and progressing upward. The pad of the thumb, with its greater sensitivity, will pick up the liver edge as the infant breathes. Generally, the liver edge will be felt 2 to 3 cm below the right costal margin. In infants with intrauterine growth retardation, the liver may not be palpable. In infants of diabetic mothers, the liver may be enlarged to as much as 4 cm below the costal margin.

Deep (and sometimes briefly painful) palpation is done to examine the bladder and the kidneys. With careful bimanual palpation, the left kidney can almost always be palpated, the examiner placing the third finger of one hand posteriorly in the lowest costovertebral angle and then trapping the left kidney against that finger with the index and third fingers of the other hand (Figure 3–1). The lower pole of the normal right kidney is only occasionally palpated, but if the right kidney is enlarged it will thus be noted.

Genitalia and Anus

The labia majora in the term female infant are enlarged and generally cover the labia minora, except in the clitoral region. The clitoris should be examined for size and palpated for diameter. Both labia should be spread, and the pink, glistening vaginal orifice should be examined for patency and discharge (usually creamy and white). An apparent imperforate hymen should be checked with a small soft catheter to see if it will slip by, because an enlarged Bartholin's gland often mimics imperforation. The fourchette should be checked for any fistula. The labia majora should be palpated briefly for masses (which, when present, are most commonly an ovary).

In the male, the penis and foreskin should be examined for hypospadias, with consideration given to the size of the penis. A hooded foreskin may be present in a first-degree hypospadias. The scrotum's rugation and size should be noted. Testes should be palpated bilaterally. Finding nonpalpable testes in any phenotypic male should raise a question of virilizing adrenal hyperplasia. Undescended testes are commonly found in males with less than 34 weeks of gestation.

The anus should be checked for patency and position. Occasionally, large fistulae are mistaken for a normal anus.

Hips

Dislocated hips are the most common hidden and quiescent anomaly, and, unfortunately, if not diagnosed until the infant (or even child) starts to walk, can result in permanent disability. The hips are examined by placing the legs in a frog-leg position, with the third fingertip on the greater trochanter and the thumb pressing laterally and down on the inside of the knee until the knee is pressed against the mat-

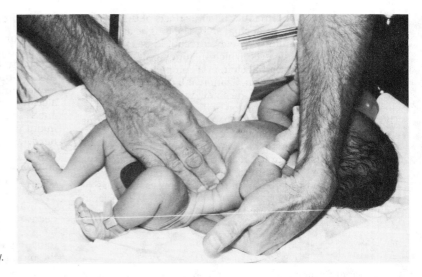

Figure 3-1. Palpation of the left kidney.

tress; meanwhile, the third finger is pushing up toward the examiner. In other words, the femoral head most commonly has dislocated following a vector that has a posterior superior and a lateral component, so to relocate it the examiner is trying to bring the femoral head back upward. The knee abducted in the frog-leg position tightens the anterior segment of the hip capsule, thus creating a fulcrum that permits the head of the femur to move back into its socket. One sign of a dislocated hip is an asymmetric crease of skin folds under the buttock (Galeazzi's sign). This sign is not helpful if there is bilateral dislocation. The possibility of undiagnosed dislocated hips should obviously be rechecked at follow-up physical examinations.

Extremities and Joints

All long bones should be palpated briefly for unexpected fractures. Joints should be assessed for range of motion and evidence of uterine deformation. The most common deformation is tibial bowing and the next most common is forefoot adduction, with a clubfoot being the most extreme. Any foot that can be corrected passively to a neutral position will usually correct spontaneously over time. Counting the fingers and toes avoids the embarrassment of being asked later, "Why does my baby have six toes?" The clavicles should be palpated for fracture, which, if present, heals spontaneously. Thought should be given to the length of the limbs; the fingers should extend as far as the lower buttocks when stretched out. Infants presenting by breech often hold their legs in bizarre positions, yet in a matter of days all returns to normal.

Head, Eyes, and Ears

Normal head circumference at term is between 33 and 38 cm. The head should be observed and palpated for the degree of molding and *caput succedaneum* (edema of the leading portion of the scalp in a vertex delivery). Occasionally, the degree of molding is marked but still benign (Figure 3–2). A caput occasionally obscures a developing cephalohematoma (the latter caused by bleeding under the outer periosteum of a parietal bone). Cephalohematomas usually do not mature until day 2 or 3 of life and, being subperiosteal, do not extend beyond the suture line as do caputs.

The parietal and coronal sutures should be examined for patency and mobility. If the head circumference is within normal limits, the diameter of the anterior fontanelle can vary from 1 cm to 5 to 6 cm. Very large anterior fontanelles may be associated with hypothyroidism. *Craniotabes*, a ping-pong ball feel over the parietal bones with pressure, is a rare but normal variant.

The eyes may be difficult to visualize because the caput edema has migrated to the lids. In subdued light, while sucking on a pacifier or being held vertically, most infants will open their eyes. The eye examination is more easily done on the day of discharge, when the integrity of the iris, presence of a red reflex, and absence of cataracts can be evaluated. Hemorrhages in the conjunctivae are common, especially after strong labor. The ears should be examined for shape and the presence of an outer canal.

Neck and Mouth

Newborn infants may look like little football players because they have such short necks, so care must be exercised

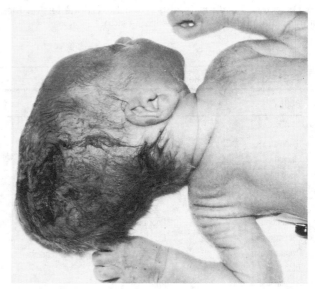

Figure 3-2. Molding of the head.

to rule out thyroid abnormalities or sinus tracts of the thyroid or of the second or third branchial arch. The tongue and gums should be checked carefully. The mouth should be examined, especially for palatal defects, which include bony clefts with an intact soft palate, a partial cleft, or a complete cleft of both the hard and soft palates. Visualization and palpation are usually necessary. *Ebstein's pearls* are small, white cysts often seen close to the midline at the junction of the hard and soft palates. They soon disappear with sucking. Abnormalities of the gums are less common, and sublingual cysts (ranulae) are unusual. If cysts are present, temporizing is worthwhile to see if vigorous sucking causes them to break spontaneously. *Asynclitism,* in which the maxillary gum line is not parallel to the mandibular gum line, is common, and extreme cases are associated with temporary feeding problems. It is often associated with arrest of descent during labor.

Skin

Normal findings and variations on the first day include tiny milia (unbroken sweat glands), most commonly found on the nose, and petechiae, usually noted above the nipple line or on the head secondary to the pressure of labor. Occasionally, 0.5- to 1-cm vesicles or pustules, often broken, with no erythematous base are seen, usually clustered around the genitalia. Petechiae scattered more generally should prompt a more complete evaluation. Jaundice on the first day should always be considered abnormal. Mongoloid or blue spots up to 10 to 15 cm in size are often noted on the trunk or thighs of non-Caucasian infants. A nevus flammeus of the upper eyelids, at the nape of the neck, or occasionally extending down to the nose and upper lip is frequently seen but will soon fade.

As part of gestational age-dating, there are helpful variations to be recognized in the general appearance of a newborn's skin. The skin during late prematurity is still quite thin, and thus that infant's color is pinker (almost red) compared with that of a postterm infant, whose epidermis is thicker and, at least in repose, appears pale with a faint pink tinge. Although there is some racial variation, *lanugo* (fine hair found especially on shoulders) is more common as prematurity increases. *Vernix caseosa,* the greasy, white, often quite copious material produced in utero by the exocrine glands, is most common after 35 weeks of gestation and is usually completely shed into the amniotic fluid after the 40th to 41st week. Postterm infants either have none left on their skin or have it only in creases in the skin.

Neurologic Examination

Neurologic assessment of the newborn usually includes evaluation of cranial nerves, peripheral motor activity, general body tone, the quality of the cry, the level of alertness, the newborn reflexes, and occasionally some of the deep tendon reflexes (Table 3–1). Body tone is most easily evaluated with the infant held up off the mattress face-down, balanced over a hand on the chest. Held thus, the normal-term infant will generally hold the arms and legs flexed, and the head, although hanging down somewhat, will have some degree of extension. With the infant in this position, the spine can be examined for anomalies such as pilonidal sinus tracts and neural tube defects. Variations of the infant's cry can be assessed for strength and quality.

Most so-called newborn reflexes, such as the Moro reflex, decrease with repetition. The sucking and rooting reflexes can be assessed with a pacifier or a well-scrubbed finger. Lightly touching the upper lip laterally elicits the *rooting response,* with the mouth opening and the head turning toward the touch. The *Moro reflex* to being startled is characterized by extension of the arms with fingers extended, flexion of the thighs, grasping of the toes, and a strong cry, followed by folding of the arms and relaxation of the hands (Figure 3–3). The Moro reflex can be elicited by dropping the end of the crib 10° to 20° or by pulling the infant by the arms slightly off the bed, followed by a sudden release. The stepping and placing responses may be difficult to elicit. The *stepping reflex* is elicited by placing and pushing the infant's feet against the mattress and then leaning the infant far forward to flex the feet up toward the tibiae. With gentle rocking from side to side, the infant may take a few clumsy steps forward. (This is possibly a fetal reflex that may assist the fetus to the vertex position before delivery and may still be functioning in the early newborn period.) The *placing response* is brought out by holding the top of the infant's feet against the edge of the crib or a similar object. The infant will then lift that leg and place the foot on the object. Normal reflexes are indicators more of peripheral than central neurologic integrity at birth, and so cannot exclude occasional severe CNS pathology.

Normal Variations

It is important for the examiner to decide whether particular variations of physical findings are within the normal range. For instance, most infants void within 24 hours and pass their first meconium stool by 48 hours, yet the great majority

TABLE 3-1. Common Reflexes of Newborns and Infants

Reflex	Newborn	2 Months	4 Months	6 Months	8 Months
Moro	Present/Complete		Fading/Partial	Absent	
Stepping	Present	Fading		Absent	
Placing	Present	Fading		Absent	
Tonic neck	Present	Fading			
Rooting	Excellent	Fading		Absent	
Sucking	Present		Fading (replaced by purposeful activity)		
Head control	Poor but present	Improving	Good		
Palmar grasp	Excellent	Fading		Absent	
Plantar grasp	Excellent	Fading		Absent	
Triceps	Present				
Patellar	Present				

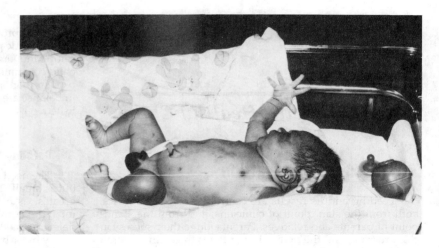

Figure 3-3. The Moro reflex.

of term infants have both urinated and passed meconium by 12 hours or earlier. Concern about cardiac findings, especially murmurs, is common. A first-day murmur associated with a heart rate of less than 160 at rest and an examination not associated with hyperdynamic activity, respiratory symptoms, or cyanosis may not require further workup. Murmurs lasting more than a day, however, especially when accompanied by other clinical symptoms, need further evaluation, including chest x-ray and electrocardiogram (ECG) evaluation. Acrocyanosis must be differentiated from general cyanosis. If the infant's tongue is pink, then general cyanosis is not present.

Respiratory variations include transient tachypnea (a rate over 60) or periodic breathing. If the tachypnea changes minute by minute and there are intervals of minutes when the rate is below 60 per minute, that is a good prognostic sign. Periodic breathing, accompanied by periods of hypoventilation, should be of no concern as long as no color change accompanies the finding. Persistent expiratory grunting, especially if the infant is not cold, requires additional evaluation. Cyanosis accompanying hard crying only is not uncommon.

CNS variations are common. For excessive irritability, the examiner must exclude problems such as previous hypoxia or trauma, hypoglycemia, drug withdrawal, or infection. If an irritable infant is easily soothed by a pacifier or by holding, the process is more likely benign. Infants may appear to be somnolent or stuporous after a long, hard labor. This behavior may wax and wane, with the infant "shutting down" for a brief period, but should generally resolve after an hour or two. A lack of motion or a decrease in motion of an arm or leg suggests nerve injury. Seizures are often difficult to diagnose and may be confused with the posturing and brief apnea some infants exhibit secondary to mucus or formula in the airway, but seizure activity usually involves the eyelids or hands and is usually clonic in nature. Also, when picked up, the infant with a seizure will usually continue such behavior. An infant's cry can be high and piercing, as might be seen with CNS involvement, or hoarse, as might be seen with vocal cord paralysis or hypothyroid, and yet be perfectly normal.

■ BREAST-FEEDING AND FORMULAS

Breast-feeding of newborns has had a resurgence in the United States, and, in many hospitals, at least 75% of mothers breast-feed. Feeding schedules should ideally be adjusted to the infant's demand. This is more easily accomplished when infants room-in with the mother, so this should be encouraged whenever feasible. Breast-feeding should begin within the first hour after birth, even in the delivery or birthing room. During the first hour, the baby is often alert, awake, and anx-

ious to suck. Infants less than 2 to 3 days old should be fed at least every 2 to 3 hours during the day and evening, and more frequently if awake and hungry. Newborns may awake frequently for a number of feeds before spacing out their next feeding to 2 to 3 hours. Within several days, they often can be so satiated by frequent day and evening feedings that they will begin to space their feedings as long as 5 to 6 hours apart at night. As the mother's milk supply builds up by day 3 or 4, more milk is taken per feeding, which lengthens the time between feedings. On the first day, the infant should nurse for only 5 to 10 minutes on a side, increasing to 15 to 20 minutes over the first 3 to 4 days and as the mother's nipples toughen. By a week of age, most breast-fed infants are on a fairly definite schedule of six to eight feedings per day.

Breast-feeding women need support and instruction by trained personnel. Women who have had cesarean deliveries may take an extra day or two to establish their milk supply. Breast-feeding and formulas are discussed in more detail in Chapter 4.

■ MATERNAL–INFANT INTERACTION

Klaus and Kennell (see Selected Readings) argue strongly that mothers should hold their babies (and nurse if they plan to breast-feed) for much of the first hour after birth, because findings in their original and subsequent studies indicated that such mothers had a stronger attachment to and interest in their infants, observable for months later. Recent data suggest that the mother's voice (especially a repetitive sequence) becomes recognized by the fetus, who can identify it postnatally. A new mother should be especially encouraged to have her infant in the postpartum room with her most of the time, which allows her to feed the infant on demand. Rooming-in provides new mothers with an increased opportunity to interact with their infants and to anticipate questions about child care. The professional staff (especially the nurses) should be available 24 hours a day to answer questions about care, bathing, and breast-feeding while the mother is still in the hospital postpartum. Cesarean section or interventions such as phototherapy can interrupt mother–infant interactions. Rooming-in phototherapy can be used if necessary, permitting a nursing mother to nurse on demand more easily. It is useful for new mothers to meet as a group with a supervising nurse or other health professional to discuss common concerns.

(Abridged from William D. Cochran, Management of the Normal Newborn, in Oski, DeAngelis, Feigin, McMillan, Warshaw: *Principles and Practice of Pediatrics, Second Edition*, J.B. Lippincott, 1994.)

Oski's Essential Pediatrics,
edited by Kevin B. Johnson and Frank A. Oski.
Lippincott–Raven Publishers,
Philadelphia © 1997

4

Feeding the Healthy Child

■ PRINCIPLES OF NUTRITION

Feeding and its results are central issues in pediatrics, both from the standpoint of clinicians, and from the standpoint of parents and relatives. Parents judge their success in child rearing, and the pediatrician judges the child's overall well-being, by growth.

Energy Substrates

Energy is needed for the metabolic functions that sustain life, for growth, and for physical activity. The rapid growth rate of the infant creates energy needs that are not matched by the healthy organism during any other part of the life span. Energy intake is the prime mover of the diet, without which other nutrients cannot be appropriately used. In ways that are not completely understood, energy intake is closely regulated through appetite in most persons, leading them to eat enough to grow during childhood and to maintain weight during adulthood.

Energy needs are expressed in kilocalorie (kcal) units. A kilocalorie is the amount of energy required to raise the temperature of 1 kg of water from 15°C to 16°C. Caloric needs can be estimated by summing energy needed for growth, which averages about 5 kcal per gram of weight gain, and for activity, which varies with the work required, with experimentally measured baseline energy needs for the maintenance of life. Such maintenance needs are age and gender specific. Besides varying with age, gender, body size, and activity, caloric needs increase with abnormal losses of nutrients in stool or urine and with fever, illness, and injury. The average needs for male and female infants, children, and adolescents are presented in Table 4–1. "Average" needs cover considerable individual variation. Deficient intake is expressed in the individual child as inadequate growth or weight loss.

Protein, carbohydrates, and fats can be used to meet caloric needs, providing for each ingested gram 4 kcal, 4 kcal, and 9 kcal, respectively. Essential nutrients, which are substances the body requires and cannot manufacture, are provided by the foods that supply these energy substrates, and the balance among them is crucial.

Protein

Protein contributes to energy intake and supplies essential and nonessential amino acids needed for protein synthesis and tissue growth and replacement. Essential amino acids are those that must be present in the diet because they are not synthesized at all or in sufficient quantities. Amino acids that are dietary essentials for adults are isoleucine, leucine, lysine, methionine, phenylalanine, threonine tryptophan, valine, and probably histidine. Cystine and tyrosine are not synthesized by infants at rates adequate to meet their needs. Infants also may need taurine. Dietary sources of these amino acids can decrease, but not eliminate, the need

for dietary methionine and phenylalanine. Good dietary sources of protein are listed in Table 4–2.

Too little protein intake results in kwashiorkor or, if total caloric intake is also low, marasmus. The average American child consumes a larger percentage of calories in the form of protein than is recommended. The long-term results of this imbalance are unknown. No safe upper limit has been established.

Carbohydrates

The need for carbohydrate as an essential nutrient exists but is small. The importance of carbohydrate to the diet is greatest as a contributor of energy calories, thereby minimizing the intake of protein and fat, both of which have deleterious effects when consumed in excess. Extreme deficiency of carbohydrate in the diet leads to ketosis.

Lactose is the primary carbohydrate in the diet of most infants, as is starch in the diet of most older children. Children also consume monosaccharides, disaccharides, and fiber, which is indigestible carbohydrate.

Fiber emphasis should begin after the first year. Good dietary sources of fiber are listed in Table 4–2.

Fat

The most common dietary fats are triglycerides, consisting of glycerol plus three fatty acids. Two fatty acids are essential dietary components. Linoleic acid, a component of cell membranes and a precursor in prostaglandin synthesis, cannot be synthesized by the body. From it, the body derives arachidonic acid. Linolenic acid, found in the nervous system, is also essential. Triglycerides containing these essential fatty acids should comprise at least 3% of the caloric content

TABLE 4-1. Recommended Energy Intake for Children and Adolescents

Age Group	Average Energy Allowance (kcal)	
	Per 1 kg of Weight	*Per Day (Rounded)*
INFANTS		
0–6 mo	108	650
7–12 mo	98	850
CHILDREN		
1–3 y	102	1300
4–6 y	90	1800
7–10 y	70	2000
ADOLESCENTS		
11–14 y females*	47	2200
11–14 y males	55	2500
15–18 y females*	40	2200
15–18 y males	45	3000

Add 300 kcal/day for pregnancy or 500 kcal/day for lactation.

Subcommittee on the Tenth Edition of the RDAs, Food and Nutrition Board, Commission on Life Sciences, National Research Council. Recommended dietary allowances, ed 10. Washington, DC: National Academy Press, 1989.

TABLE 4-2. Dietary Sources of Specific Nutrients

Protein	Fiber
Legumes	Whole Grain Bread
Fish	Cereal
Poultry	Fruits
Dairy Products	Vegetables
Meat (meat sources provide highest biologic value)	
Eggs	

of the diet. Deficiency develops rapidly in newborn infants who do not receive dietary fat. After the newborn period, deficiencies are less likely to occur. No restriction should be placed on fat and cholesterol during the first 2 years of life (Committee on Nutrition, American Academy of Pediatrics [CONAAP] Statement on cholesterol, 1992). Thereafter, the fat and cholesterol content of the diet can be decreased gradually to achieve the goal of 30% of daily calories from fat, with fewer than 10% of total calories from saturated fats and fewer than 300 mg of cholesterol.

Water

Water is an essential nutrient. It is required for growth and to replace losses through the skin, from the respiratory tract, and in urine and stool. Daily water needs begin at 125 to 145 mL/kg at term and decrease on a unit basis as a child increases in size. After a weight of 3 kg is achieved, water requirements can be calculated as 100 mL/kg to 10 kg, 50 mL/kg for each additional kg up to 20 kg, and 20 mL/kg for each 1 kg thereafter (Kelts & Jones, 1984). More detailed discussion of water and electrolyte requirements can be found in Chapter 8.

Vitamins, Minerals, and Trace Elements

Most vitamins, essential cofactors in metabolic processes, must be supplied by the diet. The characteristics of those vitamins most commonly given consideration in pediatric nutrition are described in Table 4–3. Trace elements and their dietary sources are outlined in Table 4–4.

■ FEEDING THE INFANT

Healthy term infants obtain their nourishment by sucking. They do so in a pattern that appears to encourage social interaction. After a few minutes of vigorous sucking, they settle into a rhythm of bursts of sucking followed by pauses. The feeder's behavior during these pauses is usually to stimulate the infant, and a reciprocity develops. The feeding situation appears to be one barometer of overall satisfaction in the mother–infant relationship, with maternal behavior during feeding predicting her overall parenting behavior.

Feeding Choice

For a healthy, term infant and a healthy mother who wishes to breast-feed, there is no doubt that human milk is the best food. Its composition is assumed to most closely approximate the needs of the human infant. It contains nutrients and immunologic properties at least somewhat individualized to the infant's needs.

Breast-feeding offers a unique opportunity for mother—infant bonding. In addition, breast-fed infants are somewhat protected from gastroenteritis, otitis media, early wheezing illnesses, and allergic reactions. Although the mechanism is less apparent, breast-feeding appears to confer to the child small but consistent advantages in measures of mental development (Morley et al., 1988).

However, if breast-feeding is contraindicated or not chosen, commercially prepared formulas offer an acceptable substitute.

Human Milk Nutritional Content

Recognized changes in the composition of human milk occur with time after birth. Colostrum, the milk produced during the first few days after birth, is yellowish and translucent, and is produced in small quantities. It contains cellular debris from flushed mammary glands and ducts. Colostrum is relatively rich in nonnutrient factors, such as immunoglobulins, but it is relatively poor in carbohydrate and fat (and therefore energy content) and in many vitamins. The exclusively breast-fed infant receives few calories in the first several days of life. In most cases, glycogen stores allow tolerance of this waiting period, and routine supplementation should be strongly discouraged because of its possible deleterious effect on the infant's suckling, which promotes the mother's milk supply.

Transitional milk, typical of days 6 through 10, is more milky looking and, except for having higher phosphorus content than either, has a composition that represents a progression between colostrum and mature milk. This progression continues throughout the first month of the infant's life.

Mature milk is a thin, somewhat oily, blue–white liquid higher in fat and lactose content than colostrum and lower in protein, most minerals, and in fat-soluble vitamins and immunologic elements. In contrast to cow's milk, the major protein component of human milk is whey. Human milk provides more cystine and taurine and less methionine and phenylalanine than does a cow's milk formula. Lactose is the major carbohydrate component, constituting 90% of the carbohydrate content. The fat in human milk is relatively high in oleic acid and low in short-chain fatty acids. Although the total fat content is not affected much by maternal diet, the composition is.

Human milk is rich in immunoglobulins, particularly secretory IgA. Cells in human milk include polymorphonuclear leukocytes, macrophages, and T and B lymphocytes. Freezing milk inactivates these white cells.

Several active enzymes are found in human milk, including lipase, which assists fat digestion in the infant's stomach. Practically all maternal hormones and several other proteins and peptides have been detected in milk, but their roles are largely unknown.

Vitamin and Mineral Supplementation

A breast-fed infant may require supplementation of essential vitamins and minerals. For example, infants without sufficient exposure to sunlight may become deficient in vitamin D. A daily dose of 400 IU provides optimal calcification of bone and prevention of rickets.

Fluoride at 0.25 mg/day is recommended for infants who are breast-fed and who receive ready-to-feed commercial formula or formula made from concentrate with local water containing less than 0.3 ppm of fluoride. Finally, if a breast-feeding mother adheres to a narrow vegetarian diet, her deficiency

TABLE 4-3. Vitamins

Name	Characteristics	Biochemical Action	Effects of Deficiency	Effects of Excess	Dietary Sources
Vitamin A (retinol) 1 μg retinol = 3.31 IU	Fat soluble, heat stable; bile necessary for absorption, specific binding protein in plasma; stored in liver	Component of visual purple; integrity of epithelial tissues; bone cell function	Night blindness, xerophthalmia, keratomalacia, poor growth, impaired resistance to infection	Hyperostosis, hepatomegaly, alopecia, increased cerebrospinal fluid pressure (also from 13-cis-retinoic acid)	Milk fat, egg, liver
Provitamin A: β-carotene 1/6 activity of retinol	Converted to retinol in liver, intestinal mucosa			Carotenemia	Dark green vegetables, yellow fruits and vegetables, tomato
Biotin	Water soluble; synthesized by intestinal bacteria; deficiency only with large intake of raw egg white	Coenzyme: acetyl CoA carboxylase, other carboxylases	Dermatitis, anorexia, muscle pain, pallor, alopecia	Unknown	Liver, egg yolk, milk, meat
Cobalamin (vitamin B$_{12}$)	Slightly soluble in water, heat stable only at neutral pH, light sensitive; absorption (ileum) dependent on gastric intrinsic factor; CoA part of the molecule	Coenzyme component, red blood cell maturation, central nervous system metabolism, methylmalonyl CoA mutase	Pernicious anemia; neurologic deterioration, methylmalonic acidemia	Unknown	Animal foods only: meat, milk, eggs
Folacin group of compounds containing pteridine ring, p-amino-benzoic, and glutamic acids	Slightly soluble in water, light sensitive, heat stable; some production by intestinal bacteria; ascorbic acid involved in inter-conversions; interference from oral contraceptives, anticonvulsants	Tetrahydrofolic acid the active form; synthesis of purines, pyrimidines, methylation reactions, one carbon acceptor	Megaloblastic anemia, impaired cellular immunity	Only in patients with pernicious anemia not receiving cobalamin	Liver, green vegetables, cereals, oranges
Niacin (nicotinic acid, amide)	Water soluble, heat and light stable; availability from corn enhanced by alkali; synthesized in the body from tryptophan (60:1), some by intestinal bacteria	Component of coenzymes I and II (NAD, NADP), many enzymatic reactions	Pellagra: dermatitis, diarrhea, dementia	Nicotinic acid (not the amide): flushing, pruritus, liver abnormalities	Meat, fish, whole grains, green vegetables
Pantothenic acid	Water soluble, heat stable	Component of CoA; many enzymatic reactions	Observed only with use of antagonists; depression, hypotension, muscle weakness, abdominal pain	Unknown	Most foods
Pyridoxine (vitamin B$_6$) also pyridoxal, pyridoxamine	Water soluble, heat and light labile, interference from isoniazid; pyridoxal is the active form	Cofactor for many enzymes eg, transaminases, decarboxylases	Dermatitis, glossitis, cheilosis, peripheral neuritis; in infants, irritability, convulsions, anemia	Unknown	Liver, meat, whole grains, corn, soybeans
Riboflavin	Water soluble, light labile, heat stable; ? synthesis by intestinal bacteria	Oxidation reduction, cofactor for many enzymes, synthesis of FMN and FAD	Photophobia, cheilosis, glossitis, corneal vascularization, poor growth	Unknown	Meat, milk, egg, green vegetables, whole grains
Thiamine (vitamin B$_1$)	Heat labile; absorption impaired by alcohol, requirements a function of carbohydrate intake; synthesis by intestinal bacteria	Coenzyme for decarboxylation, other reactions as thiamine pyrophosphate	Beriberi; neuritis, edema, cardiac failure, hoarseness, anorexia, restlessness, aphonia	Unknown	Liver, meat, milk, whole grains, legumes
Ascorbic acid (vitamin C)	Easily oxidized, especially in presence of copper, iron, high pH; absorption by simple diffusion	Exact mechanism unknown; functions in folacin metabolism, collagen biosynthesis, iron absorption and transport, tyrosin metabolism	Scurvy	Massive doses may lead to temporary increase in requirement predispose to kidney stones	Citrus fruits, tomatoes, cabbage, potatoes, human milk

From Barness LA (ed). Committee on Nutrition. American Academy of Pediatrics. Pediatric nutrition handbook, 2nd ed. Elk Grove Village, IL: American Academy of Pediatrics; 1993: 134–137.

TABLE 4-4. Trace Elements

Element	Biochemical Action	Effects of Deficiency	Effects of Excess	Food Sources
Zinc (Zn)	Component of many enzymes	Anorexia, diarrhea, hypogeusia, retarded growth, delayed sexual maturation, impaired wound healing, skin lesions	May aggravate marginal copper deficiency, lowers high-density lipoprotein	Seafood, liver, meat, eggs (Appendix J)
Copper (Cu)	Constituent of ceruloplasmin; component of key metalloenzymes; role in connective tissue biosynthesis	Sideroblastic anemia, retarded growth, osteoporosis, neutropenia, decreased pigmentation, glucose intolerance	Relatively nontoxic; Wilson disease, liver dysfunction	Shellfish, meat, legumes
Manganese (Mn)	Constituent of pyruvate carboxylase, superoxide dismutases, glycosyl transferases	Decreases glucose tolerance; induces short, thick limbs, spine curvature, enlarged joints, impaired otolith, ataxia, abnormal lipid metabolism	Relatively nontoxic; neurologic manifestations from industrial contamination have occurred	Nuts, whole grains, tea
Iodine (I)	Thyroid hormones	Hypothyroid, cretin, goiter	Thyrotoxicosis, goiter	Iodized salt, seaweed
Selenium (Se)	Component of enzyme glutathione peroxidase	Cardiomyopathy; animals: liver necrosis, muscular dystrophy, exudative diathesis, pancreatic fibrosis	Hair, finger nail loss, garlic odor, irritation of mucous membranes	Seafood, meat, whole grains
Chromium (Cr)	Required for maintenance of normal glucose metabolism; potentiates the action of insulin	Impairment of glucose utilization	Relatively nontoxic; humans, not well documented; animals, growth retardation, liver and kidney damage	Meat, cheese, whole grains, brewer's yeast
Cobalt (Co)	Component of B_{12}	Humans, unknown; animals, anemia, growth retardation	Relatively nontoxic; polycythemia, myocardial degeneration	Green leafy vegetables
Molybdenum (Mo)	Component of enzymes involved in production of uric acid (xanthine oxidase) and in oxidation of aldehydes and sulfides	Neurologic dysfunction	Humans, gout-like syndrome, antagonist of copper	Meats, grains, legumes

From: Barness LA (ed.). Committee on Nutrition. American Academy of Pediatrics. Pediatric nutrition handbook, 2nd ed. Elk Grove Village, IL: American Academy of Pediatrics; 1993: 126–127.

in B vitamins may be reflected in the milk she produces. The mother should receive appropriate supplements.

Breast-Feeding Techniques

In-Hospital Procedures. The mother who has just delivered should be allowed to breast-feed her healthy infant as soon as possible in the delivery or recovery room. If this is her first experience, a supportive person should be available to help her with technique. Thereafter, the infant should be put to breast as often as the baby is awake and will suckle. The infant should spend as much time as possible with the mother. Supplementation should be offered to the infant only if it is specifically indicated and should follow breast-feeding. When supplementation is necessary, the liquid can be delivered to the infant's mouth with a dropper or by small squirts from a needleless syringe so that the infant does not get accustomed to sucking on a bottle nipple. For the same reason, in-hospital use of a pacifier should be discouraged.

Engorgement. On about the third day, when the milk comes in, the breasts become swollen, firm, and often painful. This is a normal finding accompanying lactogenesis and is "cured" by allowing the baby to empty the breasts. If the firmness of the breast prevents the baby from latching on efficiently, enough milk can be hand expressed or pumped to make the breast more pliable.

Patterns and Schedules

The young infant nurses 10 or more times in 24 hours, initiating feeding every 2 to 3 hours. Because each feed may take a half hour or more, the mother spends considerable time in breast-feeding. Suckling time should be limited to a few minutes per breast during the first few days of life to prevent nipple soreness, but most mothers soon become comfortable with a pattern of letting the baby suckle about 10 minutes on one breast, burping the baby, and then allowing it to suckle as long as it cares to on the second. The next feeding is started with the breast used second at the last feeding. If all is going well, the breast-fed infant surpasses birth weight at about 2 weeks and gains at about 1 oz (28 g) per day thereafter. As the infant ages, it gradually allows more time to elapse between feeds, particularly at night; but frequent feeds are the hallmark of the early weeks and help to stimulate adequate milk production. Demands for frequent feeds recur periodically (often at about 6 weeks and 3 months) as the infant's caloric needs for growth outstrip the milk supply. Such increases in feeding stimulate consonant increases in milk production after 2 or 3 days, and then the feeds space out again. At 4 months or more, when the infant becomes acutely aware of its environment, it typically goes through a period when it is easily distracted from the breast, making it seem uninterested in feeding. At that time, the mother may need to repair to a quiet, darkened room for morning and evening feeds to ensure satisfactory intake.

Breast-fed infants who are adequately nourished urinate eight or more times a day. The urine is colorless. In the early weeks, infants produce a soft, seedy, yellow stool after almost every feeding. Hard, dry stools are not expected in a breast-fed infant with adequate intake; infrequent stools are normal only after 1 or 2 months.

Problems Specific to Breast-Feeding

Sore Nipples. If nipples are cracked and sore, the pain impairs the letdown reflex and makes feeding difficult. To avert nipple problems, mothers should keep them as dry as possible, avoid soaps, and vary the feeding position. If a sore nipple is interfering with feeding, the mother may be advised temporarily to initiate feeding on the breast that is least sore, because the infant sucks hardest initially. As a last resort, a nipple shield may be used briefly for a few feedings. After letdown has occurred, the pain decreases, and latching to the breast can be attempted.

Breast Milk Jaundice. Postnatal bilirubin levels rise more on average in breast-fed infants than in infants fed formula, and 1 or 2 in 100 breast-feeding infants suffer an exaggeration of physiologic jaundice produced by substances in breast milk that impair bilirubin degradation. If icterus in a breast-fed infant is prolonged without another explanation and the bilirubin level demands therapeutic intervention, breast-feeding can be temporarily suspended and the infant can be fed formula. The mother should pump her breasts to maintain lactation but should discard the milk. The bilirubin level should fall. After it does and breast-feeding is reinstituted (usually after about 24 hours), the bilirubin may increase slightly again but should then stabilize and decrease.

Maternal Diet. The breast-feeding mother should eat a good, balanced diet.

Although intake of alcohol and caffeine should be modest at best, no other dietary exclusions need to be recommended from the start. Nursing mothers occasionally report a pattern that appears to be infant intolerance, most often expressed as vomiting or colic, of a certain food in the mother's diet. Cow's milk is most commonly implicated. It is reasonable to avoid that food for a few days and then retry it. If similar symptoms follow, the food may be omitted from the diet during lactation. If the mother reports many exclusions, the situation should be carefully assessed, because the need for restrictions is unusual.

Substituting for and Storing Human Milk. Many mothers return to work before weaning their infant and hope to continue to breast-feed. If the workplace is supportive and provides time and equipment for pumping, exclusive human milk feeding can be continued with the mother pumping her breasts for milk for the next day's feedings. If formula or bottles of human milk are to be offered, it is best to introduce the artificial nipple after lactation is well established, usually at about 6 weeks.

Human milk can be safely stored in the refrigerator for 24 hours. It can be stored frozen in the refrigerator freezer for 30 days and in a deep-freeze for 6 months.

Between 4 and 6 months, most breast-fed infants outgrow their reliance on exclusive breast-feeding because of increasing caloric needs and because of the development of oral-motor mechanisms that allow drinking and eating. Liquids can be offered from a nursing (lidded) cup when the infant is sitting. Breast-feeding can be continued as long as desired. Offering foods in addition to human milk is not "unnatural." In hunter–gatherer societies, for example, premasticated foods are given to the infant at a early age.

When a mother is willing to continue breast-feeding as long as the child wants, a gradual weaning process takes place. The child takes a decreasing proportion of its calories from human milk, maintains suckling apparently for its comfort value for some time, and eventually loses interest in breast-feeding altogether. Weaning is accomplished in a way that is developmentally acceptable for the mother and the child.

Toxicology. Most medications ingested by or administered to the mother can be detected in breast milk. A nursing mother should avoid over-the-counter preparations and should remind a prescribing physician that she is breast-feeding. Compendia of findings for drugs in human milk should be consulted if maternal medication is indicated. A partial listing is presented in Table 4–5. Recent publications should always be consulted if there is doubt.

Contraindications to Breast-Feeding

There are relatively few circumstances for which a mother should be advised not to breast-feed although she wishes to do so. Infants with galactosemia may not be breast-fed, because galactose is contraindicated no matter what the source. Some other hereditary metabolic disorders require special formulas.

Some maternal infections can be passed to the infant through breast milk or by the close contact breast-feeding requires. Breast-feeding should probably be temporarily suspended if the mother has group B streptococcal disease, herpes simplex or syphilitic lesions involving the breast, chickenpox, pertussis, or non-B hepatitis and while cultures remain positive if the mother is being treated for active tuberculosis. Maternal hepatitis B and human immunodeficiency virus (HIV) infections are considered contraindications by many in developed countries where commercial formulas are readily available and easily used, because there is a risk (as yet unquantified in the case of HIV) of transmitting the virus through human milk.

Formula Feeding

Commercially prepared formulas are available for healthy term infants and for some infants with special needs. They are designed to satisfy the needs of the infant as nearly as current research can define them and to resemble human milk as closely as possible with current technology and nutrient sources.

Most formula-fed infants receive one of a limited number of modified cow's milk formulas intended for healthy term infants. Although parents may develop a strong brand-name preference, the formulas are basically interchangeable. The physician should be certain that the "with iron" alternative is chosen (CONAAP, Iron-fortified infant formulas, 1989). Controlled trials consistently show that formulas containing an adequate amount of iron do not cause gastrointestinal symptoms. For infants with cow's milk intolerance, there are several modified protein and lactose-free alternatives. Carnitine is now being added to some of these formulas after reports that it was lacking. Sucrose-free, corn-free, phenylalanine-free, protein-modified, and fat-modified formulas are commercially available for infants with special needs.

TABLE 4-5. Drugs and Human Milk

CONTRAINDICATED FOR THE BREAST-FEEDING MOTHER

Amethopterin, biomocriptine, cimetidine,* clemastines, cyclophosphamide, ergotamine, gold salts, methimazole, phenindione, thiouracil

CEASE BREAST FEEDING UNTIL DRUG IS EXCRETED

Radiopharmaceuticals: gallium 69 (2 wk), iodine 125 (12 d), iodine-131 (2–14 d), radioactive sodium (96 h), technetium 99m (15–72 h)

Chloramphenicol, clindamycin,† clonidine,† zomepirac†

USUALLY COMPATIBLE, BUT ADVERSE EFFECTS REPORTED OR POSSIBLE

Anesthetics, Sedatives

Alcohol, bromide, chloral hydrate, methyprylon, diazepam and flurazepam as single doses (avoid chronic use)

Antiepileptics (avoid chronic use, if possible)

Carbamazepine, ethosoximide, phenobarbital, phenytoin, primidone, thiopental, valproic acid

Antihistamines, Decongestants

Chlorpheniramine, cyproheptadine, dexbrompheniramine maleate with D-isoephedrine, diphenhydramine, brompheniramine, ephedrine, pseudoephedrine

Antihypertensives, Cardiovascular Drugs

Quinidine, reserpine

Anti-infective Drugs

Amantadine, ethambutol,† isoniazid,† methenamine, sulfas (avoid in immediate newborn period)

Antithyroid Drugs

Carbimazole, methimazole, propylthiouracil

Bronchodilators

Albuterol, isoproterenol, metaproterenol, terbutaline, prednisone in short-term use, theophylline

Diuretics (may supress lactation)

Bendoflumethiazide, chlorothiazide, chlorthalidone, furosemide, hydrochlorothiazide, methyclothiazide, spironolactone

Hormones

Estrogen/progesterone contraceptives

Muscle Relaxants

Carisoprodol

Pain Relievers

Indomethacin, salicylates†

Psychotropic Agents

Antianxiety drugs: chlordiazepoxide, clorazepate, diazepam,* hydroxyzine, meprobamate,* oxazepam, prazepam*

Antidepressants: lithium*

BREAST FEEDING NEED NOT BE INTERRUPTED

Anesthetics, Sedatives

Barbiturate, chloroform, diphenhydramine, halothane, hydroxyzine, magnesium sulfate, secobarbitol

Anticoagulants

Bishydroxycoumarin, Coumadin, heparin

Antihistamines, Decongestants, and Bronchodilators

Diphenhydramine, diphylline,* trimeprazine, tripelennamine

Antihypertensives, Cardiovascular Drugs

Atenolol, captopril, digoxin, disopyramide, guanethidine, hydralazine, methyldopa, metoprolol,* nadolol,* propranolol

Anti-infective Drugs

Cefadroxil, cefazolin, cefotaxmine, cefoxitin, cephalexin, cephalothin, chloroquine, dicloxacillin, erythromycin, gentamicin, nafcillin, nalidixic acid, nitrofurantoin, oxacillin, penicillin, tetracycline,† trimethoprim, vancomycin

Muscle Relaxants

Baclofen, methocarbamol

Pain Relievers

Acetaminophen, butorphanol, codeine, flufenamic acid, heroin, ibuprofen, mefenamid acid, meperidine, methadone, morphine, Naprosyn, oxycodone, phenylbutazone, prednisone, propoxyphene

Psychotropic Agents

Antidepressants: amitriptyline, amoxapine, desipramine, dothiepin, imipramine, nortriptyline, tranylcypromine

Antipsychotic drugs: chlorpromazine, haloperidol, mesoridazine, piperacetazine, prochlorperazine, thioridazine, trifluoperazine

*Accumulate in breast milk

†Some consider these drugs contraindicated; others do not. Refer to original sources.

Information abstracted from Committee on Drugs, American Academy of Pediatrics. The transfer of drugs and other chemicals into human breast milk. Pediatrics 1983;72:375. Marx CM. Drugs excreted in breast milk. Nutrition and Feeding of Infants and Toddlers, Appendix 7. Boston: Little, Brown, 1984:433. See sources for reported side effects and monitoring suggestions.

Infants fed one of the cow's milk or soy-based formulas fortified with iron and intended for healthy term infants need no routine vitamin, mineral, or water supplementation. Fluoride supplements should be provided to prevent dental caries if ready-to-feed formula is being used exclusively or if concentrate is being mixed with water containing less than 0.3 ppm well into infancy.

Techniques

Formula Preparation. Formulas come in three forms: powder to be mixed with water, liquid concentrate to be diluted in one-to-one volumes with water, and ready-to-feed liquids. The latter is the most expensive; the powder is generally least expensive, but it is hardest to prepare. The powder may be stored without refrigeration, but after it is mixed with water, the formula must be refrigerated. Liquid concentrate and ready-to-feed formulas must be refrigerated after opening.

Feeding. The infant should be held during feedings. Propping the bottle is dangerous during early infancy because the baby may choke on the milk. Moreover, the social aspects of feeding are as important as the nutrients. As the infant ages, the milk from a propped bottle may pool around the teeth as he or she falls asleep and cause caries, or it may be sucked into the middle ear, predisposing to otitis media.

Several bottle and nipple styles are available. Most infants nurse adequately from any of them, but if feedings are not going well, experimenting with other nipples may provide a remedy. Infants tend to swallow air and to tire with feeds if the nipple hole is too small and to choke or to consume the feeding before sucking needs are met if it is too large. If the bottle is held upside down, the milk should come out in frequent drips, not a stream. While the infant is being fed, the bottle should be held so that formula fills the nipple.

Warming. Contrary to popular belief, formula does not need to be warmed before a feeding but can be used straight from the refrigerator. Warming may cause burns. Microwave ovens, for instance, do not warm liquids evenly, and hot spots may burn the infant's mouth. If warming is deemed desirable, the bottle may be put briefly in tepid, not hot, water.

Burping. The infant should be burped after every few ounces while held in a sitting position on the feeder's lap or with abdomen against the feeder's chest and shoulder. The position should be one that allows air to escape up the esophagus. Burping is encouraged by rubbing or gently patting the infant's back.

Patterns and Schedules

Although appropriate growth rate is the most salient marker of appropriate intake, ounces become the preoccupation in formula-fed infants. The stomach capacity at birth is between 1 and 3 oz, increasing to 3 to 5 oz at 1 month, and in the first few weeks, most infants do not consume a whole 4-oz bottle. As the infant ages, fewer but larger feedings are demanded. Feedings usually take 15 to 20 minutes. Table 4–6 describes the usual ranges for number and volume of formula feedings by age. The rule of thumb is that an exclusively formula-fed infant needs 100 to 120 kcal/kg/day, which is provided by 150 to 180 mL of formula/kg/day.

Problems Specific to Bottle Feeding

Sensitivity. Some infants do not tolerate cow's milk protein. Prevalence figures for this problem vary with diagnostic criteria up to about 8% of infants. Symptoms attributed to cow's milk sensitivity include diarrhea, vomiting, abdominal pain, failure to thrive, asthma, eczema, and shock. A formula change is indicated if intolerance is suspected. About 30% of infants intolerant of cow's milk formula are also sensitive to soy protein formula. A casein hydrolysate formula or a meat-based formula can be tried. However, formulas are changed far more frequently than medically indicated; many changes are probably in response to frustration over infantile colic. Evidence has not supported a simple dietary basis for most cases of colic, but perhaps 10% or 15% do improve on a "hypoallergenic" formula based on casein or whey hydrolysate.

TABLE 4-6. Recommended Bottle Feedings for a Normal Infant by Age

Age	No. of Feedings	Volume (ml)
Birth–1 wk	6–10	30–90
1 wk–1 mo	7–8	60–120
1 mo–3 mo	5–7	120–180
3 mo–6 mo	4–5	180–210
6 mo–9 mo	3–4	210–240
10 mo–12 mo	3	210–240

Kelts DG, Jones LG. Manual of pediatric nutrition. Boston: Little, Brown, 1984:38.

Improper Dilution. Many failures to gain weight at the expected rate and some electrolyte imbalances in young infants can be traced to misunderstandings about formula preparation. The problem may be too much or too little water added to the formula. Parents may dilute formula because they cannot afford an adequate supply.

Regurgitation. Although breast-fed infants spit up, bottle-fed infants seem especially prone to this, probably because they swallow more air when they feed. Some infants tolerate regurgitation well. When regurgitation is threatening appropriate caloric intake or blocking the airway and cannot be reversed by changes in feeding technique or volume, it is labeled reflux (see Chapter 151).

Weaning. At about 5 months of age, an infant is capable of putting lips on the rim of a cup, and sometime in the last half of the first year, cup feeding of liquids can begin to replace bottle feeds. The bedtime bottle, often a source of comfort and nutrition, is usually the last to go, although the temptation to let the child take it to bed should be avoided. The child should be held during this feeding and the teeth should be cleaned after it. It is probably wise to be rid of this evening bottle by 2 years of age. Other bedtime rituals can be substituted. The toddler should not be given a bottle to carry about as a pacifier. Constant feeding can lead to caloric overload and perhaps to dental caries.

By 1 year of age, a formula-fed child should be receiving a wide variety of other nutrients, and formula can be discontinued. Modest intake of whole cow's milk can begin at this time. Milks with reduced butterfat (*eg,* low-fat or skim milk) are not recommended until a child is about 2 years of age.

Addition of Other Foods to the Diet

Nutrients are initially presented in liquid form because the infant cannot chew and swallow well. Other digestive processes, although still maturing during the first 3 months of life, are already quite good. Competence to handle food antigens matures with time, and the risk of inducing food allergies may be increased with early introduction of solids. The decision of when to begin to feed pureed and soft foods centers on the age at which they are nutritionally and developmentally appropriate. Customs have changed markedly through the years. Currently, the recommended age is 4 to 6 months.

Choice and Progression

Introduction of solids midway through the first year coincides with the time the child may have depleted iron stores and be outgrowing the iron dose available from formula or human milk. Because iron content is important, many suggest iron-fortified infant cereal as the first solid food, but only a small proportion of its iron is absorbed.

At the time of introduction of solids, most infants take five feedings a day, and nonliquid foods are introduced before the bottle or breast at one or more of these times, beginning with several spoonfuls. As a wider variety of foods are introduced and quantities increase, nonliquid foods satisfy a greater portion of the infant's hunger, and smaller volumes of formula or breast milk are taken after the meal, until they are omitted altogether at some and then all feeding times. By 2 years of age, most children are taking three small meals and two snacks a day.

■ FEEDING THE OLDER CHILD

The onset of the desire and the skill to self-feed usually become apparent by 1 year of age, and ultimate control over intake shifts to the child. Although the transfer of complete dietary independence to the child takes place gradually over many years and at different rates in different families, the parental role increasingly becomes one of providing a balanced, healthy range of appropriately prepared foods from which the child can select and of discouraging inappropriate feeding behaviors. The latter must be done in ways that do not become counterproductive.

The conversion to self-feeding ordinarily begins at the same time growth velocity is slowing and separation–individuation is a prominent developmental theme. Parents are well advised to become as dispassionate as possible about the feeding process, to avoid assigning great meaning to the consumption of any particular food at any particular meal, to avoid using food as a reward or a punishment, and to avoid insisting that portions are finished. However, it must be acknowledged that food and feeding have immense cultural and social importance and that much of family life revolves around meals.

Nutrient Requirements and Diet Planning

By the time a child is 18 to 24 months of age, the meals are drawn almost exclusively from foods eaten by the rest of the family, although the foods must be specially cooled and chopped and may need to be set aside before spices are added. Portions are small, and the young child demands between-meal snacks, as most children do throughout childhood and adolescence.

Vitamin and Mineral Supplementation

Healthy older children taking adequate calories from a well-balanced, varied diet do not appear to develop deficiencies of vitamins and minerals. There are relatively few circumstances for which supplementation is indicated.

Iron deficiency is the most common nutritional deficiency in American children, manifested by behavioral changes before anemia is apparent. Some dietary sources of

TABLE 4-7. Good Dietary Sources of Iron

Food	Serving Size	Iron (mg)
SOURCES OF HEME IRON (ABSORPTION IS 15%–30%)		
Pork chop	3 oz	3.3
Lean steak	3 oz	3
Hamburger	3 oz	2.7
Sardines	3 oz	2.5
Chicken, dark meat	3 oz	2
Lamb	3 oz	1.7
Tuna	3 oz	1.6
Ham	3 oz	1.2
Chicken, white meat	3 oz	1
Salmon or white fish	3 oz	1
SOURCES OF NONHEME IRON (ABSORPTION IS ABOUT 5%)		
Dried apricots	3 oz	4
Baked beans	½ cup	3
Baked potato with skin	1 medium	2.8
Almonds	2 oz	2.7
Lima beans	½ cup	2.1
Raisins	½ cup	2.1
Macaroni, enriched	1 cup	1.6
Bread, enriched white	2 slices	1.4
Spaghetti, enriched	1 cup	1.4
Peas	½ cup	1.2
Peanut butter	4 Tbsp	1.2
Egg	1	1
Breakfast cereal, enriched or fortified	1 oz	1–10

Modified from University of California, Berkeley Wellness Letter, August 1987;5 and from Pipes PL. Selected food sources of iron. Nutrition in infancy and childhood. St. Louis: CV Mosby, 1981:81.

iron usually acceptable to children are presented in Table 4–7, and iron intake should be emphasized throughout childhood and adolescence. If deficiency is documented or suspected, iron may be given in supplemental form at a dosage of 3 mg/kg/day. Laboratory confirmation of a response should be sought after 1 month, and supplementation should be continued for 3 or 4 months (see Chapter 120).

Children whose water supplies are not fluoridated should receive supplemental fluoride because of its well-documented anticarcinogenic effect. Optimal daily intake is thought to be about 0.05 mg/kg/day. The intake of fluoride from nonwater sources and even the intake of water are hard to quantitate and probably vary widely among people.

(Abridged from Modena Hoover Wilson, Feeding the Healthy Child, in Oski, DeAngelis, Feigin, McMillan, Warshaw: *Principles and Practice of Pediatrics, Second Edition*, J.B. Lippincott, 1994.)

Oski's Essential Pediatrics,
edited by Kevin B. Johnson and Frank A. Oski.
Lippincott–Raven Publishers,
Philadelphia © 1997

5

Immunization

The virtual disappearance of many of the once common and dreaded infectious diseases of childhood since the introduction of immunoprophylaxis with vaccines is one of the most remarkable success stories of modern medicine. To sustain these gains and reach the ultimate goal of eradicating selected diseases requires constant vigilance and meticulous attention to immunization.

■ THE IMMUNIZATION PROCESS

Immunoprophylaxis, the prevention of infectious disease with specific antibody, can be accomplished in two ways. *Active immunization* refers to delivering one or more antigens of an infectious agent to a person to stimulate the immune system to produce antibody before exposure to natural infection, thereby preventing disease. *Passive immunization* is accomplished by transferring to the person preformed antibody produced by another host. The protection persists for a limited period, disappearing as the antibody is degraded. Passive immunization can also occur naturally, by way of transplacental antibody transfer, serotherapy, or infusion of intravenous gamma globulin.

Immunization Practices

Scheduling Vaccine Administration

Scheduling of vaccines involves consideration of the age of likely exposure and age at which antibody response is likely to be adequate. The latter depends on characteristics of the immunizing antigen, the host, and the likelihood of the presence of interfering maternal antibody. Recommended schedules are those found to provide protective antibody in most recipients before the age at which disease is likely to occur. A schedule used for routine immunization of infants and children is found in Table 5–1.

Standards for Pediatric Immunization Practices

The National Vaccine Advisory Committee has developed standards for the provision of childhood immunization services. They are presented in Table 5–2.

■ IMMUNIZATION FOR CHILDHOOD DISEASES

Diphtheria

Susceptibility

Infants born of mothers immune to diphtheria are relatively immune, but this passive protection is usually lost in the first half year of life and does not prevent active immunization of 2-month-old children. Although long-lasting immunity can be induced by administering diphtheria toxoid, it is not lifelong. Natural infection is now uncommon

and is an unlikely source of resistance. Serum antibody level surveys of US adults suggest that at least 40% are susceptible. At particularly high risk are health workers, and their immunizations should not be allowed to lapse. Immunization protects against systemic disease that is caused by the exotoxin, but it does not prevent nasopharyngeal infection. Even the disease does not reliably confer immunity, and active immunization with toxoid should be initiated during convalescence.

Active Immunization

Active immunization against the manifestations of diphtheria infection is usually achieved with diphtheria toxoid combined with tetanus toxoid and pertussis bacterial vaccine (DTP). A preparation combining the toxoids with acellular pertussis vaccine (DTaP) may be given as doses four and five. Also available are DT (*ie*, diphtheria and tetanus toxoid without pertussis) and Td (*ie*, tetanus toxoid and diphtheria toxoid at reduced concentration); Td is used in older children (after the seventh birthday in the United States) and adults. All preparations are injected intramuscularly because they contain adjuvant. A typical vaccine schedule is listed in Table 5–1. If, for any reason, immunization does not proceed on schedule, the Report of the Committee on Infectious Diseases of the American Academy of Pediatrics (AAP; the Red Book) lists guidelines that should be followed.

TABLE 5-1. Immunization Schedule Conforming With Recommendations for Healthy US Children With No Additional Risk Factors

Age	Vaccine and Dose Number
Postpartum	HBVrV[1]
1–2 mo	HBVrV[2]
2 mo	DTP[1], OPV[1], PRP-OMP[1] or HbOC[1] or PRP-T[1]
4 mo	DTP[2], OPV[2], PRP-OMP[2] or HbOC[2] or PRP-T[2]*
6 mo	DTP[3], HbOC[3] or PRP-T[3]
12 mo	HBVrV[3],† Any Hib†, Varicella
15 mo	MMR[1], DTaP[4], OPV[3], Any Hib (if not give at 12 mo), Varicella (if not given previously)
18 mo	DTaP[4] and OVP[3] (if not given at 15 mo), Varicella (if not given previously)
4–6 y	MMR[2],† DTaP[3], OPV[4]†
11–12 y	MMR[2]* (if not given at 4–6 y)
14–16 y	Td booster (to follow every 10 y)

DTaP[1], diphtheria and tetanus toxoids with acellular pertussis vaccine; DTP, diptheria and tetanus toxoids with whole-cell pertussis vaccine; HBVrV, hepatitis B virus recombinant vaccine. OPV, oral poillovirus vaccine; MMR, measles, mumps, and rubella vaccines; Td, tetanus and low dose diphtheria toxoids.

* One of the following vaccines administered; PRP-OMP; Haemophilus influenzae b conjugate vaccine (polysaccharide plus outer membrane protein complex of N meningitidis B), or Oligo-CRM; Haemophilus influenzae b conjugate vaccine (olligosccharide plus diphtheria CRM197 protein).

† Final dose of the vaccine.

Adverse Reactions

A variety of local and systemic reactions may occur following DTP administration. Some adverse reactions are diminished by the use of acetaminophen during the hours immediately after vaccination. The incidence of various reactions after DTP administration is summarized in Table 5–3. Certain serious adverse events occurring in an interval after, but not necessarily caused by, vaccination are to be reported to the Vaccine Adverse Event Reporting System (VAERS); these include anaphylaxis or anaphylactic shock within 24 hours (DTP, DT, Td), encephalopathy within 3 days (DTP, DT, Td), shock–collapse or hypotonic–hyporesponsive collapse within 3 days (DTP), a residual seizure disorder (DTP, DT, Td), or any complication of one of these reactions, including death.

Contraindication

The only absolute contraindication to the administration of diphtheria toxoid is a previous systemic hypersensitivity to the vaccine or a vaccine component. In addition to the toxoids (and pertussis vaccine in the case of DTP), the preparations may contain a small amount of a mercury preservative.

Postexposure Prophylaxis

A person exposed to diphtheria by household or habitual close contact with a patient should, in addition to being cultured and receiving antibiotic prophylaxis, be given the age-appropriate preparation of toxoid (ie, DTP, DT, or Td) if a dose is due or 5 years or more have elapsed since the last dose. If the person is unimmunized, a dose should be given to initiate active immunization.

Passive Immunization

Diphtheria equine antitoxin can be obtained through the Centers for Disease Control (CDC) Drug Service, and, because of the severity of the disease, it is administered if diphtheria is strongly suspected without waiting for culture confirmation. An infectious disease specialist should be consulted. Administration of antitoxin does not preclude active immunization, which should begin during convalescence because disease does not always confer immunity.

Tetanus

Susceptibility

All unimmunized persons are susceptible, and all are candidates for active immunization with tetanus toxoid. Active immunization results in protection that persists for at least 10 years, and booster doses after complete immunization confer continued high levels of immunity. Transient immunity follows administration of human tetanus immune globulin (TIG) and of equine tetanus antitoxin (TAT). Persons who have recovered from the disease are not reliably immune and are candidates for active immunization.

Active Immunization

In most situations, tetanus toxoid should be presented in combination with other immunizing agents. Tetanus toxoid adsorbed is combined with diphtheria toxoid in high-dose (DT) or low-dose (Td) formulations, as well as combined with pertussis and diphtheria as described above. All should be injected intramuscularly. The recommended schedule for active immunization against tetanus in the United States is the same as that recommended for diphtheria (see Table 5–4).

Adverse Reactions

Local reactions are common, and systemic reactions occur with administration of DTP, but serious reactions are rarely due to the tetanus component of the vaccine. Because pertussis vaccine is more commonly implicated, these reac-

TABLE 5-2. Standards for Pediatric Immunization Practices From the National Vaccine Advisory Committee, 1992

Standard 1.	Immunization services are readily available.
Standard 2.	There are no barriers or unnecessary prerequisites to the receipt of vaccines.
Standard 3.	Immunization services are available free or for a minimal fee.
Standard 4.	Providers use all clinical encounters to screen and, if indicated, immunize children.
Standard 5.	Providers educate parents and guardians about immunization in general terms.
Standard 6.	Providers question parents or guardians about contraindications and, before immunizing a child, inform them in specific terms about the risks and benefits of the immunizations their child is to receive.
Standard 7.	Providers follow only true contraindications.
Standard 8.	Providers administer simultaneously all vaccine doses for which a child is eligible at the time of each visit.
Standard 9.	Providers use accurate and complete recording procedures.
Standard 10.	Providers coschedule immunization appointments in conjunction with appointments for other child health services.
Standard 11.	Providers report adverse events following immunization promptly, accurately and completely.
Standard 12.	Providers operate a tracking system.
Standard 13.	Providers adhere to appropriate procedures for vaccine management.
Standard 14.	Providers conduct semiannual audits to assess immunization coverage levels and to review immunization records in the patient populations they serve.
Standard 15.	Providers maintain up-to-date, easily retrievable medical protocols at all locations where vaccines are administered.
Standard 16.	Providers operate with patient-oriented and community-based approaches.
Standard 17.	Vaccines are administered by properly trained individuals.
Standard 18.	Providers receive ongoing education and training on current immunization recommendations.

TABLE 5-3. Reaction Rates in the 48 Hours After Immunization With DTP

Reactions	Occurrence/Doses
LOCAL REACTIONS	
Pain	1/2
Swelling	1/2.5
Redness	1/2.8
COMMON SYSTEMIC REACTIONS	
Fretfulness	1/1.9
Fever of 38.3°C or more	1/2.2
Drowsiness	1/3.2
Anorexia	1/5
LESS COMMON SYSTEMIC REACTIONS	
Vomiting	1/16
Persistent crying	1/32
REACTIONS CONTRAINDICATING FURTHER DOSES	
Crying for 3 or more hours	1/100
Fever of 40.5°C or more	1/330
Convulsion	1/1750
Hypotonic-hyporesponsive episode	1/1750
Encephalopathy	1/110,000
Permanent brain damage*	1/310,000

* Based on the most recent analyses of available data; the Committee on Infectious Diseases of the AAP has concluded that pertussis vaccine has not been shown to be a cause of brain damage.

(Occurrence estimates are from Cody CLJ, Baraff LJ, Cherry D, Marcy SM, Manclark CR. Nature and rates of adverse reactions associated with DPT and DT immunization in infants and children. Pediatrics 1981;68: 650 and Miller DL, Ross EM, Alderslade R, Bellman MH, Rawson NSB. Pertussis immunisation and serious neurological illness in children. Br Med. 1981;282:1595.)

tions are discussed more fully in the pertussis section of this chapter. The incidence of various reactions after DTP administration is summarized in Table 5–3.

Contraindications

The only absolute contraindication to the administration of tetanus toxoid is a previous systemic hypersensitivity response to a vaccine component. In addition to the toxoids (and pertussis vaccine in the case of DTP), the preparations may contain a small amount of a mercury preservative.

Postexposure Prophylaxis

A dose of tetanus toxoid is not necessary as part of wound management for persons with clean, minor wounds who have completed a primary series of tetanus toxoid and for whom fewer than 10 years have elapsed since the last dose. If a person who has received fewer than three doses of tetanus toxoid sustains a wound, a dose of tetanus toxoid should be administered as DTP, DTaP, DT, or Td, depending on age and indications, and the series should be completed in a timely fashion.

If a more serious wound is sustained by a previously immunized person (eg, puncture wound, avulsion, burn, frostbite, missile wound, crush wound) or a wound is contaminated with dirt, soil, human or animal feces, or saliva, a booster dose of tetanus toxoid as DT or Td should be administered if 5 years have elapsed since the last dose. If a child

younger than 7 years of age with a wound meets the 5-year criterion, she or he is, by definition, inadequately immunized and should, unless it is specifically contraindicated, receive tetanus toxoid in the form of DTP. Adequacy of immunization against other childhood diseases should be addressed.

Passive Immunization

Persons who have sustained clean, minor wounds should not receive tetanus antibody products whether or not they have been previously immunized. The only candidates for serotherapy are inadequately immunized persons with more serious wounds. Persons who have had three or more previous injections of tetanus toxoid do not need tetanus antitoxin, even for serious wounds.

Persons with serious wounds who have had fewer than three previous injections of tetanus toxoid should receive TIG. The administration of an antibody product does not eliminate the indication for immunization with toxoid. Both should be given, but in separate syringes into separate sites.

Pertussis

Susceptibility

Pertussis is highly communicable, and as many as 90% of nonimmune household contacts become infected. Unlike many other childhood diseases, there is no clear evidence that passive protection is conferred transplacentally.

Many cases are mild and undiagnosed. Infection results in prolonged immunity, but second cases occur, and cases in adolescents and adults suggest that many are incompletely immunized or that vaccine-induced immunity wanes.

The pertussis components of vaccines available in the United States are of two types. Whole-cell pertussis vaccines (P) are prepared from disrupted or otherwise inactivated *Bordetella pertussis* bacteria. Acellular pertussis vaccines (aP) contain one or more bacterial components. The purpose for developing acellular pertussis vaccines was to decrease the rate of adverse reactions associated with immunization against pertussis while retaining immunogenicity and efficacy.

Whole-cell pertussis vaccine is associated with an efficacy of about 80% after three doses, and immunity lasts at least 3 years. Infection of the immunized person results in mild disease.

Acellular pertussis vaccines have been routinely administered in Japan since 1981 to children 2 years of age or older and to some children beginning at 3 months of age since 1989. Disease rates have declined, but questions remain about whether acellular vaccines are associated with acceptable efficacy if given during infancy and whether they confer immunity comparable to that associated with whole-cell vaccine at any age.

The DTaP is licensed only for use as a fourth or fifth dose of pertussis in children who are at least 15 months but younger than 7 years of age who have had at least three doses of whole-cell pertussis vaccine. It is preferred as the fourth and fifth doses because of its lower rate of adverse reactions. It cannot be substituted for whole-cell vaccine if whole-cell pertussis vaccine is considered contraindicated.

The recommended immunization schedule is summarized in Table 5–1. If the schedule is for some reason interrupted, it is resumed where left off, not restarted. Pertussis vaccine is not usually administered to persons who are 7 or older, even if they have not received the recommended number of doses, because the risk of complications from the disease at that age is low and because adverse reactions to the vaccine are more common. The inadequately immunized older child's schedule is completed with Td.

Before the administration of each dose of pertussis (and of all multidose vaccines), the parent should be asked if there were any adverse reactions after the previous dose or doses.

Adverse Reactions

Local reactions at the site of injection (*eg*, redness, swelling, induration, tenderness, apparent pain) are common after pertussis vaccination (see Table 5–3). The frequency increases with increasing numbers of doses. Bacterial abscess indicates contamination of the preparation or inadequate procedure. Bacterial or sterile abscesses from the site of injection occur after six to ten of one million doses. Generalized symptoms, such as fever, drowsiness, irritability, persistent crying, decreased appetite, and vomiting, are fairly commonly observed within hours of vaccination, but they resolve rapidly. Children who display these local or systemic symptoms with one dose are more likely to display them with subsequent doses.

Administration of acetaminophen (15 mg/kg/dose) at the time of DTP vaccination and at 4 and 8 hours afterward decreases the incidence of common local and systemic reactions, including fever. The Advisory Committee on Immunization Practices (ACIP) recommends the use of acetaminophen at the time of vaccination and every 4 hours for 24 hours for children with a personal or family history of convulsions. Prophylaxis is recommended for children with a personal history of convulsions if the decision is made to administer DTP.

Local and mild generalized symptoms do not preclude additional doses. These appear to be less frequent with the acellular vaccines. DTaP should not be administered if DTP is contraindicated; DT should be used.

Severe adverse events associated with pertussis vaccine are uncommon or rare. These include high fever, brief convulsions associated with fever, persistent (> 3 hours) or unusual cry, and collapse with a shocklike (hypotonic–hyporesponsive) state. Other attributed associations, such as encephalopathy, "brain damage," onset of seizure disorder, infantile spasms, and sudden infant death syndrome, appear on close study to be temporally rather than etiologically associated. The risk of catastrophe in infancy from the disease appears to be much greater than from the vaccine. In the case of preparations containing pertussis vaccine, reportable events include anaphylaxis or anaphylactic shock within 24 hours, encephalopathy within 3 days, shock–collapse or hypotonic–hyporesponsive collapse within 3 days, residual seizure disorder, or any complication of these reactions, including death.

Contraindications

Children who have a disorder characterized by progressive developmental or neurologic deterioration should not receive pertussis vaccine. Examples include infantile spasms, uncontrolled epilepsy, progressive encephalopathy, and tuberous sclerosis. After the child's condition has stabilized, pertussis immunization can be considered.

Future doses of pertussis vaccine should not be administered if any of the following occurred after an administered dose:

Encephalopathy within 7 days

A convulsion with or without fever within 3 days

Persistent, unconsolable screaming or crying for 3 or more hours or an unusual, high-pitched cry within 48 hours

Collapse or shocklike state within 48 hours

Fever of 40.5°C (104.9°F) or greater, unexplained by another cause, within 48 hours

An immediate severe allergic or anaphylactic reaction to the vaccine

Postexposure Prophylaxis

Immunization and antibiotic prophylaxis should be considered for children younger than 7 years of age exposed to pertussis by close contact with a sick patient at home or in day care. Children who have had fewer than four doses of pertussis vaccine, who have not yet met usual age criteria for dose four but for whom 6 months or more have elapsed since dose three, or for whom 3 years or more have elapsed since dose four all should receive a dose of pertussis vaccine. If the child has already received at least three doses of whole-cell pertussis vaccine and is at least 15 months old, the postexposure dose can be DTP or DTaP.

Polio

Susceptibility

Unimmunized persons who have not had asymptomatic infections are susceptible to polio infection. Lifelong but type-specific immunity is conferred by natural infection. Immune mothers pass transient passive immunity to the paralytic disease to their infants.

Active Immunization

Two types of poliovirus vaccines are available: inactivated poliovirus vaccine (IPV) and oral poliovirus vaccine (OPV).

IPV is recommended only when OPV is contraindicated. It is prepared from poliovirus seed strains by formalin inactivation. Seroconversion rates are comparable to those induced by OPV. Ninety percent or more of children have antibody to all three poliovirus types after three doses.

IPV should be offered to immunodeficient infants and children (including those with human immunodeficiency virus [HIV] antibodies or proven infection), infants and children with immunodeficient or immunosuppressed household contacts, infants and children whose parents have refused OPV, unimmunized adults at risk of exposure, beginning more than 4 weeks from the date of immunization, and adults known to be unimmunized who are in close contact with a child who receives OPV and may excrete polio vaccine virus.

Candidates for immunization with OPV include normal infants and children without immunodeficient or immunosuppressed household contacts who are undergoing the routine schedule of immunizations, inadequately immunized children at risk of exposure, adults at risk of exposure who have had one or more doses of OPV or IPV, and unimmunized adults who are at risk of exposure within 4 weeks.

The recommended schedule for immunizing a normal infant against polio in the United States is summarized in Table 5–1.

Adverse Reactions

Live polio vaccine virus (OPV) rarely causes paralytic polio in a vaccine recipient or the contact of a vaccine recipient. Administration of OPV results in about one case of paralytic polio in a vaccine recipient or contact for every 2.64 million doses distributed. Most cases are among susceptible adult contacts. If susceptibility in adult contacts is recognized, they should be informed of the small risk involved. If complete immunization of the infant can be assured, it is acceptable to delay the infant's initial OPV dose until the susceptible adult is receiving the second of two monthly doses of IPV.

TABLE 5-4. Diphtheria, Pertussis, and Tetanus Immunization of US Children

Age at Presentation for the Initiation of the Series*	Candidacy for Pertussis Vaccine	Primary Series	Boosters
Early infancy	No contraindication	Initiate at age of 2 mo; give 3 doses of DTP at 2-mo intervals and a fourth dose as DTaP or DTP at 15 (or 18) mo	Give 1 dose of DTaP or DTP between ages 4 and 6 before child starts school. Follow with Td at 10-y intervals.
Older than 2 mo but younger than 7 y	No contraindication	Initiate at earliest convenience with 3 doses of DTP given at intervals of at least 4 wk and a fourth dose DTaP or DTP 6 to 12 mo later.	Give a fifth dose as DTaP or DTP between ages 4 and 6 unless the fourth dose was given after the fourth birthday. Follow the "preschool" dose with Td at 10-y intervals.
Early infancy	May have contraindication; situation likely to become clearer with passage of time	In areas where risk of tetanus in infancy is low, may delay initiation of primary series for a limited time. A decision should be made and a DTP or DT series initiated by about the first birthday.	
Early infancy	Contraindicated	Initiate at age 2 mo, give 3 doses of DT at 2-mo intervals and a fourth dose at 15 (or 18) mo	Give 1 dose of DT between ages 4 and 6 before child starts school. Follow with Td at 10-y intervals.
1 y or more, but younger than 7 y	Contraindicated	Initiate series at earliest convenience with 2 doses of DT given 2 mo apart and give a third dose 6 to 12 mo later.	Give a fourth dose between ages 4 and 6 unless the third dose was given after the fourth birthday. Follow with Td at 10-y intervals.
7 y or older	Persons 7 y or older not given pertussis vaccine	Initiate series at earliest convenience with 2 doses of Td given 1 to 2 mo apart and give a third dose 6 to 12 mo later.	Follow third dose with Td at 10-y intervals.

*If interval between doses is extended, complete the series without beginning again. DTP, DT, and Td can each be given at the same visit as OPV, IPV, Hib conjugate, HBVV, and MMR. Total doses of D or T should not exceed 6 before the seventh birthday.

No serious side effects of the currently licensed IPV have been recognized. The IPV preparation may contain minute amounts of the antibiotics neomycin, streptomycin, and polymyxin B. Theoretically, persons with sensitivity to any one of these may exhibit adverse reactions to the vaccine.

Events reportable to the VAERS after immunization against polio with OPV include paralytic poliomyelitis occurring in an immunocompetent recipient within 30 days, in an immunodeficient recipient within 6 months, or a vaccine-related case in nonrecipient at any time. Also reportable are complications or death due to poliomyelitis. Anaphylaxis or anaphylactic shock within 24 hours of receipt of IPV is a reportable event, as are resulting complications or death.

Contraindications

There is no convincing evidence that OPV or IPV is a risk during pregnancy for the mother or the fetus, but immunization of the pregnant woman is ordinarily avoided unless specifically indicated because of risk. If immediate protection against polio is needed, OPV may be administered.

Patients with immune states altered by immunodeficiency disease, by malignancy or its therapy, or by pharmacologic doses of corticosteroids should receive IPV.

OPV should be avoided for children who have household contacts of any age with immunodeficiency disease or altered immune status, or who are immunosuppressed, because live vaccine virus may be excreted by the vaccine recipient.

Measles

Susceptibility

Infants whose mothers had measles or the measles vaccine are protected during early infancy. Other persons who have not experienced the disease or been immunized are almost universally susceptible. The disease usually confers lifelong immunity. The period of immunity that follows active immunization with live measles vaccine is prolonged, but its exact duration is unknown.

Active Immunization

The recommended age for administration of measles vaccine has changed with the recognition that far too few persons responded and were protected if the vaccine was given before 1 year of age. About 85% developed antibody if the vaccine was administered at 12 months, and 95% developed antibody if given the vaccine at 15 months. Patterns may be changing now that antibody passively transferred from the mother most often represents her response to vaccine rather than natural disease. In the United States, where exposure is relatively unlikely, vaccination at 15 months has been the rule, with vaccination at 12 months recommended in communities with recent measles outbreaks. (During an outbreak, infants as young as 6 months are immunized and then reimmunized at 15 months.) High-dose vaccines intended to produce a lasting protective response at a younger age of administration are being studied in developing countries.

Measles vaccine is available as a single agent (M), in combination with rubella vaccine (MR), and in combination with mumps and rubella (MMR). Unless disease or previous immunization has been documented, the combined vaccine should be used for measles immunization. MMR can be given at the same time as other vaccines without diminished protection or increased adverse reactions.

Measles vaccination is recommended for all susceptible persons 15 months of age or older according to the schedule in Table 5–1, unless a specific contraindication exists.

Vaccinating susceptible persons before international travel is especially important, because exposure to disease in other countries accounts for many cases. Finding and vaccinating susceptible adolescents and young adults is important, because outbreaks on campuses account for a significant proportion of remaining cases. Adequate immunity at the time of pregnancy is highly desirable so that passive immunity is conferred to protect the infant during the early months of life, when the risk of complications from the disease is greatest.

Adverse Reactions

As many as 15% of persons who receive further attenuated measles vaccine develop fever, and about 5% develop a rash resembling mild measles, occurring 4 to 10 days after vaccination and lasting for 2 to 5 days. Reactions after the second dose are expected to be even less common, because many recipients are immune.

Encephalopathy associated with measles vaccine has been reported after fewer than one in one million doses. The fact that this is lower than the background incidence of encephalopathy permits the interpretation that at least some of the cases are merely temporally and not etiologically related to measles vaccine. Subacute sclerosing panencephalitis (SSPE) has been reported in children who have been immunized, and a linkage between the vaccine and SSPE cannot be ruled out. However, the incidence of SSPE has fallen, suggesting that immunization has had an overall protective effect.

Contraindications

Measles vaccine as MR or MMR should not be given to women known to be pregnant or who intend to become pregnant within 3 months. This recommendation is based on theoretic risk of passage of one of the vaccine viruses to the fetus or of spontaneous abortion, not on direct evidence. Pregnancy should be delayed for 30 days after measles monovalent vaccine (M) administration.

Because the vaccine virus is grown in chick embryo cell culture, persons with hypersensitivity to chicken products may have adverse reactions to the vaccine. These usually consist of minor urticarial reactions at the injection site. Rare, potentially life-threatening reactions to the vaccine have occurred in children with a history of anaphylactic reactions to egg ingestion. Persons with such a history should be immunized with extreme caution. Persons with nonanaphylactic reactions to eggs or with reactions to chickens or feathers are not at increased risk for severe reaction and should be vaccinated in the usual manner.

The vaccine contains small amounts of neomycin; persons with a history of anaphylactic reaction to topically or systemically administered neomycin should not receive the vaccine.

Persons who recently have received immunoglobulin, whole blood, or another antibody-containing product may not adequately respond to immunization because of passively acquired antibody. Vaccination should be deferred for 3 to 10 months depending on the dose of IgG the product is estimated to have contained (Siber et al, 1993).

Immunocompromised persons, with the exception of those with HIV infection, should not receive measles vaccine. However, persons vaccinated with live measles vaccine do not transmit the vaccine virus to others, and the presence of immunocompromised household contacts should not prevent vaccination. Unimmunized children with HIV infection, even symptomatic infection, should receive measles vaccine (MMR) because fatal cases of measles have occurred in HIV patients, but no complications of MMR immunization have been reported.

Passive Immunization

If exposure is recognized within 72 hours, the exposed person should be vaccinated in most instances. However, if exposure occurred within 6 days but more than 72 hours before recognition, immunoglobulin must be used because the interval is too short to provide protection through active immunization. Immunoglobulin given within 6 days of exposure may prevent or modify the severity of the disease.

Mumps

Susceptibility

After infection, immunity is generally lifelong. Most adults can be considered immune through natural infection, even if they have no history of clinical disease, because the incidence of inapparent infection is high.

Active Immunization

Mumps vaccine, delivered as MMR, is recommended for routine immunization of all children at 15 months unless there are specific contraindications.

Adverse Reactions

Fever occurs in about 5% of recipients of mumps vaccine, but other adverse reactions are rare. Because their incidence is below that expected for the age-specific population at large, central nervous system (CNS) events that are temporally associated do not appear to be etiologically associated. Orchitis is reported rarely.

Adverse events reportable to the VAERS after mumps vaccine administration include anaphylaxis or anaphylactic shock within 24 hours, encephalopathy with onset within 15 days, a residual seizure disorder, or any complication of these reactions, including death.

Contraindications

Patients with acute febrile illnesses should have mumps vaccine delayed until recovery.

Because of the theoretic risk of transplacental exposure to the fetus, women should not be immunized during pregnancy and should be counseled to avoid pregnancy for 3 months after administration of the vaccine.

Live mumps vaccine (MMR) should be administered only with extreme caution to persons who have exhibited anaphylactic reactions to eggs. The contraindications are those discussed for measles vaccine.

Mumps vaccine and MMR contain trace amounts of neomycin. Persons with a previous history of anaphylactic reaction to neomycin should not receive them.

Mumps vaccine should not be given to patients with immunodeficiency, except for children with HIV infection.

Postexposure Prophylaxis

Immunization after exposure does not protect contacts from infection resulting from that exposure, but it is not contraindicated because it offers future protection.

Rubella

Susceptibility

Unimmunized populations are susceptible to rubella infection. Contemporary serologic surveys in the United States suggest that 10% to 20% of young adults are susceptible, suggesting that congenital rubella syndrome should remain a topic of concern.

Efforts to eliminate congenital rubella syndrome can center on universal immunization for children of both sexes or on immunization of females before the childbearing years. Both strategies have advantages and proponents. Congenital rubella syndrome has decreased in areas using each method.

Active Immunization

Live rubella virus vaccine in use in the United States produces satisfactory antibody levels in more than 98% of recipients, with lasting, probably lifelong, immunity. Rubella vaccine is available as a single agent or in combination with measles and/or mumps vaccines (MMR, MR). It is injected subcutaneously.

Rubella vaccine is recommended for all US children given as MMR at 15 months of age, unless there is a specific contraindication.

Every effort should be made to immunize susceptible girls before the onset of puberty, and immunization of susceptible males is recommended. Because it is difficult to diagnose rubella with certainty clinically and because many infections are asymptomatic, immunization or serologic confirmation of immunity is desirable unless a date of immunization is documented.

Susceptible postpubescent females should be immunized, but only if they are not pregnant. Pregnancy should be deferred for 3 months after immunization. Women found to be serologically susceptible during pregnancy should be immunized in the immediate postpartum period. Neither breast-feeding nor the concomitant administration of Rho(D) immune globulin or blood products is a contraindication.

Rubella immunity is highly desirable before entry into educational institutions, military service, and professions in health care and day care because of the likelihood of acquiring and spreading the disease.

Adverse Reactions

Rash, fever, and lymphadenopathy follow vaccination in a few children. Less commonly, pain in peripheral joints is reported. Frank arthritis is uncommon. Joint complications appear to be more common in postpubescent females, are transient, and usually begin 1 to 3 weeks after immunization. Transient paresthesias and limb pain have been reported, as have CNS complications and thrombocytopenia, but the etiologic association has not been established.

Adverse events reportable to the VAERS after rubella vaccine administration include anaphylaxis or anaphylactic shock within 24 hours, encephalopathy with onset within 15 days, a residual seizure disorder, or any complication of these reactions, including death.

Contraindications

Pregnant women should not be given rubella vaccine. Immunocompromised persons should follow instructions including those with immunodeficiency disease, and those on immunosuppressive therapy, except children with HIV infection (who should receive MMR), should not receive rubella vaccine. Immunization should be withheld at least 3 months after the discontinuation of therapy and may be withheld longer, depending on the timing of expected recovery of immunocompetence.

Rubella vaccine need not be withheld if household contacts are pregnant or immunocompromised, because there is no evidence that the vaccine virus, although shed in small amounts from the nasopharynx, is transmitted.

Postexposure Prophylaxis

Active immunization after exposure does not prevent infection and illness from that exposure. However, exposure is not a contraindication to immunizing a person who is not pregnant for future protection. Please refer to the Report of the Committee on Infectious Diseases for discussion of the care of the patient exposed during pregnancy.

Haemophilus influenzae Type B

Susceptibility

All persons who do not have the bactericidal or anticapsular antibody acquired passively through the placenta or by previous experience with infection are considered susceptible, but children younger than 4 years of age who are in close contact with another child who has developed invasive *Haemophilus influenzae* type b (Hib) disease are at highest risk. The highest incidence of invasive Hib disease is among children between the ages of 3 months and 3 years, with a peak at 9 months. Children who have had one episode of Hib disease are at increased risk of incurring another, with a recurrence rate of approximately 1%.

Conditions that carry increased risk of Hib disease in early childhood and beyond include sickle cell disease, asplenia, antibody deficiency, and, perhaps, malignancy treated with chemotherapy.

Active Immunization

Active immunization against Hib disease should begin at about 2 months of age with one of the three vaccines licensed for use in infancy. Summary information about the

TABLE 5-5. *Haemophilus Influenzae* b Conjugate Vaccines, 1992

Vaccine Name	Manufacturer/Distributor	Protein	Schedule
ProHibit PRP-D	Connaught	Diphtheria toxoid	15 mo
HIBTITER HbOC	Lederle Praxis	Diphtheria CRM 197	2, 4, 6, 12–15 mo
PedvaxHib PRP-OMP	Merck Sharp & Dohme	Outer membrane protein complex of *N meningitidis* B	2, 4, 6, 12–15 mo
Act HIB PRP-T	Pasteur Merieux Vaccins	Tetanus toxoid	2, 4, 6, 12–15 mo

Hib conjugate vaccines is presented in Table 5–5. Hib disease at a young age does not necessarily produce immunity; children who have documented Hib infection before the age of 24 months should be immunized. Immunization status does not affect the recommendation for chemoprophylaxis with rifampin after exposure.

Adverse Reactions

Local reactions, including tenderness, erythema, and induration at the injection site, have been reported in about 25% of recipients, and systemic reactions defined as crying or fever have been reported in 10% to 15%. However, in neither category did these reactions exceed the rates in groups injected with placebo.

High fever and febrile seizures occur infrequently. Immunization is not protective immediately, and febrile illness occurring in the first few days after immunization should be evaluated.

Contraindications

Except for serious acute febrile illness, there are no known contraindications to administration of Hib conjugate vaccines for the age groups for which they are considered indicated (2 to 59 months) and for older persons at high risk.

Hepatitis B Virus

Susceptibility

Most hepatitis B virus (HBV) infections occur among adults and adolescents. The virus is transmitted by contact with infected blood products and by sexual intercourse with infected persons.

At particularly high risk of infection are children born to infected mothers. Depending on the mother's hepatitis B antigen status, the risk of perinatal infection can be as high as 85%. Even if an infant escapes perinatal infection, the risk of acquiring infection during the first 5 years of life is high. Early infection is associated with an especially high rate of chronic infection and long-term mortality from liver disease. Persons with HBV infection are also at risk for coinfection or superinfection with the hepatitis delta virus (HDV) and consequent fulminant or chronic active hepatitis.

Active Immunization

All pregnant women should be screened for the presence of hepatitis B surface antigen (HBsAg). The infants of HBsAg-positive women should receive postexposure prophylaxis with hepatitis B immune globulin (HBIG). Table 5–6 outlines the recommended schedules for HBV vaccine and HBIG administration according to age and risk status. Vaccination is an essential component of postexposure prophylaxis and has been highly effective in preventing infection and its long-term sequelae.

Although universal immunization in infancy against HBV infection is recommended, it is prudent to continue to try to immunize older persons who may be at special risk, including patients who receive blood products or dialysis frequently, patients who have had multiple sexual partners in the previous 6 months, sexually active homosexual males, household and sexual contacts of HBV carriers, children from populations with a high rate of endemic HBV infection (eg, Alaskan natives and refugees from Africa and eastern Asia) or who are traveling to such an area, people working in settings in which one or more HBV carriers attend, health care workers and others with occupational exposure to blood. Particular consideration should be given to immunizing adolescents at the time of health supervision, ideally before sexual activity is initiated.

Clinical trials estimate effectiveness to be in the range of 80% to 95%. As with other vaccines, some recipients fail to seroconvert, but, if antibody response is adequate after immunization, protection against disease appears to last at least 9 years. Booster doses are not recommended in routine settings, but the need for additional doses may be reconsidered as clinical experience through time dictates.

Adverse Reactions

When HBV vaccine is administered at the same time as DTP, there is no increase in local or febrile reactions. A possible rare association between the first dose of plasma-derived HBV vaccine and Guillain-Barré syndrome was reported (Shaw et al, 1988). No association has been observed between the recombinant preparations of the vaccine and Guillain-Barré syndrome. HBV vaccines are safe for infants, children, adolescents, and adults.

Contraindications

Pregnant and lactating women can be vaccinated, because there has been no apparent risk to developing fetuses with vaccine use. No risk is anticipated, because the vaccine does not contain live virus.

Postexposure Prophylaxis

HBIG is prepared from plasma with high titer of antibody against HBsAg but no antibodies to HIV. The preparation process excludes viable HIV. HBIG protection lasts for 3 to 6 months and is recommended only in some situations for postexposure protection (see Table 5–6). If exposure has occurred or is imminent, HBIG protection is essential in the interval between vaccination and adequate antibody response.

Varicella

Susceptibility

Susceptibility to infection with the varicella-zoster virus (VZV) is high among persons who have not had known previous infection. Studies of household exposure suggest that 80% of those without a history of chickenpox develop disease. Natural infection is thought to confer long-lasting immunity for most persons, but it may not be complete for all. Second infections occur.

It has been estimated that the complications of varicella lead to more than 50 deaths in otherwise healthy children each year. About the same number develop encephalitis associated with chickenpox. VZV infection is responsible for many physician and pharmacy visits, with the accompanying costs, and with many missed work days for parents and school days for child patients. VZV infection can cause severe disease in susceptible leukemia patients and other immunocompromised persons, in adults, and in the newborns of mothers infected late in pregnancy. Many researchers suggest that the weight of this combined burden argues in favor of active immunization.

Active Immunization

A live attenuated virus vaccine, developed in Japan, is licensed for use in the United States. The vaccine induces both cellular and humoral (antibody-mediated) immunity, both of which are important to prevent Varicella infection

TABLE 5-6. Recommended Dose and Immunization Schedule for Routine Use of the Currently Licensed Hepatitis B Vaccines by Age and Risk Status

Immunization Groups	Energix-B* Dose (mg)	Energix-B* Dose (mL)	Recombivax-HB Dose (mg)	Recombivax-HB Dose (mL)	Immunization Schedule	HBIG[†]
Infant of HBsAg-positive mother	10	0.5	5	0.5 1 mo, 6 mo[‡]	Birth (within 12 h), 12 h	Yes, within 12 h
Infant of mother whose HBsAg status is unknown	10	0.5	5[§]	0.5	Birth (within 12 h), 1–2 mo, 6 mo	Yes, if mother proves to be HBsAg positive[‖] No, if mother proves to be HBsAg negative
Infant of HBsAg-negative mother[▲]	10	0.5	2.5	0.25	Birth (before hospital discharge), 1–2 mo, 6–18 mo[¶] or 1–2 mo, 4 mo, 6–18 mo,	No
Children < 11 y	10	0.5	2.5	0.25	0, 1 mo, 6 mo	No
Adolescents 11–19 y	20	1.0	5	0.5	0, 1 mo, 6 mo or 0, 2 mo, 4 mo[#]	No
Adults ≥ 20 y	20	1.0	10	1.0	0, 1 mo, 6 mo	No
Dialysis patients** and immunocompromised persons[§§]	40	2.0[††]	40	1.0[‡‡]	0, 1 mo, 2 mo and 12 mo	No

*Also licensed for a four-dose series administered at 0, 1, 2, and 12 months. May be preferred when rapid response is sought; fourth dose cannot be omitted.

[†]HBIG, hepatitis B immunoglobulin. For infants, 0.5 mL is administered intramuscularly at a site different than the immunization.

[‡]Serologic response (anti-HBs) should be measured 3 to 9 months after completion of the vaccination series 9 to 15 months of age.

[§]Doses after the first can be 2.5 μg if mother proves to be HBsAg negative.

[‖]Administer as soon as possible, ideally within 48 hours of birth and certainly within 7 days. If mother's antigen will never be known, HBIG is probably indicated.

[¶]Longer intervals between the last two doses result in higher final anti-HBs titers.

[#]This shortened schedule can be used if compliance with follow-up is a concern.

**Annual antibody testing is recommended as is a booster dose when antibody levels decline to < 10 mIU/mL.

[††]Dose given as two 1-mL injections at different sites; four-dose schedule (0, 1, 2 and 6 months).

[‡‡]Special high-dose formulation.

[§§]Postvaccination testing should be performed at 1 to 6 months if results may affect subsequent clinical management.

[▲]Infants prematurely born of an HBsAg-negative mother should begin the HBVrV series at 2 months or a weight of 2000 g.

and, theoretically, to lower the incidence of zoster later in life. The vaccine is heat labile and must be stored frozen.

The *Varicella* vaccine is recommended for all healthy children aged 12 months to 13 years without a reliable history of *Varicella*. Children over the age of 13 with no history of *Varicella* infection may also receive the vaccine, although studies suggest that serotesting before immunization may be cost-effective in this age group. The recommended age for routine administration of the vaccine is between 12 and 18 months.

Adverse Reactions

Reactions at the injection site are common and include pain, swelling and erythema in approximately 20% of children who receive the vaccine. In otherwise healthy children, the most likely adverse reaction is the development of a varicelliform or maculopapular rash within 6 weeks of vaccination. The rash occurs in 7% of children and 8% of adolescents and adults, and may be localized at the injection site or generalized. Fever occasionally accompanies the rash. If a child develops a rash, the child should avoid contact with immunocompromised people until the rash disappears, because of a risk of transmission from vaccine recipients to susceptible individuals.

Contraindications

The *Varicella* vaccine should not routinely be administered to immunocompromised children, including children with congenital or acquired immunodeficiencies, malignancies, and those receiving immunosuppressive therapy. Children receiving high doses of corticosteroids (≥2 mg/kg/day of prednisone) for 1 month or more should receive the vaccine 1 to 3 months after steroids are discontinued. The vaccine should not be given to pregnant adolescents, because of possible effects on the fetus. Vaccinated females of childbearing age should avoid pregnancy for at least 1 month after immunization. Children whose mothers are pregnant and susceptible to *Varicella* should not be vaccinated until after delivery of the sibling. Children with anaphylactoid reactions to neomycin should not be vaccinated.

TABLE 5-7. Immunization for Special Situations

Vaccine	Indications for Use	Dosing Schedule	Side Effects
Pneumococcus	Children 2 y of age or older with sickle cell disease, functional/anatomic asplenia, nephrotic syndrome, or congenital or acquired immunodeficiency, children at risk for serious disease if they contract pneumococcal infection (diabetes, organ transplant, renal disease)	IM/SC. Administer 2 weeks or more before elective splenectomy or planned immunosuppressive therapy	Soreness, low-grade fever. Rare anaphylaxis. Contraindicated during febrile illness
Meningococcus (Quadrivalent polysaccharide vaccine for serogroups A, C, Y, and W-135; Monovalent vaccine for serogroup A)	Children 2 y of age or later with functional/anatomic asplenia, terminal complement component deficiencies, or along with rifampin chemoprophylaxis for close contacts of cases with disease caused by one of the included serogroups	2 doses SC given 3 mo apart when younger than 18 mo (use serogroup A specific monovalent vaccine for exposure to serogroup A); 1 dose for older children	Rarely mild reaction at injection site
Influenza	Use in children 6 mo of age or older who are considered at high risk for decompensation with a case of influenza (including children on chronic aspirin therapy who may be at risk for Reye's syndrome as complication of influenza)	IM. Vaccine dose and schedule vary with age and history of vaccine use	Local reactions (more common in those over age 13). Do not use in children with a history of anaphylactic reactions to eggs

■ IMMUNIZATIONS FOR SPECIAL SITUATIONS

Other vaccines that are available but reserved for special situations are listed in Table 5–7.

Hepatitis A Virus

Field studies have repeatedly shown that immunoglobulin given before exposure or early in the incubation period (15 to 50 days) protects against clinical hepatitis A virus (HAV) disease. It is 80% to 90% protective if given early, after which its value declines. The Committee on Infectious Diseases of the AAP recommends that the following patients be adminstered HAV immunoglobulin:

Household contacts of persons with serologically confirmed HAV

The infant of a mother with jaundice due to HAV at the time of delivery

TABLE 5-8. Rabies Postexposure Prophylaxis Guide, United States, 1991

Animal Type	Evaluation and Disposition of Animal	Postexposure Prophylaxis Recommendations
Dogs and cats	Healthy and available for 10 days observation	Do not begin prophylaxis unless animal develops symptoms of rabies*
	Rabid or suspected rabid†	Immediate vaccination‡ and RIG§
	Unknown (escaped)	Consult public health officials for advice
Skunks, raccoons, bats, foxes, and most other carnivores; woodchucks	Regarded as rabid unless geographic area is known to be free of rabies or until animal proven negative by laboratory tests.†	Immediate vaccination‡ and RIG§
Livestock, ferrets, rodents, and lagomorphs (rabbits and hares)	Consider individually	Consult public health officials. Bites of squirrels, hamsters, guinea pigs, gerbils, chipmunks, rats, mice, other rodents, rabbits, and hares almost never require antirabies treatment.

*During the 10-d holding period, treatment with RIG§ and vaccine should be initiated at the first sign of rabies in the biting dog or cat. The symptomatic animal should be killed immediately and tested.

†The animal should be killed and tested as soon as possible. Holding for observation is not recommended. Vaccination is discontinued if immunofluorescent test of the animal is negative.

‡See text.

§RIG = Rabies Immune Globulin (Human).

In: Peter G, ed. 1994 Red Book: Report of the Committee on Infectious Diseases. 23rd ed. Elk Grove Village, IL: American Academy of Pediatrics; 1994: 391.

Children exposed to a case of HAV in a day care setting (The reader is encouraged to consult the Red Book for specific guidelines in these cases.)

Patients known to have been exposed to contaminated water or food within 2 weeks of exposure

Travelers who spend extended time in remote areas of underdeveloped countries (The reader is encouraged to consult the Red Book for specific guidelines in these cases.)

Rabies

The decision about providing postexposure prophylaxis against rabies must be made frequently by physicians for patients with animal bites, scratches, or other contact. Important factors in the decision are the species of the animal involved and its regional history of positivity for rabies, whether the animal was captured and can be observed and then sacrificed, whether the animal was provoked, and the type and anatomic location of the exposure. Although bites from domestic animals are much more common, more wild animals are proved rabid, with seven species accounting for most cases: skunks, bats, raccoons, cattle, dogs, cats, and foxes, in descending order of importance. Rodents and rabbits are rarely rabid. Transmission is probably by way of infected secretions passed by a bite. Licks, scratches, and aerosolization may rarely transfer the virus. Table 5–8 outlines a treatment guideline from the Committee on Infectious Diseases of the AAP.

Immunizations for Travelers

Infants and children who travel to other countries should have up-to-date immunizations. Recommendations for additional vaccines are dictated by exposures likely in the country of destination and by what vaccination requirements are placed on persons who enter and return from that country. The most complete source of information for use in the United States is *Health Information for International Travel*, which is available from the Superintendent of Documents of the US Government Printing Office and which is updated annually.

(Abridged from Modena Hoover Wilson, Immunization, in Oski, DeAngelis, Feigin, McMillan, Warshaw: *Principles and Practice of Pediatrics, Second Edition*, J.B. Lippincott, 1994.)

Oski's Essential Pediatrics,
edited by Kevin B. Johnson and Frank A. Oski.
Lippincott–Raven Publishers,
Philadelphia © 1997

6

Injury Control

In industrialized countries, injury is the leading cause of death for pediatric patients who survive the perils of the first few days and months of life. Injury is also a prominent cause of morbidity and disability. It precipitates numerous emergency room visits and hospitalizations and adds substantially to health care costs. It is not an exaggeration to say that injury is now the most important health problem of childhood.

Injury causes about half of all childhood and three quarters of adolescent deaths in the United States (Table 6–1). Moreover, many of the deaths due to perinatal problems and congenital anomalies are not preventable with current knowledge. Injury deaths are.

■ PRINCIPLES OF INJURY CONTROL

Injury control is more than accident prevention. An injury is not the same as an accident. The word *accident* conveys a sense of surprise and bad luck. Although unintended, most events and the injuries they produce are predictable. For example, it is easy to foresee that a child riding a walker may fall down an unguarded stairway and be injured on the concrete floor below. These injury-producing events can be predicted and avoided, and injuries can be prevented even though accidents occur. To illustrate, seat belts do not prevent car crashes, but they do decrease injuries during a car crash.

Injury control strategies can be grouped by their temporal relation to the injury event. Some strategies are preevent phase; they reduce the likelihood that an event with injury-producing potential will occur. Some are event phase in that they reduce injury during the event. Postevent phase strategies reduce the resulting damage even after the injury has occurred. Table 6–2 lists examples of these strategies. A complete approach to injury control requires attention to all three phases.

The most effective injury control strategies are automatic. Strategies that require frequent individual action, such as buckling a seat belt, are called active. These strategies are likely to be omitted by at least some persons at least some of the time. Achieving widespread use of new active strategies appears to require the addition of incentives and removal of disincentives and may only occur after a gradual change in cultural attitudes. Some persons, often those at highest risk, are unprotected because they fail to comply.

■ INJURY RISK

Injury is a common problem. No child or adolescent can be considered free from risk. However, some patterns may be helpful in designing programs or counseling individual patients.

Demographic Issues

Throughout the life span, males have higher injury death rates than females. It is not clear whether these differences in male behavior are entirely due to socialization (*ie*, role expectations) or reflect innate behavioral characteristics specific to the male. Gender differences are greatest for fatal and other severe injuries. Because the total number of nonfatal injuries for males is only slightly greater than for females, the exaggerated differential in death rates suggests that injuries sustained by males are, on average, more serious.

If the full spectrum of injury is considered, rates are highest for both sexes during adolescence. The adolescent injury death rate is exceeded only by that for the most elderly segments of the population.

Injury death rates vary with ethnicity and economic status, with native Americans having the highest injury rates, followed by African Americans. Asian Americans have the lowest rates. Part of the differences by race can be explained by differences in socioeconomic status. There is considerable evidence that unintentional injury rates are highest in the lowest income areas. Unintentional injury death rates fall markedly as the per capita income increases. Whites and

TABLE 6-1. Causes of Death of Children in the United States, 1984

Cause of Death	<1 y No.	<1 y %	1–4 y No.	1–4 y %	5–14 y No.	5–14 y %	15–24 y No.	15–24 y %
All causes	39,580	100	7372	100	9076	100	38,817	100
Infections	1732	4	660	9	408	4	746	2
Cancer	192	<1	612	8	1287	14	2293	6
Cardiovascular disease	1084	3	411	6	470	5	1507	4
Congenital anomalies	8548	22	946	13	484	5	516	1
Perinatal problems	18,682	47	144	2	26	<1	9	<1
Injuries	1075	3	3155	43	4859	54	29,646	76

Advance Report of Final Mortality Statistics, 1984. NCHS Monthly Vital Statistics Report 1986; 35 (Suppl2):6.

blacks of the same income level have about the same death rates from unintentional injury (Baker et al, 1992).

Although homicide rates are highest where the population is most dense, unintentional injury rates are highest in the most remote rural areas. Unlike differences in injury rates by race, disparities by population density do not narrow when adjustments are made for differences in per capita income (Baker et al, 1992).

Developmental Issues

The type of injuries to which a child is most vulnerable varies with personal circumstance and with age. Age is a rough correlate of size, developmental ability, and lifestyle, which influences exposure.

Infants

The small size of infants may be the first of their developmental disadvantages predisposing to injury. With small body size comes a small airway that is easily occluded. A small body slips through small spaces that do not always permit the relatively large head to follow, resulting in entrapment injury. Infants, completely dependent on their caregivers, are handled on elevated surfaces for the caregiver's convenience, precipitating falls. In addition, their primitive motor skills do not allow them to escape danger easily, causing a relatively high rate of drownings, suffocations, and deaths from fires and burns. The combination of complete dependence, small size, and primitive motor and language skills may make the infant an easy target for inflicted injury.

Infants spend most of their time in their own homes or in the homes of substitute caregivers, and most injuries in infancy occur in the home. It is worthwhile making the home a safe (ie, childproof) environment.

An additional worry in infancy is motor vehicle occupant injury. Infants not properly restrained in a safety seat are at exceptional risk in a crash. Tests with anthropomorphic dummies suggest that unrestrained infants become missiles during crashes or are crushed between the car interior and the body of the adult who was holding them. Small size is a disadvantage.

After adolescents, infants are the pediatric age group with the highest injury death rate.

Toddlers

Toddlers are busy pushing, pulling, finding, poking, mouthing, climbing, and exploring all day long. An active toddler can exhaust even the most vigilant parent. The explosive toddler is likely to run into the street, to tumble down stairs, and to disappear in crowds. Toddlers have no impulse control. They do not understand cause and effect. Making the indoor environment a safe area for exploration is worthwhile. Although the injury death rate for the toddler does not stand out, the rate of nonlethal injuries is high.

Preschoolers

Increasingly sophisticated motor and intellectual skills combined with the desire to imitate the behavior of older children and adults bring the preschooler in contact with a whole new group of injury risks. Although skills are becoming sophisticated, judgment is not. The child of this age cannot be relied on to recognize danger. Thinking is magical. "If superheroes can fly, why not I?"

Elementary School-Age Children

The grammar school-age group is healthy. Persons of this age boast the lowest injury death rate of the life span. Perhaps this is because these children spend so much of their total time sitting at a desk! About half of deaths that occur

TABLE 6-2. Three Basic Injury Control Strategies

Stages of Prevention	Phase of Prevention	Example
Prevention of events that may cause injury	Before event	Bicycle paths separate from roads used by motorized vehicles
Prevention of injury when the event occurs	During event	Helmets for bicyclists
Prevention of unnecessary severity or disability after an injury occurs	After event	Neuroresuscitation in a pediatric trauma center

Adapted from Wilson MH. Childhood Injury control. Pediatrician. 1985;12:20. Used by permission of S Karger AG, Basel.

are due to injury, as are many urgent medical visits and hospitalizations.

More children this age die as pedestrians than as motor vehicle occupants, and bicycling injuries begin to take their toll. Children of this age are still not capable of making accurate judgments about speed and distance. Their decisions begin to be heavily influenced by the actions and opinions of their peers. Their motor skills and knowledge (*eg,* how to light a fire, how to fire a gun, how to start a lawn mower or car) far outstrip their judgment.

Early Adolescents

As they approach adolescence, children are given more freedom, spend more time without adult supervision, and range farther from home. Peer pressure exerts its most profound influence. Helmets and seat belts may be eschewed by the group. Risk taking becomes more conscious. The traffic environment poses the biggest hazard, particularly for those who ride with older adolescent friends who drive, who operate any kind of motorized vehicle themselves, or who ride a bicycle in traffic.

Older Adolescents

Adult privileges and practices are attained by older adolescents without adult experience, ability, and responsibility. The assumption of the adult behaviors of drug and alcohol use and use of weapons play an important but incompletely understood role in this age group, in which injury accounts for about 75% of all deaths. The older adolescent has the highest risk of any age group for motor vehicle occupant death and for drowning. Intentional injuries (*ie,* suicide, homicide) also take a striking toll.

■ MAJOR INJURIES

Transportation Injuries

Most children and adolescents who die of transportation-related injuries were motor vehicle occupants. Pedestrians struck by motor vehicles in traffic situations make up the second largest group. A significant number of deaths also is attributed to motorcycle and bicycle incidents. The number of deaths secondary to transportation injuries in 1986 for persons younger than 20 years of age is shown in Table 6–3. Because of their impressive numbers and severity, preventing transportation-related injuries should be a high priority.

For the US population as a whole, motor vehicle crashes cause about half of the annual 100,000 unintentional injury deaths. Injuries from motor vehicle crashes are a leading cause of death well into adulthood, and they are an important cause of permanent disability. For every death, there are at least 10 hospitalizations and 100 injuries.

The pediatric age group at highest risk is the adolescent. For older adolescents and young adults, motor vehicle crashes cause about 40% of all deaths. Although the risk of being involved in a crash is lower for the younger pediatric age groups, the case-fatality rate for motor vehicle injury is particularly high for the youngest children; if an unrestrained infant is involved in a crash, injuries are more likely to be fatal. The motor vehicle death rate in rural areas is twice that in urban areas, a difference accounted for almost entirely by motor vehicle occupant deaths. Counseling points are summarized in Table 6–4.

Injuries Not Involving Transportation

Injuries occur wherever children are—at home, at school, in places of recreation. Causes and kinds of injury are so numerous that no discussion can be exhaustive. The clinician and parent must be alert for injury potential when viewing the child's whole lifestyle and milieu. The most common unintentional injury events resulting in death (Table 6–5) are discussed in the following sections.

Drowning

Incidence. Drowning (*ie,* death from submersion) is second only to transportation injuries as a cause of unintentional injury death for children and adolescents, accounting for about 2000 deaths each year. Drowning death rates peak at 1 to 2 years of age and again in older adolescence. The increased drowning risk experienced by boys is apparent at a very early age, but it becomes even more exaggerated in adolescence when male drowning death rates are the highest of the life span and almost 10 times higher than rates for girls of the same age.

Most toddler and preschooler drownings occur when a briefly unattended child falls into a body of water. One third of these drownings, about 250 each year, take place in swimming pools, often at home. The increasing popularity of home whirlpools, hot tubs, and spas is providing a new place for young children to drown. Toddlers can drown in any amount of water that is sufficiently deep to cover the nose and mouth; diaper pail, toilet bowl, large bucket, and bathtub drownings

TABLE 6-3. Number of US Transportation-Related Injury Deaths, 1986

Category of Injury	Deaths by Age Groups in Years				
	0–4	*5–9*	*10–14*	*15–19*	*0–19*
Motor vehicle occupant	640	380	614	5664	7298
Pedestrian					
Traffic*	368	471	275	494	1608
Nontraffic	129	28	9	4	170
Motorcycle	2	11	73	583	669
Bicycle	17	126	230	152	525

*On public roads.

Data compiled from Baker SP, O'Neill B, Ginsburg M, Li G: The injury fact book, 2nd ed. New York: Oxford University Press; 1992:308.

TABLE 6-4. Age-Appropriate Injury Prevention Topics and Advice

	Advice for Prevention
0-Years	
Car crashes, falls, choking, suffocation, fires, burns, drowning, poisoning	Use a safe car seat correctly.
	Never leave infants alone on high places.
	Avoid baby walkers.
	Keep small objects, hard foods, and harmful substances out of reach.
	Never leave a child alone in or near water, hot liquids, or any heat source.
	Install a smoke detector.
	Have syrup of ipecac in the home.
	Write Poison Control Center number on the home phone.
	Know how to save a choking child.
	Lower hot water heater to 120°F–125°F.
1–2 Years	
Poisoning, falls, choking, fires, burns, drowning, car crashes	Use safety caps on medications.
	Store all toxic household products and medicines out of reach.
	Use window screens which cannot push out and gates.
	Keep toddler in an enclosed space and closely supervised when outdoors.
	Keep electrical cords and handles of pots and pans on stove out of reach and keep hot foods away from edge of table.
	Never leave child in a tub or pool.
	Use toddler car seat.
	Eliminate or safely store firearms.
2–4 Years	
Falls, fires, burns, poisoning, drowning, car crashes, pedestrian injury	Keep doors to dangerous areas locked.
	Use screens, guards, and gates.
	Teach children about watching for cars in driveways and streets and danger of following ball into street, but continue to supervise.
	Keep firearms locked up.
	Keep medicines, knives, electrical equipment, and matches out of reach.
	Arrange group swimming lessons after 3 years of age.
	Never leave child in a tub or pool.
	Use toddler car seat and then belt-positioning booster seat.
	Continue to keep syrup of ipecac in the home.
	Teach children to avoid unknown animals.
5–9 Years	
Car crashes, pedestrian injury, bicycle injury, drowning, firearms, burns	Teach pedestrian, motor vehicle, and bicycle safety.
	Do not allow bicycling on roadway before 10 years of age.
	Use seat belts and bicycle helmets.
	Continue swimming classes.
	Supervise around water.
	Keep firearms locked up.
	Avoid off-road motor vehicle use.
	Supervise use of matches.
10–15 Years	
Car crashes, pedestrian injury, bicycle injury, firearms, drowning, burns, falls	Continue rules of bicycle, pedestrian, motor vehicle safety, with good examples set by adults.
	Insist on seat belts and bicycle helmets.
	Discourage night bicycle riding and riding of off-road and other motorized vehicles.
	Discourage nonpowder firearms.
	Provide safe facilities of recreation and social activities.
	Stress the buddy system in all sports.
	Prohibit unsupervised swimming or boating.
	Discourage alcohol use.
	Eliminate or safely store firearms.
16–19 Years	
Car crashes, drowning, pedestrian injury, other motorized vehicles, firearms, suicide, homicide	Provide appropriate driver's education.
	Insist on seat belt use.
	Insist on helmets for bicycling and for riding other motorized vehicles.
	Prohibit driving or swimming when under the influence of alcohol or other drugs.
	Prohibit firearms except under the most stringent safety and training conditions.

Adapted from McIntire MS, ed. Injury control for children and youth. Elk Grove Village, IL: American Academy of Pediatrics; 1987.

TABLE 6-5. Number of US Nontransportation-Related Deaths, 1986

| Category of Injury | Deaths by Age Groups in Years | | | | |
	0–4	5–9	10–14	15–19	0–19
Drowning	754	326	323	659	2062
Fires/burns	793	292	144	153	1382
Asphyxiation					
Suffocation	250	31	66	64	411
Choking/aspiration	280	21	28	28	357
Unintentional shootings	34	57	143	238	472*
Poisoning†	93	24	30	219	366
Falls	117	22	33	150	322

*Total firearm deaths far exceed this number because firearms are responsible for many homicides and suicides.

†About 60% are due to solids or liquids, the rest to gases or vapors. Many in the 10–19 age group are classified as suicides.

Data compiled from Baker SP, O'Neill B, Ginsburg M, Li G. The injury fact book, 2nd ed. New York: Oxford University Press; 1992:308.

occur. Older children, adolescents, and adults also inadvertently fall into water and drown, and about one third of unintentional drowning deaths occur that way.

Prevention. Home water hazards should be eliminated. Children should not play in or near water without supervision. Wherever possible, fixed physical barriers should prevent young children access to water hazards. Particularly important is the requirement for unbreechable fencing around all four sides of home and public swimming pools. All persons in boats should wear personal flotation devices.

Fires and Burns

Incidence. Fires and burns cause about 1400 child and adolescent deaths each year. House fires cause most injuries. Most persons who die in house fires die of smoke inhalation and are dead before rescue and medical attention are provided. House fire death rates are highest for young children and for the elderly. Both groups are disadvantaged in at least two ways. They are less able to escape after fire breaks out, and they have high fatality rates with burn injury.

Scald and contact burns are an important cause of injury morbidity in childhood. Hot liquids, often coffee or the liquid from a tipped-over cooking pot, cause most childhood burn hospitalizations. Another major source of scald burns is hot water from the tap. Burns from contact with a hot object, including the iron, the stove, the oven, the hot comb, the grill, charcoal, a cooking pot, a heater grate, a lighted cigarette, and fireworks, are common in childhood. Although occasionally severe or permanently damaging, these burns usually affect a more limited skin area and are, therefore, more easily treated than scalds. Burns to the face, eyes, hands, and genitals are particularly likely to result in long-term developmental problems. Burns are significant sources of injury because of their terrible toll of pain, prolonged medical treatment, and permanent disfigurement.

Some contact burns and hot water scalds are inflicted by the caregiver or result from willful neglect. Often, however, the circumstances of injury remain in doubt. Some prevention strategies may protect without regard to intent. If water from the tap was not hot enough to burn infant skin, the injury would be prevented no matter what the intent.

Prevention. The greatest gains in preventing fire and burn injuries can be made by the elimination and early detection of house fires. Working smoke detectors should be on every floor of every home. Although it would have a smaller impact on mortality statistics, decreasing hot water temperature can decrease morbidity, as can measures that reduce other sources of scald and contact burns.

The severity of burns can be decreased by immediately cooling the burned skin by immersing it in cool water or applying a cool wet pack.

Asphyxiation

Incidence. A major cause of injury death during childhood is asphyxiation by choking ($\approx$350 deaths) or by mechanical suffocation ($\approx$400 deaths). The size of the asphyxiation problem is exaggerated by existing data, because the presence of regurgitated food in the respiratory tract, a common terminal finding, is included; it accounts for some of the cases coded as asphyxiation. The fact remains, however, that choking on food and on other items kills more than 200 children each year. Child fatalities are concentrated among children younger than 4 years of age, with the peak occurring in the first year. Round, firm food products (*eg*, pieces of hot dog, candy, nuts, raw vegetables, grapes) are the most common airway-blocking agents in early childhood. Children also choke on small objects like round or pliable toys (*eg*, small balls, uninflated balloons), pop tops, safety pins, coins, and pieces of makeshift pacifiers, bottle nipples, or plastic-lined disposable diapers. Older children and adults usually choke on meat.

Asphyxiation can occur when the child is trapped in an airtight space or when the child's airway is constricted from the outside, as in hanging. Crib strangulations occur when the baby's relatively small body slips between the bars and the head, too large to follow, is trapped. Current Consumer Product Safety Commission regulations for slat spacing for new cribs ($2^3/_8$ in or less) prevent such events, but old cribs must be checked.

Children are also asphyxiated in inadvertent hangings in drapery, pacifier, or toy cords; when lids fall on them as they peer inside a toy chest; when they are trapped between frame and mattress of a bed or in the folds of a mesh playpen; when nose and mouth are covered in a soft basket, pillow, beanbag, or waterbed; when, unattended, they slip out of a high chair; inside plastic bags; in old refrigerators; in excavations that collapse; or when inadvertently covered by materials such as grain in the farm environment. The likely events vary with age.

Prevention. Parents can be taught what to do if a child chokes and can be cautioned about the household choking and suffocation hazards, like foods that may block the airway of a young child and unsafe crib designs. However, the most promising prevention strategies are probably those that involve redesign and regulation of hazardous products.

Unintentional Firearm Injuries

Incidence. Children in the United States have a uniquely high risk of being shot. As with burn injuries, intent is not always easy to judge. Guns in this culture are highly available and over all age groups are responsible for 2% of all unintentional injury deaths, about two thirds of homicides, and more than half of suicides. Children can be the victims of all three. Unintentional shootings kill about 500 and severely injure many additional children and adolescents each year. Even more children and adolescents are murdered with guns. Suicide, most often accomplished with a gun, is the third leading cause of death in male adolescents, exceeded only by unintentional injuries and homicide. Nonwhite adolescent boys are more likely to be murdered with a gun than to die in any other way.

No other type of injury shows such a strong inverse association with socioeconomic status. Rates for unintentional firearm deaths are 10 times higher in low-income areas than in high-income areas and are highest in rural and remote areas. Firearm homicide is more common in urban areas than in rural areas. Males are at highest risk, with a male-to-female ratio of 6:1 for unintentional shootings and 5:1 for homicide and suicide.

Boys between the ages of 13 and 17 have the highest rates of unintentional shooting death. The most common scenario for unintentional shootings is for one child to shoot another at home with a gun kept by the parents, ostensibly for the family's safety. Although unintentional firearm deaths have been decreasing, suicides and homicides have increased for adolescents and children, respectively. The presence of a gun in the home increases the risk of adolescent suicide.

Although some fiercely assert the right of the individual to keep a gun for protection, the fact remains that a gun in the home is much more likely to kill a family member than an intruder. Children cannot be trusted to handle a gun safely, even though they quickly acquire the mechanical skill and strength to fire one. No amount of exhortation is enough to ensure they will not make a deadly error. It is not clear what effect television or toy gun play has on the number of gun injuries in this country. It is clear that guns sold as toys, those that shoot nonbullet projectiles, and nonpowder firearms are associated with high injury rates.

Prevention. Guns and children should be nowhere near each other. If parents choose to own guns, the guns should be locked away unloaded and separate from ammunition. If parents choose to allow older children to learn to shoot, it should be under the strictest training and supervision.

Acute Poisoning

Incidence. Most deaths from acute poisoning are among adults. Two pediatric age groups incur most of the childhood poisoning events: children between the ages of 1 and 4 (<100 deaths/year) and adolescents between the ages of 13 and 19 (≈250 deaths). For every death, there are more than 20 hospitalizations. Centers belonging to the American Association

of Poison Control Centers, which cover 60% of the US population, record more than 800,000 calls a year about children and adolescents. More than half of all calls to poison centers concern children, but children younger than age 5 comprise only 1% of poisoning fatalities. Most fatalities among the young are secondary to ingested drugs—aspirin, antidepressants, and cardiovascular drugs. Petroleum products make up the second largest category in the youngest age group. Caustics, although much less frequently involved, remain a source of particularly damaging ingestions.

There has been a satisfying decrease in the number of early childhood poisoning deaths. The sharpest decline followed the introduction of child-resistant packaging in 1970.

Adolescent intentional poisoning deaths (ie, suicides) have not decreased. In one state where hospitalizations of adolescents with drug ingestions were studied, aspirin and its alternatives, benzodiazepines, alcohol, and antidepressants, were the most common drugs used. More girls than boys were hospitalized. Female death rates from antidepressant overdose are higher than male rates throughout the life span, an association not found for any other kind of injury death.

Children and adolescents are not exempt from carbon monoxide poisoning from car exhaust and faulty heating systems. For all ages taken together, carbon monoxide from motor vehicle exhaust is the most common agent in poisoning deaths. There are many unintentional deaths from motor vehicle exhaust each year. Deaths peak in adolescence for females and early adulthood for males. Rates are higher in low-income and rural areas and during the coldest months. Suicidal deaths from carbon monoxide are much more common than unintentional deaths, with rates being highest for middle-age females and in high-income areas of intermediate urbanization.

Prevention. The key to preventing unintentional and intentional poisonings is to prevent access to lethal quantities of chemicals. This can be done in several ways, but the more automatic the approach (ie, the less it depends on the watchfulness of persons), the better.

Falls

Incidence. Falls are the most common cause of nonfatal injury. Every year, 1 in 20 persons receives medical care for injuries suffered in a fall. Falls are the leading cause of unintentional injury emergency room visits for children and a prominent cause of hospitalization. Falls are an important cause of brain injury.

Falls are common at all ages, but the peak incidence of medically treated falls is 1 year of age. Each year, 1 in 10 children between the ages of 1 and 3 years receives emergency treatment for a fall. Of these, about one eighth fell down stairs, and stair-related falls constitute about one quarter of hospital series. Most of the other hospitalized children fell from one surface to another.

Falls can occur on the same level (*eg*, slipping while walking on an icy sidewalk), from one surface to another (*eg*, off a bed or changing table to the floor, down stairs), from a vehicle (*eg*, a car, pickup truck, bike), or from a height (*eg*, out of an upper story window, off the slide).

Prevention. Environmental redesign has much to offer in protecting all segments of the population from falls. Falls from a height should be prevented by barriers. Where falls are predictable, forgiving surfaces should be in place to greet the child who falls.

(Abridged from Modena Hoover Wilson, Injury Control, in Oski, DeAngelis, Feigin, McMillan, Warshaw: *Principles and Practice of Pediatrics, Second Edition*, J.B. Lippincott, 1994.)

Oski's Essential Pediatrics,
edited by Kevin B. Johnson and Frank A. Oski.
Lippincott–Raven Publishers,
Philadelphia © 1997

7

Special Needs of Children With Chronic Illnesses

Caring for children with chronic physical, emotional, and social problems accounts for a substantial amount of the practicing pediatrician's time and energy. The pediatrician in training sees more than the usual number of patients with chronic, complex, multisystem disorders. These facts make it easy to focus entirely on the problem and lose sight of the broad picture. It is important to step back and consider the needs of children with ongoing problems and identify those common to all children and those that are unique.

The fact that childhood chronic illness is becoming more common attests to the success of advances in medical care. The incidence of a particular problem may remain constant, but, if survival is improved, the prevalence of that problem increases. For instance, major advances in neonatal care permit the survival of extremely-low-birth-weight infants. Even with no change in the annual number of premature births, increasing numbers of former premature infants are being cared for. There has also been a significant reduction in the incidence of certain acute diseases, such as measles, because of the success of immunizations. As the proportion of a pediatric practice committed to care for acute problems in normal children decreases, the proportion made up by children with chronic problems increases. Children with chronic problems make frequent health care visits and often have complex needs, but these needs are not always identified or met. The focus is usually on the specialized medical problem, eclipsing the rest of the child's needs. Studies have shown that these families receive little information about special schooling, behavior issues, adjustment to the handicap, future vocational or sexual potential, or support services.

During the past 20 years, children with chronic disorders have been progressively viewed as having many similar problems and needs that transcend specific diagnoses. The child and family must learn to negotiate the monolith of the health care system. They must learn how to incorporate the child's medical needs into the family's routine. They need to make the child's life as normal and similar to that of peers as possible. They need to know how to set consistent limits and reasonable expectations for behavior of all family members. They need to have their fears for their child's life and health acknowledged and understood. They must learn to deal with nosy neighbors and strangers who stare. They need to learn how to work with the medical, educational, third-party payer, and governmental bureaucracies.

In essence, this approach is a return to the concept of treating the "whole child" in the context of his or her family and community, instead of focusing on a diseased organ system.

■ MEDICAL NEEDS

All children, regardless of whether they have a chronic problem, deserve regular health maintenance care. General assessments often provide crucial pieces of information in determining how well controlled the chronic problem is. For instance, in the oxygen-dependent premature infant or the infant with congenital heart disease and congestive heart failure, inadequate weight gain signals the need for reassessment of the management plan. Does the infant need more oxygen? Does he or she need increased doses of medication or surgical intervention? Very rapid weight gain may signal worsening fluid retention. Measuring length and head circumference as faithfully as weight fluctuations offers data for deciding what is "catch-up growth" and what is fluid retention. This approach is often neglected during prolonged hospitalizations because the focus is on acute care.

Some children carry multiple diagnoses and require the care of multiple specialists. They have the extra need for coordination among specialties in scheduling visits, tests, or procedures and in combining prescribed treatments.

All children have acute problems that may or may not be related to their special problem. Fever is exceedingly common in childhood and can be due to common conditions, although the cause is not always clear before medical evaluation. In a young child with meningomyelocele, hydrocephalus, a ventriculoperitoneal shunt, and a neurogenic bladder, a fever may be due to otitis media or the current respiratory virus spreading through the community, to a urinary tract infection, or to a shunt infection. Although this child may need the services of a neurosurgeon or a urologist in the course of evaluation or treatment of this problem, he or she first needs the services of a pediatric generalist to determine the likely diagnosis and which tests or consultations are necessary.

Nursing Care Needs

The range of nursing needs of children with chronic illnesses is broad. These needs exist regardless of the setting. We are most accustomed to these needs being met by health care professionals in the hospital setting, but the same needs exist in the child's home and often in the child's school. In all of these settings, family members often take on substantial portions of these nursing functions. They may do this with the support of a visiting nurse who comes to the home periodically to assess the child's status and how successfully the recommended regimen is accomplished in the home setting. The frequency of visits varies with the child's needs from several times per week to once every few months. A child who requires more constant attention, such as a ventilator-dependent child, often receives shifts of skilled nursing care in the home or school.

Allied Health Care Needs

There are numerous health care professionals who specialize in the evaluation of particular problems, formulation of a treatment plan, and ongoing assessment of progress. They are usually based in a medical center or school, but they often make home visits as well. Allied health care workers include physical therapists, occupational therapists, respiratory therapists, speech therapists, and psychologists, all of whom may be called on to assist in the rehabilitation of children with disabilities.

Equipment

A vast array of equipment is used in the home care of children with chronic medical problems.

Monitors have become commonplace in the homes of premature infants and other children at risk because of pulmonary, cardiac, or neurologic disease. The monitor is supposed to sound an alarm when the child is apneic or bradycardic; it should be set at sensitivities that pick up the normally small breaths taken by premature infants but not so sensitive that it incorrectly interprets nonbreathing movements.

There are problems associated with monitors, including false alarms that disturb the family's sleep and may make them less responsive to future alarms, and dependence on the "security" provided by constant monitoring, making it difficult to discontinue their use after they are no longer indicated.

Equipment used to assist in positioning and ambulation can be recommended by the occupational or physical therapist. This may include specific forms for use in bed or chair, splints or braces, crutches or walkers, and wheelchairs.

Intravenous therapy is becoming more common in the home setting. Children requiring long-term intravenous medications or parenteral alimentation may have central venous catheters in place. These usually require a daily protocol of flushing the line to maintain patency and periodic local care of the site of catheter entry. Newer catheters have subcutaneous ports, reducing the frequency of line manipulation.

Special feeding programs have equipment needs. Sucking problems may require special nipples or feeding syringes. A child with fine motor problems may need specially designed eating utensils to promote independent feeding. Tube feedings require special formula and a system for delivering it. A pump is often used for prolonged feedings, such as overnight.

■ EDUCATIONAL NEEDS

All children deserve the best education possible. In 1975, the US Congress passed Public Law 94-142, the Education for All Handicapped Children Act. Its intent is to ensure access to free and appropriate education in the least restrictive environment for children with special needs. It states that these children should have a fair assessment of their learning needs, a formal written plan for the child called the *individualized educational program,* any needed supplementary aids and services, and due process procedures if the parent disagrees with school policy.

Because each child's medical and educational needs are unique, determining how best to meet these needs must be done by those who know the child best. This involves communication and teamwork among parents, teachers, physicians, and any other professionals with ongoing contact with the child.

A child with motor and intellectual deficits who also has a tracheostomy and is ventilator dependent needs special educational services, supplementary services such as physical or occupational therapy, and skilled nursing during the school day. Services may be home or center based; even children with this level of technologic dependence can often be accommodated in the public school. It requires willingness to be creative and flexible on the part of parents, school officials, and health care professionals.

■ FINANCING HEALTH CARE

Caring for a child with chronic medical problems is a significant financial burden on families. No medical insurance program pays for everything that the child needs. A combination of private or government insurance and funds from family and charitable organizations is usually needed.

Private insurers offer a multitude of medical plans that vary in cost, eligibility, and coverage. Families are usually insured as part of a group plan through a parent's place of employment. This may give the family little flexibility in the company or type of policy available. Alternatively, families may purchase an individual policy directly from an insurer, but this is expensive.

Most policies have two main sections. There is a basic plan that pays for a defined list of tests, procedures, and some medications. It usually does not pay for physician visits. The major medical portion is intended to cover costs not covered by the basic plan. However, the amount that the family has to pay (ie, the deductible) before the policy reimburses them varies, as does the proportion of the bill that is covered after the deductible is met. Some types of service may not be covered under the policy, and there is usually a lifetime limit to benefits paid. These limitations and exclusions usually make no difference to the average medical consumer, but they have substantial impact for the family of a chronically ill child who incurs medical bills totaling thousands of dollars year after year.

There are government programs that pay some or all of the cost of medical care for eligible children. The Medicaid program is funded jointly by the federal and state governments, and the benefits and eligibility requirements vary from state to state. Its purpose is to ensure access to medical care for the medically needy. One segment of this population consists of low-income patients; without Medicaid, they would be unable to obtain needed medical services. Children with chronic conditions form another population of medically needy patients. Their medical expenses are completely out of line with the family's income, assets, and ability to pay. Although eligibility requirements vary, these children may be eligible for Medicaid even though their family's income does not fall below the poverty level. The Supplemental Security Income program revised its guidelines, expanding eligibility for children with chronic health impairments.

Several states have a Model Waiver for Disabled Children that enables coverage of certain children with special needs who would normally be ineligible for Medicaid benefits. It is often used to provide high-technology care in the home for a child who would otherwise remain hospitalized indefinitely. This legislation was a major step forward in providing cost-effective care and achieving unity of the family in their own home.

Crippled Children's Services is an assistance program for children with chronic or disabling conditions funded at the state and local levels. Benefits vary from state to state but may include physician visits, laboratory testing, medications, hospitalization, and equipment.

■ BEHAVIORAL AND FAMILY ISSUES

Families have many concerns about dealing with behavior problems and discipline for their special child that frequently remain unaddressed. It is important that physicians realize how commonly parents are concerned about their children's behavior, how powerful an influence this has on family relationships and functioning, and the special risks involved for a family with a chronically ill child.

Children who undergo painful procedures, are repeatedly hospitalized, or are physically restricted due to their chronic problem may act out or become withdrawn. It is important to differentiate expectations for family behavior in routine situations from those for difficult circumstances for which the special child bears most of the burden. For instance, a child undergoing a painful procedure normally cries and resists. Adults need to support the child's ability to tolerate the procedure. This same child should not be allowed to hit his siblings or throw food or refuse to go to school; no one in the family is allowed to do that. Parents need to be reminded that much of their child is normal and needs to be treated as such.

Siblings may also be vulnerable. They may have less access to a parent's time and energy due to the chronically ill child's needs. They may feel they caused the sick child's problems or fear becoming sick, too. Parents need to recognize the importance of allowing siblings to play and to expect attention.

Vulnerable children are at increased risk for child abuse and neglect. Although it seems paradoxical that a parent who is concerned about a child's health could also do harm to the child, having a child with special needs can be stressful. For parents without successful coping strategies, anger and frustration may be vented on the perceived source, the special child.

Adult relationships, especially marriages, are stressed by a child's chronic illness. So much time and energy are consumed in caring for the child that little may be left for the spouse. Sometimes couples blame each other for the child's problems. Sometimes the illness is the last straw for a relationship that was not working well.

■ ROLE OF THE PHYSICIAN

Many of the needs of the ill child or his or her parents can be filled by the child's physician. Primary care is supposed to be accessible first-contact care, which is vitally important for children with chronic illnesses who have exacerbations or crises. The child should be followed over time to assess changes in the child's illness and developmental level. Primary care should occur with a continuous provider. The same physician seeing the child over time for well and sick visits has a better perspective for evaluating the child when ill and develops a solid and supporting relationship with the family.

The physician should be responsible for the child's overall plan of care. It is too easy for multiply involved professionals to assume that someone else is taking care of a special need. Someone needs to assume the responsibility for seeing that the needs are recognized and met. In this role, the pediatric generalist can find real satisfaction in knowing that he or she has been able to offer healing, even if there is no cure.

(Abridged from Nancy Hutton, Special Needs of Children With Chronic Illnesses, in Oski, DeAngelis, Feigin, McMillan, Warshaw: *Principles and Practice of Pediatrics, Second Edition,* J.B. Lippincott, 1994.)

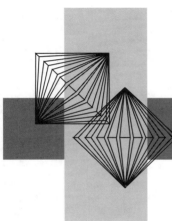

PART II

The Premature Newborn

Oski's Essential Pediatrics,
edited by Kevin B. Johnson and Frank A. Oski.
Lippincott–Raven Publishers,
Philadelphia © 1997

8

The Premature Newborn

A *premature newborn* is defined as an infant born at an estimated gestational age of less than 37 weeks. This definition is distinct from low birth weight (LBW), which describes infants with a birth weight below 2500 g, and includes appropriate-for-gestational-age (AGA) premature infants and small-for-gestational-age (SGA) premature and term infants. AGA infants may be described as moderately-low-birth-weight (MLBW; birth weight 1501 to 2500 g), very-low-birth-weight (VLBW; birth weight 1001 to 1500 g) or extremely-low-birth-weight (ELBW; birth weight 1000 g or less). Low birth weight occurs in about 7 per 100 live births in the United States, of which 82% are MLBW infants, 12% are VLBW infants, and 6% are ELBW infants.

The risk of death among MLBW, VLBW, and ELBW infants is increased over that of infants of normal birth weight and gestational age by 40 times, 200 times, and 600 times, respectively. Moreover, there may be significant morbidity among the survivors, particularly among VLBW and ELBW infants. The premature newborn infant presents the practitioner with a variety of problems that can be categorized broadly as those due to low birth weight and those due to functional immaturity.

The body composition of the LBW premature infant is characterized by low body fat, high total body water, and a large surface-area-to-body-mass ratio. These characteristics functionally translate to problems in extrauterine growth and thermoregulation.

■ EXTRAUTERINE GROWTH

With the shift from intrauterine to extrauterine existence, the constant source of nutrition from the mother is interrupted and the infant's energy expenditure increases. Thus, achieving a positive energy balance adequate to promote growth depends on the level of nutritional support relative to energy expenditure. Moreover, the quality of nutritional support dictates the composition of weight gain. Ideally, the growth of the infant would approximate fetal growth.

The energy expenditure of LBW infants depends on the basal metabolic rate, which reflects the minimum energy required for vital cellular processes such as the maintenance of transmembrane potentials, ion transport, and protein synthesis. Additional energy is expended with activity, with diet-induced thermogenesis, and in response to environmental cold stress. Typically the basal and other energy requirements can summarily be termed the *minimal energy expenditure*. Minimal energy expenditure for well LBW infants in a thermoneutral environment is 45 to 60 kcal/kg/day. Requirements for growth exceed the minimal energy expenditure: the

energy cost of growth has been estimated at 4 to 5 kcal per gram of weight gain. Thus, the energy provision above minimal energy expenditure necessary to support a weight gain of 10 to 20 g/kg/day is 40 to 100 kcal/kg/day. Although requirements vary, an adequate weight gain of 10 to 20 g/kg/day can usually be achieved by providing a total of 100 to 120 kcal/kg/day, and growth at a lesser rate can be achieved at caloric intakes of 80 to 100 kcal/kg/day.

Parenteral and/or enteral nutritional support is generally begun within the first week of life. The goals are to provide adequate calories to meet the energy requirements for growth and adequate nitrogen for protein synthesis. Net protein accretion will not occur unless positive nitrogen and caloric balance are achieved. Generally, the protein needs of premature infants can be met by providing protein at 2 to 3.5 g/kg/day, with 50% to 70% of the nonprotein calories as carbohydrate. Essential fatty acid deficiency may occur as early as 7 to 10 days of age in premature infants receiving no fat intake. Essential fatty acid deficiency is associated with dry, scaly skin, which may desquamate. Exudation may occur in the body folds, particularly in the perianal area. Minimal essential fatty acid provision is generally achieved with 0.5 g/kg of intravenous lipid twice a week. Generally, lipid infusions are tolerated well without hyperlipidemia if the infusion rate is 150 mg/kg/h or less for infants more than 1000 g of birth weight, and 50 to 100 mg/kg/h for infants less than 1000 g of birth weight. Lipid infusions are typically not begun until after 48 to 72 h of life and are better tolerated when prepared as 20% solutions.

The rate of weight gain can be related to postnatal growth curves (Figure 8–1) or to one of the intrauterine growth curves (Figure 8–2). The published intrauterine growth curves must be related to factors affecting fetal growth. These include maternal factors such as age, race, and socioeconomic status, environmental factors such as the ambient oxygen tension, and fetal-neonatal factors, which are a function of both intrinsic fetal maturation and the accelerated maturation associated with the transition from intrauterine to extrauterine life. Ideally, fetal and neonatal growth curves should relate gestational age to the composition of weight gain as well as to linear growth. However, such standards are not available, and an approximation of the postnatal curves or one of the standard intrauterine growth curves is acceptable. One must remember that the Shaffer postnatal growth curves include sick infants. Thus, these curves illustrate typical growth given current clinical standards of care and do not necessarily reflect optimum growth as might be better defined by intrauterine growth curves.

■ THERMOREGULATION

Fetal body temperature is 37.6°C to 37.8°C, and the fetus actually dissipates heat to the surrounding amniotic fluid. After delivery, the wet infant is exposed to delivery room air temperatures, which are 22°C to 25°C. As a result, significant heat losses can occur in the first few minutes after birth, resulting in a drop in body temperature of 1°C to 3°C. These losses can be diminished by drying and swaddling and placing the infant in a controlled, warm environment. In the nursery, environmental temperatures are rigorously regu-

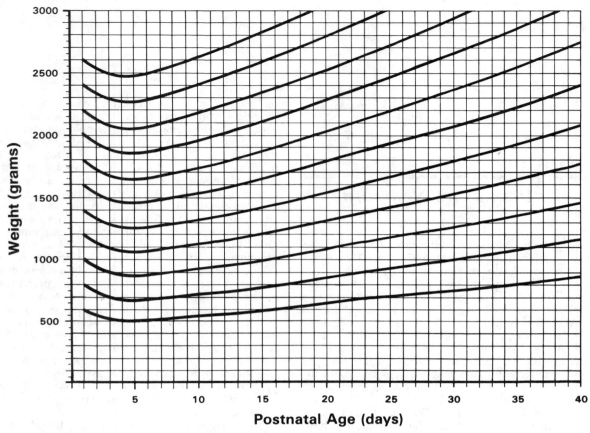

Figure 8-1. Postnatal growth grid, including growth curves for 100-g birth-weight groups. Derived from postnatal body weight changes in 385 surviving infants with birth weights of less than 2500 g. (Shaffer SG, Quimiro CL, Anderson JV, Hall RT. Postnatal weight changes in low-birth-weight infants. *Pediatrics.* 1987;79:702.)

lated to a preset skin temperature of 36.5°C to 37.0°C. This is associated with extrauterine body temperatures, which range from 36.3°C to 37.1°C in premature infants and 36.5°C to 37.5°C in term infants.

The typical response of newborn infants to environmental cold stress is to increase total specific insulation and heat production. Total specific insulation depends on the ability to regulate vasomotor tone (peripheral vasoconstriction shunting blood away from the body surface and conserving heat), on the quantity of subcutaneous fat, which acts as an insulating medium, and on the skin surface area available for heat exchange with the environment. In the last case, surface area and heat exchange are reduced by postures of flexion and increased by postures of extension. Because premature infants do not shiver, heat production depends on the ability to generate heat by chemical thermogenesis in brown adipose tissue. Brown adipose tissue differentiates from reticular cells at around 26 weeks of gestational age. At term, it constitutes 6% of the body weight and 40% of the body fat stores. However, in the LBW premature infant, brown adipose tissue may be markedly diminished or even functionally absent. VLBW infants of less than 1000 g birth weight do not exhibit a thermogenic response to lowered skin temperatures until the third week of life. Thus, VLBW premature infants may be functionally poikilothermic for days after birth, dependent on the thermal environment for the maintenance of an optimum body temperature. The ability to thermoregulate improves with advancing postnatal age, and VLBW infants have been demonstrated to have increased

subcutaneous body fat deposits and increased thermogenic potential at 3 weeks of age. Conversely, profoundly cold-stressed infants studied at autopsy have little or no residual brown fat stores.

Heat loss is a significant problem in LBW premature infants, especially during early postnatal life. Infants exchange heat via three routes: conduction, convection, and radiation. In addition, heat can be dissipated via evaporation. Modern nurseries use convection air incubators, radiant warmers, and heating mattresses to help stabilize body temperatures. In addition, attempts to decrease heat loss can be made by using a Plexiglas radiant heat shield or polyethylene blanket.

In general, the goal of thermoregulation is to balance heat production and heat loss in such a way that the infant is maintained within the thermoneutral zone. The thermoneutral zone is defined as the environmental temperature at which the infant maintains a normal body temperature at the lowest level of energy expenditure. Energy expenditure increases at environmental temperatures higher or lower than the thermoneutral zone range of temperatures. Figure 8–3 demonstrates the effects of body size and postnatal age on the ranges of temperature defining the thermoneutral zone. Smaller, less mature infants have lower heat production, less subcutaneous fat, and a higher surface-area-to-mass ratio, with higher rates of heat loss. Thus, the range of temperatures defining the thermoneutral zone for those infants is higher and narrower. Body fat stores and thermoinsulation increase with postnatal age. In addition,

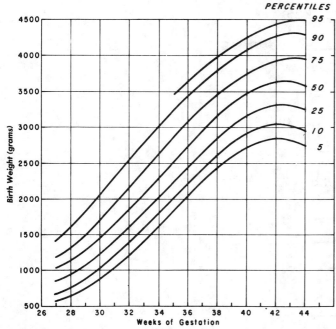

Figure 8-2. Percentile curves of fetal growth in weight in relation to gestational age (calculated to the nearest week) for a white, middle-class population. (Babson SG, Behrman RE, Lessel R. Fetal growth: live-born birth weights for gestational age of white, middle-class infants. *Pediatrics.* 1970;45:937.)

advancing neurologic maturity allows the infant increasingly to assume a posture of flexion, which reduces the surface area available for heat exchange with the environment. Thus, as the infant gets older and grows, thermoregulatory capability improves and the range of temperatures defining the thermoneutral zone is lower and wider.

■ PROBLEMS DUE TO FUNCTIONAL IMMATURITY

Although the body organ systems are morphologically identifiable early in gestation, the function of the various body organs depends on the infant's stage of development. Although much attention is given to cardiopulmonary function in the early days of postnatal life, all organ systems are immature and undergo development with advancing postconceptional and postnatal ages. Different disease states and the quality of nutritional support further complicate the picture. Moreover, functional maturation of certain organ systems occurs with the transition from intrauterine to extrauterine life. Thus, there are both developmental and transitional changes to consider in the care of the premature infant, and the associated problems are both acute and chronic. In addition to being at risk because of lung immaturity and surfactant deficiency, premature newborn infants may have decreased central ventilatory drive, particularly if born before 30 to 32 weeks of gestational age, and asphyxia exacerbates this problem. Moreover, with decreasing gestational age, ventilatory muscle mass decreases and chest wall compliance increases. Thus, even with adequate central ventilatory drive, VLBW premature infants may not be able to perform the work necessary for effective ventilation. The fluid-filled alveoli and pulmonary interstitium result in a less compliant lung, exacerbating the problem. If ventilatory

work is ineffective, alveolar surface area is diminished, with ensuing atelectasis and increased dead space ventilation. The net effect is poor respiratory gas exchange.

Most of the acute problems due to functional immaturity present in the first 72 h of life. These are outlined in Table 8–1 and are discussed in greater detail in other sections. Chronic problems of the premature infant may be secondary to specific therapeutic interventions, as with bronchopulmonary dysplasia, or may be due to the long-term consequences of metabolic immaturity, as occurs in metabolic bone disease.

Fluid and Electrolyte Balance

Infants born at less than 34 weeks of gestational age have a glomerulotubular imbalance that results in decreased free water clearance and increased urinary losses of sodium, bicarbonate, and glucose. In addition, there is a limited capacity to acidify the urine and excrete ammonia. Sodium losses may be as high as 8 to 10 mEq/kg/day, although the typical range is 2 to 3 mEq/kg/day. Bicarbonate loss may result in a metabolic acidosis unless adequate replacement is given. Most infants, term or premature, have a low urinary output in the first 24 to 36 h of life. This may be due to increased plasma concentrations of arginine vasopressin or catecholamines resulting from the stress of labor. Generally, urine output averages at least 0.5 mL/kg/h during the first 24 h of life and more than 1 to 2 mL/kg/h thereafter.

Fluid balance depends on the rates of sensible and insensible water losses relative to fluid intake. Thus, estimation of fluid needs requires measurement of ongoing urinary losses and estimation of insensible water losses, which consist primarily of evaporative water losses. Evaporative water loss consists of respiratory and transepidermal losses. Respiratory water loss generally accounts for about 33% of insensible water loss. This can be reduced to nearly zero for infants breathing humidified air from mechanical ventilators or oxygen hoods. Transepidermal water loss depends on body size, gestational age, and skin thickness. Smaller, less mature infants have higher transepidermal water losses due to their thin skin, low subcutaneous body fat deposits, and high surface-area-to-mass ratios (Table 8–2). With increased postnatal age, the stratum corneum of the skin keratinizes and is less permeable. Accordingly, by the end of the first week of life, transepidermal water losses can be reduced by 50%. The thermal environment can affect transepidermal water losses. Higher environmental temperatures or the use of radiant heat increase transepidermal water losses. These losses can be reduced by using a thin plastic cover or conductive heating mattress.

Management of fluid and electrolyte balance is a critical feature of premature newborn care and is also an area of considerable controversy. The controversy has arisen largely from the question of how fluid management relates to the development of patent ductus arteriosus (PDA). LBW infants given fluid at 160 mL/kg/day after the third day of life were found to have a higher incidence of PDA than infants given fluid at 120 mL/kg/day, whereas other investigators observed no difference in the incidence of PDA in LBW infants given 60 mL/kg/day versus 80 mL/kg/day. Animal studies have shown a vascular volume-dependent increase in circulating prostaglandins E_1 and E_2, which are associated with ductal patency. Based on the above studies, many nurseries have adopted the practice of providing fluids at 60 to 80 mL/kg/day, regardless of the infant's size and gestational age. For VLBW infants, in whom the risk of PDA is highest, this fluid intake may approximate or be consider-

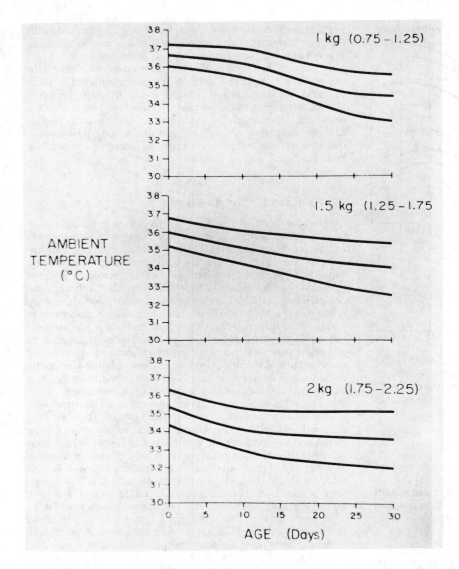

Figure 8-3. Range of ambient temperatures defining a thermoneutral environment in infants with birth weights <1250 g (upper panel), 1250-1749 g (middle panel), and 1750-2250 g (lower panel). From Bell EF, et al. *Pediatrics.* 1980;96:452.)

ably less than their ongoing evaporative water losses. Thus, the risk of dehydration and hypernatremia is increased.

There are two approaches to early fluid management of the ELBW premature infant. Both have three goals: main-taining an adequate vascular volume for effective cardiac output and renal plasma flow; avoiding vascular volume expansion; and preventing pathologic hypo- or hyperna-tremia. The first approach provides LBW infants with fluid intakes of 60 to 80 mL/kg/day; for ELBW infants nursed under radiant warmers, this may be less than their insensi-ble water loss. Close surveillance is maintained, and fluids are increased as indicated to maintain urine flow and keep the serum sodium at 150 mEq/L or less. The second approach is to provide infants with a fluid intake that approximates their estimated insensible water loss, resulting in a loss of body weight of 2% to 3% per day, up to 12% to 18% total body weight loss over the first week of life. This also results in a higher initial fluid intake per kilogram of body weight for ELBW infants than for other LBW or term infants. Again, close surveillance is maintained to ensure adequate urine flow and sodium balance. This approach must take into account the body size, gestational age, body posture, type of cradle (radiant versus convective heat source, with or without a conductive heat source), effects of postnatal age on skin thickness and transepidermal water loss, effects of radiant energy phototherapy, and other mod-ifying factors. In practice, either approach is acceptable as long as close monitoring of body weight, urinary output, and serum electrolytes is maintained.

TABLE 8-1. Problems of Premature Newborns

Acute	Chronic
Respiratory disease	Necrotizing enterocolitis
Intracranial hemorrhage	Infection
Fluid and electrolyte imbalance	Bronchopulmonary dysplasia
Thermoregulation	Metabolic bone disease
Patent ductus arteriosus	Retinopathy of prematurity
Hyperbilirubinemia	Parental support
Hypoglycemia	
Hypocalcemia	
Apnea	

TABLE 8-2. Insensible Water Loss in an Incubator or Radiant Warmer

Birth Weight (g)	Insensible Water Loss (mL/kg/day)	
	Incubator	*Radiant Warmer*
<1250	33–79	46–189
1251–1500	28–57	39–73
1501–1750	22–39	31–53
1751–2000	12–34	12–48

Adapted from Bell EF, et al. J. Pediatr. 1980; 96(3):452, 460; Bell EF, Rios GR. Pediatr Res. 1983; 17:135; Marks KH, et al. Pediatrics. 1980;66(2):228, and Baumgart S. Clin Perinatol. 1982;9(3):483.

Patent Ductus Arteriosus

In utero, the ductus arteriosus is patent, probably under the influence of circulating prostaglandins and the low oxygen tension of fetal blood. After birth, the plasma oxygen tension rises sharply, effecting a reactive vasoconstriction of the ductus arteriosus. In addition, the lung is a major site of prostaglandin catabolism, and the postnatal increase in pulmonary blood flow may result in a higher rate of prostaglandin degradation.

The ductus arteriosus remains patent in 15% to 35% of VLBW and ELBW infants. This may result in significant left-to-right shunting, with subsequent myocardial stress and pulmonary congestion. Progressive heart failure diminishes effective cardiac output and may reduce renal perfusion, glomerular filtration rate, and free water clearance. Typically, infants with a PDA have a systolic murmur and bounding pulses consistent with a wide pulse pressure. A precordial thrill may be palpable, and thoracic impulses are easily seen and are referred to as an active precordium. If heart failure ensues, tachypnea, tachycardia, and progressive respiratory distress occur, with cardiomegaly, hepatic congestion, and decreased urinary output due to poor renal perfusion.

The approach to a PDA depends on the severity of resultant symptoms. Some patients respond to fluid restriction. However, this approach should not be prolonged, because caloric deprivation may be an unavoidable complication. Pharmacologic closure may be attempted using indomethacin, an inhibitor of prostaglandin synthesis. Potential complications of indomethacin therapy include reduced glomerular filtration rate, impaired platelet aggregation, and reductions in both gastrointestinal and cerebral blood flow. Surgical closure is the final and only definitive option; however, the associated risks (transport to and from the surgical suite, effects of anesthesia, blood loss, and infection) must be considered.

Intracranial Hemorrhage

Intracranial hemorrhage may occur at any time in the first several weeks of life, but the incidence is highest in the first 72 h of life. The overall incidence of intracranial hemorrhage among LBW infants is 40% to 50%, so it is a major cause of mortality and morbidity of premature newborns (see Chapter 12).

Hypoglycemia and Hyperglycemia

Regulation of blood glucose can be a problem for both the term and the premature newborn. Blood glucose in utero is typically about 20% lower than maternal levels. Except for the smallest premature infant, most neonates have glycogen stores adequate to maintain the blood glucose for the first several hours of life. However, infants of diabetic mothers who have become hyperinsulinemic secondary to chronic exposure to high glucose levels in utero may develop hypoglycemia within the first hour after birth, and fetal distress or neonatal stresses such as asphyxia or hypothermia may deplete glycogen stores and increase the risk for hypothermia. Moreover, SGA premature infants may not be able to use available glycogen stores, predisposing them to early hypoglycemia.

Hyperglycemia can occur in sick premature infants. Although many ELBW infants can tolerate a glucose intake of 8 to 24 g/kg/day, sick ELBW infants may become hyperglycemic when receiving a glucose intake of more than 10 to 12 g/kg/day. If hyperglycemia results in severely restricted nutrient intake or in diuresis, then cautious insulin therapy should be considered.

■ CHRONIC PROBLEMS

Many of the acute consequences of prematurity have presented by 3 days of age, and ongoing management of acute problems begins to blend with anticipatory management of chronic problems. Many of the chronic problems relate to the consequences of acute disease processes and to problems with nutritional support. These include such conditions as necrotizing enterocolitis, bronchopulmonary dysplasia, and retinopathy of prematurity, which are discussed in later sections.

TABLE 8-3. Mortality and Major Neonatal Morbidity According to Birth Weight for the NICHD Neonatal Network

	Weight (g)			
	501–750	*751–1000*	*1001–1250*	*1251–1500*
Survival (%)	34	66	87	93
Morbidity among survivors (%)	56	39	25	15
Chronic lung disease (%)	26	14	7	3
Intracranial hemorrhage (%)	26	17	13	6
Enterocolitis (%)	3	8	6	4

Adapted from Hack M, Horbar ID, Malloy MH, Tyson JE, Wright E, Wright L. Very-low-birth-weight outcomes of the National Institute of Child Health and Human Development Neonatal Network. Pediatrics. 1991;82:585.

■ OUTCOME

Mortality among LBW infants, after declining sharply in the 1970s, has begun to level off. Mortality and selective morbidity rates among LBW infants are shown in Table 8–3 As mortality has declined, morbidity among the survivors has increasingly distressed health care providers. Nelson and Ellenberg associated a 10- to 33-fold increase in the risk of cerebral palsy with several factors, including birth weight of less than 2000 g, head circumference greater or less than three standard deviations from the mean, 5-minute Apgar score of less than 3, diminished activity or cry of greater than 1 day in duration, thermal instability, need for gavage feeding, hypotonia or hypertonia, apnea, or hematocrit of less than 40%. A 50-fold increase in cerebral palsy was associated with neonatal seizures or a 10-minute Apgar score of less than 3. Other studies have related LBW and the need for ventilator support to functional handicaps and an increased incidence of rehospitalization, most often related to chronic conditions that are consequences of prematurity (eg, bronchopulmonary dysplasia, posthemorrhagic hydrocephalus, failure to thrive), infections, and the need for herniorrhaphy.

However, infants of less than 1000 g of birth weight studied at 5 years of age were reported to have demonstrated an improvement in function and, in some cases, appeared to have outgrown the developmental or neurologic disability. It is likely that such "improvements" reflect difficulties in early diagnosis of developmental or neurologic abnormalities. Moreover, low socioeconomic status and decreased maternal age and experience can adversely affect motor and cognitive development. These environmental influences are not easily distinguished from the effects of premature delivery and its sequelae as causes of developmental delay.

In the final analysis, the outcome among LBW infants of more than 1000 g of birth weight is generally good in terms of both morbidity and mortality. However, the ethics and cost-effectiveness of intensive care for infants of less than 1000 g of birth weight, and particularly for those of less than 750 g of birth weight, continue to pose problems for health care providers and society at large. Hack and coworkers (1991) described a 3-year experience with 98 infants of less than 700 g of birth weight. Although overall mortality was 81%, resuscitation was attempted in only 45% of the infants. Survival among resuscitated infants was 43%. Morbidity among survivors was high and included bronchopulmonary dysplasia (70%), PDA (60%), septicemia (65%), necrotizing enterocolitis (10%), grade III or IV intraventricular hemorrhage (20%), and stage 3 or 4 retinopathy of prematurity (25%). Ninety-five percent of surviving infants demonstrated subnormal growth at term. Clearly, long-term follow-up is necessary, but these data illustrate that guidelines for resuscitation of extremely immature infants must be evaluated continually, particularly in the face of recent advances such as the use of artificial surfactant, which appears to reduce mortality although subsequent long-term neurologic morbidity among survivors is unknown.

The economic cost of providing tertiary care to the ELBW infant can be calculated, but it is not uniformly relevant to the perceived quality of life for the surviving infants and their parents. Moreover, in large public hospitals, distribution of personnel and services is severely affected, potentially affecting the care of more mature, more viable LBW infants.

(Abridged from Steven R. Mayfield, Ricardo Uauy, and Joseph B. Warshaw, The Premature Newborn, in Oski, DeAngelis, Feigin, McMillan, Warshaw: *Principles and Practice of Pediatrics, Second Edition*, J.B. Lippincott, 1994.)

Oski's Essential Pediatrics, edited by Kevin B. Johnson and Frank A. Oski. Lippincott–Raven Publishers, Philadelphia © 1997

9

Growth and Metabolic Adaptation of the Fetus and Newborn

■ THE BASIS OF DEVELOPMENTAL PATHOLOGY

Many neonatal disease processes can be explained by preterm delivery, which determines unsuccessful adaptation and progressive compromise of specific organ function. The occurrence of hyaline membrane disease in babies born before 34 weeks gestation (*ie,* before surfactant production is adequate) is a good example of developmental pathology. Table 9–1 outlines many of the normal adaptations associated with extrauterine life. Overall, these adaptive responses are integrated and mediated by the neuroendocrine system, which acts as a focal point to ensure successful adaptation.

TABLE 9-1. Immediate Neonatal Adaptations Necessary for Successful Extrauterine Life

CARDIOVASCULAR

Reduction in pulmonary vasculature resistance

Increased lung blood flow

Closure of ductus arteriosus

Separate right and left cardiac pumps

PULMONARY

Maturation of alveoli and capillary network

Development of the surfactant system (phosphatidylcholine and phosphatidylglycerol)

Rhythmic respiration

Maturation of antioxidant enzyme systems

METABOLIC-ENDOCRINE

Thermogenesis and temperature regulation

Glucose homeostasis (glycogenolysis, gluconeogenesis)

Neuroendocrine responsiveness

Enzymatic maturation for detoxification, excretion, and metabolism of fuels and substrate

NUTRITIONAL

Intermittent rather than continuous feeds

Digestion and absorption of nutrients

Excretion of acid, nitrogen, and electrolytes

Maintenance of nutrient supply for growth and development

NEURODEVELOPMENTAL

Integrated responses to environmental stimuli

Maintenance of autonomic regulation under new conditions

Activation of sensory input and processing necessary for learning

Operation of reflexes and behaviors needed for survival

TABLE 9-2. Genetic, Hormonal, and Environmental Influences on Fetal Growth

GENETIC AND FETAL FACTORS

Species, racial, gender
Congenital anomalies
Chromosomal disorders
Fetal hormones (insulin, corticosteroids, thyroid hormone, androgens)
Growth factors (IGF I and IGF II, EGF and TGF-α)

MATERNAL UTERINE ENVIRONMENT

Uterine and placental anatomy
Uteroplacental function
Human placental lactogen
Substrate fluxes and transfer
Uterine blood flow
Maternal systemic disease

MACROENVIRONMENT

Infectious agents (STORCH)
Diet and nutrition
Social and emotional stress
Drugs and smoking
Teratogens and toxins
Altitude and temperature
Ionizing radiation

Many of the neonatal consequences of obstetric problems can be avoided because of advances in prenatal and delivery room care. Thus, birth trauma and birth asphyxia are less frequent. Still, the consequences of preterm labor remain important because of poor understanding of the mechanisms responsible and of the interventions required to prevent premature deliveries. Even if premature labor and obstetric complications associated with birth were eliminated, there would still be neonatal morbidity and mortality associated with genetic disorders, congenital malformations, and environmental factors (Table 9–2).

(Abridged from Ricardo Uauy, Patricia Mena, and Joseph B. Warshaw, Growth and Metabolic Adaptation of the Fetus and Newborn, in Oski, DeAngelis, Feigin, McMillan, Warshaw: *Principles and Practice of Pediatrics, Second Edition,* J.B. Lippincott, 1994.)

Oski's Essential Pediatrics,
edited by Kevin B. Johnson and Frank A. Oski.
Lippincott–Raven Publishers,
Philadelphia © 1997

10

Fetal Evaluation and Prenatal Diagnosis

Serious birth defects, often genetically determined, complicate and threaten the lives of 3% of newborn infants. These disorders account for 20% of deaths during the newborn period and contribute to an even higher percentage of serious morbidity in infancy and childhood. The cost of neonatal intensive care is staggering; higher still are the costs of rehabilitation programs for the severely handicapped. The family tragedy is perhaps unmeasurable. With growing recognition of the frequency and importance of congenital disorders and with social trends toward a smaller family size as well as delay in beginning a family, prenatal diagnosis plays an important role in the management of many pregnancies.

■ INDICATIONS FOR PRENATAL DIAGNOSIS

The identification of a pregnancy with an increased chance of a diagnosable fetal disorder involves a search for general and specific risk factors. Counseling before prenatal diagnosis is important. The central issue is balancing the risk of an abnormal child against the risk of an investigative or interventional procedure. Prospective parents must understand the concept of excluding or establishing a specific diagnosis with a high reliability but without complete certainty. One of the most important goals in genetic counseling is to help patients understand the reproductive options available. A person's previous experience, ethnic and cultural background, and religious beliefs will affect the acceptability of prenatal diagnosis and the choices made after the diagnosis of an abnormality. Counseling should be nondirective and should concentrate on accurate presentation of all the facts and options available. Common indications for prenatal counseling and diagnosis are summarized in Table 10–1.

General Factors

It is standard practice to offer prenatal cytogenetic diagnosis to all women who at their expected delivery date will be 35 years or older. Numeric chromosome abnormalities occur with increasing frequency with advancing maternal age (Table 10–2). Testing for biochemical markers in maternal serum identifies patients at risk for certain cytogenetic and structural abnormalities. Alpha-fetoprotein, the major protein of early fetal life, is synthesized in the fetal liver and yolk sac. Open neural tube and ventral wall defects are associated with exposed fetal membrane and blood vessel surfaces, which increase the levels of alpha-fetoprotein in amniotic fluid and maternal serum. Low levels of maternal serum alpha-fetoprotein and unconjugated estriol are associated with trisomies 21 and 18.

The single marker that yields the highest detection rate for Down's syndrome is human chorionic gonadotropin, which is significantly elevated in this syndrome. The combined use of the markers human chorionic gonadotropin, unconjugated estriol, maternal serum alpha-fetoprotein, and maternal age leads to detection of about 60% of cases of Down's syndrome, with a false-positive rate of 6.6%; the use of ultrasonography to verify gestational age reduces the false-positive rate to 3.8%.

Maternal serum alpha-fetoprotein screening should be offered to women at 16 to 18 completed weeks of pregnancy. Careful evaluation of gestational age is of critical importance because maternal serum alpha-fetoprotein values increase steadily throughout the second trimester. Because of population differences of median maternal serum alpha-fetoprotein values, laboratories should provide interpretation of results that take into account the variables of race, multiple gestation, diabetes mellitus, and maternal weight. Most centers in the United States have chosen a cutoff of 2.0 to 2.5 times the median for the general population screened for neural tube defects. Invasive procedures such as amniocentesis may give rise to maternal alpha-fetoprotein elevations; therefore,

TABLE 10-1. Indications for Prenatal Testing

GENERAL FACTORS

Maternal age ≥35 at time of delivery

Maternal serum alpha-fetoprotein concentration

Triple screening (maternal serum alpha-fetoprotein, human chorionic gonadotropin, and unconjugated estriol)

SPECIFIC FACTORS

Previous child with structural defect or chromosomal abnormality

Stillbirths, neonatal deaths

Parent with structural abnormality

Parent with balanced translocation

Inherited disorders (cystic fibrosis, metabolic disorders, sex-linked recessive disorders)

Maternal medical disease (diabetes, phenylketonuria)

Teratogen exposure (ionizing radiation, anticonvulsant medicines, lithium, isotretinoin, alcohol)

Infections (rubella, toxoplasmosis, cytomegalovirus)

ETHNIC FACTORS

Disorder	Ethnic Group	Screening Test
Tay-Sachs disease	Ashkenazi Jews, French Canadians	Decreased serum hexosaminidase A
Sickle-cell anemia	Black Africans, Mediterraneans, Arabs, Indo-Pakistanis	Presence of sickling in hemolysate followed by confirmatory hemoglobin electrophoresis
Thalassemia (alpha and beta)	Mediterraneans, Southern and Southeast Asians, Chinese	Mean corpuscular volume <80 semtoliters followed by confirmatory hemoglobin electrophoresis

blood samples for screening markers should be obtained before amniocentesis is performed.

Specific Factors

After birth of one child with trisomy 21, the likelihood that a subsequent child will have a similar chromosomal abnormality is about 1%. The recurrence rate for neural tube defects is 2% to 5%, compared with a general population risk of 1 to 2 per 1000 births. The general recurrence risk of a cardiac defect is 2% to 4%, compared with the general population risk of 4 to 8 per 1000 live births. If a parent has spina bifida, congenital heart disease, or a known chromosome translocation or inversion, there is an increased chance that a child will have a related defect. Antenatal diagnosis is possible for many inborn errors of metabolism, almost all of which are transmitted in an autosomal recessive fashion. Maternal diabetes and maternal phenylketonuria are associated with an increased risk of fetal malformations. Other known teratogens include ionizing radiation, drugs, and maternal infections.

Ethnic Factors

The gene frequencies of various genetic disorders differ among geographic population groups. Carrier detection programs can be applied to different ethnic groups at risk for specific diseases (*eg*, for Tay-Sachs disease in Ashkenazi Jewish populations, hemoglobins in blacks, and thalassemia in people of Mediterranean origin). The populations involved and the methods of screening are listed in

TABLE 10-2. Maternal Age and Estimated Rates of Chromosomal Abnormalities at Time of Expected Live Birth

Maternal Age	Risk of Down Syndrome	Total Risk for Chromosomal Abnormalities
20	1/1667	1/526
25	1/1250	1/476
30	1/952	1/385
35	1/385	1/202
36	1/295	1/162
37	1/227	1/129
38	1/175	1/102
39	1/137	1/82
40	1/106	1/65
41	1/82	1/51
42	1/64	1/40
43	1/50	1/32
44	1/38	1/25
45	1/30	1/20
46	1/23	1/16
47	1/18	1/13
48	1/14	1/10
49	1/11	1/7

Modified from Hook EB. Rates of chromosome abnormalities at different gestational ages. Obstet Gynecol. 1981;58:282, and Hook EB, Cross PK, Schreinemacher MS. Chromosomal, abnormality rates at amniocentesis and in live-born infants. JAMA. 1983;249:2034.

tions involved and the methods of screening are listed in Table 10–1.

■ EFFICACY OF SCREENING METHODS

Prenatal diagnosis for chromosomal analysis is offered to women who will be 35 years or older at the time of delivery. Nearly all genetic procedures performed in the United States are performed in the 5% of women who are over 35 years of age. This approach detects only 20% of cases of Down's syndrome; the use of maternal serum alpha-fetoprotein screening in women of all ages will identify an additional 25% of cases. Use of maternal serum alpha-fetoprotein, human chorionic gonadotropin, unconjugated estriol, and maternal age will identify about 60% of cases of Down's syndrome. Clinicians using a maternal serum alpha-fetoprotein screening program can expect to detect 80% to 90% percent of fetuses with neural tube defects, almost all cases of gastroschisis, and 70% to 80% of cases of omphalocele. The use of routine ultrasound screening, including a four-chamber view of the heart, potentially can diagnose about half of major cardiac, kidney, and bladder anomalies that would not be detected with maternal serum alpha-fetoprotein screening (Table 10–3). When a targeted ultrasound examination is done to detect malformations suspected by history or screening ultrasonography in referral centers with skilled ultrasonologists, the sensitivity and specificity exceed 90%.

■ THE FUTURE

The project of mapping the human genome is expected to be completed in the next 10 to 15 years, and, as a result, molecular genetic technology is likely to be available for detection of many additional common monogenic disorders. Cost-effective screening will be available for many disorders, including cystic fibrosis. Preimplantation diagnosis is possible in certain circumstances and may allow fetal treatment before organogenesis.

A promising new technique for isolating fetal cells from maternal blood is under intensive study. The challenges of this technique include reliably separating fetal cells by identifying unique fetal cell surface antigens and modifying molecular genetic techniques such as the polymerase chain reaction so that small samples of fetal genetic material can be analyzed. It is likely that continued research into the fetal cell separation methods will make noninvasive prenatal diagnosis a reality.

(Abridged from Mary E. D'Alton, Fetal Evaluation and Prenatal Diagnosis, in Oski, DeAngelis, Feigin, McMillan, Warshaw: *Principles and Practice of Pediatrics, Second Edition*, J.B. Lippincott, 1994.)

Oski's Essential Pediatrics, edited by Kevin B. Johnson and Frank A. Oski. Lippincott–Raven Publishers, Philadelphia © 1997

11

Intrauterine Growth Retardation

Intrauterine growth retardation (IUGR), or, preferably, intrauterine growth restriction, represents a final common pathway by which genetic and environmental influences result in low birth weight for gestational age. The diverse factors that influence fetal growth and may contribute to IUGR are reviewed in Chapter 9. IUGR has been defined most commonly in the United States as a birth weight of less than the 10th percentile for gestational age. This definition probably overestimates the incidence of IUGR, because it is unreasonable to consider 10% of all births as having pathologic restriction of growth. Small infants in whom there is no evidence that adverse genetic or environmental influences are limiting growth should be spared the IUGR label, which connotes pathology, and should be defined as small for gestational age (SGA). SGA should be applied to all infants less than the 10th percentile, and IUGR generally should be reserved for infants less than the 3rd percentile, recognizing that some infants with growth restriction will fall out of this range if an insult occurs late in gestation. Thus, whereas all IUGR infants also are SGA, not all SGA infants are IUGR.

Confusion about definitions is amplified further by significant differences in the 10th percentile birth weights at each gestational age that have been published. Differences in published standards of growth have probably been influenced by racial composition, socioeconomic status of the population, and altitude above sea level when the standards were developed. The commonly used Lubchenco grids were developed in Denver, which is about 5000 feet above sea level, and may overestimate IUGR when these charts are used at sea level. What is necessary for an effective comparison between populations is the adoption of a single standard for fetal growth, for example the standards developed

---

TABLE 10-3. Sonographic Findings in Chromosomal Abnormalities

TRISOMY 21

Duodenal atresia, tracheoesophageal fistula, esophageal atresia; polyhydramnios is usual if these gastrointestinal lesions present

Cardiac abnormalities (atrioventricular canal defects, ventricular septal defects, atrial septal defects)

Hypoplasia of middle quadrant of the fifth digit

Second trimester findings: thickened nuchal fold >6 mm; ratio of actual to expected femur length, 0.91

TRISOMY 18

Intrauterine growth retardation

Polyhydramnios

Clenched hands with overlapping digits

Clubfeet, rocker-bottom feet

Cardiac abnormalities (ventricular septal defect)

Omphalocele, diaphragmatic hernia

Choroid plexus cysts

TRISOMY 13

Holoprosencephaly

Cleft lip and palate

Cardiac abnormalities (ventricular septal defect)

Polydactyly

Omphalocele

Polycystic kidneys

by Brenner from 30,772 deliveries from 21 to 44 weeks' gestational age in Cleveland. These standards include correction factors for poverty, race, and sex.

Recognition and treatment of IUGR require an understanding of the diverse etiologies that result in restricted fetal growth. The pattern of growth of the infant with IUGR often reflects the underlying condition that has resulted in growth restriction. The terms *proportionate* and *disproportionate* have been used to distinguish newborns with decreased growth potential from those with restricted growth due to fetal malnutrition.

Newborns with decreased growth potential due to conditions such as chromosomal disorders, congenital infections, or exposure to environmental toxins characteristically have body proportions that are proportionate or symmetric (*ie*, the head, length, and weight generally occur within similar percentile grids), or the head is small relative to the body, as in microcephaly. Obstetric monitoring of the fetus with decreased growth potential characteristically demonstrates decreased body growth, including that of the head, from midgestation or earlier. Fetuses with decreased growth potential are at high risk for having major malformations or congenital infection.

Newborns with fetal malnutrition have weight reduced out of proportion to length or head circumference and may exhibit a sparing of head growth during late gestation. These infants are disproportionate, with the head circumference and length closer to the expected percentiles for gestational age than those for weight. Nutritional constraints on growth are unusual before 24 to 25 weeks of gestation; in most cases, only after that time will restriction in blood supply to the fetus result in IUGR. In mild to moderate degrees of IUGR, head growth may proceed along normal percentile grids, with a decrease in body fat and restriction in length and weight (disproportionate growth). This sparing of head growth is thought to result from circulatory changes in the fetus that favor a redistribution of blood flow to the heart and brain. There may be exceptions to this general pattern. In instances of extreme nutritional restriction in the fetus with class D diabetes or other conditions that result in severely compromised uterine blood flow, even head growth may be decreased.

Infants with either proportionate or disproportionate IUGR should be evaluated carefully for conditions causing hydrocephalus or microcephaly that may also confound the measurements. Figure 11–1 summarizes the etiology of IUGR. The importance of environmental exposures such as cigarette smoking cannot be overestimated. In the developed countries of the world, cigarette smoking is perhaps the single greatest determinant of low birth weight. It has been estimated that perinatal mortality would be reduced by 15% with elimination of all cigarette smoking in pregnancy.

The pattern of postnatal growth is also important to record and follow. As a consequence of decreased growth potential, infants with proportionate growth retardation may exhibit sluggish postnatal growth even with adequate nutrition. A slow rate of postnatal growth may be seen in genetic disorders, congenital infections, or the fetal alcohol syndrome. Infants with growth retardation secondary to fetal malnutrition often exhibit rapid growth when adequate nutrients are provided in the postnatal period; this is a good prognostic finding. About 30% of nutritionally induced IUGR newborns are still below the 3rd percentile at 2 years of age.

■ MANAGEMENT

Optimal management of IUGR should begin with recognition of the problem in utero so informed decisions can be made concerning the appropriate time and method of delivery. This includes consideration of the options of cesarean section versus vaginal delivery. If biophysical data obtained during fetal monitoring show fetal distress, cesarean section may be the preferred mode of delivery. Decreased maternal weight gain and fundal growth should alert the obstetrician to the likelihood of fetal growth retardation. Ultrasonography can then confirm the diagnosis by monitoring such parameters of fetal growth as the biparietal diameter or the relationship of head size to body size.

Strategies to treat fetal growth retardation have included therapies to decrease the platelet aggregation and abnormalities in uteroplacental circulation seen in toxemia of pregnancy as well as maternal nutritional supplementation and oxygen therapy. In a promising study of 323 women at risk for fetal growth retardation, administration of 150 mg/day aspirin resulted in a 225-g newborn weight increase over the placebo group. The beneficial effect of low-dose aspirin probably related to inhibition of the synthesis of thromboxane B_2, which decreases the platelet aggregation and placental vasocclusion seen in the toxemic state.

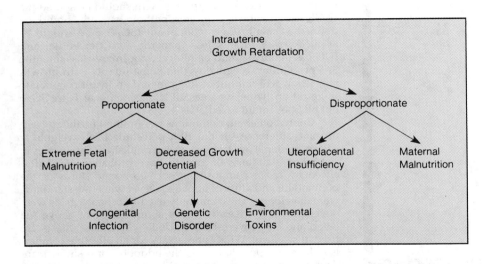

Figure 11-1. Classification of intrauterine growth retardation.

Maternal parenteral nutritional supplementation is controversial. An adverse influence was observed when short-term administration of glucose to normal patients before delivery resulted in a significant increase in lactic acid and a fall in pH. When the fetus is "adapted" to a decreased nutrient supply, there may be a potential risk to increasing nutritional intake without a corresponding increase in fetal oxygenation. Indeed, several of the changes seen in IUGR can be considered adaptations to an adverse intrauterine nutritional environment: sparing of brain growth, increased red cell mass, and small size itself, in which the size of the fetus may be appropriate to the availability of nutrients. Even early lung maturation can be considered an adaptation that improves the opportunity for a good postnatal outcome.

Important problems of the infant with IUGR secondary to intrauterine malnutrition are summarized in Table 11–1. Appropriate management can prevent many of these problems (Table 11–2). If there is birth asphyxia, support measures should be instituted immediately, including the establishment of an effective airway and the management of meconium if present. Suctioning and clearing the meconium from the airway before delivery of the thorax and establishing of the first breath, together with tracheal suction if meconium is present at the level of the cords, have greatly reduced problems associated with meconium aspiration. Meconium aspiration is rarely seen in infants of less than 35 weeks' gestation; therefore, in those infants, hypoxia per se is the major problem. An estimate of the degree of acidosis can be obtained from the cord blood pH. Hyaline membrane disease is generally less of a problem in infants with disproportionate IUGR because of the accelerated lung maturation commonly seen in these infants. Some asphyxiated newborns exhibit significant right-to-left cardiac shunting, making systemic oxygenation difficult to achieve. This is a consequence of chronic intrauterine hypoxia, which results in abnormal thickening of the smooth muscle of small pulmonary arterioles, thereby reducing pulmonary blood flow and increasing right-to-left blood flow at the atrial level or through the ductus arteriosus. Diagnosis is confirmed by measuring the disparity between preductal (right radial) and postductal (umbilical arterial) PO_2. Because acidosis and hypoxia modulate pulmonary arteriolar vasomotor tone, therapeutic efforts should be directed toward reversing these conditions. There is no clearly effective therapy, although some infants appear to improve with an induced respiratory alkalosis (pH 7.45 to 7.55). Tolazoline is often used to reduce pulmonary arterial pressure, but there is little evidence for its efficacy. Extracorporeal membrane oxygenation has had a surge in popularity in the treatment of this condition, but efficacy for this expensive and complex intervention has not been clearly established.

Apgar scores should be assigned in the delivery room, and the infant should be dried rapidly and warmed to prevent hypothermia. As soon as the infant is stable, measurements should be taken and plotted on standard growth grids. As mentioned above, the Lubchenco charts are used in most institutions, although they may underestimate IUGR because the observations were made well above sea level and may have been influenced by racial and ethnic differences in the Denver population.

A careful assessment of gestational age should be done in all infants with IUGR. The examination most commonly used is a modification of a scale developed by Dubowitz that includes physical signs involving skin color and texture, hair, breast size, plantar creases, ear form and firmness, external genitalia, and neuromuscular assessment, which measures tone, posture, and reflexes. Scores are assigned for these measures, with a total score being used to assign gestational age. This examination can be completed in about 10 minutes and has a predictive error of plus or minus 2 weeks in infants weighing more than 1000 g. It is most accurate when performed within the first 6 hours of life and by two observers.

Newborns with IUGR secondary to fetal malnutrition (eg, those with decreased uteroplacental blood flow) are disproportionate, with the head and length generally in higher percentiles than the weight. These infants frequently appear scrawny as a result of their marked decrease in subcutaneous fat. They have an alert appearance and have higher Dubowitz ratings than do premature infants with similar weights.

Infants should be examined for genetic causes of IUGR, including the presence of congenital malformations. They should also be evaluated for any stigmata of congenital infection. The examination should include weighing and examining the placenta to determine whether there are structural or vascular abnormalities contributing to IUGR.

Many of the problems of IUGR newborns relate to their markedly decreased metabolic reserves. There is a risk of perinatal asphyxia when oxygen and metabolic demands exceed the oxygen provided by the uteroplacental circulation. This underscores the need for careful biophysical monitoring of the at-risk fetus to alert the obstetrician to the presence of uteroplacental insufficiency. Hypoglycemia is found frequently in the immediate postnatal period. Hypothermia may increase oxygen and glucose requirements. Blood glucose should be measured, and a central hematocrit test should be performed to detect polycythemia. Hyperviscosity and hypoglycemia are primarily problems of the nutritionally growth-retarded newborn. Those with IUGR secondary to congenital infection, genetic disorders, or environmental insults are less likely to experience these complications.

TABLE 11-2. Management of the IUGR Infant

Gestational age assessment and careful history for drugs, and so forth

Prevent hypothermia

Check central hematocrit

Monitor blood sugar within first 45 min

Evaluate for congenital infections and congenital malformations

Chromosomal and genetic evaluation as indicated

Careful follow-up

TABLE 11-1. Problems of the IUGR Newborn

Birth asphyxia	Hypoglycemia
Meconium aspiration	Hypocalcemia
Persistent fetal circulation	Polycythemia
Hypothermia	Congenital malformation

(Abridged from Joseph B. Warshaw, Intrauterine Growth Retardation, in Oski, DeAngelis, Feigin, McMillan, Warshaw: *Principles and Practice of Pediatrics, Second Edition*, J.B. Lippincott, 1994.)

Oski's Essential Pediatrics,
edited by Kevin B. Johnson and Frank A. Oski.
Lippincott–Raven Publishers,
Philadelphia © 1997

12

Intraventricular Hemorrhage of the Preterm Infant

Intraventricular hemorrhage (IVH), or hemorrhage into the germinal matrix tissues with possible rupture into the ventricular system and parenchyma of the developing brain (Figure 12–1), remains a major problem of preterm neonates. Because the germinal matrix begins to involute after 34 weeks of gestation, germinal matrix and intraventricular hemorrhages (GMH/IVH) are lesions of preterm infants, and a recent study of 2928 neonates of less than 1500-g birth weight demonstrated an incidence of GMH/IVH of greater than 45%.

■ CLINICAL STUDIES

The incidence of GMH/IVH increases as gestational age decreases, and as many as 50% of infants less than 25 to 26 weeks' gestation have the disorder. In addition, although the incidence has been reported to vary between 20% and 40% in large cohorts of infants of less than 34 weeks' gestation, high-grade hemorrhages are found more commonly in neonates with very low birth weights. Hemorrhages have been reported within the first postnatal hour, and a significant number of hemorrhages occur by the sixth hour. About half of all preterm infants who will have GMH/IVH do so on the first postnatal day, and less than 5% have hemorrhage after the fourth to fifth postnatal days. This risk period for GMH/IVH appears to be independent of gestational age. Finally, some infants, especially those with the earliest onset of GMH/IVH, will have extension of hemorrhage over the first several postnatal days; this progression has been linked to clinical events such as pneumothoraces and seizures that are known to increase cerebral blood flow (CBF).

The clinical manifestations of GMH/IVH are varied. In a significant percentage of cases, GMH/IVH is felt to be clinically silent, although infants with major hemorrhages may experience coma, seizures, abnormal eye findings (including dilated pupils and loss of eye movements), and changes in tone and reflexes. Persistent bradycardia and apneic spells may be secondary to increased intracranial pressure or alterations in CBF to brain stem respiratory centers. Infants may have significantly elevated values of blood glucose and evidence of inappropriate secretion of antidiuretic hormone. Finally, patients with large parenchymal hemorrhages frequently experience a persistent metabolic acidosis that is unresponsive to alkali therapy or pressor agents.

■ OUTCOME STUDIES

Infants with GMH/IVH are at risk for the development of posthemorrhagic hydrocephalus (PHH) and are known to have higher incidences of neonatal seizures and periventricular leukomalacia than do infants with hemorrhage, as compared with normal infants matched for birth weight or gestational age. Finally, most investigators agree that those infants with parenchymal involvement of GMH/IVH are at high risk for neurodevelopmental handicap.

Posthemorrhagic hydrocephalus (Figure 12–2) is the combination of ventriculomegaly, diagnosed by serial echoencephalography studies, and increased intracranial pressure, defined as an opening pressure of greater than 140 mm H_2O on either lumbar puncture or, if indicated, cerebral ventricular tap. Posthemorrhagic hydrocephalus generally is a communicating hydrocephalus with a block at the level of the arachnoid villi or, less commonly, at the foramina of Luschka and Magendie in the posterior fossa. Hydrocephalus results when the blood and protein in the cerebrospinal fluid (CSF) produce a chemical arachnoiditis that may be transient or, less commonly, permanent. A small percentage of infants with IVH will have a noncommunicating hydrocephalus with a block at the level of the aqueduct secondary to an ependymal reaction similar to that of the arachnoid. Infants with the latter type of hydrocephalus will require neurosurgical intervention, whereas the treatment for neonates with communicating PHH, at least initially, is medical.

All infants with intraventricular blood require close ultrasound monitoring of ventricular size. These patients should

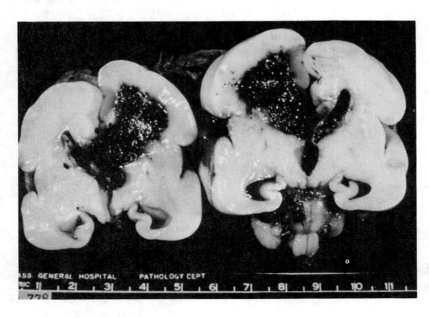

Figure 12-1. Coronal sections of the brain of a 28-week preterm infant with a large intraventricular and frontoparietal parenchymal hemorrhage.

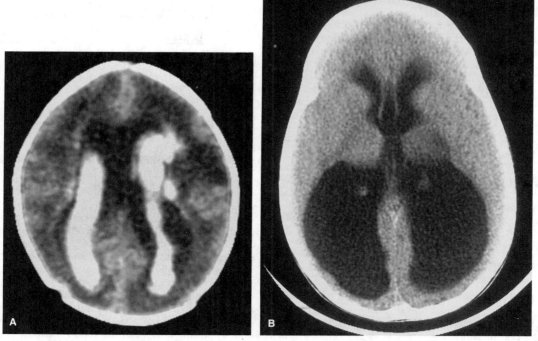

Figure 12-2. (**A**) CT scan of preterm infant of 28 weeks' gestational age with bilateral intraventricular hemorrhage. (**B**) Repeat CT, performed because of rapidly increasing occipitofrontal head circumference, lethargy, and increasing apneic spells, demonstrated ventriculomegaly. Lumbar puncture revealed an opening pressure of greater than 200 mm of water, consistent with the diagnosis of posthemorrhagic hydrocephalus.

undergo frequent head circumference measurements and cranial ultrasound examinations for determination of ventricular size. Because prolonged increased intracranial pressure may result in apnea, vomiting, lethargy, and, ultimately, optic atrophy, the intracranial pressure of infants with head circumferences crossing the expected growth curves and evidence for increasing ventricular size should be checked and, when the diagnosis is confirmed, treatment should be provided.

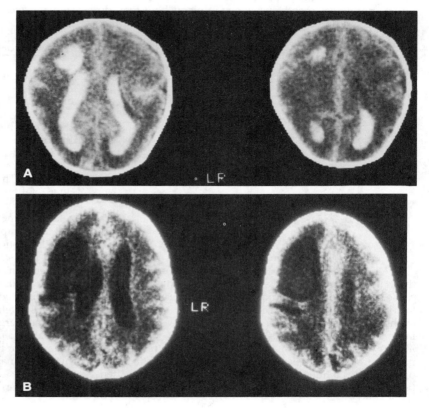

Figure 12-3. This male of 27 weeks' gestation initially was found to have a bilateral intraventricular hemorrhage with a right frontal parenchymal component (**A**). Repeat CT 12 weeks later demonstrated a large right porencephalic cyst and moderate ventriculomegaly (**B**).

In many large series of preterm neonates, the incidence of motor handicaps appears to be low. These abnormalities include spastic diplegia, hemiparesis, and, rarely, spastic quadriparesis. Most infants with spastic diplegia have neuroimaging evidence for PVL but, in general, have normal head circumferences, no evidence of seizures, and cognitive scores within the normal range. Although many investigators believe that there are no differences in the developmental outcome of infants with grades I, II, or III IVH when compared with infants with no known evidence of hemorrhage in the neonatal period, recent data suggest that the rate of cognitive deficits may increase with the grade of IVH in this patient population. Infants with parenchymal involvement of hemorrhage, or grade IV IVH, experience a wide range of outcomes; about 50% of all neonates with grade IV IVH will have motor and cognitive handicaps. For many of these children, the development of a porencephalic cyst follows resolution of the parenchymal blood, and this can be demonstrated easily both on CT scan (Figure 12–3) and with ultrasound.

■ INTERVENTION STUDIES

A variety of measures have been suggested to prevent GMH/IVH. Clearly, the most important way to prevent GMH/IVH is to prevent preterm birth. When that is not possible, transport of the mother and fetus to a regional perinatal center specializing in high-risk obstetric care is preferred; "outborn" infants have consistently higher rates of GMH/IVH than do those who are "inborn."

Neonatal care should be based on an understanding of the pathogenesis of GMH/IVH. Abrupt increases in blood pressure and, thus, changes in CBF should be avoided. Blood pressure and transcutaneous PO_2 should be monitored continuously to avoid hypotension and hypoxemia. Hypercarbia should be avoided similarly. The role of the patent ductus arteriosus, and its abrupt closure, in the genesis of IVH long has been debated, and it appears that pharmacologic closure promotes smoother changes in blood flow than do surgical procedures.

(Abridged from Laura R. Ment, Intraventricular Hemorrhage of the Preterm Infant, in Oski, DeAngelis, Feigin, McMillan, Warshaw: *Principles and Practice of Pediatrics, Second Edition*, J.B. Lippincott, 1994.)

Oski's Essential Pediatrics,
edited by Kevin B. Johnson and Frank A. Oski.
Lippincott–Raven Publishers,
Philadelphia © 1997

13

Perinatal Asphyxia

Perinatal asphyxia, or hypoxic-ischemic encephalopathy (HIE), represents "the single most important perinatal cause of neurologic morbidity" in the full-term as well as the low-birth-weight infant, occurring in 6:1000 full-term live births and in an even higher percentage of low-birth-weight infants. Follow-up studies indicate that 25% or more of infants who survive perinatal asphyxia demonstrate permanent neurologic sequelae, ranging from often subtle developmental disabilities such as learning disabilities and attention deficit disorder to more obvious problems such as

TABLE 13-1. Etiology of Perinatal Asphyxia

Time of Insult	Percentage of Total
Antepartum	20
Intrapartum	35
Intrapartum ± antepartum	35
Postnatal	10

Volpe JJ. Neurology of the newborn. 2nd ed. Philadelphia: WB Saunders; 1987.

cerebral palsy, mental retardation, pervasive developmental disorders, and seizures.

The causes of perinatal asphyxia are considered most reasonably within a temporal framework as shown in Table 13–1. About 70% of the cases of perinatal asphyxia that are seen in full-term infants are related to events occurring during labor and delivery; these include fetal distress (*eg*, abnormal fetal heart rate patterns, meconium-stained amniotic fluid, or abnormalities in fetal acid–base values), abruptio placentae, cord prolapse, and traumatic delivery.

The onset of asphyxia is followed by metabolic changes and alterations in cerebral blood flow. Metabolic consequences include an increase in brain lactate levels, a reduction in high-energy phosphate concentrations, and the release of excitotoxic neurotransmitters, which are believed to play a critical role in neuronal damage. Alterations in cerebral blood flow accompany these metabolic changes and include an initial increase in cerebral blood flow, loss of vascular autoregulation, reduction in cardiac output, hypotension, and, finally, reduction in cerebral blood flow. Circulatory changes are believed to play a more prominent role in the production of two other commonly observed pathologic changes after asphyxia: parasagittal cerebral injury and periventricular leukomalacia.

■ CLINICAL FEATURES

Perinatal asphyxia may be recognized clinically both before delivery (antepartum and intrapartum) and after delivery (Table 13–2). Recent advances in technology such as ultrasonography, electronic fetal heart rate monitoring (EFM), and direct fetal blood sampling offer the opportunity to evaluate the status of the fetus before delivery. Perinatal asphyxia may be assessed in the antepartum period by two measures: the fetal heart acceleration test (nonstress test) and the biophysical profile. The former measures the increase in fetal heart rate after fetal movement. The latter combines the nonstress test with the ultrasonographic determination of fetal breathing, fetal movements, fetal tone, and amniotic fluid volume. During the intrapartum period, the evaluation of fetal heart rate and its relationship to uterine contractions has been used to assess fetal status. Investigations indicate that such findings as decelerations in fetal heart rate after a uterine contraction (late decelerations) are related to uteroplacental insufficiency and are influenced considerably by fetal hypoxia. Similarly, decelerations in fetal heart rate beginning with or occurring shortly after the uterine contraction (variable decelerations) appear to be related to umbilical cord compression, which, if continued, can result in reduction in umbilical cord blood flow and fetal hypoxia. Finally, evaluation of fetal acid–base status by direct fetal blood sampling may provide another index reflecting the effects of perinatal asphyxia.

TABLE 13-2. Clinical Features of Perinatal Asphyxia

FETAL

Abnormal biophysical profile

Abnormal electronic fetal monitoring

   Bradycardia

   Late decelerations

   Variable decelerations leading to late decelerations

Abnormal fetal acid–base status

POSTNATAL

Evidence of asphyxia at birth

   Failure to initiate respiration

   Low Apgar scores

State of consciousness

   Ranges along a continuum from normal, to hyperalertness, through obtundation, lethargy, stupor, and coma

Evidence of damage to other organ systems

   Renal (oliguria)

   Cardiac (myocardiopathy)

   Liver (abnormal liver function test results)

Laboratory studies

   Neuroimaging abnormal

      Magnetic resonance imaging (MRI)

      Ultrasound

      Computed tomography

   Electroencephalography abnormal (*eg*, burst suppression)

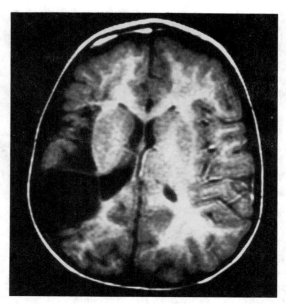

Figure 13-1. Magnetic resonance image of a full-term neonate with a right hemisphere porencephaly. In the perinatal period, the patient experienced a precipitous drop in fetal heart rate and low Apgar scores.

Although Apgar scores are by far the most widely used index of the condition of the infant at birth, a number of investigators have shown that Apgar scores are not well related to more direct measures of hypoxia such as umbilical cord pH, PCO_2 and PO_2 levels. Additional indicators of hypoxia include the involvement of other organ systems, specifically renal involvement (decreased urinary output), cardiac problems (cardiomyopathy), and liver abnormalities (abnormal liver enzyme levels). Imaging the brain may reveal evidence of those neuropathologic changes that are associated with perinatal asphyxia. Magnetic resonance imaging (MRI) is most sensitive (Figure 13–1); ultrasonography is not as sensitive, but often is able to demonstrate periventricular echodensities. MRI and ultrasound both are considerably more sensitive than is computed tomographic imaging. The association of an abnormal electroencephalogram with perinatal asphyxia carries ominous prognostic implications.

■ MANAGEMENT AND OUTCOME

The management of perinatal asphyxia is focused on diagnosing the problem as early as possible and instituting interventions designed to eliminate or at least minimize the frequency, duration, and severity of the hypoxic insult. For example, when the diagnosis of fetal distress is suspected on the basis of EFM, immediate delivery by cesarean section often is indicated. Emergent care of the infant at birth includes respiratory support, correction of acid–base abnormalities, and treatment of any organ systems that were damaged by the asphyxia (*eg*, heart, kidney). If seizures complicate the neonatal course, these should be treated as well. Pharmacotherapy

designed to minimize the central nervous system insult has been disappointing, although new medications directed at the presumed excitatory neurotoxic mechanisms are under development. The outcome of perinatal asphyxia ranges from normal, to subtle developmental disabilities such as learning disabilities and attention disorders, to more obvious and severe problems such as cerebral palsy, pervasive developmental disorder, mental retardation, and seizures, to death. Prediction of long-term outcome in any given child remains problematic, however, and the pediatrician needs to tread cautiously in this area. Reasonable predictions of outcome may need to await follow-up evaluation at 6 months or even later.

(Abridged from Bennett A. Shaywitz, Perinatal Asphyxia, in Oski. DeAngelis, Feigin, McMillan, Warshaw: *Principles and Practice of Pediatrics, Second Edition,* J.B. Lippincott, 1994.)

Oski's Essential Pediatrics,
edited by Kevin B. Johnson and Frank A. Oski.
Lippincott–Raven Publishers,
Philadelphia © 1997

14

Infant of the Diabetic Mother

About 1 in 200 pregnancies is complicated by overt diabetes; gestational diabetes develops in an additional 2% to 3% of pregnancies. This statistic refers to a patient in whom diabetes develops during pregnancy and disappears after delivery. Despite advances in perinatal care over the past 20 years, infants of diabetic mothers (IDMs)

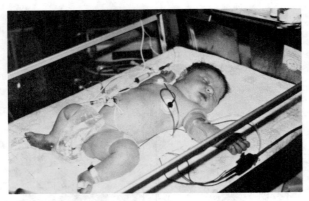

Figure 14-1. Infant of a diabetic mother.

TABLE 14-1. Problems of the Infant of the Diabetic Mother

Birth trauma and asphyxia

Hypoglycemia

Hypocalcemia

Hyperbilirubinemia

Hyaline membrane disease

Polycythemia

Renal vein thrombosis

Septal hypertrophy and myocardiopathy

Congenital malformations

remain a significant cause of perinatal morbidity and mortality.

Overt diabetes in pregnancy should be managed in a perinatal center by a high-risk pregnancy health care group that is equipped to monitor the pregnancy and has a newborn facility capable of caring for the newborn in the event of an adverse outcome. All women should be screened for gestational diabetes between the 24th and 28th weeks of pregnancy. Those who have a plasma glucose level in excess of 150 mg/dL 1 h after the oral administration of 50 g of glucose should be followed closely and have second evaluations. Insulin therapy may be required to treat gestational diabetics who have persistent hyperglycemia.

Fetal glucose levels reflect those of the mother. High levels of fetal glucose in response to maternal hyperglycemia stimulate the fetal islet to secrete insulin. Fetal islet cell volume has been shown to be proportional to maternal glucose concentrations, and macrosomia has been associated with increased insulin and C peptide levels in cord blood. Insulin functions as a fetal growth hormone, resulting in the characteristic macrosomia of IDMs. In utero, IDMs are not overgrown until some time after the 26th or 27th week; this staging may be related to the development of insulin receptors.

The risk for having a fetus with macrosomia is increased when the mean maternal glucose concentration exceeds 130 mg/dL. Measurement of glycosylated hemoglobin (HbA$_1$c) provides an important index of long-term diabetes control. Normal levels of HbA$_1$c generally are less than 8%. Many studies have demonstrated that increased perinatal morbidity is associated with elevated HbA$_1$c levels. The obstetric goal should be maintenance of fasting glucose levels below 100 mg/dL and other plasma glucose levels below 130 mg/dL.

IDMs have a characteristic appearance, with macrosomia, abundant adipose tissue, and a cherubic facial appearance; their head circumference, however, is similar to that of age-matched normal infants because insulin does not influence brain growth. A typical IDM is shown in Figure 14–1. The insulin-induced increase in glucose and amino acid transport into fetal tissues results in increased adipose tissue deposition and macrosomia. Adipose tissue of IDMs often exceeds the 16% of body weight that is fat in normal infants. The IDM has an increased glycogen content in the liver, kidney, skeletal muscle, and heart. The "growth hormone" effects of insulin result in increased linear growth.

Macrosomia may be associated with birth trauma and birth asphyxia. Perinatal asphyxia may occur in 25% of infants of insulin-dependent diabetics and correlates with maternal hyperglycemia before delivery and with maternal nephropathy. Maternal and fetal hyperglycemia during the intrapartum period may result in increased fetal oxygen requirements and place the fetus at greater risk during delivery. Nephropathy and hyperglycemia are associated with decreased placental blood flow, which may further increase the risk of asphyxia. Premature birth also is associated with birth asphyxia in IDMs.

Throughout early childhood, IDMs are large and may have increased adipose tissue. This tendency may have implications for the development of later obesity.

Problems of IDMs are summarized in Table 14–1. Despite their very large size, IDMs are functionally immature. The risk of hyaline membrane disease developing in these infants is six times that of normal infants until the 38th week of gestation. Fetal hyperglycemia and hyperinsulinism have been associated with pulmonary immaturity and decreased synthesis of surfactant phospholipids and their associated proteins. Hyperbilirubinemia also is an index of immaturity and occurs in about 20% of IDMs. Contributing factors include newborn polycythemia and hepatic immaturity.

(Abridged from Joseph B. Warshaw, Infant of the Diabetic Mother, in Oski, DeAngelis, Feigin, McMillan, Warshaw: *Principles and Practice of Pediatrics, Second Edition,* J.B. Lippincott, 1994.)

Oski's Essential Pediatrics,
edited by Kevin B. Johnson and Frank A. Oski.
Lippincott–Raven Publishers,
Philadelphia © 1997

15

Craniofacial Defects

■ CLEFT LIP AND CLEFT PALATE

Epidemiology and Genetics

The degree of cleft formation varies greatly. Minimal degrees of involvement include bifid uvula, linear lip indentations (so-called intrauterine-healed clefts), and submucous palatal cleft. Clefts may involve only the upper lip or may extend to the nostril and may be combined with defects of the hard or soft palate. Isolated palatal clefts may be limited to the uvula or they may be more extensive, cleaving the soft palate or both the soft and hard palates to just behind the incisor teeth.

A combination of cleft lip and cleft palate is more common than isolated occurrence of either. Cleft lip with cleft palate composes about 50% of the cases, with cleft lip and isolated cleft palate each constituting about 25%, generally irrespective of race. Vanderas (1987) reported that cleft lip with or without cleft palate occurs in about 1 per 1000 white births (range 0.8 to 1.6 per 1000). Frequency is higher in Native Americans (3.5 per 1000), Japanese (2.1 per 1000), and Chinese (1.7 per 1000); it is lower among African Americans (0.3 per 1000).

Isolated cleft lip may be unilateral (80%) or bilateral (20%). When unilateral, the cleft is more commonly on the left side (about 70%), but it is no more extensive. Lips are somewhat more frequently clefted bilaterally (about 25%) when combined with cleft palate. The cleft lip and palate combination is more common in men than women. About 85% of cases of bilateral cleft lip and 70% of cases of unilateral cleft lip are associated with cleft palate. Cleft lip is not always complete (ie, extending into the nostril). In about 10% of the cases, the cleft is associated with skin bridges or Simonart's bands.

Isolated cleft palate appears to be an entity separate from cleft lip with or without cleft palate. Numerous investigators have determined that siblings of patients with cleft lip with or without cleft palate have an increased frequency of the same anomaly but not of isolated cleft palate, and vice versa. The incidence of isolated cleft palate among both whites and blacks appears to be 1 per 2000 to 2500 births. It occurs somewhat more often in girls, comprising about 60% of the cases. Whereas there is a 2:1 female-to-male predilection for complete clefts of the hard and soft palate, the ratio approaches 1:1 for clefts of the soft palate only.

Cleft uvula varies in degree of completeness. Incomplete clefts are more common. The frequency of cleft uvula (1:80 white persons) is much higher than that for cleft palate with no sex predilection. The frequency in parents and siblings of probands ranges from 7% to 15%. Cleft uvula among Native American groups is high, occurring in 1 per 9 to 14 births depending on tribal group. In blacks, it is rare. Estimates are 1 per 350 to 400 births.

Risk of Recurrence

In most cases, the cleft is either isolated or associated with a constellation of anomalies that do not form a recognizable syndrome. Although more than 300 cleft syndromes or associations are recognized, Gorlin and coworkers (1990) report that they constitute a low percentage of cases. Efforts must be made to recognize a cleft syndrome, because the pattern of inheritance may be simple and the genetic risk for future affected children may then be more precise. For example, a parent with or without a cleft who has paramedian pits of the lower lip has a 50% chance of having a child with cleft lip or palate.

In the case of isolated clefts, the risk to a first-degree relative of an affected individual is 2% to 4%. This information applies only to risks for similar anomalies (ie, a parent with isolated cleft palate has no greater risk of having a child with cleft lip with or without cleft palate than anyone else, and vice versa). The risks increase as more individuals are affected. For example, if a parent and a child have clefts, the risk for a future affected sibling increases to about 10% to 12%. These and other situations are presented in detail in Table 15–1.

The severity of a facial cleft also affects recurrence risk in the offspring. For example, it has been found that if a parent has isolated unilateral cleft lip, the recurrence risk is 2.5%. If there is unilateral cleft lip and palate, the risk increases to 4%; if there is bilateral cleft lip with cleft palate, the risk is more than 5.5%.

Care of Infant With Cleft Lip or Cleft Palate

A cleft palate team—usually composed of a maxillofacial surgeon, audiologist, speech pathologist, prosthodontist, otolaryngologist, pedodontist, and geneticist—is extremely important in helping parents understand the sequential approach to therapy for the many attendant problems. The desirability of a team approach is discussed by Bardach and Morris (1990). A recommended handbook for parents is that of Moller and colleagues (1989).

Feeding usually requires considerable patience. Those with more severe clefts of the lip or palate should be fed by placing the infant in a sitting position to minimize fluid loss through the nose. Various techniques and equipment are used to feed infants with clefts, but Clarren and coworkers (1987) report that no one method is optimal for all infants. Infants with cleft lip or cleft palate swallow normally but suck abnormally. A cleft in the lip or palate generally does

TABLE 5-1. Facial Clefts—Risk of Recurrence

Parents	Siblings		Cleft Lip (Palate) %	Cleft Palate %
	Normal	*Affected*		
Normal	0	1	4.0	3.5
	1	1	4.0	3.0
	0	2	14.0	13.0
One affected	0	0	4.0	3.5
	0	1	12.0	10.0
	1	1	10.0	9.0
	0	2	25.0	24.0
Both affected	0	0	35.0	25.0
	0	1	45.0	35.0
	1	1	40.0	35.0
	0	2	50.0	45.0

Adapted from Tolarová M. Empirical recurrence risk figures for genetic counseling of clefts. Acta Chir Plast (Praha). 1972;14: 234.

not allow sufficient negative pressure. In the case of cleft lip only, breast-feeding or an artificial nipple with a large, soft base works well. For infants with cleft lip or palate, regular breast-feeding or normal bottle feeding is often not successful because they are unable to seal either their lips or their velopharynx. With cleft of the palate only, breast-feeding or normal bottle feeding usually can be carried out if the cleft is narrow or involves only the soft palate. Soft artificial nipples with large openings are more effective.

Regular bottle nipples do not work well for infants with wider palatal clefts or the Robin malformation sequence. Enlarging the nipple opening in association with a softer nipple with a large base and a long shaft often enables tongue movement to express a greater quantity of milk. One can also deliver milk directly into the mouth with a soft plastic bottle.

Children with cleft palate are prone to repeated infections of the middle ear and paranasal sinuses. The tonsils and adenoids enlarge, and chronic nasopharyngitis may lead to recurrent otitis media with resultant conductive hearing loss. Nasopharyngeal infection should be treated promptly with antibiotics. The tonsils and adenoids may play a vital role in allowing normal speech. Thus, tonsillectomy and adenoidectomy, especially in those with velopharyngeal insufficiency, may result in postoperative nasal speech.

Fria and colleagues (1987) stress the importance of assessing auditory function in infants with cleft palates. Assessment may be more accurately carried out in the infant or young child by auditory specialists.

Surgical Repair of Clefts

Closure of the lip is usually carried out between the 2nd and 10th week after birth, depending on the infant's weight and state of health. The primary purpose is to create a seal to allow normal sucking. Various techniques have been employed for repair of the lip, depending on the degree and extent of defect. In those cases in which tissue in the two lip segments is insufficient to create an acceptable lip and nostril, the surgeon may have to move small flaps of tissue from other places in the upper or, occasionally, the lower lip. For bilateral cleft lip, surgery is more difficult. The primary palate may not be attached to the secondary palate and requires repositioning. Subsequent surgery is usually required to correct nasal alar form, to compensate for uneven growth of tissue on the two sides of the lip, or to match evenly the vermilion line on both sides. This secondary surgery is best done during the teen years (Cronin and Denkler, 1988).

Surgical closure of the hard and soft palate is often done at about 18 to 24 months of age, but some surgeons prefer to wait longer. The object is to create air-tight and fluid-tight closure of the cleft and to preserve the length and mobility of the soft palate, which often involves multiple surgical operations. If insufficient tissue is available for closure by any of the many techniques available, an obturator or speech bulb is made by the prosthodontist.

■ CRANIOSYNOSTOSIS

If obliteration of sutures takes place before or soon after birth, it inhibits the growth of adjacent bones perpendicular to the course of the obliterated suture. Consequently, skull diameter is reduced in this direction. Compensatory and abnormal growth, however, proceeds in directions permitted by open sutures and fontanelles (Figure 15–1). If a single suture is involved, it is termed *simple craniosynostosis;* if multiple sutures, *compound craniosynostosis.* Early obliteration of the sagittal suture results in scaphocephaly (dolichocephaly, Figure 15–2). The skull is long and narrow and the parietal protuberances are absent. As the brain expands, the coronal and lambdoidal sutures are widened and fronto-occipital elongation takes place. In some cases, a bony crest is seen in place of the sagittal suture. In brachycephaly, the coronal sutures are prematurely fused, resulting in a short, squarish cranial configuration (Figure 15–3). Plagiocephaly refers to skewing of the skull due to premature unilateral fusion of a coronal or lambdoidal suture. Trigonocephaly describes a keel-shaped forehead due to premature fusion of the metopic suture. Acrocephaly (turricephaly) results from multiple suture closures. The highest point on the calvaria is usually near the anterior fontanelle, head form being short, high, and broad. The coronal suture is chiefly affected, although the sagittal and lambdoid sutures are frequently

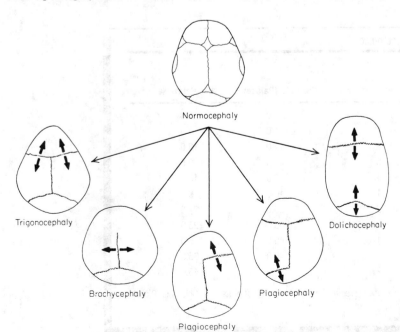

Figure 15-1. Craniosynostosis. Various skull shapes resulting from premature fusion of individual sutures or groups of sutures. (Courtesy of M.M. Cohen Jr., Halifax, Nova Scotia, Canada.)

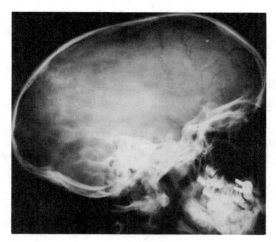

Figure 15-2. Scaphocephaly (dolichocephaly).

involved. If the anterior fontanelle and metopic suture remain open, the skull expands in abnormal directions, which results in steep frontal, parietal, and occipital bones and a high, broad, short skull. There frequently are digital impressions.

Craniosynostosis may be primary, as in simple or compound premature fusion described earlier, or it may be secondary to a known disorder, such as thalassemia, hyperthyroidism, microcephaly, mucopolysaccharidoses, or rickets. Craniosynostosis may also be syndromic.

Epidemiology and Genetics

The frequency of simple or nonsyndromal craniosynostosis is approximately 0.4 per 1000 newborns. There appears to be no racial predilection. Premature fusion of the sagittal suture is the most common type of simple synostosis, constituting approximately 55% of cases. Boys are more commonly affected 4:1 over girls. Unilateral or bilateral coronal synostosis comprises approximately 20% to 25% of cases with a slight predilection for female infants. Metopic synostosis and lambdoidal synostosis each constitute a few percent. Two or more sutures comprise 15%.

Simple craniosynostosis is usually sporadic. Of patients with coronal synostosis, about 10% are familial; of patients

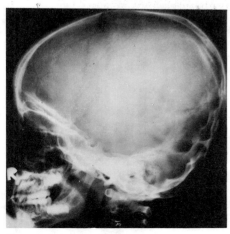

Figure 15-3. Brachycephaly.

with sagittal synostosis, about 2% are familial. In those with familial occurrence, autosomal dominant inheritance is far more common than autosomal recessive inheritance. In some kindreds, the same suture is synostosed in affected individuals, and, in others, different sutures are fused. Hunter and Rudd (1976) found that sagittal synostosis appeared to be most consistent with multifactorial inheritance, the frequency in the general population being approximately 1 in 4200, with a recurrence risk of approximately 1 in 64 siblings. Twin studies clearly indicate that single-gene inheritance does not play a large role in craniosynostosis because discordance is more frequent than concordance in monozygotic twins.

Treatment in Infancy

Treatment of craniosynostosis in infancy is controversial. The craniosynostoses represent not only diverse groups, but also extreme variables if found within each group. Opinions regarding treatment vary from conservative observation until completion of facial growth to radical extensive surgical correction in the first months of life. The existence of complications such as increasing intracranial pressure or progressive corneal exposure secondary to exorbitism often mandate early treatment.

Albin and colleagues (1985) suggest that patients with premature closure of cranial sutures be surgically treated under the age of 2 years and those patients with metopic suture closure under the age of 6 months. The operation most frequently performed for simple craniosynostosis is linear craniectomy parallel to the prematurely fused suture. Polyethylene film is inserted over the bony margins to delay secondary closure. Bilateral, premature closure of the coronal sutures is frequently accompanied by anomalies of the facial, orbital, and sphenoid bones with downward displacement of the orbital roof and overgrowth of the lesser wing of the sphenoid, the orbits being markedly reduced in size, thus causing exophthalmos. Maximum decompression of the cranial vault rather than orbital decompression is carried out. Canthorrhaphy is performed to avoid dryness of the cornea and prolapse of the globe. Complex plastic surgical treatment of severe facial deformities of craniofacial dysostoses has been described in detail by Tessier (1986). The optimal time for such operations is at 10 to 12 years of age. Bartlett and colleagues (1990) and Bruneteau and Mulliken (1992) extensively discuss surgical treatment of unilateral suture closure and plagiocephaly.

Surgical techniques are reviewed by Whitaker and colleagues (1987). In general, they conclude that asymmetric synostosis treated at younger than 1 year of age by unilateral orbital repositioning and forehead remodeling gave excellent results. No further surgery was needed in greater than 90% of patients. For bilateral or symmetric synostoses and mild upper face deformity, orbital advancement and forehead reshaping carried out within the first year of life was less satisfactory, with about 50% of patients needing another major osteotomy. For those with moderate to severe symmetric synostoses (Crouzon's disease and Apert's syndrome), extensive facial reconstruction is carried out between 7 and 14 years of age. Despite delayed and aggressive treatment, surgical outcome is less satisfactory (David & Sheen, 1990.)

(Abridged from Robert J. Gorlin, Craniofacial Defects, in Oski, DeAngelis, Feigin, McMillan, Warshaw: *Principles and Practice of Pediatrics, Second Edition,* J.B. Lippincott, 1994.)

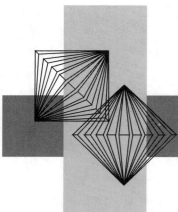

PART III

Ambulatory Pediatrics

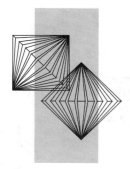

SECTION 1

Adolescent Medicine

Oski's Essential Pediatrics,
edited by Kevin B. Johnson and Frank A. Oski.
Lippincott–Raven Publishers,
Philadelphia © 1997

16

Adolescent Pregnancy and Contraception

The age at which adolescents in the United States initiate sexual activity has decreased over the past few decades. In the United States, 79.8% of males and 53.2% of females ages 15 to 19 years of age had experienced sexual intercourse in 1988.

Several factors cause difficulty for adolescents in their attempt to make responsible decisions regarding initiation of sexual activity and contraceptive behaviors. Young persons often lack adequate knowledge regarding fertility and contraception. Health services may be unavailable or difficult to access. Furthermore, adolescents may be unable to communicate with those individuals who can help them best in these decisions (*ie*, their parents, health professionals, and sexual partners). The psychological profile of an adolescent compounds the difficulty. Adolescence is characterized by risk-taking behaviors and impulsiveness.

■ EPIDEMIOLOGY

The United States has the second highest pregnancy rate among all developed countries for which data are available. Overall, 1 in 10 adolescent women becomes pregnant during adolescence. Two thirds of these pregnancies are unplanned.

■ DIAGNOSIS

Clinicians should be aware of the epidemiology of adolescent pregnancy and maintain a high index of suspicion for the condition. No method of contraception is 100% effective. The diagnosis of pregnancy may be entertained immediately because of the young woman's chief complaint or may not be suspected until much later in the evaluation. The most common diagnosis in the adolescent patient who presents with secondary amenorrhea is pregnancy. Other symptoms that suggest pregnancy include nausea, fatigue, dizziness, syncope, urinary frequency, breast tenderness, and nipple sensitivity.

The physical examination can support the diagnosis of pregnancy. On abdominal examination, a midline lower abdominal mass may be palpable after the first trimester of pregnancy. On pelvic examination, the cervix acquires a cyanotic appearance and softens, and the cervicouterine angle blurs. The uterine size should be assessed to estimate the length of gestation. At 12 weeks' gestation, the uterus is palpable at the symphysis pubis; at 20 weeks' gestation, the uterus is palpable at the umbilicus.

Laboratory confirmation of pregnancy can be made with either urine or blood measurement of human chorionic gonadotropins (HCG). Newer urine tests are extremely sensitive and can diagnose a pregnancy as early as within 7 days after conception (*ie*, 1 week before the missed menses).

■ COUNSELING

Once a diagnosis of pregnancy is confirmed, the adolescent should be informed and counseled about her options. Ideally, the young woman should be counseled by an experienced professional who can present unbiased information to assist her in her choice. If personal reasons prevent the physician from doing so, it is appropriate to refer the patient elsewhere for services. Optimally, the parents should be involved to provide support. The options are to continue the pregnancy to term and keep the baby, continue the pregnancy to term and place the baby for adoption, or obtain an abortion.

There is no easy solution for the adolescent experiencing an unintended pregnancy. Supportive counseling should allow the patient to express her feelings so she can make the best decision.

In summary, early sexual activity and resultant pregnancy continue in epidemic proportions in the United States. Health care providers must anticipate unintended adolescent pregnancy, make a timely diagnosis, and provide or refer for choice counseling.

■ ADOLESCENT CONTRACEPTION

There is a tremendous need for safe and effective methods of contraception that are acceptable to sexually active young persons. All counseling regarding contraception should include counseling regarding sexually transmitted disease (STD) and human immunodeficiency virus (HIV) infection risk reduction. An assessment made in confidence helps determine which adolescent plans to become or is sexually active. If contraception is needed, counseling regarding an appropriate method is indicated. In addition to obtaining a history and physical examination and determining which methods are contraindicated medically, it is important to elicit what method of contraception the patient desires. The choice must be acceptable to the young person and clinician. Ultimately, the patient must be comfortable with the method and be willing to use it correctly and consistently. The health care provider needs to assess the patient's level of maturity as well as ability and willingness to use a given method of contraception.

Contraceptive counseling should include a discussion of the risks, benefits, side effects, and effectiveness for the methods being considered. Effectiveness is best described in terms of percentage of typical female users who become pregnant using the stated method for 1 year. It is important to recognize that the failure rate among adolescents using any contraceptive method is much higher than the rate among older individuals. Written materials generally augment verbal instructions. Table 16–1 summarizes the methods of contraception commonly used by adolescents.

Oral Contraception

Oral contraception is one of the most frequently used methods of contraception during adolescence. Birth control pills are prepared from a combination of estrogen and progestin, which is a synthetic progesterone.

Oral contraceptives offer many advantages that make them particularly well suited for teenagers. They are extremely effective, with 3.0 pregnancies occurring among 100 women in 1 year. Of note, oral contraceptives do not provide protection against STDs or HIV infection. Thus, adolescents should be counseled to use oral contraceptives in conjunction with a barrier method, ideally condoms.

Minor side effects include symptoms that, although not dangerous, may bother the patient and therefore result in her decision to discontinue use. Frequently, patients experience nausea and, occasionally, vomiting as their bodies adjust to an altered hormonal milieu. Taking the medication with meals, especially in the evening, alleviates this condition. Adolescents commonly experience either spotting or breakthrough bleeding in the first few months of oral contraceptive use. If irregular bleeding persists, selection of a pill with higher progestational activity usually corrects the condition.

Young women benefit from frequent medical follow-up after initiation of oral contraceptives. A suggested schedule includes a visit at 6 weeks and one every 3 months thereafter. At each visit, the physician should inquire about any of the following symptoms: chest pain, headaches, visual distur-

---

TABLE 16-1. Methods of Contraception

Method	Failure Rate in Typical User (%)*	Benefits	Risk/Disadvantages
Combined oral contraceptives	3.0	Use not related to coitus; decreased risk of dysmenorrhea, breast disorders, arthritis, iron deficiency anemia, ovarian and uterine cancers, ovarian cysts	Thromboembolic phenomena, cerebrovascular accident, coronary artery disease, hepatomas, gallbladder disease, hypertension, worsening of migraines, breakthrough bleeding, amenorrhea, nausea, weight gain, acne, depression, glucose intolerance
Progestin-only pill (mini-pill)	†	Fewer metabolic complications, used for patients with hypertension, diabetes, sickle cell disease	Menstrual irregularities
Norplant	0.04	No demand after insertion, highly effective, long-lasting protection	Requires minor surgical procedure for insertion, removal; side effects—menstrual irregularities, headaches, nervousness, nausea, dizziness, dermatitis, acne, change in appetite, weight gain, breast tenderness, hirsutism, and hair loss
Condom	12.0	No major risks, low cost, nonprescription, male involvement, protects against STDs and cervical cancer	Allergy to materials (rare), loss of sensation, use with each act of coitus
Diaphragm with contraceptive cream or jelly	18.0	Protects against STDs, no major risks	Allergy (rare), toxic shock syndrome (rare), incidence of urinary tract infection, vaginal ulceration, requires motivation
Spermicide	21.0	Nonprescription, no major medical risks, some STD protection	Allergy (rare), use related to coitus
Intrauterine device	3.0	Minimal demands after insertion, secrecy	Pelvic inflammatory disease, ectopic pregnancy, infertility, dysmenorrhea, menorrhagia
Natural family planning	20.0	Natural, no risks, nonprescription	Not very effective with irregular menses, requires high motivation
Coitus interruptus	18.0	Useful when nothing else is available, no planning, no major medical risks	Less satisfying relationships

*Percentage of women who become pregnant during the first year using a specified contraceptive method.

†Lowest reported failure rate 1.1%.

From Hatcher RA, et al. Contraceptive technology 1990–1992. 15th ed. New York: Irvington Publishers; 1990.

bances, leg or abdominal pains as possible indicators of thromboembolic disorders or hepatic neoplasm. The physical examination should include measurement of weight and blood pressure. Hypertension develops in a small percentage of individuals and necessitates cessation of therapy. Pelvic examination should be performed annually and more frequently if the patient has multiple or new sexual partners or if gynecologic symptoms supervene.

Norplant Implants

Norplant is a long-acting, reversible method of contraception approved for use in the United States in 1991. It is implanted under the skin of the upper arm in a minor surgical procedure. Norplant is composed of six flexible Silastic capsules containing the progestin levonorgesterol.

Norplant is a long-lasting, highly effective contraceptive method that provides protection for up to 5 years. The failure rate in the first year of use is 0.04%. It is recommended that the capsules be removed after 5 years of use. The capsules may be removed earlier if the patient desires. Primary advantages of Norplant include its ease of use (once inserted, the patient does nothing more) and its high rate of effectiveness. Disadvantages of Norplant are that a surgical procedure is required for insertion and removal and that many women experience bothersome menstrual irregularities. Common side effects include headache, nervousness, nausea, dizziness, dermatitis, acne, change in appetite, weight gain, breast tenderness, hirsutism, and hair loss.

Barrier Methods

The commonly recommended barrier devices include condoms, diaphragms, contraceptive sponges, and vaginal spermicide. Barrier methods, especially condoms, deserve increasing attention because of their role in preventing the spread of STDs including HIV infection.

Condoms

The condom is the second most frequently used method of contraception during adolescence. Data from the 1988 Survey of Adolescent Males demonstrate that the rate of condom use has increased among 17- to 19-year-old males. Condoms have a failure rate in typical users of 12.0%. When used with spermicide, they are more effective. They are extraordinarily safe without any major medical risks. Condoms are easily available at low cost without prescription.

Diaphragm

The diaphragm is chosen by only a small number of adolescents. It is a dome-shaped rubber cup that acts as a physical barrier to conception, while jelly or cream applied to it provides spermicidal properties. Like condoms, the diaphragm protects against STDs and has no major health risks. The pregnancy rate among adult users is 18.0%. There is increased frequency of urinary tract infections.

Vaginal Spermicide

Vaginal spermicide contains a spermicidal agent, either nonoxynol-9 or oxtoxinol-9, coupled with an inert substance, foam, cream, or suppository. Vaginal spermicide can be bought without prescription and must be inserted vaginally within 1 hour of intercourse. When used alone, vaginal spermicide has a failure rate of 21.0%. Therefore, it is recommended that spermicide be used with condoms. Nonoxynol-9 has antibacterial and antiviral properties that help protect against STDs.

■ EVALUATION FOR CONTRACEPTION

Before initiating contraception, it is important to obtain a careful history and physical examination to define medical and behavioral factors relevant to contraceptive choices. It is desirable for young women to experience regular menses for 1 to 2 years before initiating oral contraceptives. This allows for establishment of mature functioning of the hypothalamic–pituitary–ovarian axis. There is no evidence that long-term fertility is compromised by early oral contraceptive use. Thus, the desired establishment of regular menses is not absolute and may be waived if no other suitable method exists and the young woman is sexually active.

Obtaining a sexual history is pertinent to the decision. A young woman or man who has not yet engaged in sexual intercourse but is feeling peer pressure might need reassurance regarding abstinence rather than contraception, whereas a young person who engages in infrequent intercourse may choose a barrier method. All individuals should be counseled regarding risks for STDs and desirability of condom use.

A complete physical examination is recommended. Particular attention is paid to blood pressure, cardiovascular system, thyroid, and breasts. Skin should be inspected for xanthomas, chloasma, jaundice, or scleral icterus. Extent of pubertal development should be assessed because hormonal contraceptives are recommended only for young women who are at Tanner sexual maturity rating stage IV or V. Abdominal examination checks for liver enlargement or tenderness. A pelvic examination should include a Papanicolaou smear as well as screening cultures for gonorrhea and chlamydia, if available. Syphilis serology should be obtained in the sexually active individual.

In summary, having identified an adolescent in need of contraceptive services, the medical assessment should include a comprehensive history, physical examination, and evaluation of the adolescent's level of maturity and needs. Ultimately, both the physician and the young patient must be satisfied with the selected method for safe and successful contraception.

(Abridged from Michele Diane Wilson, Adolescent Pregnancy and Contraception, in Oski, DeAngelis, Feigin, McMillan, Warshaw: *Principles and Practice of Pediatrics, Second Edition,* J.B. Lippin ott, 1994.)

Oski's Essential Pediatrics,
edited by Kevin B. Johnson and Frank A. Oski.
Lippincott–Raven Publishers,
Philadelphia © 1997

17

Sexually Transmitted Diseases

Sexually transmitted diseases (STDs) are generally defined as diseases that are transmitted primarily through sexual intercourse. The traditional list of STDs included syphilis and gonorrhea as the two major diseases of concern. Chancroid, lymphogranuloma venereum (LGV), and granuloma inguinale completed the list as the diseases of minor importance. The current expanded list of STDs also includes *Chlamydia trachomatis* infections, genital herpes, genital mycoplasmas, cytomegalovirus, hepatitis, bacterial vaginosis, human papillomavirus, and ectoparasitic diseases.

■ GONOCOCCAL INFECTIONS

Gonorrhea is caused by the gram-negative diplococcus *Neisseria gonorrhoeae*. The true incidence of disease is estimated to be two to three times that which is actually reported. Extrapolated to the estimated true incidence of disease, these figures translate into 1 in every 30 to 50 males and 1 in every 20 to 30 females acquiring a gonococcal infection each year.

Clinical Presentation

The clinical spectrum of diseases associated with the *N gonorrhoeae* is broad. In males, gonorrhea is frequently a cause of urethritis. Complications due to direct extension to other sites is unusual in males; however, epididymitis, prostatitis, and seminal vesiculitis can occur. In females, in addition to localized infection of the cervix, urethra, and Bartholin's or Skene's glands, there is frequently an extension to the upper genital tract causing endometritis, salpingitis, parametritis, and perihepatitis (commonly known as FitzHugh-Curtis syndrome). Extragenital mucosal infections in males and females due to *N gonorrhoeae* are commonly manifested as proctitis and pharyngitis. Rare occurrences in both sexes include meningitis, endocarditis, arthritis, and dermatitis.

Disseminated gonorrhea, or the arthritis-dermatitis syndrome, occurs primarily in females and is present in less than 1% of all patients with gonorrhea. Dissemination occurs as a result of hematogenous extension of the gonococcus from the site of entry. It is seen frequently after menstruation. Patients may note the presence of myalgia, headache, malaise, fever, or anorexia initially, but the clinical manifestations noted most frequently are the characteristic hemorrhagic or necrotic appearing skin lesions, arthralgias, tenosynovitis, and monoarticular or oligoarticular arthritis. The joints most frequently affected include the knees, elbows, ankles, wrists, and small joints of the hands or feet.

Blood cultures early in the course are positive in only 10% to 30% of cases. Gram stains of synovial fluid frequently contain an increased number of leukocytes but are positive for gram-negative diplococci in only 10% to 30% of cases, and fluid is culture positive in less than 30% of cases. Most often, the diagnosis of disseminating gonorrhea is based on the typical clinical manifestations, the recovery of the organism from a mucosal site, and the appropriate response to therapy. Hence, the cervix, urethra, pharynx, and rectum should be cultured before treatment.

Treatment

The primary goal in treating gonococcal infections is to eliminate the infection as effectively, economically, and safely as possible. Important concerns are the treatment of coexisting chlamydial infection, which is documented in one third to one half of patients with gonorrhea, and the eradication of associated diseases such as incubating syphilis. To address these concerns, therapy is directed toward a single-dose regimen to treat gonorrhea followed by a 7-day course of treatment with doxycycline or tetracycline. The treatment regimen of choice for uncomplicated gonococcal infections is ceftriaxone 250 mg given intramuscularly, in addition to doxycycline 100 mg bid or tetracycline hydrochloride 500 mg qid for 7 days to eradicate chlamydia.

Adolescents who have had recent exposure to gonorrhea should be cultured and treated as if they have infection. All teenagers with gonorrhea should have a serologic test for syphilis performed at the time of diagnosis. It is recommended that all patients with gonorrhea be offered confidential counseling and testing for human immunodeficiency virus (HIV).

In cases with complicated gonococcal infections such as disseminated gonorrhea, the usual recommendation is for hospitalization and treatment with intramuscular or intravenous ceftriaxone or a substitute. Acceptable treatment regimens can be found in the frequently updated *Sexually Transmitted Disease Treatment Guidelines* published by the Centers for Disease Control.

■ CHLAMYDIAL INFECTIONS

C trachomatis is the most commonly isolated sexually transmitted agent, causing an estimated 3 to 4 million sexually transmitted infections annually. It is most prevalent in the age group 15 to 19 years. *C trachomatis* infections are not reportable diseases; however, data from STD clinics suggest a sharp increase in incidence since 1975. *C trachomatis* has been isolated from 10% to 26% of adolescent females in teen clinics and is much more prevalent than gonococcal infection in most studies.

The most frequently noted risk factors for infection with *C trachomatis* include young age, history of multiple sexual partners, presence of other STDs, use of oral contraceptives, use of a nonbarrier method or no method of contraception, and abnormal Papanicolaou smear.

Clinical Presentation

The clinical presentation associated with chlamydial genital tract infections is similar to that of gonococcal infection. Infections commonly associated with *C trachomatis* include acute urethral syndrome, bartholinitis, cervicitis, salpingitis, nongonococcal urethritis, epididymitis, proctitis, conjunctivitis, and Reiter's syndrome.

Chlamydial infection in the female may be associated with mucopurulent cervicitis or urethritis, but frequently it is asymptomatic. Ascending infection may occur, leading to salpingitis and perihepatitis (FitzHugh-Curtis syndrome). Chlamydial salpingitis is frequently subclinical and is implicated as a significant cause of involuntary infertility.

Infants born to women with cervical chlamydial infection are at significant risk for developing chlamydial infection. About 60% to 70% of infants exposed to chlamydiae during passage through an infected birth canal become infected. The approximate risk of developing conjunctivitis is 30% to 40%; pneumonia, 10% to 20%; and asymptomatic nasopharyngeal infection, 20%.

Diagnostic Tests

Several laboratory diagnostic methods are available to identify chlamydial infections including tissue culture isolation and serologic, cytologic, and immunodiagnostic techniques. Tissue culture techniques are the most sensitive and specific methods and are the preferred method of detection.

If detection methods for chlamydia are not available, presumptive treatment for this organism should be considered when genital symptoms suggest the possibility of infection. Anyone treated for gonorrhea should receive treatment for chlamydia as well.

Treatment

Treatment regimens for chlamydial disease include doxycycline, tetracycline, or erythromycin, as an alternative. Treatment of genital infections in individuals 8 years of age or younger is erythromycin for 7 to 10 days. The recommended therapy for chlamydial conjunctivitis or pneumonia is oral erythromycin for 2 to 3 weeks.

■ SYPHILIS

Syphilis is caused by the spirochete *Treponema pallidum*. *T pallidum* is a pathogen only in humans and is transmitted from infected individuals through intimate contact. In 1991, more than 29,000 cases of primary and secondary syphilis were reported in the United States.

Clinical Presentation

The initial lesion of primary syphilis, the chancre, usually develops 14 to 21 days after the initial infection. The incubation period, however, varies from 10 to 90 days. The primary lesion usually appears as a small, solitary, round or elongated, indurated ulcer with a clean base. The chancre does not usually cause pain and, if located in an inconspicuous site, may go unnoticed. The lesions vary in size from 3 to 4 mm or 1 to 2 cm. Regional lymphadenopathy usually accompanies the chancre. The chancre usually remains stable in appearance for several weeks and, if untreated, slowly resolves.

Secondary syphilis is heralded by the presence of a generalized macular or maculopapular eruption, which, at times, can also be nodulopapular in appearance and is usually not associated with pruritus. The rash of secondary syphilis is usually concentrated on the trunk, but the characteristic lesions frequently can be found on the face, palms, and soles. The rash may be accompanied by fever or malaise. Other clinical signs of secondary syphilis include the presence of flat moist papules in the anal or genital region

referred to as condyloma lata, small patches of alopecia in the scalp, and loss of the lateral eyebrows.

When the symptoms and signs of secondary syphilis disappear, the disease is referred to as latent syphilis. Patients with latent syphilis have no signs or symptoms but may still be infectious, if untreated, for a period of several years. Approximately one third of those with latent syphilis progress to late syphilis if untreated; this condition may occur within 2 to 30 years after the original infection. The clinical manifestations are highly variable and take the form of benign late syphilis in about 50%, cardiovascular syphilis in about 30%, and neurosyphilis in about 20%.

Diagnosis

The best method for verifying the diagnosis of primary syphilis is darkfield microscopic examination of a sample of material from the chancre. If positive, this is the only test required to establish the diagnosis of primary syphilis. When darkfield examination is not available, the diagnosis usually is based on the standard serologic tests, the VDRL (Venereal Disease Research Laboratory) and RPR (rapid protein reagin), which are used for screening. Because these two nontreponemal tests are nonspecific, a positive result should be confirmed by the highly specific fluorescent treponemal antibody (FTA) test.

Treatment

The choice of treatment for primary, secondary, or latent syphilis of less than 1 year's duration is benzathine penicillin G, 2.4 million U intramuscularly at one visit. Patients who are allergic to penicillin should be treated with tetracycline for 15 days. All patients should be encouraged to return for repeat VDRL tests at 3, 6, and 12 months after treatment. All patients with syphilis should be counseled concerning the risks of HIV and be encouraged to be tested for HIV antibody.

The optimal treatment regimen for syphilis of more than 1 year's duration is less well established. Except for neurosyphilis, the suggested treatment is benzathine penicillin G, 2.4 million U intramuscularly each week for 3 successive weeks or, for those allergic to penicillin, tetracycline 500 mg qid for 30 days.

■ HERPES SIMPLEX VIRUS INFECTIONS

Infections due to herpes simplex virus (HSV) are increasingly common in the United States. The spectrum of clinical manifestations associated with this organism includes primary and recurrent genital herpes, pharyngitis, urethritis, cervicitis, proctitis, neonatal HSV infections, and possible association with cervical carcinoma.

Primary genital herpes may be caused by either type 1 (HSV-1) or type 2 (HSV-2) herpes simplex virus. In the United States, 70% to 90% of primary genital infections are caused by the HSV-2, although the two are clinically indistinguishable. Primary HSV infections may or may not produce clinically apparent symptoms. In general, first episodes of genital herpes are more likely than recurrent episodes to be associated with systemic signs and symptoms, more severe and prolonged symptoms, and increased and prolonged viral shedding. It is not uncommon for patients to experience central nervous system involvement during a primary HSV infection. Aseptic meningitis, autonomic dysfunction resulting in hyperesthesia or anesthesia, transverse myelitis, and encephalitis are frequently documented. Dissemination with viremia and widespread involvement can occur but is rare.

The clinical diagnosis of genital herpes is usually made by recognition of the characteristic lesions of grouped vesicles on an erythematous base. Both primary and recurrent HSV infections are accompanied by tender lymphadenopathy. The inguinal nodes, upon palpation, are usually mildly tender, nonfixed, and only slightly firm.

Several methods are available to document the organism including isolation by tissue culture, detection of viral antigen by direct fluorescent assay or enzyme-linked immunosorbent assay (ELISA), cytologic examination of clinical specimens, or serology. Diagnosis should be confirmed by culture if an alternative initial method of detection is used.

Symptomatic treatment for mild genital herpes usually includes good genital hygiene, topical anesthetics, cool compresses, and analgesia. Oral acyclovir is the preferred treatment in most episodes of symptomatic HSV disease. Topical therapy is substantially less effective than oral therapy. Systemic acyclovir provides partial control of the symptoms and signs of HSV infections; it accelerates healing but does not eradicate or affect the subsequent risk, frequency, or severity of recurrences. Systemic therapy prevents new lesion formation, and because of the high incidence of urethral, cervical, and oral infections, oral acyclovir is preferred in first-episode infections. All patients with first-episode genital HSV who present with active lesions should be treated. The recommended dosage is 200 mg five times per day. Although intravenous acyclovir may be more effective, it is usually reserved for those with severe symptoms or complications that necessitate hospitalization.

■ HUMAN PAPILLOMAVIRUS INFECTION

Genital warts are an STD caused by human papillomavirus (HPV). Genital wart virus infections appear to be increasing in prevalence and are rapidly becoming one of the most common STDs diagnosed. More than 50 HPV types have been characterized. Acute infections may be asymptomatic or produce exophytic or flat condylomas; chronic persistent infections may result in intraepithelial neoplasia or squamous cell carcinoma. HPV types 6 and 11 are the viral types most commonly associated with exophytic warts.

Genital warts are transmitted through intimate contact including sexual intercourse. It is unclear whether transmission rates differ for HPV types, and indirect transmission through fomites has never been demonstrated convincingly.

The standard treatment of genital warts consists of podophyllin—a cytotoxic agent that is applied to warts as a 20% solution in ethanol or tincture of benzoin and allowed to dry. It is washed off after 3 to 4 hours. Treatment is repeated once or twice a week. Treatment failures are common.

Routine screening with frequent Papanicolaou smears and close follow-up are important for those diagnosed with this infection. Examination and treatment of sexual partners is an important preventive strategy.

■ SPECIFIC STD SYNDROMES

Vaginitis/Cervicitis

Lower genital tract infections in females, which can involve the urinary tract, cervix, vulva, and vagina, produce a variety of overlapping symptoms including pruritus, dyspareunia, dysuria, and alteration of vaginal discharge. Based on symptoms only, it is difficult to distinguish among the various lower genital tract infections. Physical examination and appropriate use of simple laboratory tests often can help clarify the presumptive diagnosis of vaginitis, cervicitis, or urethritis.

Normal vaginal secretions consist of a mixture of secretions from the vaginal wall, cervical mucus, exfoliated vaginal epithelial cells, and secretions from the sebaceous, sweat, Bartholin's, and Skene's glands. With the onset of menarche and under the influence of estrogen, the vaginal epithelium becomes thicker, and increased amounts of lactic acid are produced from the glycogen-rich cells, which causes the pH to fall. The low pH, which is normally less than 4.5, fosters the growth of *Lactobacillus* species, which are the most prevalent organisms in the normal vaginal flora.

Estrogen causes changes in the cervix as well. Typically, visual inspection of the adolescent cervix reveals the presence of an ectropion or ectopy (columnar epithelium on the outer surface of the cervix) with a well-demarcated squamocolumnar junction. Many adolescents have ectopy, which gradually is replaced by squamous epithelium through the process of squamous metaplasia as the cervix matures.

The three most common types of vaginitis are bacterial vaginosis (formerly called nonspecific or *Gardnerella vaginalis* vaginitis), *Trichomonas vaginalis* vaginitis, and *Candida* vaginitis. The adolescent complaining of a vaginal discharge often has a specific etiology for her symptoms (Figure 17–1). Careful evaluation should include measurement of vaginal fluid pH, examination of vaginal fluid saline and potassium hydroxide preparations, endocervical culture or antigen detection tests for *C trachomatis* and *N gonorrhoeae*, a Gram-stained smear of endocervical secretions, and a Papanicolaou smear.

The characteristic findings of *Candida* vaginitis include vaginal and vulvar erythema, vulvar edema, pruritus, and the presence of a thick cottage cheeselike discharge. The diagnosis can be confirmed by the microscopic finding of yeast forms on a potassium hydroxide preparation or by culture. Predisposing factors include diabetes, recent use of antibiotics, immunosuppressive therapy, obesity, or use of oral contraceptives. Treatment with topical vaginal clotrimazole or miconazole usually results in relief of symptoms.

Trichomonas vaginalis vaginitis is characterized by a malodorous vaginal discharge that is homogenous and classically described as yellow-green and frothy and has a vaginal fluid pH greater than 4.5. The vagina and cervix may be erythematous, and occasionally punctate hemorrhages or strawberry spots are seen on the cervix. On examination of the saline wet preparation, flagellated organisms and polymorphonuclear leukocytes are seen. The only effective treatment for *Trichomonas vaginalis* vaginitis is metronidazole. A single 2-g dose appears to be as effective as the 7-day treatment regimen and is the preferred regimen for most adolescents.

Bacterial vaginosis is the most common cause of an abnormal vaginal discharge. Several anaerobic bacteria in addition to *Gardnerella vaginalis* are thought to be involved in this complex syndrome. This complex alteration of the vaginal flora appears to be closely linked to sexual activity, but no specific etiologic organism has been defined. The diagnosis is based on the finding of a gray homogenous discharge, a vaginal fluid pH greater than 4.5, a positive whiff test (fishy odor when KOH is added to vaginal fluid), and clue cells on the examination of a wet preparation of vaginal secretions. Metronidazole 500 mg bid for 7 days is the treatment of choice. Alternative treatment with ampicillin is less effective, and topical agents are no more effective than placebo.

Sexually active patients who present with dysuria or other urinary tract symptoms may have urethritis, cervicitis,

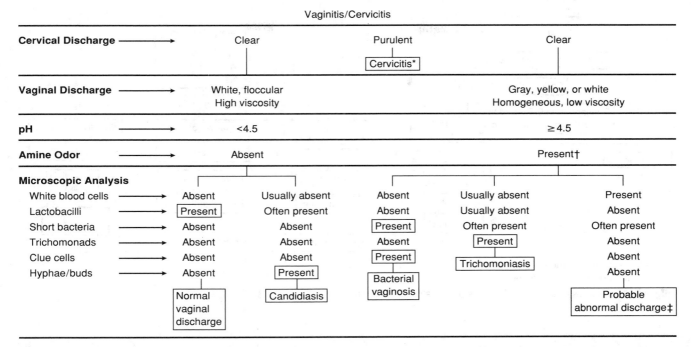

Figure 17-1. Vaginitis/cervicitis.

* Diagnosis supported by gram stain of endocervical secretion; confirm with culture and treat for *Chlamydia trachomatis* and *Neisseria gonorrhoeae.*

† An amine or "fishy" odor after addition of 10% KOH (the "whiff test") is a common feature of bacterial vaginosis

‡ Consider mixed infection

cystitis, or vaginitis. Evaluation should include microscopic examination of a clean voided urine specimen. Women without evidence of vaginitis or cervicitis but with pyuria and bacteriuria usually have a bacterial urinary tract infection. Pyuria in the absence of bacteriuria may indicate urethral infection with *C trachomatis* or *N gonorrhoeae.*

Cervicitis is most frequently associated with infection due to *C trachomatis, N gonorrhoeae,* or HSV. The presence of a mucopurulent endocervical discharge and the presence of 30 or more PMN leukocytes on a Gram-stained smear of endocervical secretions correlate highly with infection caused by these three organisms. In addition, the observation of green or yellow mucopus on a white swab (positive swab test) helps to identify this disorder. Cultures should be performed for *C trachomatis* and *N gonorrhoeae,* and treatment should include a regimen that is active against both organisms.

Pelvic Inflammatory Disease

Pelvic inflammatory disease (PID) is the syndrome resulting from the ascending spread of microorganisms from the vagina and cervix to the endometrium, fallopian tubes, and the contiguous upper genital tract structures. About 1 million women are treated each year for PID. It is a disease of young women, primarily, with adolescents 15 to 19 years of age constituting the group at highest risk when rates are adjusted for age. Although rates for women in other age groups show declines, rates for adolescents appear to be increasing.

Although the microbiologic etiology of PID is polymicrobial in nature, *C trachomatis, N gonorrhoeae,* and a variety

of anaerobic bacteria (*Peptostreptococcus, Peptococcus, Bacteroides*) are the organisms most commonly identified from tubal cultures. Mycoplasmas, *Ureaplasma urealyticum,* and facultative bacteria (most frequently *Gardnerella vaginalis, Streptococcus* species, *Escherichia coli,* and *Haemophilus influenzae*) have also been isolated from tubal cultures.

PID frequently poses a difficult diagnostic problem and may be confused with appendicitis, pyelonephritis, and a host of gynecologic problems such as ruptured ovarian cyst, ectopic pregnancy, and septic abortion. The diagnosis is particularly difficult in adolescents with milder PID in whom *Chlamydia* is more likely to be the causative agent. The suggested criteria for the diagnosis of PID include the presence of all three of the following: history of abdominal pain and presence of direct lower abdominal tenderness with or without rebound, cervical motion tenderness, and adnexal tenderness.

In addition, one or more supporting symptoms must be present. These include temperature of at least 38°C, leukocytosis (10,500 white blood cells per cubic millimeter), culdocentesis that yields peritoneal fluid containing white blood cells and bacteria, presence of an inflammatory mass noted on pelvic examination or sonography, elevated erythrocyte sedimentation rate, Gram stain of an endocervical smear revealing gram-negative intracellular diplococci suggestive of *N gonorrhoeae,* or a monoclonal directed smear from endocervical secretions revealing *C trachomatis.*

The goals of treatment are the prevention of infertility and the chronic residual of infection. To be effective, treatment should be instituted early and should cover the polymicrobial spectrum of the disease. Often the most difficult therapeutic decision for the physician is whether to hospitalize the adolescent with PID or to treat her as an outpa-

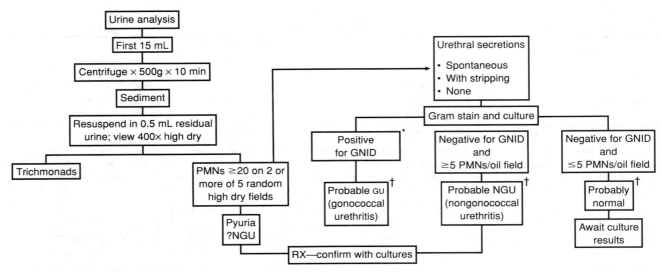

* Gram-negative intracellular diplococci
† Confirm Rx with culture results

Figure 17-2. Diagnostic patterns to determine presence of urethritis in males.

tient. Current recommendations favor aggressive inpatient treatment of this disease in the hope of preserving fertility and minimizing complications caused by noncompliance or inaccuracy of diagnosis. Although several treatment regimens are suggested, intravenous cefoxitin and doxycycline is favored because of its excellent coverage for *N gonorrhoeae*, *C trachomatis*, and the anaerobic organisms.

If patients are treated as outpatients, it is important to ensure that there is adequate follow-up within 48 hours to evaluate the clinical course. Partner treatment always should be a part of the therapeutic approach.

At least one fourth of women with acute PID experience one or more serious long-term sequelae. Involuntary infertility due to tubal occlusion is experienced by approximately 20% of young women after one episode of PID. Other sequelae include an increased risk of ectopic pregnancy, chronic pelvic pain, dyspareunia, pelvic adhesions, pyosalpinx, and the development of inflammatory masses.

The prevention of the sequelae through prompt and accurate diagnosis coupled with effective treatment should be a primary goal in the approach to adolescents with this disease.

Urethritis

Urethritis is the response of the urethra to inflammation of any etiology. Urethritis is almost always sexually acquired and is classified as gonococcal or nongonoccocal urethritis (NGU) depending on the presence or absence of *N gonorrhoeae*. Symptoms of urethritis may include urethral discharge, urinary frequency, burning on urination, and itching at the distal urethra or meatus; urethritis may also be present with no symptoms.

The incidence of urethritis is uncertain because it is not a reportable disease. It is generally appreciated that the incidence of NGU has increased despite the observed decrease in gonococcal urethritis.

C trachomatis is the most common cause of NGU. In addition, *U urealyticum* appears to be a common causative agent. Approximately 20% to 30% of patients with NGU have neither *C trachomatis* nor *U urealyticum* identified. In this group, the etiologic agent may include other bacteria including genital mycoplasmas, *Haemophilus*, *Bacteroides*, or other anaerobes; herpes simplex virus; yeasts; or parasites such as *T vaginalis*.

Most males with symptoms of dysuria or urethral discharge, especially if the exudate is purulent, spontaneous, or easily expressed and either mucoid or yellow-green in color, have urethritis (Figure 17–2). On clinical grounds, however, it is impossible to distinguish gonococcal urethritis from NGU. Moreover, a clear discharge or a small amount of mucoid discharge does not always indicate urethritis. Procedures that provide information to support the diagnosis include the microscopic examination of a Gram-stained smear of urethral secretions and the quantification of leukocytes in the centrifuged sediment from the first 10 to 15 mL of a first-voided urine specimen.

In most STD centers, the Gram stain is the procedure of choice. The presence of five or more leukocytes on a Gram-stained smear is indicative of urethritis. The findings of gram-negative intracellular diplococci is a sensitive indicator of gonococcal urethritis and correlates well with culture positivity.

The presence of pyuria (20 or more PMN leukocytes in two or more of five random fields) in the sediment of a first-catch urine specimen is a valuable aid in the diagnosis of urethritis. This noninvasive test helps identify adolescents with asymptomatic urethral infection and, therefore, may be useful in screening patients with minimal or no symptoms. All individuals with urethritis should have appropriate cultures performed for *C trachomatis* and *N gonorrhoeae* and should be treated with an antibiotic regimen to cover both organisms.

(Abridged from Hoover Adger, Sexually Transmitted Diseases, in Oski, DeAngelis, Feigin, McMillan, Warshaw: *Principles and Practice of Pediatrics, Second Edition*, J.B. Lippincott, 1994.)

Oski's Essential Pediatrics,
edited by Kevin B. Johnson and Frank A. Oski.
Lippincott–Raven Publishers,
Philadelphia © 1997

18

Hypertension

Detection of hypertension during adolescence has important implications for optimal health in later life, including the prevention of long-term cardiovascular complications and the early identification of serious disease.

By contrast, an unwarranted diagnosis of hypertension has serious negative consequences. Giving an individual the diagnosis of hypertension commits him or her to frequent medical visits, an extensive evaluation, and the cost and potential side effects of medications.

■ BLOOD PRESSURE MEASUREMENT

Blood pressure should be measured as a routine part of a yearly examination. It is important that the patient be calm, and that the blood pressure be measured with the patient seated and the arm at about the level of the patient's heart. The blood pressure cuff should have an internal bladder that completely encircles the arm and that covers a minimum of three fourths of the length of the upper arm.

After the cuff has been inflated and allowed to slowly deflate, the first heart sound or first Korotkoff sound is recorded as the systolic blood pressure. As the pressure continues to drop, the heart sounds become muffled. This point is called the fourth Korotkoff sound. Finally, the disappearance of all heart sounds is the fifth Korotkoff sound. If the fourth and fifth sounds are both heard, they should be recorded. In adolescents, the fourth Korotkoff sound is frequently not audible. Thus, the standards for diastolic blood pressures in this age group are based on the fifth Korotkoff sound.

■ BLOOD PRESSURE STANDARDS

Normal blood pressure is defined as blood pressure that is less than the 90th percentile. High normal blood pressure is defined as a blood pressure between the 90th and 95th percentile. Hypertension implies that either the systolic or diastolic blood pressure is greater than or equal to the 95th percentile. It is important to note that an individual who is either obese or unusually tall for age may have a blood pressure elevation that is normal for that individual. Only when the average of readings obtained on three different occasions is abnormal is the diagnosis of hypertension appropriate. Although 5% to 13% of adolescents are hypertensive on an initial blood pressure measure, only 1% remain persistently hypertensive on repeat evaluation.

■ TYPES OF HYPERTENSION

Common etiologies of hypertension are listed in Table 18–1. The most common "cause" of hypertension—so-called essential or primary hypertension—indicates that significant hypertension exists for which an underlying etiology cannot be found. About 90% of adolescent hypertension fits in this category. Because essential hypertension appears to have a genetic component, a family history of hypertension or a history of cardiovascular disease makes the diagnosis more likely.

■ EVALUATION OF THE ADOLESCENT WITH HYPERTENSION

When it is determined that a young person is hypertensive, a complete medical evaluation is indicated. History may elucidate any complaints resulting from the blood pressure elevation, although symptoms are rare unless the blood pressure elevations are severe (*ie,* diastolic readings above 110). Symptoms may include occipital headaches, visual disturbance, chest pain, seizures, or epistaxis. An exhaustive review of systems and a family history targeted at renal disease, hypertension, coronary artery disease, cerebrovascular infarct, or virilization will help to find a cause if one exists.

Physical examination should include a careful search for evidence of ocular or cardiac damage from longstanding or severe blood pressure elevation. Elements of the physical examination may provide clues to the etiology of hypertension. Vital signs, growth parameters, body habitus, thyroid, cardiovascular system, and abdominal examination are important in the evaluation.

■ LABORATORY EVALUATION

The extent of laboratory evaluation is determined by history and physical examination as well as by severity of hypertension. If essential hypertension is suspected based on positive family history coupled with an otherwise unremarkable history and physical examination, then laboratory assessment should not be extensive. A urinalysis is indicated to evaluate for signs of nephrosis, nephritis, or urinary tract infection. Serum electrolytes including urea nitrogen and creatinine as measures of renal function are indicated. Routine complete blood count is recommended. Anemia may suggest the presence of undiagnosed chronic illness, and hemolysis directs the investigation to include hemolytic uremic syndrome. If secondary hypertension is suspected based on history, physical examination, or severity of blood pressure elevation, more extensive evaluation is suggested.

■ TREATMENT

Treatment modalities include pharmacologic and nonpharmacologic methods. Nonpharmacologic methods are useful as either the primary therapy of patients with mild blood pressure elevation or as an adjunct to medication in cases of more severe hypertension. These methods include weight reduction, sodium restriction, and aerobic exercise.

The initial pharmacologic therapy is a single medication, usually either an angiotensin-converting enzyme (ACE) inhibitor, calcium-channel antagonist, or adrenergic blocking agent. The dose of the medication is gradually increased until the blood pressure responds, significant side effects occur, or the maximal dose is reached. If the initial medication does not adequately control blood pressure despite good compliance, another medication should be added. Usually a diuretic is added as the second medication. If the diuretic fails, a direct vasodilator, either hydralazine or pra-

TABLE 18-1. Differential Diagnosis of Hypertension in Adolescence

Essential Hypertension
Renal Parenchymal Disorders
  Acute glomerulonephritis
  Chronic glomerulonephritis
  Hemolytic uremic syndrome
  Henoch-Schönlein purpura
  Systemic lupus erythematosus
  Nephrotic syndrome
  Pyelonephritis
  Polycystic kidney disease
Obstructive Lesions
  Hydronephrosis
Renal Vascular Lesions
  Neurofibromatosis
  Renal artery thrombosis
  Renal vein thrombosis
  Renal artery stenosis
Trauma
Endocrine Disorders
  Hyperthyroidism
  Congenital adrenal hyperplasia
  Hyperaldosteronism
  Pheochromocytoma
  Turner's syndrome
  Pregnancy-induced hypertension
Cardiovascular Disorders
  Coarctation of the aorta
  Takayasu arteritis
Drug/Toxin
  Oral contraceptives
  Corticosteroids
  Anabolic steroids
  Cocaine
  Phencyclidine
  Amphetamines
  Nonsteroidal anti-inflammatory drugs
  Heavy metal or lead poisoning
Central Nervous System
  Increased intracranial pressure
Miscellaneous
  Burns
  Leg traction

zosin, is used. A fourth step is to use minoxidil as a vasodilator and a centrally acting agent rather than the ACE inhibitor or calcium-channel blocker.

■ COMPLIANCE

Compliance problems are frequently encountered in hypertensive patients of all ages and may be more severe during adolescence. The disease is usually asymptomatic and therefore not bothersome to the patient. Thus, the young person may not fully comprehend the need for treatment. In addition, medications must be faithfully taken indefinitely. Finally, bothersome side effects often outweigh perceived benefits. The medical provider may enhance compliance by careful education about the disease process and the need for treatment. Counseling patients that different medications may be used if side effects occur may be helpful.

■ CONCLUSION

A methodical approach to the diagnosis, evaluation, and treatment of hypertension results in optimal care for those in need of therapy and avoids unnecessary treatment for those who are healthy or have transient blood pressure evaluation.

(Abridged from Michele Diane Wilson, Hypertension, in Oski, DeAngelis, Feigin, McMillan, Warshaw: *Principles and Practice of Pediatrics, Second Edition*, J.B. Lippincott, 1994.)

Oski's Essential Pediatrics,
edited by Kevin B. Johnson and Frank A. Oski.
Lippincott–Raven Publishers,
Philadelphia © 1997

19

Adolescent Drug Abuse

Today's adolescent lives in a society in which use of alcohol and other drugs is prevalent and acceptable. The consequences of such use are evident. Although individuals in all other age groups have experienced an improvement in overall health status and a prolonged life expectancy, young people aged 15 to 24 years constitute the only group to experience an increase in mortality over the past decade. The major causes of mortality in this group are homicide, suicide, and unintentional injuries. A large proportion of these are associated with alcohol or other drugs.

■ DEFINITIONS

Chemical dependence can be defined as a chronic and progressive disease process that includes both the physical and psychological reliance on a chemical. It encompasses both alcoholism and dependence on other psychoactive substances. Chemical dependence is characterized by loss of control over use, compulsion, and establishment of an altered state in which one requires continued administration of a psychoactive substance to feel good or avoid feeling bad.

Substance abuse, in contrast, is characterized by a maladaptive pattern of use, indicated by continued use despite consequences or recurrent use when such use may be physically hazardous.

■ EPIDEMIOLOGY

Since 1975, the National Institute on Drug Abuse has conducted an annual nationwide survey of approximately 17,000 high school seniors on the use of alcohol, tobacco, and other drugs. Although surveys of drug use probably underestimate the magnitude of usage, they provide useful information about prevalence patterns and usage trends. Overall usage levels for many illicit drugs have declined from their peak levels during the late 1970s. Evidence continues to show, however, that the drug abuse problem among youth is a major dilemma.

Not all drugs have declined in level of use. Since the advent of "crack," a powerful and easily marketable form of cocaine, reported use in youth has been a major concern. Almost 10% of high school seniors in 1976 reported ever using cocaine. By 1985, this figure had risen to 17%. This is the highest figure yet reported for this group, and it indicates the escalating impact of this drug.

Although there has been a decrease in the reported prevalence for use of most illicit drugs, there has been relatively little change in the reported use of alcohol and tobacco, which are the major drugs of abuse. More than 90% of high school seniors in 1990 reported some experience with alcohol, 60% reported use in the past month, and 4% reported daily use. Additionally, problematic use among those who continue to use alcohol appears to be rising.

There has been a trend toward earlier initiation of use. There is also an inclination among today's youth to simultaneously use more than one drug. The earlier a person begins to drink or use other drugs, the greater the likelihood of later drug problems. Hence, potentially harmful effects are most serious in those who initiate use at a young age.

■ RISK FACTORS

Individuals who have been identified as particularly at risk for development of alcohol and other drug problems include children from families in which alcoholism or drug abuse is present. In addition, the following adolescents are at increased risk: those who experience significant problems in behavior such as aggressiveness and rebellious deviancy; those with difficulties in cognition such as learning disabilities or attention deficit disorders; those with problems in psychological well-being such as depression, isolation, and low self-esteem; and those with impaired familial functioning such as neglect, abuse, loss, and lack of close relationships. Genetics and environment also play important roles in the risk profile of an individual.

Identification and Treatment

Substance abuse should be included as a primary differential diagnosis whenever behavioral, familial, psychosocial, or related medical problems occur. As part of the routine health examination, all adolescents should be questioned about the use of cigarettes, alcohol, and other drugs. In addition, there should be an assessment of risk by reviewing risk factors and behaviors with adolescents and their parents.

A number of treatment alternatives are available for the chemically dependent adolescent. Short-term inpatient treatment, residential care, and outpatient care span the spectrum from traditional office-based care to intensive and structured day programs. Most treatment programs share beliefs that treatment begins with the interruption of use, requires continued abstinence from drugs, and sets as a goal for the adolescent the development of a drug-free lifestyle.

(Abridged from Hoover Adger, Adolescent Drug Abuse, in Oski, DeAngelis, Feigin, McMillan, Warshaw: *Principles and Practice of Pediatrics, Second Edition*, J.B. Lippincott, 1994.)

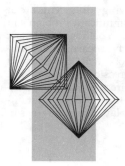

SECTION 2

Emergency Medicine

Oski's Essential Pediatrics,
edited by Kevin B. Johnson and Frank A. Oski.
Lippincott–Raven Publishers,
Philadelphia © 1997

20

Emergency Medicine Except Poisoning

Physicians in pediatric emergency departments or clinics care for children with a broad range of illnesses, from mild, nonurgent problems to life-threatening emergencies. This chapter examines the common life-threatening pediatric emergencies.

■ CARDIOPULMONARY RESUSCITATION IN CHILDREN

Every attempt should be made to identify the cause of the arrest, because special considerations may affect treatment. The most common causes are listed in Table 20–1. Trauma is the leading cause of cardiopulmonary arrest in children 1 to 14 years of age.

Children who have delayed resuscitation or present in asystole have a poor prognosis, because hypoxemia has already caused extensive damage to the brain and other vital organs. Survival is more likely if cardiopulmonary resuscitation (CPR) is started immediately, there is respiratory arrest only, the arrest is witnessed in the hospital, there is extreme bradycardia rather than asystole, or oxygen is the only necessary drug.

Basic Life Support

When first encountering a child who appears unresponsive, assess the adequacy of airway, breathing, and circulation. If a neck injury is plausible given the cause of the accident, stabilize the neck with axial traction or a Philadelphia collar, and do not attempt to extend the neck or turn it. Gently shake and call to the victim to determine if he or she is unresponsive or having respiratory difficulty. If conscious, allow the child to position his or her own airway; the child automatically assumes the best position. Position an unconscious child on a firm surface. When moving or turning the child, move the head and neck as a single unit. If a neck injury is not suspected, place a hand on the forehead and tilt the head back to a neutral position. Overextension of the neck obstructs the trachea. The fingers of the other hand are placed under the lower jaw at the chin to lift the chin off the airway. If a neck injury is suspected, use the jaw thrust without a head tilt.

After the airway is opened, verify that the child is breathing. If the child is not breathing, the rescuer must breathe for the victim. The rescuer can cover the mouth and nose of an infant with his or her mouth or pinch closed the nose of an older child and breathe mouth to mouth.

If aspiration is witnessed or strongly suspected or if an unconscious victim has airway obstruction that cannot be relieved by head tilting and jaw thrust maneuvers, the rescuer should attempt to remove the object manually only if it is visible on careful inspection. Blind finger sweeps may push a foreign body further into the airway and should be avoided.

The Heimlich maneuver is considered safe for children older than 1 year of age. With the child supine, the heel of the hand is placed in the midline between the umbilicus and rib cage and pushed rapidly inward and upward. This maneuver can be repeated 6 to 10 times. In infants under 1 year of age, alternating back blows (*ie*, four blows between the scapulae) and chest thrusts (*ie*, four compressions as in CPR) is recommended.

The adequacy of circulation is assessed by checking the pulse of a large artery, such as the carotid, brachial, or femoral. If no pulse is found, chest compressions are started immediately. In a small infant, the rescuer can encircle the baby's chest with both hands, support the back with the fingers, and compress the sternum with both thumbs.

Table 20–2 outlines breathing and circulation requirements for basic life support.

Advanced Cardiac Life Support

When a child arrives in the emergency department, an initial assessment should be done, including state of con-

TABLE 20-1. Common Causes of Cardiac Arrest

Cause	Circumstances
Traumatic	Motor vehicle injuries, burns, child abuse, firearm wounds
Pulmonary	Foreign body aspiration, smoke inhalation, near drowning, respiratory failure
Infectious	Epiglottitis, sepsis, meningitis
Central nervous system	Head trauma, seizures
Cardiac	Congenital heart disease, myocarditis
Other	Sudden infant death syndrome, poisoning, suicide, dehydration, congenital malformations

TABLE 20–2. Basic Life Support

Patient	Respirations Per Minute	Compressions Per Minute	Depth (Inches)	Where to Compress
Infant (<1 year)	20	100	0.5–1.0	Place index finger below intermammary line; press with middle and ring fingers
Child (>1 year)	15	80	1.0–1.5	Place middle and index fingers at base of sternum; place heel of hand above that and use for compression

sciousness, spontaneous respiratory effort, pulse, blood pressure, cardiac rhythm, temperature, perfusion, and pupillary responses.

Airway and Breathing

Humidified 100% oxygen should be administered to the patient immediately on arrival at the hospital or sooner if possible. If the child is unable to breathe on his own, the child will need to be intubated. Until that time, bag and mask ventilation should be administered.

Circulation

While an airway is being secured, other members of the resuscitation team should be securing intravenous access and monitoring pulse and cardiac rhythm. Intravenous access is crucial for drug and fluid administration, but it is often difficult to achieve in a child with poor circulation. The preferred methods for access are femoral vein catheterization, greater saphenous vein cutdown, or intraosseous vascular access. An intraosseous infusion is often the easiest and quickest method of access to the circulation, and it is recommended for children younger than 3 years of age.

Drugs

A variety of drugs are used to correct hypoxemia, reverse acidemia or increase coronary and cerebral perfusion pressure. The goal is to restore spontaneous circulation and stabilize the child's cardiac rhythm.

The preferred route of administration of drugs during resuscitation is intravenous bolus or infusion. If there is a delay in establishing intravenous access, epinephrine, lidocaine, or atropine may be given through the endotracheal tube. For endotracheal administration, the drug should be diluted to 5 to 10 mL, pushed in rapidly, and followed by five positive pressure breaths. All drugs and fluids may be given by intraosseous infusion. Table 20–3 outlines the drugs used commonly during an arrest.

Ventricular arrhythmias may occur in patients with congenital heart disease, myocardial disease, chest trauma, or drug ingestions. Many arrhythmias are best treated with electrical defibrillation or cardioversion (timed with depolarization of myocardial cell), which causes asynchronous depolarization of the myocardium. Use a paddle whose surface completely contacts the chest wall. Place paddles to the right of the sternum under the clavicle and on the left anterior axillary line at the apex of the heart. The initial dose for defibrillation is 2 J/kg. Subsequent doses are doubled. Stop if the rhythm converts out of ventricular fibrillation. If three shocks do not correct the rhythm, CPR should be resumed with drugs, and the patient should be assessed again for acidosis, hypoxemia, and hypothermia.

Frequent reassessment, including body temperature, is mandatory during any resuscitation.

■ PEDIATRIC TRAUMA

Most childhood trauma is mild. Lacerations are the most common injury, followed by contusions, fractures and dislocations, ingestions, and bites. Approximately 90% of life-threatening injuries are from blunt trauma, in which multiple and occult organ injuries are common, and head trauma often is involved. These children often die of shock, respiratory obstruction, or brain stem damage. The child is occasionally a victim of penetrating trauma, such as a gunshot or stab wound.

The head of a child is especially vulnerable in trauma because it is proportionately larger relative to body mass than that of an adult and because it is not well supported by strong neck muscles. Head trauma occurs in more than 80% of severely injured children. Because of the elasticity of the child's chest wall, rib and sternal fractures are rare, and an intact chest wall can mask severe crush injuries to the heart and lungs. The liver and spleen are less well protected by the chest wall than other structures. The poorly developed abdominal muscles offer little protection for the viscera, including the kidneys and bladder. Because children with stress and screaming swallow a large amount of air, gastric distention is common and may impair diaphragmatic function.

Management

Initial Assessment and Treatment

The priorities in treating a patient with trauma are to preserve or restore vital signs and to correct life-threatening injuries. To establish treatment priorities, the patient is assessed in a rapid primary survey. Any resuscitation that has begun during the primary survey is continued in the resuscitation phase. After resuscitation, the patient is thoroughly evaluated in the secondary survey, and plans are made for definitive care (ie, advanced trauma life support).

The *primary survey* (Table 20–4) is the first priority, followed by the secondary survey. Each area of the body should be completely visualized, palpated, and auscultated if appropriate. The cervical spine films are ordered, if not already done, with other appropriate radiographic and laboratory studies. After this examination is completed, the definitive care is begun.

Definitive Care

Laboratory. If trauma is minimal and physical examination results are normal, a urinalysis is necessary to rule out injury to the genitourinary system. For multiple-trauma patients, the minimal laboratory studies include type and crossmatch of blood, complete blood count (CBC), electrolytes, amylase, blood urea nitrogen (BUN), creatinine, and urinalysis. Radiographs should include the lateral cervical spine, chest, abdomen, and pelvis. Other laboratory and

TABLE 20-3. Resuscitation Drugs

Drug	Action	When Used	Route	Dose	Side Effects
Humidified oxygen	Improves arterial tension	Arrhythmias arrest	Mask ET tube	Highest FIo_2 possible 100% (adjust with Pao_2 later)	
Epinephrine	Vasoconstriction (α)	Asystole	IV	0.01 mg/kg (0.1 mL/kg of 1:10,000)	Tachycardia; VE; excessive vasoconstriction
	Inotropy (β)	Hypotension unresponsive	ET tube	0.02 mg/kg (0.2 mL/kg of 1:10,000)	
	Chronotropy (β)	Convert fine to coarse, VF for DC defibrillation, bradycardia unresponsive to atropine	IV	Start 0.1 µg/kg/minute¶ and titrate	
Sodium bicarbonate*	Reverse metabolic acidosis	Asystole (if acidotic); metabolic acidosis in arrhythmias	IV	2 mEq/kg under 2 y (½ strength under 6 mo); can repeat every 10 min 1 mEq/kg over 2 y; further doses based on BD: mEq bicarbonate $= \dfrac{\text{BD} \times \text{kg body wt} \times 0.4}{2}$	Hypersomolality; CSF acidosis; IVH in premature infants
Atropine sulfate	Accelerates sinus or atrial pacemaker	Asystole; symptomatic sinus bradycardia (hypotension, poor perfusion)	IV	0.02 mg/kg (min, 0.16 mg; max, 2 mg)	
	Increases AV conduction	Vagally mediated bradycardia (intubation); sinus bradycardia with PVCs	ET tube	Same dose	
Calcium†	Increases myocardial contractile force	Hypocalcemia Hyperkalemia Hypermagnesemia Calcium-channel blocker overdose	IV (peripheral)	Calcium gluconate, 30–60 mg; kg, IV (central) calcium chloride, 10–20 mg/kg	Bradycardia, toxicity;
Dextrose‡	Increases blood glucose	Hypoglycemia	IV	1 g/kg (25% solution)	
Dopamines§	Low dose increases shock unresponsive to fluid resuscitation; increases renal and splanchnic blood flow	Hypotension	IV	Start at 1 µg/kg/min# and titrate	Tachycardia; vasoconstriction, VE
	Intermediate dose stimulates cardiac β-adrenergic receptors				
	High dose stimulates α-adrenergic receptors				
Lidocaine	Decreases automaticity depressant	VF, VT	IV	1 mg/kg	Myocardial VT
		Sustained VA	IV	20–50 µg/kg/min** (with bolus)	
Isopreteronol	Increases HR, conduction velocity, and cardiac contractility	Symptomatic bradycardia	IV	0.1–1.0 µg/kg/min	Tachycardia
Bretylium tosylate	Prolongation of refractory period	VF, VT	IV	5–10 mg/kg followed by defibrillation	Nausea, vomiting, postural hypotension

AV, atrioventricular; BD, base deficit; CSI, cerebrospinal fluid; DC, direct current; ET, endotracheal; HR, heart rate; IV, intravenous; IVH, intraventricular hemorrhage; max, maximum; min, minimum, PVC, premature ventricular contraction; VA, ventricular arrhythmia; VE, ventricular entropy; VF, ventricular fibrillation; VT, ventricular tachycardia.

*Use sodium bicarbonate only after adequate ventilation has been established; otherwise, it causes a worsening respiratory acidosis.

†Calcium is no longer recommended for use during asystole. Calcium chloride is preferable (produces higher and more predictable calcium levels) to gluconate, but central line is needed for calcium chloride because it is sclerosing.

‡Use glucose (dextrose) in any arrest situation. Poor glycogen stores and starvation predispose infants and children to hypoglycemia.

§Low doses, 2–5 µg/kg/min; intermediate doses, 5–10 µg/kg/min; high doses; 15–20 µg/kg/min.

‖Because of its α-adrenergic activity, epinephrine is preferable to isuprel for patients in asystole.

¶Preparation of infusion: 0.6 × kg body wt = mg added to 100 mL diluent; then 1 mL/h delivered 0.1 µg/kg/minute.

#Preparation of infusion: 6 × kg body wt = mg added to 100 mL diluent; then 1 mL/h delivered 1.0 µg/kg/min.

**Preparation of infusion: 120 mg added to 100 mL diluent, then 1 mL/kg/h delivered 20 µg/kg/min.

TABLE 20-4. Trauma Surveys

Primary Survey	Resuscitation	Secondary Survey
Airway maintenance with cervical spine control	Oxygenation	Head and skull—pupils, fundi, vision, injury
Breathing	Shock therapy	Maxillofacial trauma
Circulation with hemorrhage control	Vital signs	Neck—films, pulses, crepitation
Disability—alert, verbal, painful, unconscious	Monitoring—electrocardiogram, nasogastric catheter,* urinary catheter*	Chest
Expose—undress patient		Abdomen, perineum, rectum
		Extremities—pulses, fractures
		Neurologic examination—Glasgow Coma Scale
		Radiographs, laboratory tests

*If not contraindicated.

Committee on Trauma, American College of Surgeons. Advanced trauma life support student manual 1993.

radiologic studies are dictated by the history and physical examination. Commonly, special x-ray studies such as a liver–spleen scan, computed tomography (CT) scan, and arteriography are indicated.

Head Trauma

Initial Assessment and Treatment

Although central nervous system (CNS) injury is the most common cause of pediatric traumatic death, most head trauma in children is blunt and mild. The initial evaluation includes a history of the force involved, any loss of consciousness and its duration, and a check of current vital signs and level of consciousness. Place a cervical collar if cervical spine injury is suspected. As always, primary and secondary surveys are essential.

The Glasgow Coma Scale (Table 20–5), indicating the level of consciousness, is the most important part of the neurologic examination. The scale is useful in evaluating and following the child and in predicting immediate and future outcome. A Glasgow Coma Scale score less than 5 is associated with a high probability of mortality or permanent neurologic sequelae. Children with scores of at least 6 have a better prognosis.

A more thorough physical examination includes palpation of all scalp wounds to determine depth of injury and possible depression of bone and signs of blood indicating a basilar skull fracture, including raccoon eyes, battle ears, and hemotympanum.

Skull films are rarely useful in the evaluation of head trauma in children because they are usually negative. They have a higher yield if restricted to children with at least one of the following criteria: age less than 1 year, a history of unconsciousness for at least 5 minutes, a penetrating wound, lethargy, a palpable depression, signs of a basilar skull fracture, or focal neurologic signs. Many of these children receive a CT scan, obviating the need for skull films.

Definitive Care

If there is minor head trauma with a Glasgow Coma Score of 15 and a normal neurologic examination and cranial CT, the child may be observed at home for changes in mental status, vomiting, and gross motor ability.

A child with loss of consciousness for less than 5 minutes, indicating a concussion, may need hospital admission for close observation. If there is deterioration of the Glasgow Coma Scale score or focal neurologic abnormalities, a CT scan

is obtained to look for an intracranial hemorrhage. Magnetic resonance imaging may be more sensitive than CT in detecting traumatic brain damage. Children with a longer period of unconsciousness, deteriorating examination results, or focal signs are at risk for major and sudden decompensation and need immediate treatment to reduce intracranial pressure. This treatment is outlined in Table 20–6.

Thoracic Trauma

Thoracic trauma can cause multiple threats to a child's life. More than 90% of thoracic trauma in children is blunt, resulting from motor vehicle injuries and falls. The injury from blunt trauma may be obvious, such as a tension pneu-

TABLE 20-5. Glasgow Coma Scale

Observation	Response	Score
Eye opening	Spontaneous	4
	To verbal command	3
	To pain	2
	None	1
Best verbal response	Oriented	5
	Confused	4
	Inappropriate words	3
	Incomprehensible words	2
	None	1
Best motor response	Obeys command	6
	Localizes pain	5
	Withdraws from pain	4
	Flexion to pain (decorticate)	3
	Extension to pain (decerebrate)	2
	None	1
Total		3–15

Modified from Mayer T, Matlak ME, Johnson DG, et al. The modified injury severity scale in pediatric multiple trauma patients. J Pediatr Surg. 1980;15:719.

TABLE 20-6. Initial Treatment of Increased Intracranial Pressure

Intubation with in-line traction of cervical spine*

Hyperventilation (Pco_2 20–25 mm Hg) and oxygenation

Dexamethasone, 0.5–1.0 mg/kg IV

Mannitol, 0.25–0.5 g/kg IV†

Fluids, $\frac{2}{3}$ maintenance‡

Computed tomography scan as soon as possible.

*Obtain cervical spine films first, if possible.
†If herniation is suspected.
‡If there is accompanying shock, start full fluid resuscitation.

mothorax, or more subtle, detected only during a careful physical examination. Penetrating trauma from a gunshot or stab wound usually causes significant damage, and penetrating wounds must be surgically explored.

Initial Assessment and Treatment

The initial evaluation starts with a history of the force, an assessment of vital signs, and a primary survey. Air hunger, cyanosis, tachypnea, and anxiety are signs of ventilatory insufficiency. Retractions and stridor occur with partial upper airway obstruction. If the child is not moving air well, look for airway obstruction, open pneumothorax, tension pneumothorax, or flail chest. If shock exists, massive hemothorax, cardiac tamponade, and myocardial contusion must be considered. If evidence exists of a pneumothorax, a needle thoracostomy is performed, followed by placement of a chest tube.

Chest radiography, electrocardiogram (ECG), and arterial blood gas measurement may provide clues to other seri-

ous but less apparent injuries when the physical examination is not suggestive. For example, a widened mediastinum on x-ray film indicates the possibility of aortic rupture, necessitating an emergency aortogram. Mediastinal air may indicate tracheobronchial tree rupture.

Definitive Care

Patients with penetrating trauma that enters only the superficial tissues or with mild blunt trauma may be discharged from the emergency department if no other serious injuries are detected. Management of other injuries is summarized in Table 20–7.

Abdominal Trauma

Like head and thoracic trauma, abdominal trauma in children is usually blunt and mild; most cases are due to motor vehicle injuries and falls. If the injury is penetrating, moderate or severe injuries are expected. Children with multiple trauma and severe neurologic impairment are at higher risk for intra-abdominal injury than those without coma.

Initial Assessment

An accurate abdominal examination is often difficult to obtain because of an uncooperative child producing a falsely tight abdomen or because of an unconscious child producing falsely negative examination results. In a young, alert child, it is important to establish rapport before examining the abdomen and to examine the painful area last.

Treatment

Mild injury, manifested by superficial abrasions or tenderness warrants a rectal examination and a urinalysis to

TABLE 20-7. Life-Threatening Thoracic Injuries

Injury	Physical Examination Findings	Initial Treatment
Airway obstruction (eg, foreign body, sections, severe maxillofacial trauma)	Decreased or no air movement (ventilatory insufficiency)	Suction, jaw thrust, chin lift, oropharyngeal/nasopharyneal airway intubation
Open pneumothorax	Open wound in chest	Cover hole with occlusive dressing
	Ventilatory insufficiency (if large, air passes through hole with each respiration)	Chest tube through another site
Flail chest* (ie, multiple rib fractures)	Paradoxic motion of segment of chest wall	Turn patient onto affected side to stabilize flail
		Intubate if ventilatory failure
Massive hemothorax	Decreased breath sounds	Volume resuscitation
	Dull to percussion	Chest tube
		Surgery
Tension pneumothorax	Decreased breath sounds	Needle aspiration
	Tracheal deviation	Chest tube
	Shift of point of maximum impulse	
	Hyperresonance	
Pericardial tamponade	Shock	Pericardiocentesis
	Distended neck veins	Surgery
	Decreased pulse pressure	
	Muffled heart tones	

*Because the thoracic cage is very compliant in children, significant pulmonary contusion may be present without rib fractures. Flail chest is usually combined with lung contusion and ventilation–perfusion mismatch.

screen for more significant abdominal injury. If there is a suspicion of more severe injury, diagnostic tests should be performed, including a CBC, amylase, and type and crossmatch of blood; radiography; and observation. Patients with the possibility of free blood in the abdomen need peritoneal lavage, unless abdominal surgery is imminent. Other indications for lavage are lethargy or coma with abdominal injury, thoracic injury with suspected abdominal injury, or equivocal diagnostic findings. Before lavage is performed, a nasogastric tube and urinary catheter are placed unless contraindicated.

Extremity Trauma

Care of the extremities is not part of the primary survey and resuscitation, except for control of major hemorrhage. During the secondary survey, the extremities are examined for perfusion, deformity, and function. If not treated promptly, combined vascular and bone injuries can result in limb loss.

Initial Assessment

The history should be directed to disclose the mechanism of injury, any risk of contamination, and predisposing factors such as underlying illness and previous injuries. A history of tetanus prophylaxis can be obtained after the acute care.

The limb should be inspected, with attention paid to active and passive motion, angulation, shortening, swelling, bruising, and wounds. If indicated, obtain appropriate radiographs. Neurovascular and musculoskeletal integrity may be compromised by penetrating trauma, by a compartment syndrome from blunt trauma, by dislocations, and by fractures.

Treatment

Definitive care restores alignment and peripheral perfusion. All dislocations involving loss of pulse should be reduced immediately and arteriography performed if the pulse is not restored to prevent limb loss. All fractures are immobilized by splinting or traction. Immobilization is the best treatment for pain, but pain medication may be needed. Open wounds should be debrided of gross contamination and covered with sterile dressings. Tetanus prophylaxis is administered if indicated.

Wound Care

Initial Assessment

Wound care begins with a careful history of when, where, and how the injury occurred. The type of wound, the amount of contamination in the wound, and the delay until treatment determine the management. Other important history includes tetanus immunization status, allergies (especially to local anesthesia), bleeding disorders, and medications.

Treatment

Gently wash the wound and surrounding area with soap and water or dilute iodine solution and shave area if necessary before injecting local anesthesia (Table 20–8). Explore the wound for injuries to deep tissues and structures, and remove any foreign bodies. If there is doubt about the presence of a foreign body, particularly glass, obtain appropriate radiographs.

Wounds should not be sutured if 12 hours have elapsed since injury. Face wounds may be sutured after a 12-hour delay. Other "dirty" wounds, such as animal bites and deep punctures, should not be immediately sutured; delayed primary closure may be possible after 4 or 5 days. If in doubt, leave the wound open.

TABLE 20-8. Local Anesthesia With Lidocaine

Approach

  Rule out allergy to lidocaine.

  Document sensation distal to injury.

  Topical anesthesia: ethyl chloride spray

  Inject 1 cm away from wound edge (if clean wound, can inject through wound margin).

Lidocaine concentration

Infants	0.25–0.5%
Children	0.5–1.0%
Lidocaine dose	7 mg/kg (max) with epinephrine*
	3–5 mg/kg without epinephrine
Onset	5 min
Duration	90–200 min

*Do not use epinephrine for end organs, such as digits, ears, nose, or genitalia.

Most patients with wounds do not need antibiotics. If the wound is more than 18 hours old before treatment or shows signs of infection, antibiotics should be prescribed for a short course. The patient is seen again in 24 to 48 hours to check the wound for healing and signs of infection. Sutures are removed from the face in 2 to 4 days, scalp in 5 days, extremities in 7 to 10 days, and joints in 10 to 14 days.

■ BITES

Human and nonhuman animal bites are common among children. More than half of these bites are not serious, but certain initially innocuous-looking bites can lead to serious infectious complications. Dog bites account for about 90% of nonhuman bites that require medical attention, and cat bites account for almost 10%, with rodent and rabbit bites composing the remainder.

Human and nonhuman animal bites are common among children. Most wounds are colonized by aerobic and anaerobic organisms obtained from the skin of the victim and the oral cavity of the biter. An average infected wound yields three to five organisms on culture, with the highest estimate from human bites. The most common organisms in all bite wounds are *Staphylococcus aureus*, *Streptococcus* spp, anaerobic cocci, and *Bacteroides* spp. Dog and cat bite wounds commonly carry *Pasteurella multocida* and *Pseudomonas fluorescens*.

Management

After initial care and debridement when necessary, most children with minor bite wounds can be managed as outpatients with careful follow-up. Tetanus toxoid is given if indicated, and rabies prophylaxis is considered, depending on the animal species and area. In the United States, the animals most commonly infected with rabies are skunks, raccoons, and bats, but other animals, including dogs and cats, may be infected. A final decision about whether to treat a potentially exposed patient can be made in conjunction with the local health department. Treatment consists of thorough local wound care and passive and active immunoprophylaxis. Human rabies immune globulin is given as soon as possible to cover the time during which the patient has insufficient active antibody production. At the same time, active immunization is begun with human diploid cell vaccine.

Prophylactic antibiotics are probably useful for patients with wounds at a high risk for infection. High-risk wounds include all cat and nonsuperficial human bites, dog bites more than 8 hours after injury, hand wounds, deep puncture wounds, and wounds with the potential of delayed primary closure.

Amoxicillin with clavulanic acid (Augmentin) covers all the common organisms. An alternative includes the use of penicillin in combination with a penicillinase-resistant penicillin or cephalosporin. Erythromycin can be used for patients with penicillin allergy. Additional therapy of infected wounds is guided by Gram stain and culture results.

■ BURNS

Burns are a common injury in children, exacting a large toll in terms of loss of function, deformity, pain, and psychological strain. Burn injuries are classified as thermal (ie, flame, scald, contact, inhalation), electrical, or chemical, including battery burns. Most burned children are younger than 5 years old (average, 2.5 years). Eighty-five percent of these injuries are scalds from hot tap water or liquids spilled from cooking pots. Flame, electrical, and chemical burns are less common.

Management

Initial Emergency Treatment

The emergency management of a burn patient starts with removal of all clothing and assessment of airway, breathing, and circulation. Upper airway edema from smoke inhalation burns or soft-tissue edema of the neck and face may compromise airway patency and breathing. Respiratory status must be quickly evaluated and oxygen applied. Intravenous access is established if there is inhalation injury or if more than 10% to 15% of the body surface area is burned. If there is chemical injury, start copious irrigation with water as soon as possible.

History. A detailed history of the burn injury (ie, environment of burn, materials burned, clothing worn) and the child's medical history are essential for care. For example, if the burn injury included a fall, explosion, or child abuse, there may be other serious injuries. If the child was in a fire in an enclosed space, smoke inhalation must be considered. If the burn was electrical, extensive damage may exist below the surface of the skin.

Physical Examination. The extent of the burn can be roughly estimated using the "rule of nines" shown in Figure 20–1. Another helpful rule for estimating the extent of scattered, irregular burns is that one surface of the patient's hand represents approximately 1% of body surface area.

Laboratory Studies. Laboratory and other studies to consider in the significantly burned patient are CBC, type and crossmatch of blood, carboxyhemoglobin, electrolytes, BUN, creatinine, albumin and total protein, prothrombin time, arterial blood gas, chest radiograph, and radiographs of associated injuries.

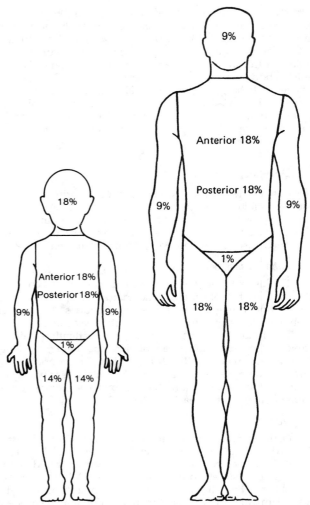

Figure 20-1. Rule of nines for child (*left*) and adult (*right*). Adapted from Scherer JC. *Introductory medical-surgical nursing.* 4th ed. Philadelphia: JB Lippincott; 1986:687.)

Definitive Treatment

Airway Management. Patients with inhalation injury have a marked increase in morbidity and mortality. The upper airway is extremely susceptible to swelling and obstruction from exposure to hot, moist air or toxic gases. Direct thermal injury from hot air is unlikely unless the heat is conveyed by steam. The subglottic airway is protected from direct injury by the larynx. Inhalation injury can damage the lower respiratory tract, resulting in pulmonary edema, aspiration pneumonia, and pneumonitis.

In the first 36 hours after an inhalation injury, management is directed at airway edema and acute pulmonary insufficiency. Diagnosis of airway or pulmonary injury should be entertained if there is a history of fire in an enclosed space or the child has facial burns, singed nasal hairs, or inflammatory changes in the pharynx or carbonaceous sputum. Humidified 100% oxygen must be applied. Positive-pressure ventilation may be necessary later to prevent pulmonary edema.

Measurement of carboxyhemoglobin level is performed early in patients involved in a fire in an enclosed space. Symptoms of mild intoxication, such as impaired judgment, headache, and decreased fine motor skills, may begin at a carboxyhemoglobin level as low as 5% in a nonsmoker, and become more severe at higher levels. Levels of 60% or more are associated with convulsions, coma, and death. The treatment is removal from the "contaminated" environment and administration of 100% oxygen. The half-life of carboxyhemoglobin decreases from approximately 4 hours in room air to less than 1 hour in 100% oxygen. Treatment with hyperbaric oxygen decreases the half-life even further, and it can be helpful in severely toxic patients.

A chest radiograph, although essential in patients at risk for respiratory complications, may show no abnormalities in the first 12 to 24 hours after injury. After initial airway management, the patient is observed for pulmonary edema and later observed for bronchopneumonia. The care is generally supportive, because prophylactic antibiotics and steroids are not of proven benefit.

Fluid Management. Fluid management in patients with burns is complex and requires attention to skin losses of water, electrolytes, and protein.

Wound Care

The burn surface is a warm, moist, protein-rich environment, and colonization with fungi and bacteria is a constant source of infection. Meticulous wound cleansing and dressing minimizes colonization and infection. With full-thickness burns, later skin grafts survive better on wounds with lower bacterial colony counts.

If cared for as an outpatient, the child should be bathed twice each day and Silvadene then applied. A burned extremity should be elevated to avoid swelling. Oral penicillin for 3 to 5 days may be helpful in preventing infection of the wound. Broad-spectrum antibiotics are contraindicated. Daily follow-up care is necessary until clean healing is ensured.

Pain Medications

If the child is anxious or restless and hypoxia is not a problem, analgesics or narcotics may be used sparingly. Morphine

(0.1 mg/kg, given intravenously) or Demerol (1 mg/kg intravenously, orally, or intramuscularly) are effective analgesics.

■ RESPIRATORY DISTRESS

Respiratory distress may result from airway obstruction, pulmonary parenchymal disease, or from processes outside the respiratory system (Figure 20–2).

Airway obstruction can be divided into upper and lower airway obstruction. The *upper airway* refers to the level above secondary bronchi, and the *lower airway* refers to the peripheral airways, which are usually less than 3 mm in diameter. Lower airway obstruction usually involves a diffuse distribution of obstruction. The differentiating characteristics are listed in Table 20–9.

Upper airway obstruction interferes primarily with inspiration. As upper airway obstruction progresses, a small increase occurs in respiratory rate, and a large increase occurs in respiratory effort, leading to dyspnea. The increased respiratory effort causes an increased negative intrathoracic pressure, manifested by retractions. Stridor, a low-pitched respiratory sound, increases. Complete obstruction above the bifurcation of the trachea causes asphyxia and death.

Lower airway obstruction interferes with expiration of air from the smaller airways, causing the expiratory phase to be prolonged. The turbulent airflow is heard as wheezing. As the obstruction increases, expiration is prolonged, and accessory muscles are used. Wheezing increases as the obstruction progresses, and then decreases as airflow becomes limited.

Foreign body aspiration, croup, asthma, and bronchiolitis are the more common causes of respiratory distress seen in a pediatric emergency department.

Foreign Body Aspiration

Foreign body aspiration is a significant health hazard in young children, particularly between the ages of 6 months and 3 years. Most foreign bodies that children aspirate are small

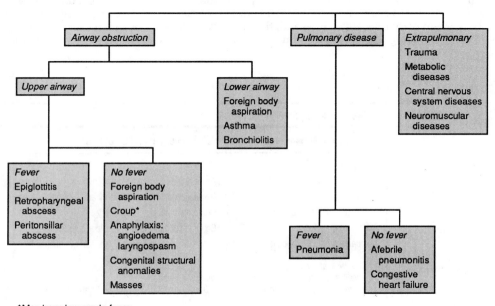

Figure 20-2. Common causes of respiratory distress.

*May have low-grade fever.

TABLE 20-9. Airway Obstruction

Upper Airway	Lower Airway
Interferes primarily with inspiration	Interferes primarily with expiration
Inspiratory stridor	Expiratory wheeze
Severe retractions	Mild retractions
Croupy or brassy cough	Prolonged expiration
Death from complete obstruction	Hacking and repetitive cough
	Patchy areas of atelectasis from areas of complete obstruction

and, rather than lodging in the trachea and causing acute obstruction and death, pass through the trachea to lodge in a main stem bronchus. These small foreign bodies, usually composed of organic matter, are not immediately life threatening.

Assessment

The child with foreign body aspiration may present with no history of aspiration and only subtle signs and symptoms, and the diagnosis is frequently missed. With delayed diagnosis, these children may present with recurrent attacks of wheezing diagnosed as asthma, pneumonia, or bronchiectasis. The diagnosis of foreign body aspiration requires a high index of suspicion and should be considered in any child with unexplained pulmonary complaints. In most children, a history of sudden onset of coughing with acute respiratory distress or subsequent coughing, wheezing, or stridor suggests the diagnosis of foreign body aspiration. The clinical symptoms depend on the location of the foreign body (Table 20–10). The most frequent physical findings are wheezing, decreased air movement, and rhonchi, all localized over the lung with the involved airway.

The most helpful supporting tests are inspiratory and expiratory or bilateral decubitus chest radiographs. Persistent air trapping on an expiratory or lateral decubitus radiograph is a common finding in foreign body aspiration. Persistent atelectasis or infiltration are other common findings. The foreign body is rarely opaque and, therefore, rarely visible on the radiograph. The chest film ranges from diagnostic to totally unremarkable. The diagnostic yield may be increased with fluoroscopy, which may show persistent lung inflation during inspiration and expiration.

Management

If the child presents to the emergency room with no air movement, the Heimlich maneuver or back blows are administered (see CPR section at the beginning of this chapter). Most aspirations are not life threatening, and a thorough history and physical examination can be obtained. If suspicion of a foreign body aspiration is supported by physical examination or radiographs, bronchoscopy is the treatment of choice for its removal. The degree of urgency depends on the location of the foreign body. If the foreign body is in the distal airways, postural drainage and percussion may be helpful.

Croup

Croup, or laryngotracheobronchitis, is a common syndrome involving inflammation or edema of the subglottic area and causing airway obstruction in the larynx, trachea, or bronchi. Croup usually affects children 6 months to 4 years old; the peak incidence is in 1- to 2-year-old children. It occurs all year, but the incidence increases in late fall and winter. There is a slight male predominance.

Most croup is viral, but it may also be spasmodic (ie, allergic) or bacterial. As many as 75% of cases of viral croup are caused by parainfluenza viruses; other viruses include respiratory syncytial virus, influenza viruses, and adenovirus. *Mycoplasma pneumoniae* can cause croup.

Assessment

Viral croup has an insidious onset after a few days of an upper respiratory tract infection. It progresses to hoarseness and the characteristic inspiratory stridor and barking cough. Symptoms wax and wane and are usually worse at night. Oral intake may be decreased.

Spasmodic croup appears as a sudden onset of severe stridor, usually at night, in a well child with no upper respiratory tract infection. The cause is thought to be allergic, but viruses may play a role.

The child with croup is usually mildly or moderately ill; he or she rarely appears to be toxic. There are usually signs of an upper respiratory tract infection and a low-grade fever. The respiratory examination shows signs of upper respira-

TABLE 20-10. Foreign Body Aspiration

Location of Foreign Body	Common Signs and Symptoms
Trachea	
Total obstruction	Acute asphyxia, marked retractions
High partial obstruction	Decreased air entry, inspiratory and expiratory stridor, retractions
Low partial obstruction	Expiratory wheezing, inspiratory stridor
Main stem bronchus	Cough, expiratory wheezing, blood-tinged sputum*
Lobar/segmental bronchus	Decreased breath sounds[†]; wheezing, rhonchi

*Usually a later finding.
[†]Localized to area of lung related to affected bronchus.
Adapted from Cotton E, Yasuda K. Foreign body aspiration. Pediatr Clin North Am. 1984;31:937.

tory obstruction: inspiratory stridor, suprasternal and intercostal retractions, and an increased respiratory rate. Children with croup have a characteristic barking cough and a hoarse voice.

There are no diagnostic laboratory tests for this illness. A lateral neck radiograph may be helpful to rule out other causes of upper respiratory obstruction, such as epiglottitis, foreign body aspiration, or retropharyngeal abscess. The lateral neck radiograph in croup usually shows a normal epiglottis, subglottic narrowing, and ballooning of the hypopharynx. On a posteroanterior neck view, there is narrowing of the air column at the top, known as the steeple sign.

Management

Most children with croup can be managed as outpatients with a cool mist vaporizer or shower mist and careful observation of fluid intake. Children with spasmodic croup respond well to most therapeutic measures. If the child has moderate or severe respiratory distress, oxygen is given.

Steroids by intramuscular or oral routes may be helpful in patients with croup. A single intramuscular injection or oral dose of dexamethasone (0.6 mg/kg) may allow significant clinical improvement during the next 24 hours. Antibiotics are not indicated unless there is evidence of bacterial disease.

Racemic epinephrine, a local vasoconstrictor given by nebulization, temporarily relieves airway obstruction by decreasing edema, especially in spasmodic croup. Because the obstruction usually returns to pretreatment level or worse in 1 or 2 hours, the child must be carefully observed.

Croup and epiglottitis may occasionally be confused with each other. Table 20–11 shows the main differentiating characteristics of these two diseases. Croup is diagnosed approximately ten times as frequently as epiglottitis.

Bronchiolitis

Bronchiolitis is a common and acute viral infection of the lower respiratory tract that causes mild or severe respiratory distress. The organism invades the epithelial cells of the bronchioles, causing sloughing of cells, edema, and increased mucus secretion. The resultant narrowing of the small airways causes uneven air trapping and overdistention of the lungs; ventilation–perfusion mismatch can lead to hypoxemia or hypercarbia.

Bronchiolitis most commonly affects infants 2 to 8 months of age but can be seen in children up to 2 years of age. Occur-

rence peaks in winter and spring. The organism in most cases is respiratory syncytial virus; others are parainfluenza viruses, adenovirus, influenza viruses, and *Mycoplasma pneumoniae*.

Assessment

The diagnosis of bronchiolitis is made by clinical presentation, age of the child, and season. After a few days of an upper respiratory tract infection, the child has an acute onset of cough, expiratory wheezing, and rales. If there is moderate or severe respiratory distress, the child may eat poorly, be dehydrated from poor oral intake, and be irritable. The chest examination reveals wheezing and rales bilaterally; these findings may change on subsequent examinations. Increased respiratory rate and, in severe disease, nasal flaring and retractions are seen.

Viral culture results from the nasopharynx are positive for as many as 50% of cases of bronchiolitis but are not available in time for diagnosis. Some laboratories have immunofluorescent techniques for viral identification. A chest radiograph shows nonspecific changes; it may show diffuse hyperinflation with patchy areas of infiltration or atelectasis. An arterial blood gas determination may be necessary for more severely ill infants.

Management

Traditional therapy for bronchiolitis is supportive and includes oral fluids, mist therapy, antipyretics, and oxygen if necessary.

Recent studies show that many children with bronchiolitis have a reversible component to their airway obstruction and benefit from a bronchodilator such as nebulized albuterol. If the child improves with a trial of a nebulized β_2-adrenergic agent or subcutaneous epinephrine, treatment with albuterol syrup for 5 to 7 days may improve the symptoms.

The early use of steroids in bronchiolitis patients in the emergency department with β_2-adrenergic drugs may improve clinical status and allow a higher percentage of these patients to go home. Antibiotics have not been beneficial.

The only specific therapy for bronchiolitis involves the use of ribavirin for respiratory syncytial virus infection in very ill or high-risk infants.

The child with bronchiolitis should be hospitalized for severe respiratory distress or if aspiration, dehydration, and secondary bacterial pneumonia are concerns. Most children are completely well in 2 to 3 weeks.

The prognosis for a child with bronchiolitis is excellent, and the complications of persistent wheezing, apnea, or superimposed bacterial pneumonia are rare. Children with bronchiolitis are more likely to have reactive airway disease or asthma in the future.

■ SEIZURES

Seizures are a common neurologic emergency; about 5% of children have at least one seizure by the age of 16 years. The more common causes of seizures are listed in Table 20–12.

Initial Treatment

The most common seizure emergency is generalized tonic clonic status epilepticus. If the level of consciousness is satisfactory, most other seizures are not medical emergencies and can, therefore, be treated while an electroencephalogram (EEG) is being monitored.

Continuous generalized tonic clonic seizures need immediate treatment to prevent life-threatening complica-

TABLE 20–11. Differentiation Between Croup and Epiglottitis

Characteristic	Croup	Epiglottitis
Age	6 mo to 4 y	2 to 8 y
Site	Subglottic	Supraglottic
Onset	Gradual history of upper respiratory infection	Rapid, usually less than 24 h
Presentation	Inspiratory stridor; hoarse, barky cough	Inspiratory stridor; high fever, toxic appearance; sits forward
Etiology	Viral	Bacterial

TABLE 20-12. Common Causes of Seizures in Children

Simple febrile seizures
Infections
    Intracranial infections—bacterial or aseptic meningitis, encephalitis
    Shigellosis
Head trauma
    Direct trauma
    Shaking injury
Metabolic abnormalities
    Hypoxia
    Hypoglycemia—insulin reaction in diabetics, alcohol ingestion
    Electrolyte disturbances or dehydration
    Hypocalcemia
    Pyridoxine deficiency
    Renal failure
    Hepatic failure
    Inherited metabolic disorders
Toxic ingestions (rule out suicide attempt)
    Alcohol
    Theophylline
Withdrawal of anticonvulsant medications
Miscellaneous
    Hypertensive encephalopathy
    Brain tumor
    Intracranial hemorrhage
    Idiopathic

tions. After advanced life support is established, and the ABCs are ensured, the seizure is stopped with anticonvulsant medication and diagnostic studies are considered.

Intravenous anticonvulsants, as shown in Table 20–13, are used for the patient in status epilepticus; they allow prompt administration and produce quick therapeutic levels. The patient should be monitored while these drugs are given, because they have significant hemodynamic and respiratory-depressant side effects.

The patient having a seizure must be protected from physical harm. The child is placed on a soft surface and restrained as necessary. Fever control is part of supportive care. Body temperature may be elevated from infection or from the seizure itself, and the fever increases metabolic demands.

Assessment

It is essential to check for conditions that need immediate therapy. The history should include questions about the current seizure, including how it started, type, and duration; previous seizures and frequency; evidence of infection; abnormal behavior; development; pica; trauma; possible ingestion; birth history; and current medications, including anticonvulsants.

The physical examination includes assessment of vital signs, evidence of injury or infection, and the general medical condition. Abnormal neurologic signs are common during and after a seizure. Serious neurologic abnormalities may indicate a problem that needs immediate further assessment and treatment by a neurologist.

The selection of laboratory studies is determined by the age of the patient, the history, and the physical examination. The traditional tests of electrolytes, calcium, and magnesium are required only if there is suspicion of a relevant abnormality. A CBC with differential is obtained if there is suspicion of infection. Other studies, such as urinalysis, anticonvulsant drug levels, toxicology screens of serum and urine, blood cultures, liver function, ammonia, and lead levels may be indicated.

Skull radiographs are rarely indicated in a child with seizures, but they may be helpful if a skull fracture is suspected and CT scanning is not available. A CT scan is helpful if there is a focal deficit, history of trauma, evidence of increased intracranial pressure, or suspicion of a mass lesion. A lumbar puncture is indicated for a child with a febrile seizure and meningeal signs; seizures often occur in children with acute bacterial meningitis. If concern exists about increased intracranial pressure, a CT scan should be done before a lumbar puncture.

After a seizure has been stopped in the emergency department, any underlying conditions that may have caused the seizure must be treated. It is often advisable to treat the seizures themselves, and a neurologist should be consulted concerning ongoing seizure management.

If the seizure cannot be controlled, cardiovascular signs are unstable, or neurologic examination results are abnormal after the seizure and immediate postictal period, the patient should be hospitalized for further observation and management. The nonemergent care of children with seizures is discussed in Chapter 208.

Management

Simple Febrile Seizure. Children commonly have seizures as a consequence of an abrupt and steep rise in body temperature. For this simple febrile seizure, several criteria must be met: age 6 months to 6 years, generalized seizure of less then 20 minutes' duration, occurrence within 24 hours of onset of the fever, normal development and neurologic examination results, and no family history of afebrile seizures. If the child and seizure meet these criteria, the child is given an antipyretic and observed. If the child looks fine, no further studies or treatment is indicated.

If the criteria are not met and the child does not look fine or is younger than 18 months, a lumbar puncture may be necessary to rule out meningitis. CNS infections are rarely found, even in the children with "atypical" or complex febrile seizures. Other laboratory studies are performed as necessary. If the seizure is atypical, treatment may be started, usually with phenobarbital. The child with a simple febrile seizure has an approximately 30% risk of recurrence.

Known Seizure Disorder. Many children presenting with seizures have chronic seizure disorders and are already on anticonvulsant medication. The seizures in these children often are due to inadequate anticonvulsant drug levels in the blood. It is important to ask whether this is a typical seizure for this patient (or does the child need further evaluation), how often the seizures usually occur (if at all), and whether he or she is taking the anticonvulsant medication. Often the patient has not been given the medication, has run out of medication, or is vomiting the medication. Management involves checking serum drug levels and loading the patient intravenously or orally. Follow-up care should be arranged with the patient's usual provider.

■ COMA

The child in coma or with an otherwise decreased level of consciousness is a common and perplexing problem for

TABLE 20-13. Drugs Used in Treating Status Epilepticus

Drug	Dose and Route	Side Effects	Comments
Lorazepam*	0.05–0.1 mg/min, IV, max 1 mL/min	Respiratory depression (unusual)	May have longer onset and longer duration than diazepam.
Diazepam†	0.2–0.5 mg/kg, IV, slow push (1 mg/kg), max 10 mg per injection	Respiratory depression, hypotension, sedation (may be prolonged)	May push larger dose slowly until seizure stops. May repeat as necessary.
Phenobarbital†	10–20 mg/kg, IV, over 5–10 min, max 120–150 mg	Respiratory depression, hypotension, sedation	Monitor serum level.
Phenytoin‡	10–20 mg/kg, IV, over 10–20 min (25 mg/min)	Arrhythmias, cardiovascular collapse, hypotension	Must be on cardiac monitor. No respiratory depression. Never use IM route. Monitor serum level. Must give directly into vein; may crystallize in solution.
Paraldehyde	100–200 mg/kg over 5 min, followed by 20 mg/kg min (10% solution)	Pulmonary edema, metabolic acidosis	Monitor serum level.

*Lorazepam is the drug of choice for child with a known seizure disorder on maintenance doses of anticonvulsant drugs.

†Do not use intravenous diazepam and intravenous phenobarbital together, because of potentiated, cardiorespiratory side effects.

‡Useful as second drug if diazepam or phenobarbital is ineffective.

the emergency physician. Coma is a state of consciousness from which the patient cannot be aroused. Terms to describe other decreased levels of consciousness, such as obtundation and stupor, are confusing, and it is more efficient and exact to describe the particulars of the state of consciousness.

Processes causing coma can be divided into three groups: supratentorial mass lesions that compress or displace brain tissue, subtentorial mass or destructive lesions that directly affect the ascending reticular-activating system (ARAS), and systemic metabolic disorders that diffusely affect the brain. These processes depress the function of both cerebral hemispheres and can produce abnormal functioning of the ARAS in the brain stem, which arouses the cerebral hemispheres. The ARAS extends from the pons up to the diencephalon.

The more common causes of coma are listed in Table 20–14.

Management

Initial Treatment

Many causes of coma are reversible without long-term morbidity if they are properly diagnosed and managed. Certain conditions that are readily treatable can cause rapid deterioration if untreated.

After initial assessment, including blood pressure and temperature, all patients receive full resuscitation, because ultimate prognosis is unknown. One hundred percent oxygen and 2 mL of intravenous 25% dextrose per kg of body weight are administered as substrates for brain metabolism. Naloxone (0.01 to 0.1 mg/kg of body weight) is given intravenously to reverse a possible narcotic overdose, and fluids are begun. The naloxone can be repeated in 2 or 3 minutes.

The patient should be undressed and checked for evidence of trauma, systemic illnesses, drug ingestion, and infection such as meningitis. After a thorough physical examination and a systematic consideration of etiologic factors, therapy is given for specific suspected causes, such as seizures, shock, infection, or increased intracranial pressure.

Assessment and Further Treatment

After initial resuscitation, it is essential to assess the important historic and physical information that may indicate at what level the brain is impaired, to choose the most likely diagnoses, and to act quickly with further informative studies and treatment. Important historic information includes description and rapidity of onset of coma, trauma, drug ingestion, medications, medical history, psychiatric history, and previous symptoms such as headache, vomiting, weakness, and seizures.

The neurologic examination starts with an assessment of level of consciousness. The Glasgow Coma Scale, based on eye opening and best motor and verbal responses, is used to standardize and communicate the level of consciousness (see Table 20–5). A modified scale, the Children's Coma Score, can be used in young children. These scales may predict future outcome.

The pattern and depth of respirations, pupillary reactions, ocular movements, funduscopic examination, and motor response to pain may help localize the level of the brain involved (Table 20–15). Cheyne-Stokes respirations (ie, alternating periods of breathing and apnea), central neurogenic hyperventilation (ie, deep, regular, and rapid respirations), and ataxic breathing (ie, respirations with irregular rate and depth) indicate a decreasing level of arousal, with ataxic breathing signaling an impending respiratory arrest. The size, reactivity, and comparison of the pupils provide information about the level of the lesion and possible lateralization. For example, if one pupil is fixed and dilated, there may be impending herniation of the temporal lobe and compression of the third cranial nerve on the side of the dilated pupil.

TABLE 20-14. Common Causes of Coma in Children

Cause	Circumstances
Trauma	Subdural and epidural hematomas, parenchymal bleeding
Poisoning/ingestions	Alcohol, barbiturates, opiates, aspirin, carbon monoxide, lead
Infectious disorders	Meningitis, encephalitis (*eg*, herpes simplex); severe systemic dysfunctions
Metabolic disorders	Hypoglycemia, diabetic ketoacidosis, uremia, electrolyte disturbances
Circulatory disorders	Shock, hypertensive encephalopathy
Respiratory failure	Airway obstruction, pulmonary disease, sudden infant death syndrome
Other	Tumors, seizures (postictal)

Adapted from Kandt RS, D'Souza BJ, Kaplan RA, et al. Disorders of the central nervous system. In Ehrlich FE, Heldrich SI, Tepas JJ, et al, eds. Pediatric Emergency Medicine. Rockville MD: Aspen Publishers; 1987; and Advanced pediatric life support course. The Johns Hopkins University School of Medicine; 1987.

Intact oculocephalic and oculovestibular reflexes signify an intact brain stem. The oculocephalic reflex (*ie*, doll's eye reflex) is performed only if no possibility of a neck injury exists. When the head is turned in one direction, the eyes should move in the other direction before returning to mid position. If there is brain stem damage, the eyes turn with the head, as on a doll.

The oculovestibular reflex (*ie*, "cold water calorics") is performed after an ear examination ensures that the tympanic membranes are intact. The head is elevated 30 degrees, and cold water is introduced into one ear canal. If the brain stem is intact, the eyes should have slow movement or tonic deviation toward the ear with the cold water. If one or both of these reflexes are preserved, the process causing coma is not in the brain stem but involves both cerebral hemispheres. The motor examination includes assessment of tone, movements, deep tendon reflexes, and gag reflex. In response to pain, the patient may have purposeful movement (*ie*, intact cerebral hemispheres), decorticate posturing (*ie*, hemispheric dysfunction), decerebrate posturing (*ie*, upper brain stem dysfunction), or flaccidity (*ie*, lower brain stem dysfunction). The arms are flexed in decorticate posturing (*ie*, point to the "core") and extended in decerebrate posturing; the legs are extended in both.

At the end of the neurologic examination, any focal findings should be evident. If there are findings such as unequal pupils, increased muscle tone, or brisk reflexes, the process is more likely a primary CNS problem. If there are no focal neurologic signs, equal and reactive pupils, and decreased muscle tone and reflexes, the process is more likely systemic, such as metabolic or toxic encephalopathy. In end-stage disease of either origin, the pupils tend to be bilaterally fixed and dilated.

The laboratory investigation is guided by the most likely diagnoses, ascertained from the medical history and physical examination. A few initial studies are routine for any comatose patient: blood glucose, arterial blood gas, electrolytes, calcium, BUN, ammonia, liver function tests, CBC, urinalysis, toxicology screens of blood and urine, ECG, and a chest radiograph. A CT scan is the best way to detect a structural or mass lesion and is often indicated to determine the cause in a patient in coma or to evaluate the severity of a known process. A lumbar puncture is performed to rule out meningitis or encephalitis, but it is contraindicated if the physician suspects a mass lesion, head trauma, Reye's syndrome, or a bleeding diathesis. If there is any suspicion of increased intracranial pressure, with or without papilledema, a CT scan should precede a lumbar puncture. If meningitis is

TABLE 20-15. Diagnosis of Level of Neurologic Lesion

Level	Pupils	Ocular Movements	Breathing Pattern	Motor Response to Pain
Thalamus	Small, reactive	Intact oculocephalic and oculovestibular reflexes	Cheyne-Stokes respiration	Increased motor tone, decorticate
Midbrain	Midposition or dilated, nonreactive	Depressed oculocephalic and oculovestibular reflexes	Central neurogenic hyperventilation†	Decerebrate
Pons	Pinpoint, nonreactive	Absent*	Central neurogenic hyperventilation; apneustic or cluster breathing	Flaccid
Medulla	Dilated, nonreactive	Absent	Ataxic	Flaccid

Absent brain stem reflexes may also be due to metabolic encephalopathy or drug ingestion.

†Also may be present with acid–base disorders, hypoxia, sepsis.

Adapted from Pascoe DJ, Grossman M, eds. Quick Reference to Pediatric Emergencies. 3rd ed. Philadelphia: JB Lippincott; 1984; and Plum F, Posner JB. The diagnosis of stupor and coma. 3rd ed. Philadelphia: FA Davis; 1980.

TABLE 20-16. Clinical Features of an Anaphylactic Reaction

Cutaneous: pruritus, urticaria, angioedema
Respiratory: bronchospasm, laryngeal edema
Circulatory: hypotension, cardiac arrhythmias
Gastrointestinal: diarrhea, abdominal pain

suspected but a lumbar puncture is contraindicated, empiric treatment should begin immediately. Other studies that may be helpful to determine the cause of coma or to localize the disease process include carboxyhemoglobin level determination, electroencephalogram (EEG), radionuclide brain scan, and cerebral arteriography.

The patient must be continually reassessed and treatment changed as indicated. With careful observation, the physician can gauge the progression of disease and the effectiveness of treatment.

■ ANAPHYLAXIS

Mechanism

Anaphylaxis is an extreme systemic allergic reaction. It is caused by hypersensitivity to a foreign substance and usually occurs within a few hours of oral or parenteral exposure to an antigen. Common causes of anaphylactic reactions include Hymenoptera stings, primarily bees and wasps; drugs, such as penicillins and local anesthetics; foods, such as nuts, seafood, and eggs; iodinated contrast media for radiologic studies; blood products; and hormones, such as insulin.

After exposure to a sensitizing antigen, IgE antibody is formed and binds to tissue mast cells. After a subsequent exposure, the antigen binds to the IgE–mast cell combinations and initiates degranulation of the mast cells, releasing preformed mediators, such as histamine, and subsequently releasing secondary mediators, such as slow-reacting substance of anaphylaxis.

The most common clinical features of anaphylactic reactions are listed in Table 20–16. Urticaria may be localized to the exposed area or be generalized; it is often accompanied by angioedema, swelling of the lower dermis and subcutaneous tissues.

Management

Assessment

The history focuses on the time immediately preceding the reaction in an effort to determine exposure to an antigen.

The physical examination focuses on vital signs; airway, including swelling and bronchospasm; circulation, including heart rate and rhythm; skin changes such as urticaria and angioedema; and CNS changes. If there are clinical signs of respiratory distress, such as voice change or dyspnea, difficulty swallowing, or circulatory collapse, treatment must proceed immediately.

Treatment

Treatment of a generalized reaction depends on the type and severity of the reaction. Treatment begins with support of the airway, circulation, and cardiac rhythm. Subcutaneous or intramuscular administration of epinephrine is the drug of

choice in most systemic reactions. This drug should relieve laryngeal edema and severe bronchospasm and can be repeated every 15 to 20 minutes. Nebulized bronchodilators, such as salbutamol or Alupent, and intravenous aminophylline are helpful for reactive airway disease. If severe airway obstruction cannot be relieved, intubation or tracheotomy may be necessary.

Anaphylaxis may include a rapid decrease in plasma volume, requiring intravenous fluid boluses for support of blood pressure. Crystalloid infusion such as lactated Ringer's solution or normal saline can be given in 20 mL/kg of body weight boluses and repeated as often as necessary. If the patient remains hypotensive, the Trendelenburg's position and an epinephrine infusion may be used.

Generalized cutaneous reactions, such as urticaria or angioedema, may be treated with intravenous, intramuscular, or oral diphenhydramine. The benefits of steroid therapy are controversial. In patients with persistent allergic urticaria, intravenous cimetidine may be of benefit.

(Abridged from Paula J. Schweich, Emergency Medicine Except Poisoning, in Oski, DeAngelis, Feigin, McMillan, Warshaw: *Principles and Practice of Pediatrics, Second Edition*, J.B. Lippincott, 1994.)

Oski's Essential Pediatrics, edited by Kevin B. Johnson and Frank A. Oski. Lippincott–Raven Publishers, Philadelphia © 1997

21

Acetaminophen Overdose

Acetaminophen is widely available. Children younger than 6 years of age and adolescents are the two groups most often associated with acetaminophen overdoses. Overdose most commonly affects children younger than 6 years of age; it is usually accidental. The amount of acetaminophen consumed by this group of patients is less than that ingested by adolescents. In the adolescent group, the overdose is either a suicide attempt or a manipulative episode. Handfuls of tablets typically are consumed.

■ PHARMACOLOGY

Acetaminophen is absorbed rapidly after an oral therapeutic dose, producing a peak plasma level between 30 and 60 minutes after ingestion. This absorption may be delayed in overdose so that peak plasma levels may not occur until 4 hours after ingestion. Approximately 94% of the drug is metabolized to the glucuronide or sulfate conjugate. Most of the remainder is metabolized through the cytochrome P-450 mixed-function oxidase system. With a significant overdose, the P-450 mixed-function oxidase becomes the major system for metabolizing acetaminophen. When the liver glutathione stores are sufficiently depleted—usually to about 70% of normal—the highly reactive intermediate metabolite binds to hepatic macromolecules and produces hepatocellular necrosis.

Clinical experience suggests that, if an adult consumes more than 7.5 g of acetaminophen as a single dose or if a child ingests 150 mg/kg of body weight, hepatotoxicity may result. Plasma acetaminophen levels are not interpretable until at least 4 hours after ingestion. The overall mortality of unselected patients with untreated acetaminophen poisoning is 1% to 2%.

■ CLINICAL COURSE

The clinical course of acetaminophen toxicity has four stages. In the first stage (ie, first 24 hours), adult and adolescent patients develop nausea, vomiting, diaphoresis, and general malaise. Children younger than 6 years of age show little diaphoresis and vomit earlier. They develop vomiting regardless of the acetaminophen level and have no symptoms unless the blood level is in the toxic range. Symptoms develop within 14 hours in patients with toxic

levels of acetaminophen. Liver enzymes are normal during this period. Lethargy is rarely seen during this stage. If lethargy develops, some other agent should be considered in addition to or instead of the acetaminophen.

During the second stage (ie, second 24 hours), most patients begin to feel better. If no treatment was received or treatment was unsuccessful, the serum glutamic-oxaloacetic transaminase (SGOT), serum glutamic-pyruvic transaminase (SGPT), bilirubin level, and prothrombin time begin to become abnormal.

During the third stage, from 48 to 96 hours after ingestion, peak abnormalities occur. SGOT levels higher than 20,000 IU/L may be seen in patients with severe acetaminophen overdoses. Examination of the liver at this point demonstrates centrilobular necrosis.

In the final stage, 7 to 8 days after ingestion, hepatic abnormalities should be at or near resolution. Renal abnormalities may be seen in acetaminophen overdose, but it is rare for a renal defect to occur without concomitant hepatic

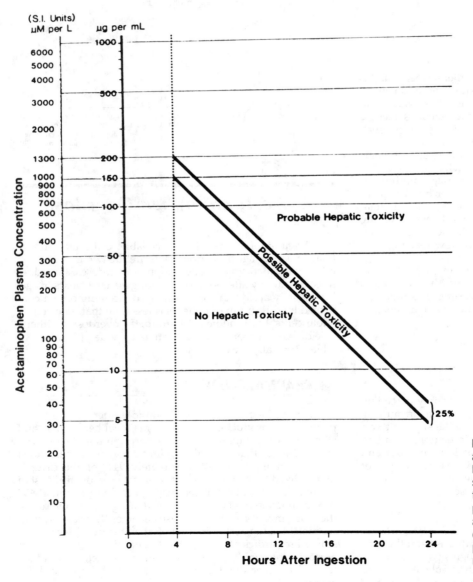

Figure 21-1. Semilogarithmic plot of plasma acetaminophen levels over time. Levels drawn less than 4 hours after ingestion may not represent peak levels. The lower solid line 25% below the standard nomogram is included to allow for possible errors in acetaminophen plasma assays and estimated time from ingestion of an overdose. (Rumack BH, Matthew H. Acetaminophen poisoning and toxicity. *Pediatrics*. 1975;55:871; reproduced with permission.)

damage. Follow-up evaluation of patients who had experienced significant hepatotoxicity reveals no sequelae clinically or on hepatic biopsy.

■ TREATMENT

Treatment consists of an initial evaluation to determine respiratory and cardiovascular status. For adolescents, the history should be interpreted with caution, because studies have shown it is impossible to differentiate potentially toxic from nontoxic overdoses based on patient history. Plasma levels should be tested no sooner than 4 hours after ingestion. A significant change in sensorium necessitates investigation into ingestions of other substances.

If the ingestion has occurred within 1 to 2 hours, initial therapy is directed at gastric emptying. Activated charcoal effectively absorbs acetaminophen if administered early. Acetaminophen ingestion is frequently associated with polypharmacy overdose, and activated charcoal may absorb these other medications. However, use of charcoal remains controversial, because in vitro studies demonstrate that charcoal binds N-acetylcysteine. Clinical studies show only variable and questionable interference by charcoal. Activated charcoal may be given in a single dose if indicated. Before using N-acetylcysteine, the charcoal is removed by nasogastric suction, or the initial dose of N-acetylcysteine is increased by 30% to 40%. The indications for the immediate use of N-acetylcysteine include a plasma level above the toxic line on the acetaminophen nomogram (Figure 21–1) or known ingestion of more than 7.5 g (150 mg/kg). N-acetylcysteine given within 8 hours of ingestion is protective, regardless of the initial plasma acetaminophen concentration. There is no further protective effect if N-acetylcysteine is given within the first 4 hours after ingestion. A dose of N-acetylcysteine should be administered if a plasma acetaminophen level cannot be obtained within 16 hours after ingestion, and N-acetylcysteine should be administered as late as 24 hours after ingestion.

In the patient with an unknown amount of acetaminophen ingestion (<7.5 g or <150 mg/kg), the plasma level is determined not earlier than 4 hours after ingestion, and the potential for toxicity is determined by the nomogram (see Figure 21–1).

Acetylcysteine is administered orally. If activated charcoal has been used, the stomach should be emptied before administration of oral acetylcysteine, because activated charcoal binds it. Baseline data should include SGOT, SGPT, bilirubin level, prothrombin time, and creatinine level. Another set of data should be drawn in at most 24-hour intervals after ingestion. Abnormalities become apparent 36 to 48 hours after ingestion, with the peak usually at 72 to 96 hours.

Although children younger than 6 years of age are unlikely to experience toxic effects, the recommendation is that any patient with a plasma acetaminophen level in the toxic range should be treated. A child accidentally consuming small amounts of children's acetaminophen can be managed safely at home if follow-up care is ensured.

(Abridged from M. Michele Mariscalco, Acetaminophen Overdose, in Oski, DeAngelis, Feigin, McMillan, Warshaw: *Principles and Practice of Pediatrics, Second Edition,* J.B. Lippincott, 1994.)

Oski's Essential Pediatrics,
edited by Kevin B. Johnson and Frank A. Oski.
Lippincott–Raven Publishers,
Philadelphia © 1997

22

Poisoning

■ GENERAL PRINCIPLES

About 100 children younger than 5 years of age die from poisoning annually in the United States. Accidental intoxication in young children is usually caused by ingestion of a single product, but multiple drugs often are ingested by the suicidal older child or adolescent.

■ DIAGNOSIS

The diagnosis of poisoning may not be obvious. The diagnosis is often not considered because of purposeful falsification by an older patient or because the young or confused patient is unable to provide an adequate history. Poisoning should be considered particularly in children younger than 5 years of age who have acutely developed disturbed consciousness, abnormal behavior, seizures, coma, respiratory distress, shock, arrhythmias, metabolic acidosis, severe vomiting and diarrhea, or other puzzling multisystem disorders. Underlying drug or ethanol intoxication should be considered in adolescent and adult victims of accidental trauma.

During stabilization, information should be obtained from family members, friends, or paramedics who have transported the patient to the hospital about the possible agent, the mode of intoxication, the maximum potential dose, and the time since exposure. If poisoning is suspected but the history is not confirmatory, information regarding the different drugs in the home should be obtained by inquiring about illnesses of the patient and other family members.

The physical examination may be particularly helpful in the case of a questionable exposure to a toxic agent. Specific physical findings may suggest a diagnosis (Table 22–1). However, most children who arrive in the emergency department with a diagnosis of poisoning are asymptomatic.

Routine laboratory tests may play an important role in the diagnosis and management of the poisoned patient. Decreased hemoglobin saturation with a normal or increased PaO_2 is found in patients with carbon monoxide poisoning or in methemoglobinemia. An increased anion gap metabolic acidosis suggests metabolites of methanol, ethylene glycol, paraldehyde, and toluene. An elevated measured serum osmolarity compared with a calculated osmolarity indicates the presence of small-molecular-weight and osmotically active compounds such as methanol, ethanol, isopropyl alcohol, mannitol, and ethylene glycol. Hypoglycemia may affect patients intoxicated by ethanol, methanol, isopropyl alcohol, isoniazid, acetaminophen, salicylates, and oral hypoglycemic agents.

Toxicology testing may be helpful in confirming the clinical diagnosis of drug intoxication. Because drug screens vary among institutions, it is important for the physician to know exactly which drugs can be detected. Toxicology screening tests generally detect a wide range of narcotics, analgesics, barbiturates, antidepressants, tranquilizers, sedative-hypnotics, and various other drugs and abused substances. Ethylene glycol, lithium, iron, cyanide, lead, and other heavy metals are agents usually not included in drug screening tests.

■ TREATMENT

The three goals of treatment are preventing further drug absorption, providing antidotal therapy, and hastening the elimination of an absorbed poison.

Basic Life Support

Attention to basic life support and emergency cardiorespiratory support must precede any diagnostic studies in the poisoned child. An adequate airway is the first priority. It can be accomplished by jaw-thrust or chin-lift maneuvers or the placement of an oral or nasopharyngeal airway or an endotracheal tube. Only endotracheal intubation protects the airway of a comatose patient lacking a gag reflex from the hazards of aspiration.

Hypotension in the poisoned child usually is associated with hypovolemia from excessive volume losses or secondary to vasodilation or capillary leak with third-space losses. Intravenous access and fluid resuscitation are important parts of the initial management of any symptomatic child.

Control of convulsions is a common problem. Seizures can result from direct toxicity or indirectly from hypoxia, hypoglycemia, and electrolyte disturbances. Anticonvulsant drugs may be ineffective. The most useful drugs are diazepam, lorazepam, phenobarbital, and paraldehyde.

Hyperthermia should be treated with cooling blankets or fans rather than antipyretic drugs. Hypothermia is treated or prevented with warming devices. Coagulopathies may occur, and blood or factor replacement therapy may be indicated.

Gastrointestinal Decontamination

Traditional principles of gastrointestinal decontamination have undergone scrutiny in recent years. Dilution was previously recommended as an initial step in management of ingestions. Several studies demonstrated that dilution actually enhances absorption of ingested toxins, and therefore it should not be employed. Standard approaches to management have included gastric emptying by emesis or gastric lavage. Evidence suggests that these techniques may not significantly improve toxin retrieval when used in the emergency room and, in the case of ipecac, may delay the effective use of more beneficial agents such as activated charcoal and N-acetylcysteine.

Ipecac may effectively remove some toxins if given within 30 minutes after an ingestion, making it valuable for home use. However, its benefits after 30 minutes in the emergency room are uncertain. Ipecac induces emesis within 30 minutes in more than 90% of children, although the contents returned may harbor minimal toxin. Absolute contraindications to the use of ipecac include the ingestion of caustic acids or alkalis, altered neurologic status or seizures, loss of airway protective reflexes, or hydrocarbon ingestions, unless the ingested distillate contains dangerous additives such as heavy metals or organophosphates.

Gastric lavage may be more effective than ipecac for removing toxins if gastric emptying is to be employed. Lavage is particularly beneficial within the first hour after ingestion and with drugs that delay gastric emptying, such as narcotics or tricyclic antidepressants. Lavage is contraindicated in alkali ingestions because of the increased risk for esophageal perforation. It should be employed cautiously in patients at risk for developing mental status changes, and endotracheal intubation should be performed first to protect the child with absent or compromised airway reflexes.

Activated charcoal effectively minimizes gastrointestinal absorption of toxins by adsorbing them onto its large sur-

TABLE 22-1. Toxidromes: Prominent Clinical Findings as an Aid to Diagnosis of the Unknown Ingestion

Drug Involved	Clinical Manifestations
Anticholinergics (atropine, scopolamine, tricyclic antidepressants, phenothiazines, antihistamines, mushrooms)	Agitation, hallucinations, coma, extrapyramidal movements, mydriasis, dry mouth, tachycardia, arrhythmias, hypotension, decreased bowel sounds, urinary retention, flushed, warm, dry skin
Cholinergics (organophosphates and carbamate insecticides)	Salivation, lacrimation, urination, defecation, nausea and vomiting, sweating, meiosis, bronchorrhea, rales and wheezes, weakness, paralysis, confusion and coma, muscle fasciculations
Opiates	Slow respirations, bradycardia, hypotension, hypothermia, coma, meiosis, pulmonary edema, seizures
Sedatives and hypnotics	Coma, hypothermia, central nervous system depression, slow respirations, hypotension, tachycardia
Tricyclic antidepressants	Coma, convulsions, arrhythmias, anticholinergic manifestations
Salicylates	Vomiting, hyperpnea, fever, lethargy, coma
Phenothiazines	Hypotension, tachycardia, torsion of head and neck, oculogyric crisis, trismus, ataxia, anticholinergic manifestations
Sympathomimetics (amphetamines, phenylpropranolamine, ephedrine, caffeine, cocaine, aminophylline)	Tachycardia, arrhythmias, psychosis, hallucinations, delirium, nausea, vomiting, abdominal pain, piloerection
Alcohols, glycols (methanol, ethylene glycol; also salicylates, paraldehyde, toluene)	Elevated anion gap, metabolic acidosis

Mofenson NC, Greensher J. The unknown poison. Pediatrics. 1974;54:337; reproduced by permission.

TABLE 22-2. Systemic Antidotes and Treatment Agents for Common Ingestions

Ingested Chemical	Antidote or Treatment
Acetaminophen	N-acetylcysteine (Mucomyst)
Benzodiazepines	Flumazenil
Carbon monoxide	Hyperbaric oxygen
Cyanide	Sodium nitrite or sodium thiosulfate
Digoxin	Digibind (antidigoxin antibody)
Iron	Deferoxamine
Isoniazid	Pyridoxine
Methanol or ethylene glycol	Ethanol
Methemoglobinemic agents	Methylene blue
Opiates	Naloxone
Organophosphates	Atropine, pralidoxime
Phenothiazines	Diphenhydramine
Warfarin	Vitamin K

are associated findings. In severe intoxications, shock and encephalopathy may ensue in this early stage. In the second phase, a deceptively stable period of ameliorated symptoms and subtle physical findings may follow for 6 to 72 hours. Some patients, however, advance to a third phase with return of gastrointestinal symptoms, metabolic acidosis, coagulopathy and overt shock, and liver dysfunction, rarely progressing to hepatic necrosis. Survivors may develop a fourth phase of gastrointestinal scarring and acute obstruction 4 to 6 weeks after ingestion.

Prediction of potential iron toxicity determines treatment. Serum iron levels should be obtained 2 to 4 hours after ingestion; after 6 hours, the liver has cleared most free iron and levels may be misleading. Empiric deferoxamine challenge with 40 mg/kg (maximum dose 1 g) administered intramuscularly can be used to demonstrate excess circulating free iron, which is chelated and excreted in the urine with a classic pink-orange "vin rose" color. Significant symptoms should encourage aggressive treatment, and abdominal radiographs should be obtained to look for tablet concretions.

Therapy for iron ingestion includes gastric lavage to remove fragments. The use of sodium bicarbonate in the lavage fluid may precipitate iron as insoluble ferrous bicarbonate and decrease absorption. Deferoxamine, an avid iron chelator, should be initiated in all cases of moderate or severe iron poisoning.

(Abridged from J.D. Fortenberry and M. Michele Mariscalco, Poisoning, in Oski, DeAngelis, Feigin, McMillan, Warshaw: *Principles and Practice of Pediatrics, Second Edition*, J.B. Lippincott, 1994.)

face area. The use of activated charcoal has risen significantly as studies have demonstrated that activated charcoal produces better toxin recovery and fewer complications than emesis or gastric lavage techniques. It should be considered as the primary means of gastrointestinal decontamination in most ingestions, with the exception of a few compounds in which its use is not effective or recommended. Nasogastric tube administration should be performed without delay if a child refuses oral intake.

■ MANAGEMENT OF SPECIFIC TOXINS

Although the preceding principles may be applied to most ingestions, an effective pharmacologic antagonist or chelating agent is available for fewer than 5% of poisonings (Table 22–2). These antidotes should be used in consultation with a local poison control center or person trained in the management of poisoning. The physician should be aware that many ingestions are nontoxic and do not require intervention.

Iron Ingestion

Iron ingestion is the most frequent cause of pediatric ingestion fatalities, accounting for 30.2% of deaths in the past 8 years reported by the American Association of Poison Control Centers. Overdoses in young children usually occur as accidental ingestions rather than intentional overdoses.

Ingested iron produces increased capillary permeability, intravascular permeability, and vasodilation on overwhelming the intestinal barrier and entering the circulation. When available free iron exceeds circulating transferrin-binding levels, toxicity of the liver and other parenchymal organs ensues. Iron intoxication usually follows four characteristic stages. The initial phase, occurring shortly after ingestion, is produced by direct effects on gastric and ileal mucosa to induce abdominal pain and vomiting. Gastrointestinal hemorrhage may occur. Fever, leukocytosis, and hyperglycemia

Oski's Essential Pediatrics, edited by Kevin B. Johnson and Frank A. Oski. Lippincott–Raven Publishers, Philadelphia © 1997

23

Oral Rehydration Therapy

Dehydration resulting from acute gastroenteritis (AGE) is the leading cause of child morbidity and mortality in the world. In the developing nations, an estimated 4 million children die annually from dehydration. In the United States, dehydration still accounts for 300 to 500 deaths per year. Although most diarrheal episodes among children in the United States are mild, the resulting physicians' visits produce substantial health care costs. In developing countries, where children are expected to have 7 to 10 episodes of AGE annually, and where significant malnutrition exists, the impact is still greater.

Oral rehydration therapy (ORT) is a powerful, simple, and inexpensive approach that is credited with saving about a million lives annually. Paradoxically, ORT is used least in the industrialized countries where much of the original basic scientific research was done. Like any therapy, ORT relies on appropriate teaching and implementation for its ultimate effectiveness. In the balance of this chapter, we will describe the pathophysiology of AGE, the mechanisms of action of ORT, and practical aspects of delivery of ORT, particularly in an industrialized world setting.

■ ORAL REHYDRATION SOLUTIONS

Limitations

Although ORT provides simple, safe, and effective therapy for the majority of children with dehydration, certain limitations exist. Physiologically, as indicated in the preceding section, oral rehydration solutions (ORS) are limited in the quantities of solute they can contain without becoming hyperosmolar and exacerbating fluid losses. Glucose-based ORS, therefore, provide good rehydration but have no effect by themselves on stool output or duration of illness. Solutions that contain complex carbohydrate molecules (see below) may overcome this barrier and provide sufficient substrate to reverse fluid losses and decrease diarrhea.

A small proportion (about 1%) of children with AGE experience carbohydrate malabsorption, heralded by a dramatic increase in stool volume with reducing substances present when ORS is given. Substances present in stool after ORS administration. In infants with carbohydrate malabsorption, if ORS is discontinued and parenteral fluids are provided, a dramatic reduction in stool output occurs.

Vomiting is often (and inaccurately) cited as a contraindication to ORT. Most children with vomiting can be successfully rehydrated if fluids are provided in small, frequent quantities. We recommend use of a 5-mL syringe or teaspoon. As tissue acidosis is corrected, vomiting generally ceases, although an occasional child may benefit from a few hours of parenteral fluids.

■ DIETARY CONSIDERATIONS

Enteral feeding, rather than fasting, during AGE has been shown to increase cell renewal in the gut and to diminish intestinal permeability. In addition, the calories provided during feeding have been shown, in a careful balance study by Brown, to contribute to improved nutritional parameters among children who were fed during diarrhea. The role of soy-based, rather than lactose-containing formulas in the setting of AGE remains controversial.

Breast-Feeding During Diarrhea

Human breast milk contains more lactose than cow's milk or milk-based formulas, and breast-feeding has, in the past, been discouraged during diarrhea. Khin-Maung-U performed a controlled trial in hospitalized children and demonstrated reduced stool output among children who received continued breast-milk feedings compared with those whose feedings were interrupted.

■ DELIVERY OF ORAL REHYDRATION THERAPY

Clinical Assessment and Management

Patients presenting for therapy of AGE should initially be examined in light of their relevant history. In patients with abdominal pain, distention, and vomiting, acute abdominal processes such as appendicitis, volvulus, and intussusception should be clinically excluded. The physical examination should be directed at the assessment of dehydration. Table 23–1 shows the accepted system for such assessment. In children and infants with uncomplicated acute watery diarrhea, we discourage the routine use of laboratory diagnostic studies. Urine specific gravity, however, may provide a useful parameter for monitoring the progress of rehydration therapy.

The management of the dehydrated child is divided into two phases: rehydration and maintenance (see Table 23–1). Replacement of ongoing losses as well as maintenance fluids must also be provided throughout the treatment period.

Rehydration Phase

In this phase, the total fluid deficit is intended to be replaced over a 4-hour period. This rapid restoration of circulating volume reverses systemic acidosis and improves tissue perfusion more successfully than the relatively slow repletion over 24 hours that has traditionally been recommended.

Children with mild or moderate dehydration should be given 60 to 80 mL/kg, respectively, over 4 hours. Patients with severe dehydration (frank or impending shock) should receive

---

TABLE 23-1. Fluid Therapy Chart

Degree of Dehydration	Signs*	Rehydration Phase† (First 4 hours, repeat until no signs of dehydration remain)	Maintenance Phase (Until illness resolves)
Mild	Slightly dry mucous membranes, increased thirst	ORS 50–60 mL/kg	Breast-feeding, undiluted lactose-free formula, ½ strength cow's milk or lactose-containing formula
Moderate	Sunken eyes, sunken fontanelle, loss of skin turgor, dry mucous membranes	ORS 80–100 mL/kg	Same as above
Severe	Signs of moderate dehydration plus one or more of the following: rapid thready pulse, cyanosis, rapid breathing, delayed capillary refill, lethargy, coma	IV or IO isotonic fluids (0.9% saline or Ringer's lactate), 40 mL/kg/h until pulse and state of consciousness return to normal, then 50–100 mL/kg of ORS based on remaining degree of dehydration‡	Same as above

*If no signs of dehydration are present, rehydration phase may be omitted. Proceed with maintenance therapy and replacement of ongoing losses.
†Replace ongoing stool losses and vomitus with ORS. 10 mL/kg for each diarrheal stool and 5 mL/kg for each episode of vomitus.
‡While parenteral access is being sought, nasogastric infusion of ORS may be begun at 30 cc/kg/h, provided airway protective reflexes remain intact.

an initial bolus of normal saline or Ringer's lactate by the intravenous or intraosseous routes at 40 mL/kg/h, until signs of shock resolve. While parenteral access is being sought, nasogastric infusion of fluid using a small (5–7 Fr) soft catheter may be initiated at a rate of 30 mL/kg/h, providing that the patient's airway protective reflexes remain intact.

At the end of each hour of rehydration, ongoing losses should be calculated and that volume added to the fluid remaining to be given. Alternatively, parents may be instructed to provide 10 mL/kg or about 4 oz of ORS for each diarrheal stool.

When the 4-hour rehydration phase is complete, clinical assessment should be repeated. If signs of dehydration persist, the rehydration phase should be repeated until fluid repletion has occurred. When rehydration is complete, the maintenance phase is begun (see Table 23–1).

Maintenance Phase

The goal during this phase is to provide fluids for replacement of ongoing losses, as well as to meet requirements for maintenance fluids to meet baseline metabolic needs. Maintenance fluid replacements should be met with breast milk on demand in breast-fed infants. Formula-fed infants should receive approximately 150 mL/kg/day of lactose-free formula where available.

Ongoing stool losses should be replaced with ORS on a 1:1 basis. In hospitals and clinics, this can be accomplished using diaper weights. At home, 10 mL/kg or 4 oz of ORS should be given for each watery stool. Parents should be instructed about the gastrocolic reflex that often results in a bowel movement immediately after a feeding and may result in poor compliance with ORT at home. Parents should be reassured that the fluid given by mouth is absorbed and is likely to exceed in quantity the amount lost in stool.

Because of their high osmotic load and low sodium content, fluids such as full-strength juices, punches, and soft drinks should *not* be recommended during AGE.

The Older Child

Toddlers and school-age children may be offered Saltine crackers and half-strength apple juice, which provides a solution of acceptable osmolality and some sodium in a safe fashion. These children should not be given soft drinks, teas, or full-strength fruit juices. Because the nutrition provided by this regimen is inadequate, children with AGE should return to a regular diet as soon as their diarrhea begins to resolve.

Feeding the Vomiting Child

Infants and children with AGE often vomit. Vomiting is exacerbated by systemic acidosis, hypokalemia, and gastric distention. Antiemetic medications may have significant adverse effects and may mask serious underlying processes, and their use is contraindicated in infants and children with diarrhea.

Once the rehydration phase has been completed and vomiting has diminished, children should be started back on regular feedings. When possible, foods high in lactose should be avoided. We have found that prescribing specific foods such as the standard BRAT (banana, rice, applesauce, toast) diet is less acceptable to families than is a careful description of foods high in complex carbohydrates and low in fats and simple sugars. Families then may make sensible choices from a wide variety of foods that are culturally acceptable.

(Abridged from Julius G. Goepp and Mathuram Santosham, Oral Rehydration Therapy, in Oski, DeAngelis, Feigin, McMillan, Warshaw: *Principles and Practice of Pediatrics, Second Edition*, J.B. Lippincott, 1994.)

Oski's Essential Pediatrics,
edited by Kevin B. Johnson and Frank A. Oski.
Lippincott–Raven Publishers,
Philadelphia © 1997

24

Eye Problems

■ CONGENITAL MALFORMATIONS

The most common abnormalities and those requiring attention or screening for associated systemic abnormalities are discussed here. Children with any of these conditions should be referred to an ophthalmologist.

Retinopathy of Prematurity

Retinopathy of prematurity (ROP) is a vasoproliferative retinopathy seen in premature infants exposed to high concentrations of oxygen for prolonged periods. Two phases are seen: an acute proliferative phase and a cicatricial phase in which scarring and tractional retinal detachment occur. More than 90% of patients with acute disease undergo spontaneous regression, and fewer than 10% of eyes develop significant cicatrization.

The most important risk factor in the development of ROP is low birth weight. The disease is rare in infants with a birth weight over 2000 g. Other risk factors are gestational age, duration and concentration of oxygen exposure, shift of the oxygen dissociation curve by transfused adult hemoglobin, sepsis, high light intensity, hypoxia, and hypothermia.

ROP results from incomplete vascularization and sprouting of new vessels from the demarcation line between vascularized and nonvascularized retina. The pathogenetic mechanisms of new vessel formation and the roles of the various agents implicated in ROP have not been fully elucidated; hypoxemia and hyperoxic damage to growing retinal vessels seem to be important factors. Fibrovascular proliferation results in traction on the normal retina, dragging of the macula and disc, and in partial or total retinal detachment in severe cases. In progressive ROP, the iris is involved, and dilated iris vessels can be seen on anterior segment examination.

Newborns at risk for ROP should be examined by an ophthalmologist after discontinuation of oxygen therapy and before hospital discharge. If ROP is discovered, examinations should be repeated frequently; significant changes may occur within days, and surgery may be indicated. If regression is documented, examinations may be done less frequently. The optimal time for examination is 6 to 10 weeks postpartum, when most cases are detected. Long-term complications of regressed ROP include high myopia and angle-closure glaucoma.

Treatment of ROP includes cryotherapy or laser surgery to the avascular retina to arrest progression of the disease. A large multicenter trial has documented the value of this therapy.

■ COMMON EYE PROBLEMS

Obstruction of the Lacrimal System

The majority (61%) of lacrimal drainage obstructions in children are developmental; others are caused by infections (24%), trauma (12%), and dysfunction (3%). Nasolacrimal duct (NLD) obstruction, most commonly caused by a failure of the distal membranous end of the NLD to open, occurs in 1.75% to 6.1% of infants and is bilateral in as many as one third of cases. NLD obstruction may be caused by blockage elsewhere in the lacrimal system or by a lack of some parts of the system, such as the puncti or canaliculi, interfering with the normal drainage of tears. Rarely, lacrimal obstruction is seen as part of the facial clefting syndromes and the Goldenhar syndrome.

Infants with lacrimal obstruction present with a "wet-eyed" appearance, persistent or intermittent tearing, and various degrees of mucopurulent discharge over the medial canthal area and lids. Pressure over the lacrimal sac area expresses whitish material from the lacrimal puncti.

Most obstructions (90%) resolve spontaneously by 18 months of age, and lid hygiene alone is the indicated treatment in most cases. Fingertip or cotton-tip applicator massage over the lacrimal sac area, with massage directed inferiorly while the upper end of the lacrimal system is blocked, may be tried for a short period; this results in increased pressure inside the system, possibly causing the distal membrane to rupture into the nose. Chronic antibiotic therapy should be avoided. Early probing after a short trial of conservative management for 2 to 4 weeks results in early patency of the system and avoids potential infections and continuous cosmetic annoyance. Infants can be probed in the office with topical anesthesia and restraint; older children are probed in the operating room under general anesthesia. Probing is successful in 90% of patients. If it fails, it may be repeated with or without silicone intubation of the lacrimal system; silicone stents are left in place for 3 to 6 months. If probing and silicone intubation fail, a dacryocystorhinostomy is performed. This provides direct drainage of tears from the lacrimal sac into the nose.

Ophthalmia Neonatorum

Conjunctivitis is the most common ocular disease of newborns, occurring in 1.6% to 12% of neonates. The cause and incidence of neonatal conjunctivitis have been altered by the routine use of silver nitrate prophylaxis. This treatment is effective in preventing gonococcal conjunctivitis, but it has no effect on *Chlamydia trachomatis*. The 1980s were marked by a dramatic increase in the prevalence of chlamydial neonatal conjunctivitis due to maternal genital chlamydial disease. The use of 1% tetracycline ointment and of erythromycin ointment, instead of silver nitrate drops, has reduced the incidence of gonococcal and chlamydial ophthalmia neonatorum.

Of 100 neonates with conjunctivitis in one study, 43 were found to have chlamydial disease; rates as high as 73% have been reported. Other causal agents in ophthalmia neonatorum include *Staphylococcus aureus, Haemophilus influenzae, Streptococcus pneumoniae, Escherichia coli, Proteus mirabilis, Klebsiella pneumoniae, Branhamella catarrhalis, Neisseria gonorrhoeae, Pseudomonas aeruginosa, Staphylococcus epidermidis, Streptococcus viridans*, and coxsackievirus A9.

The external appearance of the eye is the same regardless of the causal agent; in addition to swelling of the lids and conjunctiva, there is profuse and sometimes bloody discharge, especially if pseudomembranes are formed. The timing of the infection in relation to birth is helpful, although not diagnostic, in the determination of the causal agent. Chemical and mechanical conjunctivitis occur in the first day of life and are due to birth trauma and manipulation or to silver nitrate prophylaxis itself. Gonococcal conjunctivitis, which is acquired in the birth canal, usually manifests between days 2 and 4. The remaining organisms cause conjunctivitis at various times

after birth. *Pseudomonas* conjunctivitis is particularly aggressive and may be complicated by corneal ulceration and blindness; it is acquired in the hospital and should be suspected in infants on mechanical ventilation with other foci of *Pseudomonas* infection. Treatment consists of frequent instillations of fortified topical aminoglycoside eye drops and systemic aminoglycosides if other foci of infection are present. Gonococcal conjunctivitis and chlamydial conjunctivitis require systemic and topical antibiotic therapy.

An infant suspected of having conjunctivitis should be immediately isolated. If the infant is in the nursery, strict handwashing precautions should be observed. If the mother is found to be free of gonorrhea, the nursery staff should be checked for the disease, which may be transmitted through the hands. Conjunctival scrapings for Gram and Giemsa stains and for a direct immunofluorescent monoclonal antibody stain for *Chlamydia* should be obtained. Aerobic, anaerobic, and chlamydial cultures should all be done. Therapy should be started based on staining, with definitive culture pending. Patients suspected of having chlamydial disease should be given oral erythromycin ethylsuccinate (50 mg/kg/day in four divided doses) for 2 weeks. If erythromycin fails to clear chlamydial conjunctivitis, a 2-week course of oral trimethoprim-sulfmethoxazole and a concurrent 1-week course of topical tetracycline usually succeed.

If gonococcal conjunctivitis is suspected, the infant is admitted to the hospital and started on intravenous aqueous penicillin G potassium and saline lavage of the eyes. Parents and their sexual partners should be treated for chlamydial and gonococcal infection in the usual manner. Gram-negative bacilli indicate treatment with gentamycin sulfate ophthalmic ointment, using one application four times per day for 1 week. If gram-positive cocci or inflammatory cells without organisms are found, erythromycin ophthalmic ointment should be given four times per day for 1 week.

Bacteria may be cultured from the conjunctivae of infants with chlamydial conjunctivitis. The child with recurrent conjunctivitis should be suspected of having nasolacrimal duct obstruction (see p. 105), and patency of the lacrimal system should be tested.

Conjunctivitis

Three major categories of conjunctivitis are recognized: infectious, allergic, and traumatic or chemical. Ocular conditions that should be differentiated from simple conjunctivitis include iritis (ie, inflammation of the iris, a form of anterior uveitis), acute glaucoma, traumatic corneal abrasions, and infectious corneal ulceration. Table 24–1 lists the differentiating features of these various conditions.

In bacterial conjunctivitis, conjunctival hyperemia is marked, and there is a moderate to copious purulent discharge. The patient is usually in pain and feels as if there is a foreign body in the eye. Vision, pupillary reflexes, intraocular pressure, and corneal clarity are all normal. Staphylococcal blepharitis (ie, chronic infection or inflammation at the lid margins) is a common associated finding. Cultures may be obtained, and bilateral antibiotic eye drops or ointment should be started. Ten percent sulfacetamide or erythromycin is a good initial choice; it may be changed later, depending on culture and antimicrobial sensitivity results. Antibiotics may prevent recurrences and shorten the course of the disease somewhat, but bacterial conjunctivitis usually improves within 4 to 5 days, irrespective of treatment.

Viral conjunctivitis may involve a mild purulent discharge, but tearing and lid swelling, with or without preauricular lymphadenopathy, are the prominent features. Pho-

TABLE 24-1. Differential Diagnosis of Conjunctivitis

Finding	Acute Conjunctivitis	Allergy	Iritis	Acute Glaucoma	Corneal Abrasion/Ulcer
Pain	Mild	None	Moderate	Moderate	Severe
Tearing	Mild to moderate	Moderate	Moderate	None	Severe
Discharge	Moderate to copious	Moderate	None	None	Watery/purulent
Incidence	Very common	Very common	Uncommon	Uncommon	Common/uncommon
Vision	Normal	Normal	Mildly decreased	Decreased	Decreased
Injection	Diffuse	Diffuse	Perilimbal	Perilimbal	Diffuse
Cornea	Clear	Clear	Clear	Clear to cloudy	Clear/hazy
Intraocular pressure	Normal	Normal	Normal	Increased	Normal
Pupil size	Normal	Normal	Small	Mid-dilated	Normal
Pupillary reaction	Normal	Normal	Poor	Very poor	Normal
Culture	Causative organism	Normal	Normal	Normal	Normal/causative agent

Modified from DeAngelis C. The eye. In: DeAngelis C, ed. Pediatric primary care. 3rd ed. Boston: Little, Brown; 1984:221.

tophobia and blepharospasm (*ie*, squeezing of the lids, usually in response to light) occur if the cornea is involved. Adenoviruses are common causal agents. Primary herpetic conjunctivitis is not easily recognized unless it is accompanied by herpetic lesions on the lids. Treatment (except for herpes simplex type 1) is nonspecific; mild steroid drops may be given if inflammation and swelling are severe.

The hallmark of allergic conjunctivitis is itching. There is usually a stringy mucoid discharge. Allergic conjunctivitis may be seasonal, associated with hay fever, and the patient frequently has a history of allergic disorders. Mild vasoconstricting, decongestant drops are usually sufficient to improve symptoms in mild cases; mild steroid drops may be necessary in more severe cases. In vernal conjunctivitis, a seasonal, rather severe allergic ocular condition characterized by large palpebral conjunctival papillae and perilimbal infiltrates, 4% cromolyn sodium drops have decreased recurrence rates and shortened the course of the disease if administered frequently and prophylactically.

The classic example of a chemical conjunctivitis is that induced by silver nitrate prophylaxis (*ie*, Crede procedure) in newborns. Any chemical that reaches the ocular surface is potentially toxic; the most serious of the chemical conjunctivitides are those caused by alkali. Many common household detergents are strong alkali that can cause serious ocular injuries. An ophthalmologist should be immediately consulted in case of suspected ocular alkali burns. Until then, topical anesthetic drops should be instilled and the eye copiously irrigated for as long as possible with at least 2 L of normal saline solution or until a litmus paper test reveals a normal *p*H. Any debris or foreign bodies should be washed out of the conjunctival fornices. Because the bulk of the ocular damage occurs within the first few minutes of exposure, irrigation should be done immediately. The ophthalmologist treats the patient for the ocular surface, cornea, and lid problems that follow these potentially severe injuries.

Periorbital and Orbital Cellulitis

Periorbital cellulitis and orbital cellulitis are bacterial infections of the eyelids and orbital area. In preseptal or peri-

orbital cellulitis, the infection remains anterior to the orbital septum, a fibrous structure located in the lids that separates the orbit proper from the subcutaneous lid structures. In orbital cellulitis, the infection involves the orbit proper and may affect all orbital structures, including extraocular muscles, sensory and motor nerves, and the optic nerve. The two types may coexist, and one may lead to the other.

Bacterial organisms may gain access through the lid skin secondary to insect bites, pustules, or trauma; they may gain access through adjacent infected paranasal sinuses, upper respiratory tract, or teeth. *Staphylococcus aureus* is the most common cause of disease acquired through the lids; other causal organisms are *Streptococcus pyogenes*, *Peptostreptococcus*, *Bacteroides*, and others. *H influenzae*, which gains access to the orbit from upper respiratory tract infections, bacteremia, or sinusitis, is a leading cause of periorbital and orbital cellulitis in children. Children younger than 5 years of age are immunologically most susceptible to *H influenzae*, especially to the b serotype. Fungal orbital cellulitis (*ie*, phycomycosis, aspergillosis) is rare, usually occurring only in immunocompromised or ketoacidotic persons; the orbit is involved through extension of the disease from infected paranasal sinuses.

Proptosis and limitation of ocular motility differentiate preseptal from orbital cellulitis. Fever, lid swelling, redness, and hotness occur in orbital and periorbital infections. Computed tomography (CT) is helpful in documenting orbital involvement and delineating orbital and subperiosteal abscesses, and it is used to exclude the diagnosis of rhabdomyosarcoma.

Complications of orbital cellulitis include orbital abscess, subperiosteal abscess, cavernous sinus thrombosis, meningitis, brain abscess, and orbital apex syndrome.

Orbital cellulitis is a medical emergency, and early diagnosis and treatment are imperative. Children with this condition should be admitted, and a complete blood count and cultures of any skin lesion around the eye or nasopharynx, blood, cerebrospinal fluid, and subcutaneous aspirate should be obtained. Urine antigen studies for a variety of bacterial organisms may be helpful. Sinus x-ray films and CT films of the orbits should be obtained. An ophthalmologist should be consulted.

Periorbital cellulitis is treated with intravenous antibiotics until the periorbital induration and redness decrease. Oral antibiotics are then substituted for intravenous therapy for an additional 7 to 10 days. If a skin infection is documented in the etiology of the condition, a penicillinase-resistant penicillin (*eg*, methicillin, cloxacillin) should be administered. With the emergence of β-lactamase-producing strains of *H influenzae*, cephalosporins have become the mainstay of treatment. Cefuroxime (100 to 150 mg/kg/day in three divided doses) is preferred because of its relatively good penetration into the cerebrospinal fluid. For orbital cellulitis, intravenous antibiotics are given for 2 weeks, followed by oral antibiotics in the recovery phase. Surgical drainage of orbital abscesses may be necessary if these abscesses are localized. Surgery is necessary in the rare instance of mucormycosis.

Amblyopia

Amblyopia is loss of vision caused not by an organic ocular or visual pathway lesion but rather by disuse of one eye and predominant use of the other. The mechanism of vision loss is thought to be of central nervous system origin. This is a reversible process in younger children, and a major aim of strabismus treatment is the prevention or reversal of amblyopia in addition to the restoration of good ocular alignment. Amblyopia therapy consists of patching of the better eye to allow stimulation of the central visual centers from the deviated eye. The younger the child, the faster and more dramatic is the response to short periods of occlusion therapy. Longer periods of patching are required in older children. There is some debate about the upper limit of age at which amblyopia is still reversible; it may be around 10 years of age. Continuous patching for several weeks may be needed for children older than 7 or 8 years of age.

Congenital or infantile esotropia is not present at birth but is diagnosed in the first 6 months of life. The angle of ocular deviation is usually large, and there is little refractive error. Associated conditions include overacting inferior oblique muscles and dissociated vertical deviations, which may manifest later in childhood despite the original therapy and apparently good ocular alignment (Figure 24–1). The mainstay of therapy is early surgical intervention and ocular patching for prevention of amblyopia.

Exophoria is an intermittent outward deviation of either eye that may become evident when the affected child is tired or ill. Exophoric patients often squint in the sunlight. Treatment consists of the correction of any error of refraction and close follow-up. There is no associated amblyopia. Surgery is indicated only if fusion breaks down and the deviation exists more than 50% of the time.

■ EMERGENT EYE PROBLEMS

Emergent eye problems are often seen in the emergency room or clinic and require immediate consultation with an ophthalmologist.

Battered Child

The ophthalmologic manifestations of physical child abuse have received much attention in the literature, as have the social and medical manifestations. The spectrum of ocular problems seen in battered children is broad, and findings may be due to delayed complications of acute injuries. Gen-

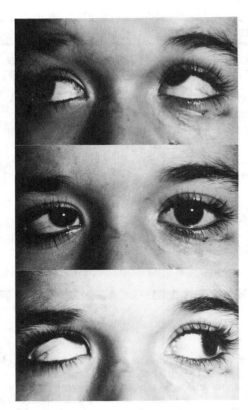

Figure 24-1. Right esotropia with overaction of the inferior oblique muscles. Notice the elevation of the abducted eye (toward the nose) in right and left gazes, indicating overaction of the inferior oblique muscles.

eral physical and social findings in physically abused children are discussed elsewhere. The incidence of ocular involvement in abused children is about 30% to 40%. Most commonly, intraocular hemorrhages are seen in the retina, vitreous, or anterior chamber. Less common findings include periorbital edema and ecchymosis, retinal detachment or dialysis, cataracts, chorioretinal atrophy, subluxated lenses, traumatic mydriasis, papilledema, subconjunctival hemorrhage, esotropia, corneal opacity, and optic atrophy. Bleeding into the optic nerve sheath may be the only finding in shaken babies. A detailed ophthalmologic examination should be part of the routine evaluation of children suspected of being physically abused.

Trauma

Ophthalmologic trauma may be divided into blunt injuries, penetrating injuries, and injuries involving the globe, orbit, adnexae, or any combination of these three. Nonpenetrating injuries to the globe include thermal, ultraviolet, electrical, and chemical burns, corneal abrasions, and contusions.

Contusions to the eyeball may result in subconjunctival hemorrhage, hyphema, iritis, iridodialysis and iris sphincter tears, subluxated lenses that may become cataractous, angle recession with delayed glaucoma, ghost cell glaucoma, vitreous hemorrhage, retinal and choroidal tears, detachment and rupture, and optic nerve injury with edema or avulsion.

Penetrating injuries to the globe may produce corneal lacerations, corneoscleral lacerations, scleral lacerations, or double-penetrating injuries. An intraocular foreign body may be retained. Lid lacerations may involve the lacrimal drainage system and may result in traumatic ptosis. Extraocular muscles may become entrapped in blow-out orbital fractures, leading to restrictive strabismus.

A detailed ophthalmologic examination by an ophthalmologist is mandatory in all cases of periocular and ocular injuries, and all of the described complications are looked for so the appropriate management plan can be instituted. Patients with suspected penetrating ocular injuries should have a protective metallic shield placed over their eyes, and no attempts should be made to open the lids forcefully; especially in the case of a young child, opening of the lids may need to be done with the patient under anesthesia. Tetanus immunization should be given, as in any penetrating injury.

Sports and work-related ocular injuries are receiving increased attention. The use of protective eyewear in athletic activities should be encouraged, especially in one-eyed children and children with compromised ocular function, a predisposition to retinal detachment, or subluxated lenses.

(Abridged from Elias I. Traboulsi and Irene H. Maumenee, Eye Problems, in Oski, DeAngelis, Feigin, McMillan, Warshaw: *Principles and Practice of Pediatrics, Second Edition*, J.B. Lippincott, 1994.)

Oski's Essential Pediatrics, edited by Kevin B. Johnson and Frank A. Oski. Lippincott–Raven Publishers, Philadelphia © 1997

25

Pediatric Dermatology

Skin complaints are common reasons for children to visit physicians. A survey performed in a pediatric clinic setting indicated that 12.8% of primary and 11.2% of secondary concerns prompting clinic visits were related to the skin. Because of the volume of skin-related problems, it is incumbent on physicians who care for children to gain some facility in recognizing and managing the most common cutaneous disorders.

■ SKIN LESIONS IN THE NEONATAL PERIOD

Pigmented Macular Lesions

Mongolian Spots

Mongolian spots is an unfortunate name for this common, benign skin discoloration. Present at birth, mongolian spots are blue-gray or blue-green in color and represent areas of dermal melanocytosis. They occur most frequently in the lumbosacral area (Figure 25–1) and over the shoulders. More than 90% of blacks and Asians have mongolian spots, whereas less than 10% of whites have them.

Macular Vascular Birthmarks

Flame Nevi

Flame nevi are the most common vascular lesions in infancy, seen in almost half of all newborns. These dull pink macules composed of distended dermal capillaries are most prevalent over the eyelids and forehead. Almost all infants with lesions on the face also have lesions on the nape of the neck and on the occiput. Facial lesions tend to fade with time, generally within the first years of life. Neck lesions, however, are likely to persist. The macules often are called salmon patches, stork bites, or angel kisses. During crying, older infants and children may demonstrate flushing in areas of previous lesions that have faded.

Melanocytic Nevi

Histologically proven congenital melanocytic nevi are present in about 1% of newborns, although four times that many have lesions resembling melanocytic nevi (see Color Figure 1). Most of the nevi are small, well defined, and flat. Considerable controversy surrounds their management. Some specialists advocate removing all congenital nevi, regardless of their size, whereas others recommend removing only those greater than 20 cm in diameter. The risk of malignant melanoma developing in a large lesion is estimated to be between 6% and 7% over the child's lifetime.

Papules and Vesicles

Milia

Multiple 1- to 2-mm yellowish-white cystic lesions, known as milia, occur in about 40% of newborns. These lesions are found most commonly over the cheeks, forehead, nose, and nasolabial folds (Figure 25–2). Much less commonly, they may be found on the trunk or extremities. Histologically, the cysts are composed of keratin and are similar to Epstein's pearls, the whitish papules noted on the palates of many newborns. Treatment is unnecessary; the cysts disappear in the first few weeks of life.

Erythema Toxicum

The erythematous macules, papules, and, sometimes, vesicles of erythema toxicum (see Color Figure 2) occur in at least half of full-term newborns; they are less common in premature infants. Generally, the lesions appear between the first 24 and 48 hours of life, and are described best as resembling flea bites. The individual lesions tend to last less than 24 hours, but new lesions can appear during the first 2 weeks of life and, occasionally, later. It may be difficult clinically to separate the lesions of erythema toxicum from those of more ominous conditions, such as staphylococcal pustulosis or herpes simplex. Identification of large patches of macular erythema surrounding the lesions is one way to recognize erythema toxicum; however, a more reliable method is to scrape the lesions and stain the contents with Wright's stain, which will reveal the predominance of eosinophils. A peripheral eosinophilia often is present as well.

Transient Neonatal Pustular Melanosis

Transient neonatal pustular melanosis is a relatively common neonatal dermatosis that was not described until 1976. The lesions, which consist of vesicopustules, ruptured vesicopustules with a collarette of scale, and small pigmented macules in the sites of previous lesions, occur in 4% to 5% of black infants and in less than 1% of white infants. The face, chin, neck, and shoulders are the most commonly affected sites. If vesicopustules are present, they disappear rapidly within 1 to 2 days. In contrast, the pigmented macules may take weeks or even months to fade. The pustules are 1 to 3 mm in diameter, usually are flaccid, and have no surrounding erythema (see Color Figure 3). Most have very

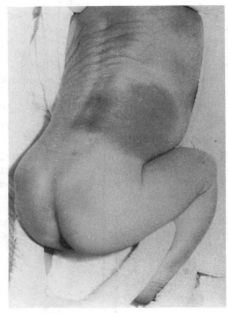

Figure 25-1. The blue-gray hyperpigmentation of mongolian spots is most common over the buttocks and back.

little content on rupturing, including perhaps a few neutrophils. The cause of this disorder is unknown, but it appears to be an entirely benign condition. A simple Gram's stain of the contents of a pustular lesion should prove most helpful in differentiating transient neonatal pustular melanosis from bacterial pustulosis. No therapy is necessary.

Miliaria

Miliaria crystallina are tiny, teardroplike, clear, fragile vesicles caused by plugged sweat ducts. They may appear shortly after birth (particularly on the forehead), have no surrounding erythema, and disappear rapidly without intervention.

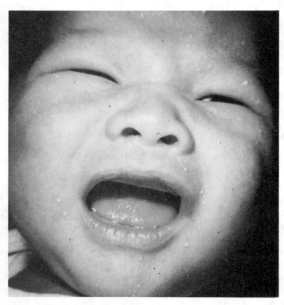

Figure 25-2. Milia on the face of a newborn.

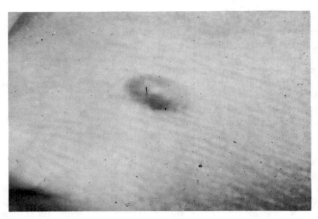

Figure 25-3. A solitary bullous lesion, due to sucking in utero, on the dorsum of a newborn's hand.

Bullous Lesions

Sucking Blisters

Infants commonly suck their hands or fingers in utero. Occasionally, a thick-walled bullous lesion on the dorsum of the hand will result (Figure 25–3) The most helpful clue to this diagnosis is observation of the infant sucking the involved area of skin after birth.

■ PAPULAR DISORDERS

Warts

Warts are among the most common skin lesions affecting children; they also are among the most frustrating, because they often are difficult to treat and control. Warts are caused by infections with human papillomaviruses, DNA viruses of which at least 15 different types have been described. Each type of human papillomavirus usually can be related to a specific clinical presentation of the wart. The highest incidence of these infections occurs in the second decade of life. Untreated warts generally have a lifespan of a few months to 5 years or more. About two thirds disappear within 2 years, but self-inoculation and spread to other persons may occur.

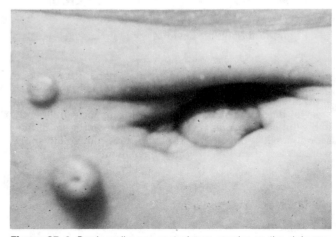

Figure 25-4. Pearly molluscum contagiosum papules on the abdomen. Note the central umbilication of the larger lesion.

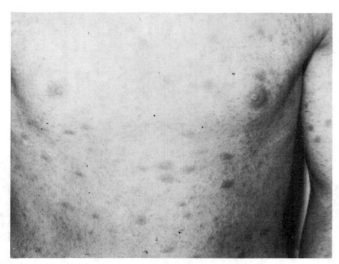

Figure 25-5. Pityriasis rosea. The diffuse erythematous papules may obscure the classic lesions, which are scattered, ovoid, pink plaques.

Molluscum Contagiosum

Lesions of molluscum contagiosum, which are caused by a DNA pox virus, are described best as pearly papules. Their size may vary from that of a pinhead to more than 1 cm in diameter. The top of the lesion is almost translucent, often revealing a whitish core known as the molluscum body. Larger lesions may have a central umbilication (Figure 25–4). The number of papules present may vary from few to hundreds. Spread by autoinoculation is common; other members of the family also can become infected through contact with the affected person.

Although some physicians recommend no treatment, the lesions have a lifespan of months to years, and parents frequently insist that something be done. If there are only a few lesions, they can be picked off or excised with a curet. Cantharidin is a potent medication that, when used by trained personnel, can be effective.

Pityriasis Rosea

Pityriasis rosea is a papulosquamos disorder, consisting of oval lesions composed of tiny papules with a fine scale. At times, individual papular lesions may be prominent. The presence of a myriad of individual papules occasionally confuses the diagnosis by making the ovoid lesions less noticeable (Figure 25–5). The disorder occurs most commonly in teenagers and young adults, but has been described in infants. The herald patch is a single, papular, erythematous lesion that enlarges over 1 to 2 days. It may precede the appearance of the more extensive rash, or it may not appear at all; its reported prevalence has varied in different series from 12% to 94%. At times, this raised lesion may be mistaken for tinea corporis. The interval between the appearance of the herald patch and the more generalized eruption is 1 to 2 weeks.

The typical ovoid lesions of pityriasis rosea have their longest axis along skin tension lines; thus, their distribution on the patient's back gives the appearance of the boughs of a pine tree. It often is helpful to view the child's rash from across the room to see the characteristic pattern. Individual lesions may have a pinkish to brownish color. Most lesions are covered by a fine, wrinkled scale (Figure 25–6).

The lengthy course of this disorder should be emphasized to the patient or the parents. The eruption develops over a 2-week period, persists for 2 weeks, and then fades over another 2 weeks. Treatment with an emollient containing menthol and phenol is helpful. No therapy will shorten the course of the eruption.

Red Papules

Papular Urticaria

Papular urticaria is a common, intensely pruritic disorder caused by hypersensitivity to insect bites. The fresh lesions are papules with an erythematous flare capped by a central punctum at the site of the bite (Figure 25–7). Lesions generally appear in crops, particularly on exposed skin surfaces. Most cases occur in the late spring and summer, but household exposure to fleas from animals can cause problems any time of year. Not all lesions have a central punctum. Linear or irregular clusters may be related to localized

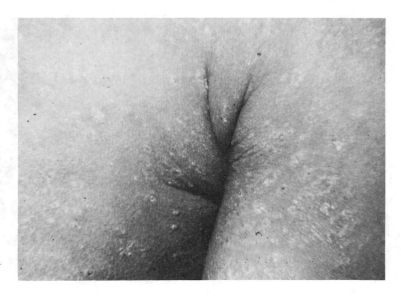

Figure 25-6. The fine scale on the ovoid plaques is characteristic of pityriasis rosea.

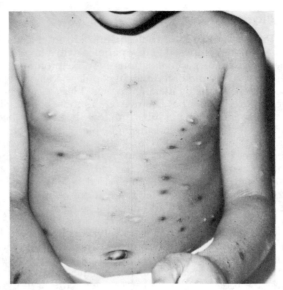

Figure 25-7. Papular urticaria. Old, hyperpigmented lesions and recent, erythematous papules with central puncta from flea bites.

reactions caused by immunoglobulins and complement released into surrounding vessels.

Fleas are the most common cause of papular urticaria. Mosquitoes and other biting insects also may produce the lesions. Secondary infections from excoriations are extremely common and, in some children, the wheals may progress to bullae. Treatment success depends on eliminating the biting insects from the child's environment. Topical antipruritic agents may be of some help. Secondary infections also need to be treated. This severe reaction to the bites lasts 1 to 2 years.

■ NODULAR DISORDERS

Red Nodules

Hemangiomas

Tumors composed of blood vessels come in various shapes, types, and sizes. They occur in 10% of all infants and generally are benign growths with an excellent prognosis. Capillary hemangiomas are tumors composed of a proliferation of endothelium-lined vascular spaces (see Color Figure 4). They generally project above the surface of the skin, are soft, and can be blanched with pressure.

Capillary, commonly referred to as strawberry, hemangiomas rarely are present at birth. Occasionally, a pink or hypopigmented macule may be seen. The lesions grow rapidly during the first 6 months of life, reach a quiescent stage when the patient is 6 to 12 months old, and then begin to regress when the child is between 12 and 18 months old. The individual lesions may be pink, red, or a mixture of the two colors. Ninety-five percent of these lesions will show complete regression by age 12 years.

Cavernous hemangiomas may not show complete regression; these tumors impart a bluish tint to the overlying skin (Figure 25–8). Hemangiomas often are mixed, with superficial capillary and deep cavernous components (see Color Figure 5).

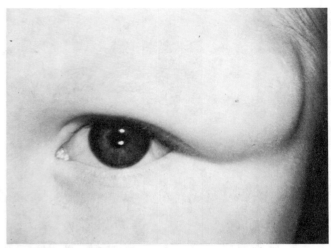

Figure 25-8. A soft, bluish cavernous hemangioma without epidermal involvement.

Pigmented Nodules

Mast Cell Disease

The most common form of mast cell disease in childhood is urticaria pigmentosa. The lesions, which are macular or slightly elevated papules and nodules that occur primarily on the trunk, may number from a few to hundreds and often appear in the first few months of life, although they can occur at any time (Figure 25–9). The most helpful clue to diagnosis is the appearance of an erythematous or urticarial flare after vigorous rubbing of the lesion (Darier's sign). In some cases, systemic symptoms, including diarrhea and gastrointestinal bleeding, may be prominent.

Fortunately, mast cell disease in children generally is benign. The younger the child is when the lesions appear, the more likely it is that they will resolve. Isolated mastocytomas usually are gone by the time the child is 10 years of age, and

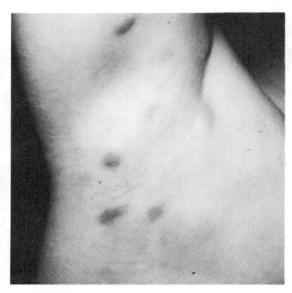

Figure 25-9. Multiple pigmented nodules of urticaria pigmentosa in the axilla. Rubbing causes an erythematous flare and swelling.

half of all cases of urticaria pigmentosa that develop early in childhood are resolved by the late teenage years.

■ VESICULAR AND BULLOUS ERUPTIONS

Disorders With Grouped Vesicles

Herpes Simplex

Whenever a localized group of small vesicles is found anywhere on the skin, the most likely cause is infection with herpesvirus hominis, a DNA virus. Most primary infections are mild and almost inapparent. The vesicles rapidly become pustular, dry, and form crusts, or the tops are removed, leaving erosions or shallow ulcerations. The most common sites of infection are the lips and genital area. In young children, symptomatic primary infections most often involve the oral cavity, where multiple vesicles on the gums and buccal surfaces rapidly erode to form ulcers. The illness is accompanied by high fever, increased salivation, refusal to drink, and swollen, fragile gingiva. When affected children suck their fingers, vesicles may appear there as well (Figure 25–10).

Recurrent herpes simplex infections are very common. The vesicles appear at the sites of previous infections at various time intervals. Often, burning or itching of the area precedes the appearance of the vesicles. The virus appears to remain dormant in the regional nerve ganglion of the affected area until some event—often illness, stress, or sunburn—triggers the clinical infection. Although most lay people recognize the "cold sore" or "fever blister" when it occurs on the lips, many fail to realize that this infection may occur on any surface of the body.

Genital herpes in children always must be viewed with suspicion of possible sexual abuse. Neonatal herpes simplex infections have high rates of morbidity and mortality, and must be recognized and treated immediately (see Color Figure 6). Unfortunately, 60% to 80% of mothers being delivered of infected babies are asymptomatic, with no history of infections. Most of the infants are infected as they pass through the birth canal. If a mother's herpes infection is primary, her infant has a 40% to 50% chance of acquiring a herpes virus infection if delivered vaginally; if the mother's lesion is recurrent, the risk is about 3%. The incubation period of natally acquired herpesvirus infections is 2 days to 3 weeks. Given that almost half of affected infants manifest no skin lesions, the absence of skin lesions does not indicate lack of infection. Neonatal herpes lesions may be localized at the site of trauma, particularly the scalp, where fetal monitors may have been applied (see Color Figure 7); they may be scattered over the skin; or they may be large areas of erosion, simulating epidermolysis bullosa. Whenever a suspicious vesicle appears on a neonate's skin, a Tzanck test should be done to reveal the multinucleated giant cells characteristic of the herpes group of viruses.

The use of acyclovir has led to a significant decrease in the morbidity and mortality associated with herpes simplex virus infections. This drug enters cells, where it is activated selectively by herpes simplex viral thymidine kinase and, in turn, specifically inhibits replication of the virus. The effectiveness of the drug depends on the timeliness of treatment initiation.

Disorders With Generalized Vesicles (Varicella)

Chickenpox is a highly contagious childhood disease caused by the same herpes group DNA virus that is responsible for herpes zoster. Infection usually follows contact with children infected with varicella, but zoster lesions are infectious also. The characteristic lesions occur in crops, with varying types present at the same time. The initial lesion is an erythematous macule/papule that becomes vesicular in a few hours. The vesicles then become pustular and umbilicated, and are covered with a crust in 1 to 2 days. Occasionally, the vesicles may appear teardroplike on an erythematous base. Mucous membrane involvement is common. Lesions initially are scattered on the trunk, face, and scalp, with the extremities becoming involved within a short time.

The incubation period of varicella is 7 to 21 days, with most cases appearing 14 days after exposure. Pruritus often is marked, and fever is common. Generally, the disease is fairly mild, except in adults, immunocompromised children, and neonates. Secondary infections are common. When large, glistening erosive lesions or bullae appear, secondary staphylococcal infection is likely. Complaints of pain in lesions usually indicate a secondary infection. Treatment of uncomplicated varicella is symptomatic. Aspirin should be avoided because of its association with Reye's syndrome. Calamine lotion and cool compresses may reduce the itching and enhance drying of the lesions. In immunocompromised patients, acyclovir may be lifesaving. If the diagnosis is in question, a Tzanck test can be performed to demonstrate multinucleated giant cells. The Tzanck preparation will not differentiate varicella from herpes simplex or herpes zoster, however; all of these show the characteristic cells.

Disorders With Linear Vesicles (Rhus Dermatitis)

Vesicles that occur in lines are characteristic of allergic contact dermatitis, which, in the United States, is caused most commonly by poison ivy or poison oak (Figure 25–11). The eruption is a delayed contact hypersensitivity reaction to a saplike material known as urushiol that is present in the plants. Trauma to the leaves of the plants releases this material, which can be transferred to the skin. The rapidity of reaction to contact depends on the sensitivity of the individual and the amount of toxin deposited on the skin. Pruritic papules and vesicles may appear in a few hours in areas of

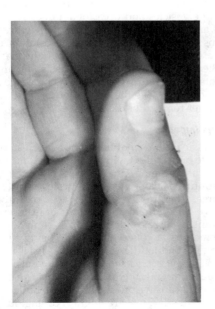

Figure 25-10. Herpes simplex infection always should be considered when grouped vesicles are present.

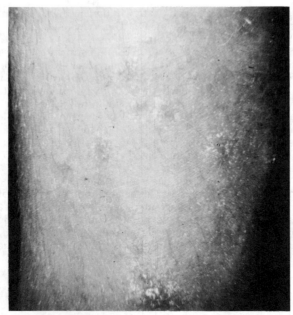

Figure 25-11. Rhus dermatitis caused by poison ivy is characterized by linear papules, vesicles, and bullae.

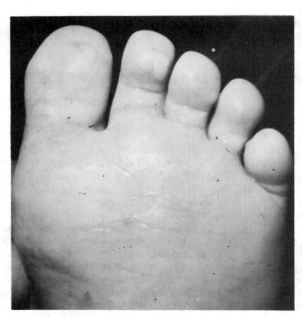

Figure 25-12. In hand-foot-and-mouth disease, vesicles are present on the hands and feet, as well as in the mouth. Note the linear configeration of these vesicles.

heavy contamination, or over a few days on skin areas where contact was minimal. The development of new lesions over a few days' time has fueled the false tale that the vesicular fluid itself spreads the lesions.

Poison ivy most frequently occurs in the summer, but it can occur at any time of year. Dried leaves, stems, and roots may release the toxic material. Burning vines may release particles into the air that affect very sensitive individuals. Scrubbing areas that are known to have come in contact with these plants can prevent the development of lesions if it is done early enough. The urushiols are bound rapidly to the skin on contact, however.

The classic lesions of rhus dermatitis are vesicles arranged in lines, but linear and nonlinear erythematous papules can be found as well. Children's faces may be edematous and erythematous, resembling the manifestations of angioneurotic edema. The arms, legs, and neck should be examined carefully for the presence of linear lesions to establish the diagnosis.

The treatment of rhus dermatitis is symptomatic. Wet compresses and calamine lotion assist in drying the lesions, and antihistamines may help relieve the pruritus. Topical steroids probably are of little benefit in extensive cases. Oral steroids such as prednisone (1 to 2 mg/kg/day) in decreasing doses over a 2-week period are indicated. As in any other pruritic disorder, care must be taken to prevent or, if prevention is not possible, to recognize secondary skin infection.

Other Vesicular Lesions With Typical Distributions

Hand-Foot-and-Mouth Disease

The characteristic feature of hand-foot-and-mouth disease is the distribution of the vesicular eruption, as per the name. This viral exanthem occurs most often in the summer months, often in mini-epidemics. The most frequent site of lesions is the mouth, where the vesicular tops are eroded rapidly, leaving ulcers. The exanthem on the hands and feet is vesicular, but the vesicles often have a curious linear or arcuate shape (Figure 25–12). The rash may appear maculopapular at the outset. Occasionally, the buttocks may be involved. Coxsackievirus A16 is associated most frequently with this disease, with occasional coxsackievirus A5 and A10 infections.

The primary disorder to differentiate from hand-foot-and-mouth syndrome is primary herpes gingivostomatitis. Treatment is symptomatic, and the course of the illness usually is benign.

Scabies

The characteristic feature of scabies is intense pruritus. Early lesions are vesicular before excoriation and lichenification of the skin. The head generally is spared, except in babies. Large vesicles and occasional bullae may appear on the palms and soles of infants and toddlers with scabies. The best means of documenting scabies infestation is to apply immersion oil, scrape the vesicles or papules with a scalpel blade, collect the oil, apply it to a glass slide, and examine the contents under a microscope for the presence of the mite or its eggs or feces. (See the section on pruritic lesions later in this chapter for further discussion.)

Bullous Impetigo

The classic lesions of bullous impetigo, a staphylococcal infection, are bullae filled with cloudy fluid surrounded by a thin margin of erythema. Characteristically, many of the bullae have ruptured, leaving dried-up lesions scattered in contiguous areas (Figure 25–13). The most recently ruptured lesions have an erythematous, shiny base resembling lacquered paint, whereas older ones are completely dry and nonerythematous, a collarette of scale being the only remnant. In infants and toddlers, the diaper area is affected most frequently. *Staphylococcus aureus* is the organism responsible for this infection, with the exfoliative toxin released locally by this bacteria causing production of the bullae.

Because the lesions are highly contagious and may spread cutaneously as well as systemically, parenteral rather than topical antibiotics are required for treatment.

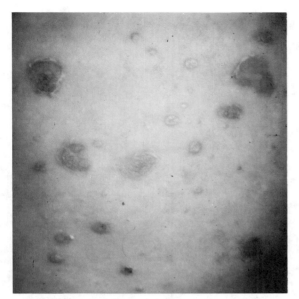

Figure 25-13. Fresh and ruptured bullous lesions of staphylococcal impetigo.

Staphylococcal Scalded Skin Syndrome

Some *Staphylococcus aureus* produce an exfoliative toxin, usually phage group II, type 70 or 71. Infections with these phage-producing strains often may be subtle, but they produce a striking picture befitting the name. The entire skin surface may be erythematous, and bullae may appear in areas of trauma or in areas that are rubbed or simply touched (see Color Figure 8). The separation of skin at sites of trauma is known as Nikolsky's sign. Affected children are in extreme pain. A characteristic feature is crusting in a radial pattern (sunburst) around the mouth, nose, and eyes (Figure 25–14). The mucous membranes are not involved, which may help distinguish this illness from Stevens-Johnson syndrome.

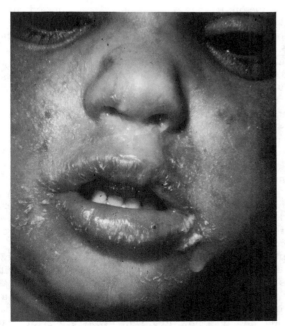

Figure 25-14. The purulent nasal discharge is the likely site of infection in this child with staphylococcal scalded skin syndrome. Note the early perioral scaling.

The skin separation in staphylococcal scalded skin syndrome is intraepidermal rather than deeper, at the epidermal basement membrane, as occurs in toxic epidermal necrolysis (TEN). In the latter disorder, there usually is mucous membrane involvement and no sunburst of crusting around the mouth and eyes. With or without antibiotic treatment, improvement occurs within 3 to 5 days. Antibiotic therapy should be used to prevent recurrences of the problem. Occasionally, dehydration is a major complication because of the loss of cutaneous covering.

■ VESICULOPUSTULAR LESIONS

Impetigo

Bacterial infections of the skin are the most common dermatologic condition for which children are brought to physicians. Superficial infections account for the great majority of these infections, and impetigo is the most common pyoderma. The prevalence of impetigo varies with the season of the year, occurring most often in the warm summer months among individuals with poor hygiene and crowded living conditions. Impetigo previously was divided into two types, each with a typical clinical picture and different bacterial etiology. An increasing number of studies have found that *Staphylococcus aureus* is the primary agent responsible for most impetigo, however, whether the lesion is golden crusted (which type used to be caused by group A β-hemolytic streptococcus) or bullous (which type always has been staphylococcal in origin).

The crusted lesions of impetigo have little surrounding erythema, but local lymphadenopathy is common (Figure 25–15). The lesions tend to spread locally, and scratching, particularly of insect bites, may result in widespread lesions. Family members often are infected as well. Any area of the body may be involved, and any break in the skin (*eg*, abrasions, excoriations, lacerations, burns) may provide access.

When group A β-hemolytic streptococci were the most common bacteria responsible for impetigo, secondary nonsuppurative complications, such as poststreptococcal glomerulonephritis, were common in some areas of the United States and other countries. Acute rheumatic fever, however, never has been reported to follow impetigo.

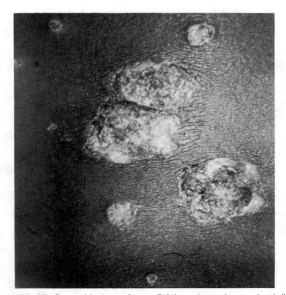

Figure 25-15. Crusted lesions of superficial pyoderma in a perioral distribution.

When impetigo is widespread, systemic therapy usually is indicated. Until reports of a change in the bacterial cause of impetigo appeared, crusted lesions were treated with penicillin and bullous impetigo was treated with an antistaphylococcic antibiotic. The trend at present is to treat all impetigo as if the infection were caused by *S aureus*. Mupirocin, a topical antibiotic cream, may be used effectively when the lesions are not widespread.

Candidiasis

Yeast infections are caused most commonly by *Candida albicans*, a dimorphic fungus that occurs in both budding and mycelial phases. *Candida* thrives in warm, moist places; the diaper area of infants, which can be likened to a tropical rain forest, is an ideal site for proliferation (Figure 25–16). Characteristically, the inguinal creases are involved in candidal infections, which produce a confluent erythema, often with maceration and fissuring. The earliest lesions of *Candida* are small vesicopustules on an erythematous base. The lesions enlarge and tend to become confluent. Their roofs then are lost rapidly, leaving the red base. Other common sites of candidal infection include the axillae, the neck in young infants, and the corners of the mouth.

Infants commonly have "thrush," which appears as adherent, cheesy plaques of candidal infection in the mouth. Infection of the nails and paronychia also may develop in young children who suck their fingers or in individuals who immerse their hands in water for extended periods on a regular basis. Outside the neonatal period, overt candidal infections are uncommon. The presence of *Candida* might suggest the presence of diabetes mellitus, hypoparathyroidism, Addison's disease, an altered immunologic response to infection, acquired immunodeficiency syndrome, or malignancy.

Cutaneous infection with *Candida* usually can be treated effectively with drying and the application of an anticandidal agent, such as nystatin (Mycostatin).

■ SCALING AND DRY LESIONS

Atopic Dermatitis

Atopic dermatitis, a common skin condition better known among lay people as eczema, affects about 4% of the pediatric population. The cause is unknown but seems to be

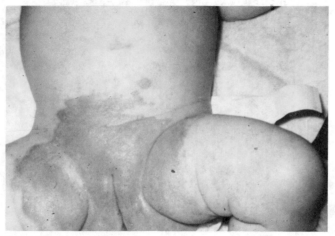

Figure 25-16. Candidal infection is characterized by involvement of the inguinal creases and satellite pustules.

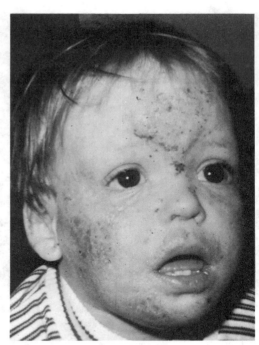

Figure 25-17. Typical morphology and facial distribution of infantile atopic dermatitis.

multifactorial; heredity plays a role, modified by environmental factors. The basic problem seems to be a sensitivity of the skin to numerous stimuli, all of which produce pruritus. An apt description of atopic dermatitis is "an itch that rashes." If the itch can be controlled, the rash usually will not develop.

Atopic dermatitis is rare in infants less than 2 months of age, primarily because the "itch–scratch" mechanism does not mature until around 3 months of age. Onset of the rash occurs before the age of 1 year in 60% of affected children and before the age of 5 years in 85%. The rash of atopic dermatitis most often appears as dry patches, but sometimes it is eczematoid (weeping), particularly on the cheeks and the extensor surfaces of the arms and legs (Figure 25–17). Dry patches may occur on much of the body surface. Lesions may become hyperpigmented, especially in black individuals, from the scratching and rubbing. In toddlers, the rash characteristically appears in the popliteal and antecubital fossae, although other areas are involved as well. In adults, the periorbital and neck areas often are affected. The skin of most patients generally is dry, and the decreased humidity of the environment that is associated with heating in the winter commonly accentuates the problem.

In addition to appearing dry and somewhat scaly, the skin of individuals with atopic dermatitis is thickened or has undergone lichenification (Figure 25–18), and normal skin markings are accentuated (Figure 25–19). Scratching commonly results in secondary infections, particularly with staphylococci. The presence of infection, which may be occult, often leads to accentuation of the pruritus with a resultant flare in the rash.

The major and minor criteria used to diagnose atopic dermatitis are listed in Table 25–1. Because this disorder is chronic and relapsing, treatment involves a great deal of teaching and explaining to the parents and child, as well as prescribing of medications. Given that ichthyosis commonly accompanies atopic dermatitis, other medications may be

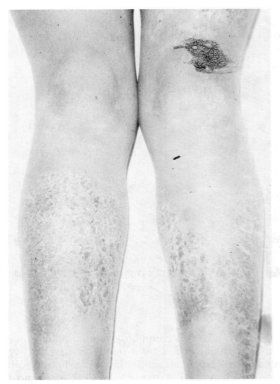

Figure 25-18. Lichenous plaques of atopic dermatitis involving both lower legs.

TABLE 25-1. Diagnostic Criteria for Atopic Dermatitis

I. All of the following
  A. Pruritus
  B. Typical morphology and distribution
    1. Facial and extensor involvement in infants
    2. Flexural lichenification in children
  C. Tendency toward chronic or chronically relapsing dermatitis
  D. II or III below

II. Two or more of the following
  A. Personal or family history of atopic disease (asthma, allergic rhinitis, atopic dermatitis)
  B. Immediate skin test reactivity
  C. White dermographism or delayed blanch to cholinergic agents
  D. Anterior subcapsular cataracts

III. Four or more of the following
  A. Xerosis/ichthyosis/hyperlinear palms
  B. Pityriasis alba
  C. Keratosis pilaris
  D. Facial pallor/infraorbital darkening
  E. Dennie-Morgan infraorbital fold
  F. Elevated serum IgE
  G. Keratoconus
  H. Tendency toward nonspecific hand dermatitis
  I. Tendency toward repeated cutaneous infections

Hanifin JM, Lobitz WC Jr. Newer concepts of atopic dermatitis. Arch Dermatol. 1977;113:63.

necessary to give the skin a relatively normal texture and appearance.

Factors that may precipitate pruritus in atopic skin include soaps; sweating and, conversely, exposure to cool air; certain materials, especially wool and synthetic fibers; and stress. Well-controlled studies have demonstrated food sensitivity in as many as 5% of affected children. The foods most frequently implicated are eggs, milk, wheat, peanuts, soybeans, and chicken. The role of inhalants (pollen, mold, and dust mites) is not clear.

Atopic skin also is prone to viral infections; herpes simplex may spread rapidly and extensively over the entire skin surface, resulting in severe disease and even death (Figure 25–20). Molluscum contagiosum also can be extensive on atopic skin. Interestingly, atopic children are less prone than are normal children to contact dermatitis.

Fifty percent to 80% of children with atopic dermatitis go on to have allergic rhinitis or asthma. Although the skin of the majority of children improves by adulthood, it tends to remain "sensitive," especially to winter dryness and soaps, throughout their lives.

The keys to treatment, in addition to education, are avoidance of precipitants (particularly drying soaps), use of emollients to keep the skin moist, and application of corticosteroids to reduce the inflammation and pruritus. Nonfluorinated steroids should be used to circumvent adrenal suppression and skin atrophy, which may occur with stronger medications. Topical fluorinated steroids should be applied only to the most severely affected areas for the shortest possible time, and they never should be used on the face or perineum. Hydrocortisone may be added to an emollient to produce a 1% concentration. A potent oral antipruritic agent such as hydroxyzine should be prescribed in doses large enough to reduce the pruritus, which results in the

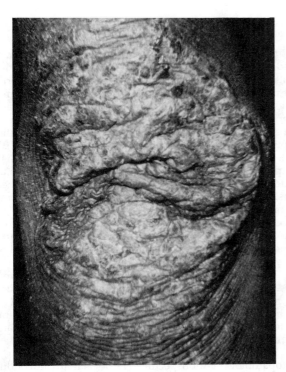

Figure 25-19. Dramatic lichenification from chronic scratching in atopic dermatitis.

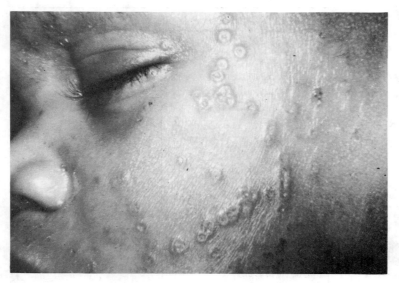

Figure 25-20. Children with atopic dermatitis are susceptible to the development of widespread cutaneous herpes simplex.

"itch–scratch–itch" cycle. A large dose at bedtime will help to reduce scratching during sleep.

If there is any suspicion of possible secondary bacterial infection, an antistaphylococcic antibiotic should be administered by mouth. In severe cases of recalcitrant atopic dermatitis, children may need to receive daily doses of antibiotics. As the rash improves, the frequency of application of steroid medications and the use of antipruritic agents may be reduced. Emollients, however, often need to be continued, particularly after bathing.

Atopic dermatitis may be confused with seborrheic dermatitis in young infants, or with "dandruff" in older children and adults. Scabies, which also is characterized by pruritus, should be differentiated easily from atopic dermatitis by the presence and distribution of the papulovesicular lesions and the short duration of the skin condition. Allergic or contact dermatitis also usually has a shorter course than does atopic dermatitis.

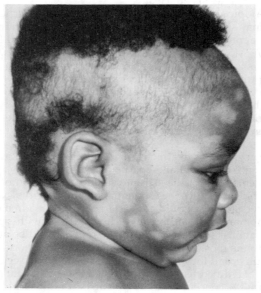

Figure 25-21. Note the facial depigmentation and scalp hair loss without prominent scaling in this child with seborrheic dermatitis.

Pityriasis Alba

Pityriasis alba is a common, asymptomatic skin condition that is characterized by a relatively distinct hypopigmented patch or patches with minimal to no fine scale. The lesions, which generally are round to oval, occur most commonly on the face and less often on the neck, upper trunk, and proximal extremities. Most cases seem to appear after sun exposure in children between the ages of 3 and 16 years. Individual lesions last 1 to 2 years. Although the lesions commonly occur in atopic individuals, the cause is unknown. The response to topical steroids and emollients is not good. The differential diagnosis includes tinea corporis, tinea versicolor, vitiligo, and psoriasis.

Seborrheic Dermatitis

Seborrheic dermatitis is a common skin condition with a predilection for two pediatric age groups, infants and adolescents. In infants between 2 and 10 weeks of age, seborrheic dermatitis generally begins on the scalp, producing a greasy, yellowish scale. The base may or may not be erythematous. Commonly, the scaling extends down the forehead to involve the eyebrows, nose, and ears. In black individuals, significant depigmentation may accompany the rash (Figure 25–21). The scale may be barely perceptible, and the rash generally is not pruritic. The diaper area also may be involved; in this area, which usually is infected with *Candida,* there is an erythematous, diffuse rash involving the creases. Without treatment, seborrheic dermatitis clears by 8 to 12 months of age. Intertriginous areas need to be treated with a mild steroid combined with an anticandidal agent. Continued "dandruff" of the scalp should suggest other disorders, including tinea capitis, atopic dermatitis and, rarely, histiocytosis X.

In adolescents, the scaling most commonly occurs on the scalp, eyebrows, eyelashes, nasolabial folds, postauricular crease, and presternal and interscapular regions. A mild tar-based shampoo usually keeps the scalp involvement under control. Mild (0.5% to 1%) hydrocortisone will aid in clearing other areas of the skin.

The etiology of seborrheic dermatitis is not clear; the histopathology is nonspecific. The idea that the condition has something to do with sebaceous glands is supported by development of the dermatitis in areas with the highest density of these glands. The appearance of seborrheic dermatitis in infants probably reflects the effect of transmitted maternal sex hormones on these glands; reappearance of the condition during puberty occurs with the resurgence of sex hormones.

Tinea Versicolor

The characteristic clinical presentation of tinea versicolor is the asymptomatic, gradual appearance and spread of hyperpigmented and hypopigmented areas on the neck, chest, and back. The lesions of this common fungal disorder are relatively discrete, are irregular in shape, and may be red, brown, or whitish. The macules may be ovoid or coin shaped and have a fine adherent scale. Pruritus is uncommon. Most cases occur after puberty, but facial lesions in infants have been described, probably resulting from contact with affected mothers.

The diagnosis may be confirmed by microscopic examination of the scale (to which potassium hydroxide has been added) for the presence of the budding cells and hyphae of *Pityrosporum orbiculare,* which give a spaghetti-and-meatball appearance. A Wood's light examination in a totally dark room should reveal a yellow to yellow-blue fluorescence, unless the patient has bathed in the previous 6 to 12 hours.

Treatment of tinea versicolor consists of selenium sulfide lotion applied in various therapeutic routines. Although this usually produces good results, relapses of the infection are common. Ketoconazole, 200 to 400 mg orally every month, also is effective.

Psoriasis

The fact that psoriasis often has its onset in childhood is not commonly known. It is estimated that 10% of cases begin before the patient is 10 years of age and that 35% begin by 20 years of age. The cause of the condition is not known, although it is clear that hereditary factors play a role. Trauma to the skin is a common precipitant in susceptible individuals.

The clinical lesions usually are distinctive, with well-demarcated papules or maculopapular lesions covered with a scale (see Color Figure 9). Larger lesions form characteristic plaques with distinct borders, a silvery scale, and an erythematous base. The scale tends to build up in layers, and its removal may cause a bleeding point (Auspitz' sign). The papules enlarge to form plaques. The distribution usually is symmetric, with plaques commonly appearing over the knees and elbows because they are sites of repeated trauma. The Koebner phenomenon (*ie,* the appearance of rash at sites of physical, thermal, or mechanical trauma) often is evident. The scalp frequently shows a thick, adherent scale; the nails often demonstrate punctate stippling or pitting, or become discolored and crumbly; and the palms and soles may show scaling and fissuring.

A variety of inciting factors in addition to trauma have been associated with the appearance of psoriatic lesions. An interesting one in children is the development of guttate psoriasis, a condition characterized by multiple, small, teardrop-like lesions associated with group A β-hemolytic streptococcal infection (Figure 25–22). Other agents implicated are sunburn, drug eruptions, and viral infections. The histologic picture is one of hyperproliferation of the epidermis.

The course of psoriasis is unpredictable. Treatment consists of the application of a good lubricant. For small areas of involvement, fluorinated steroids may be successful; tars also may help. Exposure to sunlight, with care taken not to burn the skin, seems to be the best therapy. Oral psoralens

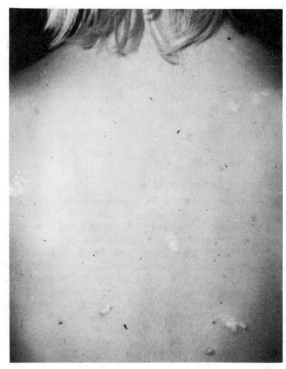

Figure 25-22. The sudden widespread appearance of small, scaly plaques is characteristic of guttate psoriasis.

combined with ultraviolet light and methotrexate therapy rarely are indicated for use in children.

The differential diagnosis in childhood includes uncommon disorders such as pityriasis rubra pilaris, parapsoriasis, and lichen planus. Occasionally, atopic dermatitis may be confused with psoriasis, but psoriasis is not pruritic.

Café au Lait Spots

Discrete macular areas of light brown pigmentation that are present at birth or develop shortly thereafter are common "birthmarks." They usually are seen as an isolated finding, especially among members of darkly pigmented races. The presence of multiple café au lait spots may provide an important cutaneous clue to von Recklinghausen's disease (neurofibromatosis). The presence of five or more café au lait spots greater than 0.5 cm in diameter in a child or six or more café au lait spots greater than 1 cm in diameter in an adult should prompt careful examination for other findings of this autosomal dominantly inherited disorder with protean features.

The presence of café au lait spots (rarely exceeding five or six in number) may be associated with other syndromes as well, including Russell-Silver syndrome, multiple lentigines, ataxia-telangiectasia, tuberous sclerosis, Fanconi's anemia, and Turner's syndrome.

Vitiligo

The lesions of vitiligo are much lighter than those of the disorders listed above. Many or all of the pigment cells in the skin have been destroyed. The cause of vitiligo is unknown. It probably is not an autoimmune disorder, as once suspected, although individuals with autoimmune disorders are more prone than normal to this disorder. It is more common than most people suspect; as much as 2% of the general population may have vitiligo, and 50% of those have the problem before the age of 20 years.

The lesions usually are bilateral and symmetric, commonly appearing around body orifices (Figure 25–23). The most frequent sites of involvement are the face, backs of the hands and wrists, umbilicus, and genitalia. Halo nevi are common in individuals with vitiligo. Topical steroids result in the return of normal color to the skin in about 20% of treated patients. Treatment with PUVA (psoralens and ultraviolet A light) should be reserved for older children. Care must be taken to protect the depigmented skin from sunburn.

Purpuric Lesions

Henoch-Schönlein Purpura

The rash of Henoch-Schönlein purpura is classically purpuric, but early on, it may appear urticarial or maculopapular. The characteristic distribution of the rash helps determine the diagnosis. The rash is located primarily from the buttocks on down the lower extremities. The upper extremities are involved less frequently, the face even less commonly, and the trunk only rarely. The characteristic lesion is that of a vasculitis (ie, palpable purpura), but the purpuric lesions may be macular and small or large, and, in severe cases, they may develop necrotic centers. Striking areas of edema involving the scalp, hands, feet, scrotum, or other areas may appear.

Individuals with Henoch-Schönlein purpura generally have associated disorders. A periarticular arthritis occurs in more than two thirds of the cases. Abdominal pain, gastrointestinal bleeding, and glomerulonephritis also are common. The purpuric lesions may appear in waves. One third of the cases resolve within 2 weeks, another third in 2 weeks to 2 months, and the remaining third in 2 to 6 months. It seems that the leukocytoclastic vasculitis of Henoch-Schönlein purpura may be precipitated by a variety of infections and exposures. Group A β-hemolytic streptococcal infections, *Mycoplasma*, varicella, hepatitis B, food allergens, insect bites, and exposure to cold have been implicated. Therapy is mainly supportive, although gastrointestinal bleeding and severe joint pain may respond to courses of systemic steroids.

■ PRURITIC LESIONS

Contact Dermatitis

In allergic contact dermatitis, in contrast to primary irritant contact dermatitis, pruritus is a prominent feature. Rhus dermatitis, which includes poison ivy, is the most frequently recognized of the allergic contact group. The characteristic feature of this eruption is the appearance of vesicles and vesicular papules in a linear distribution. The rash may be localized with groups of erythematous papules and vesicles, may have widely scattered lesions, or, on occasion, may be limited to the face, which appears swollen. A history of contact with eruption-producing plants is helpful to the diagnosis. The linear vesicles, or papules if the lesions are early, may be subtle. Pruritus often is severe. Contrary to common belief, the vesicular fluid does not spread the rash. The rapidity of appearance of the rash depends on how sensitive the affected person is to the toxin and how much of the toxin has reached the skin. In sensitive individuals, areas of significant exposure may show a rash within hours, whereas areas of minimal toxin exposure may not show a rash for days. (Lesions might not develop in less sensitive individuals until several days or a week later.)

Rhus dermatitis should not be confused with atopic dermatitis, which is a chronic disorder. Atopic dermatitis usually begins in early childhood and has a morphology and distribution much different from those of poison ivy. In addition, individuals with atopic dermatitis usually do not react to exposure to poison ivy.

Other contact rashes may create problems in diagnosis. Some are localized to areas that indicate the underlying problem. Contact dermatitis from metal, for example, develops in areas where metal comes in contact with the skin (*eg*, on fingers with rings, wrists with watches, the neck with necklaces, earlobes with earrings). Cosmetics occasionally produce less obvious rashes. Eyelid dermatitis from fingernail polish is common.

Foot dermatitis in children often is mistaken for tinea pedis; however, prepubertal children rarely have tinea infections of their feet. If the rash involves the dorsum of the foot, an allergic contact dermatitis is likely. The reactions are caused primarily by rubber antioxidants and potassium dichromate leather-tanning agents. If the dermatitis is on the weight-bearing surface, the cause may be unclear, but contact dermatitis usually can be ruled out. Atopic dermatitis develops eventually in some children with chronic foot dermatitis.

Treatment of contact dermatitis involves removal of the cause of the outbreak. A topical steroid may aid in relieving the pruritus and inflammation. Oral antihistamines may be needed in extensive cases. Oral steroids, which sometimes are indicated in severe cases of contact dermatitis, should be given in decreasing doses over a 10- to 14-day course.

Pediculosis

The human louse has a field day with children. Pediculosis capitis is an extremely common problem and a difficult one to eradicate, despite the best efforts of schools, health agencies, and physicians. The human head louse is an obligate human

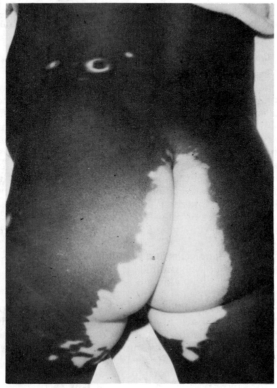

Figure 25-23. In vitiligo, depigmentation with distinct borders frequently involves the perineum.

parasite; it cannot survive away from its host for more than 10 days in the adult form or for more than 3 weeks as a fertile egg. The insect, which is 2 to 4 mm in length and ivory, rarely is seen. Nits, the egg sacs of lice, are the usual sign of infestation. Firmly cemented to the hair shaft, usually within 1 cm of the scalp, they resemble dandruff but cannot be picked off easily.

Pediculosis capitis usually results in pruritus of the scalp. Common accompaniments to the scratching are folliculitis and impetigo. The lice are spread easily through close contact, toilet articles such as combs and brushes, and clothing, especially hats. Treatment may be difficult, especially in young children, who may be reinfested by playmates. Lindane and pyrethrin shampoos are the standard forms of therapy. It is important to treat other family members and close contacts as well. Black individuals rarely are infested with head lice; the reason for their resistance is not known.

Pediculosis corporis is a much less common problem in the United States. These lice live in the seams of clothing and feed on the skin, producing small, red papules and wheals. To rid the clothing of the lice, it must be sterilized or at least have a hot iron run over the seams.

Pubic lice usually are acquired through contact during sexual intercourse; thus, sexual abuse must be considered in the case of pubic lice in a child. Although the lice usually cling to pubic hair, in young children, they may attach to body hair. Nits may be found in the eyelashes as well. The primary symptom is pruritus, and excoriations are common in heavy infestations. The nits on hair shafts are seen more commonly than is the louse itself, which is broader and shorter than are head and body lice. Infestation sometimes is manifested by the appearance of bluish-gray, faint purpuric lesions. Known as maculae caeruleae or taches bleuâtres, these spots are sites of feeding by the louse. Treatment consists of a 6- to 8-hour application of pyrethrin or lindane to affected areas.

Scabies

Epidemics of scabies seem to occur in 30-year cycles. A peak in cases occurred in the United States in the 1970s, but the infestation still is prevalent. The culprit, *Sarcoptes scabiei*, is a 0.2- to 0.4-mm female mite that burrows into the stratum corneum, where it deposits eggs and excrement. The clinical picture, which usually develops 4 to 6 weeks after infestation, is thought to be the result of sensitization to the mite and its products. A person can have mites on the body and transmit them to others without having symptoms and signs of the disorder.

The pruritus of scabies usually is intense and unremitting. A characteristic feature is that it seems worse at night, perhaps as a result of a rise in skin surface temperature and increased activity of the scabies mites. The lesions of scabies are papules, tiny vesicles, and pustules. Most are excoriated and, in long-standing cases, lichenification may be extensive. Burrows (*ie*, linear tracks) are not seen commonly in children. The distribution of lesions usually is from the neck down, although young infants and children can have scalp and even facial lesions. Characteristically, the lesions are most intense on the hands, particularly the webs of the fingers in older children and adults, and the palms and soles in infants; on the wrists; in the axillae; on the belt line; on the gluteal cleft; and around the nipples and genitalia in adults and older children. Scabies in babies can produce nodular/vesicular lesions on the palms and soles that can mimic pyoderma. Secondary infections occur frequently.

Although the clinical picture may be typical of scabies, it always is prudent to try to identify the mite in a scraping from one of the lesions. A simple technique is to choose a nonexcoriated, fresh vesicle or papule, place a drop of immersion oil on it, scrape it with a scalpel blade to open it, collect the oil from the skin, place the oil on a glass slide with a cover-slip on top, and look for the mite, eggs, or feces.

Treatment of scabies usually can be accomplished effectively by the application of 5% pyrethrin cream to the entire body surface, including the head in infants. The pyrethrin cream should remain on for 8 to 12 hours and then be washed off. One treatment usually is effective, although some prefer a second application 10 to 14 days later. Lindane, applied as a 1% concentration, is also effective and should remain on the skin for 6 to 8 hours. The pruritus may take a week or more to resolve after treatment. All family members must be treated at the same time. Failure to treat close contacts, such as babysitters, grandparents, aunts, and uncles, often results in reinfection. Many contacts may be infested despite a seeming absence of lesions.

The use of lindane on children has been the subject of much concern and debate. A review of reported cases of toxicity, however, has shown the preparation to be safe if it is not ingested or used inappropriately. Lindane is not recommended for use on pregnant women, however. Ten percent crotamiton is much less effective. Two applications, 24 hours apart, are recommended before the agent is washed off 48 hours later. Benzoyl benzoate, 12.5% to 25%, is effective but difficult to obtain. A 6% to 10% precipitate of sulfur in petrolatum hardly ever is used because of its unpleasant odor. Clothing worn and bedding used by the family before treatment should be washed or stored for 72 hours before reuse to prevent reinfestation by mites.

Scabies can affect families at all socioeconomic levels. Its presence denotes contact with a source. Although the contact generally requires intimate exposure, epidemics can occur in hospital settings, where nurses and physicians care for children and adults with undiagnosed scabies. Simple handwashing after patient contact prevents infection of health care providers.

■ DIFFUSE ERYTHEMA

Scarlet Fever

In the past, scarlet fever was manifested by a finely papular rash on an erythematous background that felt like sandpaper to the touch. Recently, however, the disease seems to have become much milder. Although still common, it frequently is not diagnosed because of a lack of typical features. The slapped cheek appearance is not common. Pastia's lines (*ie*, the erythematous accentuation of flexural creases), circumoral pallor, and even severe pharyngitis are seen infrequently. Most cases feature a fine, rough, papular rash predominantly over the bridge of the nose and face, shoulders, and upper chest. In fair-skinned individuals, the erythematous base may be present.

The rash of scarlet fever is produced by sensitization to those strains of group A β-hemolytic streptococci that produce an erythrogenic toxin. Because prior exposure to the toxin is required, it is rare to see this disorder in children less than 2 years of age. The incubation period is only 24 to 48 hours. It is important to warn parents that their child's hands and feet may show significant sheets of desquamation in 7 to 14 days.

Toxic Shock Syndrome

The typical skin eruption in toxic shock syndrome is a diffuse sunburnlike erythema. The other features of this serious illness, however, should separate it readily from scarlet fever and scalded skin syndrome. Early symptoms include a temperature higher than 38.9°C (102°F), bulbar conjunctival hyperemia, oropharyngeal and vaginal hyperemia, hypotension, a strawberry tongue, and striking palmar and plantar erythema and edema. There is evidence of multiple organ system involvement as well. The kidneys, muscles, central nervous system, gastrointestinal tract, and hematopoietic system all may be involved. Desquamation of the hands and feet develops 1 to 2 weeks after the illness.

The toxic shock syndrome is a medical emergency often requiring major medical life support. Hypotension leading to death is common. The toxin responsible for the disorder is produced by *S aureus* organisms. The disease occurs most frequently in young women using vaginal tampons during their menstrual period, but other infections also may be responsible, including osteomyelitis, cellulitis, and burns.

Drug Photosensitivity

Drug reactions to light have been divided into two types, toxic and allergic. Toxicity reactions occur after a single exposure and appear to be an exaggerated sunburn. Immediate reactions may occur with sulfonamides, phenothiazines, griseofulvin, and some tetracyclines. Delayed phototoxicity may follow the systemic administration of furocoumarins or psoralens. Most photoallergic reactions occur after topical contact with chemical agents. Early signs are pruritus and eczema, which appear within 24 hours after the chemical and light exposure. Drugs in this category include sulfonamides, griseofulvin, hydrocortisone, benzocaine, coal tar, and phenothiazines. In reactions caused by the combination of drugs and light, the distribution of the rash, which is confined to sun-exposed areas, is an important diagnostic clue. Treatment consists primarily of removal of the offending agent and of the sun exposure.

■ ANNULAR LESIONS

Tinea Corporis

Superficial fungal infections probably are the most readily identified annular lesions of the skin. The ringlike lesions are recognized by most lay people, although not all ringed lesions are tinea. Because the infection of nonhairy areas of the skin by dermatophytes is limited to the epidermis, only the most superficial layers of the skin are involved. The rings generally are erythematous. As the inflammation spreads, the active infection in the center of the lesions is destroyed, and this area clears, resulting frequently in the picture of an advancing border with central clearing. The border generally is scaly and slightly elevated, and, on close inspection, is seen to contain microvesicles and pustules (Figure 25–24). The lesions, which may be single or multiple, are not always round. Bizarre shapes and, occasionally, a coalescence of lesions may be noted, and borders may not be continuous. Targetlike lesions may occur as a result of reinfection or failure of clearing of the central part of the lesion. Tinea corporis usually is asymptomatic, although pruritus may be present.

The organism responsible for most cases of tinea corporis is *Trichophyton tonsurans. Microsporum canis, Microsporum audouini,* and *Trichophyton mentagrophytes* infections also are seen. Treatment consists of application of one of the topical antifungal agents, such as clotrimazole, haloprogin, or miconazole. Application twice a day for 2 to 3 weeks after the lesion clears usually is sufficient. The diagnosis may be con-

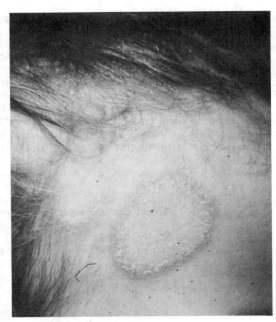

Figure 25-24. Annular lesion of tinea corporis with a raised border and scaling on the forehead.

firmed by potassium hydroxide preparations. Because tinea corporis occurs on nonhairy skin, the lesions do not fluoresce with a Wood's lamp. The three lesions most frequently confused with tinea corporis are granuloma annulare, the herald spots of pityriasis rosea, and dry nummular eczema.

Granuloma Annulare

The uninitiated almost always mistake granuloma annulare for tinea corporis. Granuloma annulare is an inflammatory disorder characterized by the eruption of papules, which may be superficial or subcutaneous, in a ringed arrangement. The initial papule enlarges outward and the center clears, sometimes seeming depressed (Figure 25–25). The key to differentiation from tinea corporis is close inspection of the borders. In granuloma annulare, the surface of the lesion is devoid of scale, vesicles, or pustules; skin markings are normal. In tinea, the border of the lesion is scaly, with microvesicles and pustules, and the color of the lesions varies from skin tone to erythematous. The lesions of granuloma annulare are asymptomatic, being neither pruritic nor tender.

The cause of granuloma annulare is unknown. Some believe that it represents a delayed type of hypersensitivity. Most lesions resolve spontaneously within 2 years, but some may last for decades. In adults, an association with diabetes mellitus has been reported, but this has not been noted in children. About half of all individuals with granuloma annulare have a single lesion. The lesions most frequently appear on the distal extremities. Deep-seated lesions can appear to be attached to the periosteum of bone, particularly the tibia. On biopsy samples, these lesions resemble rheumatoid nodules, but there is no association with connective tissue diseases. The nodules regress in 6 weeks to 6 months.

Urticaria

Hives, or wheals, are common in both children and adults. The lesions represent a localized vasodilation and transudation of fluid from capillaries and small blood vessels. Hives are transient, lasting less than 24 hours. They are lightly erythematous and may have central clearing, creating an annular pattern. Stasis of blood in the center of lesions frequently creates an appearance of purpura. Pruritus is a common feature.

Urticaria is a manifestation of the release of mediators from cutaneous mast cells, which increase vascular permeability. Histamine, kinins, and prostaglandins are among the mediators released. Urticaria may be caused by drugs, foods, inhalant allergies, infections, and arthropod bites and stings. Other agents include contactants, internal diseases, psychogenic factors, genetic abnormalities, and physical agents. Given the wide variety of possible agents, it often is difficult to pinpoint the cause of urticaria.

Infections that may cause urticaria include those with group A β-hemolytic streptococci, hepatitis virus, and Epstein-Barr virus. Physical agents that may result in urticaria include heat, cold, pressure, light, water, and vibration. Cholinergic urticaria is a fairly distinctive form manifested by the appearance of 2- to 3-mm papules surrounded by large erythematous flares. These flares are very pruritic and follow the onset of perspiration.

Uncovering the cause of chronic urticaria, defined as urticaria of at least 6 weeks' duration, is particularly difficult. In most series, the cause of the problem has been uncovered in less than 20% of the cases. Urticarial lesions that persist for more than 24 hours should raise the suspicion of urticarial vasculitis. A skin biopsy of one of the lesions will be diagnostic.

Treatment of urticaria depends on the extent and severity of the condition. Acute episodes that threaten vital functions should be treated with epinephrine as well as with antihistamines. Systemic steroids are indicated occasionally. Usually, an antihistamine alone is satisfactory therapy until the problem resolves.

Syphilis

The brownish to dull red macules and papules of secondary syphilis may appear annular and resemble pityriasis rosea. The lesions generally are discrete and follow lines of cleavage on the trunk, similar to pityriasis rosea. Reddish brown lesions on the palmar and plantar surfaces should be a clue to this diagnosis in sexually active patients. The rash appears 6 to 8 weeks after the primary syphilitic lesion, and it may last from a few hours to months.

Hair Loss

Tinea Capitis

As mentioned previously, hair loss always should suggest the possibility of tinea capitis. The hair loss may be localized to one spot and be associated with scaling of the scalp or, less frequently, it may be associated with microvesicles at the advancing borders of the hair loss. More commonly, the scalp may look relatively unaffected except for the hair loss and the presence of black dots, which represent broken-off, infected hairs. There may be many patches of hair loss or a diffuse thinning of hair. If the cause of hair loss is not clear, a fungal culture is indicated.

Alopecia Areata

The hallmark of alopecia areata is the appearance of well-circumscribed, round or oval patches of complete or

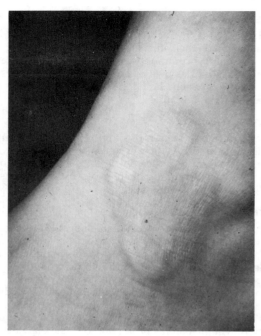

Figure 25-25. A granuloma annulare lesion on the ankle. Note the lack of epidermal involvement.

relatively complete hair loss. The scalp appears normal, without scale or scarring. The lesions tend to appear rapidly and may be single or multiple. Hair at the periphery of the lesions can be pulled out easily. Alopecia areata totalis is total loss of scalp hair; alopecia universalis is the complete loss of body hair.

Alopecia areata is much more common than most physicians realize. In reviews of dermatology clinics, as many as 2% of new patients have been found to have this disorder. The cause is not known, although an autoimmune phenomenon is suspected. Psychiatric disturbances used to be considered the underlying cause.

Alopecia areata rarely occurs in patients less than 4 years of age, but almost half of the cases appear in those less than 20 years of age. The course is totally unpredictable. Factors associated with a poor prognosis for eventual recovery include extensive alopecia in areas other than the scalp; occurrence in association with atopic dermatitis; the presence of nail changes, such as pitting; prepubertal onset; and ophiasis, the loss of hair in a swath above and behind the ears and across the occiput. The prognosis is good for most older children and adults. Hair may regrow in some places, however, only to be lost in others. Regrown hair often is light or even white.

The treatment of alopecia areata is disappointing. A wide variety of therapies have been tried with little sustained effect. Hair regrown during a course of systemic steroids is lost again when the steroids are discontinued. Local injections of triamcinolone into the scalp usually result in hair regrowth in injected areas, but the procedure is painful and the regrowth temporary. Topical irritants of various types were in vogue for some time, but rarely are effective. The key to treatment is careful, empathic education of the patient and the parents. Support groups of similarly affected patients are increasingly common in large communities and offer a great deal of help for both patients and parents. Artificial hairpieces often help patients maintain a positive body image.

Traction Alopecia

The hair loss in traction alopecia is secondary to prolonged tension on the hair shaft, usually from braiding of the hair. Traction most commonly produces hair loss at the margins of the scalp or as oval or linear areas in part lines (Figure 25–26). Permanent hair loss may result if pressure is maintained for a long time.

Pressure Alopecia

Pressure alopecia is most common in young infants, who lie prone and rub their occiputs on the bedding. Such hair loss occasionally indicates a lack of stimulation by the parents. Persistent rubbing of the scalp by any means may result in hair breakage and loss.

Trichotillomania

Hair loss as a result of trichotillomania, the pulling out of one's own hair, often assumes bizarre shapes and irregular patterns (Figure 25–27). The hair loss in this condition is never complete. A key feature distinguishing this from other forms of alopecia is the lack of scalp lesions and the presence of broken hairs of different lengths within the lesions. Body hair from other areas also may be lost, especially from the eyebrows or eyelashes. Rarely will a child admit to hair pulling, and rarely will the parents have noticed such behavior.

In young children, hair pulling usually represents a fairly benign reaction to stress. With time, most children discontinue the habit spontaneously. A short haircut and grease applied to the hair may help discourage the activity. In older children and adolescents, trichotillomania may reflect a more serious psychological problem. An attempt should be made to uncover the cause of the stress. Open discussion with the child and the parents may lead to resolution of the problem.

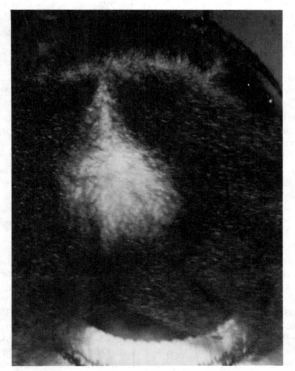

Figure 25-26. Traction alopecia over the midline of the occiput as a result of braiding.

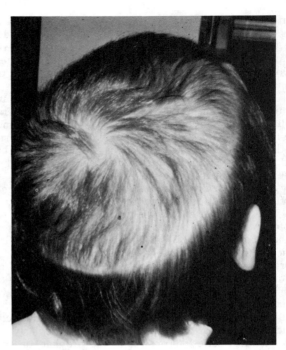

Figure 25-27. Alopecia with various hair lengths in an unusual configuration is characteristic of trichotillomania.

■ DIAPER DERMATITIS

Almost all children in diapers have a rash in the covered area at some point during their diaper-wearing years. In most cases, the irritation is minimal and can be treated effectively with any of a host of available creams, ointments, and powders. As many as 10% of children, however, have a problem rash that leads to consultation with a physician. Diaper dermatitis is not a life-threatening condition, but it may produce discomfort for the infant and it certainly causes anxiety for the parents.

The etiology of diaper dermatitis is multifactorial. The rash may take on a number of forms and must be differentiated from a variety of other conditions. The basic problem is the diaper. If infants did not wear diapers, there would be no diaper rashes; in countries where diapers are not worn, diaper dermatitis is almost unheard of. Diapers protect us and the environment from the urine and stools of infants. As barriers, however, they also impede the evaporation of moisture from the skin. The stratum corneum becomes edematous and increasingly susceptible to friction from the diaper. Friction leads to maceration, which allows other irritants and bacteria (especially *Candida*) to gain a foothold and create even more inflammation.

Ammonia used to be thought to play a major role in diaper dermatitis. Bacteria capable of producing ammonia from urea are present in the perineal areas of most infants. Although ammonia will not initiate diaper dermatitis, it will aggravate the condition. In contrast, *Candida* may be able to initiate an inflammatory response in the skin and produce a diaper dermatitis.

Diaper dermatitis can be grouped into two major categories: primary irritant and candidal. Primary irritant diaper dermatitis, also called generic diaper dermatitis, is characterized by varying degrees of erythema and papules, often with a shiny, glazed surface. The creases tend to be spared; primarily involved are the convex surfaces, which are directly in contact with the diaper. *Tidemark dermatitis* is the name given to the form that features chafing from the recurrent wet–dry effect of urine contact. Nodules and ulcerations of the convex surfaces occur only rarely, usually as a result of prolonged contact of the skin with soiled diapers.

Candidal diaper dermatitis, caused by infection with the yeast *Candida albicans,* is characterized by the appearance of the rash in the inguinal and other creases, with erythema, superficial erosions, and numerous bright red satellite pustules and erosions. Infantile seborrheic dermatitis also may produce a diaper dermatitis involving the inguinal creases; however, although seborrhea may play a role, treatment should be aimed at eradicating the secondary *Candida* infection that usually is present.

The treatment of diaper dermatitis would be easier if diapers could be removed. Realities of daily life and societal pressures make such removal difficult for any length of time. Nevertheless, in recalcitrant cases, that may be the recommended treatment. Wet diapers always should be removed quickly. The perineum then should be washed gently with mild cleansing agents, these agents should be rinsed off thoroughly, and the whole area should be dried completely before a new diaper is put on. In primary irritant dermatitis, a number of soothing ointments, most of which contain zinc oxide, are available to protect the skin and decrease friction on it from diapers. Persistence of any diaper dermatitis for more than 48 to 72 hours indicates secondary infection with *Candida;* in such cases, an antifungal agent specific for this yeast should be used. Treatment of candidal diaper dermatitis requires use of the above measures, as well as application of an antifungal agent and a mild hydrocortisone cream to treat the inflammation. In some cases, it may be wise to use a separate antifungal agent and hydrocortisone product to be applied alternately every 2 hours with each diaper change.

Talcs and cornstarch may be used to protect the skin and absorb excess fluid. Parents must be warned that talc can be inhaled by the infant, however, resulting in respiratory problems. Cornstarch does not enhance candidal growth, contrary to common belief.

Whether cloth or disposable diapers are less likely to result in dermatitis is a moot concern. Some infants seem to react to the detergents used to clean cloth diapers; others react to certain types of disposable diapers. The plastic covering on disposable diapers may cause irritation of the skin. Elastic bands in disposable diapers and plastic covers for cloth ones may result in contact dermatitis in susceptible infants. Disposable diapers with absorbent gels will hold a greater amount of fluid and pull it away from the skin.

Although most diaper dermatitis is the result of primary irritant dermatitis or *Candida,* other disorders also may cause rashes in the diaper area. Impetigo, a bacterial infection, is common in the diaper area. Bullous impetigo, characterized by blisters that rupture rapidly and leave moist areas of erythema or dried lesions with collarettes of scale, is the most frequent bacterial infection found in the diaper region. This infection is caused by *Staphylococcus aureus* and, therefore, is treated best with oral antistaphylococcic antibiotics. Folliculitis and furunculosis may occur, particularly on the buttocks. Recurrent staphylococcal furuncles generally resolve once the child no longer wears diapers. Tinea corporis occasionally masquerades as diaper dermatitis. An advancing border of microvesicles, crusting, and erythema usually is present. The lesions may not be as clearly ringlike as they are on other body areas.

Psoriasis also may occur in the diaper area, because the skin at this site is subjected to repeated irritation. Because of the moisture produced by diapers, the thick, silvery, adherent scale typical of psoriasis may not be clearly evident. Allergic contact dermatitis also may mimic diaper dermatitis. Parents may apply a variety of ointments and creams that contain sensitizing agents to the skin of the perineum, only to create a worsening dermatitis. It is important to obtain a complete list of all medicaments used in this area.

Herpes simplex infections usually can be distinguished readily by the presence of grouped vesicles, but, occasionally, larger areas of erosion may simulate diaper dermatitis. Acrodermatitis enteropathica typically produces vesiculation and erosions around the mouth and nose, in the perineum, and on the acral surfaces (*ie,* hands and feet). Affected infants are irritable, usually have diarrhea and failure to thrive, and lose their hair. Infants with histiocytosis X may have an erythematous, papular/nodular, and, occasionally, ulcerative rash in the diaper area, particularly in the inguinal creases. The rash may mimic a candidal infection but does not respond to appropriate treatment for such an infection. The scalp may be affected with a scaly rash, frequently with underlying petechiae. Scabies may result in a diaper dermatitis, but the infestation has signs of involvement in other areas as well and, therefore, is not difficult to diagnose. Finally, child abuse or neglect needs to be considered in cases of suspicious lesions of the perineum or severe, unattended diaper dermatitis.

A discussion of diaper dermatitis is not complete without mention of granuloma gluteale infantum. This is a rare, but worrisome-looking disorder characterized by red-purple nodules occurring in any portion of the diaper area, most commonly on the abdomen and upper thighs. The lesions are asymptomatic and are firm or soft and elastic. They usually develop in children who have had preceding irritant dermatitis. Although the cause is not known, many cases seem to occur in children who previously were treated with moderate- to intermediate-potency topical steroids. The lesions sometimes suggest lymphomatous nodules.

■ ACNE

Acne undoubtedly is the most common skin problem of adolescents. Unfortunately, it often is relegated to a minor position in most medical school curricula. Acne is not a life-threatening illness, but its impact on adolescents in their formative years is significant. The scars on the face are only a superficial reflection of the psychological scars, which may run much deeper. The magnitude of sales of over-the-counter medications for acne are an indication of the importance of this problem to adolescents.

Pathogenesis

The pathogenesis of acne is not clearly understood. Many factors seem to contribute to development of the lesions. Development of acne starts in the sebaceous gland, a large, multilobular gland that empties into a relatively long canal containing a vellus hair, the follicle for which lies at its base. The concentration of sebaceous follicles is highest on the face, chest, and back, areas that commonly develop acneiform lesions. At puberty, the sebaceous glands are stimulated by androgens to increase in size and lipid production, resulting in an increase in the oiliness of the skin.

Dihydrotestosterone, a product of testosterone, is the most potent androgen end-organ effector. Dihydrotestosterone is formed primarily in cells located within the sebaceous glands. An important event along the path to acne is obstruction of the sebaceous follicle unit. For some reason, sebum and keratin from the shedding of cells lining the follicle stick together to form plugs. The plugs, called comedones, are invaded by bacteria, especially *Propionibacterium acnes*. The primary role of bacteria in the pathogenesis of acne may be the production of lipases, which hydrolyze the triglycerides of sebum into free fatty acids and other extracellular products, which, in turn, stimulate an inflammatory response (chemotaxis), leading to the rupture of the pilosebaceous unit. The presence of lipids outside the sebaceous follicle causes a further inflammatory response and the production of the papular pustules of acne. All these factors act in concert to produce the lesions of acne.

Acne vulgaris, or common acne, begins with the appearance of comedones, usually in early adolescence (Figure 25–28). Blackheads, or open comedones, represent sebaceous follicles whose orifices at the skin surface are patulous. The blackhead is not composed of dirt, contrary to popular belief; rather, it represents discoloration of the sebaceous plug by melanin. Blackheads are unsightly, but they are not typical precursors of inflammatory lesions.

The closed comedo, or whitehead, is more likely to become inflamed. In these lesions, the opening of the sebaceous follicle is tiny, and a plug of sebum pushes the skin up in a small mound. Rupture of the follicular wall is likely to cause the lesion to become inflammatory and to produce papulopustules in an attempt to clean up the "oil spill." Generally, the follicular wall re-forms; the neutrophils, macrophages, and other debris from the inflammation are expelled or cleared; and the lesion eventually recedes.

Deeper lesions, or nodules, may develop when the products of inflammation take longer to clear and fibrous tissue is laid down. Scars may result from the formation of this fibrous tissue. Nodules of inflammation may coalesce to form large lakes of pus, resulting in cystic lesions, which heal slowly, frequently become reinflamed, and may form sinus tracts. In acne conglobata, a severe, disfiguring form of acne generally occurring in adolescent males, a maze of channels may form in the dermis; the skin surface is distorted by large, purplish mounds as well as by a myriad of pustules and blackheads (Figure 25–29).

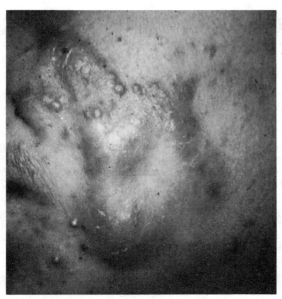

Figure 25-29. Large cysts and pustules are characteristic of acne conglobata, a severe form of acne.

Treatment

The treatment of acne begins with education. It is important that the adolescent understand as much as possible about the pathogenesis of the problem. Old myths should be discarded, particularly the relationship between "junk" food and acne. It must be made clear that the medications used to treat acne take time to work and sometimes must be changed or combined.

The most commonly used medication is benzoyl peroxide, which appears to have three modes of activity: a sebostatic effect; mild comedolytic activity; and a strong inhibitory effect on bacteria. Most over-the-counter acne medications contain benzoyl peroxide. Unfortunately, the adolescent usually does not read the directions carefully, uses too much or too strong a concentration, and gives up after a short time because of irritation from the medication or lack of rapid response.

Retinoic acid A, a metabolite of vitamin A, is another excellent topical medication for acne. In addition to having a strong comedolytic effect, this medication increases superficial blood flow, enhancing clearing of existing lesions. Antibiotics long have played a role in acne therapy. Tetracycline and erythromycin reduce the surface concentration of bacteria and, equally importantly, decrease the surface content of free fatty acids. Their primary beneficial effect may be their ability to depress the chemotaxis of leukocytes, thereby reducing the pustular inflammatory response to follicular injury. Topical antibiotics are a more recent addition to the armamentarium of acne therapy.

A key to success in treating acne is development of a partnership with the patient. Most physicians should be able to treat the great majority of their patients with acne. Failure of therapy generally is the result of a lack of understanding of the disorder. Adolescents expect overnight cures and must be made to understand that it often will take 4 to 6 weeks before treatment effects much change.

Topical medications often are used only on papulopustules. They should be used on the entire surface involved in acne, however, to keep all sebaceous follicles open. Care should be taken not to apply too much of the topical med-

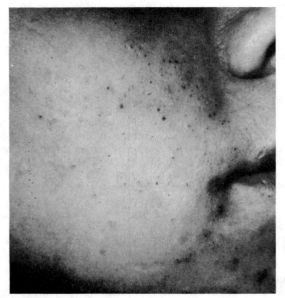

Figure 25-28. Comedones predominate in this teenager with acne.

ication. The fact that a little bit is good does not mean that a lot is better; excessive application leads to dryness and irritation of the skin, which often causes the patient to discontinue the medication.

In 1982, a derivative of vitamin A, isotretinoin, was approved by the United States Food and Drug Administration for oral use in cases of severe cystic acne. It has proved to be a highly effective agent. Unfortunately, it is expensive and has many annoying side effects, and its long-term effects are unknown. It also is a highly teratogenic agent.

■ DRUG REACTIONS

One of the main difficulties in dermatologic differential diagnosis is deciding whether a rash is drug induced. Obviously, if the child is not taking a medication currently or has not received one recently, this is not a possibility. All too frequently, however, a febrile child is prescribed an antibiotic and later erupts in a rash. Is it an allergic reaction? Should the antibiotic be discontinued? The answers often are difficult to determine. The difficulty lies in the fact that drug rashes can resemble almost any other kind of cutaneous eruption. Skin biopsies generally are nonspecific and provide no help in determining the cause of the problem.

In studies of types of drug reactions, four cutaneous types have been found to make up almost 90% of the rashes. About half of the rashes associated with drug reactions are similar to exanthems. These lesions may be maculopapular, morbilliform (similar to measles), macular, or scarlatiniform. They have no characteristic features that distinguish them easily from viral or bacterial exanthems. Penicillins, sulfonamides, trimethoprim sulfa, and erythromycin all are capable of producing this type of reaction.

The rash associated with ampicillin presents a special diagnostic problem. This rash may be allergic or, more commonly, nonallergic. The latter is not a true hypersensitivity reaction and is morbilliform and blotchy. It usually begins 5 to 10 days after ampicillin is initiated and resolves despite continuation of the drug. The difficulty lies in deciding which one of these reactions the rash represents. An extensive, erythematous, maculopapular rash develops in more than 80% of children and adults with infectious mononucleosis who receive ampicillin. This rash does not indicate penicillin allergy.

The difficulties associated with differentiating drug reactions from exanthems probably has resulted in a significant number of cases in which patients erroneously were designated as being allergic to a drug because they erupted with viral exanthems while receiving antibiotics.

Urticarial eruptions account for about 25% of drug eruptions. These reactions are IgE mediated, and their onset generally is sudden, usually occurring hours or days after drug exposure. The individual wheals are transient, but the entire process may last for 4 to 6 weeks. Penicillins, sulfonamides, barbiturates, and acetylsalicylic acid are drugs well known to cause this type of reaction.

Fixed drug reactions in children are less common than in adults; they are localized to a small area rather than being generalized, as usually is the case with drug reactions. The lesions are discrete, violaceous plaques that often are single or few in number and generally are asymptomatic. If the same drug is administered again, the rash will appear in the exact same spot. As many as 10% of drug reactions are of the fixed type.

Reactions resembling erythema multiforme, which feature concentric rings, or targets, occasionally with bullous or purpuric centers, account for 5% of drug reactions. Sulfonamides, penicillins, hydantoin, barbiturates, and griseofulvin have been implicated in this type of drug reaction. Infections and some systemic disorders can cause a similar eruption, however.

Other forms of drug reactions run the gamut of cutaneous lesions. Photosensitive dermatitis, vasculitic lesions with palpable purpura, vesicular/bullous eruptions, exfoliative lesions, erythema nodosum, and eczematous contact type reactions all have been described. The child with a rash who is receiving a medication will continue to present diagnostic problems until sensitive and reliable tests for drug allergy are developed.

(Abridged from Walter W. Tunnessen, Jr., Pediatric Dermatology, in Oski, DeAngelis, Feigin, McMillan, Warshaw: *Principles and Practice of Pediatrics, Second Edition*, J.B. Lippincott, 1994.)

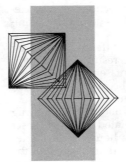

SECTION 3

Upper Airway Infections

Oski's Essential Pediatrics,
edited by Kevin B. Johnson and Frank A. Oski.
Lippincott–Raven Publishers,
Philadelphia © 1997

26

The Common Cold

Respiratory illness accounts for more than half of all acute disabling conditions in adults annually in the United States, and for an equal percentage of child outpatient visits to health care providers. The common cold, almost always caused by a virus, is the most common of the specific disorders. Most of the medical literature regarding the etiology, epidemiology, pathophysiology, and treatment of the common cold derives from studies performed in adults, with more occasional reports in children providing the bases for extrapolation to pediatrics. There is no specific association of any respiratory syndrome with a particular agent. Depending on the pathogen, the age of the patient, and the immunologic experience of the host, all respiratory pathogens can cause undifferentiated upper respiratory tract illness. Laboratory techniques are not available or cannot be applied practically for specific diagnosis in most instances of upper respiratory tract illnesses. A careful clinical history, including epidemiologic information, combined with physical examination can result in a reasonably accurate prediction of the cause of any particular episode.

■ ETIOLOGIC AGENTS

Initially believed to be caused by either a single virus or a group of viruses, the common cold now is recognized to be associated with more than 200 viruses, occasional bacteria, protozoa, and *Mycoplasma.*

Table 26–1 gives an abbreviated list of the agents that cause the common cold and their relative prevalence in children. Rhinoviruses and coronaviruses have even more importance in adults; symptoms of the common cold are the classic manifestations of these viruses.

Factors related to the host, pathogen, and environment that are gleaned from the child's history indicate the likelihood of causative agents in upper respiratory illness and provide an approach to the delineation of specific causes (Table 26–2) Although rhinoviruses are the most frequent cause of the common cold overall, the role of other agents can be suggested by consideration of the information listed in Table 26–2. Season (Table 26–3) age, and prior immunologic experience have the most important influence on cause. For example, disease resulting from respiratory syncytial

virus and parainfluenza viruses is most common and most severe in patients who are less than 3 years of age. Infection occurs less commonly and with milder symptoms (frequently those of the common cold) with increasing age.

Rhinoviruses belong to the family of picornavirus, included among enteroviruses. They are RNA viruses with a diameter of 15 to 50 nm. They are ether stable, but, unlike other enteroviruses, are inactivated in 3 to 4 hours by a *p*H level of 3. More than 100 distinct serotypes are known, and recent data suggest that new serotypes are not evolving; rather, a large pool of antigenically stable rhinoviruses exists.

Rhinoviruses are found in nasal secretions and are not found in stool specimens. Peculiar requirements for growth limit attempts at isolation in research laboratories. Most serotypes grow only in human cell lines, and some fastidious strains grow only in organ culture of human tracheal or nasal epithelium. No rapid antigen detection systems are available.

■ EPIDEMIOLOGY

Children normally experience two to eight colds per year. The peak age of occurrence is the second 6 months of life. The incidence does not fall significantly until the child is well into school age. The number of respiratory illnesses is increased during day care exposure in infancy.

TABLE 26-1. Etiologic Agents of the Common Cold in Children

Agent	Prevalence*
VIRUSES	
Rhinoviruses	+++
Parainfluenza viruses	++
Respiratory syncytial virus	++
Coronaviruses	+
Adenoviruses	+
Enteroviruses	+
Influenza viruses	+
Reoviruses	+
OTHER	
Mycoplasma pneumoniae	+
Bordetella pertussis	+

* +++ indicates most prevalent cause; ++ indicates prevalent cause; + indicates occasional cause.

TABLE 26-2. Use of Historical Information to Differentiate Among Causes of Nonspecific Upper Respiratory Illnesses

Factor	Typical for Rhinovirus	Examples of Factors Typical for Other Etiologies	
Age	School age	Toddler	Parainfluenza viruses
		School age	*Mycoplasma pneumoniae*
Season	Fall, spring	Winter	RSV, influenza
		Summer	Adenoviruses
Immunization status	Any	Incomplete	*Bordetella pertussis*
		Incomplete	Mumps
Sibling	School age	Infant	RSV
		Adolescent	Adenoviruses
		Toddler	Parainfluenza viruses
Illness in contacts	Common cold	Bronchiolitis	RSV
		Croup	Parainfluenza viruses
		Conjunctivitis	Adenoviruses
		Exudative pharyngitis	Adenoviruses, Epstein-Barr virus
		Ulcerative enanthema	Enteroviruses
Incubation period	3–5 d	2 wk	*Mycoplasma pneumoniae*
			Bordetella pertussis
Acquisition	Home	Hospital	RSV, influenza viruses
		Day care	All agents
Community epidemic	Common cold	Parotitis	Mumps
		Hand-foot-and-mouth disease	Enteroviruses
		Aseptic meningitis	Enteroviruses
		Febrile upper respiratory tract infection	Influenza viruses, adenoviruses

RSV, respiratory syncytial virus.

Viruses causing the common cold spread from person to person by means of virus-contaminated respiratory secretions. Kissing is an inefficient way to transmit rhinoviruses. They are transmitted by sneezing, by nose blowing and wiping, or from secretions that are on environmental surfaces. Recipients become infected by touching one of these sources and then inoculating their nose or conjunctiva.

■ CLINICAL MANIFESTATIONS

The common cold syndrome has been defined as that which most typically follows rhinovirus infection, its most frequently occurring cause. Throat irritation, sneezing, and nasal stuffiness are the primary complaints on the first and second days of illness; rhinitis, watering eyes, and, sometimes, hoarseness and cough follow on the second to fourth days of illness. Fever is absent or low grade. Chilliness, headache, and myalgia can be present early in the illness. Cough and nasal discharge are the most persistent complaints. Typically, illness caused by rhinoviruses lasts for 6 to 7 days. Nasal symptoms tend to be more prominent and throat and systemic symptoms less prominent in upper respiratory tract illness caused by rhinovirus compared to that caused by other viruses. The large number of rhinovirus types is associated predictably with variable symptoms and degrees of discomfort.

The symptoms described above are typical for older children and adults. Young infants are more likely to have a temperature of 38°C or 39°C, irritability, and restlessness. Nasal obstruction can interfere with sleeping and eating.

Complications of the common cold are those associated with extension of the virus to the lower respiratory tract and an increase in local susceptibility to bacterial infection by

TABLE 26-3. Seasonal Peaks of Respiratory Tract Pathogens

Fall	Rhinoviruses
	Parainfluenza viruses
	Group A *Streptococcus*
Winter	Respiratory syncytial virus
	Adenoviruses
	Influenza viruses
	Coronaviruses
Spring	Rhinoviruses
	Parainfluenza viruses
	Group A *Streptococcus*
Summer	Adenoviruses
	Bordetella pertussis
	Enteroviruses

indigenous flora. Additionally, in children with hyperreactive airways, mild viral upper respiratory illnesses and their complications incite episodes of asthma.

■ TREATMENT AND PREVENTION

Treatment of the common cold is supportive. No antiviral agent effective against rhinovirus is available. The use of nasally applied or systemically administered decongestants has not been shown to be beneficial; they should be used infrequently in children and not at all in infants less than 6 months of age. Acetaminophen can be used occasionally to relieve fever or discomfort, but it should be used rarely for cold symptoms in infants less than 6 months of age. Aspirin should not be given because it is implicated causally in influenza-associated Reye's syndrome, and assigning viral causes to nonspecific upper respiratory illnesses is difficult.

The relief of nasal obstruction is the most important focus of supportive care. Comfortable environmental temperature and humidity should be maintained.

(Abridged from Sarah S. Long, The Common Cold, in Oski, DeAngelis, Feigin, McMillan, Warshaw: *Principles and Practice of Pediatrics, Second Edition*, J.B. Lippincott, 1994.)

Oski's Essential Pediatrics, edited by Kevin B. Johnson and Frank A. Oski. Lippincott–Raven Publishers, Philadelphia © 1997

27

Paranasal Sinusitis

Acute infection of the paranasal sinuses is a common complication of allergic or infectious inflammation of the upper respiratory tract. About 1% to 5% of upper respiratory infections are complicated by acute sinusitis. As adults average two to three colds per year and children average six to eight, sinusitis is a problem commonly seen in clinical practice.

The four paired paranasal sinuses are the ethmoid, maxillary, sphenoid, and frontal sinuses. All but the frontal sinuses are present at birth. The frontal sinuses develop from the anterior ethmoid sinuses, and become clinically important after the 10th birthday. The maxillary and ethmoid sinuses are the principal sites of sinus infection in young children.

■ ANATOMY

The anatomic relationship between the nose and the paranasal sinuses is shown in Figure 27–1. The nose is divided in the midline by the nasal septum. From the lateral wall of the nose come three shelflike structures, the inferior, middle, and superior turbinates. The position of the outflow tract of the maxillary sinus, high on the medial wall of the nasal cavity, impedes gravitational drainage of secretions and accounts for the frequency of involvement of the maxillary sinuses when upper respiratory tract inflammation becomes complicated by bacterial superinfection.

■ CLINICAL PRESENTATION

In most children with acute or chronic sinusitis, the respiratory symptoms of nasal discharge, nasal congestion, and cough are prominent. During the course of an apparent viral upper respiratory tract infection, there are two common clinical presentations that suggest a diagnosis of acute sinusitis.

The first, most common clinical situation in which sinusitis should be suspected is when the signs and symptoms of a cold are persistent. Nasal discharge and daytime cough that continue beyond 10 days and are not improving are the principal complaints. Most uncomplicated upper respiratory tract infections last for 5 to 7 days. The lack of improvement in respiratory symptoms beyond the 10-day mark suggests that a complication has developed. The nasal discharge may be of any quality (thin or thick; clear, mucoid, or purulent) and the cough (which may be dry or wet) usually is present in the daytime, although it often is noted to be worse at night. The persistence of daytime cough frequently is the symptom that brings a child to medical attention. The child may not appear ill and, usually, if fever is present, it will be low grade. When the complaint of malodorous breath is accompanied by respiratory symptoms (in the absence of exudative pharyngitis, dental decay, or nasal foreign body), it is a clue to the presence of sinus infection. Facial pain rarely is present, although intermittent, painless, morning periorbital swelling may have been noted by the parents. In this case, it is not the severity of the clinical symptoms, but their persistence that calls for attention.

The second, less common presentation is a cold that seems more severe than usual: the fever is high (above 39°C), the nasal discharge is purulent and copious, and associated periorbital swelling or facial pain may be present. A less common complaint is headache (a feeling of fullness or a dull ache either behind or above the eyes.) Occasionally, there may be dental pain, either from infection originating in the teeth or referred from the sinus infection.

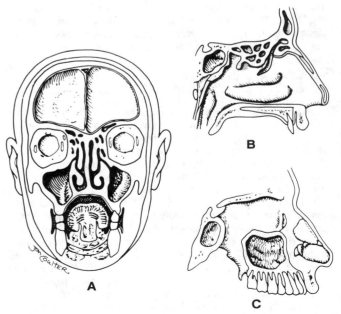

Figure 27-1. Anatomy of the parasinal sinuses.

■ DIAGNOSIS

Physical Examination

On physical examination, the patient with acute sinusitis may have mucopurulent discharge present in the nose or posterior pharynx. The nasal mucosa is erythematous; the throat may show moderate injection. The cervical lymph nodes usually are not enlarged significantly or tender. None of these characteristics differentiates rhinitis from sinusitis. Occasionally, there will be either tenderness as the examiner palpates over or percusses the paranasal sinuses, appreciable periorbital edema (soft, nontender swelling of the upper and lower eyelid with discoloration of the overlying skin), or both. Malodorous breath in concert with nasal discharge or cough suggests bacterial sinusitis.

In general, for most children less than 10 years old, the physical examination is not very helpful in making a specific diagnosis of acute sinusitis. If the mucopurulent material can be removed from the nose and the nasal mucosa is treated with topical vasoconstrictors, however, pus may be seen coming from the middle meatus. The latter observation, or the presence of periorbital swelling or facial tenderness, probably is the most specific finding in acute sinusitis.

Radiography

The radiographic findings most diagnostic of bacterial sinusitis are the presence of an air–fluid level in, or complete opacification of, the sinus cavities. An air–fluid level is an uncommon radiographic finding in children younger than 5 years of age who have acute sinusitis; however, mucosal swelling may be appreciated and is suggestive of sinus disease. A normal radiograph suggests, but does not prove, that a sinus is free of disease.

Computed tomography (CT) scans are superior to plain radiographs in the delineation of sinus abnormalities. However, they are not necessary in children with uncomplicated acute sinusitis and should be reserved for the evaluation of recurrent, chronic, or complicated sinus infections.

Sinus Aspiration

Aspiration of the maxillary sinus can be performed in children who are older than 2 years of age to establish the precise cause of a sinus infection. Indications for sinus aspiration in patients with suspected sinusitis include clinical unresponsiveness to conventional therapy, sinus disease in an immunosuppressed patient, severe symptoms such as headache or facial pain, and life-threatening complications such as intraorbital or intracranial suppuration at the time of clinical presentation.

■ MICROBIOLOGY

The bacteriology of sinus secretions similar to that found in otitis media (Table 27–1). The predominant organisms are *Streptococcus pneumoniae*, *Moraxella catarrhalis*, and nontypeable *Haemophilus influenzae*. Both *H influenzae* and *M catarrhalis* may produce β-lactamase and, consequently, may be ampicillin resistant. Anaerobic isolates and staphylococci rarely are recovered. Several viruses, including adenoviruses, influenza viruses, parainfluenza viruses, and rhinoviruses, have been recovered from maxillary sinus aspirates. The performance of nasal, throat, or nasopharyngeal cultures is of no value in patients with acute sinusitis because the results are not predictive of the bacterial isolates within the maxillary sinus cavity.

The microbiology of chronic sinusitis differs slightly from that of acute sinusitis. Anaerobes of the respiratory tract, viridans streptococci, and, occasionally, *Staphylococcus aureus* are found in addition to the aerobes of acute sinusitis.

■ DIFFERENTIAL DIAGNOSIS

The major symptoms that prompt consideration of the diagnosis of acute sinusitis are persistent or purulent nasal discharge and persistent cough. Alternative diagnoses to consider for patients with purulent nasal discharge are simple viral upper respiratory infection, group A streptococcal infection, adenoiditis, and nasal foreign body. Nasal foreign body usually is characterized by unilateral nasal discharge, which is purulent, bloody, and strikingly foul smelling. Patients who have persistent cough may have reactive airways disease, *Mycoplasma pneumoniae* bronchitis, cystic fibrosis, and gastroesophageal reflux.

■ TREATMENT

The objectives of antimicrobial therapy for acute sinus infection are achievement of a rapid clinical cure, sterilization of the sinus secretions, prevention of suppurative orbital and intracranial complications, and prevention of chronic sinus disease.

The relative frequency of occurrence of the various bacterial agents suggests that amoxicillin is an appropriate drug for most uncomplicated cases of acute sinusitis (Table 27–2). In areas where ampicillin-resistant organisms are prevalent,

TABLE 27-1. Bacteriology of Acute Sinusitis

Bacterial Species	Prevalence (%)
Streptococcus pneumoniae	25–30
Moraxella catarrhalis	15–20
Haemophilus influenzae	15–20
Streptococcus pyogenes	2–5
Anaerobes	2–5
Sterile	20–35

TABLE 27-2. Antimicrobial Agents for Sinusitis

Antimicrobial Agent	Dosage
Amoxicillin	40 mg/kg/d in 3 divided doses
Erythromycin/ sulfisoxazole	50/150 mg/kg/d in 4 divided doses
Sulfamethoxazole/ trimethoprim	40/8 mg/kg/d in 2 divided doses
Cefaclor	40 mg/kg/d in 3 divided doses
Amoxicillin/ clavulanate	40 mg/kg/d in 3 divided doses
Cefuroxime axetil	250 or 500 mg/d in 2 divided doses

or when disease is more severe, several alternative regimens are available, including the combination agent sulfamethoxazole/trimethoprim (Bactrim, Septra), most second- and third-generation cephalosporins, the combination of erythromycin/sulfisoxazole (Pediazole), the combination of amoxicillin and potassium clavulanate (Augmentin), and the new macrolides, clarithromycin (Biaxin) and azithromycin (Zithromax). Antimicrobials should be prescribed for a minimum of 10 to 14 days; some patients may benefit from an additional 7 days if they are not fully recovered after 2 weeks of therapy. Because appropriate antimicrobial therapy results in prompt clinical improvement within 48 to 72 hours, additional pharmacologic agents, such as antihistamines or decongestants, usually are not necessary.

Irrigation and Drainage

Irrigation and drainage of the infected sinus may result in dramatic relief from pain for patients with acute sinusitis. Drainage procedures usually are reserved for those who fail to respond to medical therapy with antimicrobial agents or those who have a suppurative intraorbital or intracranial complication. If an episode of acute sinusitis cannot be treated effectively by medical therapy alone or by medical therapy and simple sinus puncture, more radical surgery may become necessary.

Surgical Therapy

Most current surgical efforts involve using an endoscope to enlarge the natural meatus of the maxillary outflow tract by excising the uncinate process and the ethmoidal bullae and performing an anterior ethmoidectomy. A pilot study assessing the safety and efficacy of endoscopic sinus surgery in children with chronic sinusitis reported that 71% of the patients were considered normal by their parents 1 year after the operation. Endoscopic surgery in children is promising but requires further study.

■ COMPLICATIONS

Complications of sinus disease may cause both substantial morbidity and occasional mortality. Major complications result from either contiguous spread or hematogenous dissemination of infection. A complete list of the major complications of sinusitis is provided in Table 27–3.

Orbital Complications

Orbital complications are the most common serious complication of acute sinusitis and, despite antimicrobial therapy, may lead to loss of vision and severe morbidity. The usual presenting feature of sinus-related orbital complications is a "swollen eye." It is essential to establish the severity of the cellulitis clinically so appropriate decisions can be made regarding specific therapy and the need for surgical drainage. With early involvement (stage I), the inflammatory edema is confined to the medial aspect of the upper or lower eyelid. There is gradual onset of lid swelling, minimal skin discoloration, and low-grade or no fever. No proptosis, visual impairment, or limitation of extraocular movement is observed. This is not an actual infection of the orbit, but,

TABLE 27-3. Major Complications of Sinusitis

ORBITAL	INTRACRANIAL
Inflammatory edema (preseptal or preorbital cellulitis)	Epidural abscess
Subperiosteal abscess	Subdural empyema or abscess
Orbital abscess	Cavernous or sagittal sinus thrombosis
Orbital cellulitis	Meningitis
Optic neuritis	Brain abscess
OSTEOMYELITIS	
Frontal (Pott's puffy tumor)	
Maxillary	

rather, swelling caused by impedance of the local venous drainage. As such, it must be distinguished from a much more virulent form of periorbital or so-called preseptal cellulitis caused by *H influenzae* type b. The septum is a connective tissue reflection of periosteum that inserts into the eyelid and provides an anatomic barrier protecting the orbit. Both "inflammatory edema" and *H influenzae* type b preseptal infection involve tissues anterior to the orbital contents. *H influenzae* type b periorbital cellulitis, however, is characterized by an abrupt onset, rapid progression, and severe systemic toxicity. The markedly swollen and tender periorbital tissue has a violaceous, almost hemorrhagic discoloration, the texture of the skin is altered, and the subcutaneous tissue is indurated. *H influenzae* type b is recovered frequently, and *S pneumoniae* less often, from blood cultures and tissue aspirate. Because most *H influenzae* organisms isolated from sinus aspirates are nontypeable, the relationship, if any, of these acute bacteremic *H influenzae* type b infections to sinusitis is unclear. Other entities to distinguish from inflammatory edema include an infected periorbital or blepharal laceration, insect bite, contact allergy, conjunctivitis, dacryocystitis, and eczematoid dermatitis.

Treatment and Outcome

Children with stage I disease occasionally can be treated carefully as outpatients by the usual regimen for acute sinusitis, provided the parents are cooperative and can return for reevaluation readily. The antimicrobial agent selected must provide an antibacterial spectrum that includes β-lactamase–producing *H influenzae* and *M catarrhalis*. Careful follow-up is essential to detect progression of infection and the need for hospitalization. If the infection has progressed beyond stage I, then hospitalization and intravenous antibiotics are mandatory. The choice of antibiotics is guided by knowledge of the usual bacteriology of acute sinusitis. Surgical drainage is required if there is a subperiosteal or an orbital abscess, but orbital cellulitis may respond to antimicrobial agents without surgical intervention. The prognosis for patients with stage I and II disease usually is excellent if diagnosis and appropriate therapy are carried out promptly, but residual visual loss as a result of infection of the optic nerve may complicate orbital abscesses. Severe neurologic sequelae or death may follow cavernous sinus thrombophlebitis.

(Abridged from Ellen R. Wald, Paranasal Sinusitis, in Oski, DeAngelis, Feigin, McMillan, Warshaw: *Principles and Practice of Pediatrics, Second Edition*, J.B. Lippincott, 1994.)

Oski's Essential Pediatrics,
edited by Kevin B. Johnson and Frank A. Oski.
Lippincott–Raven Publishers,
Philadelphia © 1997

28

Pharyngitis

Children and young adults visit physicians more often for sore throats than for any other problem or symptom. Technically, pharyngitis is an inflammatory illness of the mucous membranes and underlying structures of the throat.

■ ETIOLOGY

The etiologic agents involved in nasopharyngitis most often are viruses, with adenovirus types 7a, 9, 14, and 15 being the most common. Influenza and parainfluenza are the other major viral agents. Rhinovirus and respiratory syncytial virus infections are not associated often with objective pharyngeal findings.

Pharyngitis (including tonsillitis and tonsillopharyngitis) can be caused by a diversity of infectious agents. In normal, healthy children, more than 90% of all cases of pharyngitis are caused by the following organisms, listed in order of decreasing frequency of occurrence: group A β-hemolytic streptococci; adenoviruses; influenza viruses A and B; parainfluenza viruses 1, 2, and 3; Epstein-Barr virus; enteroviruses; *Mycoplasma pneumoniae*; and *Chlamydia pneumoniae.*

Other β-hemolytic streptococci, especially groups C and G, also have been isolated from children and young adults with pharyngitis. Other, less common bacterial sources of pharyngitis include *Archanobacterium haemolyticum,* formerly called *Corynebacterium haemolyticum,* an organism that is more likely to infect teenagers and young adults, and also can cause a scarlatiniform rash. *Neisseria gonorrhoeae* should be considered in adolescents who are sexually active or are known to have been exposed, and possibly in abused children.

Among viral causes, adenovirus is the most prevalent. A recent study has found viruses to be responsible for 42% of all cases of pharyngitis in a group of children, aged 6 months through 17.9 years, with acute exudative tonsillitis. Adenovirus was responsible for 19% of the cases, followed by Epstein-Barr virus. Two children (2%) had infections with herpes simplex virus, and five children had infection with *M pneumoniae.*

■ CLINICAL PRESENTATION

Nasopharyngitis tends to be more common in younger children. The presentation can be variable, depending on the agent. Fever usually is present. Infection with adenovirus may be associated with conjunctivitis and exudative pharyngitis, whereas infection with influenza A or B frequently is associated with more severe systemic complaints. The onset of pharyngitis can be acute, with fever and the complaint of sore throat. The child also may have headache, nausea, vomiting, and, occasionally, abdominal pain. Physical examination usually reveals moderate to severe pharyngeal erythema and tonsillar enlargement, and varying degrees of cervical adenitis. The erythema can be associated with follicular, ulcerative, and petechial lesions, as well as areas of exudate. Follicular tonsillitis is fairly characteristic of adenoviral infections, and ulcerative lesions usually are observed with enteroviral infections. Pharyngitis in children is almost entirely acute and self-limited, lasting from 4 to 10 days, depending on the cause.

Streptococcal pharyngitis can have significant suppurative complications, including peritonsillar abscess and bacteremia.

■ DIFFERENTIAL DIAGNOSIS

Because of the numerous organisms that can cause pharyngitis and the significant overlap among them in clinical presentation and findings, it is difficult to make a specific diagnosis based on physical findings alone, such as the presence of exudate. The age and clinical status of the patient and the time of year should be taken into account. Age may be the most important factor in predicting the causative agent, with viral tonsillitis being most common in patients younger than 3 years of age and group A β-hemolytic streptococci found most often in children 6 years of age or older. The presence of rhinitis also is more suggestive of a viral infection. In adolescents and adults, viral infection with *M pneumoniae* and *C pneumoniae* is more likely.

■ SPECIFIC DIAGNOSIS

Because infection with group A streptococci can have significant suppurative and nonsuppurative complications, streptococcal disease must be excluded in all instances of acute pharyngitis. If the child is young (less than 3 years of age) or has obvious viral infection such as pharyngoconjunctival fever (adenovirus) or herpangina, antibiotic therapy is not needed and, therefore, cultures are not indicated.

The only way to make a definite diagnosis of group A streptococcal infection is to identify the organism in the pharynx by culture. Recent confirmation that early treatment of severe streptococcal pharyngitis hastens recovery has made rapid diagnosis of this condition desirable. Even "routine" culture methods may have problems with sensitivity. The use of a single blood agar plate culture for the diagnosis of streptococcal pharyngitis has only 72% sensitivity compared to a two-plate culture method when the plate is read at 2 days. A number of rapid, nonculture antigen detection kits are available for the diagnosis of streptococcal pharyngitis. Although these tests appear to be very specific, they often lack sensitivity.

■ TREATMENT

Because the majority of episodes of pharyngitis are viral and self-limited, specific therapy is not indicated except for a streptococcal pharyngitis. Generally, either intramuscular benzathine penicillin or a 10-day course of oral penicillin or another antibiotic such as erythromycin will be about 90% effective.

(Abridged from Margaret R. Hammerschlag, Pharyngitis, in Oski, DeAngelis, Feigin, McMillan, Warshaw: *Principles and Practice of Pediatrics, Second Edition,* J.B. Lippincott, 1994.)

Oski's Essential Pediatrics,
edited by Kevin B. Johnson and Frank A. Oski.
Lippincott–Raven Publishers,
Philadelphia © 1997

29

Peritonsillar and Retropharyngeal Abscesses

A deep neck abscess is a collection of pus in a potential space bounded by fascia. These potential spaces are areas of least resistance to the spread of infection. An infection may begin with a minimal area of cellulitis and progress to a deep neck abscess, which then may extend to invade adjacent potential spaces; these frequently encompass vital structures in the neck. Destruction or dysfunction of these structures represent the major complications of deep neck infections.

PERITONSILLAR ABSCESS (QUINSY)

A peritonsillar abscess is circumscribed medially by the fibrous wall of the tonsil capsule, and laterally by the superior constrictor muscle. The cause of peritonsillar abscesses is not constant; they may follow any "virulent" tonsillitis, with extension through the fibrous tonsil capsule. Peritonsillar abscesses are rare in young children. They are most common in late adolescence and in the early part of the third decade.

■ CLINICAL MANIFESTATIONS

The patient's recent history may include a sore throat with occasional unilateral pain, malaise, low-grade pyrexia, chills, diaphoresis, dysphagia, reduced oral intake, trismus, and a muffled "hot-potato voice." Trismus results from irritation and reflex spasm of the internal pterygoid muscle. Impaired palatal motion from edema contributes to the muffled voice.

On physical examination, there is minimal to moderate toxicity, dehydration, and drooling. Inspection of the oropharynx may be compromised by trismus. The soft palate is displaced toward the unaffected side, is swollen and red, and frequently contains a palpable fluctuant area. The edematous uvula is pushed across the midline. The displaced tonsil and its crypts rarely are coated with exudate. The breath is fetid, and there is ipsilateral, tender cervical adenopathy. Indirect laryngoscopy reveals supraglottic and lateral pharyngeal edema. The white blood cell count is elevated, with a predominance of polymorphonuclear leukocytes.

■ TREATMENT

Aspiration of the fluctuant mass with an 18-gauge needle commonly confirms the diagnosis of peritonsillar abscess, especially if the pus is located in the superior pole. Aspiration along with intravenous antibiotics has been found to be very effective treatment.

Untreated peritonsillar abscess may point, with spontaneous rupture, or extend to the pterygomaxillary space, with potentially fatal complications.

RETROPHARYNGEAL ABSCESS

The anterior wall of the retropharyngeal space is the middle layer of the deep cervical fascia, which abuts the posterior esophageal wall (the superior pharyngeal constrictor muscle). The deep layer of the deep cervical fascia circumscribes the posterior wall of this potential space. Inferiorly, these two fasciae fuse to limit the depth of this pocket at a level between the first and second thoracic vertebrae. A retropharyngeal abscess can erode inferiorly through the junction of these fasciae to extend posteriorly into the prevertebral space. Subsequently, pus in the prevertebral space can descend inferiorly below the diaphragm to the psoas muscles.

The retropharyngeal space contains two paramedian chains of lymph nodes that receive drainage from the nasopharynx, adenoids, and posterior paranasal sinuses. These structures are prominent in early childhood and undergo atrophy at puberty. Retropharyngeal abscesses are most common in young children and are thought to be secondary to suppurative adenitis of these retropharyngeal nodes. Other sources of infection are penetrating foreign bodies, endoscopy, trauma, pharyngitis, vertebral body osteomyelitis, petrositis, and dental procedures. In adults, tuberculosis and syphilis were common causes of retropharyngeal abscesses in the era before antibiotics.

■ CLINICAL MANIFESTATIONS

The symptoms of retropharyngeal abscess frequently begin insidiously after mild antecedent infection. Airway stridor from edema, cellulitis, or an obstructing mass is common. Laryngeal edema may cause dyspnea and tachypnea. Dysphagia, drooling, and odynophagia may occur. There is no trismus, but a stiff neck secondary to muscle tenderness may be present, along with an ipsilateral tender cervical adenopathy. In adults, the symptoms may be milder. Chest pain may reflect mediastinal extension. Early in the course, there is midline or unilateral swelling of the posterior pharynx. Later, gentle palpation may demonstrate a large fluctuant mass in the posterior pharynx. Vigorous palpation should be avoided because the abscess may rupture into the upper airway.

■ TREATMENT

The administration of intravenous antibiotics combined with incision and drainage is the treatment of choice for retropharyngeal abscess. If the mass is small, a peroral incision made with the patient in Rose's position (supine, with the neck hyperextended) may provide some drainage, but there is a slight risk of aspiration. If the mass is large or if there is persistent fever after peroral drainage, an external incision is preferred. A tracheostomy may be required if there is risk of compromising the airway.

Posterior mediastinitis can result from the spread of infection from the retropharyngeal area into the prevertebral space. Other complications may be seen when the abscess extends to the parapharyngeal space and involves the great vessels and cranial nerves.

■ MICROBIOLOGY OF DEEP NECK ABSCESSES

Group A streptococci (*Streptococcus pyogenes*) and *Staphylococcus aureus* have been considered to be the organisms most frequently associated with pharyngeal space infections. Several recent studies, however, have demonstrated the presence of oral anaerobes in the majority of these infections.

Obtaining adequate cultures is of the greatest importance. The optimal material for culture is an aspirate of the pus obtained at operation. Throat swabs or swabs of the abscess obtained after drainage usually are inadequate because of contamination with normal oropharyngeal flora. A Gram's stain of the exudate provides important clues to the bacterial cause. A Gram's stain showing a mixture of organisms suggests a mixed aerobic–anaerobic infection.

Antibiotic therapy is most effective in conjunction with adequate surgical drainage. Resolution of some peritonsillar and retropharyngeal infections may occur without drainage when therapy is initiated at an early stage of infection, before suppuration occurs. Penicillin and ampicillin probably are adequate antibiotic therapy, but the frequent presence of penicillin-resistant bacteria such as *S aureus* and *Bacteroides* species may warrant the administration of antimicrobial agents that are effective against these organisms, such as clindamycin, amoxicillin/clavulanic acid, ticarcillin/clavulanic acid, ampicillin/sulbactam, or metronidazole in combination with an antistaphylococcic β-lactam. The newer, expanded-spectrum oral cephalosporins such as cefixime, quinolones, and new macrolides do not have adequate gram-positive or anaerobic coverage to enable them to be used alone for these infections.

(Abridged from Paul E. Hammerschlag and Margaret R. Hammerschlag, Perionsillar, Retropharyngeal, and Parapharyngeal Abscesses, in Oski, DeAngelis, Feigin, McMillan, Warshaw: *Principles and Practice of Pediatrics, Second Edition*, J.B. Lippincott, 1994.)

Oski's Essential Pediatrics,
edited by Kevin B. Johnson and Frank A. Oski.
Lippincott–Raven Publishers,
Philadelphia © 1997

30

Otitis Externa

Under normal circumstances, the external auditory canal is protected from infection by a physical barrier of squamous epithelium and a chemical barrier provided by the acidic *p*H of cerumen. Factors that disrupt these barriers, such as trauma, excessive cleansing or wetting, and high temperature and humidity, predispose to development of otitis externa.

■ CLINICAL MANIFESTATIONS

A history of swimming or diving, or of repetitive ear cleansing with soapy water and cotton-tipped swabs often is elicited. Most patients are seen for evaluation of ear pain, itching, and fullness. Pain is exacerbated by manipulation of the pinna or tragus, a feature that is useful in differentiating between otitis externa and otitis media. Purulent discharge may be present in the external auditory canal. The canal walls are diffusely erythematous and edematous. Ipsilateral cervical lymph node enlargement may be noted, but fever usually is absent.

■ DIAGNOSIS

Generally, the diagnosis of otitis externa is made on clinical grounds. A microbiologic diagnosis helps to guide antibiotic therapy for otitis externa. A nasopharyngeal calcium alginate swab is used to obtain purulent material from the auditory canal for routine bacterial cultures and Gram's stain. Special stains and cultures for fungi, mycobacteria, or viruses may be indicated under unusual circumstances. The most common causative agents are *Staphylococcus aureus*, *Pseudomonas aeruginosa* and other gram-negative bacilli, and group A *Streptococcus*. Infections frequently are polymicrobial. Varicella zoster virus may produce external otitis with ipsilateral oral vesicles and facial nerve paralysis.

■ TREATMENT

After cultures are obtained, the auditory canal can be flushed with 3% saline or 2% acetic acid and dried with a cotton-tipped applicator. A suspension of polymyxin B-neomycin-hydrocortisone (Cortisporin) is instilled in the canal four times daily, generally for 10 to 14 days. Swelling may be so severe initially that drops will not enter the auditory canal. In these cases, Cortisporin cream may be placed in the canal on a wick and removed in about 24 hours when inflammation has subsided. Cutaneous sensitivity to neomycin, with local signs and symptoms mimicking those of otitis externa, is a potential complication of therapy with Cortisporin. Prevention of recurrent otitis externa may be accomplished by use of 2% acetic acid ear drops after swimming.

(Abridged from Mark W. Kline, Otitis Externa, in Oski, DeAngelis, Feigin, McMillan, Warshaw: *Principles and Practice of Pediatrics, Second Edition*, J.B. Lippincott, 1994.)

Oski's Essential Pediatrics,
edited by Kevin B. Johnson and Frank A. Oski.
Lippincott–Raven Publishers,
Philadelphia © 1997

31

Otitis Media

Otitis media is one of the most common infectious diseases of childhood. In one large study, 33% of pediatric office visits for illness of any kind were attributable to disease of the middle ear (acute otitis media or otitis media with effusion). Infants and young children are at highest risk for the development of otitis media, with a peak prevalence between 6 and 36 months of age. Two of every three children have at least one episode of otitis media before their first birthday.

Otitis media occurs more commonly in boys than in girls, and is particularly prevalent among Eskimos and Native Americans, and among children with cleft palate or other craniofacial defects. A familial predisposition to otitis media may exist in some cases. Other implicated predisposing factors include lower socioeconomic group status, bottle-feeding in the horizontal position, bottle-feeding versus breast-feeding, day care center attendance, and atopy. In general, the highest rates of otitis media are observed in the winter months, coinciding with the peak incidence of respiratory viral infections.

Either obstruction or abnormal patency of the eustachian tube may lead to the development of otitis media. Intrinsic (*eg,* inflammation secondary to infection or allergy) and extrinsic (*eg,* tumor or adenoid enlargement) types of mechanical eustachian tube obstruction are recognized. Functional obstruction, caused by persistent collapse of an abnormally compliant eustachian tube, an abnormal active opening mechanism, or both, is common in young children and individuals with cleft palate. An abnormally patent, or patulous, eustachian tube, which is found commonly among Native American populations, permits reflux of nasopharyngeal secretions into the middle ear. Reflux, aspiration, or insufflation of nasopharyngeal bacteria into the middle ear on any basis leads to mucoperiosteal inflammation and otitis media.

TABLE 31-1. Bacterial Etiology of Acute Otitis Media in Children*

Bacterial Isolate	Prevalence (%)
Streptococcus pneumoniae	31
Haemophilus influenzae	22
Moraxella catarrahalis	7
Group A *Streptococcus*	2
Enteric gram-negative bacteria	1
Staphylococcus aureus	1
Other	3
No bacterial isolate	33

Based on cultures obtained by needle tympanocentesis.

ACUTE OTITIS MEDIA

■ CLINICAL MANIFESTATIONS

The classic description of acute otitis media is of a child with upper respiratory tract infection who suddenly develops fever, otalgia, and hearing loss. A classic presentation, however, may be the exception rather than the rule. Fever and hearing loss are inconstant features of the disease, and otalgia may not be reported. In many young children in particular, otitis media must be inferred on the basis of nonspecific symptoms (*eg,* fretfulness or irritability, anorexia, loose stools) and subtle findings suggestive of middle ear disease (*eg,* scratching or tugging at the ear). Otitis media must be excluded before any child is labeled as having fever without localizing signs, or fever of undetermined origin.

The appearance of the tympanic membrane is key to the diagnosis of acute otitis media. All wax and debris must be removed from the external canal before examination. Otoscopy usually reveals a hyperemic, opaque tympanic membrane with distorted or absent light reflex and indistinct landmarks. A red appearance of the drum may be noted if the child is agitated or if inadequate illumination is provided; this is not evidence of otitis media in the absence of other findings. Adequate assessment of tympanic membrane mobility requires pneumatic otoscopy, using an ear speculum large enough to occlude the external canal completely. Decreased mobility of the drum results from either eustachian tube dysfunction or middle ear effusion.

■ ETIOLOGIES

The approximate prevalence rates of various bacterial agents of otitis media beyond the neonatal period are shown in Table 31–1. Most *Haemophilus influenzae* isolates from the middle ear are nontypeable; only a minority are type b. Many *H influenzae* strains and most strains of *Moraxella catarrhalis* produce β-lactamase and, therefore, are resistant to ampicillin and penicillin. Studies assessing the role of viruses have found a low rate of isolation from middle ear fluid, with respiratory syncytial virus and influenza viruses being most common.

■ TREATMENT

A number of agents that are active against the common bacterial pathogens of otitis media are available (Table 31–2).

As a rule, children younger than 1 month who have otitis media should be admitted to the hospital. Cultures of blood, cerebrospinal fluid (CSF), and middle ear fluid should be obtained, and parenteral antibiotic therapy should be initiated. If blood and CSF cultures are sterile after 72 hours and the infant appears well, with disease limited to the middle ear, therapy may be completed with an oral antibiotic that is active against the middle ear isolate.

Oral amoxicillin is a reasonable first choice for the treatment of otitis media in older infants and children. An alternative agent may be needed if there is no response to therapy in 72 to 96 hours, or if a resistant organism is cultured from middle ear fluid. Cefuroxime axetil, cefixime, cefpodoxime proxetil, and amoxicillin/clavulanate are considerably more expensive than are other alternative antibiotics. Antibiotic ear drops are of no value in acute otitis media. Supportive therapy, including acetaminophen and local heat, may be helpful in children with acute otitis media. Sedation should be avoided.

Ideally, children with acute otitis media should be reexamined at the end of therapy to document resolution of tympanic membrane inflammation. Complete resolution of middle ear effusion may require 2 to 3 months.

■ RECURRENT ACUTE OTITIS MEDIA

Recurrent episodes of acute otitis media occur commonly. Underlying susceptibility to middle ear infection is important in the development of recurrent otitis media; recurrences represent reinfection more often than recrudescence or relapse. Early development of otitis media caused by *Streptococcus pneumoniae* seems particularly likely to predispose to recurrent otitis media.

Several strategies have been employed for the prevention of recurrent acute otitis media. Antibiotic prophylaxis with amoxicillin (20 mg/kg once daily) or sulfisoxazole (75 mg/kg/d in two divided doses) is reasonable in the child who has at least three episodes of acute otitis media within 6 months or four episodes in 1 year. Prophylaxis generally is continued for 3 to 6 months, at which time the antibiotic is discontinued and the child is observed. Pneumococcal vaccine may benefit individual children, but it is least efficacious in infants, the group at highest risk for recurrent disease. Myringotomy with tympanostomy tube insertion is an option for patients who fail to respond to antibiotic prophylaxis. Adenoidectomy may be of benefit for selected patients.

TABLE 31-2. Antimicrobial Therapy for Acute Otitis Media

Age of Patient	Drug	Dosage*
Less than 1 mo	Ampicillin and Gentamicin	200 mg/kg/d IM or IV in 4 divided doses
		7.5 mg/kg/d IM or IV in 3 divided doses
1 mo to 15 y	Amoxicillin	40 mg/kg/d po in 3 divided doses
	or	
	Trimethoprim/sulfamethoxazole	8–10 mg/kg/d trimethoprim po in 2 divided doses
	or	
	Erythromycin/sulfisoxazole	40 mg/kg/d erythromycin po in 3 divided doses
	or	
	Cefuroxime axetil	250–500 mg/d po in 2 divided doses
	or	
	Cefixime	8 mg/kg/d po in 1 dose
	or	
	Cefpodoxime proxetil	10 mg/kg/d po in 2 divided doses
	or	
	Amoxicillin/clavulanate	40 mg/kg/d po in 3 divided doses

*IM, intramuscularly; IV, intravenously; po, orally.

The relative efficacies of the various strategies for prophylaxis, alone and in combination, are unknown.

■ OTITIS MEDIA WITH EFFUSION

After an episode of acute otitis media, 10% of children have middle ear effusion that persists for 3 months or longer (chronic otitis media with effusion). Clinically, otitis media with effusion is characterized by a sensation of fullness in the ears, muffled hearing, and tinnitus. Pneumatic otoscopy usually reveals an opaque tympanic membrane with decreased mobility.

Bacteria are recovered from one third to one half of all middle ear fluid specimens obtained at myringotomy in cases of otitis media with effusion. The bacteriology closely mimics that of acute otitis media. It is not known whether the bacteria have a direct pathogenic role, but an initial course of antibiotic therapy similar to that used for acute otitis media seems warranted. Oral decongestant–antihistamine combinations and corticosteroids have not been found to be effective in the treatment of persistent middle ear effusion. Evaluation for respiratory allergy, obstructive adenoid enlargement, immune deficiency, or anatomic abnormalities such as submucous cleft palate may be necessary in patients whose disease does not respond to treatment.

For patients whose condition fails to respond to medical therapy, myringotomy with tympanostomy tube insertion may prevent subsequent accumulation of middle ear fluid and improve hearing. Tympanostomy tubes also are used to prevent structural middle ear damage and cholesteatoma in selected cases. Tonsillectomy is not efficacious in the treatment of otitis media with effusion.

■ COMPLICATIONS

Serious complications of otitis media are uncommon when appropriate medical therapy is initiated promptly. Extracranial complications include serous or purulent labyrinthitis, mastoiditis, osteomyelitis of the temporal bone, and facial nerve paralysis. Intracranial complications are subdivided into meningeal and extrameningeal complications. Epidural and subdural abscess, meningitis, lateral sinus thrombosis, and otitic hydrocephalus are reported meningeal complications of otitis media. Lateral sinus thrombosis is characterized by high temperature, chills, signs and symptoms of increased intracranial pressure, and septicemia with embolization. The mortality rate is about 25%. Otitic hydrocephalus may follow acute otitis media by several weeks, and usually is associated with impaired intracranial venous drainage. Hydrocephalus commonly subsides spontaneously. Extrameningeal complications of otitis media include brain abscess and petrositis.

(Abridged from Mark W. Kline, Otitis Media, in Oski, DeAngelis, Feigin, McMillan, Warshaw: *Principles and Practice of Pediatrics, Second Edition*, J.B. Lippincott, 1994.)

Oski's Essential Pediatrics,
edited by Kevin B. Johnson and Frank A. Oski.
Lippincott–Raven Publishers,
Philadelphia © 1997

32

Mastoiditis

Inflammation of the mucoperiosteal lining of the mastoid air cells usually accompanies otitis media. Clinically evident suppurative infection, or mastoiditis, develops when inflammation causes progressive swelling and obstruction to drainage of exudative materials from the mastoid. Mastoiditis is uncommon in this era of effective antibiotic therapy for otitis media, but it remains a potentially life-threatening disease requiring prompt recognition and appropriate treatment.

■ CLINICAL MANIFESTATIONS

Children with mastoiditis almost invariably have otitis media concomitantly. Classically, the child with acute mastoiditis presents with fever, otalgia, and postauricular swelling and redness. Swelling typically occurs over the mastoid process, pushing the earlobe superiorly and laterally, but in infancy, it may occur above the ear, displacing the pinna inferiorly and laterally. The clinical presentation of acute mastoiditis may be quite subtle, particularly in the child who has received oral antibiotic therapy for otitis media (so-called masked mastoiditis). Mastoiditis should be considered in a patient with otitis media that is unresponsive to antibiotic therapy.

■ DIAGNOSIS

In some cases, the diagnosis of mastoiditis can be made with confidence on clinical grounds alone. Plain roentgenograms may show coalescence of mastoid air cells and loss of normal bony trabeculations. Computed tomography sometimes is helpful in cases in which clinical findings and plain roentgenograms are equivocal or nonspecific.

A bacteriologic diagnosis is highly desirable in cases of mastoiditis. Tympanocentesis obtained through an intact tympanic membrane yields bacteriologic information that correlates well with specimens obtained from the mastoid bone itself. Common causative agents of acute mastoiditis include *Streptococcus pneumoniae*, group A *Streptococcus*, *Staphylococcus aureus*, and *Haemophilus influenzae*. *Mycobacterium tuberculosis* rarely causes chronic mastoiditis today, but it should be considered if there are suggestive epidemiologic or historic features in the case.

■ TREATMENT

Patients with acute onset of symptoms and no evidence of intracranial or local extracranial complications of mastoiditis usually are treated initially with myringotomy and parenteral antibiotics alone. Signs of increased intracranial pressure or meningeal irritation signal complications of mastoiditis, such as meningitis, brain abscess, epidural abscess, subdural empyema, or venous sinus thrombosis. A postauricular fluctuant area implies subperiosteal abscess formation. Because of proximity to the mastoid bone, other local structures may be involved by infection, producing facial nerve paralysis, jugular venous thrombosis, or internal carotid artery erosion and hemorrhage. Lack of appropriate response to medical therapy or development of complications necessitates mastoidectomy and possibly other surgical interventions.

The initial selection of specific antibiotic therapy is made empirically, with some guidance provided by Gram's stain of specimens from the middle ear or mastoid. In acute mastoiditis, a combination of a penicillinase-resistant penicillin (such as nafcillin or oxacillin) and one of the third-generation cephalosporins (such as cefotaxime or ceftriaxone) is reasonable. Provided complications have not occurred, and if it is feasible on the basis of the organisms' susceptibility to oral agents, the course of therapy can be completed orally once signs of acute inflammation have subsided. The minimum course of therapy for mastoiditis is 21 days, and it may be longer if complications of infection have occurred. For patients discharged on oral antibiotic therapy, careful monitoring of compliance and documentation of bactericidal activity in serum are desirable.

(Abridged from Mark W. Kline, Mastoiditis, in Oski, DeAngelis, Feigin, McMillan, Warshaw: *Principles and Practice of Pediatrics, Second Edition*, J.B. Lippincott, 1994.)

Oski's Essential Pediatrics,
edited by Kevin B. Johnson and Frank A. Oski.
Lippincott–Raven Publishers,
Philadelphia © 1997

33

Epiglottitis/Supraglottitis

Supraglottitis is an inflammation of the structures above the glottis, including the epiglottis, arytenoepiglottic folds, and arytenoids. The most common site of involvement is the epiglottis.

■ ETIOLOGY

Haemophilus influenzae type b causes more than 90% of all supraglottitis involving the epiglottis. This, undoubtedly, will change, however, consequent to the increased use of *H influenzae* type b conjugate vaccines in infancy. Rarely, other organisms, including *Staphylococcus aureus*, *Streptococcus pyogenes*, and *Streptococcus pneumoniae*, have been documented. Viral causes, specifically parainfluenza virus and herpesviruses, have been reported to cause supraglottitis in individual cases.

■ EPIDEMIOLOGY

Although supraglottitis resulting from infection with *H influenzae* type b can occur at any time from infancy to adulthood, it most often affects children between 2 and 7 years of age. Epiglottitis is unique among illnesses caused by *H influenzae* type b in that it characteristically develops in older children; infection with this bacterial species usually is seen in those aged 3 months to 3 years. Cases occur year-round, and boys and girls are affected equally. When *S pyogenes* causes supraglottitis, the children most often are of early school age and their illness occurs during the winter and early spring.

■ CLINICAL MANIFESTATIONS

The child with typical epiglottitis usually has an abrupt onset of sore throat and dysphagia. High temperature (39°C to 40°C) generally is noted almost simultaneously. Within a short time, evidence of toxemia and respiratory distress develops. The youngster appears extremely anxious and prefers to remain sitting up, usually leaning forward with the chin hyperextended. The respiratory effort is slow and labored; drooling as a manifestation of dysphagia begins. Cough, hoarseness, and stridor are belated symptoms if they occur at all. The interval from the onset of clinical symptoms until appearance at the emergency department because of fever and progressive respiratory distress generally is less than 12 hours.

■ DIAGNOSIS

If the diagnosis of epiglottitis is unclear but suspected and the degree of respiratory distress is moderate, a lateral neck radiograph can be performed. The characteristic finding in cases of epiglottitis is the so-called thumb sign, reflecting the dimensions of the swollen epiglottis. In addition, there may be ballooning of the hypopharynx as a nonspecific indication of upper airway obstruction (Figure 33–1).

When a child has classic signs and symptoms of epiglottitis, the diagnosis is straightforward and should be confirmed in the operating room under direct vision when intubation of the airway is accomplished. In these cases, a lateral neck radiograph may delay airway establishment. The tentative diagnosis of epiglottitis constitutes a medical emergency. Every effort is made to keep the child calm and comfortable; manipulations are kept to a minimum. Under no circumstance is the child placed in the supine position. Parents are encouraged to accompany the youngster until definitive treatment is accomplished. After very rapid assembly of a team that includes an otolaryngologist, an anesthetist, and a pediatrician, direct inspection of the upper airway should be undertaken (in a setting in which intubation can be accomplished) to confirm the diagnosis. After the airway has been secured, a blood culture and a surface culture of the epiglottis should be performed. Blood culture results almost always are positive for *H influenzae* type b.

■ DIFFERENTIAL DIAGNOSIS

When a child presents with acute onset of fever, dysphagia, and labored respirations, diagnostic considerations include laryngotracheobronchitis with secondary bacterial infection (bacterial tracheitis), uvulitis, diphtheria, and retropharyngeal or peritonsillar abscess. Severe laryngotracheobronchitis occasionally can be caused by parainfluenza or influenza viruses without bacterial superinfection; however, patients with uncomplicated viral croup usually have a more indolent presentation, with lower-grade fever and slower progression of respiratory distress. In croup, barking cough and hoarseness are prominent, the respiratory rate is rapid, and the patient spontaneously assumes the supine position.

If the child is cooperative, inspection of the mouth and throat should be undertaken gingerly, without a tongue blade. This may reveal a peritonsillar abscess, uvulitis, or a diphtheritic pharyngeal membrane. Diphtheria is a rare infection seen only in certain geographic areas of the United States. A history of immunization against diphtheria and the absence of a pharyngeal membrane on physical examination make the diagnosis unlikely. A lateral neck film can help to diagnosis a retropharyngeal abscess.

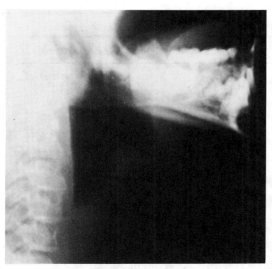

Figure 33-1. Lateral neck radiograph showing a positive "thumb" sign and ballooning of the hypopharynx.

■ COMPLICATIONS

The most serious complication of supraglottitis is complete airway obstruction leading to respiratory arrest and hypoxia before arrival at the hospital. Potential therapeutic complications of supraglottitis include aspiration, tube dislodgment, irritation or erosion of the trachea, and extubation. Pneumomediastinum and pneumothorax also may occur. Pulmonary edema may complicate epiglottitis either before or after artificial airway placement.

■ TREATMENT

The most important component of treatment of epiglottitis is securing the airway. This can be accomplished by nasotracheal intubation or tracheostomy, depending on the facilities available at the receiving hospital. In general, intubation is accomplished with a tube that is slightly smaller than that which ordinarily would fit the airway. After the child has been intubated successfully, intravenous antimicrobial agents are initiated. Extubation generally can be accomplished in 24 to 48 hours. Prompt defervescence generally occurs after the initiation of appropriate antimicrobial treatment; oral medication can be used to complete a 7- to 10-day course of therapy as soon as extubation has been accomplished and oral intake is ensured. The index case should receive rifampin to eradicate colonization with *H influenzae* type b if there are susceptible children in the household or child care setting. Intimate contacts of the child with epiglottitis also may require rifampin prophylaxis if they are susceptible to invasive *H influenzae* type b disease.

(Abridged from Ellen R. Wald, Epiglottitis/Supraglottitis, in Oski, DeAngelis, Feigin, McMillan, Warshaw: *Principles and Practice of Pediatrics, Second Edition*, J.B. Lippincott, 1994.)

Oski's Essential Pediatrics, edited by Kevin B. Johnson and Frank A. Oski. Lippincott–Raven Publishers, Philadelphia © 1997

34

Croup

The term *croup* describes a clinical syndrome characterized by a barking cough, hoarseness, and inspiratory stridor.

ACUTE LARYNGOTRACHEITIS

The term *croup* usually refers to acute laryngotracheitis, a respiratory disease that is prevalent in preschool children. Acute laryngotracheitis is seen in children of any age but is most common between the first and third years of life; boys are affected more often than are girls. The causative agents are respiratory viruses exclusively, and the illness frequently occurs in epidemic patterns. The viruses most frequently implicated are parainfluenza 1 and 3, but influenza A and B, respiratory syncytial virus, parainfluenza 2, adenoviruses, and *Mycoplasma pneumoniae* also may cause croup. In summertime croup, the enteroviruses (coxsackievirus A and B and echovirus) are the usual cause.

■ PATHOPHYSIOLOGY

Transmission of the causative virus is by the respiratory route, either direct droplet spread or hand-to-mucosa inoculation. After acquisition, primary viral infection involves the nasopharynx. Viral replication ensues, producing nasal symptoms, and infection spreads locally to involve the larynx and trachea.

■ CLINICAL MANIFESTATIONS

The usual onset of croup is with the signs and symptoms of a common cold: coryza, nasal congestion, sore throat, and cough, with variable fever. The cough becomes prominent, with a barklike quality (akin to that of a puppy or seal), and the voice becomes hoarse. Many children with this syndrome do not ever visit a physician. The child may begin to have evidence of respiratory distress, however, with the onset of tachypnea, stridor (when agitated or crying), nasal flaring, and suprasternal and intercostal retractions. The increase in respiratory distress prompts a visit to the physician or emergency department. Usually, the illness peaks in severity over 3 to 5 days and then begins to resolve. Most characteristically, the signs and symptoms worsen in the evening.

In typical cases of acute laryngotracheitis, the diagnosis is made easily on clinical grounds and no radiographs or blood tests are required. If an anteroposterior radiograph is performed, a so-called steeple sign may be seen as a consequence of subglottic swelling. Indications for hospitalization, which is undertaken in about 10% of children with laryngotracheitis, include the presence of stridor, anxiety or restlessness, cyanosis, or retractions at rest. Children for whom close follow-up cannot be arranged or whose families cannot provide the necessary observation and care also should be admitted to the hospital.

As laryngeal inflammation increases and secretions accumulate, respiratory distress increases and complete obstruc-tion may occur. Almost always, this progression is gradual and is signaled by slowly increasing respiratory rate and effort, increased stridor at rest, and pallor or cyanosis. Agitation increases and air entry is poor. In about 5% of hospitalized patients, intubation is required to overcome the respiratory obstruction. Children who have a deteriorating respiratory status should be monitored in an intensive care unit (ICU) by staff who are skilled in the care of pediatric patients.

One of the most important principles of treatment of patients with croup or other upper airway problems is minimal disturbance. Any stimulus that upsets the child will result in crying, which causes hyperventilation and an increase in respiratory distress. The parents should be encouraged to hold and comfort the child whenever possible, and invasive procedures should be kept to a minimum.

Treatment strategies for acute infectious laryngotracheitis have included mist, racemic epinephrine, and corticosteroids. Although not shown to be of demonstrable benefit, mist therapy has been considered standard management. Racemic epinephrine, in use since 1971, is a potentially lifesaving therapy in patients with croup who are in moderate to severe respiratory distress. Administration results in rapid clinical improvement; by its β-adrenergic vasoconstrictive effects on mucosal edema, racemic epinephrine increases the airway diameter.

The use of steroids in acute laryngotracheitis has been controversial for 3 decades. They appear to offer neither great benefit nor excessive risk when used for a short period. There seems to be a subgroup of patients (perhaps those with spasmodic croup) who may benefit from steroid use, although they are not easy to identify before treatment. Accordingly, some investigators recommend that, if the clinical syndrome of croup is severe enough to warrant the use of racemic epinephrine, a single dose of steroids (dexamethasone 0.30 to 0.50 mg/kg per dose) should be employed as a test dose. Although steroids do not have an immediate effect, improvement within 6 hours of their use suggests efficacy, and a repeat dose may be given. If no improvement is noted in 6 hours, subsequent doses are withheld. Antibiotics are not indicated in the routine treatment of children with this croup syndrome.

Most patients who are hospitalized for acute laryngotracheitis are treated with supportive therapies (mist and, occasionally, oxygen and intravenous fluids) and can be discharged in a few days. If intubation is required, the nasotra-

TABLE 34-1. Differential Diagnosis of Acute Infectious Obstruction in the Region of the Larynx

Category	Epiglottitis	Acute Laryngotracheitis	Laryngotracheobronchitis	Spasmodic Croup
Prodrome	Usually none or mild upper respiratory infection	Usually upper respiratory symptoms	Usually upper respiratory symptoms	None or minimal coryza
Age	1–8 y	3 mo–3 y	3 mo–8 y	3 mo–3 y
Onset	Rapid; 4–12 h	Gradual	Variable	Sudden, always at night
Fever	High (19.5°C)	Variable	Usually high	None
Hoarseness/barking cough	No	Yes	Yes	Yes
Dysphagia	Yes	No	No	No
Toxic appearance	Yes	No	Yes	No
Microbiology	Blood culture positive for *Haemophilus influenzae* type b	Viral infection	Viral infection with bacterial superinfection	Viral infection with allergic component

Modified from Cherry JD. Croup. In: Feigin RD, Cherry JD, eds. Textbook of pediatric infectious diseases. *2nd ed. Philadelphia: WB Saunders; 1987.*

cheal tube frequently must remain in place for 3 to 4 days until an air leak develops around it, reflecting subsidence of the inflammation. Hospitalization for several days after extubation is desirable to ensure respiratory stability and the reintroduction of oral feeding.

SPASMODIC CROUP

Acute spasmodic croup is a clinical entity seen in exactly the same age group and during the same season, and is caused by the same viruses, as is acute infectious laryngotracheitis. Typically, children experiencing an episode of acute spasmodic croup go to sleep well or with the mildest of upper respiratory infections. They awaken in the night with a barking cough, hoarseness, inspiratory stridor, and variable degrees of respiratory distress. They always are afebrile. Most patients respond to mist therapy, provided by the bathroom shower or a cool-water vaporizer. Occasionally, the night air inhaled en route to the hospital is sufficient to reduce the dyspnea. Although most episodes are mild to moderate, airway support occasionally is required. Recurrences may be observed during the same evening or on the subsequent two to three nights.

This condition may be differentiated from infectious laryngotracheitis endoscopically. Whereas examination of the mucosa in the former reveals an erythematous, inflamed, velvety appearance, the mucosa is pale and boggy in the latter. Although viral cultures yield the same agents as in laryngotracheitis, the mucosal appearance and clinical course suggest an allergic component of the pathophysiologic process. This group of patients usually benefits from racemic epinephrine if the degree of respiratory distress mandates its use. Likewise, these patients may do well with corticosteroid therapy, reflecting either the allergic nature of the process or the natural history of a self-limited disease.

■ DIFFERENTIAL DIAGNOSIS

The differential diagnosis in patients who have upper airway obstruction includes both infectious and noninfectious problems. A common noninfectious cause is foreign body aspiration. Foreign body aspiration occurs most often in children 2 to 4 years of age. A history of an abrupt onset of symptoms should arouse concern about this diagnosis. Endoscopy is diagnostic and therapeutic in this situation.

The remaining causes of acute infectious obstruction in the region of the larynx are contrasted in Table 34–1. Laryngitis is not included because it rarely presents difficulty in differential diagnosis.

(Abridged from Ellen R. Wald, Croup, in Oski, DeAngelis, Feigin, McMillan, Warshaw: *Principles and Practice of Pediatrics, Second Edition*, J.B. Lippincott, 1994.)

Oski's Essential Pediatrics,
edited by Kevin B. Johnson and Frank A. Oski.
Lippincott–Raven Publishers,
Philadelphia © 1997

35

Cervical Lymphadenitis

Cervical adenitis is inflammation of one or more lymph nodes of the neck. In children, the most common causes of cervical lymph node enlargement exceeding 10 mm are reactive hyperplasia in response to an infectious stimulus in the head or neck and infection of the node itself. Self-limited cervical lymph node inflammation occurs in association with upper respiratory tract infection as the lymphatic channels drain proximally affected sites. In 80% of children with acute cervical adenitis, the submaxillary, submandibular, and deep cervical nodes are inflamed, because these are the routes by which much of the lymphatic drainage of the head and neck proceeds. Malignancy is the second most common cause of lymph node enlargement in children, but neoplasia constitutes a minority of neck masses. Children with malignant lesions tend to have systemic complaints and firm, nontender nodes that are located characteristically in the posterior triangle or supraclavicular regions.

■ EPIDEMIOLOGY

Although patients at any age may be affected, the majority of children with cervical adenitis are 1 to 4 years of age. This age restriction and peak in incidence reflects the prevalence of infections caused by *Staphylococcus aureus,* group A *Streptococcus,* and atypical mycobacteria. The sexes are affected equally, with two exceptions. Some studies indicate a female predominance for granulomatous lymphadenitis caused by atypical mycobacteria, and young infants with the cellulitis-adenitis syndrome caused by group B *Streptococcus* are predominantly male (75%). There is no racial predilection for acute bacterial cervical adenitis (Table 35–1). A history of dog or cat contact, bite, or scratch may be a helpful clue in suggesting specific causative agents, such as *Pasteurella multocida, Toxoplasma gondii,* or the gram-negative pleomorphic rod that causes cat-scratch disease (CSD). Similarly, a history of a minor inoculation wound of the skin proximal to affected cervical lymph nodes should suggest the possibility of soil organisms such as *Nocardia brasiliensis,* atypical mycobacteria, and gram-negative enteric organisms. Finally, the human immunodeficiency virus (HIV) should be added to the list of agents causing cervical adenopathy, and, because most HIV-infected children are infected perinatally, the epidemiology reflects that of the mothers.

■ CLINICAL MANIFESTATIONS

Cervical adenitis may be classified according to its mode of presentation as acute, in which symptoms are of less than 2 weeks in duration, or subacute to chronic (Table 35–2). The causative agents tend to fall into one of these two categories, although there may be overlap. Overall, about three fourths of all the infections have an acute presentation. The duration of lymph node swelling is less than 2 days in half of all children with acute adenitis, and less than 1 week in the majority of them. Acute bilateral cervical adenitis generally is associated with upper respiratory tract viral infection

TABLE 35-1. Differentiation of Bacterial and Mycobacterial Cervical Adenitis

Clinical Characteristics	Bacteria	Atypical Mycobacteria	*Mycobacterium tuberculosis*
Onset	Acute (<2 wk)	Subacute to chronic	Subacute to chronic
Age (y)	1–4*	1–4	All
Rate	All	White	Black, Hispanic, or Asian
Regional node distribution	Unilateral	Unilateral	Unilateral or bilateral
Local tenderness	Mild to marked	Usually absent	Usually absent
Exposure to adult with tuberculosis	Absent	Absent	Present
Abnormal chest radiograph appearance	Never	Never	Sometimes
Mantoux test (PPD-S) result >15 mm induration	Never	Rare	Often

Seventy percent to 80% of cases.

Modified from Butler KM, Baker CJ. Cervical lymphadenitis. In: Feigin RD, Cherry JD, eds., Textbook of pediatric infectious diseases. 3rd ed. Philadelphia: WB Saunders; 1992:221.

or with streptococcal pharyngitis. Lymph nodes may be tender, but none of the other signs of inflammation are found. Exanthem and focal findings such as gingivostomatitis are features that suggest either a respiratory viral or a streptococcal cause.

Children with acute unilateral cervical lymphadenitis generally have a paucity of systemic manifestations. A history of upper respiratory tract symptoms such as sore throat, earache, coryza, or impetigo can be elicited from one fourth to one third of patients. The infected node usually ranges in diameter from 2.5 to 6.0 cm, is tender, and exhibits varying degrees of warmth and erythema. *S aureus* and group A *Streptococcus* are the causative agents in 50% to 90% of infections. Less commonly, other bacteria residing in the oropharynx are implicated (see Table 35–2). Streptococcal adenitis occurs in younger children, is accompanied more often by generalized adenopathy, has a shorter duration of symptoms (4 versus 10 days), and is less likely to suppurate than are nodes infected by *S aureus*. Concomitant lymphadenopathy at other sites is observed in as many as one third of children with acute unilateral cervical adenitis, most commonly in association with a generalized viral process or a group A streptococcal infection. Hepatomegaly or splenomegaly is rare, however, and, if found, should suggest a generalized process (*eg*, HIV infection, Epstein-Barr virus, tuberculosis, reticuloendotheliosis, and so forth).

Table 35–2 lists common causes of cervical adenitis. The most common causes of subacute to chronic cervical adenitis are mycobacteria, cat-scratch bacillus, *Nocardia*, and Epstein-Barr virus. Nontuberculous adenitis has an age distribution similar to that of acute bacterial adenitis, and almost invariably is unilateral and localized to a single submandibular or tonsillar node. Although marked erythema may develop, these masses are "cold" and there is less tenderness than would be expected given the degree of erythema. Mantoux skin testing is a helpful discriminator between atypical and typical mycobacterium, because the diameter of the reaction usually exceeds 15 mm when infection is caused by *M tuberculosis*, whereas reactions of smaller diameter commonly are found in children with infection caused by atypical mycobacteria.

Cat-scratch disease is a lymphocutaneous syndrome in which regional lymph nodes proximal to the subcutaneous inoculation of the cat-scratch bacillus become inflamed. Fever, persisting for as long as 1 week, occurs in 25% of children, but constitutional symptoms of malaise, anorexia, and headache are mild or absent in the majority of them. In 15%

(range, 10% to 30%), the lymph nodes suppurate. Adenitis usually resolves within 2 weeks to 2 months, but it may persist for a more protracted interval in a minority of children (up to 20%).

■ DIFFERENTIAL DIAGNOSIS

Noninfectious causes of cervical adenitis include a variety of benign and malignant entities (Table 35–3). Location is a helpful distinguishing feature, because about half of all masses located in the posterior triangle are malignant tumors, whereas masses found in the anterior triangle, with the exception of those involving the thyroid, tend to be benign. Masses that extend across the sternocleidomastoid muscle to involve both the anterior and the posterior triangles should be viewed as potentially malignant. Finally, age is a discriminator to some extent, because lymphoreticular malignant tumors occur more frequently among older children, in contrast to the infectious causes that predominate in children 1 to 4 years of age.

Lymphoid neoplasms and neuroblastoma constitute two thirds of all malignant neck masses seen in children (see Table 35–2). Lymphomas, both Hodgkin's and non-Hodgkin's, are more common than is neuroblastoma in older children, whereas neuroblastoma is the most common malignant lesion in young children. Kawasaki disease deserves special mention, as it is a common cause of unilateral anterior cervical adenitis for which the causative agent is undefined. This syndrome is diagnosed by clinical criteria that include persistence of fever for longer than 5 days and the presence of other major features (conjunctivitis, truncal exanthem, oral manifestations, and involvement of the hands and feet).

Congenital lesions of the neck may simulate cervical adenitis. The most common of these is the thyroglossal duct cyst, which may be distinguished by its midline location and movement with tongue protrusion. These cysts may become infected secondarily, and even may progress to frank suppuration. The existence of a pit, dimple, or draining sinus along the anterior margin of the sternocleidomastoid muscle serves to differentiate between branchial cleft cyst and cervical adenitis, although the distinction may be difficult if the cyst becomes infected secondarily. Cystic hygromas are soft masses that transilluminate, aiding in their differentiation from inflammatory or malignant neck masses.

TABLE 35-2. Infectious Agents or Diseases Associated With Cervical Adenitis

Agent or Disease	Frequency*	Onset Acute (A) or Subacute to Chronic (S)	Generalized Adenopathy
BACTERIAL			
Staphylococcus aureus	+++	A	−
Group A Streptococcus	+++	A	+
Anaerobes	+++	A/S	−
Cat-scratch disease bacillus	+++	S	−
Atypical mycobacteria	+++	S	−
Mycobacterium tuberculosis	++	S	±
Nocardia brasiliensis	++	S	−
Gram-negative enteric organisms	++	A	−
Group B Streptococcus†	++	A	−
Pasteurella multocida	++	A	+
Haemophilus influenzae	+	A	−
Yersinia pestis	+	A	+
Actinomyces israelii	+	A	−
Diphtheria	+	A	−
Tularemia	+	A	−
Syphilis	+	S	+
Anthrax	+	A	−
VIRAL			
Epstein-Barr virus	+++	A/S	+
Herpes simplex	+++	A	−
Cytomegalovirus	+++	A/S	+
Adenovirus	+++	A	−
Varicella	++	A	+
Enterovirus	+++	A	+
Human herpes virus-6	+	S	+
Measles	+	A	+
Mumps	+	A	−
Rubella	+	A	+
Human immunodeficiency virus	+	S	+
FUNGAL			
Histoplasmosis	+	S	+
Cryptococcus	+	S	−
Aspergillosis	+	S	−
Candida	+	S	−
Coccidioides	+	S	−
Sporotrichosis	+	A	−
PARASITIC			
Toxoplasma gondii	+	S	+

*Key: +++, common; ++, uncommon; +, rare.
†Neonates and young infants only.

Modified from Butler KM, Baker CJ. Cervical lymphadenitis. In: Feigin RD, Cherry JD, eds. Textbook of pediatric infectious diseases. 3rd ed. Philadelphia: WB Saunders; 1992:224.

■ DIAGNOSIS

As stated previously, a detailed history to ascertain the duration of the illness (acute or subacute to chronic), the presence or absence of associated systemic symptoms, animal exposures, preceding trauma, contact with an adult with tuberculosis, the presence of maternal risk factors for HIV infection, drug usage (especially phenytoin [Dilantin]), ingestion of unusual substances (undercooked meat, unpasteurized milk), or recent travel may yield important diagnostic clues regarding the cause of cervical adenitis. The physical examination reveals the location of the adenitis (anterior or posterior triangles), the presence of dental disease, noncervical lymphadenopathy, oropharyngeal or

TABLE 35-3. Noninfectious Causes of Cervical Adenitis

Causes	Frequency*	Associated With Generalized Adenopathy
NEOPLASM		
Hodgkin's disease	++	+
Lymphosarcoma, rhabdomyosarcoma	++	−
Non-Hodgkin's lymphoma	++	+
Neuroblastoma	++	+
Leukemia	+	+
Metastatic carcinoma	+	−
Thyroid tumor	+	−
COLLAGEN VASCULAR DISEASE		
Lupus erythematosus	+	+
Juvenile rheumatoid arthritis	+	+
MISCELLANEOUS		
Kawasaki disease	+++	+
Drug-associated	++	+
Sarcoidosis	+	+
Histiocytosis X	+	+
Reticuloendotheliosis	+	+
Sinus histiocytosis with massive lymphadenopathy	+	+

*Key, +++, common; ++, uncommon; +, rare.

Modified from Butler KM, Baker CJ. Cervical lymphadenitis. In: Feigin RD, Cherry JD, eds. Textbook of pediatric infectious diseases, 3rd ed. Philadelphia: WB Saunders; 1992:225, and from Margileth AM. Cervical adenitis. Pediatr Rev. 1985;7:13.

skin lesions, and evidence of generalized or localized involvement.

In patients with acute infection, needle aspiration of the largest or most fluctuant affected node is the best way to establish a specific cause. In 60% to 88% of patients with acute cervical adenitis caused by aerobic agents or mycobacteria, a causative agent is recovered by this diagnostic maneuver. Only inflamed nodes should be aspirated, however. These need not be fluctuant, and the clinician should make sure that the cervical mass is not a vascular structure.

If purulent material is not obtained, cultures for aerobic bacteria are negative, and the patient fails to respond to antibiotics that are active against staphylococci and streptococci, the following laboratory evaluation should be considered: throat culture; Mantoux intradermal purified protein derivative (PPD) test; complete blood count; antistreptolysin O test; rapid plasma reagin test for syphilis; and serologic tests for Epstein-Barr virus, cytomegalovirus, toxoplasmosis, human herpesvirus 6, HIV, tularemia, *Brucella*, histoplasmosis, and coccidioidomycosis. Intradermal (Mantoux) testing for *M tuberculosis* with 5 TU of tuberculin always should be done in patients with subacute or chronic adenitis; induration greater than 15 mm is strongly suggestive of infection with *M tuberculosis*, whereas smaller reactions are more consistent with atypical mycobacterial infection. Patients with a PPD reaction exceeding 10 mm should undergo a chest radiograph and be subjected to further questioning about exposure to tuberculosis in the recent past. Cat-scratch disease is generally diagnosed based on clinical findings; however, serologic tests for *R hensalae*, the organism felt to cause the disease, are becoming available.

If the evaluation outlined above does not reveal the cause of the adenopathy and it persists, enlarges, or is hard or fixed to adjacent structures, excisional biopsy should be considered strongly.

■ TREATMENT

Many infants and children with cervical lymphadenopathy accompanying viral infections of the respiratory tract never see a physician because of the self-limited nature of these infections. In others, cervical adenitis resolves during the course of antimicrobial therapy given for a primary diagnosis of otitis media, streptococcal pharyngitis, or impetigo of the face or scalp. Another group of patients has acute inflammation of cervical lymph nodes as the primary site of infection; in these, empiric antimicrobial therapy without prior needle aspiration may be given. If no clinical response occurs within 48 hours, however, aspiration should be performed. This empiric therapy should be directed against *S aureus* and group A *Streptococcus*.

In children with acute suppurative cervical adenitis, surgical drainage is key to appropriate resolution. Some patients have progression of local inflammation and persistence of systemic symptoms despite oral antimicrobial therapy. These children require parenteral therapy. Antimicrobial therapy can be modified once a causative agent is identified (*eg*, group A streptococcal infection can be treated with penicillin G or V) and may need to be modified if there is an obvious primary infectious focus, such as a dental abscess, in which therapy active against anaerobic organisms is mandatory.

Clinical improvement in bacterial adenitis is expected within 48 to 72 hours of the initiation of treatment, but the size of the node or nodes usually does not regress at this stage, and low-grade fever may persist. Regression of lymph node enlargement is slow. As a general guideline, however, significant enlargement that persists beyond 4 to 8 weeks demands exclusion of an underlying disorder and consideration of excisional biopsy.

■ OUTCOME

Cervical adenitis generally resolves without complication when the infection is caused by agents that are susceptible to antimicrobial therapy (staphylococci and streptococci). Delay in diagnosis or initiation of therapy, however, may prolong the clinical course. In this situation, complications or sequelae may occur, including sinus tracts (mycobacteria and CSD), abscess formation, cellulitis and bacteremia (*S aureus* and group A *Streptococcus*), acute glomerulonephritis (group A *Streptococcus*), and disseminated infection (*M tuberculosis*). Untreated suppurative cervical adenitis usually drains exteriorly; rarely, this process may extend internally, producing thrombosis of the jugular vein, rupture of the carotid artery, mediastinal abscess, or purulent pericarditis. Compression of the esophagus or larynx also has been described.

These complications, with the exception of abscess formation, are rare. In children with abscess, appropriate drainage and specific antimicrobial therapy result in prompt resolution of signs and symptoms, and relapse is rare. In the unusual patient with repeated adenitis caused by *S aureus*, chronic granulomatous disease should be excluded.

The availability of effective antibacterial and antituberculous agents has resulted in an excellent prognosis for almost all children with cervical adenitis. Without surgical excision, however, 84% of those with atypical mycobacterial infection have ongoing morbidity. Appropriate surgical intervention as sole therapy produces cure in 92% to 98% of patients.

(Abridged from Carol J. Baker, Cervical Lymphadenitis, in Oski, DeAngelis, Feigin, McMillan, Warshaw: *Principles and Practice of Pediatrics, Second Edition*, J.B. Lippincott, 1994.)

Oski's Essential Pediatrics, edited by Kevin B. Johnson and Frank A. Oski. Lippincott–Raven Publishers, Philadelphia © 1997

36

Herpangina

Herpangina is a specific, common, acute, febrile viral illness that usually occurs in epidemic form in young children in the summer and fall in temperate climates. Although the clinical symptoms and signs were referred to in 1906, the name *herpangina* was introduced in 1920 to distinguish the clinical entity. Although coxsackieviruses of group A were the first known, and thought to be the only, causative agents, it is apparent now that infection with coxsackieviruses of group B and many echoviruses can result in herpangina. At least 24 enteroviral agents have been isolated in epidemic or sporadic cases of herpangina.

■ PATHOPHYSIOLOGY

In experimental infection with coxsackievirus A4 in rhesus monkeys, oropharyngeal lesions typical of herpangina developed 2 to 7 days after inoculation. Transmission in humans of the viruses that cause herpangina is fecal–oral or oral–oral. Airborne transmission probably occurs, but is less common. Virus can be isolated from throat and fecal specimens in the acute phase of illness, and from fecal specimens for weeks after recovery.

■ CLINICAL MANIFESTATIONS

The diagnosis of herpangina is suggested by the presence of lesions in the oropharynx. Herpangina usually is manifested by the sudden onset of fever with no prodrome or only a few hours of anorexia or listlessness. Temperature varies from normal to 41°C, and onset can be accompanied by a seizure. Headache, backache, sore throat, and dysphagia are noted by older patients. The oropharyngeal lesions usually are present at the onset of fever or occur in the subsequent 24 hours. The characteristic lesion evolves from a small papule to a 1- to 2-mm vesicle with surrounding erythema and then to an ulcer. Lesions remain discrete and enlarge to only 3 to 4 mm over 3 days. The sites of the lesions are characteristic in their involvement of the anterior tonsillar pillars, tonsils, soft palate, uvula, and pharyngeal wall. Occasionally, posterior buccal surfaces and the tip of the tongue are involved. Features differentiating herpangina from other diseases with enanthems are shown in Table 36–1.

■ TREATMENT AND PREVENTION

No specific antiviral therapy is available for the treatment of herpangina due to enteroviruses. Treatment is focused on maintaining comfort and adequate hydration, and on observing patients for the involvement of other organ systems. The prognosis is excellent, except in rare instances when herpangina is associated with hepatitis, encephalitis, or myocarditis, or with disseminated disease in the neonate. Oral secretions and feces are infectious during acute phases of the illness, and virus can be recovered from feces for weeks after symptoms abate. Asymptomatic infected individuals probably are the primary sources for the spread of infection. Care with handling diapers, good handwashing practices, and attention to personal hygiene limit the spread of these viruses.

(Abridged from Sarah S. Long, Herpangina, in Oski, DeAngelis, Feigin, McMillan, Warshaw: *Principles and Practice of Pediatrics, Second Edition*, J.B. Lippincott, 1994.)

TABLE 36–1. Features Differentiating Herpangina From Other Diseases with Enanthems

Disease	Etiology	Occurrence	Character of Oral Lesion(s)	Site of Oral Lesion(s)	Number of Lesions	Size of Lesions	Other Features
Herpangina	Coxsackieviruses, echoviruses	Acute	Vesicles, ulcers with erythema	Anterior pillars, posterior palate, and pharynx	1–5	1–2 mm	Dysphagia
Herpes stomatitis	Herpes simplex 1	Acute	Vesicles, shallow ulcers	Gingival/buccal mucosa, tongue, lips	Any	>5 mm, coalescent	Drooling, nodes
Hand-foot-mouth	Coxsackieviruses, enterovirus 71	Acute	Vesicles, shallow ulcers	Tonsillar fauces, buccal mucosa, tongue	Any	1–3 mm, coalescent	Vesicles on hands and feet, maculopapular rash
Aphthous stomatitis	Unknown	Acute, recurrent	Ulcers with rim of erythema, gray exudate	Buccal mucosa, lateral tongue	1–2	>5 mm	Pain, no fever
Behçet's syndrome	Unknown	Chronic, recurrent	Ulcers with rim of erythema, gray exudate	Any	1–5	>5 mm	Ulcers of genital mucosa, uveitis
Stevens-Johnson syndrome	Many, unknown	Acute	Ulcers, hemorrhagic ulcers, pseudomembranes	All, lips	Confluent	Confluent	Systemic illness, rash, drug history
Mucositis (ulcerative gingivitis)	Neutropenia, chemotherapy, bacteria	Chronic	Ulcers, exudate, pseudomembranes	Gingiva, buccal mucosa	Confluent	Confluent	Fetid breath, pain, other gastrointestinal mucosal lesions
Kawasaki disease	Unknown	Acute	Erythema, strawberry tongue	Diffuse	—	—	Prolonged fever, rash, conjunctival hyperemia, cracked lips
Toxic shock syndrome	Staphylococcus aureus toxin	Acute	Erythema, strawberry tongue	Diffuse	—	—	Erythroderma, conjunctival hyperemia, hypotension
Streptococcal pharyngitis	Group A Streptococcus	Acute	Erythema, exudates, strawberry tongue, palatal petechiae	Tonsils, pharynx	—	—	Sore throat, dysphagia
Adenoviral pharyngitis	Adenoviruses	Acute	Follicles, erythema, exudate	Tonsils, pillars, pharynx	—	—	Dysphagia, nodes, conjunctivitis
Epstein-Barr pharyngitis	Epstein-Barr virus	Acute	Exudate, palatal petechiae	Tonsils	—	—	Nodes, fatigue, splenomegaly

Oski's Essential Pediatrics,
edited by Kevin B. Johnson and Frank A. Oski.
Lippincott–Raven Publishers,
Philadelphia © 1997

37

Pharyngoconjunctival Fever

Pharyngoconjunctival fever is an acute viral illness defined by the presence of fever, conjunctivitis, and pharyngitis. It occurs in epidemic and sporadic fashion. Several distinct serotypes of adenovirus are causative agents. Pharyngoconjunctival fever has been associated most often with adenovirus type 3, followed by adenovirus type 7. Sporadic disease has been associated with more than 11 different antigenically distinct adenoviruses.

■ EPIDEMIOLOGY

Pharyngoconjunctival fever occurs in large community epidemics (usually associated with public swimming facilities), in local outbreaks (such as in hospitals, schools, and camps), and sporadically. It is primarily a disease of school-age children. The increase in frequency noted in outbreaks that occur in the summer probably reflects the risk of conjunctival inoculation in swimming pools. Water that was chlorinated inadequately was implicated in one epidemic of adenovirus disease.

Conjunctival infection usually is the result of direct inoculation. The same serotypes of adenovirus that cause pharyngoconjunctival fever associated with swimming pool outbreaks rarely cause sporadic cases of conjunctivitis.

■ PATHOPHYSIOLOGY

The route of inoculation of adenoviruses causing pharyngoconjunctival fever determines the pathophysiologic sequence. Biopsies of conjunctivae in infected volunteers reveal, predominantly, infiltration of lymphocytes in the submucosa. Biopsy material from tonsils and involved lymph nodes reveals hypertrophy and hyperplasia of the lymphoid tissue, with congestion and edema of connective tissue. Primary infection, regardless of the clinical syndrome, generally confers protection against clinical illness caused by that strain. Adenoviruses do not destroy the cells they infect in vivo.

■ CLINICAL MANIFESTATIONS

Patients with pharyngoconjunctival fever have fever, pharyngitis (hoarseness, sore throat, cough, or local signs of pharyngeal inflammation), and conjunctivitis (eye pain, itching, excessive tearing, hyperemic conjunctival). Fever is abrupt in onset and the temperature is greater than 39.2°C (102.6°F) in more than 50% of patients. Throat complaints range from mild irritation to severe pain and dysphagia. Tonsils usually are enlarged, and about one third of patients have follicular exudates. Conjunctival abnormalities are more severe than are symptomatic complaints. Disease usually is bilateral. Itching, aching, and soreness are common; photophobia, exudate, and keratitis occur less frequently. Conjunctivae are erythematous and edematous. The palpebral conjunctiva appears granular, and 1- to 3-mm yellow-gray collections of lymphocytes on hyperemic epithelium sometimes are visible (so-called follicles).

Compared to other viral respiratory illnesses, adenoviral infections are quite protracted. High fever generally is sustained for 4 to 5 days. Although eye findings improve by the end of the first week of illness, symptoms of burning or irritation and dryness of the throat, as well as general malaise, persist into the second week. The peripheral white blood cell count frequently is elevated, and an increase in polymorphonuclear leukocytes may be noted. Conjunctival swabs, throat swabs, and nasal wash specimens are excellent sources of virus for isolation.

■ DIFFERENTIAL DIAGNOSIS

The differential diagnosis is not problematic, because the triad that leads to the appellation is unique. Epidemic hemorrhagic conjunctivitis, caused by coxsackievirus A24 and enterovirus 70, is associated with subconjunctival hemorrhages ranging in size from small petechiae to large blotches. Chemosis and hyperemia of the bulbar conjunctivae, serous discharge, and fine corneal erosions also can be observed. In addition, patients usually are febrile and have preauricular lymphadenopathy. Conjunctivitis caused by herpes simplex virus is much more serious and usually is distinguished by its unilateral involvement, vesicular lid lesions, corneal involvement, and preauricular lymphadenopathy. The hallmark of bacterial infections of the conjunctivae, such as those caused by *Haemophilus influenzae,* *Streptococcus pneumoniae,* and *Neisseria gonorrhoeae,* is purulent exudate. The history and physical examination should separate patients with pharyngoconjunctival fever from those with cat-scratch disease, Newcastle disease, or allergic conjunctivitis.

■ TREATMENT AND PREVENTION

No specific form of therapy shortens the course of pharyngoconjunctival fever. The prophylactic use of antibiotics administered topically has no proven efficacy. Steroid-containing ophthalmic ointments should not be used. If purulent conjunctival discharge appears, culture to exclude a bacterial cause should be performed. The prognosis for complete recovery is excellent. Even when keratitis occurs, permanent scarring is rare.

Swimming pools are the predominant sources of epidemics of pharyngoconjunctival fever. Appropriate chlorination, adequate water filtration systems, and exclusion of infected individuals can eliminate this as a source of infection. Care in handling secretions of infected individuals, scrupulous handwashing, and careful personal hygiene habits should be practiced to reduce transmission in hospitals, within families, and in camps.

(Abridged from Sarah S. Long, Pharyngoconjunctival Fever, in Oski, DeAngelis, Feigin, McMillan, Warshaw: *Principles and Practice of Pediatrics, Second Edition,* J.B. Lippincott, 1994.)

SECTION 4

Orthopedics

Oski's Essential Pediatrics,
edited by Kevin B. Johnson and Frank A. Oski.
Lippincott–Raven Publishers,
Philadelphia © 1997

38

Sports Medicine

Pediatricians involved in primary care encounter sports medicine on a daily basis. In most practices, at least one patient each day is involved in athletic pursuits and brings to the physician an agenda related to sports participation. Athletically inclined children and their parents ask difficult questions that are different from those of other patients seeking primary medical care. Recent advances made in the diagnosis and treatment of medical problems in athletes have provided answers to many of those questions.

■ THE PREPARTICIPATION HEALTH INVENTORY

Children should have a yearly health checkup with a primary care health provider that includes a preparticipation health inventory for those patients who participate in sports activities. Most states require that athletes obtain a physician's statement of approval before they participate in sports activities, and this preparticipation visit provides an opportunity to address many health issues that may not come up at visits made for injuries.

The goals of a preparticipation health inventory vary somewhat from those of a routine health inventory in a nonathlete. In addition to assessing general health and diagnosing treatable conditions, it is important to identify conditions that may interfere with athletic participation or worsen as a result of it, especially any condition that may cause sudden death. Education related to the prevention of athletic injuries also should be included in the inventory process.

Areas of Highest Yield

The history and orthopedic examination portions of the preparticipation inventory yield the most useful information. Most important in the history are questions pertaining to past injuries and to risk factors for sudden death. It is important to question athletes regarding any family history of premature, nonaccidental death, and about fainting or dizziness with exercise. Some of the cardiac causes of sudden death in the young athlete can be prevented (Table 38–1). The low prevalence of these problems in the general population makes it difficult to justify the cost of an electrocardiogram and echocardiogram for every athlete.

A good orthopedic screening examination can be performed in 90 seconds by primary care physicians as part of a general physical examination. The orthopedic screening examination is outlined in Table 38–2. If there is a history of any injury or a positive finding on the orthopedic screening examination, a more thorough evaluation is necessary.

■ MANAGEMENT OF ATHLETIC INJURIES

Heat Cramps

Heat cramps are painful and forceful muscle contractions that usually occur in the gastrocnemius or hamstring muscles. They probably are not related to electrolyte balance or inadequate salt intake, but to heat, dehydration, and lack of training. Treatment includes rest and the ingestion of copious amounts of cold water.

Heat Syncope

Heat syncope is a term often used to describe a phenomenon that is common in runners in which they stop running at the end of a race and experience hypotensive syncope as a result of venous pooling. This is not life-threatening but is indicative of hypovolemia and the redistribution of blood volume that is caused by sweating and mild hyperthermia. Treatment is rest and the ingestion of generous amounts of cold water.

Heat Exhaustion

Heat exhaustion is manifested by pale skin color, vasoconstriction, dizziness, visual disturbances, syncope, and a moderately elevated rectal temperature (38°C to 40°C, or 101°F to 105°F). As with muscle cramps, treatment involves rest and rehydration. Ice packs and a fan may speed recovery. In some cases, intravenous fluid therapy may be required because of nausea and vomiting. Most authorities recommend 0.5% normal saline, which approximates the composition of the sweat that has been lost.

Heat Stroke

The presence of central nervous system (CNS) symptoms such as delirium, convulsions, and coma is indicative of heat stroke. A rectal temperature greater than 41°C (106°F) characteristically is seen in acute exercise-induced heat stroke. In the

TABLE 38-1. Cardiac Causes of Sudden Death in Young Athletes

Cardiomyopathy

Hypertrophic cardiomyopathy*

Congenital heart disease

Anomalous left coronary artery

Aortic rupture*

Hypoplastic coronary arteries

Prolonged QT syndrome*

Unknown

Causes of death that are potentially preventable through detection of a family history of sudden, unexplained death or symptoms during exercise.

absence of exercise, heat stroke is associated with the absence of sweating and the presence of warm, flushed skin. The young, exercising athlete with heat stroke, however, usually still is sweating profusely and has peripheral vasodilation. The CNS symptoms are more specific for heat stroke and indicate a medical emergency. Heat stroke can be fatal if it is not treated. The athlete should be packed in ice bags applied to the head, neck, and groin areas. Intravenous fluids (0.5% normal saline) should be administered as soon as possible, and immediate transport to a hospital is imperative. Because heat stroke may cause multisystem failure, the athlete may require admission to the hospital for observation.

Susceptible Individuals

Certain types of individuals are at greater risk for sustaining heat injury, including those who are obese, poorly

trained, dehydrated, or not used to heat. Athletes who wear uniforms that cover most of the body are more susceptible to heat illness, because of their inability to lose heat through evaporation. Age also is a risk factor, primarily for young children and the elderly. Anyone with a history of heat stroke is at risk for recurrence.

In addition to identifying risk factors, unlimited water should be provided to the athletes. Salt tablets should not be used, because they increase the risk of hypernatremia. Sweat is hypotonic, and athletes are depleted primarily of water.

■ COMMON MEDICAL ILLNESSES IN ATHLETES

Common Viral Infections

Few scientific data exist regarding common viral illnesses in relation to the ability of a child to participate in sports activities. The objective finding of fever is helpful. Excellent studies have shown increased cardiopulmonary effort and reduced exercise capacity in response to fever. Fever also is associated with poor tolerance of orthostatic stress, poor tolerance of submaximal exercise, and abnormal temperature regulation. For these reasons, fever should preclude participation in most instances.

Exercise-induced chest tightness or cough should alert the physician that reactive airways may be impairing the athlete's performance. Treatment with albuterol can safely provide marked improvement in symptoms. Additional agents such as cromolyn or a corticosteroid may be necessary for adequate treatment of the athlete with symptoms caused by bronchospasm.

■ DERMATOLOGIC CONCERNS IN ATHLETES

Few skin problems disqualify athletes from playing sports, but contagious skin infections do rule out competi-

TABLE 38-2. The Orthopedic Screening Examination

Athletic Activity (Instructions)	Observation
Stand facing examiner	Acromioclavicular joints; general habitus
Look at ceiling, floor, over both shoulders; touch ears to shoulders	Cervical spine motion
Shrug shoulders (examiner resists)	Trapezius strength
Abduct shoulders 90 degrees (examiner resists at 90 degrees)	Deltoid strength
Rotate arms fully externally	Shoulder motion
Flex and extend elbows	Elbow motion
Arms at sides, elbows 90 degrees flexed, move wrists into pronation and supination	Elbow and wrist motion
Spread fingers; make fist	Hand or finger motion and deformities
Tighten (contract) quadriceps; relax quadriceps	Symmetry and knee effusion; ankle effusion
"Duck walk" four steps (away from examiner with buttocks on heels)	Hip, knee, and ankle motion
Back up to examiner	Shoulder symmetry; scoliosis
Knees straight, touch toes	Scoliosis, hip motion, hamstring tightness
Raise up on toes, raise heels	Calf symmetry, leg strength

Garrick JG. Sports medicine. Pediatric Clin North Am. 1977;24:737.

tion in sports that involve close contact, such as wrestling or rugby. Impetigo and herpesvirus infections are seen most commonly, although scabies also is contagious enough to warrant disqualification. Impetigo and herpes infections can spread through a team quickly unless the athletes and coaches are cognizant of the importance of early diagnosis and treatment. With aggressive treatment, the amount of time lost from participation can be minimized.

■ COMMON INJURIES INVOLVING THE HEAD AND NECK

Concussions

Concussions occur frequently in contact sports, and determining an athlete's ability to return to play afterward can be difficult. The diagnosis of a concussion should be made in any athlete who sustains a transient loss of cognitive ability as a result of trauma to the head. The mildest form of concussion is commonly referred to as the "ding," and it consists of a few seconds of confusion, loss of balance, and "seeing stars." This can be brief enough to go undetected by teammates and coaches.

Criteria for return to play after concussion are similar to those after other injuries; the athlete must pass a functional examination. The most sensitive examination is a test for memory. In addition to asking simple information about the athlete's address or events that took place earlier in the day, it is helpful to have a teammate discuss the higher cognitive aspects of the game. If the athlete stumbles when being asked questions about the game plan or the assignments, then return to competition is forbidden.

Once an athlete has received a concussion, his or her risk of sustaining another concussion is increased. Traditionally, physicians have disqualified athletes from participating in a sport when they have sustained three concussions. The "three concussions and you are out" rule may be appropriate in some cases, but every patient must be approached individually.

Brachial Plexus Injuries

Many spectators of football, ice hockey, or wrestling are familiar with the athlete who comes off the field dangling or shaking an arm. Frequently, this athlete has sustained an injury commonly known as a "burner" or "stinger," which is a stretch of the brachial plexus. The burning pain with associated shoulder and arm weakness usually abates in a few minutes; in a few instances, weakness may persist for a few days to a few months. This injury is thought to be caused by a blow that hyperextends the neck, or causes lateral flexion of the neck away from the side of the injury, with or without a concomitant blow to the shoulder. Traction of the brachial plexus produces paresthesias in the shoulder, radiating down the arm and frequently into the hand. The athlete may complain of pain in the area of the trapezius muscle, but the injury seldom, if ever, should be associated with true neck pain.

Any persistent weakness disqualifies an athlete with a brachial plexus injury from further sports activity. The trapezius pain frequently persists beyond the paresthesia and need not disqualify an athlete from competition. The cause of trapezius pain probably is significant stretching of the muscle at the time of the injury. The athlete should be reexamined 24 to 48 hours after injury, because neuronal dysfunction resulting from edema may be delayed. Appropriate cervical spine films, including anteroposterior (AP),

lateral, oblique, and flexion and extension lateral views, should be taken the first time any athlete sustains this injury, to ascertain whether congenital anomalies are present.

■ INTRODUCTION TO ORTHOPEDIC INJURIES

In general, musculoskeletal problems are the most common reason for athletes to seek medical attention. Athletes are likely to delay seeking care until significant disability is present because they are taught to deny pain at an early age. In other words, most athletes tend to disregard minimal injuries and to obtain health care only when something is seriously wrong. Although the majority of injuries are exacerbated and recovery is prolonged by continued participation in a sport, there are some injuries that do not preclude participation and with which the athlete may play safely in the presence of pain.

Definitions

The terms *strain* and *sprain* frequently are used incorrectly; often, the former is meant to suggest a minor injury and the latter to indicate a more significant injury. A sprain is defined accurately as any injury to a ligament or joint capsule. A strain is any injury to a muscle.

Treatment Modalities

Cryotherapy often is administered effectively by placing ice cubes in a resealable plastic bag and applying the bag to the site of injury. The application of ice reduces edema and inflammation by causing vasoconstriction. Maximal vasoconstriction is produced in 15 to 20 minutes. Heat should not be applied to any acute injury for at least 72 hours, because the vasodilation it produces may increase bleeding and edema.

Anti-inflammatory medications are used liberally in sports medicine in an effort to reduce inflammation and edema in patients with acute and chronic injuries. Although they have not been studied well for use in soft-tissue injuries in athletes, these agents seem to be especially helpful during the rehabilitation period.

■ BACK INJURIES

Muscle Strain

Probably the most likely cause of low back pain in young athletes is an acute or chronic muscle strain. This tends to occur in children who have a functional hyperlordosis of the lumbar spine in the standing position. The athlete usually has loss of flexibility and benefits from regular back exercises that increase flexibility. Significant hamstring muscle tightness also is a common finding and contributor. A flexibility program should include these muscles.

Spondylolysis

Spondylolysis is another significant cause of low back pain in the adolescent athlete. Young athletes who participate in sports that involve repetitive hyperextension of the low back, such as gymnastics, may sustain stress fractures of the pars interarticularis of the lower lumbar spine. While bending, these patients frequently can touch their toes or even put their palms on the floor with their knees extended, yet most will have marked hamstring tightness. The spondylolysis may be unilateral or bilateral. When radiographs are ordered, they always should include oblique views; these may provide the only means of detecting this lesion (Figure 38–1).

Evaluation of Back Pain

The examination of the athlete with low back pain should begin with careful observation of the individual standing as well as walking. Assessment of range of motion should be performed in the standing position. The presence of pain with flexion, extension, or lateral movement should be noted. The athlete also should be asked to twist in both directions to see whether this produces pain; pain produced with this maneuver is suggestive of spondylolysis or disc protrusion. Pain that occurs when the patient extends the back while standing on one leg ("single leg hyperextension test") also is suggestive of spondylolysis.

Radiographs of the spine should be performed in most cases. In a patient with acute low back pain and no history of trauma, it may be reasonable to wait for 2 weeks after the injury before obtaining radiographs, because the pain often will resolve within that interval. Studies of back pain in children and adolescents, however, have shown that the yield of pathology on plain radiographs is much higher than that in adults with low back pain. If the history and physical examination are suggestive of spondylolysis, oblique views of the lumbosacral spine should be obtained to look for a pars interarticularis defect. A technetium bone scan may be necessary to confirm the clinical suspicion of acute spondylolysis.

Treatment of Back Pain

In general, even when the cause of low back pain is unclear, a trial of rest, anti-inflammatory medication, and a back exercise program is helpful. It is important to help the athlete understand that back pain usually does not resolve quickly, and that the exercise program probably is the most important part of the treatment.

■ GLENOHUMERAL DISLOCATION

Anterior shoulder dislocations are far more common than are posterior dislocations, and they have a high recurrence rate no matter how they are treated. There still is a great deal of controversy regarding the best method of conservative management of these injuries. Recent studies document that the recurrence rate is no different between patients treated with an early functional rehabilitation program that is begun as soon as the patient can tolerate it and those who are rigidly immobilized for 3 weeks. Return to competition is not allowed in either case until there is full range of motion and essentially equal strength in comparison with that of the uninjured shoulder.

■ FINGER INJURIES

The most common injury involving the hand is the finger sprain. Sometimes called a "jammed" finger, it usually is the result of hyperextension of the proximal or distal interphalangeal joint. The sprain may produce moderate swelling and tenderness, with some limitation of motion. Careful palpation of the finger reveals tenderness about one or both of the collateral ligaments and, frequently, tenderness over the volar plate (palmar ligament). Flexion and extension should be examined carefully at each joint in the finger.

Finger sprains are treated in a position of function, with splints applied for comfort. As soon as it is comfortable, the finger should be taken out of the splint to allow for range-of-motion exercises. If the finger is left in the splint indefinitely, the fibrosis that occurs after hematoma can cause stiffness and loss of motion. Splints should be used to protect the finger from further injury as long as any tenderness remains over the joint. One of the easiest and most comfortable methods used to splint the sprained finger is by buddy taping (taping the injured finger to the adjacent finger).

■ LEG AND KNEE INJURIES

Femoral Stress Fracture

If a young running athlete has persistent vague thigh pain, a femoral stress fracture should be considered strongly. Usually seen in high-mileage distance runners, the injury can be overlooked for weeks. The aching pain occurring with exercise has an insidious onset, and the physical examination often is nonlocalizing or the pain appears to be muscular in origin. If the pain has persisted for several weeks, the

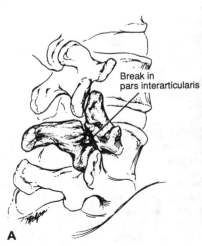
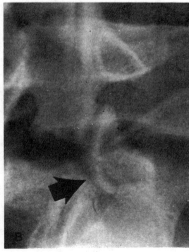

Break in pars interarticularis

Figure 38-1. (**A**) Anatomy and (**B**) radiographic evidence of spondylolysis. *Spondylolysis* is a break in the continuity of the pars interarticularis, which can be seen as a lucency on one of the oblique radiographs.

A

periosteal reaction may be seen only on oblique radiographs. If the results of plain radiographs are negative, a technetium bone scan is necessary to make the diagnosis.

Medial Collateral Ligament Sprains

In contrast to ankle injury, knowledge of the mechanism of injury can be helpful in determining the diagnosis of the acutely injured knee. The medial collateral ligament (MCL) sprain probably is the most common knee ligament injury to occur in contact sports. It occurs with valgus stress, such as happens with a blow to the lateral aspect of the knee. If the injury is mild, it may not produce much immediate disability, and the athlete may be able to continue to play for several more minutes. With significant bleeding and inflammation over the ligament, the athlete usually has a limp and must leave the game or practice.

In patients with an isolated MCL injury, examination of the knee reveals a trace to mild effusion. There is point tenderness over the MCL, often at the middle portion of the ligament. Full extension may be limited because it stretches the MCL, and the ligament is more relaxed at 30 degrees of flexion. Pain is produced with stress of the MCL, which is examined best with the patient lying supine and the knee in 20 to 30 degrees of flexion. With the table supporting most of the weight of the leg, the femur is stabilized with one hand and the ankle is grasped with the other hand. Outward stress is applied gently to the ankle to produce valgus stress to the knee, and the severity of the sprain is graded according to the degree of laxity noted. The knee should be examined for other ligament injury as well.

Radiographs should be performed to rule out a fracture. If the physes are open, stress radiographs must be taken. The MCL sprain is treated in a fashion similar to the ankle sprain. Rest for 2 to 3 days and the use of crutches often will provide pain relief, along with anti-inflammatory medication, ice, compression, and elevation. As with the ankle sprain, rehabilitation is the key to ensuring a quick return to competition. Even with a third-degree sprain, rehabilitation is vital, and MCL injuries no longer are treated surgically unless another injury is involved. The criteria for an athlete's return to play are similar to those for ankle sprain. The athlete must have no pain, full range of motion, strength equal to at least 85% of that of the uninjured leg, and no swelling, and he or she must have completed the running program without pain or limp (Table 38–3).

Anterior Cruciate Ligament Sprain

In contrast to the MCL sprain, an anterior cruciate ligament (ACL) sprain produces swelling of the knee in the first several hours after the injury occurs. Bleeding from the ligament usually produces a tense hemarthrosis. The ACL sprain almost always is a third-degree sprain, meaning that the ligament is disrupted completely.

The ACL tear usually is a noncontact injury caused by hyperextension of the knee or sudden deceleration of the leg with the foot flexed. Frequently, the athlete hears a loud pop. The injury is very painful, and the athlete seldom is capable of continuing to play.

If the athlete is evaluated on the field, stability testing for the ACL injury is extremely important. In the absence of bleeding or inflammation, the athlete will have less guarding and the examination will be more accurate. Several hours after the injury, the knee is very tender and swollen, and the

---

TABLE 38-3. The Running Program*

1. Jog ½ to 1 mile. Stop immediately if you are limping or if there is pain. Wait until tomorrow to start the program again. If there is no pain or limp during your jog, you may proceed to:
2. Six to eight 80-yard sprints at half speed. If no pain or limp, then do:
3. Six to eight 80-yard sprints at three-quarter speed. If no pain or limp, then do:
4. Six to eight 80-yard sprints at full speed, followed by 4 to 6 full speed starts. If no pain or limp, then do:
5. Six to eight 80-yard cutting sprints (changing directions) every 10 yards at half speed. Then do:
6. Six to eight 80-yard cutting sprints at full speed.

After every workout, ice should be applied immediately to the injured area. (Do not stand around.)

Once you can perform all the above tasks with no pain and minimal swelling, you may return to competition. If you short-cut this program, you are only fooling yourself, and are risking reinjury or possibly a more serious injury and a much longer time out of competition.

This running program can be given to the athlete so the criteria for return to competition are clear and the athlete can work toward a goal.

---

athlete may object to any movement of the knee, which makes examination difficult. The large, tense effusion that is seen 24 hours after the injury is grossly bloody on aspiration. More than 85% of all acute tense hemarthroses are caused by ACL disruptions. (Patella dislocations are the second most common cause of acute hemarthroses.)

On physical examination, the most important test to perform is the Lachman test. The traditional anterior drawer test, performed with the knee at a 90-degree angle, is not very reliable. The Lachman test is an anterior drawer test with the knee held in 20 to 30 degrees of flexion. One hand is placed on the femur to stabilize it, the other hand is used to grasp the proximal tibia, and anterior stress is applied (Figure 38–2). Loss of ACL integrity allows excessive anterior motion, compared to motion in the normal knee. Any hamstring spasm will negate the results of this test. Occasionally, the athlete may injure the MCL in addition, and examination for this injury should be performed also.

Radiographs should be performed, especially in an adolescent with open physes who may have a tibial plateau fracture instead of an ACL tear. (This is an avulsion fracture of the ACL, and it requires urgent attention from an orthopedic surgeon.) For an ACL tear, treatment with a knee immobilizer, crutches, and pain relief is reasonable; a surgical consultation should be obtained within the next several days. Arthroscopy or magnetic resonance imaging often is used to examine the menisci, because a meniscus tear also will be demonstrated in 30% to 40% of patients with ACL tears.

Treatment of the acute ACL tear in most, but not all, cases requires surgery. A patient with an ACL-deficient knee is likely to have recurring instability and probably is at risk for early traumatic arthritis. Recent surgical advances have led to excellent results in patients who have chosen surgical stabilization. Careful evaluation and discussion with the athlete about his or her preference are critical. Cast immobilization of an isolated ACL tear is to be condemned; it does not allow for healing and only adds to muscle atrophy and prolongs the rehabilitation process.

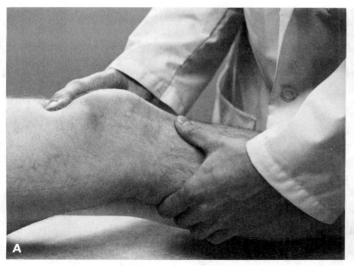
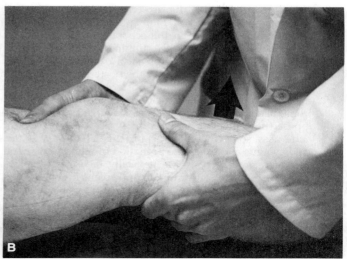

Figure 38-2. Lachman test. With the patient supine, the knee is flexed to 20 degrees to 30 degrees. (**A**) While the femur is stabilized with one hand, the tibia is grasped with the other hand. (**B**) When pulled anteriorly in the absence of the interior cruciate ligament, the tibia moves excessively anteriorly.

Patellofemoral Stress Syndrome

The most common complaint heard in most sports medicine clinics is that of chronic patellar pain. Sometimes known as chondromalacia, this entity also is called runner's knee, peripatellar pain syndrome, patellalgia, and patellofemoral stress syndrome (PFSS). Chondromalacia is an inappropriate term for most of these chronic pain conditions, because it is a specific pathologic diagnosis. When patients with this problem are examined surgically, no abnormality of the articular surface is found in more than 50% of them. The most appropriate term for the condition is PFSS. This syndrome is a common problem in athletes who run; many chronic injuries to the lower extremity occur in distance runners or in athletes who participate in sports that involve running, such as soccer.

The origin of the pain in patients with PFSS is thought to be subchondral stress or synovial inflammation. Patients typically have a history of dull, achy knee pain that is difficult to localize. Movement of the knee may be associated with a clicking or popping sound. The pain is worse with activity, especially running and going up and down stairs. Exacerbations may occur with prolonged sitting, especially in the back seat of a car with the knees fully flexed. The pain also is brought on or aggravated by any trauma to the patella. There may be "giving way" of the knee, which commonly is associated with pain. There usually is no history of swelling. The history or presence of swelling should prompt consideration of another diagnosis.

On physical examination, firm palpation of the patella often reveals tenderness over the medial facet. This may require some medial displacement of the patella with palpation of its undersurface medially. There also may be tenderness over the lateral facet of the patella or at any point along the patellofemoral joint line. Compression of the patella in the femoral groove produces pain, which sometimes is called a positive compression test result.

Radiographs should be performed in any athlete with more than 4 to 6 weeks of pain. Any history or evidence of swelling also warrants radiography. AP, lateral, tunnel, and patellar views should be obtained for complete evaluation of the knee.

The treatment of PFSS usually is not surgical. Modification of activities to avoid full flexion of the knee and stress of the patellofemoral joint is imperative. A strengthening program for the quadriceps mechanism and a stretching program, especially for the hamstring muscles, often improve the patient's symptoms. In the athlete with excessive foot pronation, treatment should include the use of flexible orthoses. Judicious use of ice and anti-inflammatory medication usually is helpful. The athlete should be warned that patellar pain tends to be chronic, with exacerbations and remissions. The pain can be a lifelong problem, depending on the patient's activities. The goal is to educate the athlete regarding means of controlling the pain and still being able to enjoy some degree of athletic activity.

Osgood-Schlatter Disease

In skeletally immature athletes with open tibial physes, swelling and point tenderness at the tibial tubercle are indicative of Osgood-Schlatter disease, which is associated with running and jumping in these individuals. This condition probably represents tiny stress fractures in the apophysis, and it is associated with a rapid growth spurt. Ice, anti-inflammatory medication, and a decrease in activity help the young athlete to manage this problem. The only permanent sequela is a prominence of the tibial tubercle, which rarely represents a cosmetic problem. Immobilization through the use of a knee immobilizer or crutches occasionally is necessary in patients who have severe pain. A few athletes continue to play until they are unable to walk without a limp. Regardless of the severity of the condition, the long-term prognosis is excellent and chronic pain or disability is uncommon.

Shin Splint Syndrome

Lower leg pain is a common reason for a young runner to seek medical attention. The most common cause of this pain is shin splint syndrome, which also is known as medial tibial stress syndrome and posterior tibialis tendinitis. The athlete complains of achy pain that increases gradually in intensity throughout the exercise regimen. The pain improves greatly with rest. Shin splints often are related to overtraining, especially in the school-age athlete who has not been doing much distance running before cross-country or track season begins. On physical examination, there is marked diffuse tenderness over the posteromedial aspect of the tibia at the insertion of the posterior tibialis and soleus muscles (Figure 38–3). The tenderness with shin splint syndrome usually is present over the distal half of the tibia, as opposed to a tibial stress fracture, which tends to produce tenderness somewhere in the proximal half of the tibia. Ankle valgus and excessive pronation of the foot frequently are seen on gait analysis. Mechanically, the excessive pronation stresses the posterior tibialis and soleus muscles at their origin at the posterior medial aspect of the tibia. Treatment of the excessive pronation with better footwear or flexible orthoses usually is key to producing resolution and preventing recurrences. Rest, ice, and anti-inflammatory medication also speed recovery. Frequent calf stretches, which stretch all the ankle plantar flexor muscles, also are helpful. Athletes usually do not have to stop running completely, but must decrease significantly the intensity and duration of their workouts.

Ankle Sprains

The most common acute injury to the lower extremity is the ankle sprain. The athlete usually reports twisting the ankle but may not remember the details of the injury. There may be an audible pop at the time of the injury. Unlike in other sports injuries, knowledge of the mechanism of injury of an ankle sprain is not very helpful. A fair amount of swelling often is noted, with disruption of the ankle ligaments as a result of bleeding. About 90% of ankle sprains are of the lateral ligaments, caused by inversion of the ankle or a combination of inversion and plantar flexion of the ankle. A small percentage are medial sprains involving eversion of the ankle.

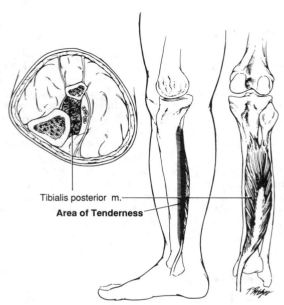

Figure 38-3. Shin splint syndrome. The pain and tenderness may be present throughout the entire posteromedial aspect of the tibia, corresponding to the fascial attachment of the tibialis posterior (and soleus) medially on the tibia.

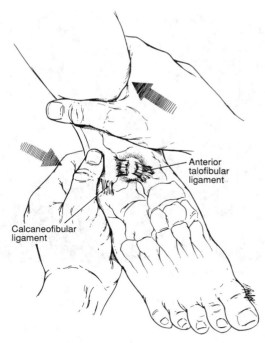

Figure 38-4. Anterior ankle drawer sign. To test the integrity of the anterior talofibular ligament, the tibia is stabilized with one hand and the calcaneus and talus are grasped with the other. With the ankle in slight plantar flexion and internal rotation, the talus is given traction anteriorly. Excessive motion with this maneuver with a poor end point is a *positive drawer sign*, and implies a third-degree sprain of the anterior talofibular ligament.

Physical examination of the ankle involves the application of applied surface anatomy. Careful palpation of the structures reveals the maximal area of tenderness to be over the ligaments. If any bony tenderness is present, a fracture should be suspected and radiographs should be obtained. Stability testing may be difficult to perform if the athlete is seen a day or two after the injury, because of marked pain and muscle spasm. The most common ankle sprain involves one or both of the lateral ligaments, which are the anterior talofibular and the calcaneofibular ligaments. The anterior talofibular ligament is examined with the anterior ankle drawer test. With the tibia stabilized with one hand and the calcaneus grasped with the other hand, traction is placed on the talus anteriorly (Figure 38–4). Increased laxity, as compared to laxity in the uninjured ankle, implies that at least a second-degree sprain has occurred. If there is a poor end point (ie, a marked diminution in resistance to stress of the ligament), a third-degree sprain of that ligament has occurred. Inversion testing with the ankle in slight plantar flexion tests the calcaneofibular ligament. Comparison to the patient's uninjured ankle is imperative, because ligament laxity varies a great deal from athlete to athlete. Eversion testing with the ankle in a neutral position reveals any instability of the deltoid ligament. In some ankle sprains, there may be a great deal of pain but no increased laxity. Careful palpation may reveal tenderness over the deltoid ligament, the lateral ligaments, and anteriorly over the inferior tibiofibular ligament. This type of sprain at first may appear to be minor because there is no appreciable ankle laxity, but the sprain also involves a tear of the interosseous membrane between the tibia and the fibula. Sometimes descriptively called the "ring-around-a-rosy" or "high" sprain, this injury usually takes longer to rehabilitate than do other, mild sprains.

Radiographs should be performed in any ankle injury that produces more than minimal swelling or pain with weight bearing. AP, lateral, and mortise views should be included to enable adequate assessment of the ankle mortise. Careful examination of the talar dome radiographically is important because any small fracture seen on the radiograph is indicative of a larger chondral defect.

Treatment of the ankle sprain initially is designed to minimize the hematoma and swelling. The mnemonic RICE is a helpful way to remember rest, ice, compression, and elevation as the important modalities with which to achieve this goal. Most athletes benefit from 48 to 72 hours of avoidance of weight bearing through the use of crutches. Compression bandages take many different forms, but a snug elastic wrap will suffice.

The second aspect of treating an ankle sprain concerns resolution of the hematoma. This involves range-of-motion exercises, along with protective weight bearing. An ankle sprain will resolve much more quickly with the help of a physical therapist or an athletic trainer who can direct an exercise program.

Protective taping has been shown to be effective in preventing recurrent ankle sprain. Because tape can be expensive and many young athletes do not have access to a coach or trainer who is skilled in ankle taping, a lace-up

ankle brace will help to prevent recurrences. High-top shoes probably are helpful in giving the ankle some stability. Surgical intervention rarely is indicated for third-degree ankle sprains. Surgery should be considered in an elite ballet dancer or gymnast, however, because athletes engaging these types of activities are less tolerant of ankle instability.

■ CONCLUSION

Sports medicine has become an important area of concern in ambulatory pediatrics because the young athletic patient expects the same care that is provided to college and professional athletes. It is important to recognize that the ability to return quickly to play and competition frequently is first on the agenda of the athlete who is seeking medical care. The most common injuries confronting the pediatrician often require the help of a physical therapist or trainer to instruct the athlete in a proper rehabilitation program. Rehabilitation frequently shortens the time that is necessary for the athlete to spend away from competition and maximizes his or her safety on returning to the sport.

(Abridged from Gregory L. Landry, Sports Medicine, in Oski, DeAngelis, Feigin, McMillan, Warshaw: *Principles and Practice of Pediatric, Second Edition*, J.B. Lippincott, 1994.)

Oski's Essential Pediatrics,
edited by Kevin B. Johnson and Frank A. Oski.
Lippincott–Raven Publishers,
Philadelphia © 1997

39

Bone, Joint, and Muscle Problems

■ DEVELOPMENTAL DYSPLASIA OF THE HIP

The normal hip develops from a common anlage resulting from reciprocal contact between the femur and a cetabulum during growth. Loss of this contact results in dysplasia of the femur or acetabulum.

The cause of congenital dislocation of the hip in an otherwise normal child is multifactorial. Mechanical factors play a role, and the frequency of developmental dysplasia of the hip (DDH) is increased greatly in fetuses with breech presentation (a factor in 30% of all cases of DDH), in first-born children, and in infants with oligohydramnios. Hormonal factors may play a role because there is generalized ligamentous laxity around the time of birth caused by increased circulating estrogens and relaxin. The incidence of DDH is sixfold greater in girls than in boys. Evidence for hereditary control of these and other factors lies in the fact that more than 20% of patients have a positive family history.

Physical examination remains the key to the diagnosis of DDH. The signs in the newborn period usually include instability without significant fixed deformity; in later months, untreated dislocation becomes more fixed and there is less instability and more limitation of certain motions.

Specifically, Barlow's and Ortolani's signs should be sought in the newborn. These signs are considered to be positive when the hip can be dislocated and relocated, respectively. The child should be relaxed when the tests are performed, and only one hip should be examined at a time. The pelvis should be enclosed and stabilized with one hand, while the femur is controlled with the other hand, with fingers placed on the greater and lesser trochanters (Figure 39–1). With adduction and pressure directed posteriorly, the femur can be felt to slide in a posterosuperior direction over the rounded limbus in the abnormal hip (Barlow's sign, see Figure 39–1A) and then back in with abduction, causing a dull clunk to be heard (Ortolani's sign, see Figure 39–1B). Thus, these signs indicating dislocation and relocation are alternate phases of the same process of hip instability.

About 60% of all unstable hips seen in newborns normalize spontaneously within the first 2 to 4 weeks after birth as perinatal laxity resolves. If the hip remains dislocated, it can be relocated on examination in less than 15% of patients by the time they are 6 months of age. Findings of asymmetry, such as limitation of abduction and of full extension (see Figure 39–1C), as well as apparent shortening of the femoral segment are more sensitive at this time.

Radiographs should not be used commonly before 6 months of age because of a lack of apparent bony changes during this time, except in infants with teratologic conditions; physical examination remains more reliable. Ultrasonography is indicated if the neonatal examination is abnormal or questionable, as well as to guide initial treatment. After 6 months of age, plain films may show cephalad and lateral migration of the femur with a break in Shenton's line (Figure 39–2), delayed appearance of the femoral ossific nucleus, a shallow and more vertical acetabulum, and later formation of a false acetabulum.

Treatment involves different measures at different ages. The aim of all therapy is to restore contact between the femoral head and the acetabulum. Because of the high percentage of

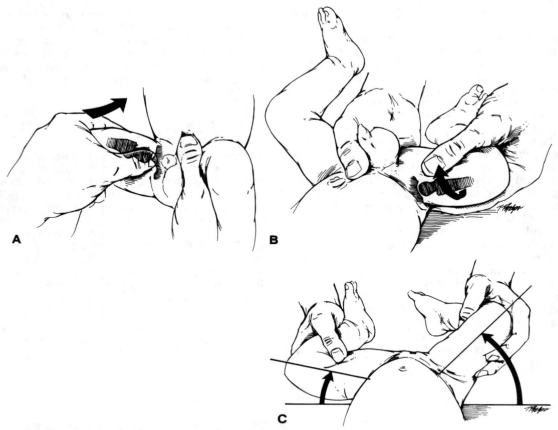

Figure 39-1. Barlow and Ortolani tests, performed with fingers on the lesser and greater trochanters, examining only one hip at a time. (**A**) *Barlow test:* adduction and posterior pressure may produce a "clink" of subluxation or dislocation. (**B**) *Ortolani test:* abducting and "lifting" hip back into place. (**C**) In children older than age 3 to 6 months, Barlow and Ortolani tests often will be negative despite dislocation because of diminished laxity; the most important finding in this age group may be limitation of abduction.

patients who experience spontaneous improvement of lax hip capsules in the early perinatal period, most orthopedists recommend observing a hip that is subject to subluxation and reexamining it 3 to 4 weeks after birth. Dislocated hips should be treated at the time of diagnosis. If the hip remains unstable, an abduction–flexion device such as a Pavlik harness may be used. This allows some motion while it promotes the appropriate femoral acetabular contact. The alignment should be checked by radiography in 1 to 2 weeks. The brace is worn until the results of clinical and radiologic examinations are normal, an interval that is equal to about one to two times the child's age at diagnosis. If treatment is begun after the child has reached 6 months of age, he or she usually is too large and strong to tolerate the brace. At that point, reduction must be preceded by traction to bring the femoral head down toward the acetabulum, decreasing the muscle forces that could contribute to avascular necrosis. If closed reduction is unsuccessful, open reduction should be carried out. This involves tightening the lax superior capsule and releasing the tight psoas tendon and inferior capsule, allowing the femoral head to be brought down to its appropriate location.

If there is extensive distortion of the bones (*ie,* a shallow acetabulum or a rotated femur), a femoral or pelvic osteotomy as well as open reduction might be indicated. This is more common in patients who are more than 2 years of age.

The earlier that treatment is carried out, the better is the resultant hip development and the safer is each of the steps in treatment. Thus, careful, methodical, early screening can decrease the need for complex orthopedic procedures later on.

■ TRANSIENT (TOXIC) SYNOVITIS OF THE HIP

Transient (toxic) synovitis of the hip is a diagnosis of exclusion; it is a self-limited condition that represents the most common cause of an irritable hip in children. The usual clinical presentation is a painful limp or hip pain of acute or insidious onset, usually occurring unilaterally. The most common age range for the condition is 2 to 6 years, but it has been described in patients ranging from 1 to 15 years in age. Males are affected more often. There is spasm on testing of hip range of motion, particularly with internal rotation. The temperature, white blood cell count, and erythrocyte sedimentation rate may be normal or slightly elevated. The cause of the condition is unknown; an immune mechanism or viral infection is postulated. The differential diagnosis should include septic arthritis, osteomyelitis, and Legg-Calvé-Perthes disease, which usually is associated with a subchondral crescent of lucency or further changes in the femoral head on radiography. Juvenile monoarthritis, rheumatoid arthritis, and slipped capital femoral epiphysis (SCFE) also should be considered. Admission to the hospital, observation, and possible early aspiration should be undertaken if septic arthritis cannot be ruled out. Treatment consists of bed

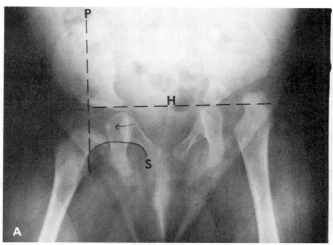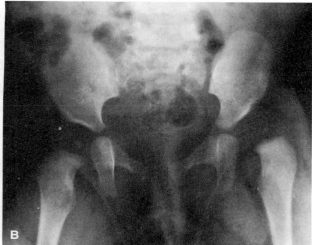

Figure 39-2. (A) Radiographic examination of congenitally dislocated hip. The femoral head ossific nucleus should be within the lower inner quadrant formed by Perkin's vertical line (P) at the outer edge of the acetabulum and Hilgenreiner's horizontal line (H). The nucleus appears at age 5 months, on the average. *Shenton's line* is the arc of the femoral neck, which should continue smoothly into the pubic ramus. This is a teratologic hip dislocation; note extreme height and rounded false acetabulum. **(B)** A more subtle example of congenital dislocation of the left hip.

rest with analgesic agents provided as needed for 2 to 7 days. Therapy sometimes can be accomplished on an outpatient basis with frequent follow-up if the diagnosis is clear. Persistence of the symptoms beyond 1 week should prompt reevaluation, although bed rest for as long as 1 month occasionally has been required.

■ LEGG-CALVÉ-PERTHES DISEASE (COXA PLAVA)

Legg-Calvé-Perthes disease first was differentiated from tuberculosis within a decade after the popularization of radiography, but its cause still is unknown. The condition is characterized by ischemic necrosis of the proximal femoral epiphysis with later resorption. The amount of the femur that is rendered ischemic varies and affects the outcome. Ischemia is followed by reossification with or without col-

lapse of the femoral head. Legg-Calvé-Perthes disease usually, but not exclusively, affects children between 4 and 8 years of age. Males are affected four times as often as are females. As a group, these patients have slightly shorter stature and delayed bone age compared to their peers. Fifteen percent of all cases are bilateral.

The clinical presentation of this disorder usually is a limp (*ie*, an abductor lurch) with minimal pain of either short or long duration. The pain is not as acute or severe as that of transient synovitis or septic arthritis. Motions that are especially limited include internal rotation and abduction. Internal rotation is performed with the patient supine and the hip flexed, and the angle to which the leg may be rotated laterally is measured. These movements may be resisted by mild spasm or guarding. In the earliest stage, radiographic results may be normal or reveal slightly smaller size of the affected femoral epiphysis compared to the contralateral side as a result of its failure to grow after becoming avascular. Later,

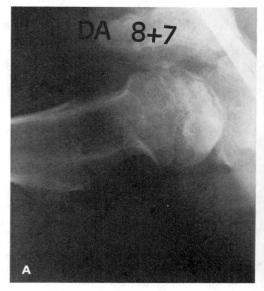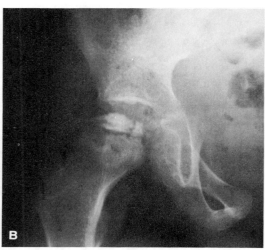

Figure 39-3. (A) Early Legg-Calvé-Perthes disease, showing subchondral "crescent." **(B)** Later, there is resorption and apparent collapse of the femoral head.

there may be a narrow crescentic lucency, seen best on the lateral view, which is the result of a tiny fracture of the subchondral bone. This reveals the extent of bone involved (Figure 39–3A). In some cases, revascularization may occur without collapse, but in others, revascularization of the femoral head is accompanied by progressive resorption and deformation, often with lateral and superior migration (see Figure 39–3B). Reossification follows, and the femoral head continues to grow. Whether this further growth occurs spherically depends on the patient's age, the amount of collapse, and the method of treatment.

The differential diagnosis should include transient synovitis, septic arthritis, hematogenous osteomyelitis, various types of hemoglobinopathy, Gaucher's disease, hypothyroidism, and the epiphyseal dysplasias. The latter two conditions often are temporally symmetric bilaterally, whereas Legg-Calvé-Perthes disease is not.

Treatment follows two principles: functional containment of the femoral head within the acetabulum and maintenance of range of motion. During the vulnerable phase, the avascular portion of the femoral head is less likely to become severely deformed and is more likely to reconstitute spherically if it is contained within the "mold" of the acetabulum by abduction. Children younger than 6 years of age who have involvement of less than half the femoral head may be observed without active treatment if a full range of motion is preserved, because this signals containment and patients in this age group have a good prognosis. Aggressive treatment is indicated for patients who have involvement of more than half the femoral head or are more than 6 years in age.

Containment may be achieved by the use of an orthosis or by surgery. Orthoses produce abduction with or without internal rotation. The most commonly employed orthosis is the Scottish Rite brace, which does not extend below the knees (Figure 39–4). Containment should be documented radiographically. The child is allowed to perform any activity that is possible in the brace. The orthosis should be worn until early reossification is seen. Surgical treatment is used if an orthosis is not desirable because of the size of the child, the anticipated duration of wear (as long as 18 months in an older child), or lack of acceptance. Either a femoral osteotomy to redirect the involved portion within the acetabulum, or an innominate osteotomy or shelf procedure may be performed. The femoral osteotomy may cause slight shortening and an increased likelihood of a limp, but it can be controlled more precisely. The two procedures produce about equal results.

■ SLIPPED CAPITAL FEMORAL EPIPHYSIS

Slipped capital femoral epiphysis (SCFE) is a disorder of the growth plate that occurs near the age of skeletal maturity; it involves a three-dimensional displacement of the epiphysis posteriorly, medially, and inferiorly. In other words, the femur is rotated externally from under the epiphysis. The cause is unknown but may involve mechanical as well as biologic factors. Slipped capital femoral epiphysis usually occurs without severe sudden force or trauma. Mechanically, there is increased stress as a result of obesity in most affected children and abnormal retroversion (posterior rotation) of the femoral head and neck. The periosteum at this age is thin and less able to resist the shearing forces. Possible biologic causes include delayed growth plate maturation and hormonal factors, which may account for the associated obesity. Increased growth hormone levels have been associated with decreased physeal shear strength, and hypothyroidism has been found in some cases. Slipped capital femoral epiphysis usually occurs during the growth spurt, and before menarche in girls. The condition is rare, with a frequency of 1:100,000 to 8:100,000. It is more common in males and in blacks. About one fourth to one third of all affected children have bilateral involvement but usually not simultaneously.

The clinical presentation varies with the acuity of the process. Most children have a limp and varying degrees of aching or pain. The discomfort may be in the groin but often is referred to the thigh or knee. Many patients are dismissed for an apparent knee complaint with no obvious cause only to have the true hip pathology discovered later with worsening of the slip. This paradoxic distribution of pain is attributed to referral within the femoral nerve distribution, which involves both the hip and knee joints. Some patients have acute, severe pain and inability to walk or move the hip. Again, abduction, internal rotation, and flexion are the motions that are most limited. A characteristic finding is external rotation of the hip with flexion, which is caused by the preexisting retroversion and the slip itself (Figure 39–5). There may be apparent limb shortening as a result of the proximal displacement of the metaphysis.

The earliest radiographic findings are widening and irregularity of the growth plate and osteopenia of the femur. Later, there is displacement of the epiphysis. This is seen best on the frog-leg lateral view of the pelvis. A line on the anteroposterior (AP) view drawn through the upper margin of the narrowest portion of the neck should intersect at least 20% of the epiphysis (Figure 39–6). This is an important point, because, with remodeling during chronic slipping, there may not be a step-off at the junction of the epiphysis and metaphysis. The severity of the slip is graded as mild (<33%), moderate (33% to 50%), or severe (>50%). Later changes may include avascular necrosis of the epiphysis or chondrolysis (ie, joint space narrowing).

Treatment centers on preventing further slippage, usually by placing the patient immediately at bed rest and

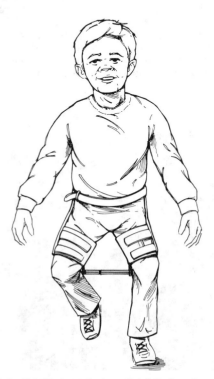

Figure 39-4. Scottish Rite brace for Legg-Calvé-Perthes disease produces containment by abduction and allows free knee motion.

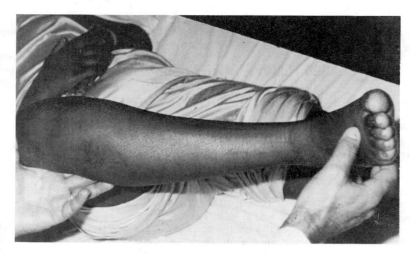

Figure 39-5. In slipped capital femoral epiphysis, the hip rotates externally as it is flexed by the examiner.

obtaining a prompt orthopedic consultation. Surgery is intended to stabilize the upper femur and cause the growth plate to close. Realignment of the slip is not safe in chronic cases, because the forces necessary to accomplish realignment may produce avascular necrosis by disrupting the blood supply to the epiphysis. The gold standard of treatment is pin fixation in situ. Long-term follow-up reveals some remodeling of the slip. The pins should not penetrate

the joint. Open epiphysiodesis using bone graft avoids the risk of pin penetration and produces faster growth plate closure, but it is a longer surgical procedure and requires cast stabilization in acute slips. Osteotomy of the proximal or distal neck to correct the deformity has been performed occasionally, but it carries a high risk of avascular necrosis. The contralateral side should be monitored for SCFE and should be pinned early if symptoms occur. Long-term follow-up

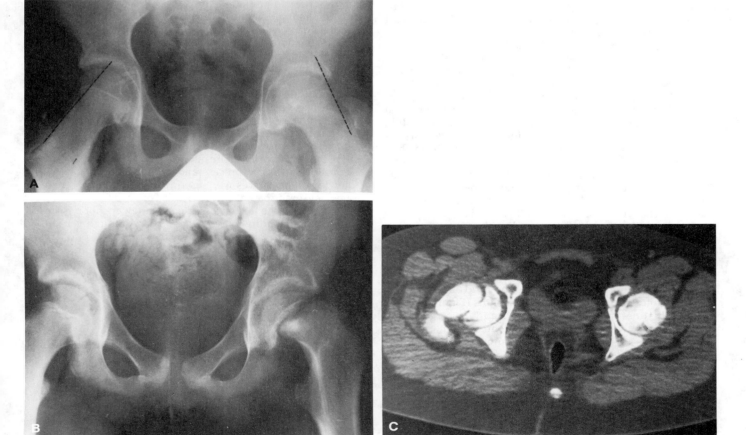

Figure 39-6. Radiographic findings in slipped capital femoral epiphysis. (**A**) A line drawn along the superior-lateral femoral neck intersects less than the normal 20% of the epiphysis on the left (affected) side. (**B**) A more severe slip, showing that the femoral neck subluxates laterally, and superiorly with respect to the epiphysis. (**C**) CT scan shows the direction of the slip most clearly.

reveals no early degenerative change unless chondrolysis or avascular necrosis occur; each has an incidence of 1% to 5%.

■ INCREASED FEMORAL ANTEVERSION

Increased femoral anteversion is one of a spectrum of torsional deformities that affect the alignment of the knee and foot with the body. The differential diagnosis of toeing-in includes this as well as internal tibial torsion and foot deformities such as metatarsus adductus (Table 39–1). Increased anteversion of the femur is defined as an increase in the angle between the plane of the femoral neck and the plane of the posterior femoral condyles (Figure 39–7). This normally is about 30 degrees at birth and declines to 15 degrees by 10 years of age. The increasing pressure of the anterior hip capsule, as the child loses the physiologic flexion contracture, causes the change. Increased femoral anteversion persists in some neuromuscular conditions, presumably as a result of lack of these remodeling forces. The type discussed here is isolated idiopathic femoral anteversion.

On physical examination, the patient appears to toe-in unless compensatory external tibial torsion is present. The patellae also face medially ("squint"). Internal rotation of the hip is much greater than external rotation in both flexion (supine) and extension (prone). Anteversion usually is not clinically significant unless external rotation at the hip is less than 15 degrees.

Radiographically, the femoral head and neck appear to be relatively straight on an AP film with the patella forward. This is a one-plane projection of a three-plane deformity. Computed tomography (CT) is best for measuring femoral anteversion directly.

The natural history of femoral anteversion is benign. In a few patients, it may contribute to patellar malalignment. Anteversion later in life has been found to be unrelated to arthritis of the hip or knee. Anteversion does not impair function. Treatment of increased anteversion consists of observation at least until the patient is 8 years of age and restriction from W-sitting, which may impair remodeling. The child instead should sit in the tailor position. Cables and bars are not effective in derotating the femur, and no orthotic method of treatment affects anteversion. In fact, most cases need no treatment. Femoral osteotomy, proximally or distally, is the only truly effective therapy. It should be performed rarely, however, and only in children more than 8 years of age who have functional disability as a result of patellar malalignment or, rarely, a persistent concern regarding their appearance.

■ GENU VARUM

Genu varum, or "bowed leg" of up to 20 degrees is normal in children until the age of 18 months (Figure 39–8). It normally does not increase significantly after walking begins. After the age of 24 months, genu valgum develops. Radiographs are indicated if genu varum is present after this age or is progressive after the age of 1 year, if it is unilateral, if it appears to be severe, or if it occurs in a high-risk group such as obese black children who walk early. Radiographic findings of benign genu varum include symmetric bowing of the tibia and femur, a normal-appearing physis without narrowing or step-off, and a generalized, rather than focal, outward angle.

Treatment involves observation to verify resolution. Measurement of the angle on physical examination should be performed with the child standing and may also be accomplished by measurement of the distance between the femoral condyles or of the AP tibiofemoral angle. These methods are not as accurate as are radiographs, but they are a practical way of observing change in patients when the presumptive diagnosis is physiologic genu varum.

The differential diagnosis of physiologic genu varum includes Blount disease, rickets, post-traumatic growth plate disturbance, enchondromatosis, achondroplasia, and other skeletal dysplasias.

■ GENU VALGUM

Genu valgum of the knee is normal after 2 years of age, reaches a mean of 12 degrees at 3 years of age, and remains constant at a mean of about 7 degrees in boys and 9 degrees in girls after 8 years of age. Night bracing may be helpful in children with angulation exceeding 20 degrees. If it remains greater than 15 degrees at 10 years, early growth plate stapling or later osteotomy of the affected region may be indicated to prevent patellofemoral problems and degenerative changes. Valga of the proximal tibia often follows medial metaphyseal fractures but frequently corrects spontaneously.

■ INTERNAL TIBIAL TORSION

Internal tibial torsion is the most common cause of toeing-in in children between 1 and 3 years of age. Tibial torsion is determined by measuring the angle between the foot and the thigh with the ankle and knee positioned at 90 degrees. The foot normally rotates externally with age (Figure 39–9). The differential diagnosis includes metatarsus adductus, femoral anteversion, and neuromuscular disorders. To make these distinctions, the foot as well as the hip should be examined (see Figure 39–9, A, B, and C). Tibial torsion improves naturally with growth, but this often takes years. Because of our improved knowledge of the benign natural history of this condition, bracing with devices such as the Denis-Browne bar is used only rarely now. Studies have shown that external braces cannot apply significant rotational force to the tibia, because it is taken up in the foot, knee, and hip joints. The improvement that previously was attributed to the brace is primarily the result of normal growth patterns. Correction is a slow process and often frustrates parents. Knowledge that braces were used heavily in the past, reinforced by grandparents and friends, often drives anxious parents to visit the doctor to make sure they are not missing a golden opportunity to avoid problems. Although very little evidence exists regarding the efficacy of a brace or of any orthotic method, it is a very widely used treatment. Some feel that its main value lies in preventing turning-in of the leg during sleep in the prone position, facilitating spontaneous correction. Minor persistent internal torsion has not been shown to be detrimental.

■ FLATFOOT (PES PLANOVALGUS)

The condition called flatfoot must be divided into flexible and rigid types. The flexible type is very common in children and usually causes no symptoms. Development of the arch of the foot occurs spontaneously during the first 8 years of life in most children. The arch of the foot is restored when weight bearing is relieved. Inward–outward motion is normal. In contrast, rigid flatfoot may be caused by tarsal coalition, a vertical talus, neuromuscular imbalance (which occasionally also may be flexible), or arthritis of the foot. These conditions should be considered in the differential diagnosis.

TABLE 39-1. Differential Diagnoses of Common Pediatric Symptoms

The following are presented to guide in the use of this chapter and in the selection of references for further reading.

DIFFERENTIAL DIAGNOSIS OF LIMP

A. *Pain*
- Septic arthritis/ osteomyelitis
- Transient synovitis
- Juvenile rheumatoid arthritis
- Migratory polyarthritis (immunologic)
- Legg-Calvé-Perthes disease
- Slipped capital femoral epiphysis
- Meniscus tear
- Idiophatic chondriolysis of the hip
- Osgood-Schlatter disease
- Imparted fracture
- Spinal disorder

B. *Weakness*
- Congenital dislocation of the hip
- Myopathy
- Polio
- Cerebral palsy/myelomeningocele
- Spinal cord compression

C. *Limitation of Motion*
- Legg-Perthes disease/slipped capital femoral epiphysis (old)
- Posttraumatic muscle contracture
- Posttraumatic joint contracture

D. *Leg-length Inequality*
- Idiophatic hermihypertrophy
- Posttraumatic malunion or growth plate closure
- Neuromuscular
  - a. Cerebral palsy
  - b. Polio
- Neurofibromatosis
- Congenital limb deficiency
- Ollier's disease
- Arteriovenous malformation

KNEE PAIN

A. *Musculotendinous*
- Patellofemoral stress syndrome
- Osgood-Schlatter disease
- Patellar/quadriceps tendinitis
- Iliotibial band syndrome

B. *Bony–Cartilaginous*
- Meniscus tear
- Discoid meniscus
- Osteochondritis dissecans
- Tibial spine fracture/physeal injury

C. *Miscellaneous*
- Infection
- Tumor
- Connective tissue disorder
- Hip disorder

CHILDHOOD BACK PAIN

A. *Developmental/Acquired*
- Scheuermann's kyphosis
- Spondylolysis/ spondylolisthesis
- Herniated nuleus pulposus
- Fracture of vertebral body
- Muscle strain

B. *Infectious*
- Vertebral body osteomyelitis
- Discitis
- Tuberculosis

C. *Neoplastic*
- Osteoid osteoma
- Osteoblastoma/osteosarcoma
- Leukemia/lymphoma
- Eosinophilic granuloma
- Ewing's sarcoma/neuroblastoma
- Spinal cord tumor

INTERNAL ROTATION OF THE LOWER EXTREMITY: TOEING-IN

A. *Femoral*
- Anteversion
- Muscular/capsular

B. *Tibial Torsion*

C. *Metatarsus Adductus*

D. *Clubfoot, Partially Treated*

E. *Neuromuscular Disorder*

FLATFOOT

A. *Flexible/Idiopathic*

B. *Tarsal Coalition*

C. *Juvenile Rheumatoid Arthritis*

D. *Congenital Vertical Talus*

E. *Marfan Syndrome*

F. *Neuromuscular Disorder*

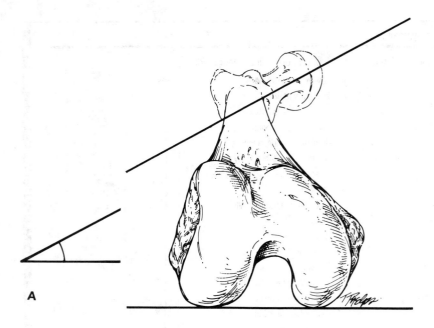

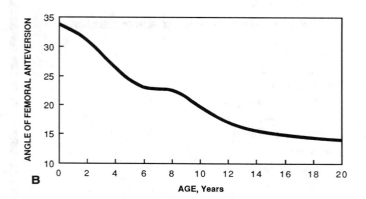

Figure 39-7. (A) Femoral anteversion is defined as the rotation of the femoral neck forward (in comparison with the distal condyles), as seen in this view down the axis of the femur. **(B)** The curve shows the normal decrease in femoral anteversion with age.

The cause of the usual type of flexible flatfoot is ligamentous laxity with mild secondary bony changes. No primary muscle abnormality exists. Occasionally, a tight heel cord may contribute by pulling the foot into greater outward angulation. Treatment is not indicated in asymptomatic cases of flexible flatfoot; prospective studies have shown that no orthotic or shoe configuration can produce a lasting change in pediatric flatfoot. Such devices may be indicated for rigid or neuromuscular flatfoot but not in asymptomatic children who have flexible flatfoot. The heel cord should be stretched if it is tight. Rarely is soft-tissue reconstruction or osteotomy indicated.

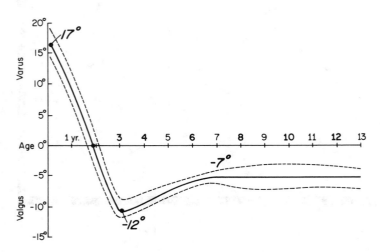

Figure 39-8. Normal change in the tibiofemoral angle during growth. (Reproduced with permission from Salenius P. Development of the tibiofemoral angle in children. J Bone Joint Surg 1975;57A:260.)

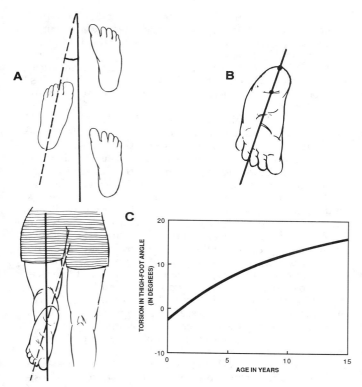

Figure 39-9. Assessment of torsional deformities. (**A**) Angle of progression: the angle between the foot and the line of gait—summation of femoral, knee, tibial, and foot relationships. (**B**) Assessment of metatarsus adductus. The heel bisector normally falls between second and third toe space. (**C**) Thigh–foot angle, and its variation with age. This is a reflection of tibial torsion.

General principles that a physician should stress to parents when asked about shoes are summarized in an article by Staheli. In short, shoes are primarily for protection; "corrective shoes" have no effect on flatfoot; and shoes should be flat, flexible, porous, and high-topped to prevent them from slipping off the foot. These characteristics are available in most reasonably priced footwear found in regular shoe stores.

■ DISCITIS

Discitis may present in a wide variety of ways. Severe back pain with limitation of back movements is common in older children, whereas younger children simply may refuse to walk or may limp. The cause of this disc inflammation is variable, but bacterial infection is suspected most commonly. The vascular anatomy of the growing disc varies from that of the adult, and the common bacteremias of childhood can infect the disc more readily than the vertebral body itself. About 50% of these children have positive blood culture results at the time of their acute pain, with the most common organism identified being *Staphylococcus aureus*. Despite this, milder forms of discitis often appear to resolve without the need for antibiotics.

The most striking finding on physical examination in patients with discitis is marked stiffness of the spine that is notable with attempts at flexion. Fever often is present. The results of the neurologic examination are normal. In the early stages, radiographs of the spine appear normal. Usually, a few weeks after the onset of pain, narrowing of a single disc

may be seen on radiography. The sedimentation rate and white blood cell count often are elevated. A technetium 99m bone scan virtually always reveals increased uptake at the involved level and should be performed whenever discitis is suspected. If the bone scan results are positive and the age and clinical presentation are typical, needle aspiration or open biopsy of the involved disc generally is not necessary.

Treatment decisions in cases of discitis revolve around whether to use antibiotics or a body jacket brace or cast. If a positive blood culture result has been obtained, antibiotics should be used for 3 to 6 weeks. We prefer to use antibiotics in children who have a positive bone scan result, even if no bacteremia has been demonstrated. Bed rest should be instituted at the time of presentation to decrease the spasm. If the spasm persists for more than a few days, a body jacket brace or cast will allow for immobilization and ambulation on a limited basis. It is extremely rare for discitis to develop into vertebral osteomyelitis with local bone destruction.

■ SCOLIOSIS

Scoliosis is a lateral curvature of the spine. The two forms of scoliosis are postural and structural. Postural scoliosis results from spinal factors outside the spine, such as leg length discrepancy. In these cases, if the leg lengths are equalized or if the child sits, the spine becomes straight, indicating that no structural change has occurred. Structural scoliosis is of greater concern, because it involves not only a lateral spinal curvature, but also a rotation of the vertebrae involved in the lateral curve.

Although numerous conditions are associated with scoliosis, the most common groups include idiopathic (80%), congenital (5%), neuromuscular (10%), and miscellaneous (5%) disorders. The miscellaneous disorders encompass connective tissue disorders, genetic diseases, and other, less common, conditions.

Congenital scoliosis is present at birth, although the diagnosis often is not made at that time (Figure 39–10). It

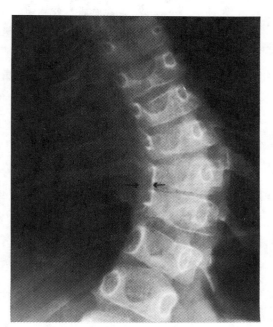

Figure 39-10. Congenital scoliosis results from incomplete vertebral segmentation in utero. Genitourinary abnormalities are frequently associated with these bony deformities.

may be associated with other birth defects or present as an isolated condition. Because the genitourinary system arises embryologically from the same region as does the spine, about 30% of children with a congenital spinal deformity have an associated genitourinary abnormality. The most common anomaly is unilateral renal agenesis, so a sonogram or intravenous pyelogram should be performed on all patients who have congenital scoliosis or kyphosis. Although active treatment of unilateral kidney absence may not be necessary, appropriate cautioning against the child's participation in contact sports that may lead to kidney injury is important. The treatment of congenital scoliosis consists of serial radiographic follow-up to determine whether the deformity is worsening. If no curve progression occurs, further treatment generally is not needed. If worsening of 5 to 10 degrees or more is documented, surgical fusion is necessary, no matter what the child's age. Brace treatment may be useful to prevent worsening of curves above or below the congenital scoliosis, but it seldom is successful or indicated for the congenital scoliosis.

Neuromuscular scoliosis is associated with a wide variety of neurologic or muscular diseases, such as cerebral palsy (CP), muscular dystrophy, and poliomyelitis. Spinal curvature that is secondary to muscular imbalance classically is C-shaped and extends to include the pelvis (Figure 39–11) which is not usually the case in idiopathic scoliosis. Scoliosis is present more often and tends to worsen most quickly in patients who do not walk because of their neuromuscular disease. With continued progression, sitting balance becomes impaired further and it may be necessary for the child to use one arm or hand to assist in sitting. Treat-

ment centers on preservation of sitting ability and pulmonary function. Although brace wear often is useful, surgical fusion frequently is indicated to preserve function.

Idiopathic scoliosis generally is found in otherwise healthy children. Although idiopathic scoliosis requiring treatment is about eight times more frequent in girls than in boys, the incidence of mild curves is about equal between the sexes.

A family history of curvature of the spine is found in as many as 70% of all children with scoliosis, although the exact mode of inheritance has not been determined definitely. Although the cause of idiopathic scoliosis remains elusive, a combination of growth asymmetry and postural imbalance is believed to be important. Minor abnormalities in the postural control center in the brain stem have been demonstrated in children with mild scoliosis. Once the curve begins to develop in response to this impaired postural feedback, growth asymmetry likely occurs. Growth is slower where increased pressure is exerted on the growth areas. Because there is more pressure on the concave growing areas than on the convex side, the convexity grows more quickly, leading to increasing curve size. This theory accounts for the observation that curves worsen most during the rapid adolescent growth spurt, which is the time when most of these curves are diagnosed. Muscles, discs, and bone appear to be normal in the young patient with idiopathic scoliosis.

The key to early detection of scoliosis is careful assessment of the entire trunk for asymmetry. The child should be examined with the back clearly exposed. The examination should include evaluation of shoulder height, scapula position and prominence, waistline symmetry, and levelness of the pelvis (Table 39–2). Asymmetry in any of these areas may indicate a scoliosis (Figure 39–12). To define further whether a structural scoliosis is present, the child should be examined bending forward (Figure 39–13). Viewed from the caudal aspect, prominence of the thoracic ribs can be detected readily, whereas further bending or viewing from the head down is better for suspected lumbar curves. Both thoracic and lumbar regions should be checked. This "forward-bending" test is very sensitive in demonstrating the vertebral rotation that takes place in a structural scoliotic curve. It is possible to measure the amount of rib hump by means of an inclinometer placed at the apex of the curve with the child bending forward. If the inclinometer measurement is 5 degrees or less,

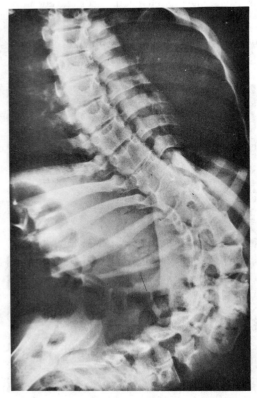

Figure 39-11. Sitting anteroposterior radiograph of a child with cerebral palsy and severe scoliosis. Note the C-shaped curve and the pelvic tilt characteristic of neuromuscular scoliosis.

TABLE 39-2. Spinal Deformity Evaluation

Examine in swimming suit or similar clothing so back is exposed.

Observe asymmetry on trunk examination; shoulder height, scapular height, waistline equality, levelness of pelvis, leg length difference, forward bending, both side and front/back.

Measure rib prominence with inclinometer (optional).

Assess skeletal maturity (eg, age of menses onset).

Obtain standing posteroanterior radiograph of the spine if asymmetry is seen.

Measure using Cobb method.

Recommend follow-up or treatment.

None if the curve is less than 25 degrees and growth is complete.

If growth remains and the curve is less than 25 degrees, obtain repeat radiographs in 4 to 15 mo (see text).

If scoliosis more than 25 degrees is seen and growth remains, consider a brace.

If scoliosis more than 40 degrees is seen, consider surgery.

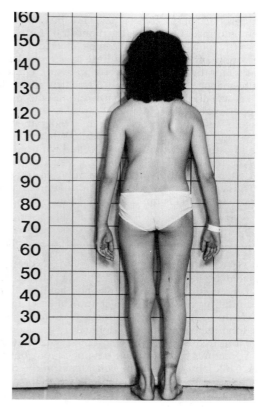

Figure 39-12. In examining for scoliosis, asymmetry of the trunk (shoulders, scapular height, waist area, pelvic height) should be noted carefully.

the scoliosis rarely is significant and radiographs usually are not needed. If the inclinometer reading exceeds 7 degrees, standing posteroanterior and lateral radiographs are indicated for better assessment.

Because no active treatment is needed until the curve reaches 25 degrees, the time estimate for a follow-up radiograph, once the diagnosis has been made, is 25 minus the present curve magnitude. This provides an estimate of the number of months that may pass until another radiograph is indicated. For example, if a child has a scoliosis of 15 degrees, waiting about 10 months before repeating the posteroanterior radiograph to check for progression is appropriate. This time estimate is based on the premise that, during the adolescent growth spurt, annual curve progression is 5 to 10 degrees or about 1 degree/month.

Completion of growth or skeletal maturity can be assessed most accurately with bone age radiographs of the hand and wrist. From the clinical standpoint, girls who have been menstruating for 2 years essentially have completed their spinal growth.

The treatment of scoliosis is based on three fundamental principles:

1. Curves more than 25 degrees are likely to increase if the child is still growing.
2. Curves of 40 to 50 degrees are likely to increase even after growth is complete.
3. Some degree of clinical pulmonary restriction may begin to be noted in thoracic curves of more than about 75 degrees.

If a child is skeletally mature and has a curvature of less than 25 degrees, no further evaluation or treatment of scolio-

sis is needed. If the scoliosis is 25 degrees or more and the child is still growing, brace treatment generally is recommended and is successful in about 80% of the patients who actually wear the brace as prescribed. Spinal exercises alone will not be successful in stopping curve progression. Once the brace treatment begins, it is continued until growth is complete. The brace usually is worn 18 to 23 hours daily. Physical activity is not limited by scoliosis, and affected children often can participate in sports activities while wearing their brace. Brace wear is considered to be successful if it prevents further progression rather than providing correction of the curve; long-term follow-up studies have shown that the final size of the curve is virtually the same as before brace treatment begins. Although children and parents often are dismayed by our inability to straighten the spine nonoperatively, if curves can be kept at less than 35 to 40 degrees by the time growth is completed, most cases of scoliosis will not worsen in adult life. If the thoracic curve is greater than 50 degrees or the lumbar curve is greater than 40 degrees at the time growth is completed, progression usually will continue at a rate of about 1 degree annually and surgery often will be required.

Surgical treatment is recommended for curves that are greater than 40 degrees, particularly in a child who is not fully grown. The surgical treatment usually employed consists of instrumentation of the curved area of the spine, combined with posterior spinal fusion of the instrumented area (Figure 39–14, *A* and *B*). Correction of the scoliosis generally is about 50%. Failure of fusion occurs in only about 1% of teenagers. Fusion is complete by 6 months after surgery, at which time the teenagers can return to almost all physical activities, except tackle football, wrestling, and gymnastics. They should be encouraged to return to activity, including physical education class in school, to deemphasize the psychological potential for disability after this surgery.

If the thoracic scoliosis exceeds 50 degrees, patients commonly have diminished vital capacity and residual lung volumes on pulmonary function testing. Arterial blood gas levels and forced expiratory volume in 1 second are normal except in children with severe curves. Vital capacity is decreased further if a thoracic lordosis is associated with the scoliosis. Even with surgical correction of the scoliosis, pulmonary function

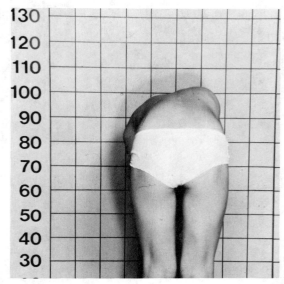

Figure 39-13. The forward bending examination will detect even very small curvatures. The prominence is produced by chestwall asymmetry, caused by vertebral-body rotation in the curved segment of the spine.

postoperatively will change little because of the persistence of chest wall or rib deformities that have occurred as a result of the scoliosis. Therefore, scoliosis should be prevented from progressing to this point if possible.

■ TORTICOLLIS

Torticollis most commonly is present at or near the time of birth and results from a contracture of one of the sternocleidomastoid muscles. The child's head will be tilted toward the side of the contracture, with the chin rotated away from the contracted side, because the origin of the contracted muscle is on the mastoid process. The cause of torticollis is not well defined, but the incidence is higher in children with breech presentation and forceps delivery.

Torticollis may present later in childhood after an upper respiratory infection or trauma. Torticollis that occurs after an upper respiratory infection is thought to result from retropharyngeal edema that leads to malposition at the atlantoaxial level, causing a rotatory deformity. Similarly, after muscular neck trauma, the child may have a persistent torticollis for several days or weeks, secondary to an unsuspected rotatory subluxation at the atlantoaxial level. If torticollis from either of these causes persists, the child should be treated with traction, followed by either bracing or atlantoaxial fusion. The likelihood that surgical fusion will be necessary increases with the duration of symptoms, so prompt treatment is required.

■ FIBROUS DYSPLASIA

Fibrous dysplasia is a disorder in which bone formation in the medulla and cortex is altered, and the marrow contains much fibrous tissue. Radiographically, the bone has a uniform "ground glass" consistency, and the cortex is thin and often deformed. One bone (the monostotic form) or several bones (the polyostotic form) can be affected. Pathologic fractures occur often but usually heal in a normal period. Proximal femoral ("shepherd's crook") bowing is the most difficult to manage. Deformities and fractures of the lower extremities usually require internal fixation, whereas those in the upper extremities require casting.

Irregular café au lait spots occur in 30% of patients with the polyostotic form of fibrous dysplasia. When polyostotic lesions and café au lait spots are associated with precocious puberty, the condition is called Albright's syndrome. Other types of endocrinopathy (thyroid, parathyroid, or adrenal problems) may occur. Malignant transformation to fibrosarcoma or osteosarcoma is rare.

■ OSTEOGENESIS IMPERFECTA

Osteogenesis imperfecta encompasses a spectrum of diseases that are the end result of defects in collagen or proteoglycan synthesis. These result in bones that have thin cortices and multiple fractures. Short stature, blue sclerae, middle ear deafness, abnormal dentition, and thin skin may coexist. Inheritance usually is dominant, occasionally is recessive, but frequently is the result of spontaneous mutation. Tiny fractures occur to cause bowing of long bones and scoliosis. Child abuse should be considered in the differential diagnosis, and the absence of pelvic deformities or wormian cranial bones in children who are subjected to abuse may be helpful.

Aids to mobility and preventive bracing can be very helpful in preventing fractures. Occasionally, intramedullary rods that elongate with growth are needed. Fortunately, the frequency of fractures diminishes with age.

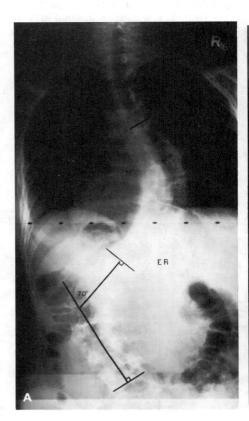

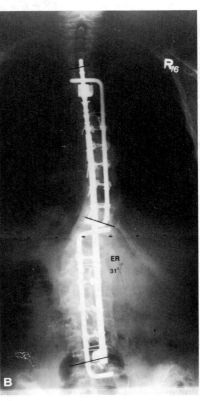

Figure 39-14. A standing posteroanterior radiograph of the spine is the correct film to use in quantitating the magnitude of scoliosis. (**A**) The Cobb method of measurement is used routinely, and is obtained as shown on this radiograph. (**B**) This is the postoperative result after spinal correction and fusion in the same patient.

■ HEMATOGENOUS OSTEOMYELITIS

The incidence and presentation of hematogenous osteomyelitis are changing following the introduction of newer imaging and treatment methods, but certain principles remain constant. The summary presented here should be coupled with that provided in the chapter regarding infectious diseases to illustrate the spectrum of treatment philosophies.

Acute hematogenous osteomyelitis by definition includes processes that have been operating for a week or less at the time of diagnosis. After infancy, this condition occurs more frequently in males than in females, presumably because trauma plays a role in increasing susceptibility. The peak ages of occurrence are infancy (less than 1 year) and preadolescence (9 to 11 years). The incidence declines in adulthood because of the change in vascular supply of bone. The most commonly affected sites are the femur and tibia, each of which accounts for one third of all cases, followed by the humerus, calcaneus, and pelvis. Any bone may be affected, however. The metaphysis is the region most often involved, and spread may occur from this point to involve any other portion. Rarely, the process may begin in the epiphysis.

Unlike septic arthritis, the organisms involved in hematogenous osteomyelitis vary slightly with the age of the patient (Figure 39–15). In all age groups, the predominant organism is *Staphylococcus aureus*, although *Streptococcus pneumoniae* and *Haemophilus* must be considered. *Staphylococcus* is associated with a higher recurrence rate than other organisms. *Salmonella* should be considered in patients with sickle cell anemia, although *Staphylococcus* still is more common in these patients. Blood culture results during the acute phase are positive about 40% to 50% of the time, and direct cultures of pus or bone are positive only 60% to 80% of the time. This may be the result of prior antibiotic use, errors in sampling or processing, or autoeradication of the organism.

Clinical diagnosis remains key despite the availability of new imaging techniques. The child may appear well or may have systemic involvement ranging from malaise to shock. Often, refusal to bear weight is an early symptom. The very earliest sign is fever and local bone tenderness, followed later by a fluctuant mass if a subperiosteal or soft-tissue abscess has developed. Spread to adjacent joints should be ruled out by palpation and range of motion evaluation.

Radiographs at the earliest stage may show soft-tissue swelling. Osteopenia or lysis may appear after 7 to 10 days, followed by new bone formation at the borders of the process. Bone scanning has been used widely in the past 2 decades, but the subtleties of its use have been recognized only recently. The tracer that is used most widely is technetium 99m methylene diphosphonate because of its speed, cost, and sensitivity (Figure 39–16). Immediate scans for flow and blood pool should be obtained, as well as later skeletal images. Results of the scan may be normal in the very early stages. It should be repeated after 48 hours if clinically indicated.

Cold or photopenic areas are important because they may indicate avascular sites, especially when they are accompanied by adjacent areas of increased uptake. Cellulitis may cause confusion but usually does not show bony localization on delayed images. The overall accuracy of nuclear imaging is about 60% to 90%. It may be much lower in neonates, however, according to some reports. Gallium citrate may be sensitive, but it requires a minimum of 24 hours; indium-labeled white cell studies require similar amounts of time, including preparation of the tracer. Because of the above-mentioned limitations, radionuclide scans should not be relied on in all instances, especially when the clinical diagnosis is clear. These studies have their greatest value when localization for aspiration is difficult. The role of magnetic resonance imaging (MRI) has yet to be defined.

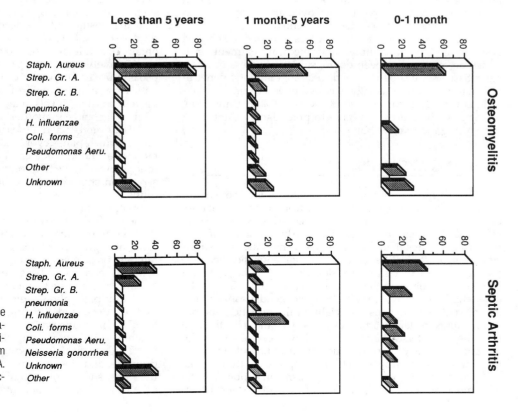

Figure 39-15. Frequency of occurrence of organisms involved in acute hematogenous osteomyelitis and septic arthritis in three age groups. (Drawn from table, with permission, from Jackson MA. Management of the bone and joint infections. *Pediatr Orthopaed.* 1982;2:315.)

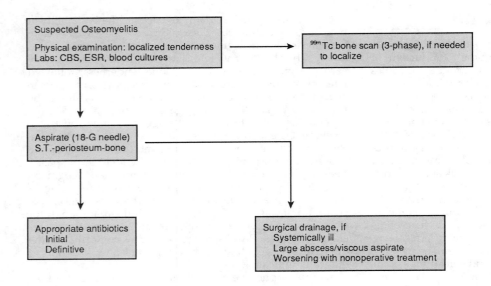

Figure 39-16. Diagnosis and treatment algorithm for hematogenous osteomyelitis.

Aspiration is indicated in all cases to identify the pathogen and in some cases to decompress localized purulence.

Treatment involves the delivery of an appropriate antibiotic to all infected tissue. Therefore, avascular abscesses may require surgical decompression if aspiration cannot accomplish this. Antibiotic therapy can be divided into initial and definitive periods. In the initial phase, broad-spectrum antibiotics, including antistaphylococcic agents such as nafcillin or oxacillin, are indicated. Vancomycin should be used if resistance is suspected. In neonates, an aminoglycoside should be added. In children younger than 3 years of age who have osteomyelitis associated with septic arthritis, chloramphenicol or cefuroxime may be used to cover *Haemophilus influenzae*. In the definitive period, the most effective, least toxic antibiotic that is effective against the isolated organism should be given for 4 to 6 weeks. It may be administered by the oral route if the patient is clinically improved and compliant, and if adequate blood levels can be documented.

Surgery is reserved for those cases in which the child is systemically ill or worsening under medical treatment, or in which an abscess has been demonstrated. Abscess or avascular tissue should be removed to allow antibiotic penetration, and the wound usually is closed over a drain. Complications include recurrence (20% overall; 6% at 6 months), minor growth acceleration, growth plate damage, and fracture through weakened bone.

■ SEPTIC ARTHRITIS

Slightly more common than hematogenous osteomyelitis, septic arthritis may have more disastrous long-term consequences if effective treatment is delayed. Most cases occur in infants and younger children, with nearly half of all affected patients being less than 3 years of age. A high index of suspicion for septic arthritis should be maintained in sick neonatal patients because they show few signs. The hip is the joint most commonly involved in the infant compared to the knee in the older child. The spread may be from the bloodstream or from an adjacent osteomyelitis, especially in the hip and shoulder where the capsular insertion extends over the growth plate onto the metaphysis. Many theories have been advanced for the pathogenesis of joint destruction, including alteration of joint fluid by toxins from both the neutrophils and the bacteria.

The spectrum of causative organisms in septic arthritis is somewhat broader than that of hematogenous osteo-

myelitis (see Figure 39–15), which may be related to the greater frequency of this condition. Overall, *S aureus* still is the most common causative organism. In patients between 1 month and 5 years of age, however, *H influenzae* is more common than *Staphylococcus*. The streptococci, *Escherichia coli, Proteus,* and other organisms also should be considered. The yield of organisms from aspiration is about 60% to 80%.

Clinical findings vary with the age of the patient. In the infant, there may be fever, failure to feed, and tachycardia. Subtle changes in position may serve as clues, as well as unilateral swelling of an extremity or a joint, asymmetry of soft-tissue folds, and pain with range of motion. In the older child, the signs are more localized.

Aspiration with a large needle should be performed if any reasonable suspicion of septic arthritis exists, both for diagnosis and, in some cases, for treatment. In deep joints such as the hip, radiopaque dye should be injected to confirm the position of the needle, especially if the aspirated fluid is normal. This ensures that joint fluid actually was obtained, and it also helps to distinguish joint infection from septic involvement of the bursa underneath the nearby psoas muscle. The white cell count in fluid obtained from patients with septic arthritis ranges from 25,000 to 250,000. Elevated lactate levels may be helpful in cases in which white cell counts are borderline.

The differential diagnosis includes toxic synovitis of the hip, in which pain, fever, leukocytosis, and spasm are more moderate and do not escalate on serial observations. At times, however, the two conditions are indistinguishable and aspiration should be performed. Rheumatoid arthritis, cellulitis, traumatic synovitis, and the migratory multiple arthralgias of rheumatic fever should be considered. A sympathetic effusion also may occur from adjacent osteomyelitis.

The role of arthrotomy versus aspiration in confirmed cases of septic arthritis is controversial. The key feature is removal of deleterious enzymes and restoration of effective synovial perfusion. Because the decision not to operate requires the ability to monitor and aspirate repeatedly as needed, it probably is preferable to use arthrotomy in joints that are deep and difficult to assess such as the hip and shoulder, in young patients who are difficult to examine, and when the fluid obtained is viscous.

The surgical procedure should include irrigation, drainage, and closure. This may be done arthroscopically in the knee, shoulder, and ankle. Direct instillation of antibiotics has no benefit. Some investigators feel that the femoral metaphysis should be drilled whenever the hip is aspirated to decompress any possible femoral osteomyelitis.

Early effective treatment is very important. The chance of achieving good results declines dramatically if treatment is initiated after the symptoms have been present for 4 days. Antibiotics should be continued for 4 to 6 weeks. Controversy exists regarding whether the joint should be immobilized or treated with continuous passive motion; however, the latter is practiced less commonly. Contractures should be prevented, and abduction of the hip decreases the likelihood of dislocation. Complications include permanent destruction of cartilage and, in the hip, avascular necrosis with resorption or overgrowth of the femoral head. Complications are more frequent in young infants.

Gonococcal arthritis also occurs in children. It usually becomes evident after the systemic and febrile phase of the illness and should be distinguished from the more common gonococcal migratory multiple arthralgia or tenosynovitis. An average of two to three joints are affected, most commonly the wrists and knees. Treatment is aspiration and closed irrigation followed by 3 days of intravenous penicillin and 4 days of ampicillin or amoxicillin. Oral treatment alone with one of these drugs for 7 days is acceptable in compliant patients after a loading dose has been given.

(Abridged from Paul D. Sponseller, Bone, Joint, and Muscle Problems, in Oski, DeAngelis, Feigin, McMillan, Warshaw: *Principles and Practice of Pediatrics, Second Edition*, J.B. Lippincott, 1994.)

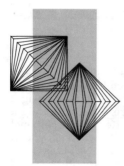

SECTION 5

Failure to Thrive

Oski's Essential Pediatrics,
edited by Kevin B. Johnson and Frank A. Oski.
Lippincott–Raven Publishers,
Philadelphia © 1997

40

Failure to Thrive

Failure to thrive (FTT) is a problem common in pediatric practice and accounts for 1% to 5% of all referrals to children's hospitals or tertiary centers. In a rural primary care setting, 10% of children in the first year of life have had FTT. Failure to thrive occurs more frequently among children living in poverty.

■ ORGANIC VERSUS NONORGANIC ETIOLOGIES

The distinction between organic causes of FTT and nonorganic or psychosocial etiologies has limited usefulness. In the child with congenital heart disease or other chronic disease, the nonorganic or environmental factors also may contribute to FTT and should not be overlooked. Likewise, the child within an emotionally disturbed family also may have an organic problem. One third to more than 50% of cases of FTT investigated in tertiary care settings and almost all the cases in primary care settings have nonorganic etiologies. About one fourth of all cases have involved a combination of organic and psychosocial factors.

■ APPROACH TO THE SIGNS AND SYMPTOMS

A careful, thorough history and physical examination (Table 40–1) of the child whose only sign may be a diminished

weight allow a logical, rational approach to ordering of laboratory tests and other investigations. Observation of the infant and of the interaction of the child with the guardian or parent, and an assessment of the social and environmental factors yield valuable information regarding the psychosocial milieu. In the absence of evidence for an organic problem in the initial history and physical examination, subsequent laboratory investigation is unlikely to reveal an organic cause.

History

The pediatric history of the patient who fails to thrive should include an elicitation of symptoms suggesting organic diseases. A detailed environmental assessment is essential. Adverse psychosocial circumstances are known to have an association with diminished weight gain and growth in infancy.

The history should include a detailed dietary and feeding history, including information related to breast-feeding in the breast-fed infant. Deficient caloric intake due to increased losses of nutrients in the stool (malnutrition or diarrhea), vomiting or regurgitation, or impaired utilization can be clarified. If a psychosocial problem is suspected, caution should be used when interpreting a dietary history, because parental guilt may result in inaccuracies.

The psychosocial history should include an assessment of the family composition (absent parents), employment status, financial state, degree of social isolation (absence of a telephone or of nearby neighbors), and family stress. Poverty indicators including eligibility for the Supplemental Food Program for Women, Infants and Children (WIC) should be sought. Maternal factors relating to the pregnancy, such as planned or unplanned pregnancy, use of medications for illness, substance abuse, physical or mental illness, postpartum depression, or inadequate breast milk, may be significant. Assessment should be made of levels of knowledge about parenting and about how to provide an

TABLE 40–1. Clinical Approach and Management for Failure to Thrive

Approach	Immediate Support	Long-Term Support
Careful history	Nutritional support (plot daily intake and weights)	Frequent follow-up visits (well-child maintenance, plot heights and weights, developmental assessment)
Thorough physical examination (plot height and weight on curves)	Team approach (pediatricians, nurses, social workers, developmental specialists, community service workers, health educators, child-life worker-volunteers) or temporary/permanent foster home	
Observation of infant's behavior		
Psychosocial evaluation (family and environmental factors)	Treatment of uncommon underlying organic illness	
Judicious approach to laboratory testing, radiology, and imaging		

adequate diet. Predisposing factors in the infant are intrauterine growth retardation, perinatal stress, prematurity, chronic disease, and frequency of intercurrent illness such as diarrhea, vomiting, or otitis media. In the dynamic interaction between the parent and the child, factors in the child, such as being "difficult" or chronically ill or giving diminished feedback, may contribute to the overall problem. Questions regarding the child's sleep pattern, other behaviors, and the amount of time spent alone may be helpful.

Family members' heights and weights, their history of illness, and any developmental delay in family members that may contribute to slow growth or constitutional short stature should be included in the assessment. Support systems available to the family and frequency of changes of home address should be examined. Initially, parents may avoid mentioning psychosocial problems such as marital discord; discussions of such issues should take place during several visits. These conversations should be conducted in a nonthreatening manner, demonstrating concern and compassion.

Simple Observation

The infant's behavior can give valuable clues regarding his or her ability to interact appropriately for age. Behavioral features suggestive of psychosocial or environmental deprivation may include avoidance of eye contact, absence of smiling or vocalization, and a lack of interest in the environment. The negative response of the child to cuddling, and an inability to be comforted, may indicate a problem. The child may exhibit repetitive motions such as head banging or self-stimulatory activity such as anogenital manipulation, or may be relatively immobile, with infantile posturing. The infant may be withdrawn and socially unresponsive, even to the mother, and actually may look away from her. Some infants inappropriately seek affection from strangers. Historically, these behaviors have been described in institutionalized infants who suffer from lack of care and affection.

Observing the mother feeding the child may be helpful. Does she cuddle the infant or merely "prop" the bottle? Does she allow sufficient time for feeding? The parents' level of concern may be inappropriate if they are eager to relinquish the child to the health team quickly. Observing the parents' interactions with each other will indicate whether they are supportive of each other.

Physical Examination

Accurate assessment of the child's height, weight, and head circumference is essential. In the child younger than 2 years, the recumbent length rather than the standing height should be obtained carefully. This figure, along with weight and head circumference, should be plotted on the National Center for Health Statistics (NCHS) growth charts and related to previous measurements. The NCHS growth charts are gender specific and appropriate for all races and nationalities. Attention to the percentile curves of length, weight, and head circumference may give valuable clues as to the etiology of FTT. When all measurements are below the third percentile, the incidence of organic disease has been noted to be 70%. Gastrointestinal disorders are more common when only the weight is below the third percentile. The single assessment of height and weight may have limited usefulness without an indication of whether the child's pattern is deviating from the percentile or of how far below the curve the measurement may be. In intrauterine growth retardation, the child initially is small for height and weight; weight gain and growth velocity may be adequate, yet continue to be below the third percentile. Also, 3% of the normal population has had growth patterns at or below the third percentile (constitutional short stature). Therefore, determining the median age for the child's length (height or length age) and the median age for the child's weight (weight age) may be useful.

The complete developmental assessment is important. Careful evaluation should be made for dysmorphic features (clinical or genetic syndromes) and for signs of central nervous system (hypotonia or spasticity), pulmonary, cardiac, or gastrointestinal (swallowing disorders, gastroesophageal reflux) disorders. Isolated defects in the soft or hard palate may indicate a feeding problem.

Signs of neglect may be indicated by a diaper rash, impetigo, flat occiput, poor hygiene, protuberant abdomen, lack of appropriate behavior, and inappropriate infantile postures. Child abuse may result in bruises and fresh lesions or healed, unexplained scars. Notation of drooling and bowel habits is essential.

■ MANAGEMENT

Most experience in the evaluation and initial management of FTT has been in the inpatient setting in tertiary centers. Exhaustive investigations for organic causes and prolonged hospitalizations to evaluate family dynamics and poor infant weight gain have resulted in inefficiencies and often the lack of a diagnosis.

Laboratory Investigation and Evaluation

A careful history and physical examination in the child with FTT may suggest clues to organic disease in the child who has received an organic diagnosis. The search for organic disease should be guided by the signs and symptoms found in the initial examination. Laboratory studies not suggested on the basis of the initial examination rarely are helpful. Simple routine testing, including hematocrit, urinalysis and culture of urine, blood urea nitrogen, calcium, electrolyte levels, human immunodeficiency virus (HIV) enzyme-linked immunosorbent assay (ELISA) antibody test, and Mantoux tuberculin skin testing, is appropriate. Additional testing, radiographs, and imaging may be indicated specifically by the clinical examination.

In the past, hospitalization was considered essential to demonstrate rapid weight gain in the child with FTT, to distinguish between organic and nonorganic etiologies. However, although immediate, rapid weight gain suggests evidence for a nonorganic cause of FTT, failure to gain weight does not rule out the nonorganic etiology. Children in whom the initial history and physical examination suggest an organic basis for FTT can either be admitted to an acute care hospital or be evaluated as outpatients, if indicated. The child who has no evidence of organic disease or who may have a combination of organic and psychosocial problems can be evaluated and supported in either outpatient or inpatient settings.

Effective evaluation, whether inpatient or outpatient, requires involvement of the parents from the beginning with the support provided by an interdisciplinary program. In addition to the pediatrician, the program may involve social workers, nurses, developmental specialists, nutritionists, child-life workers, psychiatrists, and workers from social and educational services in the community. The low self-esteem that many parents have suggests that the health care providers should not focus blame, but should work with the strengths of the family to encourage development of a nurturing environment.

The many possible causes of FTT are listed in Table 40–2.

Nutrition and Growth Recovery

Nutritional requirements for the healthy infant younger than 1 year are an average of 100 kcal/kg of body weight per

TABLE 40–2. Causes of Failure to Thrive

	Inadequate Caloric Intake			
Weight Gain During Refeeding	No Weight Gain During Refeeding	Inadequate Appetite or Inability to Eat Large Amounts	Inadequate Caloric Absorption: No Weight Gain During Refeeding; Increased Losses	Increased Caloric Requirements
Inappropriate feeding technique	Psychosocial problems*	Psychosocial problems (apathy)*	Psychosocial problems (refeeding diarrhea, intercurrent illnesses, rumination, regurgitation)*	Hyperthyroidism
Disturbed mother–child relationship	Maternal–infant dysfunction, economic deprivation	Cardiopulmonary disease	Malabsorption—diarrhea (lactose intolerance, cystic fibrosis, cardiac disease, malrotation, inflammatory bowel disease, milk allergy, parasites, celiac disease)	Cerebral palsy
	Mechanical problems	Hypotonia		Malignancy
	Insufficient lactation in mother	Anorexia or chronic infection or immune deficiency diseases (AIDS or AIDS-related complex)		Chronic systemic disease (juvenile rheumatoid arthritis)
	Cleft palate	Endocrine disorders (hypothyroidism, diabetes insipidus)	Vomiting or "spitting up" or diarrhea	Chronic systemic infection (UTI, tuberculosis, toxoplasmosis)
	Nasal obstruction			
	Sucking or swallowing dysfunction (CNS, neuromuscular, esophageal motility problems)	CNS tumors	Intestinal tract obstruction (pyloric stenosis, hernia, malrotation, intussusception, chalasia)	
		Genetic syndromes		
	Regurgitation (gastroesophageal reflux)	Metabolic conditions (lead toxicity, iron deficiency, zinc deficiency)	CNS problems—increased intracranial pressure (subdural hematoma)	
	Malformation	Anemia		
	Congenital syndromes (alcohol, phenytoin drugs)		Chronic metabolic problems (hypercalcemia, storage diseases, and inborn errors of metabolism such as galactosemia, methylmalonic acidemia, renal acidosis, diabetes mellitus, adrenal insufficiency)	
	Genetic syndromes (Turner)			

Environmental causes are the most common source of problems.

day. A child who fails to gain weight normally and whose weight is below the third percentile will not experience "catch-up," and, therefore, a caloric intake that is higher than normal is required. In such cases, intake requirements may be 50% higher than normal, or 150 kcal/kg/day. A higher caloric intake may be needed when the infant's normal energy requirements in the state of good health are considered.

Malnourished infants require extra concern because of the anorexia that may accompany the malnutrition state. The anorexia occurs early in the process and may last for up to a week. Malnutrition can result in transient malabsorption during the refeeding process. Environmental deprivation can result in the physiologic changes of hypopituitarism. The response of these secondary changes to treatment should be observed.

■ FOLLOW-UP AND PROGNOSIS

Close follow-up and frequent contact with the health care team are essential for reinforcing nutritional recommendations and psychosocial support. Involvement with the family by community social service workers, visiting nurses, and nutritionists is important. Although the prognosis with respect to weight gain and growth is good, one fourth to one half of infants with FTT remain small. The possibility that caloric deprivation in infancy will produce severe, irreversible developmental deficits is the reason why treatment should begin expeditiously. Cognitive function is below normal in half of the children with FTT, and a high incidence of behavior problems is found on follow-up. Whether these findings are a direct result of the FTT or of the contribution of continued adverse social circumstances is not known. The families need education and community services to help them to cope and to provide a nurturing environment for the children.

(Abridged from Rebecca T. Kirkland, Failure to Thrive, in Oski, DeAngelis, Feigin, McMillan, Warshaw: *Principles and Practice of Pediatrics, Second Edition,* J.B. Lippincott, 1994.)

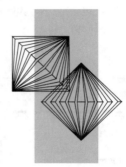

SECTION 6
Sudden Unexplained Death and Apparent Life-Threatening Events

Oski's Essential Pediatrics,
edited by Kevin B. Johnson and Frank A. Oski.
Lippincott–Raven Publishers,
Philadelphia © 1997

41

Sudden Infant Death Syndrome

Sudden infant death syndrome (SIDS) is what remains after a thorough postmortem examination fails to reveal a cause of death; in other words, it is a diagnosis of exclusion. It is defined as "the sudden death of an infant under 1 year of age which remains unexplained after a thorough investigation, including a performance of complete autopsy, examination of the death scene, and review of the clinical history."

■ EPIDEMIOLOGY

Most deaths caused by congenital anomalies occur during the first week of life, leaving SIDS as the most common single cause of death between 7 days and 365 days of age. Each year between 5200 and 5500 infants die of SIDS in the United States, making the overall incidence about 1.4 SIDS deaths/1000 live births.

Sudden infant death syndrome is uncommon during the first week of life. Most deaths occur between 1 and 5 months, peaking at about 3 months postnatal age. Males have a higher incidence of SIDS in all racial groups (female:male ratio, 1:1.6). The reason for sex differences in SIDS is unknown.

■ RISK FACTORS

A variety of potential risk factors have been considered in SIDS victims. Table 41–1 outlines many recognized risk factors.

■ PATHOGENESIS

The cause or causes of SIDS are unknown. The search for the causes of SIDS has been further complicated by the study of so-called infants at risk or high-risk infants, because identification of groups that are at risk is a matter of dispute. Some investigators have proposed that abnormal respiratory control underlies SIDS in most cases. Other proposed mechanisms include nasal/oral occlusion or suffocation of an infant, abnormal pulmonary surfactant, the long QT syndrome, hypersensitivity to vagal stimulation, underlying metabolic abnormalities, increased somnogenic substances, or combinations of factors that affect children at vulnerable times.

TABLE 41-1. Reported Risk Factors for Sudden Infant Death Syndrome (SIDS)

MATERNAL RISK FACTORS	POSTNEONATAL FACTORS
Cigarette smoking during pregnancy*	History of cyanosis or apnea
Drug use during pregnancy	History of diarrhea or vomiting in 2 weeks before SIDS death
Inadequate prenatal care*	
Lack of breast feeding*	History of listless/droopy in 2 weeks before SIDS death
Low education level*	**PRENATAL (PREGNANCY) FACTORS**
Mother unmarried*	Anemia*
Multiparity*	Low prepregnancy weight
Young maternal age (<20 years)*	Poor weight gain
Young maternal age with first pregnancy (<20 years)*	Urinary tract infection
	Venereal disease
NEONATAL RISK FACTORS	**SOCIOECONOMIC RISK FACTORS**
Cyanosis	Crowded living conditions*
Fever	Dwelling in poor state of repair
Hypothermia	Family problems
Irritability	Multiple child deaths in one family (no known medical cause)
Poor feeding	
Respiratory distress	Poor family finances
Tachycardia	**MISCELLANEOUS RISK FACTORS**
Tachypnea	Previous SIDS death in family
NEWBORN RISK FACTORS	Previous SIDS infant older than 6 months
Black race, Native Americans*	Multiple births (eg, twins)
Low Apgar score (<7)	
Low birth weight*	
Male sex*	
Prematurity*	
Small-for-gestational-age*	

*Widely accepted, general agreement among investigators.

■ GROUPS PROPOSED TO BE AT INCREASED RISK

Traditional groups said to be at increased risk include premature infants, subsequent siblings of SIDS victims, survivors of apparent life-threatening events (ALTE), and recently infants of substance-abusing mothers. Prematurity is a potent risk factor for SIDS and one of the few that is not in dispute.

Siblings of SIDS Victims

If a physiologic abnormality is operative in SIDS, it could be hereditary (eg, defects in metabolism). If family factors, child care practices, or environmental factors play a role, these would probably be similar for subsequent siblings of a SIDS victim. Finally, if intentional injury is a factor in a particular SIDS case, subsequent siblings in the same family are likely to be at increased risk. A family in which multiple SIDS deaths occur should be investigated for all of these possibilities.

The literature on the risk to a subsequent sibling after one SIDS death is unclear at present. Some studies describe an increased risk of recurrent SIDS, whereas others say there is no increased risk. A 1990 article by Guntheroth and colleagues reported a recurrence rate of 13/1000 live births among a group of 385 subsequent siblings, but also found a similar recurrence rate among siblings of non-SIDS infant

deaths. They concluded that the overall recurrence risk for SIDS is low but still significant.

■ PREDICTION

At present, SIDS risk cannot be predicted for an individual infant. No test, including a pneumogram or polysomnography, is useful for determining SIDS risk. No test can predict SIDS risk for a family or a subsequent sibling. No test can determine which infants should use home apnea monitoring or when a home monitor can be appropriately discontinued. However, we *can* predict increased risk for groups such as premature infants, infants of smoking mothers, and so forth, opening the door for a variety of preventive interventions.

■ MANAGEMENT

As Mandell and colleagues have described in several articles, the management of SIDS is the management of the surviving parents and the extended family, surviving siblings, and subsequent siblings. The parents and siblings have no warning and are frequently in a state of shock when they come into contact with the medical system. Parents often cannot believe what has happened. They may become hostile and angry, guilty, and self-blaming.

TABLE 41-2. Indications for Home Monitoring

MONITORING RECOMMENDED FOR:

Any infant perceived to be at increased risk of unexpected sudden death, including:

Infants with one or more severe apparent life-threatening events (CPR or vigorous stimulation required)

Subsequent siblings in family with SIDS case

Symptomatic premature infants (abnormal apnea or bradycardia at time of discharge)

Infants with central hypoventilation

Infants on supplemental oxygen

NOT RECOMMENDED FOR:

Normal infants

Asymptomatic premature infants

INDIVIDUALIZE CASE-BY-CASE FOR:

Infants who have experienced less severe apparent life-threatening events

Infants who have bronchopulmonary dysplasia

Infants who have tracheostomies

Infants of substance-abusing mothers

The reaction of a surviving sibling to SIDS in the family should not be overlooked. Young children do not understand. Older siblings are suddenly deprived of the role of older brother or older sister, often with devastating results. Surviving siblings may feel responsible, thinking that something they did caused the baby's death. Others deny their feelings. The pediatrician should anticipate these problems, inform parents, and, if necessary, counsel the children. Professional counseling may be necessary.

TABLE 41-3. Discontinuing Home Monitoring

Monitoring may be discontinued when the infant is no longer thought to be at increased risk of sudden death.

SUGGESTED CRITERIA FOR DISCONTINUATION OF MONITORING (ASSUMING GOOD COMPLIANCE WITH MONITOR USAGE):

No significant apparent life-threatening event (no color change, no CPR or vigorous stimulation required) for 2 or 3 consecutive months

Infant has tolerated at least one viral infection without significant alarms or events

FACTORS THAT MAY AFFECT DECISION:

Not sure if alarms are "true" or "false"

Infant on medication to treat apnea (*eg*, theophylline)

Infant on medication related to indication for monitoring (*eg*, bethanechol for gastroesophageal reflux)

Age of infant

Other indications to continued (*eg*, infant on supplemental oxygen)

Family's anxiety level

TESTING (PNEUMOGRAM, POLYSOMNOGRAPHY):

Obtaining a normal pneumogram is unnecessary.

Polysomnography (sleep study) is unnecessary.

Documented monitoring is the best way (currently) to distinguish "true" from "false" alarms.

The pediatrician's role extends to when the parents decide to have subsequent children. One should anticipate that the birth of a subsequent child will raise many concerns and questions. A danger for the subsequent sibling is overprotection or the "vulnerable child" syndrome. The pediatrician can evaluate any actual risk and advise the parents appropriately. The articles by Mandell and colleagues provide a wealth of useful information concerning SIDS and the family.

■ HOME MONITORING

The question of home monitoring is still unsettled. Home cardiorespiratory monitoring, as currently used in the United States, is intended to improve the outcome of any infant perceived to be at increased risk of sudden death. However, after decades, home monitoring has not decreased the incidence of SIDS. In 1986, the Consensus Development Conference on Infantile Apnea and Home Monitoring found that there were no reports of scientifically designed studies of the effectiveness of home monitoring on ALTE, subsequent siblings of SIDS victims, premature infants, or other pathologic conditions, and in 1997 this remains true. Current recommendations are summarized in Tables 41–2 and 41–3, and the reader is referred to the summary statements of the 1986 NIH conference report.

TABLE 41-4. Possible Approaches to Prevention of Sudden Infant Death Syndrome (SIDS)

RISK REDUCTION

Abandon recommendation of prone sleeping position for all infants (prone sleeping position still recommended for infants with specific clinical indication)

Recommend side-lying or supine sleeping position for healthy infants

Advocate better and more standardized policy concerning death scene investigation

Better educate public about dangers of over-the-counter remedies to young infants

Decrease parental smoking, before and after birth of child

Decrease parental drug use (*eg*, crack cocaine smoking), before and after birth of child

Improve access to and use of postnatal medical care

Improve prenatal care (anemia, smoking, nutrition)

Improve recognition of and services for dysfunctional families at risk for intentional injury of infants

Improve services to young mothers living in poor socioeconomic conditions

Improve targeting of very high risk groups (*eg*, Native Americans with very high maternal smoking rates)

Improve understanding of child care practices that may increase SIDS risk

PHYSIOLOGIC COMPONENT

Improve diagnosis of metabolic disorders leading to SIDS

Increase understanding of possible sources of postnatal vulnerability

Increase understanding of the role of infant sleeping position in increasing SIDS risk

INCREASE EFFICACY OF HOME MONITORING

Improve compliance with monitor use

Improve monitoring technology

Improve selection of candidates for monitoring

■ PREVENTION

Possible strategies for SIDS prevention are listed in Table 41–4. For the most part, these involve improving the general health and well-being of mothers and infants. Major risk factors such as maternal smoking, prematurity, and infant sleeping position present the pediatric community with a tremendous opportunity for preventive intervention.

(Abridged from John L. Carroll and Gerald M. Loughlin, Sudden Infant Death Syndrome, in Oski, DeAngelis, Feigin, McMillan, Warshaw: *Principles and Practice of Pediatrics, Second Edition*, J.B. Lippincott, 1994.)

Oski's Essential Pediatrics,
edited by Kevin B. Johnson and Frank A. Oski.
Lippincott–Raven Publishers,
Philadelphia © 1997

42

Apparent Life-Threatening Events

Infants who are unexpectedly discovered with some combination of pallor, hypotonia or hypertonia, cyanosis, apnea, and bradycardia, usually leading to vigorous stimulation or resuscitation by the caretaker, are often perceived by the person who witnesses the event to be at significant risk of dying. Such episodes are now called *apparent life-threatening events* (ALTE), a term that, like SIDS, describes a clinical syndrome that may result from a multitude of disorders. ALTE describes a complex of observations and events that are perceived by the child's caretaker to be life-threatening (Table 42–1).

■ ETIOLOGY

The term ALTE merely describes a manner of presentation for many different disorders (Table 42–2). In most studies of ALTE, a possible cause of the event is discovered in about 50% or more of cases.

■ APPROACH TO THE INFANT WITH AN ALTE

The goal of the initial approach to the patient is to rule out treatable causes of life-threatening events, in order to minimize the number of infants left in the idiopathic category. This can be done in about half of the cases.

A detailed history of the event must be obtained. Table 42–3 summarizes the important features of this history.

An accurate description of the intervention required to reestablish normal respirations is very important. Recovery spontaneously or with minimal intervention (ie, touching the infant) is reassuring and may suggest that what was witnessed was most likely a normal physiologic event. Information about the time required to reverse the event and the infant's mental and physical status after the event is also important.

Establishing a potential relationship between feeding and the apnea event is useful. Dysfunctional swallowing is a common problem in preterm infants, but also can be seen in term infants. Reflex apnea and bradycardia can be triggered not only by aspiration but also by reflux of formula into the nasopharynx. Apnea may be central or obstructive.

In the physical examination (see Table 42–3), signs of acute illness such as sepsis and meningitis should be sought. Assessment of growth and development, along with a focus on cardiac, neurologic, and respiratory systems, is necessary to identify subtle signs of chronic conditions that may predispose to life-threatening events.

Laboratory Studies

The minimum evaluation should include a complete blood count with differential, looking for either anemia or polycythemia and signs of acute infection. A hematocrit in the high 30s or 40s in an infant aged 2 to 3 months whose hematocrit should be at physiologic nadir suggests underlying chronic hypoxemia. Measurement of blood glucose (if the infant has not been fed recently) and some measure of acid–base status should also be obtained. A low serum bicarbonate level suggests that the event may have been severe enough to result in a metabolic acidosis, or may suggest the presence of an underlying metabolic disorder.

Based on results of these tests, the history and physical examination, or subsequent observations, other studies may be indicated (Table 42–4). However, these tests are not necessary for all infants with life-threatening events because their yield without specific indications is generally low.

Similar logic must be applied to decision making regarding other tests, such as the electroencephalogram (EEG) and electrocardiogram (ECG). If an initial workup is negative and the infant is stable, it is appropriate to defer additional testing pending the child's subsequent clinical course.

Assessment of Cardiorespiratory Patterns

Stimulated by the hypothesis that some aberration of cardiorespiratory control was involved in a significant number of ALTEs, attempts have been made to record heart rate

TABLE 42-1. History of Infants With Unexplained Apparent Life-Threatening Events

Symptom	% of Infants
Apnea	82
Pallor	70
Limpness	60
Cyanosis	48
Pallor and limpness	47
"Lifelessness"	41
Coldness	16
Not clear if breathing	14
Stiffness	11
Staring/rolling eyes	10
Shallow breathing	4

Modified from Dunne KP, Matthews TC. Near-miss sudden infant death syndrome: clinical findings and management. Pediatrics. 1987;79:889.

TABLE 42-2. Some Causes of Apparent Life-Threatening Events

Cardiac disease	CNS neoplasm
Respiratory disease	CNS structural abnormalities
Upper airway obstruction	Seizures
Gastroesophageal reflux	Infection
Laryngeal chemoreflex apnea	Metabolic disorders
Anemia	Poisoning
Hypoventilation syndromes	Prematurity

and respiratory rate over extended periods in these infants to identify underlying abnormalities in cardiorespiratory control that may predict recurrences.

Documented monitoring may be quite helpful and has been found to be useful in situations in which parents report recurrent alarms. An extended home recording may provide both extremely useful information about the nature of these spells and corroboration of the parents' reports. It also provides information on compliance with use of the monitor.

Polysomnography

Alternatively, cardiorespiratory patterns can be studied with standard nocturnal polysomnography in a sleep labo-

TABLE 42-3. ALTE Diagnostic Evaluation

HISTORY

Detailed description of the event from all observers: infant asleep or awake; position infant found in; duration of event; action required to terminate event; association with feeding, choking, formula in nose, body movement; infant's state after event

Perinatal history: labor and delivery, neonatal respiratory problems

Review of systems: infection, feeding, weight gain, vomiting, diarrhea, diet

PHYSICAL EXAMINATION

Vital signs

General appearance, growth parameters

HEENT: fontanelle, eye grounds, nose, mouth and throat

Neck: masses, rigidity

Chest: respiration rate, respiratory noises, signs of upper airway obstruction

Cardiac: rate, rhythm, murmurs

Abdomen

Neurologic examination: developmental milestones, tone, reflexes, strength, sensorium, affect

Feeding and sleep patterns

SCREENING LABS

Hgb/Hct

Acid-base status

TABLE 42-4. Other Studies Possibly Indicated in Children with ALTE

Study	Possible Diagnosis
Chest radiography	Respiratory symptoms, screen for cardiac disease
Barium swallow	Dysfunctional swallowing, gastroesophageal reflux, upper airway obstruction
EEG	Seizure disorder
ECG and echo	Rule out cardiac disease or cor pulmonale
pH probe	Suspicion of gastroesophageal reflux
Sleep studies (pneumograms or polysomnograms)	Unusual apnea, recurrent alarms, need to assess oxygenation, obstructive apnea

ratory. The following parameters are monitored: respiration (using abdominal and thoracic strain gauges in conjunction with a monitor of nasal and oral airflow), oxygenation (by pulse oximetry), ECG, EEG, and sleep state; activity during sleep usually is also recorded by videotape.

Limitations of polysomnography include the fact that it is more disruptive to usual routines. Studies are performed in strange surroundings, and many more wires are attached to the infant than in the home setting. These studies are also more expensive.

Studies of cardiorespiratory patterns cannot be used to predict subsequent risk for SIDS. However, if used judiciously, these studies can provide important information useful in the management of infants who have recurrent ALTE or recurrent alarms while on home monitoring.

■ MANAGEMENT

An infant who experiences a severe ALTE should be monitored in a hospital for 48 hours after the event. Hospitalization allows for a period of close observation. All infants should be placed on both cardiac and respiratory monitors and should be easily observable by the medical and nursing staff. This initial monitoring must be done carefully, because undocumented false alarms will lead to increased anxiety for the family and may lead to additional and unnecessary studies.

Many parents are frightened by these events and are concerned about the future; a brief hospital stay gives the appropriate medical and other support personnel enough time to talk with the family and to establish relationships that will form the basis for continuity of outpatient support. Furthermore, if a decision is made to initiate cardiorespiratory monitoring, there will be enough time to train the family in the use of the monitor and cardiopulmonary resuscitation (CPR).

(Abridged from Gerald M. Loughlin and John L. Carroll, Apparent Life-Threatening Events, in Oski, DeAngelis, Feigin, McMillan, Warshaw: *Principles and Practice of Pediatrics, Second Edition*, J.B. Lippincott, 1994.)

Oski's Essential Pediatrics,
edited by Kevin B. Johnson and Frank A. Oski.
Lippincott–Raven Publishers,
Philadelphia © 1997

43

Obstructive Sleep Apnea Syndrome

The obstructive sleep apnea syndrome (OSAS) is an important cause of morbidity in children. If left untreated, it can result in cor pulmonale, neurologic impairment, and even death.

Obstructive apnea is defined as the cessation of airflow at the nose and mouth, despite continued respiratory effort, secondary to airway obstruction. This is distinct from central apnea, where cessation of airflow is associated with absent respiratory effort. Many children with OSAS exhibit continuous partial airway obstruction, associated with hypoxemia and hypoventilation, rather than complete airway obstruction; this has been termed *obstructive hypoventilation.*

The prevalence of OSAS in the pediatric age group is unknown. The peak incidence, mirroring the peak incidence of adenotonsillar hypertrophy, is at 3 to 6 years of age, but OSAS can occur at any age, from the neonatal period on. In children, OSAS occurs equally among boys and girls.

■ PATHOPHYSIOLOGY

Obstructive sleep apnea syndrome results from a combination of abnormal neuromuscular control and anatomic narrowing of the upper airway. During wakefulness, the patient with a narrow airway can compensate by augmenting upper airway muscle tone. However, during sleep there is a decrease in ventilatory drive and in neuromuscular tone, facilitating upper airway collapse.

■ HISTORY

Most children present with a history of snoring and difficulty breathing during sleep. The onset is usually insidious. Children with OSAS have persistent, loud snoring that often can be heard outside the bedroom. During sleep, the child has labored breathing, retractions, and paradoxical inward motion of the chest wall during inspiration. During periods of complete obstruction, the child can be observed to be making respiratory efforts, but no snoring is heard and no airflow is detected. Obstructive episodes are usually terminated by gasping, motion, or arousal. The child sleeps restlessly and may adopt bizarre sleeping positions, such as sleeping in a seated position or with the neck hyperextended. Enuresis is common. Diaphoresis, pallor, or cyanosis may be present. The appearance of the child during sleep can be so alarming that it is not unusual for parents to maintain bedside vigils, or to continually stimulate or reposition the child throughout the night. Despite this, many parents do not volunteer a history of their child's sleep symptoms unless specifically asked. Most parents can mimic their child's breathing pattern when asked to do so.

■ PHYSICAL EXAMINATION

In most children with OSAS, the physical examination during wakefulness is entirely normal. This commonly leads to a delay in diagnosis because the physician often does not have the opportunity to see the child asleep.

Physical examination should include an assessment of the child's growth. Failure to thrive or, conversely, obesity may be present. Allergic stigmata, mouth breathing, adenoidal facies, midfacial hypoplasia, retro/micrognathia, or other craniofacial abnormalities may be present. The patency of the nares should be assessed. The pharynx should be evaluated for tongue size, palatal integrity, oropharyngeal diameter, redundant palatal mucosa, tonsil size, and uvula size. The lungs are usually clear to auscultation. Cardiac examination may reveal signs of pulmonary hypertension such as an increased pulmonic component of the second heart sound and a right ventricular heave. Neurologic examination should be performed to evaluate muscle tone, developmental status, behavior, and excessive daytime somnolence.

■ COMPLICATIONS

Patients with severe OSAS can have failure to thrive. Neurobehavioral complications, which result from sleep fragmentation and nocturnal hypoxemia, include hyperactivity, personality changes, excessive daytime sleepiness, poor school performance, and developmental delay. Seizures, asphyxial brain damage, and coma have been reported. Pulmonary hypertension is a common complication of OSAS and can progress to cor pulmonale and congestive heart failure. This resolves following successful treatment of OSAS. Respiratory arrest and sudden death have been reported.

■ DIAGNOSTIC TESTS

The diagnosis of OSAS should be established by polysomnography (sleep study). Polysomnography provides objective measures of severity and provides a baseline for those children whose condition does not resolve postoperatively.

■ TREATMENT

Most children are cured by adenotonsillectomy. Obstructive sleep apnea syndrome results from the relative size and structure of the upper airway components, rather than from the absolute size of the tonsils and adenoids. Therefore, both the tonsils and adenoids should be removed, even if one or the other appears to be the primary abnormality. Children with OSAS are at risk for postoperative complications, including upper airway edema, pulmonary edema, and respiratory failure. Perioperative deaths have been reported, so the patient should be monitored closely in the postoperative period. The OSAS may not resolve fully until 6 to 8 weeks after surgery.

■ PROGNOSIS

Most children experience a dramatic resolution of their symptoms following adenotonsillectomy. However, the natural course and the long-term prognosis of pediatric OSAS are unknown. Children with treated OSAS may be at risk for recurrence during adulthood.

(Abridged from Carole L. Marcus and John L. Carroll, Obstructive Sleep Apnea Syndrome, in Oski, DeAngelis, Feigin, McMillan, Warshaw: *Principles and Practice of Pediatrics, Second Edition,* J.B. Lippincott, 1994.)

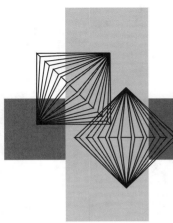

PART IV

The Sick or Hospitalized Patient

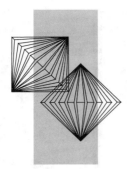

SECTION 1

Intensive Care

Oski's Essential Pediatrics,
edited by Kevin B. Johnson and Frank A. Oski.
Lippincott–Raven Publishers,
Philadelphia © 1997

44

Acute Renal Failure

Acute renal failure (ARF) is defined as an abrupt decline in the renal regulation of water, electrolyte, and acid–base balance of sufficient magnitude to result in the retention of nitrogenous waste. Renal failure is potentially fatal but often is reversible if a prompt, accurate diagnosis is made and close attention is paid to the wide variety of predictable and preventable complications. Oliguria is defined as urine output of below 0.5 mL/kg/h or below 300 mL/m²/day.

■ DIAGNOSIS

The renal failure indices listed in Table 44–1 can be helpful in distinguishing between oliguric patients with decreased perfusion to the kidneys and those with intrinsic renal failure. Clinical conditions associated with a decreased effective intravascular volume in children include both dehydration secondary to vomiting, diarrhea, or nasogastric drainage, and the peripheral pooling of fluid. Children with myocardial failure may have an adequate blood volume but diminished cardiac output, with a consequent decrease in their renal blood flow. Therapy in these children is aimed at improving cardiac function.

Patients with intrinsic renal failure manifest an acute decrease in glomerular filtration rate (GFR) and paralysis of tubular function. A decrease in GFR is reflected by a progressive increase in both the blood urea nitrogen (BUN) and the serum creatinine concentrations. The rate of BUN change is not a specific index of the level of the GFR because it can be affected by a variety of factors, including catabolic rate, protein load, and medications.

Clinical conditions associated with the development of ARF include hypotension, shock, renal ischemia, nephrotoxicity, drug toxicity, hyperuricemia, asphyxia, and sepsis. In children, more than 50% of ARF cases can be attributed to acute parenchymal disorders such as glomerulonephritis and hemolytic-uremic syndrome. Most ARF in the newborn period is secondary to major perinatal insults. More than 60% of neonatal ARF is reported to be secondary to perinatal asphyxia, hypoxia, and sepsis.

Nonoliguric ARF has been described in association with the nephrotoxic aminoglycoside antibiotics. The presentation is that of a gradual onset of nonoliguric renal failure that frequently is preceded by polyuria and decreased urine osmolality. In patients with nonoliguric renal failure, clinical studies show more normal urinary indices, a lower BUN, and a higher measured GFR, as well as fewer complications and lower mortality rates.

Once the diagnosis of ARF is made, all aspects of patient care must be monitored closely. Survival and return of renal function in 1 to 3 weeks are likely if the patient does not succumb from the underlying disease process or suffer from infectious, metabolic, or hemorrhagic complications of ARF or its treatment. The basis of therapy is careful monitoring of fluid and electrolyte balance, nutritional management directed at preventing a catabolic state, and meticulous care to avoid infections. The physiologic consequences of ARF include edema, pericarditis, electrolyte abnormalities including acidosis, anemia, thrombocytopenia, coagulopathy, gastrointestinal bleeding, poor nutrition, and sepsis.

■ TREATMENT

The first step when treating a patient with oliguria is a careful assessment of volume status. Physical examination may reveal hypovolemia (dry mucous membranes, tachycardia, "tenting" of the skin) or volume overload (peripheral edema, rales, gallop rhythm, hypertension, liver enlargement). A chest radiograph should be taken, looking for pulmonary edema or cardiomegaly, and an electrocardiogram (ECG) should be performed, looking for changes associated with hyperkalemia. Neither diuretics nor vasopressors should be given until the adequacy of circulating volume has been ascertained.

The rapid intravenous administration of 0.5 g/kg of mannitol should result in a urine output of more than 0.5 mL/kg within 1 hour. Mannitol may cause hypervolemia and pulmonary edema in patients who cannot excrete it, so it is best to avoid its use if there is any question of incipient volume overload or congestive heart failure. Furosemide also may be given, not only as a provocative test to generate urine production but also to attenuate ARF due to its vasodilating and natriuretic properties. Furosemide should be given to euvolemic patients in a dose of 1 mg/kg intravenously. If there is no response within 30 minutes, incrementally higher doses up to 10 mg/kg have been used, although the risk of ototoxicity increases dramatically. The use of these agents may have deleterious effects on renal blood flow and GFR if intravascular volume is inadequate.

Low-dose dopamine also has been advocated to improve urine output in adults with ARF. Dopamine increases renal blood flow, GFR, and sodium excretion independently of its effects on cardiac output. Other inotropic agents, such as epinephrine and norepinephrine, should be avoided because these agents reduce renal blood flow even in the face of increased systemic blood pressure.

TABLE 44-1. Clinical Evaluation of Acute Renal Failure

	Volume Depletion/ Decreased Renal Perfusion	Acute Renal Failure
	(Adolescents/Children)	(Adolescents/Children)
U_{Na} (mEq/L)	<10	>50
FE_{Na} (%)*	≤1	>2
U_{osm} (mOsm/L)	≥500	≤300
U/P_{osm}	≥1.5	0.8–1.2
BUN/Cr	>20	Progressive increases in both

*FE_{Na} % ≠ $(U/P)_{Na}$ ÷ $(U/P)_{(Cr)}$ × 100.

Once fixed renal failure occurs, conservative management should be used. This includes normalizing intravascular volume, systemic blood pressure and renal blood flow, sodium and potassium levels, and acid–base balance, and minimizing accumulation of nitrogenous wastes by restricting protein intake moderately while maximizing caloric intake. Prophylaxis for gastrointestinal bleeding should be initiated. Special care must be taken to avoid infectious complications.

Strict attention to physical examination, an accurate record of input and output, and daily weight and serum sodium determinations will maintain correct fluid balance. Fluid administration, both oral and parenteral, should be restricted to the sum of insensible losses (400 mL/m²/day) plus measured urine output and any other losses (eg, gastrointestinal, respiratory, evaporative secondary to burns). Hyponatremia can occur in the patient with volume overload; management entails further fluid restriction. Hyponatremia also can be seen in the patient with increased urinary sodium excretion who is in the diuretic phase of recovering ARF. Sodium replacement then is indicated.

Hyperkalemia is often encountered in ARF patients. Hyperkalemia is a life-threatening complication of ARF and must be treated promptly to avoid cardiac toxicity. ECG changes range from the mild (peaked T waves) to the ominous, including widened QRS complex and arrhythmias. Measures to decrease serum potassium levels rapidly include sodium bicarbonate, insulin and glucose, and 10% calcium gluconate solution. Sodium polystyrene sulfonate (Kayexalate) is an ion-exchange resin and reduces the total body burden of potassium. Dialysis may be necessary to control hyperkalemia. Continuous ECG monitoring and repeated glucose and potassium determinations should be done as therapy proceeds.

A consequence of impaired renal function is retention of hydrogen ions, sulfate, and phosphate and development of a mild metabolic acidosis with an increased anion gap. If acidosis is severe or contributing to the development of hyperkalemia, or if the patient's respiratory compensation is impaired, sodium bicarbonate can be given.

Hypertension is frequently a complication in children with ARF. Volume overload is often an inciting event and must be addressed early in the management.

Children with ARF are usually catabolic. High rates of catabolism lead to increased accumulation of potassium, phosphate, and urea, and may necessitate earlier dialysis. If calories are supplied and the breakdown of endogenous proteins is spared, the need for dialysis may be delayed. Because of fluid restriction in these patients, it often is difficult to provide adequate calories without the use of parenteral hypertonic glucose, amino acids, and intralipids. Once the patient is no longer oligoanuric or is on an artificial kidney, fluid administration may be liberalized, and nutritional management becomes easier and safer. Enteral alimentation should be initiated as soon as clinically feasible.

There are six indications for dialysis: volume overload with evidence of pulmonary edema or hypertension refractory to pharmacologic therapy; hyperkalemia despite conservative measures; severe metabolic acidosis (pH < 7.20); BUN above 150, or lower if rising rapidly; neurologic symptoms secondary to uremia or electrolyte imbalance; and calcium/phosphorus imbalance (hypocalcemia with tetany or seizures in the presence of a very high serum phosphate).

Both peritoneal dialysis and intermittent hemodialysis have been used for many years in children in ARF, but often these modes of therapy have been less than optimally effective in the critically ill child. Hemodialysis is difficult to maintain in the patient with cardiovascular instability, and its intermittent mode of administration makes removal of extravascular fluid difficult without causing further fluctuations in blood pressure. Effective peritoneal dialysis also requires an adequate cardiac output, which may not be present in these children, and peritoneal dialysis can lead to respiratory embarrassment.

Recently there has been an opportunity to use continuous renal prosthetic therapy in both adults and children. Two of these modes, slow continuous ultrafiltration (SCUF) and continuous arteriovenous hemofiltration (CAVH), are gaining widespread use. With these therapies, patients who are oligoanuric can receive the drugs and nutrients they need without fear of causing fluid excess. In addition, both of these modes are characterized by ease of application and hemodynamic stability, so therapy is instituted earlier. Both require the insertion of arterial and venous catheters. The driving pressure supplied by the arterial bed provides the flow through the dialysis membrane.

In most series of childhood ARF, mortality is associated with the irreversible nature of the underlying disease rather than the renal failure itself. Treatment modalities are largely supportive, and successful therapy requires meticulous attention to the details of the clinical setting.

(Abridged from M. Michele Mariscalco, Acute Renal Failure, in Oski, DeAngelis, Feigin, McMillan, Warshaw: *Principles and Practice of Pediatrics, Second Edition,* J.B. Lippincott, 1994.)

Oski's Essential Pediatrics,
edited by Kevin B. Johnson and Frank A. Oski.
Lippincott–Raven Publishers,
Philadelphia © 1997

45

Hemolytic-Uremic Syndrome

The hemolytic-uremic syndrome (HUS), first described in 1955, is characterized by the triad of nephropathy, thrombocytopenia, and microangiopathic hemolytic anemia. HUS is a heterogenous group of disorders that have a common end result.

■ PATHOGENESIS

The pathogenesis of HUS can be explained by several mechanisms. The anemia is most likely secondary to hemolysis, caused by mechanical destruction of erythrocytes by fibrin strands in small renal vessels. Thrombocytopenia is present universally and is secondary to peripheral destruction. The nephropathy is characterized by glomerular capillary endothelial injury and thickening. As a result of the thickening of the endothelial space, the capillary narrows, predisposing to capillary thrombosis.

■ EPIDEMIOLOGY

Hemolytic-uremic syndrome is largely a disease of infants and children. The syndrome is endemic in Argentina, southern Africa, and the western United States. There is no predilection for either sex. In southern Africa, it is more common in white children. Age of onset is between 2 months and 8 years in most cases and is usually less than 5 years.

There is no one causative factor, and etiologic agents may be viral (coxsackieviruses, echoviruses, influenza viruses, Epstein-Barr virus), bacterial (*Shigella, Salmonella, Streptococcus pneumoniae, Escherichia coli* 0157:H7), or drugs (oral contraceptives and cyclosporin A) and complement abnormalities. There seems to be a genetic predisposition.

■ CLINICAL FEATURES

The syndrome typically has a prodrome of diarrhea or an upper respiratory illness. The diarrhea may be bloody. The prodrome occurs 5 days to 2 weeks before the onset of the classic syndrome.

At initial examination, the child is pale and irritable, with petechiae and edema. Dehydration may be present if there is severe diarrhea. Hypertension also is common.

The mildly affected patient may have only anemia, thrombocytopenia, and azotemia. The severely affected patient has the complications of metabolic derangement, including hyperkalemia, metabolic acidosis, hypocalcemia, and hyponatremia or hypernatremia. Seizures, coma, and stroke may occur. Cardiac failure may result from hypertension, volume overload, or severe anemia. Bleeding also may be present in the severely affected patient.

Laboratory features include hemoglobin concentrations of 2 to 10 g/dL, platelet counts of less than 100,000/mm³, and an increased prothrombin time due to consumption of Factors II, VII, IX, and X. A decrease in fibrinogen and an increase in fibrin split products also appears early in the illness.

■ TREATMENT

Management of the HUS patient is mainly supportive. The aim of red-cell transfusions during the period of hemolysis should be to prevent heart failure and not to return the hematocrit to normal. Meticulous attention to the sequelae of renal failure is essential. Thrombocytopenia may be severe but only rarely results in significant bleeding; therefore, platelets should not be given unless clearly needed to stop bleeding or in anticipation of invasive procedures.

■ PROGNOSIS

The prognosis for the most common forms of HUS is good. Most studies report 3% to 5% mortality, and another 3% to 5% of patients experience chronic renal disease.

(Abridged from Penelope Terhune Louis, Hemolytic-Uremic Syndrome, in Oski, DeAngelis, Feigin, McMillan, Warshaw: *Principles and Practice of Pediatrics, Second Edition,* J.B. Lippincott, 1994.)

Oski's Essential Pediatrics,
edited by Kevin B. Johnson and Frank A. Oski.
Lippincott–Raven Publishers,
Philadelphia © 1997

46

Fever Without Localizing Signs

Fever is one of the most common pediatric complaints. In the first few years of life, fever is second only to routine care as the cause of office or clinic visits. Between 5% and 20% of febrile children have no localizing signs. Fever without localizing signs (FWLS), like febrile illness in general, is most common in children less than 5 years old, with a peak prevalence between 6 and 24 months of age. We define FWLS as unexplained fever of relatively brief duration, arbitrarily less than 5 or 7 days. If the unexplained fever persists longer than 5 to 10 days, it is commonly referred to as fever of undetermined origin (FUO). Although overlap exists between FWLS and FUO, the differential diagnosis and the clinical approach are quite different for children with FWLS or FUO.

In many cases, FWLS resolves spontaneously without a specific diagnosis being established. In other cases, a relatively minor infectious process, either focal (eg, otitis media, pharyngitis) or nonfocal (eg, varicella, roseola), becomes apparent as the cause for the fever. Examples of infections with long prodromal periods, during which fever may be the only manifestation, are roseola, cytomegalovirus infection, typhus, and typhoid fever. Not all cases of FWLS are due to acute infectious diseases; some cases herald the onset of chronic disorders. However, because FWLS is, by definition, of relatively brief duration, and because so many children with self-limited viral infections present with FWLS, the percentage of children with FWLS who have serious persistent infections or other inflammatory conditions such as juvenile rheumatoid arthritis is much lower than that of children with FUO. Rarely, FWLS in an infant or child represents a drug reaction, an allergic or hypersensitivity disorder, or heat illness. In recent years, a number of young children presenting with FWLS have manifested features of Kawasaki syndrome after a few days. It is not known whether Kawasaki disease is an infectious disorder.

■ OCCULT BACTEREMIA

Except in the very young infant, most serious infections can be recognized by a careful history and physical examination. However, a small but significant percentage of children with bacteremia cannot be identified by the ordinary clinical examination alone. These children have occult bacteremia, which we define as the presence of a positive blood culture in a child who looks well enough to be treated as an outpatient and in whom the positive result is not anticipated. Specifically, the child does not have any soft-tissue infection or local infection that ordinarily would be associated with bacteremia, (eg, pneumonia or epiglottitis), but he or she may have a minor infection such as otitis media. Although only about 5% of children with FWLS have occult bacteremia, somewhat more than 50% of the children with occult bacteremia come from the pool of children with FWLS (Figure 46–1).

The organism most frequently responsible for occult bacteremia is *Streptococcus pneumoniae*, the second most common organism is *Haemophilus influenzae* type b, and salmonellae and *Neisseria meningitidis* make up most of the remaining small percentage. The predominance of pneumococcus is related to age. In series that focus on children from 3 to 24 months of age, *S pneumoniae* generally accounts for more than 80% of the cases of occult bacteremia; in series that include febrile children of all ages, *S pneumoniae* is found to account for only 60% to 70% of the cases of occult bacteremia. Because *S pneumoniae* is the predominant cause of occult bacteremia, it is not surprising that many of the characteristics of occult bacteremia associated with *S pneumoniae* are statistically true for occult bacteremia in general—peak prevalence between 6 and 24 months, association with high fever and high leukocyte count, and association with the absence of evident focal soft-tissue infection. These criteria are met much less consistently in cases of occult bacteremia due to *H influenzae*, *N meningitidis*, and salmonellae.

Initially, occult bacteremia was believed to be a disease of the underprivileged, because it first was described in inner-city hospitals serving mostly indigent patients. Subsequent studies have shown that occult bacteremia occurs with essentially the same frequency in the middle- and upper-class populations as it does in the underprivileged. No racial, geographic, or socioeconomic predilection for occult bacteremia is apparent. Although the exact prevalence of occult bacteremia in different series of outpatients varies, figures generally have been in the range of 3% to 6% of significantly febrile young children. The actual prevalence appears to vary more with the selection criteria for study than with the geographic or socioeconomic base of the study population. The highest frequency of occult bacteremia is in children younger than 2 years. Children with FWLS are more likely to be bacteremic than are children with minor outpatient infections. In one series, blood cultures were obtained from all febrile children under the age of 2 years presenting to the emergency department. The prevalence of bacteremia in children with infections such as otitis media and pharyngitis was 1.5%; in those with FWLS, the prevalence was 3.9%. It is unfortunate that the authors chose to include children with evidence of upper respiratory tract infections in the FWLS group, because children with upper respiratory infections have a lesser prevalence of bacteremia. In one series, febrile children with evidence of upper respiratory tract infections had a prevalence of occult bacteremia of 3%, in contrast to those with FWLS, for whom the prevalence was 9%.

Although it is clear that most patients with high fever do not have bacteremia and that some patients with bacteremia are afebrile, a trend exists for higher fever to be associated with a greater risk of bacteremia. This trend is most pronounced for *S pneumoniae*.

About 75% of children with occult bacteremia recover completely. Of the remaining 25%, some 5% develop purulent meningitis and another 5% develop other significant soft-tissue infections such as periorbital cellulitis or osteomyelitis. The remaining 15% are found to have persistent bacteremia at the time of reexamination; most of these patients do well with treatment. The 5% figure for subsequent bacterial meningitis has been remarkably consistent from series to series. However, because the risk of subsequent meningitis is greater with *H influenzae* bacteremia than with *S pneumoniae* bacteremia, it is possible that the relatively recent introduction of routine *H influenzae* immunization in infancy will decrease the number of cases of occult bacteremia due to *H influenzae* and, therefore, decrease the overall incidence of meningitis following occult bacteremia.

■ DIAGNOSIS

Many of the diagnostic studies used to evaluate children with FWLS are directed at excluding the presence of bacteremia. Failure to identify bacteremic children accurately subjects them to the potentially adverse sequelae of undiagnosed and untreated bacteremia. Conversely, the indiscriminate use of diagnostic tests represents unnecessary effort, expense, and discomfort for the patient.

Several investigators have suggested that careful clinical evaluation of children with FWLS may permit the selection of a subgroup of patients who appear well and have a small or negligible risk of bacteremia or other serious bacterial illnesses. These clinical features include the child's appearance (eg, normal hydration, lack of apparent toxicity, and lack of distress) and behavior (eg, alert, playful, eating and drinking well). The studies on which this suggestion is based, however, all involved the full spectrum of febrile chil-

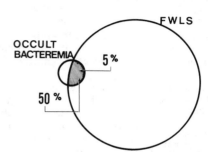

Figure 46-1. Numeric interrelationship of fever without localizing signs (FWLS) and occult bacteremia. Many more cases occur of FWLS than of occult bacteremia. Only 5% of the cases of FWLS have occult bacteremia (*shaded area*), but more than 50% of the patients with occult bacteremia have FWLS.

TABLE 46-1. Risk of Occult Bacteremia

	Low Risk	High Risk
Age	>3 years	<2 years
Temperature	<39.4°C (<103°F)	>40°C(>104°F)
WBC (per mm³)	>5,000 and <15,000	<5,000 or >15,000
Observational variables	Normal	Abnormal
Other		History of contact with *Haemophilus influenzae* or *Neisseria meningitidis*
		History of bacteremic illness
		Immunologic impairment

dren presenting to the emergency department; none focused specifically on children with FWLS. It is likely that a child with bacteremic pneumonia or bacteremic meningitis would look and act more ill than would a child with occult bacteremia. Although these clinical features can be helpful, they are not completely accurate.

Febrile children without localizing signs of infection who are at greatest risk of bacteremia are those between 6 and 24 months of age with temperatures above 39.4°C (103°F). These children should be considered for diagnostic laboratory studies. In addition, diagnostic studies to exclude bacteremia or other serious bacterial diseases (*eg*, meningitis) may be indicated routinely in the febrile neonate and in immunocompromised hosts, where the consequences of unrecognized infection can be devastating.

Two types of laboratory tests are used in the evaluation of a child for bacteremia: indirect tests, such as the white blood cell (WBC) count and erythrocyte sedimentation rate (ESR), which reflect the body's response to infection, and direct tests, such as blood culture and rapid tests for the detection of bacterial antigens, which detect the organism itself. Indirect laboratory tests, such as the WBC count, serve only as screening tests to identify a subgroup of children at high risk of bacteremia. These tests cannot diagnose specific children as bacteremic. In a population with low prevalence of a disease—as is the case with febrile children and bacteremia—even a sensitive and specific screening test will have a low positive predictive value. In other words, the test might identify most bacteremic children accurately, but it would not discriminate between these few patients and the many children with positive test results but without bacteremia. For children with FWLS, a WBC count of 15,000/μL or greater has sensitivity and specificity of about 85% and 75%, respectively, for the detection of bacteremia. The positive predictive value, however, is only about 15%. Nevertheless, the WBC count is the most widely used and probably the most practical screening test available. Other screening tests, such as the ESR and WBC morphology, suffer from the same low positive predictive value that affects the WBC count. Whether rapid tests for bacterial antigens eventually will prove useful as screening tests for occult bacteremia remains to be determined.

Blood culture is an important diagnostic tool in the child with FWLS. It is technically easy to perform and, unlike screening tests, is a direct and precise means of diagnosing bacteremia. Reserving blood culture for children deemed to be at high risk for bacteremia by clinical criteria and by the finding of a WBC count above 15,000/μL will result in substantial cost savings.

Other laboratory tests may be indicated in certain situations. Young infants, in particular, may fail to manifest signs of meningeal irritation even in the presence of confirmed bacterial meningitis, so a high index of suspicion for that dis-

ease must be maintained and a lumbar puncture performed if any concern for meningitis exists. Urinalysis is indicated in the female infant with unexplained fever to exclude "occult" urinary tract infection. Beyond the neonatal period, boys with unexplained fever appear to be at low risk of urinary tract infection. In infants, pneumonia often does not produce obvious auscultatory findings, although some clue to pulmonary involvement (cough, tachypnea, retractions) almost always is present, and a chest roentgenogram may be necessary to exclude that diagnosis. Chest roentgenogram is not indicated routinely for all infants and children with FWLS but should be considered for young infants and those patients with very high fever, signs of toxicity, or markedly elevated WBC counts.

■ ANTIBIOTIC TREATMENT

Expectant antibiotic therapy may be justified for the child with FWLS and high fever, WBC count above 15,000/μL, or risk factors for serious bacterial disease (Table 46–1). Several retrospective studies as well as prospectively collected data from one study of occult bacteremia show that children treated expectantly with antibiotics at the time of the initial visit fare better than do those who do not receive antibiotic therapy. Children who appear seriously ill, and those with underlying diseases predisposing to serious bacterial infection (*eg*, immunodeficiency states, sickle-cell disease), should receive an initial course of parenterally administered antibiotics in the hospital. In most other cases, expectant therapy may be given on an outpatient basis.

Antibiotic therapy should be directed against the most common bacterial pathogens, *S pneumoniae* and *H influenzae* type b. Amoxicillin (40 to 60 mg/kg/day) is a reasonable choice. In areas with a high prevalence of *H influenzae* type b resistant to ampicillin, reasonable alternative therapy includes erythromycin-sulfisoxazole, trimethoprim-sulfamethoxazole, or amoxicillin-clavulanic acid. A single injection of ceftriaxone in a dose of 50 to 75 mg/kg will theoretically provide coverage against the common pathogens causing occult bacteremia without concern about compliance or vomiting; studies to evaluate such a regimen currently are underway. Penicillin V does not have useful activity against *H influenzae*.

Regardless of therapy, careful follow-up care is essential, and the child should be reevaluated immediately if the clinical condition deteriorates, if signs or symptoms of serious focal infection develop, or if the blood culture yields a pathogen.

■ CLINICAL MANAGEMENT

Decisions regarding diagnostic investigation and expectant antibiotic therapy should be based on careful analysis of all available data and thoughtful weighing of the risks and cost/benefit ratio for each patient. The physician should be cognizant of the costs of diagnostic procedures and expectant therapy. Cost includes not only the dollar amount of the tests and the medication, but also the physical and emotional trauma of blood drawing, the side effects of antibiotics, and the time and distress involved in clarifying false-positive results, lost specimens, and laboratory errors. On the benefit side are possible decreased morbidity (*eg,* prevention or early detection of subsequent meningitis and other serious bacterial illness) and mortality (low in all series). Table 46–1 serves as a framework for assessing the risk of bacteremia in the individual patient.

(Abridged from Mark W. Kline and Martin I. Lorin, Fever Without Localizing Signs, in Oski, DeAngelis, Feigin, McMillan, Warshaw: *Principles and Practice of Pediatrics, Second Edition,* J.B. Lippincott, 1994.)

Oski's Essential Pediatrics,
edited by Kevin B. Johnson and Frank A. Oski.
Lippincott–Raven Publishers,
Philadelphia © 1997

47

Fever of Undetermined Origin

The definition of fever of undetermined origin (FUO) in children has evolved over the past few decades so that a prolonged period of documentation of fever and in-hospital workup no longer are required as criteria for use of this label. These rigid criteria arose primarily from studies in adults and were appropriate in earlier days when our understanding of this entity was primitive and modern diagnostic technology was unavailable. It now is acceptable to use the term FUO to describe the condition of children who are febrile for 8 or more days and in whom careful history, physical examination, and preliminary laboratory evaluation fail to reveal probable cause for the fever. Youngsters who have been febrile without explanation for fewer than 5 days should be considered as having fever without localizing signs, which carries a different set of diagnostic probabilities as well as a different clinical diagnostic approach (see Chapter 46). Youngsters evaluated between the fifth and seventh day of fever constitute an overlap group and must be approached with thought given to both entities.

■ GENERAL PRINCIPLES

Most children with FUO do not have rare or exotic diseases. This finding has been true even in series from major pediatric referral centers. For example, in a series of 100 children evaluated at the Children's Hospital Medical Center in Boston, only three had diseases that would be considered rare—undefined vasculitis, Behçet's syndrome, and ichthyosis.

Although the relative frequencies are somewhat different, the three most commonly identified causes of FUO in children are the same as in adults—infectious diseases, connective tissue disorders, and malignancies. Although the prognosis in children is somewhat better than in adults, FUO often represents a serious condition even in children. Infection, the leading cause of FUO at all ages, is even more common in children than in adults, accounting for more than 50% of the cases in some reports. Connective tissue diseases occur with approximately the same frequency in both pediatric and adult series, and neoplasms are a less common cause of FUO in children than in adults.

The percentage of specific etiologies in different reports varies with factors such as criteria for inclusion in the study, availability of diagnostic expertise, and classification of patients with probable but uncertain diagnoses. In many cases of FUO in children, a specific diagnosis is never established and the condition resolves spontaneously.

■ INITIAL APPROACH TO CLINICAL EVALUATION

The clinical approach to the child with FUO must be organized and individualized for each patient. A diagnostic evaluation may be initiated in the office or clinic for the child beyond early infancy who has been febrile for 7 to 14 days and who looks well. Conversely, a young infant or child who has been febrile for a more prolonged period, or a youngster who appears significantly ill should be hospitalized for evaluation. Hospitalization is useful not only for the purpose of expediting laboratory tests, but it also provides an important opportunity for continued history taking, repeated physical examination, and constant observation.

Documentation of prolonged or recurrent fever helps to exclude certain relatively acute infections such as viral influenza and group A streptococcal pharyngitis. The child's age affects both the probability of certain disorders and the urgency with which workup is undertaken. Young infants present a more urgent problem; bacteremia and meningitis cannot be safely excluded without appropriate cultures. Neonates and young infants also are susceptible to certain organisms such as group B streptococci and *Listeria monocytogenes,* which are rare in older patients. On the other hand, *Neisseria gonorrhoeae* as a cause of prolonged fever usually is seen in adolescents. Connective tissue diseases are more common in older children; Pizzo and colleagues reported an incidence of connective tissue disease about four times greater in children over 6 years of age than in those younger than 6 years. The patient's sex also is relevant. Autoimmune disease is more common in girls, and certain immunologic deficiencies, such as Bruton's agammaglobulinemia and classic chronic granulomatous disease, are restricted to boys. Pelvic inflammatory disease, of course, occurs only in girls.

The patient's history should be searched carefully for any possible clues, however trivial or remote. A history of transfusion or the use of blood products would raise the possibility of a variety of transmitted viral and parasitic agents, including human immunodeficiency virus (HIV). Animal contact always is important. Dogs may harbor brucellosis or leptospirosis, and cats are vectors for cat-scratch fever and toxoplasmosis. Birds are a source of ornithosis and histoplasmosis. Rodents carry tularemia, leptospirosis, *Spirillum minus,* and *Streptobacillus moniliformis.* A history of travel, even in the distant past, is notable. Endemic diseases in Africa, India, and Asia include malaria, amebiasis, and schistosomiasis, which may be manifest months to years after returning from an endemic area. Coccidioidomycosis is endemic in the southwestern portion of the United States.

■ IN-HOSPITAL EVALUATION

Inpatient evaluation of the child with FUO can be seen as three processes proceeding simultaneously: follow-up of all diagnostic clues, screening tests, and observation and reexamination.

Follow-Up of All Potential Clues

The most important aspect of the evaluation of a youngster with FUO is meticulous and complete follow-up of all potential clues, however insignificant they may appear. The results of the history and physical examination and all available laboratory data must be scrutinized closely for any abnormalities or positive features. Pizzo and coworkers noted that failure to use existing laboratory data correctly occurred in one half of the cases in their series and was a major reason for failure to establish the proper diagnosis before hospitalization. A history of an episode of abdominal pain or diarrhea even weeks before the onset of the fever may be a clue to an enteric infection or an intra-abdominal abscess. The slightest tenderness over the sinuses or mastoid area may be indicative of underlying chronic infection. Even a mild peripheral eosinophilia may be a clue to parasitic infection, immunodeficiency, or occult malignancy. Perseverance in following each potential clue is the most efficient and cost-effective method of evaluating a youngster with FUO.

Screening Tests

When there are no clues to guide the workup, the physician must rely on an initial battery of screening tests. Even when clues are present, it is not unreasonable to proceed with some preliminary screening tests while following up on specific clues. Screening tests include those that detect organ dysfunction as well as those that identify specific diseases. Basic screening tests to evaluate organ function and to look for clues as to which systems may be involved include serum levels of hepatic enzymes and alkaline phosphatase, renal function tests such as blood urea nitrogen and creatinine, urine analysis, chest roentgenogram, and complete blood count. The erythrocyte sedimentation rate (ESR) is a useful test in assessing the severity of tissue inflammation but generally is of little help in identifying specific diagnoses, although a normal ESR does weigh against diseases characteristically associated with high ESRs, such as inflammatory bowel disease. The electroencephalogram (EEG) and electrocardiogram (ECG) are unlikely to yield useful information in the absence of specific findings pointing toward these systems and, therefore, are not cost-effective as screening tests. A lumbar puncture should be considered in every child with FUO but need not necessarily be performed in all patients.

Screening tests for certain specific diseases should be done in all children hospitalized for the evaluation of FUO: blood culture, tuberculin skin test, urine culture, febrile agglutinins, serum rheumatoid factor, and antinuclear antibody titers. Because they are invasive, expensive, or infrequently positive, other screening tests should be considered as second-stage tests and generally not ordered at the time of admission unless there are specific indications or unless basic laboratory investigation had been completed before hospitalization. Such tests include bone marrow aspiration, abdominal ultrasound or computed tomography (CT) examination, gallium scan, bone scan, radiographic skeletal survey, and roentgenograms of the sinuses and mastoid.

Observation and Reexamination

Hospitalization should be used as an opportunity to obtain additional historical data from the patient and parents, and even other family members who may visit. It is surprising how often parents will recall a pertinent event, such as travel or animal exposure, or relevant family history only after days in the hospital. The patient must have a relatively complete physical examination at least daily, but obviously it is unnecessary to repeat items such as funduscopic examination, detailed neurologic examination, or rectal examination every day unless specifically indicated. Often, pulmonary rales, cardiac murmurs, skin rashes, areas of tenderness, pain on motion of a joint, and even abdominal masses will appear during the hospitalization. All available data should be reviewed continually for clues that were not initially apparent. The pattern of fever should be observed. A high spiking fever once or twice a day may be a clue to an occult abscess or to the systemic form of juvenile rheumatoid arthritis (JRA). The patient should be examined during an episode of fever; the rash of JRA may be present only at this time.

A youngster who looks well, has no tachycardia, and does not feel warm at the time of alleged fever may have factitious fever. In the age of the electronic thermometer, it has become routine for the nurse to remain at the bedside during the temperature measurement, making it difficult for the patient or parent to factitiously elevate the temperature reading. However, it still is possible to influence the oral reading by ingesting hot liquids before the temperature measurement. The ingenuity of these patients or parents in falsifying temperature readings and feigning illness is extraordinary, and undoubtedly such individuals will find ways to circumvent modern technology.

The response to antipyretic agents should be noted. Lack of response may indicate factitious fever or a central nervous system (CNS) basis for the fever. Temperature elevations secondary to neurologic dysfunction often are unresponsive to antipyretic drugs. Children with recurrent periodic fever frequently respond poorly or not at all to antipyretic drugs.

■ ETIOLOGY

Infectious Causes

In the United States, the most common infectious diseases implicated in children with FUO include brucellosis, tularemia, tuberculosis, salmonellosis, diseases due to spirochetes (leptospirosis, rat-bite fever, syphilis), rickettsial infections, cytomegalic inclusion disease, infectious mononucleosis, hepatitis, and HIV infection. The most common causes of localized infection that may present as FUO include sinusitis, otitis media, tonsillitis, urinary tract infection, osteomyelitis, and occult abscesses, including those of the subdiaphragmatic, hepatic, pelvic, or perinephric region.

Brucellosis

The presentation of brucellosis as a disease that causes FUO is explained by the nonspecificity of its symptomatology and by the chronicity of the untreated infection. Physicians tend to ignore the possibility of this disease and often neglect to ask for a history of exposure to animals or animal products.

Leptospirosis

Leptospirosis is caused by a family of organisms of which multiple serogroups and serotypes exist. Transmission of infection from animals to humans may follow direct contact with the blood, tissue, urine, or organs of infected animals, or indirectly by exposure to an environment contaminated by leptospires. The organism may be acquired from soil or from fresh water after ingestion. Reports suggest that leptospirosis is not rare. Most infections are no longer associated with occupational exposure; rather, urban and suburban cases are now more prevalent than are cases reported from rural areas.

The clinical manifestations of leptospirosis are not specific. A variety of laboratory tests are available, but appropriate handling and collection of specimens are imperative. In many cases, it is impossible to establish a definitive diagnosis because of negative culture results and failure to demonstrate a rise in antibody titer to these organisms. These factors do not exclude the possibility of active infections, because the organism may not be in the specimens that have been cultured. Moreover, the antibody titer may have peaked before the collection of an acute-phase specimen, and antibiotic therapy can suppress the development of positive titers or delay their appearance.

Salmonellosis

Salmonella spp have been found as contaminants in most food products in recent years. The nonspecificity of signs and symptoms that may be associated with salmonellosis is one reason why it is associated with FUO in children. Repetitive blood and stool cultures are most helpful in establishing a diagnosis; serologic evidence of infection also should be sought.

Tularemia

Francisella tularensis may be acquired from contact with a variety of animal species, as well as from mosquitoes, lice, fleas, ticks, flies, and contaminated water. The organism may penetrate mucous membranes and unbroken or broken skin. It also may be inhaled or swallowed. It is crucial to ask patients and their parents not only about the ingestion of rabbit and squirrel meat, but about other animal contact and a history of tick bite.

Tuberculosis

Tuberculosis is a common cause of FUO in children. Nonpulmonary tuberculosis presents as FUO more frequently than does pulmonary tuberculosis. Fever of undetermined origin is most common with disseminated tuberculosis that involves the peritoneum, pericardium, liver, or genitourinary tract. Active disseminated tuberculosis has been documented in children with normal chest radiographs and negative tuberculin test results. Funduscopic examination may reveal choroid tubercles in these individuals. The bone marrow and liver are involved frequently in children with miliary tuberculosis. Liver specimens and bone marrow aspirates should be obtained and processed for morphologic evaluation and appropriate cultures. Gastric aspirates should be cultured in patients suspected of having miliary tuberculosis, even in the presence of a normal chest roentgenogram. Culture material must be prepared by the newer, rapid culture techniques that can provide an answer within 7 to 10 days. The demonstration of acid-fast organisms on smears of gastric secretions does not necessarily indicate *Mycobacterium tuberculosis* infection because nontuberculous *Mycobacterium* spp may be present in the gastric contents of normal individuals.

Bacterial Endocarditis

Infective endocarditis is an infrequent cause of FUO in children. Acute bacterial endocarditis tends to be explosive in onset. Subacute bacterial endocarditis is rare in infants,

increasing in frequency with advancing age. The absence of a cardiac murmur does not exclude the possibility of endocarditis and is particularly common when infection involves the right side of the heart. Endocarditis also may occur in the absence of positive blood culture results, particularly in association with the following factors: right-sided cardiac lesions; use of antibiotics for an undefined febrile illness; prolonged duration of disease; infection by organisms that are not readily apparent on culture, such as *Brucella* spp or *Coxiella burnetii;* and inadequate culture methods for the detection of an infection with anaerobic organisms. Associated laboratory findings include anemia, leukocytosis, and elevated ESR. Five or six blood cultures should be obtained both aerobically and anaerobically over a period of several days. Echocardiograms may reveal vegetations, but negative study results do not exclude endocarditis.

Bone and Joint Infections

Infections of the bones and joints usually can be diagnosed clinically but occasionally may present as FUO. This situation is more common with osteomyelitis than with septic arthritis. Infection of the pelvic bones most often is implicated in this regard. Radioisotopic bone scanning is more sensitive than radiographic examination of the bones.

Liver Abscess and Other Hepatic Infections

Pyogenic liver abscesses are encountered most frequently in the immunocompromised child, but they also may be seen in the normal child. In some children, fever is the only finding. Blood cultures are usually sterile, and liver function tests are within normal limits. Hepatomegaly and right upper quadrant abdominal tenderness may be present in some patients. Diagnosis can be established by examination of the liver by ultrasound, by CT scan, or by radioisotopic scanning techniques. Bacterial hepatitis as well as cholangitis can occur in the absence of jaundice.

Granulomatous hepatitis is a syndrome characterized by granuloma formation within the liver, rather than a specific disease. In many cases, the specific etiology is never determined. Most cases have been reported in adults, but examples in children have been seen. Diagnosis can be established only by liver biopsy.

Intra-abdominal Abscesses

Subphrenic, perinephric, and pelvic abscesses all may present as FUO. A history of intra-abdominal disease, abdominal surgery, or vague abdominal complaints should heighten suspicion that an intra-abdominal collection of pus may be present. The organisms involved most commonly include *Escherichia coli,* anaerobic flora, *Staphylococcus aureus,* and streptococci.

Perinephric abscesses generally develop during the course of bacteremia, and fever may be the only sign. *S aureus* is the organism most often recovered. Urinalysis generally is normal; the intravenous pyelograph may fail to demonstrate a mass. Both pyuria and mass effect on radiographic study of the kidney are late findings. The results of examination by ultrasound or CT scan may be positive earlier in the course of infection.

Deep pelvic abscesses are an important cause of FUO in children. Possible sources of deep pelvic abscesses in children include osteomyelitis of the pelvic bones, previously infected skin lesions with associated lymphadenitis, mesenteric salmonellosis, pelvic thrombophlebitis, and appendiceal infection. Careful pelvic and rectal examinations are important in suspecting or diagnosing pelvic abscesses. Ultrasound examinations and CT scanning may be used to help confirm the diagnosis.

Viral Infections

Infection by most viruses produces an illness that is self-limited and brief, but hepatitis viruses, cytomegalovirus, Epstein-Barr virus, and certain arboviruses are exceptions to the general rule. In all of these disorders, the symptomatology may be variable and signs and symptoms nonspecific. Thus, these viral infections should be considered in the differential diagnosis of patients with FUO.

Upper Respiratory Tract Infection

Infections of the upper respiratory tract and related organs frequently present as FUO. Although obvious symptoms and signs might be expected, the complaints are often trivial and thus ignored. Physical findings may be absent even in cases of mastoiditis or sinusitis. Thus, chronic or recurrent pharyngitis, tonsillitis, peritonsillar abscess, and otitis media should be considered in the differential diagnosis of patients with FUO.

Immunodeficiency

A variety of immunodeficiency states, both congenital and acquired, can present as FUO. HIV infection may present as FUO before specific signs or symptoms of individual organ systems are noted. In other patients, malaise, listlessness, fever, and generalized lymphadenopathy are noted, but the precise etiology is not considered. Diagnosis can be established by serologic evaluation for HIV infection.

Parasitic Infections

Malaria should be considered in children as a cause of FUO. In addition to fever, splenomegaly usually is present. A history of travel to endemic areas should be sought. Several months may pass between infection and the onset of symptoms. If an appropriate mosquito vector is present, infection may be transmitted from an individual who has visited an endemic area to one who has not. Malaria also may be acquired by blood transfusion or by the use of needles and syringes contaminated by the parasite. Demonstration of the organism on appropriately stained thin or thick smears of blood is diagnostic.

Toxoplasmosis, caused by *Toxoplasma gondii*, should be considered in any child with persistent fever. Supraclavicular or cervical lymphadenopathy is present in most cases, but fever is sometimes the only manifestation. The diagnosis is established by demonstrating a rising serologic titer. Antibody to *T gondii* is so common that demonstration of a single high titer alone is not diagnostic of acute infection. Demonstration of *Toxoplasma* spp in tissue secretions or body fluids is highly suggestive, but the organism may persist in tissue for years. Therefore, isolation of the parasite is not absolutely diagnostic of acute toxoplasmosis.

Connective Tissue Diseases

Connective tissue disorders and vasculitis are the second leading cause of FUO in children. Within this group of disorders, JRA accounts for most cases in all pediatric series. Although all three clinical forms of this disorder—acute systemic, pauciarticular, and polyarticular—may be associated with fever, the acute systemic form is most likely to present as FUO. The classic fever pattern in this disorder is one or two temperature spikes daily. Most serologic test results for rheumatoid factor are negative in children with the acute systemic form of JRA, so the disease can be difficult to diagnose. The diagnosis often is made clinically by observation over a prolonged period. A therapeutic trial of a nonsteroidal anti-inflammatory drug can be useful both in controlling the symptoms and in confirming the diagnosis.

Malignancy

Malignancies are the third most frequent cause of FUO in children. The most common is the leukemia-lymphoma group and, less often, neuroblastoma; rarely, other cancers such as hepatoma, rhabdomyosarcoma, and atrial myxoma may present as unexplained fever.

Factitious Fever

Factitious fever always must be considered in the evaluation of a child with FUO. When the patient is an infant or young child, it is a parent or other caretaker who is fabricating. In bizarre cases, the parent actually may induce fever by injecting the child with infectious or noxious materials. In the case of the older child or adolescent, it is the patient who is falsifying information. In most cases, factitious fever can be excluded by having the nurse or physician stay in the room as the temperature is taken. Occasionally the temperature must be taken rectally to ensure that the youngster has not ingested or rinsed the mouth with hot liquids before the temperature measurement. In rare cases, measuring the temperature of a freshly voided urine specimen may be helpful.

Periodic Disorders

Familial Mediterranean fever is an exceedingly rare, autosomal recessive disorder seen mostly in Arabs, Armenians, and Sephardic Jews. It is characterized by acute episodes of fever and inflammation of serosal tissue such as the peritoneum, pleura, or joint synovia. Attacks occur at irregular intervals.

Reimann and McCloskey called attention to a group of disorders characterized by recurrent episodes of fever at fairly regular intervals. At first the febrile attacks tend to occur 3 or 4 weeks apart, but, as the illness persists, the interval between attacks often lengthens to 5 or 6 weeks. Between episodes, the patient is normal and asymptomatic. Some patients in the series had neutropenia at the time of fever, suggesting a relationship to the entity of cyclic neutropenia. Others had arthralgias or evidence of peritoneal inflammation. Marshall and coworkers described 12 children with periodic fever, pharyngitis, aphthous stomatitis, and no hematologic abnormalities. The nature of most of these periodic disorders remains unknown.

Other Causes

Other causes of FUO include serum sickness, drug reactions, inflammatory bowel disease, thyrotoxicosis, Behçet's syndrome, histiocytosis, sarcoidosis, ectodermal dysplasia, diabetes insipidus, chronic brain syndrome, subdural hematoma, and immunodeficiency.

Mucocutaneous lymph node syndrome (Kawasaki syndrome) should be considered in the differential diagnosis of any young child with FUO but usually can be diagnosed or ruled out by the presence or absence of clinical features. Occasionally, however, fever and irritability may be the only findings for up to 10 days. The cause of this presumably infectious disease has not been determined.

Infrequently, the apparent FUO is only an exaggerated normal circadian temperature pattern, a misinterpretation of normal temperature readings in infants or young children, which may be as high as 38°C (100.4°F), or an unfortunate (but not remarkable) series of self-limited viral infections.

Finally, in up to one quarter of all the cases of FUO in children, no definite diagnosis is ever established. Most of these cases resolve spontaneously.

(Abridged from Martin I. Lorin and Ralph D. Feigin, Fever of Undetermined Origin, in Oski, DeAngelis, Feigin, McMillan, Warshaw: *Principles and Practice of Pediatrics, Second Edition*, J.B. Lippincott, 1994.)

Oski's Essential Pediatrics,
edited by Kevin B. Johnson and Frank A. Oski.
Lippincott–Raven Publishers,
Philadelphia © 1997

48

Pathogenesis of Fever and Its Treatment

Fever often is defined simply as an elevation of body temperature above normal, or above an arbitrary upper limit. However, a more exact definition would be an elevation of body temperature as part of a specific biologic response mediated and controlled by the central nervous system (CNS). This definition distinguishes fever from other types of elevated body temperature such as heat stress and heat illness.

■ PATHOPHYSIOLOGY

Fever is one of a large array of responses elicited by chemical mediators involved in the inflammatory process. The most important substance currently identified as mediating the febrile response is interleukin-1 (IL-1), a polypeptide, or group of peptides, synthesized by blood monocytes, phagocytic cells lining the liver and spleen, and other tissue macrophages. IL-1 also is the major currently identified mediator of the acute phase inflammatory response. Before its widespread metabolic, endocrinologic, and hematologic effects were recognized, IL-1 was called *endogenous pyrogen*. In addition to fever, IL-1 or related mediators increase the synthesis of acute phase proteins by the liver, decrease serum iron and zinc levels, provoke leukocytosis, and accelerate skeletal muscle proteolysis. IL-1 also induces slow-wave sleep, perhaps explaining the somnolence and lethargy frequently associated with a febrile illness.

Fever is the result of a highly coordinated series of events that begins peripherally with the synthesis and release of IL-1 by phagocytic cells in the blood or tissues. Molecules of IL-1 enter the blood and are carried to the CNS, where they induce an abrupt increase in the synthesis of prostaglandins, especially prostaglandin E_2, in the region of the anterior hypothalamus. This increase results in elevation of the set point (or reference point) of the thermostat mechanism in this area of the brain. The temperature control region of the anterior hypothalamus then reads the current body temperature as too low in comparison to the new set point and initiates a series of events to elevate body temperature to

a height equal to the new set point. This adaptation involves an augmentation of heat production by increased metabolic rate and increased muscle tone and activity. It also involves decreased heat loss, primarily through diminished perfusion of the skin. Body temperature rises until a new equilibrium is achieved at the elevated set point.

The question often posed is, "Is fever a friend or a foe?" A more appropriate question would be, "Under what conditions is fever beneficial and under what conditions is it harmful?" Little doubt exists that, biologically, fever has some role in defending the host against infection and possibly against other diseases as well. However, it may be that fever is a less important protective mechanism in higher animals with well-developed immunologic systems, such as mammals, than in those with more primitive immunologic systems, such as fish and reptiles.

The growth or survival of a few pathogenic bacteria or viruses is impaired at temperatures in the range of 40°C (104°F). Many pathogenic bacteria require iron for their growth, and it has been shown that fever is associated with a decrease in serum iron and increase in serum ferritin, resulting in minimal levels of free iron in the blood. Because these bacteria have an enhanced need for iron at high temperatures, it has been suggested that this response is a coordinated host defense mechanism to deprive bacteria of free iron when they need it most.

Fever may have undesirable effects other than the immunologic changes described earlier. Fever often makes patients uncomfortable. It is associated with an increased metabolic rate, increased oxygen consumption and carbon dioxide production, and increased demands on the cardiovascular and pulmonary systems. For the normal child, these stresses are of little or no consequence. However, for the child with an underlying disorder, especially of the heart or lungs, these increased demands may be significantly detrimental.

Fever clearly can precipitate febrile convulsions in susceptible children between 6 months and 5 years old. Although these seizures generally are benign, they are disturbing to the parent and child and may lead to invasive procedures such as lumbar punctures as well as considerable expense. Experiments in monkeys demonstrated a deleterious effect of fever on injured cerebral tissue. Clasen and colleagues introduced a standardized insult to one cerebral hemisphere in each experimental animal. Half of the animals were maintained in the euthermic state and half were maintained at a core temperature of 40°C (104°F) for 2 hours after the injury. All animals were then killed. A 40% increase in edema was found in the traumatized hemisphere of the hyperthermic animals compared with the euthermic animals. Bleeding also was more profuse in the experimental group.

■ TREATMENT

Although our current state of knowledge does not permit dogmatic pronouncements regarding the symptomatic treatment of fever, we can make some reasonable recommendations. Clearly, fever need not always be treated and body temperature need not always be restored completely to normal. I advocate treating high fever (40°C [104°F] or greater), fever in children at risk for febrile convulsions, fever in children with underlying neurologic or cardiopulmonary disease, and any situation in which there is consideration of a component of heat illness. Until more data are compiled, the treatment of fever when necessary to establish patient comfort should not be condemned.

Once a decision is reached to treat the patient's fever symptomatically, the choice of a specific therapeutic modality should be based on several considerations. Because fever is the result of an elevation of the set point in the hypothalamic thermoregulatory center, the most rational way to treat fever is to restore this set point to normal; agents such as aspirin, acetaminophen, ibuprofen, and naproxen work on this basis. Aspirin and acetaminophen have been studied extensively and are equally effective at similar doses. Ibuprofen and naproxen are newer agents that appear to be of about the same effectiveness as aspirin or acetaminophen, but at lower dosages and perhaps with longer duration of action.

Under certain circumstances, it is necessary or advisable to use external cooling, generally by sponging, as a means of reducing body temperature, either in addition to or instead of antipyretic drugs (Table 48–1). External cooling is the treatment of choice for heatstroke and other forms of heat illness. However, in cases of fever, external cooling is indicated only in specific situations. External sponging is advisable in any situation in which suspicion exists that the cause of the elevated temperature may be a form of heat illness. Some patients with infection also have a component of heat illness from overwrapping, dehydration, or drugs.

For the previously well child with a non–life-threatening febrile illness, sponging adds little other than patient discomfort. Sponging with tepid water plus acetaminophen is only slightly more rapid in its antipyretic effect than is acetaminophen alone. Sponging with ice water is more rapid, but obviously more uncomfortable, and is indicated only when treating heat illness. Sponging often is useful in patients with neurologic disorders, because many of these children have abnormal temperature control and respond poorly to antipyretic agents. Sponging also would be preferable to antipyretic agents in children with hypersensitivity to these agents and in patients with severe liver disease. As mentioned above, in very young infants, the half-life of aceta-

TABLE 48-1. Use of External Cooling in Treating Elevated Temperature

Cooling Method	Indications
Tepid sponging *instead of* antipyretic drugs	Very young infants
	Severe liver disease
	History of hypersensitivity to antipyretic drugs
Tepid sponging *plus* antipyretic drugs	High fever (>40°C[>104°F])
	History of febrile seizures, neurologic disorders, or brain damage
	Infection plus suspicion of overheating or overwrapping
	Septic shock*
Cold sponging *alone*	Heat illness

May require cold sponging

minophen is prolonged, and sponging may be preferable to use of this agent.

Sponging should be done with tepid water (generally around 30°C [85°F]). Rubbing alcohol should not be used because its fumes are absorbed across the alveolar membrane and possibly across the skin as well, resulting in CNS toxicity.

(Abridged from Martin I. Lorin, Pathogenesis of Fever and Its Treatment, in Oski, DeAngelis, Feigin, McMillan, Warshaw: *Principles and Practice of Pediatrics, Second Edition*, J.B. Lippincott, 1994.)

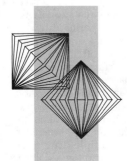

SECTION 2
Bacterial Infections

Oski's Essential Pediatrics,
edited by Kevin B. Johnson and Frank A. Oski.
Lippincott–Raven Publishers,
Philadelphia © 1997

49

Sepsis and Septic Shock

United States Supreme Court Justice Potter Stewart once wrote, "I can't define obscenity; but I know it when I see it." Most pediatricians would believe that statement could equally well be applied to "sepsis," "septic shock," and the related life-threatening systemic infections that occur in children.

In the last decade, intensive study has led to an improved understanding of the basic biochemistry and pathophysiology of serious infection. Fundamental to this new knowledge is the discovery that a great variety of illnesses—including noninfectious conditions such as immune-mediated organ injury, multiple trauma, and malignancy—have in common with infection the endogenous production of certain key inflammatory mediators that result in similar physiologic consequences.

■ TERMINOLOGY

A vigorous debate is underway among subspecialists in infectious diseases and critical care medicine regarding the terminology that should be used to classify serious infections. The American College of Chest Physicians and the

Society of Critical Care Medicine recently convened a consensus task force to consider appropriate terminology for sepsis. Their classification system is a start in the process of organized thought about these potentially life-threatening events. Their proposed definitions include the following:

- *Systemic inflammatory response syndrome (SIRS).* The systemic inflammatory response to a variety of severe clinical insults. The response is manifested by two or more of the following conditions:
- Temperature >38°C or <36°C
- Heart rate >90 or >2 SD above normal for age
- Respiratory rate >30 or >2 SD above normal for age or $PaCO_2$ <32 mm Hg
- WBC >15,000 cells/mm³, <5,000 cells/mm³, or >10% immature (band) forms
- *Infection.* Microbial phenomenon characterized by an inflammatory response to the presence of microorganisms or the invasion of normally sterile host tissue by those organisms.
- *Bacteremia.* The presence of viable bacteria in the blood. *Viremia, fungemia,* and *parasitemia* are the terms to be used when the corresponding organisms are isolated.
- *Sepsis.* The systemic response to documented infection. (Sepsis = SIRS + infection).
- *Severe sepsis.* Sepsis associated with organ dysfunction, hypoperfusion, or hypotension. Hypoperfusion and perfusion abnormalities may include, but are not limited to, lactic acidosis, oliguria, or an acute alteration in mental status.
- *Septic hypotension.* A blood pressure <2 SD below normal for age, associated with sepsis.
- *Septic shock.* Sepsis with hypotension that persists after adequate fluid resuscitation, along with the presence of perfusion abnormalities that may include, but are not limited to, lactic acidosis, oliguria, or an acute alteration in mental status. Patients who are on inotropic or vasopressor agents may not be hypotensive at the time that perfusion abnormalities are measured.
- *Multiple organ dysfunction syndrome (MODS).* Presence of altered organ function in an acutely ill patient such that physiologic homeostasis cannot be maintained without intervention.

Unlike the situation in adult medicine, SIRS and sepsis as defined above are common "problem statements" in pediatrics. Although the categories apply well to older children and adolescents, there is a need for clearer diagnostic criteria for SIRS in infants and younger children (we have made a few modifications for the purposes of this chapter). Pediatric patients compensate well for shock states with tachycardia and vasoconstriction, so septic shock and MODS by these definitions become relatively uncommon (and ominous) clinical entities. Note that the term *septicemia* is no longer used, in favor of categories with a definable physiologic status. The term *multiple organ system failure* has now been replaced by "MODS." The term *sepsis syndrome* has now been replaced by "severe sepsis." This is the category that should serve as an early warning of a life-threatening pediatric infection.

■ ETIOLOGY

Sepsis and the various septic syndromes are typically caused by bacterial infections of an advanced nature. Con-

trary to popular belief, the majority of patients with sepsis do *not* have documented bacteremia. This was a major reason for the recent changes in definitions, although the probability of positive blood cultures increases as one progresses down the classification list to septic shock and MODS. Even with negative blood cultures, however, bacterial etiology can generally be established by positive Gram stains and cultures of purulent exudates, characteristic alterations in hematologic parameters, tests for the presence of capsular polysaccharide antigens, or clinical responses to empiric antimicrobial therapy.

The common, and some of the unusual, bacterial etiologies of sepsis in the previously normal child are presented in Table 49–1, according to the presence or absence of a focal source and according to the presence of accidental or surgical alterations in integumentary and mucosal barriers. A working knowledge of these organisms and the clinical settings in which they are most likely to present provides a rational basis for organism identification and selection of an empiric antibiotic regimen. The causes of neonatal infections are discussed comprehensively in Chapter 50. It is important to recall that sepsis of a critical nature, even in a previously normal child, should prompt consideration of an important defect in host defense. For example, meningococcemia should suggest an abnormality in the terminal complement pathway.

The encapsulated organisms—*Streptococcus pneumoniae, Neisseria meningitidis,* and *Haemophilus influenzae,* type b—are the most common causes of sepsis (and bacteremia) of occult origin. These organisms are most frequent in children aged 3 months to 5 years and correspond to the nadir in transplacentally acquired maternal IgG antibodies. Such infections are commonly preceded by a viral upper respiratory illness that results in a mucosal portal of entry for the organism (for example, meningococcemia preceded by influenza).

A focus of infection should always be sought in patients with occult bacteremia. Frequently, the identity of a bloodstream isolate can provide a clue to the origin. *Staphylococcus aureus* bacteremia, for example, should always suggest the possibility of osteomyelitis, endocarditis, or pericarditis.

In sepsis of focal origin, likely bacterial etiologies are suggested by the site of the infection and often are determined by normal flora of a contiguous surface. Urinary tract infections, for example, often are caused by enteric flora. First episodes generally are due to antibiotic-susceptible *Escherichia coli.* Recurrent episodes separated by periods of prophylactic antibiotics—to the extent that prophylaxis has altered enteric flora—will be due to *Klebsiella* spp, *Enterobacter* spp, or *Pseudomonas aeruginosa* with multiple-drug resistance. Sepsis associated with bacterial enteritis generally is caused by salmonella, shigella, or *Yersinia enterocolitica. Salmonella* enteric fever often is associated with bacteremia. Shigellosis, on the other hand, rarely is bacteremic but may be associated with sepsis and septic shock, especially if *Shigella dysenteriae* is involved.

Disruption of skin or mucosal barriers may be accidental or surgical. Bite wounds can be associated with unusual oral pathogens, depending on the source. Dog bites, for example, generally are inoculated with staphylococcus and oral anaerobes but may also be contaminated with *Pasteurella multocida* or *Capnocytophaga* DF-2. The latter two species often are associated with bacteremia and sepsis. Infections affecting surgical sites generally involve normal flora at the site of operation that contaminate surgically damaged tissue. Sepsis complicating craniofacial surgery, for example, is caused by the normal flora of the skin, scalp, and upper respiratory mucosal surfaces, including staphylococci, *Haemophilus* spp, *S pneumoniae,* and oral anaerobes.

TABLE 49-1. Bacterial Etiologies of Sepsis
in Previously Normal Pediatric Patients, by Apparent Source

OCCULT

Streptococcus pneumoniae, Haemophilus influenzae
type b, Neisseria meningitidis, Staphylococcus aureus

FOCAL SOURCE

Skin and musculoskeletal: S aureus, Streptococcus pyogenes,
H influenzae type b

Respiratory tract: S pneumoniae, H influenzae, S aureus,
oral anaerobes,* S pyogenes

Gastrointestinal tract: Salmonella spp., Shigella spp., Yersinia
enterocolitica

Peritoneum: Enteric gram negative rods†, enteric anaerobes‡,
Enterococcus faecalis

Heart or pericardium: S aureus, h influenzae type b

Urinary tract: enteric gram negative rods

Genital tract: Neisseria gonorrhoeae, enteric anaerobes

Meninges: H influenzae type b, N meningitidis, S pneumoniae

ACQUIRED BARRIER DISRUPTION

Abdominal surgery or penetrating trauma: Enteric gram negative rods,
enteric anaerobes, Enterococcus faecalis

Cardiac surgery: Staphylococci§, multiply-resistant gram negative rods‖

Orthopedic surgery or compound fracture: Staphylococci

Craniofacial surgery: Staphylococci, S pneumoniae, H influenzae, oral
anaerobes

Vascular access device-related: Staphylococci, multiply-resistant gram
negative rods, Acinetobacter spp., Candida albicans

Burn wounds: S pyogenes, Pseudomonas aeruginosa

BITE WOUNDS

Human: Eikenella corrodens, staphylococci, oral anaerobes

Dog: Capnocytophaga canimorsus (DF-2), Pasteurella multocida,
staphylococci, oral anaerobes

Cat: P multocida, oral anaerobes

Rat: Streptobacillus moniliformis, Spirillum minus

Flea: Yersinia pestis

Tick: Francisella tularensis

*Peptostreptococcus, Fusobacterium spp., Bacteroides melaninogenicus,
Veillonella.

†Eschericia coli, Klebsiella spp., Enterobacter spp.

‡Bacteroides fragilis, Clostridium perfringens, Clostridium septicum,
Fusobacterium spp.

§Staphylococcus aureus, coagulase-negative staphylococci.

‖Enterobacter spp., Pseudomonas aeruginosa, Klebsiella spp.,
Xanthomas maltophilia, Serritia marcescens.

Sepsis has a broad differential diagnosis, as summarized in Table 49–2. Included are nonbacterial infections, such as viral, rickettsial, and spirochetal infections, as well as responses to bacterial products, such as vaccines. Although it is not a final diagnosis, sepsis is an appropriate problem statement for such conditions. Shock states that may be confused with septic shock include tachyarrhythmia with cardiogenic shock (often triggered by acute febrile illness) and gastroenteritis with hypovolemic shock (also commonly associated with fever). The former is particularly important to recognize, because aggressive fluid resuscitation can lead to deterioration rather than improvement in cardiovascular status.

■ PATHOGENESIS

Septic shock has in the past been considered synonymous with "endotoxin shock." Lipopolysaccharides purified from the cell membranes of a variety of gram-negative organisms such as E coli, Salmonella, Pseudomonas, and N meningitidis are capable of eliciting the characteristic picture of sepsis in experimental animals. Accidental infusion of contaminated intravenous fluids containing large amounts of endotoxin (but without viable organisms) has been found to trigger septic shock in humans. Experimental infusion of low doses of endotoxin in volunteers elicits characteristic physiologic and laboratory changes. Antiendotoxin antibodies in pooled sera or in the form of specific monoclonal antibodies can block the response and improve outcome in critically ill patients. Thus, there is no question that endotoxin is one of the trigger mechanisms of sepsis.

Other organisms can clearly produce septic syndromes either by virtue of their production of exotoxins or by sheer force of numbers. Staphylococcal and group A streptococcal toxic shock syndromes are both potentially lethal conditions whose clinical picture is caused by the circulation of well-characterized exotoxins from the site of an occult infection. Bacteremia infrequently accompanies these conditions. Although the clinical features differ somewhat, toxemias arise in association with Shigella dysenteriae dysentery and with the acute hemorrhagic colitis caused by verotoxin-producing E coli 0157. Their exotoxins are biochemically similar and lead to the hemolytic uremic syndrome. Like staphylococcal and streptococcal toxic shock, blood cultures are generally negative. Finally, it has been found in experimental animals that high level intravenous infusion of even relatively nonvirulent gram-positive bacteria, such as Staphylococcus epidermidis, can induce the physiologic changes of sepsis and septic shock. Thus, endotoxins can no longer be considered the common pathway of sepsis and septic shock.

It is now recognized that septic shock results from the sequential release of endogenous mediators. These substances, referred to as cytokines, are products of monocytes, macrophages, T-lymphocytes, endothelial cells, mast cells, polymorphonuclear leukocytes, and an increasingly lengthy list of other cell types. These substances are the signals that comprise the inflammatory cascade. Presumably these substances evolved as part of the mechanisms for controlling relatively localized infections or trauma. When a human host is confronted by a more massive challenge, however, it appears that these substances may be produced excessively—leading to a response so vigorous so as to be potentially fatal. One of the most extensively studied substances in the inflammatory cascade is tumor necrosis factor (TNF), a product of the monocytes and macrophages. Injection of TNF in experimental animals completely mimics the clinical response (fever, hypotension, coagulopathy, multiple organ failure, and death) seen after injection with endotoxin, but with a reduced latency time. Circulating levels of TNF may correlate with prognosis, as has been demonstrated in meningococcal disease.

Other mediators appear to be responsible for other familiar elements in the sequence. The interleukins (particularly IL-1, IL-2, and IL-6) mediate hypotension and fever. Hageman factor (factor XII) and platelet-activating factor (PAF) mediate coagulopathy. Interferon-gamma (IFN-γ) activates macrophages. The colony-stimulating factors (G-CSF and GM-CSF)

TABLE 49-2. Differential Diagnosis of Sepsis

INFECTION

Viral illness (influenza, enteroviruses, dengue hemorrhagic fever, disseminated herpes)

Encephalitis (arbovirus, enterovirus, herpes)

Rickettsial infection (Rocky Mountain spotted fever, *Ehrlichia*, Q fever)

Spirochetal infection (syphilis, relapsing fever; Jarisch-Herxheimer reaction)

Vaccine reaction (pertussis, whole-virus influenza, typhoid)

CARDIOPULMONARY

Pneumonia (bacterial, viral, mycobacterial, fungal, pneumocystis)

Pulmonary emboli

Congestive heart failure

Arrhythmia (with cardiogenic shock)

Pericarditis (with pericardial tamponade)

Myocarditis

METABOLIC-ENDOCRINE

Adrenal insufficiency (adrenogenital syndrome, Waterhouse-Friderichsen syndrome, steroid withdrawal)

Diabetes insipidus

Diabetes mellitus

Inborn errors of metabolism (organic acidosis, urea cycle, carnitine deficiency)

Hypoglycemia

Reye syndrome

GASTROINTESTINAL

Gastroenteritis with hypovolemic shock (viral, bacterial, parasitic)

Malrotation with midgut volvulus

Intussusception

Appendicitis or appendiceal abscess

Peritonitis (spontaneous, perforation, dialysis)

Hepatitis

Hemorrhage

Hematologic

Anemia (sickle cell, blood loss, nutritional)

Splenic sequestration crisis

Leukemia, lymphoma

NEUROLOGIC

Intoxication (drugs, carbon monoxide, intentional or accidental overdose)

Intracranial hemorrhage

Trauma (child abuse, accidents)

Guillain-Barré syndrome

Myasthenia gravis

OTHER

Collagen-vascular disease (systemic lupus erythematosus, juvenile rheumatoid arthritis)

Anaphylaxis (food, drug, insect sting)

Kawasaki syndrome

Erythema multiforme

Hemorrhagic shock–encephalopathy syndrome

Heatstroke

Malignant hyperthermia

---

stimulate production of phagocytic cells. The integrins (CD11 and CD18) and the intercellular adhesion molecules (ICAM-1 and ICAM-2) control leukocyte migration. Endothelium-derived relaxing factor (nitric oxide) is a potent vasodilator of the microcirculation. The complement system produces substances (C3a and C5a) that are the major chemotactic stimuli for leukocytes. The list of mediators is ever increasing, with a clear picture of the complete sequence only beginning to emerge.

The consequence of the release of these mediators is the development of sepsis. Progression to septic shock and multiorgan system dysfunction or failure depends on the pathogens involved and the degree to which the host mediators and effector cells are capable of localizing and killing them. The most prominent physiologic features of septic shock are fever and cardiovascular compromise or collapse. The cardiac response to sepsis is characterized by an initial increase in cardiac output followed by a period of poor myocardial performance probably due to one or more myocardial depressant factors. The effect of sepsis on the vascular bed is complex but is characterized by direct injury to the endothelium. This results in alterations in vascular tone and capillary leak. The alterations in tone result in decreased systemic vascular resistance, abnormal perfusion patterns to various organ systems, and may lead to organ dysfunction or complete organ failure. The capillary leak allows the egress of fluid and proteins from the vascular system and results in hypovolemia and the severe edema often encountered in severe cases.

The effects of compromised perfusion and capillary leak are unique to each organ system. Mortality rate is directly proportional to the number of organs that fail. Capillary leak and intrapulmonary right-to-left shunting may lead to the adult respiratory distress syndrome. Decreased renal perfusion initially leads to oliguria. In the presence of uncorrected hypotension, acute tubular necrosis may supervene. Decreased cerebral circulation leads to confusion, disorientation and obtundation. Compounding these changes is the frequent development of disseminated intravascular coagulation, which can further reduce perfusion or, by depletion of clotting factors, lead to major hemorrhage.

■ CLINICAL MANIFESTATIONS

Recognition of the septic child is difficult. The pediatrician's fundamental dilemma is how to detect the child with a potentially life-threatening infection among the many children with self-limited or readily treated infections that are not life-threatening. An awareness of the presence of predisposing conditions to infection in an individual child is probably the most helpful guide. Unfortunately, not all seriously ill children have identified defects in their host defenses, particularly in infancy.

Most children with sepsis have obvious and significant elevated temperatures. In the very young and in advanced disease, however, temperatures may actually be in the hypothermic range. Rigors and hyperthermia (temperature >41°C [105.8°F]) imply bacteremia.

Behavioral changes may be helpful indicators of serious illness. Four of the six items on the Yale Observational Scale—quality of cry, reaction to parent stimulation, state variation, and response to social overtures—are behavioral. The child with febrile illness, a weak cry, poor responsiveness, no smile, and lack of facial expression is likely to be septic. These changes in most cases reflect compromised cerebral circulation; occasionally they indicate complicating meningitis.

Table 49-3. Recommended Dosage Schedule for the Antimicrobial Agents Most Frequently Used in Empiric Treatment of Pediatric Patients With Sepsis

Agent	Dosage (mg/kg/d) and Intervals of Administration	Maximum Daily Dosage	Most Common Target Organisms
Amikacin	30 div q 8 hr	—*	Hospital gram-negative rods
Ampicillin	100–300 div q 4–6 hr	10–12 g	Community encapsulated organisms
Ampicillin/sulbactam†	150–200 div q 4–6 hr	10–12 g	Community encapsulated organisms, anaerobes
Amphotericin B	0.5–1.5 once daily	—*	Invasive fungal infection
Aztreonam†	75–150 div q 6 hr	6–8 g	Hospital gram-negative rods
Cefotaxime	150–200 div q 6 hr	8–10 g	Community encapsulated organisms
Ceftazidime	100–150 div q 8 hr	4–6 g	Hospital gram–negative rods
Ceftriaxone	50–100 div q 12–24 hr	2 g	Community encapsulated organisms
Cefurozime	100–200 div q 6 h	4–6 g	Community encapsulated organisms, staphylococci
Chloramphenicol	75–100 div q 6 h	2–4 g*	Rickettsiae, salmonella
Clindamycin	30–40 div q 8 hr	2–4 g	Anaerobes, community staphylococci
Flucytosine	100–150 div q 6 hr	—*	Invasive fungal infections (with ampho B)
Gentamicin	5–7.5 div q 8 hr	—*	Community gram-negative rods
Imipinem/Cilastatin†	60–100 div q 8 hr	2–4 g	Hospital gram-negative rods, anaerobes
Metronidazole	30 div q 6 hr	2–4 g	Anaerobes
Mezlocillin	200–300 div q 4–6 hr	18-24 g	Hospital gram-negative rods
Nafcillin	150–250 div q 4–6 hr	8–12 g	Community staphylococci
Tetracycline	20–30 div q 8–12 hr	1–2 g	Rickettsiae
Ticarcillin	200–300 div q 4–6 hr	18–24 g	Community pseudomonas
Tobramycin	5–7.5 div q 8 hr	—*	Hospital gram-negative rods
Trimethoprim/Sulfamethoxazole	8–20 trimethoprim div q 12 hr	1–2 g*	Salmonella, Shigella, pneumocystis
Vancomycin	40 div q 6–12 hr	2–4 g*	Hospital staphylococci

*Serum concentration and/or toxicity desirable.

†Not licensed by FDA for pediatric use (< age 12). Use should be limited to critical illness with high probability of resistant microorganisms.

Although changes in respiratory pattern generally point to pulmonary disease, tachypnea and acrocyanosis also may reflect metabolic acidosis and poor peripheral perfusion—both characteristic of sepsis.

A careful evaluation of circulatory adequacy is important. Measurement of blood pressure is basic, but it should be recognized that children often compensate well for early shock states, so that blood pressure may be in the normal range. Note, however, that difficulty in measuring a child's blood pressure is more likely to be a reflection of marginal circulation than it is of a technical problem with the blood pressure apparatus. Even if measured blood pressure is in the normal range, circulatory inadequacy is usually manifested by cool extremities, acrocyanosis, absent or diminished peripheral pulses, and capillary refill times of >3 seconds. Although it is said that "warm shock" may be seen early in sepsis, this is relatively unusual in children.

Cutaneous manifestations of sepsis may be externally helpful as warning flags. Between 8% and 20% of patients with fever and petechiae have a serious bacterial infection, and 7% to 10% have meningococcemia or meningococcal meningitis. Purpuric lesions or ecchymoses of the distal extremities (purpura fulminans) raise these probabilities even higher. Diffuse erythroderma in the presence of fever and shock should suggest toxic shock syndrome.

■ LABORATORY ABNORMALITIES

Laboratory manifestations of sepsis include positive blood cultures and positive cultures from other sites such as urine, cerebrospinal fluid, stool, joint or bone aspirates, exudates, abscesses, and cutaneous lesions. Continuing efforts should be made to identify the site of origin of a septic process, using multiple cultures of multiple sites if necessary. Blood cultures that are persistently positive in spite of treatment imply resistant organisms or an endovascular origin of infection.

Hematologic parameters are useful in initial and continuing evaluation. Leukocytosis is the norm; leukopenia is more prognostically ominous. Often leukopenia is the initial response, with remarkable leukocytosis the paradoxic response to successful therapy. Elevated band counts, toxic granulation, and Döhle bodies imply bacterial sepsis. Thrombocytopenia implies the presence of disseminated intravascular coagulation, which should be confirmed with documentation of prothrombin time, partial thromboplastin time, fibrinogen levels, and the presence of fibrin split products. Band counts (decreasing) and platelet counts (increasing) are useful serial studies implying successful treatment.

Metabolic acidosis, manifested by decreased serum bicarbonate, pH, and increased serum lactate, is a frequent biochemical manifestation of diminished end-organ perfusion.

Persisting metabolic acidosis during therapy is an ominous indicator of inadequate tissue oxygen delivery. Compensatory respiratory alkalosis is a common early abnormality. Prerenal azotemia or uremia is the usual manifestation of diminished renal perfusion and acute tubular necrosis, respectively. Hypoalbuminemia often develops during management of severe sepsis, the consequence of both a catabolic state and capillary leak of colloid into the interstitium.

■ THERAPY

The cornerstones of treatment for sepsis and septic shock are eradication of the infecting organisms and maintenance of adequate oxygen and nutrient delivery to vital organs. After recognition of the situation, an orderly—but rapid—sequence of initial interventions to achieve these goals is mandatory.

Patients with severe sepsis should be monitored for all five vital signs: respiration, heart rate, blood pressure, temperature, and oxygen saturation (by pulse oximetry). An adequate airway and peripheral oxygen saturation are top priorities. If abnormal, they should be immediately supported by oxygen administration and, if necessary, by an endotracheal tube and mechanical ventilation.

Circulation also should be assessed rapidly and, if marginal or inadequate, vascular access must be achieved by peripheral or central venous catheter or by the intraosseous route. Initial blood cultures should be obtained when access is achieved. If cardiogenic shock can reasonably be excluded, then 20 to 40 mL/kg of normal saline should be administered as bolus infusions.

Initial empiric antibiotic therapy is then indicated by the parenteral route. An assessment of probable etiology should be made, with consideration of the likely infecting organisms as presented in Table 49–1. The other key element in antibiotic choice is the likelihood of encountering resistance, the two major determinants of which are whether the infection was acquired in the hospital and whether the patient has received recent antimicrobial therapy. In the former instance, knowledge of previous bacterial isolates from a hospitalized child may be very helpful. In the latter, one can suspect an overgrowth phenomenon requiring an alternative drug or combination. The parenteral antibiotics most frequently used in treatment of sepsis, their dosages, and their usual indications are summarized in Table 49–3. Sepsis that is occult and of community origin is appropriately treated with cefuroxime, cefotaxime, or ceftriaxone. Cefuroxime has superior activity against staphylococci, but should not be used if the physician has not excluded the presence of meningitis. Nosocomial sepsis is best treated with multiple agents. Vancomycin, a third-generation cephalosporin, and an aminoglycoside are a commonly used combination.

The goals of initial empiric antimicrobial therapy are clearing of the bloodstream, penetration to infected sites, and control of the progress of the infectious process. With more definitive microbiologic data, regimens should be changed to the specific drugs of choice for the organisms isolated—as single agents or synergistic combinations depending on identity. Gram-positive organisms often are treated effectively with single agents; gram-negative rods are best managed with combinations. With the exception of children with bacterial meningitis, corticosteroid therapy is not beneficial. Clarification of the source of a problem may mandate surgical drainage or removal of hardware as therapeutic adjuncts. When a source or infecting organism is not defined or results are delayed, modification of regimens may be necessary based on clinical response criteria alone.

The elements of supportive care after intensive care unit admission include continued monitoring of vital signs and oxygen saturation (see Chapter 41). In addition, invasive monitoring of central venous pressure and arterial pressure generally are indicated. Pulmonary artery (PA) catheters are used aggressively in adult critical care, but more selectively in pediatric patients. Multiple organ system dysfunction, in which the pressure demands of mechanical ventilation may adversely affect cardiovascular performance, is the usual setting in which PA catheters are considered. They enable rational management of intravascular volume status, ventilator settings, and pressor infusions.

Management of pressor infusions, adult respiratory distress syndrome, acute tubular necrosis, and disseminated intravascular coagulation are discussed elsewhere in this book. Subspecialist consultation and team management of septic shock are essential. Conflicting priorities are common in managing these complex patients. One common situation is the need for administration of multiple blood products, total parenteral nutrition, and numerous drugs and infusions—in the face of pulmonary edema, marginal myocardial performance, and renal failure. This situation may be handled readily by the use of slow continuous ultrafiltration (SCUF) or continuous arteriovenous hemofiltration (CAVH), which can maintain euvolemia despite massive infusion volumes. Because they are continuous, they are much more physiologic approaches than intermittent hemodialysis.

Another major issue is maintenance of adequate nutrition. Sepsis mediators create a hypermetabolic state that rapidly depletes body stores and exceeds the caloric content of conventional intravenous fluids. Early and aggressive parenteral nutrition is necessary to keep up with these demands and to provide sufficient calories to promote tissue regeneration and healing.

The most exciting recent advances in therapy for sepsis and septic shock involve the use of monoclonal antibodies directed against gram-negative endotoxin or receptor antagonists of the mediators of the sepsis inflammatory cascade. Monoclonal antibodies against lipopolysaccharides have shown some promise in clinical trials, but only in population subgroups who have proven gram-negative infection. Their benefit may be mitigated by the fact that they are administered at a time at which pathogenic pathways are already far advanced. Perhaps more promising is the possibility of using recombinant proteins that closely resemble the naturally occurring antagonists of TNF and IL-1, or monoclonal antibodies directed against these mediators. Such products are in advanced clinical trials in adult patients. Extension of these studies to pediatric patients is in the near future.

■ PREVENTION

Dramatic reductions in the incidence of invasive *H influenzae* type b disease are the welcome result of the widespread use of polysaccharide conjugate vaccines in infancy. Meningococcal and pneumococcal polysaccharide vaccines also have had an impact on the incidence of invasive infection in high-risk children older than age 2. Conjugate vaccines are under development and may permit immunization of young infants in the future.

(Abridged from Kenneth M. Boyer and William R. Hayden, Sepsis and Septic Shock, in Oski, DeAngelis, Feigin, McMillan, Warshaw: *Principles and Practice of Pediatrics, Second Edition*, J.B. Lippincott, 1994.)

Oski's Essential Pediatrics,
edited by Kevin B. Johnson and Frank A. Oski.
Lippincott–Raven Publishers,
Philadelphia © 1997

50

Bacterial and Viral Infections of the Newborn (Sepsis Neonatorum)

The terms *neonatal sepsis* and *sepsis neonatorum* refer to invasive bacterial infections that involve primarily the bloodstream in infants during the first month of life. As a "compromised host," the neonate does not localize infection well, and invasion of the meninges occurs in about 10% to 25% of bacteremic infants. The incidence of neonatal sepsis in the United States varies from 1 to 10 per 1000 live births, with an average of 2 or 3 per 1000. Although these infections are relatively uncommon, they may be associated with case fatality rates of 15% to 30% and substantial morbidity in surviving infants. The pediatrician must be familiar with the etiologic agents, pathogenesis, and clinical manifestations of neonatal sepsis so appropriate cultures may be obtained and effective antimicrobial therapy may be initiated promptly.

■ ETIOLOGY

Although the incidence of neonatal sepsis has varied little over the years, the predominant pathogens have varied considerably from one decade to the next (Table 50–1). In the 1970s, group B streptococcus emerged and has persisted into the 1990s as the predominant pathogen in most US nurseries. The virulence of the group B streptococcus, however, has decreased in recent years. Within the United States, there has been an unexplained year-to-year as well as geographic variation in the reported rates of group B streptococcal infections. Yearly incidence of neonatal group B streptococcus infection may vary in the presence of stable maternal colonization rates for unknown reasons. Replacement of the gram-negative enteric bacilli and *Pseudomonas* spp by the group B streptococcus as the predominant pathogen in Latin American and Asian nurseries has lagged behind the pattern observed in North American nurseries by several years.

Although group B streptococcus and *Escherichia coli* account for 60% to 70% of all infections, several other pathogens are noteworthy. *Staphylococcus aureus*, *Klebsiella-Enterobacter*, *Serratia*, *Salmonella*, and *Pseudomonas* spp are most frequently isolated from infants with late-onset infections, especially during nosocomial outbreaks. Aminoglycoside-resistant strains of gram-negative bacilli and methicillin-resistant *S aureus* (MRSA) are particularly difficult to eradicate from nurseries for low-birth-weight infants. The incidence of *Listeria monocytogenes* is highly variable with temporal clustering related to maternal infection associated with foodborne outbreaks.

Several other pathogens have come to the forefront during the past decade. In a study by Broughton and colleagues (1981), the non-group D, α-hemolytic streptococcus was cited as second only to the group B streptococcus as an etiology of neonatal sepsis. This organism is less virulent than most of the other neonatal pathogens. There is a low incidence of shock and meningitis, and a case fatality rate of only 9%. Group D streptococci, both enterococcal and nonenterococcal (*Streptococcus bovis*), have been associated with clinical illness indistinguishable from early-onset disease caused by the group B streptococcus as well as late-onset nosocomial infections. *Streptococcus pneumoniae*, *Neisseria meningitidis*, *Haemophilus influenzae*, and groups A, C, and G streptococci are respiratory tract pathogens that occasionally colonize the maternal genital tract and cause early-onset neonatal sepsis. Pneumonia associated with these pathogens may be clinically indistinguishable from uncomplicated hyaline membrane disease. Friesen and Cho (1986) report that, in contrast to *H influenzae* infections in infants beyond the first month of life, only 20% of such infections in the neonate are due to type B organisms. The remaining cases are associated with nontypable strains (56%), other types (D and C, 9%), or strains of unknown type (15%). The reported overall case-fatality rate for neonatal *H influenzae* infections is 55%. *S pneumoniae* is more likely to be associated with meningitis in the neonate than are other respiratory tract pathogens.

Coagulase-negative staphylococci and *Candida* spp have been isolated more often from septic, premature infants who have prolonged stays in the intensive care unit and who receive parenteral hyperalimentation through a central venous catheter and repeated courses of broad-spectrum

TABLE 50-1. Pathogens Most Frequently Associated With Sepsis Neonatorum

Years	Most Frequent	Other
1928–1932	β streptococcus	*Staphylococcus aureus, Escherichia coli*
1933–1943	Group A streptococcus	*E coli*
1944–1957	*E coli*	*Pseudomonas aeruginosa*
1958–1965	*E coli (S aureus*)*	*Pseudomonas* spp., *Klebsiella-Enterobacter*
1966–1978	Group B streptococcus	*E coli, Klebsiella-Enterobacter*
1979–1990	Group B streptococcus, *E coli*	Coagulase-negative staphylococci, MRSA*†, gram negatives, enterococcus, *Candida*

*Nosocomial outbreaks in some nurseries.

†Methicillin-resistant S aureus.

Adapted from Freedman RM, Ingram DL, Gross E, et al. A half century of neonatal sepsis at Yale, 1928–1978. Am J Dis Child 1981;135:140.

TABLE 50-2. Nonspecific Signs of Sepsis

Temperature instability	Hypotension
Respiratory distress	Tachycardia
Feeding intolerance	Apnea and bradycardia
Vomiting	Irritability
Abdominal distention	High pitched cry
Diarrhea	Lethargy
Jaundice	Weak suck
Pallor	Convulsions
Skin rash, petechiae	Bulging of full fontanelle

antibiotics. *Candida* spp are associated with 5% to 10% of late-onset infections in low-birth-weight nurseries, whereas coagulase-negative staphylococci now account for more than 30% of late-onset infections. These two pathogens may cause right-sided endocarditis associated with catheter placement in the right atrium. The significance of anaerobes isolated from blood cultures of neonates remains unclear. Most anaerobic bacteremias are self-limited in the absence of a focal infection. *Bacteroides* and *Clostridium* spp may be associated with serious life-threatening disease, especially when peritonitis, fasciitis, or meningitis is present.

Overall case fatality rates have decreased from 90% in the 1930s to 15% to 25% in the 1980s and 1990s. This decrease is a result of earlier recognition of the nonspecific signs of sepsis and improved supportive care of the overwhelmed infant as well as development of more active antimicrobial agents.

■ CLINICAL MANIFESTATIONS

The clinical signs of bacterial infection in the neonate are presented in Table 50–2. These signs are distinctively non-specific and may be associated with viral infections or with noninfectious disorders. Because the neonate is an impaired host, the clinical course is unpredictable and usually rapidly progressive. The presence of any of these signs alone or in combination is an indication for complete evaluation to rule out sepsis.

■ DIAGNOSIS

Whenever bacterial infection of the neonate is suspected, cultures of blood, cerebrospinal fluid, urine, and infected body fluids that are normally sterile or an aspirate from an infected soft tissue site or bone should be obtained before initiating antimicrobial therapy. The optimal amount of blood for culture is 0.5 to 1.0 mL, but 0.2 mL may be adequate. Blood should be drawn from both a peripheral site and the central venous catheter when one is in place. Blood cultures should not be obtained from the umbilical cord at delivery or from umbilical catheters beyond the time of initial placement because of the high rates of contamination. Microorganisms isolated only from blood obtained through a catheter when peripheral venous blood cultures are sterile are more likely to represent colonization than septicemia.

Several laboratory tests have been evaluated for their usefulness in rapid detection of the neonate with bacterial infection. Those evaluated either singly or in combination with a defined scoring system include the leukocyte count

and differential count, platelet count, C-reactive protein level, erythrocyte sedimentation rate, haptoglobin level, IgM level, leukocyte alkaline phosphatase level, fibronectin level, nitroblue tetrazolium test, elastase-α-proteinase inhibitor level, and limulus lysate test for detection of endotoxin. No single test alone or in combination with others is superior to the leukocyte count and differential count as a reliable indirect indicator of bacterial infection. After correction of the Coulter leukocyte count for the presence of nucleated red blood cells, the absolute total neutrophil count and the ratio of immature-to-total neutrophils (I:T) are compared with normal standards for age (Figures 50–1 and 50–2). Neutropenia is more likely than neutrophilia to be associated with neonatal sepsis. Pregnancy-induced hypertension or asphyxia in the absence of infection, however, may produce neutropenia. The neutropenia of infection does not persist for more than 36 hours, whereas the neutropenia observed with noninfectious conditions may persist through the first 3 postnatal days. Similarly, neutrophilia may be associated with maternal fever before delivery or hemolytic disease of the newborn. Other noninfectious conditions that may affect

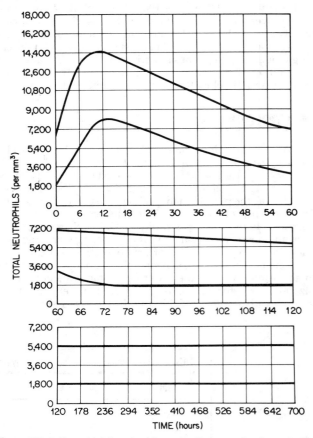

Figure 50-1. Normal total neutrophil counts after correction for nucleated red blood cells in neonates from birth to 700 hours of age. Formula for correction is as follows:

$$WBC = WBC_{cc} \times \frac{100}{NRBC + 100}$$

where WBC = corrected white blood cell counts; WBC$_{cc}$ = Coulter counter white blood cell count; NRBC = nucleated red blood cells. (Adapted from Manroe BL, Rosenfeld CR, Weinberg AG, Browne R. The neonatal blood count in health and disease. I. Reference values for neutrophilic cells. *J Pediatr.* 1979;95:89. Reprinted from House Staff Nursery Manual, Division of Neonatal-Perinatal Medicine, Southwestern Medical School. Revised 1985.)

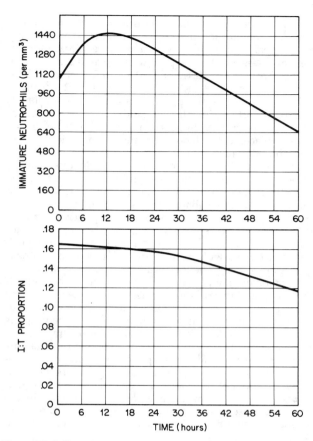

Figure 50-2. Normal total immature neutrophil counts and ratios of immature to total neutrophils (I:T) in neonates from birth to 60 hours of age. All bands and cell forms less mature than bands are classified together as immature neutrophils. (Adapted from Manroe BL, Rosenfeld CR, Weinberg AG, et al. The differential leukocyte count in the assessment and outcome of early onset group B streptoccocal disease. *J Pediatr.* 1977;91:632. Reprinted from House Staff Nursery Manual, Division of Neonatal-Perinatal Medicine, Southwestern Medical School. Revised 1985.)

TABLE 50-3. Factors Affecting Neonatal Neutrophil Values

Complication	ATN	ATI	ATI/ATN	Duration
Maternal hypertension	↓			72 h
Asphyxia	↑↓			24 h
Periventricular hemorrhage	↓			120 h
Hemolytic disease	↑	↑	↑	>28 d
Maternal fever	↑	↑	↑	24 h
Stressful labor	↑	↑	↑	24 h
Pneumothorax	↑	↑	↑	24 h
Surgery	↑	↑	↑	24 h
>6-hour oxytocin induction	↑	↑	↑	120 h

ATN, *absolute total neutrophil count;* ATI, *absolute total immature neutrophil count*

House Staff Nursery Manual *Division of Neonatal-Perinatal Medicine, Southwestern Medical School, Dallas, TX, revised 1985.*

symptoms are a manifestation of infection or that the asymptomatic infant is at high risk for developing infection within the first few hours of life. Because of the increased risk of infection and the subtlety of clinical manifestations of infection in premature infants, antimicrobial therapy should be initiated in the premature infant with only a single obstetric or clinical risk factor. In contrast, the asymptomatic term infant with only obstetric risk factors presents more of a dilemma. An approach to the early management of such infants is suggested in Figure 50–3. The goal of this scheme

the normal neutrophil values are presented in Table 50–3. The most useful indicator of bacterial infection is an I:T ratio of 0.16 or more. An I:T ratio of 0.8 or more indicates depletion of bone marrow reserves and a poor prognosis for survival. It is important to repeat the leukocyte count and I:T ratio determinations after 8 hours because studies in both animals and human infants demonstrate that the leukocyte count may be normal at the onset of group B streptococcal sepsis but becomes abnormal during the next 4 to 8 hours. No laboratory test result should ever negate a clinical impression of sepsis.

Chest roentgenogram should always be obtained as part of the diagnostic evaluation of the infant with suspected sepsis. Other radiographic studies may be indicated by the specific clinical condition. Sonography, computed tomography, and magnetic resonance imaging are the most useful imaging techniques in this age group. Technetium and gallium scans are rarely indicated in the neonate.

■ THERAPY

The decision to initiate antimicrobial therapy in the neonate is based on the likelihood that an infant's clinical

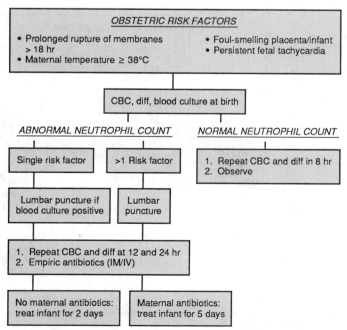

Figure 50-3. Recommended approach to diagnostic evaluation and treatment of the asymptomatic term (≥36 wk, 2200 g) infant with history of obstetric risk factors. *CBC*, complete blood count; *diff*, differential blood count; *IM*, intramuscularly; *IV*, intravenously. (Adapted from Engel WD, Sumner J, Lyttle B, Siegel JD. *Abstract Pediatr Res.* 1986;20:395A.)

is to identify and treat all infected infants but to avoid excessive investigation and treatment of uninfected infants. It must be emphasized that such an approach is applicable only to asymptomatic term infants whose mothers do not have chorioamnionitis or sepsis in the peripartum period. Omission of a lumbar puncture in asymptomatic infants with only a single risk factor is unlikely to jeopardize the diagnosis of meningitis because term infants with in utero meningitis are symptomatic. If, however, the blood culture is positive, the lumbar puncture should be performed to be certain that meningitis has not developed. Furthermore, development of symptoms is an indication for immediate completion of the sepsis workup with lumbar puncture and initiation of antimicrobial therapy.

The usual duration of treatment for most uncomplicated bacterial infections is 7 to 10 days. Longer courses of therapy are indicated for the treatment of meningitis and septic arthritis/osteomyelitis. The intravenous route of drug administration is preferred, but similar amounts of drug (area under the curve) may be delivered after intramuscular injections in infants with adequate muscle mass and stable cardiovascular function. Bacterial disease is documented by culture in approximately 10% of infants with suspected sepsis. Therefore, a 7- to 10-day course of antimicrobial therapy often is completed in infants whose bacterial cultures are negative at 48 hours when there is no other explanation for the infant's clinical condition and an apparent response to therapy has occurred.

Infants who are treated with vancomycin or aminoglycosides require initial determination of serum creatinine and peak and trough serum levels after 24 hours of therapy. Once a stable dosage schedule has been established and the infant has shown a good clinical response, trough levels only may be followed to monitor for toxicity. If renal function is changing, repeated peak and trough levels may be required. Optimal serum levels are as follows: vancomycin or amikacin, peak 20 to 30 μg/mL, trough less than 10 μg/mL; gentamicin or tobramycin, peak 6 to 8 μg/mL, trough less than 2 μg/mL.

Provision of general supportive care to the septic infant is of utmost importance in optimizing the outcome. The need for ventilatory support, volume expansion with fresh frozen plasma, replacement of blood or platelets, correction of electrolyte and other metabolic abnormalities, and early initiation of hyperalimentation must be determined. In recent years, attention has been directed toward enhancement of the neonate's deficient host responses. Exchange transfusion with fresh whole blood (less than 24 hours) may improve outcome by providing several different deficient components: granulocytes, specific antibody, complement, and fibronectin. Granulocyte transfusion has been beneficial for treatment of a small number of infants with bone marrow depletion of the neutrophil storage pool. The logistical problems associated with identification of infants with bone marrow depletion and collection of granulocytes from volunteers when needed makes this modality impractical for routine use. Furthermore, neutropenia resulting from increased margination of neutrophils by endotoxin is not improved by granulocyte transfusion. Administration of intravenous immunoglobulin preparations may improve neutrophil use and prevent bone marrow depletion as well as provide specific deficient antibodies and improved opsonophagocytosis. A beneficial effect has been demonstrated when immunoglobulin is given early in the course of disease in animal models. Very large doses, however, may cause a blockade of neutrophil receptors that are

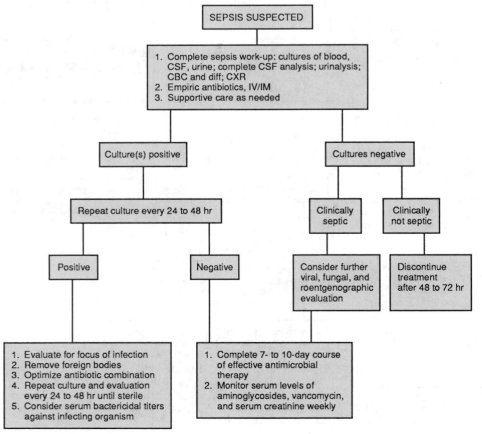

Figure 50-4. Recommended approach to the diagnostic evaluation and treatment of the neonate with suspected sepsis. *CBC*, complete blood count; *CSF*, cerebral spinal fluid; *CXR*, chest x-ray examination; *diff*, differential blood count; *IM*, intramuscularly; *IV*, intravenously.

necessary for opsonization and phagocytosis of group B streptococci. The optimal immunoglobulin preparation (IgM versus IgG or specific high-titer monoclonal antibody versus lower-titer broad-spectrum antibody) has not been determined. Further studies are required to demonstrate efficacy and safety before such immunologic enhancement measures become routine.

An approach to the evaluation and treatment of neonates with suspected sepsis is shown in Figure 50–4.

(Abridged from Jane D. Siegel, Bacterial and Viral Infections of the Newborn (Sepsis Neonatorum), in Oski, DeAngelis, Feigin, McMillan, Warshaw: *Principles and Practice of Pediatrics, Second Edition*, J.B. Lippincott, 1994.)

Oski's Essential Pediatrics, edited by Kevin B. Johnson and Frank A. Oski. Lippincott–Raven Publishers, Philadelphia © 1997

51
Neonatal Meningitis

■ EPIDEMIOLOGY

The incidence of neonatal bacterial meningitis is about 0.5 cases per 1000 live births. The rates vary according to nursery and predisposing maternal and infant risk factors. There is a preponderance of male infants with meningitis caused by gram-negative enteric bacilli, but the ratio of male-to-female cases is comparable to that for group B streptococcus. The incidence of meningitis in low-birth-weight infants is about three times that of infants with birth weight greater than 2500 g. The other risk factors associated with an increased incidence of neonatal septicemia and meningitis include premature or prolonged rupture of membranes, maternal fever or chorioamnionitis, and traumatic delivery.

Causes of Meningitis

   Common:
      Escherichia coli
      Group B streptococci
   Less Common:
      Listeria monocytogenes
      Group D streptococci
   Enterobacter spp
      Salmonella spp
      Citrobacter diversus
   Staphylococcus spp
      Candida spp
      Neisseria meningitidis
   Streptococcus pneumoniae
      Haemophilius influenzae type b

■ CLINICAL MANIFESTATIONS

The clinical manifestations of meningitis in the newborn infant are often nonspecific and indistinguishable from those of septicemia. Meningitis should always be considered when the diagnosis of septicemia is suspected. The cardinal signs of meningitis in older children, such as stiff neck, Kernig's and Brudzinski's signs, are absent in most infants.

The most frequent signs are temperature instability, respiratory distress, irritability, lethargy, and poor feeding or vomiting. Seizures occur in 40% of newborn infants. Other signs include a bulging fontanelle, hyperactivity or hypoactivity, alteration of the level of consciousness, tremor, twitching, apnea, stiff neck or opisthotonos, hemiparesis, and cranial nerve palsy. Some patients will present with a severe protracted state of shock. Group B streptococcal infection also may present as hydrocephalus without other signs of infection.

■ DIAGNOSIS

The diagnosis of meningitis is based on examination and culture of the cerebrospinal fluid (CSF). In most instances, a lumbar puncture should be performed at the time of the sepsis workup. In a critically ill child, however, the lumbar puncture can be postponed until the cardiorespiratory condition is stable. Although CSF cultures may be sterile in the infant who has received antibiotics before diagnosis, examination of CSF for cellular and biochemistry values and for antigen detection is almost always indicative of the diagnosis of meningitis. Causes of meningtitis are listed at the beginning of this chapter.

A Gram-stained smear of CSF should be made for all infants, because grossly clear fluid with only a few cells can contain many bacteria. Gram-stain or acridine orange smear of CSF reveals bacteria in at least 80% of infants with culture-proven meningitis. Because of the low concentrations of organisms (ie, 10^3 CFU/mL of CSF), most Gram-stain smears of CSF from infants with *L monocytogenes* meningitis do not reveal bacteria.

The CSF laboratory findings in the neonate differ from those in older children (Table 51–1); this difference may be a result of an increase in the permeability of the blood–brain barrier (ie, cerebral capillary endothelial cells). By 1 month of age, an infant's leukocyte count should be in the range of 0 to 5 cells/mL. An overlap exists in the different cellular and biochemical characteristics between the infants with and without meningitis. Fewer than 1% of infants with proven meningitis, however, have an initial CSF examination that is completely normal. It is important to determine simultaneously obtained blood and CSF glucose concentrations because low CSF glucose can reflect concurrent hypoglycemia, and a CSF-to-blood glucose ratio of less than 0.6 (60%) should be considered abnormal. The CSF leukocyte count is elevated in most newborns with meningitis, and polymorphonuclear leukocytes are preponderant except in some patients with listerial meningitis. The protein concentration may not be elevated at the time of diagnosis. Cerebrospinal fluid changes characteristic of bacterial meningitis associated with sterile cultures may occur in association with anaerobic infection, most commonly *Bacteroides fragilis, C diversus* brain abscesses, or subarachnoid hemorrhage.

Blood culture specimens should be obtained in every patient; 85% of neonates with bacterial meningitis have positive blood culture results at the time of presentation. Counterimmunoelectrophoresis or latex agglutination for group B streptococci and *E coli* K1 antigens in CSF and concentrated urine can be performed to facilitate a rapid diagnosis of infection. The sensitivity of these tests can be increased by evaluating specimens from more than one source with detection of the antigen in 65% to 95% of patients with culture-proven infection.

■ THERAPY

After CSF and blood cultures are obtained, antibiotic therapy should be initiated promptly with ampicillin plus

TABLE 51-1. Normal Values for Cerebrospinal Fluid (CSF) Examination in Neonates

	Term		Preterm*	
Leukocyte count/μL	7	(0–32)†	8	(0–29)
Percent of polymorphonuclear leukocytes	61%		57%	
Protein (mg/dL)	90	(20–170)	115	(65–150)
Glucose (mg/dL)	52	(34–119)	50	(24–63)
CSF: blood glucose ratio	51%	(44%–248%)	75	(55%–105%)

*Preterm less than 38 weeks' gestation.

†Mean (range)

Adapted from Sarff LD, Platt LH, McCracken CH Jr. Cerebrospinal fluid evaluation in neonates: comparison of high-risk infants with and without meningitis. J Pediatr. 1976;88:273.

cefotaxime or with a combination of ampicillin and an aminoglycoside such as gentamicin or amikacin in meningitis dosages. Therapy should be adjusted depending on results of cultures and of susceptibility testing. For group B streptococcal or *L monocytogenes* infection, 14 days of ampicillin therapy is adequate in the uncomplicated patient. The addition of an aminoglycoside to ampicillin has been suggested by some authors because of synergistic activity against group B streptococci and *Listeria* spp, especially if the strain demonstrates in vitro tolerance (*ie*, a 32-fold difference between the minimal inhibitory concentration and minimal bactericidal concentration). However, no clinical studies have proven superiority of one regimen over another.

Supportive care of the newborn is similar to that of the septic infant. Careful neurologic examination should be performed daily and the head circumference measured. Seizures should be controlled with intravenously administered phenobarbital or dilantin. The serum electrolytes should be followed for detection of hyponatremia as a result of inappropriate secretion of antidiuretic hormone; fluid restriction is instituted if this condition develops. Some newborns with group B streptococcal meningitis develop diabetes insipidus during the course of the illness. Serum concentrations of aminoglycosides in the newborn period are unpredictable, especially for the low-birth-weight premature infant, and should be routinely determined to achieve therapeutic concentrations and avoid toxicity. Every infant should have a brain-stem–evoked response audiogram at discharge or within 6 weeks after discharge from the hospital to detect hearing impairment as early as possible.

■ PROGNOSIS

Despite improvement in intensive care facilities and excellent in vitro activity of the third-generation cephalosporins, meningitis in the neonatal period is still a devastating disease. The case-fatality rate remains about 15% to 30%, depending on causative pathogen, predisposing risk factors, and availability of intensive care facilities.

A poor outcome is associated with presence of coma at admission, persistent seizures, low-birth-weight, ventriculitis, duration of positive CSF culture results, very low or very high CSF leukocyte count, protein concentration higher than 500 mg/dL, and presence of brain abscess. High concentrations of the K1 antigen of *E coli*, of interleukin 1-β, and of the polysaccharide of group B streptococci in the initial CSF specimen have been inversely correlated with clinical outcome and with severity of the disease.

For group B streptococcus, about 15% to 20% of survivors have major sequelae including spastic quadriplegia, profound mental retardation, hemiparesis, deafness, or blindness. Hydrocephalus develops in 11% of cases, and 13% have a seizure disorder. Survivors without major sequelae on physical examination, however, seem to function within normal limits and comparably with their siblings.

Sequelae are found in 35% to 50% of survivors of gram-negative meningitis. Ten percent have severe sequelae as defined by failure to develop beyond the age at which the disease occurred or required custodial care. About 25% to 35% have mild to moderate sequelae, which many times do not interfere with adequate, albeit delayed, development. Hydrocephalus develops in one third of patients. The prognosis of infants with brain abscesses is generally poor.

(Abridged from Marc H. Lebel, Meningitis, in Oski, DeAngelis, Feigin, McMillan, Warshaw: *Principles and Practice of Pediatrics, Second Edition*, J.B. Lippincott, 1994.)

Oski's Essential Pediatrics,
edited by Kevin B. Johnson and Frank A. Oski.
Lippincott–Raven Publishers,
Philadelphia © 1997

52

Escherichia coli

Escherichia coli inhabits the human gastrointestinal tract and accounts for the largest proportion of the facultative aerobic, gram-negative bacteria in fecal flora.

At least five different classes of diarrhea-associated *E coli* are recognized. Enteropathogenic *E coli* (EPEC) cause disease by adherence to the intestinal mucosa, and enterotoxigenic *E coli* (ETEC) adhere to the small bowel by a different mechanism and elaborate enterotoxins. Enteroinvasive *E coli* (EIEC) invade the mucosa of the colon. Enterohemorrhagic *E coli* (EHEC) cause grossly bloody diarrhea by adhering to the colonic mucosa and producing cytotoxins that are referred to as Shiga-like toxins. Enteroadherent or enteroaggregative *E coli* are a class of diarrhea- associated *E coli* that adhere to Hep-2 tissue culture cells but do not belong to EPEC serotypes.

These five classes of *E coli* are important causes of diarrhea in children around the world and are among the most common causes of endemic diarrheal disease of children in developing countries, where diarrheal illnesses are the leading cause of morbidity and mortality. Except for EHEC, these classes of *E coli* are less frequently associated with sporadic episodes and with outbreaks of diarrheal disease in the United States than in developing countries.

ENTEROPATHOGENIC *ESCHERICHIA COLI*

Infection with EPEC usually occurs in children younger than 2 years of age and results in acute or chronic diarrhea. In developing countries, EPEC strains are a common cause of endemic pediatric diarrheal disease, but in industrialized countries EPEC is a less frequent cause of diarrhea. In the United States, outbreaks have occurred in hospitals and day care centers, but community outbreaks and sporadic cases have been described.

■ CLINICAL MANIFESTATIONS

Children with EPEC infection often develop chronic, watery diarrhea. Most patients are younger than 2 years of age, with the majority being younger than 1 year. The diarrhea is often severe (*ie,* 10 to 20 stools a day) and lasts 10 days to 2 weeks if untreated. Dehydration is common and is the most important complication. Vomiting and fever occur in about 60% of these children. Fecal leukocytes and gross blood usually are not present in stool, but occult blood is sometimes found.

■ DIAGNOSIS AND TREATMENT

Diagnosis of infection due to EPEC is a problem for clinicians. EPEC infections are diagnosed based on isolation of *E coli* belonging to a serogroup considered to be an EPEC strain. Because these strains are biochemically the same as strains of *E coli* that are part of the normal flora, identification is established by serotyping the isolate.

Therapy involves management of dehydration by oral administration of a fluid and electrolyte solution and eradication of the organism. Agents effective for treatment of these infections include trimethoprim-sulfamethoxazole (TMP-SMX), to which EPEC may be resistant, systemically administered aminoglycosides, and the fluoroquinolones, which are approved for use only in adults.

ENTEROTOXIGENIC *ESCHERICHIA COLI*

ETEC cause disease in animals and humans, particularly in travelers and in infants and young children in tropical, developing countries.

■ CLINICAL MANIFESTATIONS

ETEC infection is characterized by secretory diarrhea. Stool specimens are watery and do not contain blood or fecal leukocytes. Fever is rare. As with most diarrheal diseases, dehydration is the major complication, especially in infants. The severity of ETEC disease varies widely. Mortality is almost always associated with dehydration, usually in smaller, malnourished infants.

■ DIAGNOSIS AND TREATMENT

The diagnosis of ETEC infection can only be accomplished by isolation of *E coli* from stool and demonstration that the isolate has the ability to produce enterotoxin or contains the genes encoding for enterotoxin production. If ETEC infection is suspected, *E coli* should be isolated and sent to a reference laboratory for evaluation.

Treatment of patients with ETEC infection consists of rehydration and eradicating the organism by administration of antimicrobial agents. ETEC-induced dehydration is usually managed with oral rehydration solutions. Studies of adult travelers and children have shown that antimicrobial agents such as TMP-SMX and fluoroquinolones in adults are effective in treating patients with ETEC diarrhea.

ENTEROINVASIVE *ESCHERICHIA COLI*

EIEC strains are a cause of diarrhea and dysentery in children in developing countries and have been implicated in foodborne outbreaks in industrialized countries. The *Shigella*-like EIEC cause disease indistinguishable from shigellosis.

■ CLINICAL MANIFESTATIONS

EIEC infection is similar to that seen with *Shigella*. Much of what is known about clinical disease is based on challenge experiments in adult volunteers and from outbreaks. Stool specimens are grossly bloody and contain mucus and fecal leukocytes. Fever is a common finding.

■ DIAGNOSIS AND TREATMENT

Definitive diagnosis of EIEC infection can be difficult. It is necessary to isolate *E coli* from stool and demonstrate that the strain has the ability to invade epithelial cells.

Little is known about the treatment of patients with EIEC disease, because the infection is usually not diagnosed. Because antimicrobial agents have shortened the course of illness and reduced the severity of shigellosis, it seems reasonable that similar antimicrobial therapy would be appropriate for diarrhea caused by EIEC.

ENTEROHEMORRHAGIC *ESCHERICHIA COLI*

In 1982, there were two large outbreaks of diarrhea associated with the consumption of hamburgers. The signs and symptoms of disease were unique and consisted of grossly bloody diarrhea with little or no fever. This clinical syndrome, called hemorrhagic colitis, was later associated with a rare *E coli* serotype, O157:H7. EHEC strains also are associated with hemolytic uremic syndrome and thrombotic thrombocytopenic purpura.

The prevalence of EHEC infection varies among regions. *E coli* O157:H7 is a common enteric pathogen in Canada and parts of the northern United States, but it appears to have a worldwide distribution. These *E coli* strains have caused food-borne outbreaks in schools, child day care centers, nursing homes, and communities. EHEC strains produce high concentrations of cytotoxins, referred to as Shiga-like toxins (SLT) or verotoxins, which inhibit protein synthesis and cause cell death.

■ CLINICAL MANIFESTATIONS

A spectrum of disease is caused by these organisms. The illness usually begins as a watery diarrhea, which may or may not develop into grossly bloody diarrhea. Fever affects 20% to 50% of patients, and severe abdominal pain is typical. Barium studies have shown a characteristic "thumbprint" pattern in the transverse colon of some patients. This is often a relatively severe illness, and many patients require hospitalization. After infection with O157:H7, children may develop hemolytic uremic syndrome. Adults can sometimes develop thrombotic thrombocytopenic purpura as a sequela of EHEC infection.

■ DIAGNOSIS AND TREATMENT

The recovery of *E coli* O157:H7 from stool specimens depends on the timing of collection and antibiotic status of the patient. Recovery of organisms is optimal early in the course of illness in patients who have not received antimicrobial agents. The clinical laboratory can screen for *E coli* O157:H7 by using MacConkey agar base with sorbitol substituted for lactose.

Little is known about the effect of antimicrobial therapy on clinical outcome or on the development of hemolytic uremic syndrome. Antimotility agents are thought to amplify morbidity and should not be used.

(Abridged from John J. Mathewson and Larry K. Pickering, *Escherichia coli,* in Oski, DeAngelis, Feigin, McMillan, Warshaw: *Principles and Practice of Pediatrics, Second Edition,* J.B. Lippincott, 1994.)

Oski's Essential Pediatrics, edited by Kevin B. Johnson and Frank A. Oski. Lippincott–Raven Publishers, Philadelphia © 1997

53

Haemophilus influenzae

Haemophilus influenzae is a fastidious, gram-negative, pleomorphic coccobacillus that is responsible for serious systemic and local infections in children.

■ MICROBIOLOGY

In the United States, approximately 20,000 cases of systemic *H influenzae* type b infection occurred yearly before the introduction of the *H influenzae* type b protein conjugate vaccines. Most cases were bacterial meningitis. The estimated annual age-specific attack rate of *H influenzae* type b infection was 100 cases per 100,000 children younger than 5 years of age.

Certain risk factors for systemic *H influenzae* type b infections have been identified. Black, Hispanic, and Native-American children have higher rates of infection than do white, non-Hispanic children. Children younger than 4 years of age who are household contacts of a patient with *H influenzae* type b disease, children with underlying immune deficiencies and anatomic or functional asplenia are more likely to develop systemic *H influenzae* infections. Other risk factors for invasive *H influenzae* type b infections are socioeconomic in nature, such as day care attendance, crowded households, frequent infections, and socioeconomic status.

Breast-feeding for infants between 2 and 5 months of age appears to be a relatively protective factor.

Unencapsulated *H influenzae* are common inhabitants of the upper respiratory tract under normal conditions in children and adults. *H influenzae* type b can be isolated from as many as 5% to 7% of young children at any time.

Invasive disease due to *H influenzae* type b frequently follows a viral upper respiratory infection, which may disrupt mucosal barriers and interrupt the normal activity of respiratory cilia.

For local infections caused by unencapsulated strains, a preceding viral upper respiratory infection frequently disrupts the normal physiologic clearance mechanisms and permits invasion of the sinuses or middle ear by normal respiratory flora (*eg, S pneumoniae,* nontypable *H influenzae, Moraxella catarrhalis*).

■ INFECTIONS CAUSED BY *HAEMOPHILUS INFLUENZAE* TYPE B

After *H influenzae* type b bacteremia develops, invasion of most sites in the body can occur, but certain sites of infection predominate. Table 53–1 lists diseases associated with common sites of infection.

■ INFECTIONS CAUSED BY NONTYPABLE *HAEMOPHILUS INFLUENZAE*

Upper Respiratory Tract Infections

Unencapsulated *H influenzae* is second only to *S pneumoniae* as a cause of acute otitis media and acute sinusitis in children. In older children and adults, nontypable *H influenzae* is associated with bronchitis. A syndrome of concomitant purulent conjunctivitis and otitis media due to nontypable *H influenzae* occurs in young children. Spread among family members is common.

Miscellaneous Infections

Bacteremia, meningitis, lung cyst, thyroglossal duct cyst infection, rectal abscess, septic arthritis, and cerebrospinal fluid (CSF) shunt infections may be caused by nontypable *H influenzae.* Systemic infections due to unencapsulated *H influenzae* occur predominantly in immunocompromised hosts. Invasive infections due to non-type b *H influenzae* should prompt an investigation for an underlying anatomic or immune defect.

TABLE 53-1. Common Sequelae From *H influenzae* type b Infection

Site	Comments
Meningitis pneumonia	Concomitant otitis media, meningitis, epiglottitis are common
Septic arthritis	Primarily large joints (knee, hip, ankle, elbow)
Cellulitis	Typically in children younger than 2 years of age, especially in the buccal soft tissues or periorbital region
Pericarditis	Children between 2 and 4 years of age, with antecedent URI
Epiglottis cervical adenitis	May also cause glossitis, uvulitis, tracheitis

■ DIAGNOSIS

Cultures of blood, CSF, and other body fluids and sites yield *H influenzae* type b in most children with invasive infections. Gram stain of appropriate specimens frequently demonstrates the characteristic pleomorphic coccobacilli of *H influenzae*. Polysaccharide antigen is detected readily by latex agglutination in a variety of body fluids, especially CSF, urine, and serum. Because antigen may be detected in urine for as long as 1 month after some *H influenzae* type b vaccines, it is not a reliable predictor of systemic infection in this instance.

■ TREATMENT

Approximately one third of *H influenzae* strains isolated from systemic infections are resistant to ampicillin, through production of the β-lactamase enzyme. Several classes of antibiotics have excellent activity against *H influenzae* isolates. Cefuroxime, cefotaxime, and ceftriaxone are parenteral cephalosporins with proven efficacy in the treatment of systemic *H influenzae* type b infections. Ampicillin- and chloramphenicol-resistant strains remain susceptible to these cephalosporins. Trimethoprim-sulfamethoxazole, cefaclor, cefixime, cefuroxime axetil, erythromycin-sulfisoxazole, and the combination of amoxicillin and clavulanic acid (a β-lactamase inhibitor) are oral agents useful for treating upper respiratory infections due to ampicillin-resistant *H influenzae* type b.

■ PREVENTION

The development of the *H influenzae* type b protein conjugate vaccines is one of the most important recent advances in preventive pediatrics. The American Academy of Pediatrics and the Centers for Disease Control recommend routine immunization with the HbOc or PRP-OMP vaccine beginning at 2 months of age. The vaccine administration schedules are different because of differences in the kinetics of antibody response to HbOc or PRP-OMP.

In areas where the *H influenzae* type b protein conjugate vaccines are administered routinely to infants, the incidence of systemic *H influenzae* type b disease is declining dramatically.

(Abridged from Sheldon L. Kaplan, *Haemophilus influenzae*, in Oski, DeAngelis, Feigin, McMillan, Warshaw: *Principles and Practice of Pediatrics, Second Edition*, J.B. Lippincott, 1994.)

Oski's Essential Pediatrics, edited by Kevin B. Johnson and Frank A. Oski. Lippincott–Raven Publishers, Philadelphia © 1997

54

Group B Streptococcal Disease

Until two decades ago, Lancefield group B streptococci were recognized infrequently as human pathogens. This organism was better known as a cause of epidemics of bovine mastitis. Sporadic reports of puerperal sepsis and occasional neonatal infection with group B streptococcus in humans surfaced during the 1930s and 1940s but remained largely academic until the early 1970s, when reviews documented a dramatic increase in the incidence of neonatal sepsis caused by group B streptococcus. Since then, it has emerged as the single most common bacterial pathogen responsible for neonatal sepsis and meningitis. The reasons for this shift in patterns of neonatal infection are unclear despite considerable advances in our understanding of bacteriologic and immunologic properties of the organism and the pathophysiology, treatment, and prevention of the infections it causes.

■ BACTERIOLOGY AND EPIDEMIOLOGY

Streptococcus agalactiae, or group B streptococcus, is a facultative, encapsulated, gram-positive diplococcus that produces a narrow zone of β-hemolysis on sheep blood agar surrounding flat, grayish white, mucoid colonies. Nonhemolytic and α-hemolytic strains have been isolated infrequently from humans but rarely cause systemic infection.

All strains of group B streptococcus share the group B-specific cell wall carbohydrate antigen originally defined by Lancefield. The strains may be classified into seven serotypes based on capsular polysaccharides (type-specific antigens) and a surface protein, c. The polysaccharide antigens are designated Ia, Ib, II, III, IV, and V. Strains possessing both the Ia polysaccharide antigen and c protein antigen are designated Ia/c. The c protein is found on all type Ib and some type II, III, IV, and V strains. Surface proteins identified as R and X antigens are found on some strains but do not seem to be associated with virulence. Nontypable strains are uncommon.

Group B streptococci may be recovered frequently from the lower genital tract of pregnant women, but their presence is rarely associated with symptoms before delivery. Recent studies indicate that the lower gastrointestinal tract may be the true reservoir for the microorganism and that genital colonization may represent contamination from this site. Reported carriage rates of group B streptococci in parturients vary from 4% to 40%. Variations are due not only to differences in age, socioeconomic status, and geographic location, but also to the site and number of culture specimens taken and to differences in bacteriologic method for growth and isolation. Some factors not influencing colonization rates include marital status, number and frequency of sexual partners, use of oral contraceptives, presence of vaginal discharge, and active gonococcal infection. Some controversy concerns the effect of ethnic background, but Hispanic women may have lower carriage rates than white and black women when other factors influencing colonization are controlled.

Transmission of group B streptococci to the neonate can occur whenever a delivering mother harbors the organism. Exposure may occur by ascending infection through ruptured or sometimes intact amniotic membranes or by surface contamination as the infant descends through the birth canal. Vertical transmission accounts for asymptomatic infection (or colonization) in 42% to 72% (mean, 58%) of infants born to mothers carrying group B streptococci at delivery. Mothers with "heavy" colonization documented by semiquantitative culture techniques are more likely to transmit the organism to their infants. Similarly, their infants are more likely to develop group B streptococcal disease. Of infants born to women whose culture results are negative at delivery, about 8% become colonized with group B streptococci. The rate of asymptomatic neonatal infection is increased by prolonged (more than 18 hours) rupture of membranes, maternal fever during the early (12 to 48 hours) postpartum period, and preterm delivery. Despite the high rate of transmission and colonization in newborns, overall only 1% to 2% of infants born to colonized mothers develop serious infection. Initial colonization may persist for weeks to months at various mucous membrane sites, but acquisition of the organism by neonates after hospital discharge is uncommon.

Clinically and epidemiologically, neonatal group B streptococcal infection can be divided into two distinct syndromes based on age of onset. Early-onset disease appears within the first 7 days of life and occurs in 1.3 to 3.7 of 1000 live births. Maternal factors increasing risk for early-onset disease are similar to those for neonatal colonization: prolonged rupture of membranes, preterm delivery, multiple births, intrapartum infection, and, perhaps, black race and age less than 20 years. Late-onset disease, that which occurs after 7 days of age, is documented in several studies to affect 0.6 to 1.7 of 1000 live births. The obstetric complications commonly accompanying early-onset disease are not factors associated with the later presentation of infant group B streptococcal infection. In both subsets of neonates, however, deficiency of maternally derived IgG antibody directed against group B streptococcal capsular polysaccharide increases the risk for invasive disease.

The distribution of serotypes has both epidemiologic and clinical significance. In surveys of large numbers of colonized adults, children, and neonates, the major serotypes are represented equally. Colonized neonates reflect the serotype of their mothers in all but the rare infant who acquires group B streptococci from nursery personnel or the community. Serotypes I (including Ia, Ib/c, and Ia/c), II, and III each account for approximately one third of the cases of early-onset disease not involving the central nervous system. Types IV and V account for only a few cases. Serotype III causes 80% to 90% of cases of group B streptococcal meningitis, regardless of age, and 90% of late-onset disease, irrespective of clinical presentation. In all, serotype III is responsible for two thirds of cases of group B streptococcal disease.

■ CLINICAL PRESENTATIONS

The frequency of neonatal group B streptococcal infection in the 1970s led to the recognition of two distinct clinical presentations based on age at onset of symptoms (Table 54–1). Early-onset infection usually appears at or within a few hours of birth. The highest attack rate is observed in preterm infants born to women with known obstetric factors posing risk for neonatal sepsis. Clinical syndromes include bacteremia without a focus, pneumonia, and meningitis. Pneumonia and meningitis typically are accompanied by bacteremia. It has been estimated that blood cultures are sterile, however, in about 10% of cases of these focal infections. Respiratory signs such as tachypnea, grunting, retractions, and cyanosis or an unexpected apneic episode in a previously well neonate, especially at term, are the first clues of illness in most infants, regardless of the primary focus of infection. Poor perfusion or "cold shock" is a presenting finding in about one fourth of cases and may be found at birth in infants with in utero onset of infection. Nonspecific symptoms such as lethargy, poor feeding, tachycardia, jaundice, and temperature instability most often occurs in the term infant without respiratory symptoms.

Forty to fifty percent of neonates with early-onset group B streptococcal infection have pulmonary involvement. One third of these infants demonstrate radiographic evidence of congenital pneumonia with distinct infiltrates, and about one half have findings typical of hyaline membrane disease. Among remaining infants, some have increased vascular markings compatible with the radiographic diagnosis of transient tachypnea of the newborn, a few exhibit small pleural effusions or pulmonary edema, and occasionally the initial chest radiograph is normal. Recent reports describe neonates with early-onset group B streptococcal sepsis manifested by respiratory distress, persistent fetal circulation (or persistent pulmonary hypertension), and a normal radiograph.

TABLE 54-1. Comparison of Early and Late Onset Group B Streptococcal Infection in Neonates

	Early Onset	Late Onset
Mean age at onset of symptoms	8 h	27 d
Incidence	1.3–3.7/1000 live births	0.6–1.7/1000 live births
Maternal obstetric risks for sepsis	Common	Uncommon
Common clinical presentations	Pneumonia (40%); meningitis (12%); bacteremia without focus (45%)	Bacteremia without focus (50%); meningitis (35%); osteomyelitis arthritis (5%)
Common serotypes	I (Ia, Ib/c, Ia/c) II III	III (85%)
Case-fatality rate	8%–16%	2%–10%

Group B streptococcal meningitis is clinically indistinguishable from bacteremia with or without pulmonary involvement. For this reason, lumbar puncture for cerebrospinal fluid (CSF) studies is always required for accurate diagnosis and appropriate therapy. Recent reports indicate that this focus of infection has decreased frequency from about 25% to 12% of cases. Although seizure activity may develop in half of neonates with group B streptococcal meningitis, it is rarely the presenting symptom. Prolonged seizure activity or coma is associated with poor outcome, as is the occurrence of shock, neutropenia, or a CSF protein level greater than 300 mg/dL.

Late-onset group B streptococcal infection is observed in infants from 8 days to 12 weeks of age and has diverse clinical manifestations. The mean age at onset is 24 days. The obstetric and early neonatal course is usually uneventful. Some infants exhibit only fever and mild irritability; others have a few hours of illness culminated by septic shock and death. As with early-onset infection, infants may present with bacteremia without a focus or may have localization to the central nervous system, skeletal system, soft tissues, or a variety of other foci.

When first described, the most frequent clinical manifestation of late-onset group B streptococcal infection was meningitis, which accounted for 85% of cases. Recently, however, bacteremia without a focus is an increasingly common presentation, perhaps reflecting earlier diagnosis and therapy as familiarity with this disease increases. Infants with late-onset group B streptococcal syndrome have comparatively fewer respiratory symptoms than their early-onset counterparts, but a preceding or concurrent upper respiratory infection is noted in 20% to 30%. Subdural effusions occur in almost one fourth of infants, but these are rarely symptomatic. More serious intracranial complications such as obstructive ventriculitis, subdural empyema, and brain abscess are rare.

Infants with nonmeningeal focal late-onset infections regularly have accompanying bacteremia. The exception is osteomyelitis. The somewhat older age at onset (mean, 31 days) and the finding of a lytic bone lesion at presentation suggest that this form of infection may be acquired during a self-limited early-onset group B streptococcal bacteremia. Group B streptococcal osteomyelitis follows an indolent course with few systemic symptoms. Decreased use of the involved extremity and pain with passive movement are typical findings. Infants often have a relatively long history before diagnosis (mean, 9 days). Unlike other pathogens causing neonatal osteomyelitis, group B streptococcus has a predilection for the proximal humerus; the femur is the second most common site involved. Rarely is more than a single bone involved. Up to 70% of infants have accompanying pyarthrosis of the adjacent joint. Group B streptococcal septic arthritis without osteomyelitis occurs exclusively in the lower extremities and usually involves the hip joint. Onset of illness is acute (mean duration of symptoms before diagnosis, 1.5 days), and concurrent bacteremia is usual. Functional impairment after antimicrobial and surgical therapy is uncommon.

A variety of foci of late-onset group B streptococcal infection have been reported, but these are uncommon when compared to bacteremia without a focus, meningitis, and bone and joint infection. Infants with facial or submandibular cellulitis due to group B streptococci have been described, as have other soft tissue infections including necrotizing fasciitis, omphalitis, and scalp and breast abscesses. Otitis media alone or in association with facial cellulitis or meningitis also occurs. Endocarditis, pericarditis, myocarditis, endophthalmitis, urinary tract infection, pleural empyema, pneumonia, and peritonitis are rare.

■ DIFFERENTIAL DIAGNOSIS

The clinical manifestations of early-onset group B streptococcal infection resemble those of neonatal sepsis due to other pathogens. In the preterm infant, the clinical and radiographic distinction between group B streptococcal pneumonia and hyaline membrane disease at onset of illness is impossible. Helpful features suggesting group B streptococcal pneumonia in this kind of patient are maternal risk factors for sepsis, apnea, and shock within the first 24 hours of life, an Apgar score of less than 5 at 1 minute, neutropenia, and cardiomegaly or pleural effusion by chest radiograph. None of these features, however, is specific for group B streptococci, and each may be observed with other etiologic agents causing early-onset neonatal pneumonia. Because clinical findings alone cannot identify the 10% to 15% of infants with meningeal involvement, each infant with suspected or proven group B streptococcal sepsis requires a lumbar puncture.

The differential diagnosis for late-onset group B streptococcal infection somewhat depends on the focus of infection. Infants who have bacteremia without a focus may present with nonspecific symptoms and fever, and they may be thought to have a viral illness. Only a high index of suspicion and collection of a blood culture specimen provide a specific diagnosis. In infants with meningitis, a presumptive diagnosis may be made if CSF is abnormal or the Gram-stained smear reveals gram-positive cocci in pairs or short chains. If the CSF Gram-stained smear is negative, other etiologic agents causing meningitis in early infancy must be considered including *Listeria monocytogenes*, *Escherichia coli*, and viral agents as well as agents affecting older infants (*Haemophilus influenzae* type b, *Streptococcus pneumoniae*, and *Neisseria meningitidis*). The relative lack of systemic symptoms in an infant with a metaphyseal lytic bone lesion, especially of the humerus, strongly suggests group B streptococcal osteomyelitis. Until group B streptococci are isolated from a bone aspirate or biopsy sample of the affected area, however, other etiologic agents such as *Staphylococcus aureus* and gram-negative enterics must be contemplated. The diversity of clinical presentations of late-onset group B streptococcal infection requires that it be appreciated as a possible etiologic agent in unknown infection at any site in infants 1 to 12 weeks of age.

■ COMPLICATIONS AND SEQUELAE

Complications of infant group B streptococcal infection range from negligible functional deficits in infants with septic arthritis to profound neurologic consequences of severe meningitis. The mortality rate for early-onset infection ranges from 8% to 16% and for late-onset disease from 2% to 6%. Factors associated with a fatal outcome in early-onset infection include prematurity, shock, neutropenia, apnea, a 5-minute Apgar score of less than 6, pleural effusion, and an initial blood *p*H of less than 7.25. Those factors related to death or permanent neurologic sequelae following meningitis are hypotension, a peripheral leukocyte count less than 4000/mm^3, coma, status epilepticus, and a CSF protein greater than 300 mg/dL. Three series report sequelae in survivors of group B streptococcal meningitis up to 8 years after illness. Major neurologic sequelae including global mental retardation, spastic quadriplegia, uncontrolled seizures, cortical blindness, deafness, hydrocephalus, and hypothalamic dysfunction occurred in 17% to 21%. Less severe sequelae such as spastic or flaccid paresis of one limb, speech and language delay, controlled seizure disorders, unilateral deafness, and mild cortical atrophy seen by computed tomography (CT) of the head were found in about 20%. The decreasing mortality rate found in many centers may result in a somewhat higher sequelae rate. Despite this significant mortality and morbidity, nearly 70% of the survivors of group B streptococcal meningitis function at or near their age-expected level.

One unusual complication of group B streptococcal sepsis is the unexplained association of early-onset infection with acquired right-sided diaphragmatic hernia. It has been hypothesized that insufficient diaphragmatic motion predisposes infected infants to the development of pneumonia and that subsequent respiratory effort leads to herniation.

Relapse or recurrence of infection of both the early- and late-onset type have been reported in a few infants. Inadequate dose or duration of antimicrobial therapy is one explanation for relapse. In a few cases, however, circumstances (maternal mastitis, undrained brain abscess, or congenital heart disease in an infant with endocarditis) may predispose infants to recurrence. In the majority, the reason for recurrence is inapparent. The opportunity for recurrent infection with optimal therapy exists in most patients, because intravenous antibiotics do not eliminate mucous membrane infection with group B streptococci nor do most infants develop protective immunity after recovery from sepsis or meningitis.

■ TREATMENT AND PREVENTION

Group B streptococcal isolates remain uniformly susceptible to penicillin G. They also are susceptible in vitro to first-, second-, and third-generation cephalosporins, semisynthetic penicillins, and vancomycin. Resistance of group B streptococci to the aminoglycosides, colistin, bacitracin, trimethoprim-sulfamethoxazole, and metronidazole is uniform.

Aggressive supportive measures are responsible for much of the increased survival in infants with invasive group B streptococcal infection. Improved ventilatory care has eased management of respiratory distress secondary to group B streptococcal pneumonia. Evidence of poor perfusion and metabolic acidosis can be treated with both volume expansion and infusion of pressor agents, and seizure activity can be controlled with anticonvulsants. Modern monitoring equipment makes anticipation of these consequences of group B streptococcal infection less problematic. Less conventional adjunctive therapies have been explored in many centers. Granulocyte transfusions in neutropenic infants, infusion of human intravenous immunoglobulin, and extracorporeal membrane oxygenation (ECMO) are among the therapeutic modalities being investigated. So far, none shows clear therapeutic advantages, and all are investigational.

Efforts to prevent neonatal group B streptococcal infection have aimed either to decrease frequency of group B streptococcal exposure of infants at birth or to alter the infant's immune status. Most widely investigated are attempts to eradicate maternal genital colonization. Courses of oral ampicillin or penicillin in colonized women (with or without concurrent treatment of sexual partners) during the third trimester of pregnancy have been ineffective in decreasing colonization at delivery. Further, this approach is impractical because to ensure "prophylaxis" for the infants at highest risk for sepsis, antibiotics would have to be initiated at the beginning of the third trimester and continued until delivery. Use of intravenous ampicillin during labor in women known to carry group B streptococci eliminates infant colonization without disturbing maternal genital flora. Because a large number of women are colonized with group B streptococci during pregnancy, the risk of anaphylactic reactions is significant compared to the number of infant cases that might be prevented. Treatment of high-risk

infants in the delivery room with intramuscular penicillin G has not been shown to be effective either, because so many of these infants are already bacteremic when prophylaxis is given. An analysis of maternal risk factors for infant group B streptococcal sepsis was performed at one urban hospital to determine which obstetric groups were most likely to benefit from intrapartum chemoprophylaxis. Seventy-four percent of neonates who developed early-onset infection had at least one of these risk factors: birth weight less than 2500 g, rupture of mother's membranes more than 18 hours before delivery, and maternal intrapartum fever. In this group, the attack rate for group B streptococcal sepsis was estimated at 45.5 per 1000 live births. Additional maternal risk factors identified by other investigators include multiple pregnancy, preterm (less than 37 weeks) labor, group B streptococcal bacteria, and perhaps black race and age less than 20 years.

The first study to document the efficacy of maternal intrapartum prophylaxis in preventing group B streptococcus-associated early-onset disease and maternal morbidity was reported in 1986. Women at 26 to 28 weeks gestation had lower vaginal and anorectal cultures for group B streptococcus. Group B streptococcus-positive women who had preterm labor or rupture of membranes more than 12 hours before delivery were randomized to receive routine care or intravenous ampicillin until delivery. Women with intrapartum fever also received ampicillin. Five of 79 infants born to untreated women but none of 85 born to ampicillin-treated women developed group B streptococcal sepsis (p = 0.02). A similar study from Madrid confirmed the efficacy of this approach. Others have restricted intrapartum maternal prophylaxis to group B streptococcus-colonized women who present with preterm labor. Excellent outcome for mother and infant were reported. Additional studies provide evidence that when selective prophylaxis is indicated, ampicillin should be administered at least 4 hours before delivery (if possible) to achieve sufficient concentrations in the placental circulation and the amniotic fluid to kill group B streptococcus. Screening for group B streptococcus during pregnancy by culture of lower vagina and anorectum appears to be an effective method to identify women who, if they develop risk factors associated with neonatal sepsis, could be given intrapartum prophylaxis. Although some controversy regards selection of high-risk women, previous delivery of a sibling with invasive group B streptococcus disease always warrants intrapartum maternal chemoprophylaxis in subsequent pregnancy. Management of newborns born to mothers receiving chemoprophylaxis should be based on the infant's clinical findings and gestational age; routine treatment is not always necessary in healthy-appearing, term neonates.

Immunoprophylaxis is the optimal "permanent" method for prophylaxis against early-onset disease, and it is the only proposed method for prevention of late-onset infection. Type-specific IgG serum antibody directed against the capsular polysaccharides of group B streptococcus in excess of 2 to 3 $\mu g/mL$ appears to correlate with protective immunity. Purified native group B streptococcal polysaccharides have been shown to be safe and variably immunogenic as vaccines in nonimmune adults. These antigens induce antibodies primarily of the IgG class that readily cross the placenta. Vaccine nonresponders do exist and their numbers vary by serotype. Thus, protein-polysaccharide conjugates may be better candidates for widespread use as vaccines. Clinical studies in progress must be followed by multicenter efficacy trials before immunoprophylaxis can be recommended.

(Abridged from Carol J. Baker, Group B Streptococcal Disease, in Oski, DeAngelis, Feigin, McMillan, Warshaw: *Principles and Practice of Pediatrics, Second Edition,* J.B. Lippincott, 1994.)

Oski's Essential Pediatrics,
edited by Kevin B. Johnson and Frank A. Oski.
Lippincott–Raven Publishers,
Philadelphia © 1997

55

Anaerobic Infections

Organisms of the genus *Clostridium* are characterized as anaerobic, gram-positive, spore-forming bacilli, although there are a few exceptions to each of these characteristics. Clostridial spores are found worldwide and are ubiquitous in soil, dust, street dirt, and human and animal feces.

CLOSTRIDIUM TETANI

■ ETIOLOGY AND EPIDEMIOLOGY

Tetanus is an ancient disease, the clinical course and prognosis of which have changed little over centuries. The disease is caused by the exotoxin tetanospasmin, a potent neurotoxin that is lethal to humans at a dose of less than 150 μg. Because the spores of *C tetani* are ubiquitous and are resistant to heat and disinfection, they can readily contaminate wounds. Most tetanus occurs in patients without a history of apparent wound contamination, although puncture wounds and grossly contaminated, ragged lacerations commonly are characterized as tetanus prone.

The incidence of tetanus varies widely throughout the world; recent figures in the United States reveal 50 to 100 cases reported annually, with an average incidence of 0.03 cases per 100,000 persons.

■ CLINICAL MANIFESTATIONS

Generalized Tetanus

The most common form of clinical tetanus, generalized disease may occur after relatively minor injuries and commonly follows wounds not characterized as tetanus prone. Although the onset may be insidious, the typical initial complaint of trismus is seen in 50% of cases. Common complaints include pain and difficulty with swallowing, unilateral or bilateral neck stiffness, and stiffness of other muscle groups. The finding of trismus is so characteristic of tetanus that this diagnosis must be strongly considered when a patient presents with this complaint.

With progression of the disease, additional muscle groups become involved; perhaps the most striking is paraspinal musculature involvement. Tonic spasm of these muscles may result in severe opisthotonos. Tetanic contractions progress over the course of several days; recruitment of additional muscle groups and significant worsening of symptoms are to be expected after the initial presentation.

The effect of tetanospasmin on the autonomic nervous system results in characteristic cardiovascular instability, manifest as labile hypertension, tachycardia, or tachyarrhythmias.

Neonatal Tetanus

Tetanus in the newborn is a generalized form of the disease that warrants special comment because of its importance worldwide and the potential for its occurrence in the United States. Infants delivered vaginally to mothers who have not been immunized are at significant risk for neonatal tetanus. Birth practices in developing countries, such as applying mud or feces to the umbilical stump, greatly increase risk and can be considered responsible for a large proportion of the many cases seen throughout the world in recent years. The mortality rate in these cases is high, with infants dying of complications such as pneumonia and pulmonary hemorrhage, central nervous system (CNS) hemorrhage, and laryngeal spasms.

The risk of neonatal tetanus in the United States should not be dismissed, particularly in unusually contaminated deliveries and if the maternal immunization status is uncertain. Passive immunization should be administered in these circumstances.

■ DIFFERENTIAL DIAGNOSIS

Tetanus is uncommon in developed nations, where immunization and hygiene practices have largely eliminated the disease. The classic presenting complaint of trismus and of muscle spasms, stiffness, and pain with dysphagia and cranial nerve weakness can be seen in other conditions, although the classic picture is sufficiently characteristic to support the diagnosis of tetanus. Other conditions that can mimic some manifestations of tetanus include viral encephalomyelitis, Bell's palsy, hypocalcemic tetany, and dystonic reactions to phenothiazines. These other conditions are relatively easily differentiated from tetanus by specific laboratory or radiographic evaluations or by the clinical course. The absence of altered consciousness in tetanus is an important point of differentiation from CNS infections.

It is difficult to confirm a specific diagnosis of tetanus by routine laboratory tests. Gram stains and anaerobic cultures of wounds reveal the characteristic gram-positive bacilli with terminal spores in as many as one third of tetanus patients. Although positive wound cultures may support the diagnosis in patients with clinical disease suggestive of tetanus, a positive culture from a contaminated wound in the absence of symptoms does not indicate that tetanus intoxication will develop.

■ MANAGEMENT AND PROGNOSIS

Without specific confirmatory laboratory tests, the clinician must institute appropriate treatment based on the clinical diagnosis. The goals of therapy are to eradicate and neutralize *C tetani* and its toxin and to provide appropriate supportive care, which is often a more complex task than the medical treatment.

Specific therapy should include intramuscular administration of tetanus immune globulin (TIG) to neutralize circulating toxin before it binds to neuronal cell membranes. Antitoxin given early in the disease may prevent spread of the toxin within the CNS.

Additional specific therapy should include antimicrobial therapy for *C tetani*, preferably penicillin G. The cephalosporins are not reliably active against *C tetani*.

Local wound care, including surgical debridement, is essential. Foreign bodies must be removed and wounds irrigated well and left open.

An important aspect of treatment is initiation of active immunization with tetanus toxoid. Patients must be immunized to prevent further disease, because the amount of toxin required to produce disease is far less than that needed to stimulate immunity.

CLOSTRIDIUM BOTULINUM

■ ETIOLOGY AND EPIDEMIOLOGY

Botulism represents acute neurologic disease caused by another potent clostridial toxin, elaborated by *Clostridium botulinum*. Botulinal toxin is the most potent poison known, causing death in mice that receive as little as 10 pg. Disease is caused in humans by less than 100 ng.

Botulinal toxin acts at the neuromuscular junction, where it inhibits the release of acetylcholine, producing a flaccid paralysis. There is no effect on the CNS or on mentation, although the earliest effect is seen on the cranial nerves. Progression of paralysis occurs in a characteristic descending fashion, ultimately affecting the entire peripheral nervous system. Respiratory failure is the major cause of death, as the paralytic effect of the toxin reaches the muscles of respiration.

Botulinum spores are common in soil, dust, lakes, and other environmental matter and can contaminate fruits, vegetables, meats, and fish. Honey has become recognized as a potential source of *C botulinum* spores and one form of botulism.

Ingestion of *C botulinum* spores may lead to generation of toxin in the intestine of susceptible hosts and to botulism. This mechanism is operative in infantile botulism, which has been linked to the addition of honey (a natural, unpasteurized product) to infant formula. This form of botulism, which represents two thirds of reported cases in the United States, first was recognized and still predominates in the western United States among families favoring "natural" food products, although it is now recognized throughout the country.

■ CLINICAL MANIFESTATIONS

The clinical manifestations of botulism are related in some measure to age, with considerably less specific symptoms in infants than in older patients. The typical patient with botulism presents 18 to 48 hours after ingestion of tainted food, with cranial nerve dysfunction manifested by diplopia, dysphagia, and difficulty speaking. Patients remain lucid, and are typically afebrile. Additional signs may include pupillary dilatation, vertigo, tinnitus, and dry mouth and mucous membranes. The descending progression of paralysis in botulism occurs at various rates. The major manifestation is respiratory embarrassment, which may appear gradually or suddenly. If progression is slow, repeated measurements of tidal volume and other pulmonary function tests may be useful to predict the need for ventilatory support.

Involvement of the gastrointestinal tract may begin with abdominal pain, bloating, cramps, diarrhea in approximately one third of patients; however, these complaints are quickly replaced by constipation or obstipation.

Botulism in infants may present suddenly with respiratory failure, and infant botulism has been implicated in some cases of apparent sudden infant death syndrome. More commonly, weakness and flaccidity are insidious, with slow progression from poor feeding and constipation to weakness,

hypotonia, and respiratory insufficiency. Most parents describe a weak cry and diminished movement. Ptosis, loss of gag reflex, and poor head control are common findings.

The typical duration of symptoms exceeds 1 month, and full recovery from weakness and fatigability may require as long as 1 year.

■ DIFFERENTIAL DIAGNOSIS

The clinical constellation of acute onset of symmetric descending flaccid paralysis, initially involving cranial nerves but sparing mentation and unassociated with fever, should be considered botulism, regardless of whether a history of tainted food can be obtained. The entities most frequently confused with botulism are Guillain-Barré syndrome, myasthenia gravis, cerebrovascular accidents, other paralytic food poisonings, and some drug toxicities. Infectious encephalomyelitis may be confused with botulism in older children. Infant botulism is easily mistaken for septicemia, hypoglycemia, encephalitis, Werdnig-Hoffmann disease, or congenital myopathies.

Electromyography may reveal suggestive changes in the form of diminished amplitude of muscle action potentials or brief, small, abundant motor-unit action potentials. Absence of these changes, however, does not rule out the diagnosis of botulism. Electrophysiologic studies may help in identifying other possible diagnoses, such as primary myopathy. Routine hematologic and biochemical testing does not produce diagnostically useful findings, although changes suggesting acute infection may direct the clinician's attention toward some other condition.

■ MANAGEMENT AND PROGNOSIS

Management of botulism is primarily supportive. Because the only available antitoxin is of equine origin and, therefore, carries a significant risk of serum sickness, every effort should be made to substantiate the diagnosis, including electromyogram (EMG), Gram stain, and culture of any infected wounds and an exhaustive history of food intake in the previous 7 to 10 days.

Treatment with penicillin G has been advocated to eradicate *C botulinum* from wounds and to treat enteric infection in infant botulism. Survivors ordinarily recover without neurologic or neuromuscular sequelae, although full recovery may require many months. Weakness and easy fatigability are prolonged.

■ PREVENTION

Boiling home-preserved foods for 10 minutes before consumption inactivates the toxin. Neither microwaves nor the temperatures commonly achieved in microwave ovens are adequate to kill *C botulinum* spores or inactivate the toxin. Home-preserved foods should be cooked in traditional equipment.

Prevention of infant botulism appears simple: eliminate honey and other uncooked or inadequately preserved foods from the diets of young infants. *C botulinum* spores have been recovered from corn syrup, although no cases have implicated this source. Breast-feeding apparently diminishes the severity of infant botulism, although cases have occurred in breast-fed infants receiving honey in supplemental feedings. Adhering to standard recommendations for infant feeding practices can eliminate this risk.

CLOSTRIDIUM DIFFICILE

Antibiotic-associated colitis is a potentially serious diarrheal illness that has been shown conclusively to be caused by toxigenic *C difficile*. Specific antitoxin neutralizes the toxic effect and prevents the disease.

C difficile produces two toxins, A and B, both of which cause disease. The prevalence of *C difficile* in the gastrointestinal flora seems to vary widely depending on patient age, underlying disease, and history of hospitalization or antibiotic usage. Carriage rate in asymptomatic neonates and infants may reach 50%, but the organism exists in fewer than 2% of older children and adults without diarrheal disease.

Symptomatic *C difficile* colitis is unusual in pediatric patients, although one investigator suggested that this organism is second only to *Salmonella* as a cause of bacterial diarrheal disease in the United States. Whatever host factors play a role in protecting newborns and infants probably influence the incidence of symptomatic infection throughout childhood.

■ CLINICAL MANIFESTATIONS

Some degree of watery diarrhea, infrequently with blood or mucus, develops in virtually all patients. The extent of other abdominal complaints or systemic symptoms varies from mild to severe. The disease may be fatal. Abdominal pain, cramps, and lower quadrant tenderness are common, as are fever and leukocytosis. Severe dehydration and vascular collapse are rare at any age and virtually unheard of in children, but they should be considered. The duration of symptoms in those with mild disease not requiring specific therapy generally ranges from 7 to 10 days after discontinuation of the instigating antibiotic. More prolonged symptoms or significant toxicity may indicate specific antimicrobial intervention. Additional complications may include toxic megacolon, intestinal perforation, and arthritis.

■ DIFFERENTIAL DIAGNOSIS

C difficile pseudomembranous enterocolitis must be differentiated from all the other infectious causes of diarrheal disease. A history of having received antibiotics in the 4 to 6 weeks before onset with the detection of *C difficile* toxin in fecal samples strongly supports the diagnosis of *C difficile* colitis. Sigmoidoscopic examination revealing characteristic pseudomembranous plaques confirms the diagnosis. In extremely ill patients, necrotizing enterocolitis and toxic megacolon should raise the question of Hirschsprung's disease, and the abdominal pain and tenderness of *C difficile* colitis may occasionally mimic peritonitis.

■ MANAGEMENT AND PROGNOSIS

Overall, the prognosis is excellent, with most patients recovering after discontinuation of the instigating antibiotic, with replacement of fluid and electrolytes as needed. In patients whose symptoms are more severe or prolonged, treatment with oral vancomycin is effective.

Retreatment with vancomycin is indicated for relapses. Metronidazole has been used with some success in adult patients, although there is not a sufficient pediatric experience on which to base recommendations. Cholestyramine, an ion-exchange resin, has been used in patients with a chronic low-grade disease or multiple relapses to suppress symptoms over several weeks while normal bowel flora are reestablished.

■ PREVENTION

C difficile colitis is an endogenous infection that is induced to produce symptoms by antibiotic therapy. There are few means by which to predict in whom it may occur, and no active or passive immunity has been shown to be protective. Epidemiologic studies of *C difficile* in hospitals have demonstrated that this organism is spread within health care institutions and that outbreaks can occur with relative ease. Because patients in hospitals may be at significant risk by virtue of prior antibiotic treatment and underlying disease, every effort should be made to prevent spread of *C difficile* within the hospital setting. Patients who are known to be excreting *C difficile* should be maintained in enteric isolation.

■ NONCLOSTRIDIAL ANAEROBIC INFECTIONS

When sought, anaerobes have been found to cause 5% to 10% of all clinically significant bacteremic episodes in infants and children. Other infections, such as peritonitis, abscesses, and a variety of soft-tissue infections, are also caused by anaerobes. Although anaerobic infections occur less frequently in children than in adults, they should be considered in high-risk situations or cases of unexplained clinical sepsis.

The common clinical syndromes in children that may be caused by nonclostridial anaerobic organisms are listed in Table 55–1.

(Abridged from Lisa M. Dunkle, Anaerobic Infections, in Oski, DeAngelis, Feigin, McMillan, Warshaw: *Principles and Practice of Pediatrics, Second Edition*, J.B. Lippincott, 1994.)

TABLE 55-1. Infections Commonly Associated With Anaerobic Bacteria

ASSOCIATED WITH ORGANISMS INDIGENOUS TO UPPER HALF OF BODY

Brain abscess

Sinusitis

Chronic otitis

Parapharyngeal abscess

Dental abscess and periodontitis

Ludwig's angina

Branchial cleft cyst infection

Human bite wound infection

Necrotizing pleuropulmonary infection

Septicemia secondary to any of the above

ASSOCIATED WITH ORGANISMS INDIGENOUS TO LOWER HALF OF BODY

Peritonitis and peritoneal abscess

Abdominal surgical wound infection

Ascending cholangitis

Cellulitis, particularly perirectal

Blood infection after gastrointestinal disease or immunocompromise

Oski's Essential Pediatrics,
edited by Kevin B. Johnson and Frank A. Oski.
Lippincott–Raven Publishers,
Philadelphia © 1997

56

Campylobacter and Helicobacter

CAMPYLOBACTER

Campylobacter has been shown to be one of the leading causes of bacterial enteritis in the world. The incidence of diarrhea due to *Campylobacter jejuni* in the United States parallels that of *Salmonella* and surpasses that of *Shigella*. Type B gastritis has been associated with chronic infection with *Helicobacter pylori*.

■ EPIDEMIOLOGY

Animals serve as the reservoir for *C jejuni* and *C coli*, which have been isolated from the gastrointestinal tracts of cattle, sheep, pigs, and numerous commercially raised fowl. Contamination of meat during slaughter may be the way bacteria enter the human food chain. The main source of *C jejuni* and *C coli* infection in humans is poultry, although pet dogs, cats, and hamsters are potential sources. Transmission occurs by the fecal–oral route through contaminated food and water or by direct contact with fecal material from infected animals or people.

In the United States, *C jejuni* is thought to be the cause of 5% to 8% of all episodes of infectious enteritis, twice the rate of isolation of *Salmonella* and five times greater than that of *Shigella*. The annual incidence of *Campylobacter* diarrhea has been estimated to be 1 in 1000 in the general population, similar to figures found in the United Kingdom. *C jejuni* has a bimodal age distribution, with peaks in children younger than 5 years of age and in people 15 to 29 years of age.

■ PATHOGENESIS

After ingestion, *C jejuni* are rapidly killed by hydrochloric acid, indicating that gastric acid is an effective barrier against infection. If the organisms survive the gastric milieu, they must attach to the intestinal mucosa for the infection to persist. From there, the organisms are capable of causing illness by three postulated mechanisms. The first involves cell attachment and production of an enterotoxin, similar to cholera toxin, with subsequent secretory diarrhea. Second, like *Shigella*, the bacteria can penetrate and proliferate within the intestinal epithelium, causing cell damage and death, which can be manifested as bloody diarrhea. In the third mechanism referred to as translocation, the bacteria may penetrate the epithelial lining without cellular damage and proliferate in the lamina propria and mesenteric lymph nodes, reaching the bloodstream to cause extraintestinal infection such as mesenteric adenitis, arthritis, meningitis, and cholecystitis.

■ CLINICAL MANIFESTATIONS

Acute diarrhea is the most common clinical presentation, and more than 90% of the cases are caused by *C jejuni*. After an incubation period of 1 to 7 days, patients typically experience prodromal symptoms of fever, headache, and myalgia. Diarrhea, accompanied by nausea, vomiting, and abdominal cramps, usually occurs within 24 hours, with stools that vary from loose and watery to grossly bloody.

Abdominal pain affects more than 90% of patients older than 2 years of age, and it can be severe enough to mimic appendicitis. Acute colitis with bloody stools, tenesmus, and low-grade fever has been reported. When this symptom complex occurs in an adolescent, the illness can easily be confused with ulcerative colitis, and it is important to exclude *C jejuni* if a diagnosis of inflammatory bowel disease is suspected. Immunoreactive complications such as Guillain-Barré and Miller-Fisher syndromes, reactive arthritis, Reiter's syndrome, and erythema nodosum have been described.

■ DIAGNOSIS

Clinical diagnosis of *Campylobacter* diarrhea is difficult because of the variation in the clinical presentation, from watery to grossly bloody diarrhea. However, when it occurs as inflammatory diarrhea, with bloody stools, fever, and abdominal pain, *Campylobacter* should always be considered first in the differential diagnosis. A microbiologic diagnosis is needed to differentiate this from other causes of colitis, such as *Salmonella, Shigella, Escherichia coli* 157:H7, or *E histolytica*. Direct examination of stool with Wright stain often shows the presence of fecal leukocytes. A Gram stain of stool may show spiral and curved organisms, which may lead to a tentative diagnosis.

TABLE 56-1. Treatment of *Campylobacter* and *Helicobacter* Infections

Species	Antibiotic Therapy	
	Children	Adults
C fetus	Aminoglycoside or chloramphenicol	Aminoglycoside or chloramphenicol or cefotaxime
C jejuni/C coli	None or erythromycin, 40 mg/kg/d in 4 divided doses for 5 d	None or erythromycin, 250 mg 4 times each day for 5 d or ciprofloxacin
H pylori	Bismuth subsalicylate plus amoxicillin plus metronidazole	Bismuth subsalicylate plus amoxicillin plus metronidazole

■ TREATMENT

Rehydration and correction of electrolyte abnormalities are the mainstay of treatment for patients with *C jejuni* enteritis. There is debate over the use of antimicrobial agents in uncomplicated infections. When antibiotic therapy is indicated, erythromycin has been the recommended agent because most *Campylobacter* strains are susceptible. Several placebo-controlled studies have shown erythromycin therapy to be of no clinical benefit if given late in the course of disease, although it does decrease fecal shedding of the organism. Excretion of the organism can persist for 2 weeks to 3 months in immunocompetent hosts not treated with antibiotics. If antibiotic therapy is initiated early in the illness, reduced excretion of the organism and rapid resolution of symptoms occur (Table 56–1).

HELICOBACTER

H pylori has been implicated as a cause of type B gastritis and an important contributing factor in the pathogenesis of peptic ulcer disease and gastric carcinoma.

■ EPIDEMIOLOGY

H pylori has been isolated from patients with gastrointestinal tract symptoms and asymptomatic persons from different parts of the world. It is a ubiquitous pathogen, with prevalence rates that differ among populations and ethnic groups. Seroepidemiologic studies in different countries have shown an age-related increase in the prevalence of antibodies to *H pylori*.

Transmission of *H pylori* to humans is not well understood. The importance of crowding has been suggested by several studies, which have consistently shown that the chance of *H pylori* infection is greater in crowded conditions. Several studies have demonstrated a clustering of *H pylori* infection in families, with a significantly higher proportion of infected household members when a child is found to be colonized with this organism, suggesting that there may be person-to-person spread of the infection. *H pylori* also may be transmitted by animals, as suggested by the higher prevalence of infection among slaughterhouse workers.

■ CLINICAL MANIFESTATIONS

Three clinical entities have been associated with *H pylori* infection: acute active gastritis; chronic gastritis, duodenitis and peptic ulcer, and asymptomatic gastritis.

Acute Active Gastritis

After infection, symptoms may initiate with epigastric pain, nausea, and vomiting that may last for a few days. Patients may improve rapidly and remain asymptomatic. The *p*H of gastric juice is usually neutral or alkaline as a result of a decrease in gastric acid output. This hypochloridia may persist for several weeks and may present with halitosis and mild gastrointestinal tract disturbances.

Chronic Gastritis, Duodenitis, and Duodenal Ulcer

The triad of antral gastritis, duodenitis, and duodenal or gastric ulcer seen by endoscopy is associated with chronic and more severe gastrointestinal tract symptoms. Children may present with severe chronic and recurrent abdominal pain, anorexia, and failure to thrive or with persistent vomiting. Occasionally, hematemesis may be the first symptom.

If *H pylori* infection is associated with chronic gastritis alone, the only symptom may be recurrent abdominal pain or symptoms associated with nonulcerative dyspeptic (NUD) syndrome or, occasionally, chronic diarrhea associated with NUD. Frequent endoscopic findings are nodular antritis and pyloric hyperemia, although it is not unusual to observe normal gastric mucosa with histologic findings of active gastritis.

Asymptomatic Gastritis

The frequency of asymptomatic gastritis is unknown, but, according to seroepidemiologic studies in which a high prevalence of antibodies has been found in the general population, it does not seem to be a rare event, particularly in older children and adults. There are no explanations for the absence of symptoms, although factors related to the pathogen and to the host have been postulated.

■ DIAGNOSIS

For isolation of *Helicobacter* species from clinical specimens, at least two homogenized biopsies from the gastric antrum should be placed in a selective and enriched medium at 37°C under microaerobic conditions for 2 to 5 days.

■ TREATMENT

Treatment is indicated only in symptomatic children in whom *H pylori* infection has been confirmed by culture or serology.

The required high concentrations of antibiotics in the gastric mucosa can be achieved with metronidazole, the new fluoroquinolones (which are not US Food and Drug Administration approved for people younger than 18 years old), newer macrolides with long half-lives, and bismuth salts (*eg*, colloidal bismuth subcytrate, bismuth subsalicylate). Antibiotics should be acid resistant, such as those just described and amoxicillin.

Treatment should be given for long periods. The highest eradication rates occur after 4 weeks of treatment, although high rates of side effects are expected and treatment compliance limits long-term regimens. Monotherapy with bismuth salts or amoxicillin is ineffective. The combination of several antimicrobial agents has proved more efficacious than the use of single-drug regimens. Triple therapy for 2 weeks is recommended.

(Abridged from G.M. Ruiz-Palacios, Robert W. Frenck, Jr., and Larry K. Pickering, *Campylobacter* and *Heliobacter*, in Oski, DeAngelis, Feigin, McMillan, Warshaw: *Principles and Practice of Pediatrics, Second Edition*, J.B. Lippincott, 1994.)

Oski's Essential Pediatrics,
edited by Kevin B. Johnson and Frank A. Oski.
Lippincott–Raven Publishers,
Philadelphia © 1997

57

Diphtheria

Diphtheria is an acute infectious disease caused by the bacteria *Corynebacterium diphtheriae*, a gram-positive, nonmotile, nonsporulating, pleomorphic bacillus. Symptoms follow production and elaboration of a toxin that is an extracellular protein metabolite of toxigenic strains of *C diphtheriae.*

■ EPIDEMIOLOGY

Diphtheria is encountered in every country of the world. In countries where infants and children are immunized routinely, diphtheria occurs relatively more frequently in adults.

Diphtheria is acquired by contact with a person with the disease or by contact with a carrier. The bacteria can be transmitted by droplets during conversation with an infected or colonized person or when an infected person coughs or sneezes. Infection of the skin with *C diphtheriae* may predispose to respiratory tract colonization and infection. Dust and fomites also serve as vehicles of transmission.

■ PATHOGENESIS AND PATHOLOGY

C diphtheriae can enter the nose or mouth, where they may remain localized on the mucosal surfaces of the upper respiratory tract. The skin, ocular, or genital mucous membranes can serve as sites of localization. After an incubation period of 2 to 4 days, lysogenized strains may elaborate toxin.

Toxin is adsorbed initially to the cell membrane, and it then penetrates the membrane and interferes with protein synthesis. Protein synthesis ceases because the toxin produces an enzymatic cleavage of nicotinamide adenine dinucleotide, with the subsequent formation of an inactive transferase, adenosine diphosphoribose.

Necrosis of tissue is most notable in the area of colonization. The local inflammatory response, coupled with the necrosis, causes a patchy exudate that can be removed in the early stages of disease. As toxin production increases, the area of infection becomes deeper, and a fibrinous exudate develops. A black or gray adherent membrane is formed that contains inflammatory cells, erythrocytes, and epithelial cells. The membrane sloughs spontaneously during the recovery period. Edema of soft tissues in the area beneath the membrane and in surrounding areas may be extensive. Secondary bacterial infections develop, usually due to group A β-hemolytic streptococci. The membrane and edematous tissue may impinge on the airway, causing suffocation.

Toxin produced at the site of infection can spread hematogenously or enter the lymphatic system. Toxin reaches the bloodstream readily from the pharynx and tonsils when they are covered by diphtheritic membrane. *C diphtheriae* may also contaminate wounds, producing a gray ulcer with a membranous base that has sharply defined edges.

Diphtheria toxin can damage any organ, but lesions of the heart, kidneys, and nervous system have been described most frequently. Diphtheria antitoxin is capable of neutralizing circulating toxin or toxin that is adsorbed to cells but is ineffective after cell penetration has occurred. Myocarditis may be observed 10 to 14 days after the onset of illness. Nervous system manifestations of disease generally do not appear until 3 to 7 weeks after the onset of disease.

The most striking pathologic findings are toxic hyaline degeneration of various organs and tissues, with associated necrosis. Cardiac findings include mononuclear cell infiltration and fatty accumulation in muscle fibers in the conducting system and generalized edema and mononuclear cell infiltration. If the patient survives, cardiac muscle regeneration and interstitial fibrosis are seen. Fatty degeneration of myelin sheaths, toxic neuritis, liver necrosis, acute tubular necrosis of the kidney, and adrenal hemorrhage have also been reported.

■ CLINICAL MANIFESTATIONS

The symptoms and signs of diphtheria depend on the immunization status of the host, the site of infection, and whether toxin has disseminated by the bloodstream to other organs and tissues.

The incubation period varies from 1 to 6 days. Diphtheria is classified clinically by the anatomical location of the initial infection and of the diphtheritic membrane (*eg,* pharyngeal, laryngeal, nasal, tonsillar, conjunctival, skin, genital). Several anatomical sites may be involved concomitantly.

■ DIAGNOSIS

The diagnosis of diphtheria is based on clinical findings. Definitive diagnosis depends on the isolation of *C diphtheriae* on appropriate media. Direct smears of diphtheritic lesions are generally unreliable, and identification by fluorescent antibody technique is reliable only in the hands of experienced personnel.

Leukocyte counts may be normal or elevated. Anemia may occur on rare occasions as a result of rapid hemolysis. Examination of cerebrospinal fluid may reveal a minimal elevation of protein or a mild pleocytosis in patients who have diphtheritic neuritis. Hepatic toxicity resulting from the diphtheria toxin may be reflected by hypoglycemia. An elevated blood urea nitrogen suggests the possibility of acute tubular necrosis. Electrocardiographic studies may reveal ST and T wave changes or dysrhythmias suggestive of myocarditis.

■ TREATMENT

Treatment of diphtheria is based on neutralization of free toxin and eradication of the organism by the use of antibiotics. The only specific antitoxin is of equine origin. Antitoxin should be administered on the basis of the size and site of the membrane, the degree of toxicity, and the duration of illness.

Antitoxin should be given intravenously as quickly as possible and in sufficient doses to neutralize all free toxin. A single dose is usually given to avoid risking sensitization from repeated doses of horse serum.

Penicillin and erythromycin are effective against most strains of *C diphtheriae.* Clindamycin, amoxicillin, and rifampin in appropriate dosages may also be effective. The carrier state has been treated effectively with oral benzathine penicillin G or erythromycin.

Bed rest is important and is recommended for a period of 2 to 3 weeks. An electrocardiogram (ECG) should be obtained two to three times each week for the first 6 weeks to detect myocarditis as quickly as possible.

A high-calorie liquid or soft diet should be provided and adequate hydration maintained. Secretions must be suctioned. Laryngeal diphtheria that progresses to obstruction may require release by tracheostomy.

Immunization always is indicated after recovery of the patient with diphtheria. Almost 50% of the patients with diphtheria fail to develop adequate immunity after recovery from their infection and remain susceptible unless immunized.

■ COMPLICATIONS

Despite the use of antibiotics, complications remain the greatest cause of morbidity and mortality associated with diphtheria. Complications include respiratory obstruction, myocarditis, paralysis of the soft palate, ocular paralysis, diaphragmatic paralysis, hypotension, and cardiac failure.

■ PROGNOSIS

The prognosis depends on the virulence of the organism, the immunization status of the host, the location and extent of the diphtheritic membrane, and the rapidity with which treatment is initiated. Diphtheria caused by the gravis strains carries a poor prognosis. The more extensive the diphtheritic membrane, the more severe is the disease. Although there are few laboratory parameters that indicate the severity of diphtheria, megakaryocytic thrombocytopenia and leukocytosis greater than $25,000/mm^3$ have been associated with a poorer outcome.

If specific treatment is provided on the first day of disease, mortality is less than 1%. Delaying treatment until day 4 is associated with a 20-fold increase in mortality.

■ PREVENTION

Prevention is accomplished by active immunization. The immunizing agent for children younger than 6 years is diphtheria toxoid, given in combination with tetanus toxoid and pertussis antigen (DTP). Primary immunization should be carried out by giving DTP vaccine at 2, 4, and 6 months of age, with booster doses at 18 months and again at 4 to 6 years.

(Abridged from Ralph D. Feigin, Diphtheria, in Oski, DeAngelis, Feigin, McMillan, Warshaw: *Principles and Practice of Pediatrics, Second Edition*, J.B. Lippincott, 1994.)

Oski's Essential Pediatrics,
edited by Kevin B. Johnson and Frank A. Oski.
Lippincott–Raven Publishers,
Philadelphia © 1997

58

Cat-Scratch Disease

Cat-scratch disease is a subacute, regional lymphadenitis syndrome that occurs following cutaneous inoculation. Contact with cats, in the form of a scratch by claws or teeth, is associated strongly with the illness, although cases without known cat contact have been reported. Two newly described bacterial organisms, *Bartonella henselae* and *Afipia*

felis, have been incriminated as causes. Complications of the disease occur, but it generally has an indolent chronic course for 2 to 3 months, followed by spontaneous resolution.

■ ETIOLOGY

Bartonella henselae was first identified in 1990 in adult acquired immunodeficiency syndrome (AIDS) patients with two unique opportunistic infections, bacillary angiomatosis and bacillary peliosis hepatitis. Children with cat-scratch disease frequently develop specific antibodies against this organism, which has been cultured from affected lymph nodes and also from the blood of epidemiologically related cats. In addition, *B henselae*-specific DNA sequences have been amplified from cat-scratch skin test antigen.

■ EPIDEMIOLOGY

Cat-scratch disease is transmitted by cutaneous inoculation. In the great majority of cases, a history of a cat scratch, often by a kitten less than 6 months old, can be elicited. Play may be more frequent with kittens than with older cats, and they are less likely to have been declawed. Interestingly, bacillary angiomatosis in adult patients with AIDS is frequently associated with a history of cat scratch.

Cat-scratch disease is more common in children than in adults, with the peak in case numbers falling between the ages of 5 and 14 years. Clustering of cases within families has been noted frequently, generally in association with the acquisition of new pets. Veterinarians as an occupational group appear to have a greater likelihood of exposure to the disease. An increased prevalence of skin test reactivity among veterinarians and asymptomatic relatives within family case clusters indicates that some infections may be subclinical.

■ CLINICAL MANIFESTATIONS

After an incubation period ranging from 3 to 30 days (usually between 7 and 12 days), one or more red papules measuring 2 to 5 mm in diameter develop at the site of cutaneous inoculation, often within the line of a previous cat scratch. Although they often are overlooked, a careful search uncovered such primary lesions in more than 90% of affected patients in one series. They persist until the development of lymphadenopathy, which generally occurs in 1 to 4 weeks.

Chronic lymphadenitis is the hallmark of cat-scratch disease, most frequently affecting the first or second sets of nodes draining the site of inoculation. Intervening lymphangitis does not occur. The sites affected most frequently, in decreasing order, are the axillary, cervical, submandibular, preauricular, epitrochlear, femoral, and inguinal lymph node groups. Involvement of more than one lymph node group, either within the same regional drainage or at an unrelated site, is present in 10% to 20% of cases. At a given site, about one half of all cases will involve a single node and the other half will involve multiple nodes.

Affected nodes usually are tender, and the overlying skin becomes warm, red, and indurated. Between 10% and 40% of the nodes eventually suppurate, occasionally with formation of a sinus tract to the skin surface. The duration of lymph node enlargement is 4 to 6 weeks, with persistence of up to 12 months in exceptional cases. Nodes that have drained to the skin surface frequently produce some residual scarring. The majority of patients lack constitutional symptoms. Elevated temperatures are documented in about 30%

of patients and, when present, are generally in the range of 38°C to 39°C (100.4°F to 102.2°F). Other nonspecific symptoms may include malaise, anorexia, fatigue, and headache.

A distinctive manifestation of cat-scratch disease is Parinaud's oculoglandular syndrome. The site of primary inoculation is the conjunctiva of one eye or the eyelid. Mild to moderate conjunctivitis accompanies the primary lesion. Preauricular lymph nodes are the corresponding regional site of adenopathy. The involved preauricular nodes may be within the substance of the parotid gland, but exocrine tissue typically is not involved. Although the oculoglandular syndrome may be induced by other agents, notably *Francisella tularensis,* the most common cause appears to be cat-scratch disease.

The most serious complication of cat-scratch disease is involvement of the central nervous system in the form of encephalopathy or encephalitis. High fever and convulsions develop within 6 weeks of the onset of lymphadenopathy, followed by alteration in the level of consciousness, headache, and muscle weakness. The cerebrospinal fluid is normal or shows minimal pleocytosis or elevated protein content. Electroencephalograms reveal diffuse slowing or focal abnormalities in most patients. Recovery has occurred without residua in nearly all the well-documented cases in the literature. A few patients had a prolonged convalescence and required anticonvulsant therapy for persistent seizure foci. The incidence of encephalopathy is low, but it can be the presenting manifestation of cat-scratch disease.

Osteolytic bone lesions have been noted in several well-documented cases. In one affected patient, biopsy of the lesion in the ilium revealed a granulomatous reaction typical of cat-scratch disease. In all the reported cases, the involved bone site was anatomically remote from the site of primary inoculation, suggesting hematogenous spread.

Granulomatous hepatitis is another newly recognized systemic manifestation of cat-scratch disease, and it may present as fever of unknown origin with or without lymphadenopathy. The reported cases have shown characteristic multiple hypodense lesions in the liver on computed tomography scanning.

Other rare complications that have been ascribed to cat-scratch disease include erythema multiforme, thrombocytopenic purpura, mesenteric lymphadenitis, pneumonia, arthralgia, neuroretinitis, iritis, urethritis, lymphedema, thyroiditis, and nontraumatic atlanto-axial dislocation (Grisel syndrome).

■ DIAGNOSIS AND DIFFERENTIAL DIAGNOSIS

A number of criteria for the diagnosis of cat-scratch disease have been proposed. In a typical patient with lymphadenopathy that has been present for 3 or more weeks, three of the following four criteria confirm a diagnosis of cat-scratch disease:

1. A history of animal contact about 2 weeks before the onset

2. Negative culture, skin test, and serologic test for other causes of lymphadenopathy

3. A positive skin test with cat-scratch antigen

4. Lymph node or other biopsy material revealing histopathologic features consistent with cat-scratch

disease, especially if pleomorphic bacilli are demonstrable by Warthin-Starry silver impregnation staining.

Serologic testing for *Bartonella henselae* may be helpful and is available from the Viral and Rickettsial Zoonoses Branch, Centers for Disease Control and Prevention.

The differential diagnosis of cat-scratch disease can include virtually all known causes of lymphadenopathy. As a general rule, the diagnosis is favored by chronicity, unilateral occurrence, tenderness, and characteristic sites of involvement, such as axillary, epitrochlear, and preauricular nodes. Cervical, femoral, inguinal, and generalized lymph node involvement is less specific for cat-scratch disease and necessitates more care in differential diagnosis.

The most common diagnoses in 85 patients with adenopathy and negative cat-scratch skin tests in one series were pyogenic lymphadenitis or abscess (29 patients), benign or malignant neoplasm (12 patients), and cervical adenitis caused by mycobacteria (10 patients). Malignant neoplasm can be ruled out definitively only by biopsy. Other conditions, such as tularemia, toxoplasmosis, plague, and Kawasaki disease, must be considered because of the need for specific therapy.

■ TREATMENT AND PROGNOSIS

Controlled studies have not shown any specific antimicrobial agents to affect the course of cat-scratch disease. Uncontrolled experience, however, suggests that rifampin, ciprofloxacin, gentamicin, and trimethoprim-sulfamethoxazole may have some efficacy. The treatment of affected patients is primarily expectant. Suppurative nodes are treated best by needle aspiration, which should be repeated if necessary. Aspirated pus should be cultured, with an emphasis on the recovery of pyogenic organisms and mycobacteria. Surgical excision of affected nodes generally is unnecessary, but is indicated when there is uncertainty about the diagnosis or an atypical or prolonged course. Incision and drainage should not be done because this leads to prolonged drainage and scar formation. Most patients with cat-scratch disease have a benign course. Systemic symptoms usually last less than 2 weeks. Affected nodes may be painful for several weeks and remain enlarged for a number of months. Patients with such complications as encephalopathy, thrombocytopenic purpura, or bone lesions generally have a more prolonged course, but also have a good long-term prognosis. Reinfection appears to be rare.

■ PREVENTION

The only preventive approach to cat-scratch disease might be to avoid cats, particularly aggressive play with young kittens. There seems to be no indication for destroying a family pet to which cases of cat-scratch disease have been attributed, because the capacity for disease transmission appears to be transient. Declawing such a pet might be considered, however.

(Abridged from Kenneth M. Boyer, Cat-Scratch Disease, in Oski, DeAngelis, Feigin, McMillan, Warshaw: *Principles and Practice of Pediatrics, Second Edition,* J.B. Lippincott, 1994.)

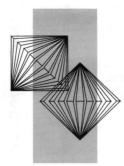

SECTION 3

Viral Infections

Oski's Essential Pediatrics,
edited by Kevin B. Johnson and Frank A. Oski.
Lippincott–Raven Publishers,
Philadelphia © 1997

59

Congenital and Perinatal Infections

CYTOMEGALOVIRUS

Cytomegalovirus (CMV) has worldwide distribution and is the most common cause of congenital infections. CMV occurs in 0.4% to 2.4% of all live births. Acquisition of CMV is nearly always asymptomatic in the immunocompetent host. Seroprevalence studies indicate that an inverse relationship exists between socioeconomic status and development of infection. CMV seropositivity in women of childbearing age varies in the United States from 45% in higher socioeconomic groups to 70% in crowded areas with substandard living conditions; this figure increases to nearly 100% in developing countries. Two likely sources of primary CMV infection for pregnant women are infected sexual partners and young children in day care centers. High rates of infection have been observed among young children in Israeli kibbutzim and in day care centers in Sweden and the United States, where the rate of viruria may be as high as 70% among children aged 2 to 3 years. Serologic studies demonstrate a 30% seroconversion rate among parents whose children shed CMV as compared with no seroconversions among parents whose children do not excrete the virus.

■ TRANSMISSION

Perinatal transmission of CMV can occur in utero, at delivery, or after delivery. In utero infection occurs transplacentally during maternal viremia. Primary CMV infection acquired during pregnancy is associated with a 30% to 40% risk of congenital infection with more severe fetal effects when maternal infection occurs in the first half of pregnancy. However, symptomatic disease is present in only 10% to 15% of these infants. CMV can also be transmitted to the fetus after reactivation of latent infection in the mother. About 1% to 3% of infants born to women who are seropositive before becoming pregnant are infected in utero, but they do not have clinically apparent disease at birth. Trans-

mission of CMV to the newborn infant also occurs at the time of delivery from contact with infected cervical secretions. In the postpartum period, maternal–infant transmission of CMV occurs during breast-feeding because 20% to 40% of seropositive women shed CMV into their breast milk. Asymptomatic infection occurs in 60% of infants fed infected breast milk. Breast-feeding is, therefore, an effective means of providing passive–active immunization of the young infant.

An important iatrogenic source of CMV infection is transfusion of blood from a seropositive donor to a seronegative infant. The incidence is 10% to 30% and usually occurs in infants who weigh less than 1300 g. The risk of infection is related to the volume of transfused blood, the number of donors, and elevated complement fixation titers to CMV in donor blood. Horizontal transmission of CMV in a neonatal intensive care unit has been documented, but is rare.

■ CLINICAL MANIFESTATIONS

Cytomegalic inclusion disease (CID) is the most serious but least common manifestation of congenital CMV infection. This syndrome is characterized by multiorgan involvement with the reticuloendothelial and central nervous systems most frequently affected. Typical clinical features of CID include intrauterine growth retardation, hepatosplenomegaly, jaundice, petechiae or purpura, microcephaly, chorioretinitis, and cerebral calcifications (Table 59–1). These features may also occur singly or in combinations.

Hepatomegaly with direct hyperbilirubinemia and mild elevation of serum transaminase levels are the most common abnormalities noted in the newborn period. Giant cell transformation with associated extramedullary hematopoiesis or large inclusion-bearing hepatocytes characteristic of CMV infection are present on pathologic examination of the liver. Hepatitis usually resolves in the first year of life, and development of cirrhosis is rare. Splenomegaly is common and may be the only abnormality present at birth.

Thrombocytopenia with petechiae is usually transient but may persist through the first year of life. "Blueberry muffin spots" are discrete, well-circumscribed lesions often mistaken for purpura; they represent dermal erythropoiesis in the more severely affected infants (Color Figure 10).

Central nervous system (CNS) infection with CMV can result in encephalitis with seizures and an elevated protein content in the cerebrospinal fluid (CSF). Cerebral calcifications occur in less than 10% of infected infants and date the maternal infection to the first trimester of pregnancy. The calcifications usually occur in the periventricular areas (Figure 59–1) and are best visualized by ultrasonography. Arrested brain growth results in microcephaly, and obstruction of the fourth ventricle may result in hydrocephalus.

TABLE 59-1. Frequency of Clinical Findings in Infants With Congenital Infections

Clinical Findings	Congenital Infection				
	Rubella	Toxoplasma	CMV	Syphilis	HSV
Intrauterine growth retardation	[+++]	±	++	++	+
Reticuloendothelial system					
Jaundice	+	++	[+++]	+++	−
Hepatitis	±	+	+++	+++	+
Hepatosplenomegaly	+++	++	[+++]	[+++]	+
Anemia	+	+++	++	+++	−
Thrombocytopenia	++	±	[+++]	++	−
Disseminated intravascular coagulation	−	−	±	−	−
Adenopathy	++	++	−	++	−
Dermal erythropoiesis	+	−	+	−	−
Skin rash	−	+	−	[++]	[+++]
Bone abnormalities	++	−	±	[++]	−
Eye					
Cataracts	[++]	±	−	−	−
Retinopathy	++	+++	[+]	±	[+++]
Microphthalmia	+	±	−	−	+
Central nervous system					
Microcephaly	+	±	++	−	+++
Meningoencephalitis	++	+++	+++	++	[+++]
Brain calcification	±	[++]	[++]	−	+
Hydrocephalus	−	[++]	±	±	++
Hearing defect	++	+	[++]	+	−
Pneumonitis	++	+	+	+	−
Cardiovascular					
Myocarditis	+	−	±	±	−
Congenital defect	[+++]	−	−	−	−

±, rare; +, 5% to 20%; ++, 20% to 50%; +++, more than 50%, □, prominent feature of particular infection; CMV, cytomegalovirus; HSV, herpes simplex virus.

Ocular defects include chorioretinitis (Color Figure 11), strabismus, optic atrophy, microphthalmia, and cataracts.

The most common manifestation of congenital CMV infection is sensorineural hearing loss resulting from direct viral invasion of the inner ear. It occurs in 15% of infants with symptomatic congenital infection and in about 5% of those with otherwise asymptomatic infection at birth. The hearing loss may be unilateral and unsuspected until the second year of life. All infants with congenital CMV require evaluation of hearing with brain stem auditory-evoked responses.

A diffuse interstitial pneumonitis occurs in less than 1% of newborns with CID. Bone abnormalities in CMV infection consist of longitudinal radiolucent streaks in the metaphysis of long bones ("celery stalk" appearance), particularly the distal femur and proximal tibia (Figure 59–2). Generalized osteopenia with irregular metaphyseal fragmentation has also been described. Defective enamelization of the deciduous teeth occurs in 40% of symptomatic newborns and in 5% of infants with asymptomatic infection at birth.

Attempts have been made to implicate CMV in cardiovascular, genitourinary, gastrointestinal, musculoskeletal anomalies, and particularly inguinal hernias in males, but the teratogenicity of CMV remains in doubt.

Of infants with asymptomatic congenital CMV infection, more than 90% have no apparent sequelae and only rarely manifest severe neurologic impairment. In contrast, severe intellectual and sensory deficits are consistently observed in infants and children with chorioretinitis, microcephaly, and intracranial calcifications. Symptomatic infants without CNS abnormalities at birth are at less risk for development of neurologic and developmental abnormalities.

Cytomegalovirus infection acquired at delivery is manifested by an afebrile pneumonia in 50% of exposed infants or, rarely, hepatitis or encephalitis after an incubation period of 4 to 12 weeks (mean, 8 weeks). In premature infants, CMV pneumonitis is associated with development of chronic lung disease. Late neurologic sequelae are not associated with perinatally acquired infection.

Transfusion-acquired CMV infection in low-birth-weight infants may be severe and is characterized by a gray ashen pallor, respiratory distress, pneumonia, hepatosplenomegaly, hepatitis, atypical lymphocytosis, thrombocytopenia, and hemolytic anemia; it has a 10% mortality rate.

■ DIAGNOSIS

All infants with congenital CMV infection have high titers of virus in their urine and pharynx at birth. Viruria and pharyngeal shedding appear after an incubation period of 4 to

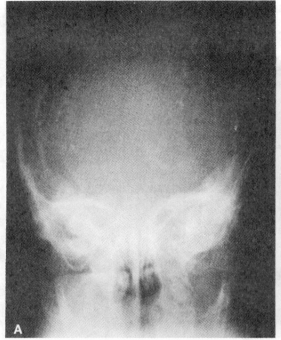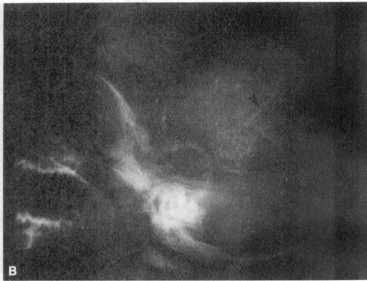

Figure 59-1. Anteroposterior (**A**) and lateral (**B**) skull roentgenograms demonstrating cerebral calcifications (*arrows*) lining the ventricles in a neonate with congenital cytomegalovirus infection. (Courtesy of Guido Currarino, MD, Dallas, Texas.)

12 weeks in infants infected with CMV perinatally. Viral excretion in the urine may persist for years, but the titer decreases markedly after 3 months. Pharyngeal shedding is not as prolonged. The diagnosis of congenital and perinatal CMV infection is best confirmed by isolation of the virus from the urine (Table 59–2). Recently, culture of saliva was as sensitive as urine for detection of congenital CMV infection. Characteristic cytopathologic developments occur within 2 weeks of inoculation of the specimen onto a human fibroblast monolayer. CMV may be identified in tissue culture after 24 to 48 hours of incubation by the shell-vial technique, which uses a monoclonal antibody to detect early CMV antigen. To diagnose congenital CMV infection accurately, cultures should be obtained within the first 2 weeks of life. After 3 weeks, viral shedding can occur from either congenital or postnatally acquired infection. CMV has been detected in the urine by electron microscopic study using the pseudoreplica method, which permits detection of herpesvirus particles within 15 to 30 minutes. This technique detects virus in 95% of specimens with high infectivity titers (greater than or equal to 10^4/mL); sensitivity is decreased when specimens are stored at 4°C.

Serologic studies have a limited role in the diagnosis of congenital CMV infection. The presence of CMV-specific IgG antibody denotes passively transferred maternal antibodies. On serial determinations, antibody titers to CMV in most congenitally infected infants show either a rapid or gradual decline to low levels between 4 months and 2 years of age. A minimum of infected infants demonstrate persistence of the high initial titer. An increase in titer has not been demonstrated in these infants despite continued shedding of the virus. False-negative antibody levels determined by the complement fixation method have been seen in infected infants. Although the CMV-IgM immunofluorescent test detects 76% of congenitally infected infants, a false-positive rate of 21% is documented. Enzyme-linked immunosorbent assays (ELISAs) that are commercially available for measurement of CMV-IgG and CMV-IgM have improved sensitivity and specificity. To interpret test results, the accuracy of the specific kit used must be known.

No effective antiviral agents are available for treatment of congenital CMV infection. There is an ongoing clinical trial with ganciclovir for treatment of congenital CMV infection; preliminary results have noted an exacerbation of chorioretinitis in some infants treated with ganciclovir.

■ PREVENTION

Handwashing after exposure to urine or saliva from young infants is the most effective means of preventing primary CMV infection in pregnant women. Transfusion-acquired CMV infection is eliminated by administration of CMV antibody-negative blood products to infants less that 1500 g in birth weight. Frozen deglycerolized red blood cells are a suitable alternative because they lack viable leukocytes. CMV vaccine ultimately may be the best preventive strategy, but vaccine development remains investigational.

HERPES SIMPLEX VIRUS

The estimated rate of occurrence of neonatal herpes simplex virus (HSV) infection in the United States is about 1 per 5000 to 7500 deliveries per year. Most neonatal infections are due to HSV-2 with some 25% to 30% due to HSV-1. More than 50% of infants who develop HSV infection are born to women who are asymptomatic for genital infection with HSV at the time of delivery and have neither a history of genital herpes nor a sexual partner with genital HSV infection. The frequency of asymptomatic shedding of HSV at the time of delivery varies from 0.2% to 1%.

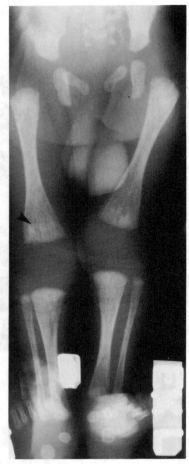

Figure 59-2. "Celery stalk" appearance of the femur (*arrow*) and tibia associated with congenital rubella, cytomegalovirus, and syphilis. Alternating bands of longitudinal translucency and relative density represent a disturbance of normal bone metabolism. (Courtesy of Guido Currarino, MD, Dallas, Texas.)

TABLE 59-2. Methods of Diagnosis of Congenital and Perinatal Infection

	Isolation of Organism	Antigen Detection	Measurement of Antibody
Cytomegalovirus	++	–	+
Herpes simplex virus	++	+	+
Varicella-zoster	±	–	++
Epstein-Barr virus	±	–	++
Rubella	±	–	++
Toxoplasmosis	±	–	++
Syphilis	±*	±	++
Human immunodeficiency virus	±	+	++
Hepatitis			
A	±	–	++
B	–	++	++
Delta	–	++	++
C	–	–	++
Neisseria gonorrhoeae	++	–	–
Chlamydia trachomatis	±	++†	++‡
Mycoplasmas	++	–	±

+, alternative method but usually less helpful; ++, preferred method; ±, possible, but may not be performed routinely by clinical laboratories; –, not available.

*Spirochetes visualized by darkfield examination of suspected lesions.

†Preferred for conjunctivitis.

‡Preferred for pneumonia.

■ TRANSMISSION

Acquisition of HSV by the infant can occur in utero, during delivery, or after birth. In utero infection with HSV accounts for about 10% of cases. Transmission occurs either transplacentally during a maternal viremia or by an ascending route from an infected maternal genital tract. The virus may pass through microscopic tears in the amniotic membranes to produce infection in infants delivered by cesarean section with intact membranes. HSV has been isolated from the blood of a pregnant woman with primary HSV infection, as well as from amniotic fluid, placenta, cord blood, and fetal tissue obtained at the time of spontaneous abortion. In utero acquisition of HSV is also suggested by reports of congenital malformations in infants born to women with genital herpes infection during pregnancy.

Transmission of HSV to the newborn infant usually occurs at delivery. Risk of neonatal infection is higher with primary maternal HSV infection than with recurrent infection (50% versus 4%) because of the infant's prolonged exposure to large quantities of virus in the absence of protective neutralizing antibody (Table 59–3). Prematurity, duration of rupture of amniotic membranes greater than 4 hours, and use of a scalp electrode for fetal heart rate monitoring also increase risk of HSV infection. Infants are at risk for developing disease after exposure to HSV infection in the first month of life.

Postpartum transmission of HSV to the newborn infant may occur after contact with a maternal breast lesion during breast-feeding, after endotracheal suctioning for meconium aspiration by a physician with herpes labialis, and from contact with other family members with active herpes labialis lesions. Nosocomial transmission of HSV in newborn nurseries has been documented by restriction endonuclease analysis of viral isolates, but it is rare.

TABLE 59-3. Maternal Genital Herpes Infection and Risk of Perinatal Transmission

	Genital Herpes Simplex Virus Infection	
	Primary	*Recurrent*
Risk of perinatal transmission	50%	3% to 5%
Site of viral shedding	Cervix	Labia
Duration of viral shedding	3 wk	2–5 d
Quantity of virus shed	Large	Small
Neutralizing antibody	Absent	Present

■ CLINICAL MANIFESTATIONS

Clinical manifestations of intrauterine HSV infection are present at birth or within the first 24 hours of delivery. Skin vesicles with scars are common. Seizures, microcephaly, hydranencephaly, porencephaly, intracranial calcifications, microphthalmia, hepatomegaly with or without splenomegaly, and abnormalities on bone roentgenograms may be seen. The adrenal gland is frequently involved, and chorioretinitis either is present at birth or develops in the first week of life.

Neonatal HSV infection acquired at birth is categorized by extent of disease: disseminated disease with or without evidence of CNS, skin, eye, and mouth involvement; CNS disease (encephalitis) with or without skin, eye, and mouth involvement; and localized infection of the skin, eye, and mouth without visceral organ or CNS involvement (see Table 58–2).

Disseminated disease accounts for 20% to 50% of neonatal HSV infection. There has been a recent decline in the incidence of disseminated disease. This decrease is probably a result of prompt diagnosis and treatment of localized infection before dissemination occurs. The average onset of illness is between 9 and 11 days of life and the principal organs involved are the liver and adrenal glands. About 50% of infants manifest CNS involvement and 90% manifest skin, mouth, or eye lesions. The presenting signs and symptoms are nonspecific and include fever, lethargy, irritability, anorexia, vomiting, respiratory distress, apnea, jaundice, seizures, and, in the most severe cases, shock with disseminated intravascular coagulation. Elevated transaminase levels and direct hyperbilirubinemia with or without hepatomegaly are common. Splenomegaly is often present. Pneumonitis, pleural effusion, and roentgenographic lesions in long bones occur rarely. Without therapy, case-fatality rate exceeds 80%; pneumonitis and disseminated intravascular coagulopathy are associated with an increased risk of death among infants with disseminated infection. Most survivors develop psychomotor retardation and ocular defects.

CNS disease accounts for about 30% of neonatal HSV infections. Clinical manifestations typically occur at 11 to 17 days of life and include lethargy, irritability, bulging fontanelle, focal or generalized seizures, opisthotonos, decerebrate posturing, and coma. Examination of the CSF reveals an elevated leukocyte count with a predominance of lymphocytes and an elevated protein content. Red blood cells are occasionally present, indicating hemorrhagic brain involvement. A normal cell count and protein concentration, however, may be found on the initial lumbar puncture. Mortality in untreated infants with localized CNS disease is 40% to 50%. Most survivors have neurologic sequelae consisting of seizures, spastic quadriplegia, chorioretinitis, microcephaly, hydrocephaly, porencephalic cyst, and psychomotor retardation.

Localized diseases of skin, eye, and mouth occur in 20% to 40% of infants with HSV infection. The hallmark of neonatal HSV infection is the discrete vesicular lesions that occur in 90% of infants with localized infection (see Color Figures 6 and 7). The vesicles usually appear first on the presenting part of the body that was in direct contact with the virus during delivery. About 70% of untreated infants who present with skin vesicles develop disseminated infection or have progression of disease to involve the eyes or CNS. Although infants with skin lesions suffer recurrences during the first 6 months of life, recurrences after 1 month of age are generally not associated with further clinical progression of disease. Ulcerative lesions of the mouth, tongue, or palate occur less commonly. Ocular involvement with HSV is manifested by keratoconjunctivitis, uveitis, chorioretinitis, cataracts, and retinal dysplasia. Sequelae of ocular HSV infection include corneal ulceration, microphthalmia, optic atrophy, and blindness. Some 10% of infants with localized infection of the skin, eyes, or oral cavity have subclinical involvement of the CNS as manifested by the development of severe neurologic impairment. Three or more skin recurrences in the first 6 months of life are associated with an increased risk of abnormal development.

■ DIAGNOSIS

The preferred diagnostic method is isolation of HSV from skin vesicles, buffy coat, brain tissue, CSF, stool, urine, throat, nares, or conjunctivae (see Table 58–1). HSV can also be isolated from duodenal aspirate in infants with hepatitis. Typing of HSV is not routinely performed, although recent evidence suggests that neurologic outcome may be better with neonatal encephalitis due to HSV-1 as compared with that due to HSV-2. When mucocutaneous lesions are present, scraping from the base of a vesicle may reveal intranuclear inclusions and multinucleated giant cells by Tzanck test or Wright's stain in 60% to 70% of cases; specific HSV antigen may be detected by immunofluorescence in 70% to 80% of cases.

Traditionally, diagnosis of HSV encephalitis in the absence of mucocutaneous lesions is confirmed by biopsy test of brain tissue because HSV is isolated from the CSF in only 30% to 50% of cases. Recent experience demonstrates usefulness of the electroencephalogram, technetium brain scan, computed tomography (CT), and magnetic resonance imaging (MRI) for identification of infants with HSV encephalitis. The characteristic electroencephalographic abnormality is a periodic slow and sharp wave discharge; more commonly, multiple independent foci of periodic activity are present. Technetium brain scan may demonstrate increased perfusion to the involved brain area. CT scan may be normal early in the course of the disease with characteristic abnormalities appearing 3 to 5 days later. The most frequently observed findings in the acute phase are patchy areas of low attenuation in both cerebral hemispheres, or hemorrhage or calcification in the thalamus, insular cortex, periventricular white matter, and along the corticomedullary junction. Late findings include multicystic encephalomalacia and ventriculomegaly as a result of brain atrophy and destruction. MRI is more sensitive in detecting early abnormalities in the periventricular white matter and in defining the extent of parenchymal lesions. Positive findings in any neurodiagnostic study provides enough evidence to initiate antiviral therapy. Recently, HSV DNA in CSF of patients with HSV encephalitis has been detected by polymerase chain reaction; this technique holds promise for identification of infected infants.

Serology is not helpful acutely because antibody may not yet be present with primary maternal infection, and, when present, antibody to HSV in neonates may be maternal. Increase in antibody titers in the convalescent phase indicates neonatal infection. Routine serologic methods do not distinguish reliably between antibodies to HSV-1 and HSV-2.

■ TREATMENT

Two antiviral agents, acyclovir and vidarabine, have decreased the mortality rate and improved the outcome of neonatal HSV infection. Antiviral therapy is initiated when the characteristic clinical features are present or when the neonate with overwhelming sepsis and negative bacterial cultures does not respond to broad-spectrum antibiotics. HSV may be recovered from brain biopsy specimens even after 24 to 48 hours of antiviral therapy. Acyclovir (10 mg/kg body wt every 8 h) or vidarabine (15 to 30 mg/kg body wt over 12 h) is administered intravenously for 10 to 14 days. A 21-day course may be required for treatment of encephalitis; there is increasing recognition of early relapse after shorter duration of therapy. Moreover, acyclovir at doses as high as 60 mg/kg/d may be more effective for treatment of encephalitis. Although there is no difference in mortality rates in infants who receive either the 15 or 30 mg/kg body wt/day dosage of vidarabine, a significantly lower percentage of infants who receive the higher dosage have progression of disease while on therapy. Ocular HSV infection requires topical antiviral medication with either 1% trifluridine or 3% vidarabine in addition to parenteral therapy. Treatment with acyclovir may prevent development of neutralizing antibody with relapse of disease after therapy is stopped. Acyclovir is the preferred drug, however, because of the insolubility of vidarabine and the large fluid volume required for vidarabine infusion. The mortality rate with disseminated disease has been reduced from 75% in untreated infants to 57% in infants treated with either acyclovir or vidarabine; 40% of these infants are normal at 1 year of age. Among infants with CNS disease, mortality is about 15%, and 35% are normal on follow-up examination at 1 year of age. No deaths have occurred among treated infants with localized infection of the skin, eye, or oral cavity, and 90% of infants are normal at 1 year follow-up examination. About 2% of infants treated with antiviral therapy for 10 to 14 days have recurrence of infection leading to CNS disease. Relapse of HSV encephalitis also has been reported after a 10-day course of vidarabine or acyclovir therapy.

A beneficial effect of human immunoglobulin that contains a large concentration of anti-HSV antibody has been observed in animal models when administered early in the course of disease. Clinical efficacy in humans has not been demonstrated.

■ PREVENTION

Delivery of the infants of pregnant women with active genital herpes by cesarean section within 4 to 6 hours of rupture of amniotic membranes is the only intervention shown to prevent neonatal HSV infection. Results of antepartum genital HSV cultures from pregnant women with a history of genital herpes do not predict the infant's risk of exposure to HSV at delivery. Even if asymptomatic, infants born by vaginal delivery or cesarean section after prolonged rupture of membranes in the presence of active genital herpes lesions should have appropriate cultures for HSV taken 24 to 36 hours after delivery. Virus present at this time represents active replication and invasive infection, whereas virus isolated from mucous membrane cultures obtained at birth merely reflects surface contamination. If the mother has primary genital herpes and the infant is premature or has had invasive instrumentation or skin laceration during delivery, prophylactic or "anticipatory" antiviral therapy is recommended. If the mother has recurrent genital herpes and no other risk factors are present, antiviral therapy is withheld until culture results are known or clinical signs of disease develop. Antiviral therapy is initiated if HSV is isolated from any infant culture. This approach is widely recommended, but its efficacy is unproved. Infants born to women with active genital herpes should be in contact isolation in the nursery or should room with the mother. Careful handwashing before handling the infant should be stressed to the mother to prevent postpartum transmission. Breast-feeding is contraindicated only if the mother has vesicular lesions on the breast. Delay of circumcision for approximately 1 month for infants at highest risk of disease may be warranted.

Nursery personnel with oral and genital HSV lesions are at low risk of transmitting infection to infants as long as their lesions are covered. They must practice strict handwashing when handling infants. Personnel with herpetic whitlow should not have direct patient-care responsibilities until the lesions have healed.

VARICELLA-ZOSTER VIRUS

Varicella-zoster virus (VZV) is a member of the herpesvirus family and is the etiology of two clinical syndromes—chickenpox (varicella) and shingles (zoster). Primary infection usually occurs in childhood. It is rare for healthy adults to develop chickenpox; 90% of adults with no history of clinical chickenpox have evidence of previous infection when tested serologically. An increased risk exists, however, for development of pneumonia in adults with chickenpox. The incidence of maternal varicella is reported to be 0.7 per 1000 pregnancies. Zoster is a result of reactivation of the latent VZV and does not have a viremic phase in normal hosts.

■ PATHOGENESIS

The neonate whose mother has never had VZV infection is at risk of acquiring varicella either transplacentally during the viremic phase of maternal chickenpox or postnatally by airborne transmission or direct contact with an acutely infected person in the neonatal nursery or at home. Transplacental transmission occurs in 25% of cases. Maternal varicella infection occurring between weeks 8 and 20 of gestation may be associated with a characteristic fetal varicella syndrome (Table 59–4). Varicella in the second and third trimester rarely is associated with birth defects. In a prospective study of 43 pregnancies complicated by varicella and 14 pregnancies complicated by herpes zoster, the congenital varicella syndrome occurred in 1 (9.1%) of 11 infants of women with first trimester varicella and in none of the infants whose mothers were infected in the second and third trimesters. The most frequently observed features of fetal varicella syndrome are cutaneous scars in a dermatomal distribution, limb hypoplasia and paresis, and eye lesions. The characteristic segmental distribution suggests that these lesions result from fetal zoster after in utero varicella infection. No evidence supports an association between maternal

---

TABLE 59-4. Characteristic Features of Fetal Varicella Syndrome

Skin lesions: unilateral cicatricial lesions that correspond to dermatome distribution

Neurologic: limb paresis/paralysis, hydrocephalus/cortical atrophy, seizures, delayed development, sphincter dysfunction

Eye: chorioretinitis, anisocoria, nystagmus, microphthalmia, cataract

Skeletal: hypoplasia of extremities, digits

Gastrointestinal and genitourinary anomalies

Failure to thrive

varicella and chromosomal damage, spontaneous abortion, or prematurity. Some infants with congenital VZV infection are normal at birth but develop zoster during the first few years of life without an episode of postnatal varicella. The usual latency of several decades is, therefore, not maintained after intrauterine exposure to VZV. Fetal infection rarely occurs in association with an episode of maternal zoster during pregnancy because of the presence of large concentrations of antibody and the absence of maternal viremia.

Infants whose mothers develop chickenpox within the 21 days before delivery have a 25% chance of developing chickenpox in the early neonatal period. Because a large inoculum of virus is transmitted directly to the fetus during maternal viremia, the usual incubation period of 10 to 21 days in older children is decreased to 9 to 15 days in the neonate. When the maternal rash develops 6 to 21 days before delivery, sufficient quantities of maternal antibody are produced and delivered to the fetus to protect against postnatal development of severe chickenpox. Those infants whose mothers develop chickenpox fewer than 5 days before delivery or within 2 days after delivery are at risk of increased morbidity and mortality.

Development of chickenpox after exposure during the neonatal period is unusual in the infant whose mother is immune because of the placental transfer of antibody. VZV antibody levels are low or undetectable in infants of birth weights less than 1000 g or less than 25 weeks' gestation; therefore, such infants should be considered unprotected until antibody titers are determined. Rarely, infection occurs despite the presence of maternal antibody, but clinical disease is mild. Infants of susceptible mothers are not protected, but they generally do not develop serious disease after postnatal exposure.

■ DIAGNOSIS

The diagnosis of VZV infections is based on characteristic clinical findings. Several methods of laboratory confirmation are available. Multinucleated giant cells or cells containing eosinophilic intranuclear inclusions identified in scrapings from the base of a vesicle indicate the presence of a herpesvirus. Virus is present in vesicular fluid during the first 3 days of illness, but VZV is difficult to isolate in the viral diagnostic laboratory; therefore, cultures are not routinely performed. IgG and IgM antibodies may be detected in serum by the fluorescent antibody to membrane antigen (FAMA) or by ELISA methods. The ELISA test is preferred for its increased sensitivity. Congenital VZV infection may be diagnosed during gestation by detecting IgM antibody to VZV in fetal blood obtained by percutaneous umbilical blood sampling. After birth, the diagnosis is confirmed by presence of IgM antibody to VZV at birth or persistence of VZV-specific IgG antibody after 1 year of age.

■ TREATMENT AND PREVENTION

Acyclovir 45 mg/kg/day intravenously in three divided doses is administered for 5 to 7 days for treatment of severe disease in the neonate. Vidarabine 10 mg/kg body wt/day is an alternative agent, but an increased fluid load is required because of its relative insolubility.

Varicella-zoster immunoglobulin (VZIG) is recommended for susceptible pregnant women who have significant exposure to chickenpox. The recommended dose is 125 U/10 kg body wt (maximum 625 U). It is advisable first to confirm maternal susceptibility by measuring antibody to

VZV. If antibody is not present, VZIG should be administered as soon as possible but not longer than 96 hours after exposure. It is uncertain whether prevention of clinical disease in the mother protects the fetus. A decision concerning termination of pregnancy must be made by the woman and her physician, taking into consideration the risk of having a malformed infant. The live, attenuated VZV vaccine administered to susceptible women before pregnancy may prove to be the most effective method for prevention of congenital varicella syndrome.

VZIG (125 U) is administered to neonates whose mothers develop chickenpox within 5 days before or 2 days after delivery because of the increased morbidity and mortality observed when infants develop chickenpox within the first 10 days of life. Although VZIG is not completely protective against infection, clinical disease is generally less severe. These infants must still be considered potentially infective and are maintained in strict isolation until 21 days of age if hospitalization is required. VZIG is not routinely administered to full-term infants exposed to chickenpox postnatally because the risk of complications is not increased. VZIG is recommended after exposure of neonates of less than 28 weeks' gestation or other premature infants who are seronegative.

EPSTEIN-BARR VIRUS

Sporadic case reports suggest an association of Epstein-Barr virus (EBV) with congenital infection. EBV is the most prevalent herpesvirus worldwide, and seroconversion usually occurs by 3 years of age in primitive societies or in crowded living conditions. In the United States, acquisition of antibody may be delayed until age 15 years in women from lower socioeconomic backgrounds and until late in the third decade in women from middle to upper socioeconomic backgrounds. Primary EBV infections rarely occur during pregnancy because of nearly universal seropositivity of women of childbearing age. Large prospective studies of more than 12,000 pregnant women in France, Canada, and the United States demonstrate seronegativity rates of less than 5%. Most studies demonstrate no seroconversions during pregnancy. Seroconversion during pregnancy is not associated with intrauterine infection. Nearly universal presence of maternal antibody is probably protective against transmission by blood transfusion during the neonatal period.

Reactivation of a primary EBV infection in association with the relative immunodeficiency of pregnancy could provide another opportunity for intrauterine infection. Because the titers of antibodies to the EBV early antigen (anti-EA) increase as additional amounts of EBV-associated antigens are released during reactivation, a prospective study by Fleisher and Bolognese (1983) compared the incidence of anti-EA in 200 pregnant women to that in 200 control patients. Anti-EA was present in significantly more pregnant women than control participants, 55% versus 22% to 32%, P less than .005. In this study, however, no difference was noted in the incidence of low-birth-weight, congenital anomalies, or jaundice in infants whose mothers had EBV reactivation during pregnancy compared with those who did not. No evidence of intrauterine infection was found in those infants born to women with reactivation and available for testing. Another study of 719 women in France, however, demonstrated a lower incidence of anti-EA (16%), but there was a significant association between reactivation and pathologic outcome.

Several case reports have attempted to associate intrauterine EBV infection with congenital anomalies. Most are inconclusive because of absence of complete serologic studies or because of simultaneous infection with another viral agent known for association with a congenital infection syndrome. The manifestations of EBV infection in utero are micrognathia, cryptorchidism, central cataracts, hypotonia, thrombocytopenia, persistent monocytosis, proteinuria, and multiple areas of metaphysitis present at birth. Serologic and virologic studies failed to detect any other infectious agents. EBV-specific serologic studies were performed at 22 days of age with the following evidence of intrauterine infection: IgM antiviral capsid antigen (anti-VCA) 1:40; IgG anti-VCA 1:640 (maternal 1:80); anti-EA 1:10; and anti-Epstein-Barr nuclear antigen (anti-EBNA) less than 2. At 5 months of age, the EBNA was detected in 18% of lymphocytes that spontaneously persisted in culture for 3 months. A case report by Weaver and coworkers (1984) describes an infant with extrahepatic biliary atresia and onset of jaundice at 5 days of age and who at 3 weeks of age demonstrated IgM-VCA greater than 1:10 and IgG-VCA 1:640; IgG-VCA was 1:320 at 1 year of age.

When a clinical diagnosis of infectious mononucleosis is made in a pregnant woman, serologic confirmation should be obtained with acute and convalescent determinations of IgM-anti-VCA, IgG-anti-VCA, anti-EA, and anti-EBNA. Acutely, IgM-anti-VCA, IgG-anti-VCA, and anti-EA are elevated; anti-EBNA is absent and does not appear for 3 to 6 months. At birth, the infant should be carefully evaluated; most infants are unaffected. If in utero infection with EBV is suspected, acute and convalescent serologic measurements as well as spontaneous lymphocyte transformation studies should be obtained.

SYPHILIS

Congenital syphilis, a result of fetal infection with *Treponema pallidum,* is a major public health problem in the United States. From 1977 through 1990, there was a steady increase in the incidence of primary and secondary syphilis among women in the United States Subsequently, the num-

ber of cases of early congenital syphilis reported to the Centers for Disease Control and Prevention (CDC) increased from 108 in 1978 to more than 4000 cases in 1991 (Figure 59–3). The majority of reported cases are from large urban areas such as Detroit, Houston, Los Angeles, Miami, and New York City. At Parkland Memorial Hospital in Dallas, the incidence of congenital syphilis also has increased steadily from 1980 through 1989; 0.2 cases per 1000 live births were reported in 1980, 0.6 cases per 1000 live births in 1982, 1.3 cases per 1000 live births in each of the years 1984 through 1987, and 1.7 cases per 1000 live births in 1989.

A major contributor to the increase of syphilis is the exchange of illegal drugs (notably crack cocaine) for sex with multiple partners whose identities are not known. Partner notification, a traditional syphilis-control strategy, is impossible to implement. The recent decrease in early syphilis (see Figure 58–3) has been attributed to novel intervention programs aimed at identification and treatment of these high risk individuals. The dramatic increase in the number of cases of congenital syphilis is due to both an increase in actual cases and the use of revised reporting guidelines. Beginning in 1989, the surveillance definition for congenital syphilis was broadened. The new definition includes not only all infants with clinical evidence of active syphilis, but also asymptomatic infants and stillbirths born to women with untreated or inadequately treated syphilis. Use of the new surveillance case definition increases the number of confirmed/presumptive cases of congenital syphilis by almost four times.

■ TRANSMISSION

Pregnant women with primary or secondary syphilis are at highest risk of delivering infected infants. Transmission of infection to the fetus usually occurs transplacentally from maternal spirochetemia, but the neonate also can be infected through contact with a genital lesion at the time of delivery. Although congenital infection can occur anytime during gestation, the risk of fetal infection increases as the stage of pregnancy advances. The theory that the Langhans' cell layer of the cytotrophoblast forms a placental barrier against fetal infection before the 18th week of pregnancy was

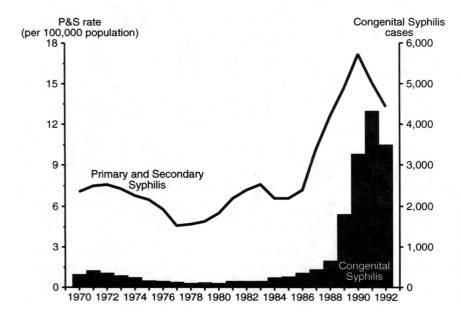

Figure 59-3. Case rates of primary and secondary syphilis among women and congenital syphilis cases in the United States, 1970 to 1992. The rate of congenital syphilis has steadily increased since 1983. The surveillance case definition for congenital syphilis changed in 1989; 1992 cases are projections based on reporting through June 1992. (Centers for Disease Control, Atlanta, Georgia, Public Health Service, 1991.)

disproved by demonstration of spirochetes in fetal tissue from spontaneous abortion at 9 and 10 weeks' gestation. Also, electron microscopy demonstrates the persistence of the Langhans' cell layer throughout pregnancy.

■ CLINICAL MANIFESTATIONS

Syphilis during pregnancy is associated with premature delivery, spontaneous abortion, stillbirth, nonimmune hydrops, perinatal death, and two characteristic syndromes of clinical disease, early and late congenital syphilis. Early congenital syphilis refers to those clinical manifestations that appear within the first 2 years of life. Those features that occur after 2 years are designated as late congenital syphilis. The clinical manifestations and laboratory findings of early congenital syphilis may be present at birth or may be delayed for several months if the infant remains untreated (see Table 58–2). The physical signs are a direct result of active infection and inflammation.

Infants with congenital syphilis may be growth-retarded at delivery. Hepatitis with hepatosplenomegaly occurs in 50% to 90% of affected infants. Splenomegaly does not occur without liver enlargement. Extramedullary hematopoiesis is seen in both the liver and spleen. About one third of infants have direct and indirect hyperbilirubinemia and elevated transaminase levels. Liver abnormalities may require more than a year to resolve, but they rarely lead to cirrhosis. Generalized nontender lymphadenopathy occurs in 20% to 50% of cases, with characteristic involvement of the epitrochlear nodes. A Coombs' test-negative hemolytic anemia is common. The peripheral leukocyte count can show either leukopenia or leukemoid reaction. Thrombocytopenia with petechiae and purpura occurs in about 30% of infants and may be the sole manifestation of congenital infection.

Mucocutaneous lesions are specific for congenital syphilis and occur in 40% to 60% of affected infants. The rash of congenital syphilis is usually maculopapular and located on the extremities. The lesions are initially oval and pink but then turn coppery brown and desquamate. Desquamation occurs mainly on the palms and soles. A characteristic vesicular bullous eruption known as pemphigus syphiliticus may develop with erythema, blister formation and eventual crusting as healing occurs (Color Figure 12). Nasal discharge associated with rhinitis or snuffles is initially watery, but it becomes thick, purulent, and even blood-tinged (Color Figure 13). Nasal discharge and vesicular fluid containing large concentrations of spirochetes are highly infectious. Rarely,

mucous patches of the lips, tongue and palate, and condyloma lata in the perioral and perianal areas may occur.

Bone roentgenograms show skeletal abnormalities consisting of osteochondritis, periostitis, and osteitis in 80% to 90% of infants (Figures 59–4 and 59–5). These abnormalities tend to be multiple and symmetric, with the lower extremities involved more often than the upper extremities. The long bones (tibia, humerus, femur), the ribs, and the cranium are principally affected. Rarely, bone lesions may be painful or have superimposed fractures resulting in pseudoparalysis of the affected limb (pseudoparalysis of Parrot). Osteochondritis involves the metaphysis and is evident roentgenographically about 5 weeks after fetal infection. Typical findings are metaphyseal demineralization and a radiodense band below the epiphyseal plate that represents a widened and enhanced zone of provisional calcification. An underlying zone of osteoporosis is evident as a radiolucent band. Bilateral demineralization and osseous destruction of the proximal medial tibial metaphysis is referred to as Wimberger's sign (see Figure 58–5). The classic transverse sawtoothed appearance of the metaphysis (see Figure 58–4) is often not seen on the plain roentgenogram but is evident on xeroradiography of long bones of stillborn infants with congenital syphilis. Periostitis requires 16 weeks for roentgenographic demonstration and consists of multiple layers of periosteal new bone formation in response to diaphyseal inflammation. Osteitis is the "celery stalk" appearance of long bones (see Figure 59–2) resulting from involvement of the medullary canal with resultant diaphysitis. After several months, complete healing of the affected bones occurs even without antibiotic therapy.

Neurosyphilis occurs in 40% to 60% of infants with congenital syphilis. Two types of CNS involvement are described. Acute syphilitic leptomeningitis occurs in early infancy. Chronic meningovascular syphilis with progressive hydrocephalus, cranial nerve palsies, and cerebral infarction secondary to endarteritis usually presents toward the end of the first year of life. CSF examination reveals pleocytosis with an elevated protein content and positive serologic test results for syphilis.

Ocular findings include chorioretinitis, cataract, glaucoma, and uveitis. Nephrosis with generalized edema, ascites, and proteinuria usually occurs at 2 to 3 months of age as a result of immune complex deposition in the renal glomeruli. Other uncommon manifestations include pneumonia alba, myocarditis, pancreatitis, and inflammation and fibrosis of the gastrointestinal tract leading to malabsorption and diarrhea.

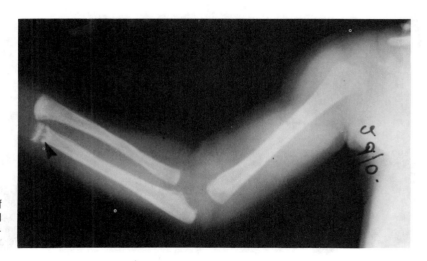

Figure 59-4. Saw-toothed appearance of the metaphysis of the distal radius (*arrow*) of an infant with early congenital syphilis. The lucent area represents syphilitic granulation tissue. (Courtesy of Guido Currarino, MD, Dallas, Texas.)

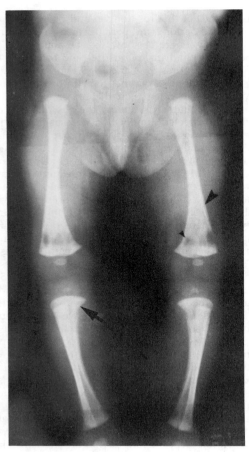

Figure 59-5. Bony lesions of early congenital syphilis: symmetric periostitis (*large arrow*); radiolucent metaphyseal area of osteochondritis (*small arrowhead*); bilateral metaphyseal defects on the upper medial aspect of the tibia, Wimberger's sign (*arrow*). Similar changes may occur at the upper ends of the humeri. (Courtesy of Guido Currarino, MD, Dallas, Texas.)

The clinical manifestations of late congenital syphilis result from ongoing inflammation or from scars caused by infection of early congenital syphilis. Development of the characteristic lesions is prevented by treatment during pregnancy or within the first 3 months of life. Infants with late congenital syphilis are not infective.

Dental stigmata result from the inflammatory response to *T pallidum* infection in the developing permanent teeth during late gestation. The affected permanent upper central incisors (Hutchinson's teeth) are small, widely spaced, barrel shaped, and notched, with thinning and discoloration of the enamel (Figure 59–6) The first 6-year lower molars (mulberry or Moon's molars) may also be affected. The top surface has many small cusps instead of the usual four. Enamelization is defective. Infection before the 18th week of gestation may result in involvement of deciduous teeth, which then are misshapen, hypoplastic, and prone to dental caries.

The sequela of periostitis of the skull is frontal bossing, of the tibia is saber shins, and of the clavicle is Higoumenakis' sign with sternoclavicular thickening. Clutton's joints, or painless synovitis and hydrarthrosis without involvement of the adjacent bones, is rare. Osteochondritis affecting the otic capsule may lead to cochlear degeneration and fibrous adhesions resulting in eighth-nerve deafness, for which steroid treatment may be beneficial.

The sequelae of syphilitic rhinitis include rhagades and short maxilla with a high palatal arch. If the inflammation of the nasal mucosa extends to the underlying cartilage and bone, perforation of the palate and nasal septum occurs, resulting in a "saddle nose" deformity.

Late ocular manifestations include uveitis and interstitial keratitis. Interstitial keratitis usually appears at puberty and is not affected by penicillin therapy. Although steroid treatment may be beneficial, keratitis resolves spontaneously after 18 to 24 months. Possible sequelae of CNS infection include mental retardation, hydrocephalus, seizure disorder, cranial nerve palsies, paralysis, and optic nerve atrophy.

■ DIAGNOSIS

The diagnosis of congenital syphilis is established by the observation of spirochetes in body fluids or tissue or by serologic testing. *T pallidum* may be identified by darkfield microscopy, fluorescent antibody or silver stain of mucocutaneous lesions, nasal discharge, vesicular fluid, amniotic fluid, placenta, or tissue obtained at autopsy. A diagnosis of congenital syphilis is also suggested by a large, pale, firm placenta, which on microscopic examination, reveals immature villi, vasculitis, and diffuse fibrosis. Serologic tests for syphilis are classified into nontreponemal tests and treponemal tests. Nontreponemal tests include the Venereal Disease Research Laboratory (VDRL) tests and the rapid plasma reagin test. Treponemal tests include the fluorescent treponemal antibody-absorption (FTA-ABS) test and microhemaggluti-

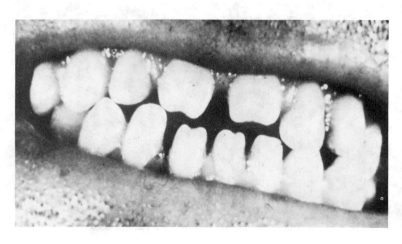

Figure 59-6. "Hutchinson's teeth" in a child with late congenital syphilis. The small, widely spaced, notched upper central incisors may be detected by radiography while deciduous teeth are in place. (Courtesy of George H. McCracken, Jr., MD, Dallas, Texas.)

nation assay for *T pallidum* antibody (MHA-TP). A diagnosis of congenital syphilis is supported by an infant's nontreponemal antibody level that is at least four times greater than that of the mother's serum. Measurement of total cord IgM levels and results of specific fluorescent treponemal IgM (FTA-ABS-IgM) tests have not proved useful in the diagnosis of congenital syphilis. Elevated cord IgM levels can result from other congenital infections as well as from noninfectious abnormalities. Rheumatoid factor, which occurs frequently in congenital syphilis, interferes with the interpretation of FTA-ABS-IgM test results by producing as many as 35% false-positive results. A 10% false-negative rate also is reported with the use of this test. Recent studies using Western blot analyses of highly purified IgM fractions of sera from infants with congenital syphilis suggest that fetal IgM reactivity with a membrane lipoprotein of *T pallidum* having an apparent molecular mass of 47 kd may accurately identify both symptomatic and asymptomatic infants with congeni-

tal syphilis. Similar IgM reactivity to the 47-kd antigen also has been found in the CSF of infants with congenital syphilis.

Recently, a polymerase chain reaction (PCR) technique was developed to detect specific *T pallidum* DNA in tissues and body fluids. Preliminary studies with PCR on amniotic fluid, neonatal serum, and CSF yielded sensitivities of 100%, 80%, and 71%, respectively, with a specificity of 100%. Combined use of IgM immunoblotting and PCR ultimately will aid in early identification of infected infants, regardless of clinical status.

A practical approach to the evaluation of infants born to mothers with reactive serologic tests for syphilis is presented in Figure 59-7. Testing of all pregnant women with reactive serologic tests for syphilis for antibody to the human immunodeficiency virus (HIV) is strongly recommended. Any infant with clinical findings suggestive of congenital syphilis requires a complete diagnostic evaluation, including

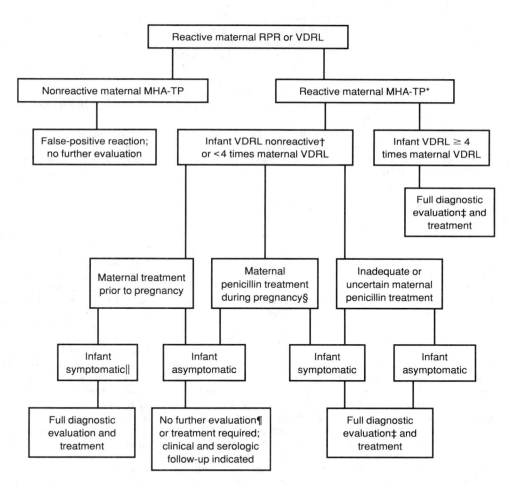

* Testing for HIV antibody recommended.

† Infant's VDRL may be nonreactive due to low maternal VDRL titer, prematurity, or recent maternal infection.

‡ Includes CBC, platelets, retic, LFT (ALT, AST, Bili T&D), long bone x-rays, and CSF examination for cell count, protein, and quantitative VDRL; eye exam if symptomatic.

§ Maternal treatment within 4 weeks of delivery is considered inadequate treatment of the infant.

‖ Women who maintain a VDRL titer ≤ 1:2 beyond 1 year after successful treatment are considered serofast. Symptomatic infants born to women believed to be serofast represent aternal reinfection.

¶ Full diagnostic evaluation of infants if maternal titers have not declined fourfold after appropriate therapy in a mother with early syphilis; no treatment is required if work-up is negative and follow-up is certain.

Figure 59-7. An approach to the evaluation of infants born to mothers with reactive serologic tests for syphilis. *MHA-TP,* microhemagglutination assay for *Treponema pallidum* antibody; *RPR,* rapid plasma reagin test; *VDRL,* Veneral Research Laboratory test.

serum VDRL test, bone roentgenograms, and CSF examination for cell count protein content and VDRL test. The diagnosis of congenital neurosyphilis is difficult to establish. Diagnosis is based on CSF examination that shows a reactive result to the VDRL test, pleocytosis (greater than or equal to 25 leukocytes/mm³), and an elevated protein content (more than 150 mg/dL). The presence of red blood cells in the CSF as a result of a traumatic lumbar puncture can produce a false-positive serologic reaction. Also, a reactive CSF VDRL test may be due to passive transfer of nontreponemal IgG antibodies from serum into the CSF. Examination of the CSF for IgM reactivities to specific *T pallidum* antigens and *T pallidum* DNA by PCR may prove more useful for diagnosis of congenital neurosyphilis.

Infants with reactive serology at delivery should have serial quantitative nontreponemal tests performed until the test results show nonreactivity. Similarly, infants who are seronegative but whose mothers acquired syphilis late in gestation should be followed with serial testing after penicillin therapy is instituted. Follow-up for these infants can be incorporated into routine pediatric care at 2, 4, 6, 12, and 15 months. In infants with congenital syphilis, nontreponemal serologic tests become nonreactive within 12 months after appropriate treatment. Uninfected infants usually become seronegative by 6 months of age. Infants with persistently low, stable titers of nontreponemal tests require retreatment. A reactive treponemal test at 12 to 15 months of age when the infant has lost all maternal antibody confirms the diagnosis of congenital syphilis. Infants with abnormal CSF findings should have a repeat lumbar puncture performed at 6 months after therapy. A reactive CSF VDRL test result or an abnormal protein content or cell count at that time is an indication for retreatment.

■ TREATMENT AND PREVENTION

Congenital syphilis is effectively prevented by prenatal screening and penicillin treatment of infected women, their sexual partners, and their newborn infants. The decision to treat an infant for congenital syphilis is based on the clinical presentation, previous serologic test results and treatment of the mother, and the results of serologic testing of the infant and mother at the time of delivery. Treatment at birth is required for the following situations: the infant is symptomatic, maternal treatment was inadequate or unknown, the mother was treated with drugs other than penicillin, the mother was treated within 4 weeks of delivery, or adequate follow-up care of the infant is uncertain. Symptomatic infants or asymptomatic infants with abnormal results of CSF examination should be treated with either aqueous crystalline penicillin G (50,000 U/kg intravenously every 12 hours for the first week of life, followed by every 8 hours beyond 7 days of age) or aqueous procaine penicillin G (50,000 U/kg intramuscularly once daily) for a minimum of 10 days. Asymptomatic infants with a normal CSF examination and normal laboratory evaluation can be treated with a single intramuscular injection of benzathine penicillin G at a dosage of 50,000 U/kg. If the risk of infection in the asymptomatic infant is significant and adequate follow-up cannot be ensured, the 10-day course of aqueous or procaine penicillin is recommended by the CDC, regardless of results of the CSF examination. Failure of a single injection of benzathine penicillin in the treatment of congenital syphilis has been reported. Treatment failures have been attributed to the inability of penicillin to adequately penetrate and achieve treponemicidal concentrations in certain sites such as the aqueous humor and CNS.

RUBELLA

Rubella first was recognized in 1814 as a mild exanthematous disease distinct from scarlatina, roseola, and urticaria and responsible for large epidemics. In 1941, an Australian ophthalmologist, Norman McAlister Gregg, made the association between congenital cataracts and a history of rubella early in pregnancy. His was the first description of the variety of defects now known as the congenital rubella syndrome. Isolation of the rubella virus in tissue culture in 1962 was soon followed by the development of live, attenuated vaccines. Since licensure of the vaccine in the United States in 1969, the total number of cases of rubella annually reported in the United States had declined by 99% to 0.23 per 100,000 population in 1986. In 1988, an all-time low of 225 cases of rubella was reported to the Centers for Disease Control (CDC). In 1989, however, the number of reported cases nearly doubled. In 1990, cases tripled to 0.4 per 100,000 population. In 1990, outbreaks were classified into two categories: outbreaks in which cases occurred in or were linked to settings where unvaccinated adults congregate (*eg*, prisons, colleges, workplaces) and outbreaks among children and adults in religious communities with low levels of rubella vaccination coverage (*eg*, Amish).

■ PATHOGENESIS

Transplacental transmission of the rubella virus occurs during the viremic phase of primary maternal infection in the week before the onset of rash. The exact rate of transmission is controversial, and most rates reported in early studies are probably underestimates. Placental infection rates of 85% to 91% with fetal infection rates of 45% to 50% have been reported. In a 1982 prospective study of virologically confirmed rubella during pregnancy in England, Miller and colleagues found fetal infection rates of 90% when symptomatic maternal rubella occurred during the first 12 weeks of gestation, 25% to 30% during the second trimester, and 53% during the third trimester. Fetal viremia results in disseminated infection with persistence of the virus throughout fetal life and into postnatal life. Gestational age at the time of infection, the quantity of virus delivered to the fetus, the ability of the fetus to limit replication, and strain variation in virulence determine the risk for malformations. Sallomi (1966) reported the incidence of anomalies according to gestational age when maternal infection occurred as follows: weeks 1 to 4, 61%; weeks 5 to 8, 26%; weeks 9 to 12, 8%; weeks 13 to 16, 1% to 4%; weeks 17 to 20, 0.5% to 2%; weeks 21 to 40, less than 1%. Most studies report no defects after maternal infection later than 18 to 20 weeks' gestation. Congenital infection after maternal reinfection is rare, but both congenital rubella syndrome and late-onset rubella syndrome are reported. Rubella virus may be transmitted to the susceptible newborn in breast milk or by the respiratory route, but postnatal disease is usually not severe.

Several mechanisms of fetal damage have been proposed. The rubella virus has both a mitotic inhibitory and cytolytic action on fetal cells that is selective for cells from different tissues. Depressed mitotic activity results in intrauterine growth retardation, a diminished number of cells per organ, and specific malformations of organs. Cytolytic action on cells resulting in necrosis may occur in organs with normal architecture and development, but the virus persists within cells. Examples of this mechanism of action are damage to the organ of Corti associated with deafness, myocarditis, hepatitis, and interstitial pneumonitis.

Vasculitis of the placenta decreases the fetal blood supply, resulting in intrauterine growth retardation; vasculitis of the fetus results in vascular anomalies. Circulating immune complexes containing rubella viral antigens have been identified in the acute phase of the late-onset rubella syndrome.

■ CLINICAL MANIFESTATIONS

Spontaneous abortion, stillbirths, and major organ defects are associated with congenital rubella infection. Maternal disease before implantation (just before and 3 weeks after the last menstrual period) may result in fetal infection. Although some investigators report no adverse effects associated with infection this early, an increased incidence of spontaneous abortion during this period is likely. Multiple-organ defects are most likely to result from maternal infection before completion of organogenesis in the first 12 weeks of gestation. The most commonly observed intrauterine defects are as follows:

1. Auditory. Sensorineural hearing loss of varying degrees is present in nearly all patients. Deafness occurs in 50% of patients as one of several defects or as an isolated defect associated with infection beyond 12 weeks' gestation. All infants with congenital rubella require evaluation of hearing with brain stem auditory-evoked responses.

2. Cardiac. Patent ductus arteriosus with or without pulmonary artery or pulmonic valvular stenosis, aortic stenosis, and ventricular septal defect.

3. Ophthalmologic. Cataract, pigmentary retinopathy, and microphthalmia.

4. Neurologic. Central auditory imperception, delayed development, microcephaly, and hypotonia.

5. Growth. Intrauterine and postnatal growth retardation.

Clinical manifestations related to persistent infection that may be present at birth include thrombocytopenia, hepatitis, jaundice, dermal erythropoiesis or "blueberry muffin spots" (see Color Figure 1), osteopathy with the characteristic "celery stalk" lesions (see Fig 58–2), meningoencephalitis, interstitial pneumonitis, and myocarditis. These lesions may resolve, but when present in combination with severe malformations, the risk for mortality is increased.

Some infants with intrauterine infection have few or no symptoms at birth but develop severe multisystem disease after a latent period of several months. The most notable manifestations of this late-onset rubella syndrome are a generalized interstitial pneumonitis associated with cough, tachypnea, and cyanosis, chronic rubelliform rash, chronic diarrhea, recurrent infections associated with defects of both the humoral and cell-mediated immune system, and progressive neurologic deterioration. Finally, endocrine abnormalities associated with an increase in autoantibodies may be observed. Insulin-dependent diabetes mellitus, hypothyroidism, and thyrotoxicosis manifest at several years of age in children with congenital rubella infection.

■ DIAGNOSIS

The diagnosis of congenital rubella infection is confirmed by isolation of the virus from the nasopharynx, urine, buffy coat, stool, CSF, or cataract. Eighty percent of infected infants excrete the virus at birth and for as long as 1 or 2 years. Viral isolation is often impractical because the tissue culture cells required for isolation of the rubella virus are not usually available in routine virology laboratories. Demonstration of rubella-specific IgM antibody at birth and an increase in the infant's IgG titer over 3 to 6 months with stable or decreasing maternal IgG titers provides serologic confirmation of the diagnosis. Not all infants with congenital rubella infection have IgM present at birth; therefore, absent rubella-specific IgM does not exclude the diagnosis. The traditional hemagglutination inhibition and fluorescence immunoassay tests have been replaced by kits that use latex agglutination and ELISA techniques. Sensitivity and specificity of the method employed by the individual laboratory should be verified before interpreting the results of serologic testing.

■ PREVENTION

Active immunization with live, attenuated rubella virus vaccine is the most effective means of prevention of congenital rubella syndrome. The only vaccine available for use in the United States—the RA 27/3, a strain grown in human embryonic lung tissue culture—is immunogenic in more than 89% of recipients and provides long-term protective immunity that is probably lifelong. The strategy of immunizing all infants at 15 months of age is more efficacious for decreasing the incidence of congenital rubella syndrome than a selective strategy that calls for routine immunization of prepubescent girls and women of childbearing age only. Women who are identified during pregnancy as nonimmune should be immunized in the postpartum period. Vaccine virus shed by the mother does not cause disease in the neonate. Postpartum immunization is not a contraindication for breast-feeding.

Immunization with rubella vaccine is contraindicated during pregnancy, and it is recommended that a woman not conceive during the 3-month period after immunization. Since 1971, the CDC has maintained a register to monitor the risks to the fetus of exposure to live, attenuated rubella virus vaccine within the 3 months before or the 3 months after conception. Data collected from more than 500 infants whose mothers received a rubella vaccine during this high-risk period show that vaccine viruses can cross the placenta and infect the fetus but do not produce the defects of congenital rubella syndrome. The rate of isolation of vaccine virus from the products of conception is only 3% for the currently used RA 27/3 vaccine as compared with 20% for the Cendehill and HPV-77 vaccines used before 1979. Serologic evidence exists for subclinical intrauterine infection in 1% to 3% of infants born to susceptible vaccinees for all vaccines used. The theoretical maximum risk for the occurrence of congenital rubella syndrome after immunization is 1.2%. This is considerably less than the 20% to 50% risk associated with maternal infection with wild-type rubella virus during the first trimester of pregnancy and no greater than the 2% or 3% risk of major birth defects occurring by chance alone. Thus, although pregnancy remains a contraindication to rubella immunization, inadvertent administration of rubella vaccine during the first trimester of pregnancy should not be considered an indication to interrupt the pregnancy.

If a nonimmune pregnant woman is exposed to rubella during the first trimester of pregnancy, serial IgM and IgG rubella antibody studies should be performed to determine if infection has occurred. Termination of pregnancy is considered if infection occurred during the first 12 weeks of pregnancy. If termination of pregnancy is not an option, immune globulin 0.55 mL/kg administered within 72 hours of exposure may prevent or modify infection in an exposed, susceptible person. Protection is not complete even in the absence of clinical disease in the mother because infants with congenital rubella have been delivered by women who received immune globulin shortly after exposure.

Infants with congenital rubella are considered contagious and are maintained in blood and body fluid isolation. Only health care workers known to be seropositive should be permitted to care for such infants. Pregnant personnel and visitors who are not known to be immune should be restricted from contact with infants with congenital rubella.

TOXOPLASMOSIS

Toxoplasma gondii is an intracellular parasite with a worldwide distribution. The cat family is the definitive host for this organism. Nonfeline mammals or birds ingest infective oocysts from contaminated soil. Tissue cysts then accumulate in the organs and skeletal muscle of these animals. The possible routes of transmission from animal to human are direct contact with cat feces, ingestion of undercooked meat containing infective cysts, and ingestion of fruits or vegetables that have been in contaminated soil. Infection may be passed from human to human by the transplacental route and rarely by transfusion of infected leukocytes or transplantation of infected organs or bone marrow. Most human infections are asymptomatic, and significant disease develops when reactivation occurs in association with suppression of the immune system. Toxoplasmosis is now an important opportunistic infection in patients with the acquired immunodeficiency syndrome (AIDS). Encephalitis develops in 30% of previously infected AIDS patients.

The prevalence of chronic or latent infection with *T gondii* varies widely among different adult populations throughout the world. Seropositivity increases with age. In the United States, overall seropositivity of pregnant women is 32%, with variation from 16% for the 15- to 19-year age group to 50% for women 35 years of age or older. In contrast, the overall seropositivity rate for women in France is 87% with variation only from 80% at age 15 to 19 years to 96% at 35 years of age and older. The incidence of congenital toxoplasmosis in the United States is estimated to be 1.3 of 1000 live births as compared with a rate of 3 to 10 of 1000 live births in Paris, Vienna, and the Netherlands.

■ PATHOGENESIS

Congenital *Toxoplasma* infection occurs only during maternal parasitemia associated with primary infection. Clinical signs are present in 10% of infected adults, but transplacental transmission results from asymptomatic as well as symptomatic maternal infection. No cases have been reported to occur in subsequent pregnancies of women who gave birth to congenitally infected children. Chronic infection is not associated with infertility or spontaneous abortion. Although the actual rate of fetal infection increases as pregnancy advances, the severity of clinical manifestations is greatest when maternal infection is acquired during the first trimester. Overall, the risk of transmission without treatment is 30% to 50% with variations of 25% in the first trimester, 54% in the second trimester, and 65% in the third trimester. The risk of severe manifestations of infection decreases from 75% in the first trimester to 0% in the third trimester.

■ CLINICAL MANIFESTATIONS

Stillbirth and death in the early neonatal period are the most severe results of congenital infection. Most infants born with congenital *Toxoplasma* infection are asymptomatic in the neonatal period with severe disease at birth in only 10% of infants. Long-term follow-up of asymptomatic infants reveals chorioretinitis in as many as 85% and severe neurologic sequelae in 10% to 20%. At birth, these infants are indistinguishable from those who are asymptomatic. Infants with generalized congenital toxoplasmosis may have clinical syndromes indistinguishable from those associated with other agents of congenital infection. The CNS is always involved in symptomatic infants. The prominence of neurologic abnormalities is indicative of toxoplasmosis. The classic triad of hydrocephalus, chorioretinitis, and intracranial calcifications can be accompanied by fever, maculopapular or petechial rash, hepatosplenomegaly, jaundice, convulsions, and abnormal CSF (xanthochromia and mononuclear pleocytosis). Markedly elevated protein concentrations (more than 1 g per 100 mL) in ventricular fluid and hydrocephalus may be explained by periaqueductal and periventricular vasculitis with necrosis that are specifically associated with toxoplasmosis. Intracranial calcifications are distributed diffusely throughout the brain (Figure 59–8) in contrast to the periventricular pattern associated with cytomegalovirus. Severely affected infants may also have myocarditis, pneumonitis, thrombocytopenia, and nephrotic syndrome.

■ DIAGNOSIS

T gondii may be isolated from the placenta, amniotic fluid, CSF, or blood by inoculation into mice or tissue culture using human fibroblasts. Because these techniques are available only in research laboratories, routine diagnosis is made serologically. The Sabin-Feldman dye test is considered the gold standard to which all newer tests are compared. This test is performed only in reference laboratories because of the requirement for viable *Toxoplasma* organisms. Commercially available methods for measuring specific IgG and IgM antibodies to *T gondii* include indirect immunofluorescent antibody, direct agglutination tests, and ELISAs. Immunoblot techniques are being evaluated. ELISAs are preferred over the previously used immunofluorescent antibody tests for their improved sensitivity and specificity. It is important to know what test method is used for antibody determination, because there is considerable variation in reliability of commercially available kits. For example, the "double-sandwich" or antibody-capture ELISA technique for detection of IgM antibodies has substantially greater sensitivity and specificity than the conventional IgM ELISA technique.

The presence of IgM antibodies or rising titers of IgG antibodies in a pregnant woman are indicative of acute infection. Serial determinations are needed because IgG antibodies may remain elevated at high titer for long periods with chronic infection. Daffos and coworkers (1988) demonstrated the ability to diagnose infection during gestation in 39 (93%) of 42 fetuses studied in France using a combination of the following studies: culture specimens of amniotic fluid and fetal blood obtained from the umbilical cord under ultrasound guidance, presence of *Toxoplasma*-specific IgM and nonspecific measures of infection (leukocyte count and differential, platelet count, total IgM level, lactic dehydrogenase level, and Γ-glutamyltransferase level) in fetal blood, and ultrasound examination of the fetal brain. Absence of IgM in fetal blood does not exclude the diagnosis of congenital infection because production of IgM may be delayed

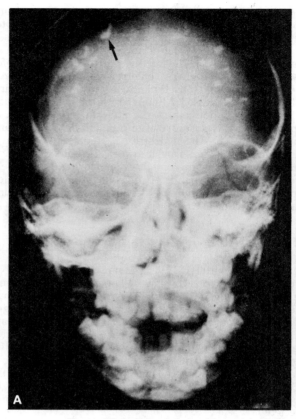
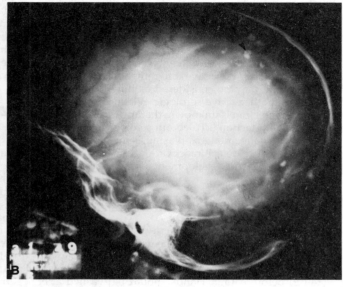

Figure 59-8. Anteroposterior (**A**) and lateral (**B**) skull roentgenogram demonstrating diffuse cerebral calcifications (*arrows*) in an infant with congenital toxoplasmosis. (Courtesy of Guido Currarino, MD, Dallas, Texas.)

until after birth due to the immaturity of the immune system and possible inhibition of synthesis by maternal IgG. This extensive prenatal evaluation may be helpful in making decisions concerning interruption of pregnancy and prenatal therapy.

Postnatally, the diagnosis of congenital toxoplasmosis may be proved by isolation of the organism from the placenta or by serial determinations of specific IgM and IgG antibody levels in the infant and mother. Initially, low IgG titers and absent IgM antibody in mother and baby suggest infection before pregnancy and do not require continued follow-up. The presence of IgM antibody in the first 3 months of life and increasing IgG in the infant during the first year of life support a diagnosis of congenital toxoplasmosis. Specific IgM antibody in the CSF is diagnostic of congenital *Toxoplasma* infection.

■ TREATMENT

Large studies of several hundred women with well-documented acute toxoplasmosis acquired during pregnancy have demonstrated the efficacy of treatment with spiramycin during pregnancy for the prevention of severe fetal abnormalities. Spiramycin is a macrolide antibiotic that is active against *T gondii* in animal experiments. It does not consistently cross the placenta; therefore, therapeutic benefits are attributed to its action within the placenta. Spiramycin is readily available in most countries, but in the United States, it must be obtained from the Food and Drug Administration by special request. A 3-week course of spiramycin (2 to 3 g/d in four divided doses) repeated at 2-

week intervals until delivery resulted in significantly more normal children: 76% versus 44%, *P* less than .001. The addition of pyramethamine and a sulfonamide to the treatment regimen of a mother with a prenatal diagnosis of congenital infection may have a beneficial effect on fetal outcome, but additional data are needed before a recommendation for routine addition of these drugs can be made.

Evaluation of postnatal treatment of congenitally infected infants is difficult because of the variations in outcome of infection and disease associated with *Toxoplasma* infection. Postnatal treatment has no effect on the severe damage that has occurred before delivery, but it may prevent progression of disease and allow healing of tissues that are not irreversibly damaged. Long-term follow-up care is necessary because sequelae of congenital infection such as chorioretinitis may not appear for several years. The organism is never completely eradicated, and tissue cysts persist for life, especially in the eye and CNS. The incidence of late adverse sequelae may be reduced significantly in treated children; treatment is recommended for both asymptomatic as well as symptomatic children with a confirmed diagnosis of congenital *Toxoplasma* infection. The combination of pyramethamine and sulfadiazine is the preferred regimen because of synergism against *Toxoplasma* organisms. The usual dose of pyramethamine is 1 mg/kg/day in two divided doses administered daily initially but decreased to 3-day intervals because the half-life of the drug is 4 or 5 days. For infants with severe disease, a daily loading dose of 2 mg/kg/day for the first 2 or 3 days may be beneficial. Sulfadiazine or trisulfapyrimidines, 50 to 100 mg/kg/day, are given in two divided doses. Sulfisoxazole should not be used because it is less effective in in vitro studies. Folinic acid, 5 mg twice a week, is also administered because pyramethamine is a potent folic acid antagonist.

The optimal duration of therapy has not been established. Infants with proven congenital infection should receive an initial 21-day course of pyramethamine, sulfadiazine, and folinic acid followed by a 4- to 6-week course of spiramycin, 100 mg/kg/day in two to three divided doses. No additional therapy is given for infants whose mothers acquired primary *Toxoplasma* infection during pregnancy but do not have serologic evidence of congenital infection. Infants with confirmed congenital infection should receive alternating courses of these two regimens for the remainder of the first year of life. In the presence of active inflammation (*eg,* chorioretinitis, CSF protein ≥100 mg/dL), the addition of prednisone, 1 to 2 mg/kg/day, may be beneficial. The prednisone is tapered after the active inflammation has resolved. Spiramycin alone may be considered as initial therapy for infants whose mothers have serologic evidence of infection but the date of infection is unknown; therapy is discontinued when congenital infection is ruled out serologically.

Infants with congenital toxoplasmosis must be followed for several years to detect reactivation and evaluate the extent of neurologic and developmental sequelae.

■ PREVENTION

Prevention of primary infection during pregnancy is the most effective means of protecting the unborn infant. Several practices are effective measures for the susceptible pregnant woman. Meat should be frozen at −20°C (−4°F) or cooked at 60°C (140°F) before eating. Hands should be washed after handling uncooked meat. Fruits and vegetables should be washed before eating. Cat feces should be avoided, and gloves should be worn when handling cat litter boxes. Cat litter boxes should be disinfected daily with boiling water left in place for 5 minutes. Boxes should be cleaned by someone other than the pregnant woman.

Serologic screening of women before pregnancy or early in pregnancy may be a cost-effective means of prevention in areas of the world with high rates of congenital toxoplasmosis. When primary infection occurs, interruption of pregnancy or treatment of the pregnant women with spiramycin or the combination of pyramethamine and sulfadiazine should be considered.

HEPATITIS VIRUSES

■ HEPATITIS A

Maternal infection with hepatitis A virus (HAV) in early pregnancy may result, on rare occasions, in prematurity and spontaneous abortion. It has not been associated with increased rates of congenital malformation or intrauterine growth retardation. Pregnant women with HAV hepatitis generally do not transmit the infection to their offspring because the associated viremia is transient and low grade.

These infants, however, are at risk of acquiring infection during delivery if the mother has jaundice or had acute hepatitis within the prior 2 weeks. Most infected infants are asymptomatic and exhibit only mild elevations in transaminase levels. Rarely does nausea, vomiting, anorexia, fever, jaundice, and dark urine occur in infancy. Detection of anti-HAV IgM acutely and persistence of anti-HAV IgG beyond 1 year of age are diagnostic of neonatal infection. Because

transmission of hepatitis A to the neonate is rare, routine serologic studies are not recommended for the asymptomatic infant. It is recommended, however, that exposed infants receive 0.02 mL/kg of immune globulin as soon as possible after delivery. The infant is potentially infectious for 6 weeks and is maintained in enteric isolation if hospitalized during this period. Strict handwashing when handling soiled diapers is stressed. Although nosocomial transmission of hepatitis A is not common, a multinursery outbreak of hepatitis A from exposure to asymptomatically infected premature infants has been described. Hepatitis A rarely is transmitted to neonates by transfusion of blood products obtained from an asymptomatic donor during the transient viremic phase of hepatitis A infection. A live, attenuated hepatitis A virus vaccine has been developed and is being evaluated in clinical trials.

■ HEPATITIS B

Hepatitis B virus (HBV) is a 42-nm, double-shelled DNA virus. The inner core consists of hepatitis B core antigen, hepatitis B e antigen (HBeAg), DNA, and DNA polymerase. The outer shell is composed of hepatitis B surface antigen (HBsAg). In about 5% to 10% of adults with acute HBV hepatitis, a chronic HBsAg carrier state develops. HBeAg is found in the serum of some individuals who are HBsAg-positive. Ninety percent of infants delivered of women who are positive for both HBsAg and HBeAg become infected. If the HBsAg-positive mother is HBeAg-negative or has antibody to HBeAg, only 25% or 12% of infants, respectively, become infected.

Vertical transmission of HBV occurs when the mother has acute hepatitis B during the third trimester or within the first 2 postpartum months, or if the mother is a chronic HBsAg carrier. About 5% of neonatal hepatitis B infection is transmitted transplacentally, presumably as a result of leakage of infected maternal blood into fetal circulation. HBV infection is not associated with congenital defects or fetal malformations. Ninety-five percent of neonatal infections occur at the time of delivery from the infant's exposure to infected maternal blood or cervical and vaginal secretions. If perinatal infection does not occur, the infant may be at risk for subsequent infection from close contact with household members who are infected or who are chronic carriers.

Neonatal infection usually is asymptomatic with only mild elevation of transaminase levels, although chronic active hepatitis B with or without cirrhosis, chronic persistent hepatitis, and fatal fulminant hepatitis can occur. Infected infants usually do not become HBsAg-positive until several weeks after birth. About 90% of infants infected perinatally become chronic HBV carriers, and one in four infants who become chronic carriers develops cirrhosis or hepatocellular carcinoma. There is a 275-fold increase in the risk of developing hepatocellular carcinoma during the third and fourth decades in chronic carriers. This risk is greatest for carriers who acquired the infection perinatally.

Effective prophylaxis of HBV infection has been possible since licensure of the first hepatitis B virus vaccine in 1982. Both the highly purified vaccine prepared from human plasma (Heptavax B, licensed but no longer produced in the United States) and the recombinant DNA vaccines (Recombivax-HB, Engerix-B) are safe, are highly immunogenic in neonates, and have an efficacy of about 90%. The Centers for Disease Control and Prevention (CDC) suggests that universal screening of all pregnant women for HBsAg is cost-effective and is the most suitable strategy for control of perinatal HBV transmission. Prenatal questioning designed to identify women in high-risk groups in urban populations fails to detect about 50% of those who are HBsAg-positive. Moreover, prenatal screening allows prompt institution of neonatal prophylaxis after delivery and minimizes risk of delivery room attendants' exposure to the mother's infective blood and body fluids.

The CDC recommends a combination of passive immunization with hepatitis B immune globulin (HBIG) and active immunization with hepatitis B virus vaccine for all newborns whose mothers are HBsAg-positive, regardless of the HBeAg or anti-HBe status. HBIG (0.5 mL) is administered intramuscularly as soon as possible after delivery, preferably within 12 hours. HBIG efficacy decreases markedly if treatment is delayed beyond 48 hours. Hepatitis B virus vaccine is administered intramuscularly at a separate site at birth or within 7 days, and administration is repeated at 1 and 6 months after the first dose. HBsAg may be detected for 24 hours after a dose of vaccine. An HBsAg-positive result at any other time indicates a vaccine failure, and the infant should not receive additional doses of HBIG or vaccine. Testing for HBsAg and measurement of anti-HBs are recommended at 9 months of age or later to determine the efficacy of therapy. The presence of anti-HBs indicates successful prophylaxis and immunization. Although the efficacy of booster doses in infants is not known, infants who are negative for anti-HBs and HBsAg should receive another dose of vaccine and be retested. Protection from immunization persists for at least 5 years. Household members and sexual contacts of HBsAg-positive mothers should be screened, and, if no evidence exists of previous HBV infection, they should also be immunized.

Infants delivered by HBsAg-positive women are bathed as soon as possible after delivery to remove all maternal blood and secretions. Intramuscular injections should be delayed until bathing is completed. These infants are placed on blood and body fluid precautions. Those infants who remain in the hospital and later require surgical procedures should be tested for HBsAg. Infants who have received both active and passive prophylaxis may be breast-fed.

Both the American Academy of Pediatrics and the CDC have recommended universal immunization of all infants with hepatitis B virus vaccine in an effort to control hepatitis B virus infections. The first dose of hepatitis B virus vaccine should be administered to newborns before hospital discharge, the second dose at 1 to 2 months of age, and the third dose at 6 to 18 months of age. An alternative schedule of the three doses administered at 2, 4, and 6 to 18 months concurrently with other routine vaccines, may be used for HBsAg-negative infants not vaccinated at birth. For premature infants and ill infants in the first few days of life, hepatitis B virus vaccine may be delayed until hospital discharge, if the mother is not HBsAg-positive.

■ DELTA HEPATITIS

Hepatitis D virus (delta virus) is a 35- to 37-nm RNA virus with an internal protein antigen (delta antigen) coated with HBsAg. Because it requires HBV for replication, hepatitis D may occur as a coinfection with acute HBV hepatitis or as a superinfection of an HBsAg carrier. The route of transmission is similar to HBV. It is diagnosed by detection of delta antigen in serum during acute infection and by the appearance of delta antibody. Vertical transmission has been reported, but the risks to the infant are undefined. Infants who become HBsAg carriers as a result of perinatal infection are also at risk of delta infection. No product is available to prevent delta infection in HBsAg carriers either before or after exposure.

■ HEPATITIS C

Most cases of non-A, non-B (NANB) hepatitis recently have been attributed to hepatitis C virus (HCV) infection. HCV is a single-stranded RNA virus closely linked to the family of *Flaviviridae,* which includes the arboviruses of yellow fever and Dengue fever. Seroepidemiologic studies show that approximately 1% of volunteer blood donors screen positive for anti-HCV antibody. Transmission of HCV occurs after transfusion of infected blood products, intravenous drug use, sexual intercourse, occupational injury with blood-contaminated needles, and human bites. Intrafamilial transmission also has been documented. Because about half of all cases of HCV infection have no identifiable risk factor, other modes of transmission seem to exist. Perinatal transmission has been documented; although its frequency is not fully known, it may play a role in sustaining a reservoir of HCV infection in the general population. Studies also suggest that vertical transmission from an HCV-antibody–positive mother to her newborn infant may be enhanced by the presence of maternal and infant coinfection with the human immunodeficiency virus.

Infants born to HCV-antibody–positive mothers should have serial measurements of serum alanine aminotransferase levels and HCV antibody for at least the first 15 months of age. Tests for HCV antibody include ELISA and a recombinant immunoblot assay (RIBA), both of which measure IgG antibody to recombinant HCV antigens. A polymerase chain reaction assay has been developed for detection of viral RNA. Infected infants can develop a chronic hepatitis. In adults, half of all HCV infections appear to be chronic; in 20% of patients, the disease progresses to cirrhosis. Moreover, HCV is implicated as a cause of hepatocellular carcinoma. HCV infection may benefit from use of interferon alpha.

No preventive strategy is available. Immune serum globulin (0.06 mL/kg) may be useful in preventing HCV infection after accidental exposure to blood from a patient with hepatitis C, but efficacy has not been established, and its use for prevention of vertical transmission is not routinely recommended.

Transmission of NANB hepatitis by blood transfusion may be prevented by screening donors for antibody to HCV, elevated serum alanine aminotransferase levels, and antibody to the hepatitis B core antigen.

■ HEPATITIS E (EPIDEMIC OR ENTERICALLY TRANSMITTED NON-A, NON-B HEPATITIS)

Another agent has been described in waterborne epidemics of NANB hepatitis in several areas of Southeast Asia, North Africa, and Mexico. The viral agent appears to be a small RNA virus of the family calcivirus with similar characteristics of the picornaviridae, which include enterovirus type 72, the hepatitis A virus. Transmission occurs by the fecal–oral route similarly to that of hepatitis A. Epidemic NANB hepatitis occurs more frequently during pregnancy, particularly in the second and third trimester according to research by Khuroo and coworkers (1981). The attack rate in the first, second, and third trimesters is reported to be 9%, 19%, and 19%, respectively, with an overall rate of 17% during pregnancy. This statistic compares to a rate of only 2% in similarly exposed men and nonpregnant women of child-bearing age. Pregnant women with acute epidemic NANB hepatitis in the third trimester are also at higher risk for developing fulminant hepatic failure, which is associated with a case-fatality rate as high as 75%.

No serologic test has been developed. Prophylactic therapy with immune serum globulin has not been shown to be effective. The only preventive measures available are good sanitation and avoiding ingestion of potentially contaminated food and water.

NEISSERIA GONORRHOEAE

The prevalence of gonococcal infection during pregnancy varies from 0.6% to 7.6%. The highest rates are found in single, low-income, nonwhite women younger than 30 years old. Gonococcal infection during pregnancy has been associated with septic abortion, chorioamnionitis, premature rupture of membranes, delayed delivery after rupture of membranes, and premature delivery.

■ TRANSMISSION

Transmission of *Neisseria gonorrhoeae* to the newborn infant can occur in utero, during delivery, or after birth. In utero acquisition occurs via an ascending route after rupture of amniotic membranes. More commonly, neonatal infection occurs at delivery from passage through an infected birth canal. About 30% of infants born vaginally to infected mothers become colonized with *N gonorrhoeae*. Horizontal transmission via fomites and by nursery personnel also is documented.

■ CLINICAL MANIFESTATIONS AND DIAGNOSIS

Conjunctivitis is the most frequently observed clinical manifestation of gonococcal infection in newborns. Although *Chlamydia trachomatis* is the most common cause of ophthalmia neonatorum, *N gonorrhoeae* is important because it can cause severe eye damage. Gonococcal conjunctivitis typically appears 2 to 5 days after birth and produces an acute, purulent, bilateral conjunctivitis with lid edema and chemosis. If treatment is delayed, the cornea may ulcerate and scar with loss of visual acuity. Ultimately, the eye may perforate, resulting in panophthalmitis and loss of the eye. Presumptive diagnosis of gonococcal conjunctivitis may be made by Gram stain of the conjunctival exudate, which demonstrates gram-negative intracellular diplococci. The diagnosis must be confirmed by isolation of the organism on selective media, especially because *Moraxella catarrhalis* has a similar appearance on Gram stain. Other bacterial pathogens associated with conjunctivitis in the neonate that may be visualized on Gram stain are *Haemophilus* spp, *Staphylococcus aureus*, enterococcus, and *Streptococcus pneumoniae*. *Pseudomonas aeruginosa* may cause conjunctivitis with severe complications in debilitated neonates.

Not only the conjunctiva but also the pharynx, umbilicus, urethra, vagina, and rectum can serve as a focus of local or disseminated disease. Disseminated infection is usually manifested by septicemia, meningitis, or septic arthritis that typically involves multiple joints. Cutaneous gonococcal lesions in infants are rare, but gonococcal scalp abscess at the site of previous placement of a scalp electrode has been described.

■ TREATMENT

Infants with gonococcal ophthalmia should be hospitalized and placed in contact isolation for 24 hours after initiation of parenteral antibiotic therapy. Because of the increased incidence of both penicillinase-producing and chromosomally mediated resistant strains of *N gonorrhoeae*, for empiric therapy the CDC recommends ceftriaxone administered intravenously or intramuscularly at a dosage of 50 mg/kg/day (maximum 125 mg). Laga and colleagues claim that a single dose of ceftriaxone may be sufficient, but therapy is usually continued for 5 to 7 days. Alternatively, cefotaxime can be used. Hourly irrigation of the infected eye with saline until the purulent discharge resolves is an important part of effective therapy. If the organism is susceptible to penicillin, aqueous crystalline penicillin G administered intravenously at a dosage of 100,000 U/kg/day in two to four divided doses also is effective. Duration of therapy is at least 7 days for disseminated infection and at least 10 days for meningitis.

All *N gonorrhoeae* isolates should be tested for β-lactamase production and for chromosomally mediated resistance, which occurs to penicillin, tetracycline, erythromycin, cephalosporins, spectinomycin, and other aminoglycosides. Identification of plasmid-mediated high-level tetracycline resistance (minimal inhibitory concentration greater than or equal to 16 μg/mL) is of epidemiologic importance because of the propensity of these resistant strains to acquire other resistance determinants. The prevalence of these strains in a community influences the choice of agent used for topical prophylaxis as well as for treatment of disease.

■ PREVENTION

Ophthalmic prophylaxis in the immediate postpartum period with either 1% silver nitrate, 0.5% erythromycin ointment, or 1% tetracycline ointment is effective in preventing gonococcal ophthalmia. Even with topical prophylaxis, some infants born to mothers with untreated gonococcal infection may develop gonococcal ophthalmia or disseminated disease. These infants should, therefore, receive a single intramuscular injection of ceftriaxone. If the isolate is known to be susceptible to penicillin, a single intramuscular injection of penicillin G (50,000 U for a full-term infant and 20,000 U for a low-birth-weight infant) may be administered. The optimal preventive measure is diagnosis and treatment of maternal gonococcal infection before delivery.

CHLAMYDIA TRACHOMATIS

Chlamydiae are bacteria that possess both RNA and DNA but are incapable of producing adenosine triphosphate outside of cells. Therefore, these organisms are obligate intracellular pathogens that require tissue culture cells for growth in the laboratory. Of the two species, *Chlamydia psittaci* and *Chlamydia trachomatis*, only the latter is a genital pathogen associated with neonatal infection. *C trachomatis* has 15 serotypes divided into two groups: oculogenital serovars A to K and lymphogranuloma serovars L-1 to L-3. Oculogenital serovars are divided into trachoma serovars A to C, which cause hyperendemic blinding trachoma in the Far East, and genital serovars D to K, which result in genital neonatal infections.

The rate of cervical colonization with *C trachomatis* during pregnancy varies from 2% to 37%. The highest rates are found in young, unmarried, nonwhite women of lower socioeconomic status. Chlamydial infection during pregnancy is usually asymptomatic. Pregnant women with cervical chlamydial infection who have IgM antibody against *C trachomatis*, however, may be at increased risk for premature rupture of amniotic membranes and delivery of low-birth-weight infants.

■ TRANSMISSION

Chlamydial infection of the newborn infant occurs most often at delivery, secondary to passage through an infected cervix. Neonatal infection after delivery by cesarean section reflects an ascending route of infection. Transplacental transmission is doubtful because *C trachomatis* is not associated with abnormalities present at birth that are characteristic of other congenital infections, and IgM antibody directed against *C trachomatis* has not been detected in umbilical cord blood.

About two thirds of infants delivered vaginally by mothers colonized with *C trachomatis* develop IgM antibody or exhibit a persistence or rise in IgG antibodies to *C trachomatis* beyond 9 to 12 months of age. About 28% to 66% of exposed infants are colonized in the conjunctivae, 15% to 20% in the nasopharynx or throat, 8% to 14% in the vagina, and 14% to 20% in the rectum. Initial colonization with *C trachomatis* occurs in the conjunctiva and pharynx, and the rectum and vagina usually become colonized in the second through sixth months of life. Of infants colonized with *C trachomatis*, 50% to 75% develop conjunctivitis, and 11% to 29% develop pneumonia.

■ CLINICAL MANIFESTATIONS

Conjunctivitis

C trachomatis is the most common cause of ophthalmia neonatorum in developed countries where it causes 13% to 74% (mean, 29%) of neonatal conjunctivitis. Onset is usually 5 to 14 days after birth. Clinical illness ranges from a mild mucoid discharge in the medial canthus without significant conjunctival erythema to a profuse, purulent bilateral discharge with lid edema, severe chemosis, and edematous, friable conjunctivae. In the most severe cases, the clinical findings are indistinguishable from those associated with *Neisseria gonorrhoeae*. Subconjunctival lymphoid hypertrophy and follicular conjunctivitis rarely occur in the neonatal period. Some 19% to 83% of infants with conjunctivitis have nasopharyngeal carriage of *C trachomatis* when first examined.

Gram stain examination of the ocular discharge reveals both polymorphonuclear leukocytes and mononuclear cells. A Giemsa stain examination of a conjunctival scraping that contains a large number of epithelial cells detects chlamydial inclusions in the cytoplasm of the epithelial cells in 50% to 90% of cases.

Untreated chlamydial conjunctivitis resolves spontaneously after several weeks to months. Ocular carriage of the organism may persist for 2½ years. Occasionally, chlamydial conjunctivitis results in mild conjunctival scars with punctate keratitis and micropannus. Normal visual acuity is preserved in most cases.

Pneumonia

C trachomatis accounts for 15% to 73% of afebrile pneumonia in infants 3 to 11 weeks of age. There is often a history of conjunctivitis or mucoid rhinorrhea, followed by gradually worsening tachypnea and a characteristic staccato cough. Most infants are afebrile or have mild temperature elevations. Infants may present with apnea in the absence of other signs of respiratory involvement, or they may develop apnea during the course of the pneumonia. Auscultation of the chest reveals diffuse rales with few wheezes. Hyperexpansion and diffuse bilateral interstitial or alveolar infiltrates are present on chest roentgenogram. Lobar consolidation and pleural effusion are unusual. Blood gas values typically show mild hypoxia but not CO_2 retention. Total leukocyte count is usually normal, but 50% to 70% of infants have eosinophil counts greater than $300/mm^3$. Serum levels of IgM, IgG, and IgA are usually elevated. Untreated infants gradually improve after 5 to 7 weeks of illness. About half of affected infants will have middle ear abnormalities, with *C trachomatis* isolated from some middle ear aspirates.

Chlamydial pneumonia in premature infants may be severe and require mechanical ventilatory support resulting in chronic lung disease. Children hospitalized for chlamydial pneumonia in early infancy have an increased risk of developing long-term pulmonary sequelae such as asthma, chronic cough, and abnormal pulmonary function tests.

The clinical significance of vaginal and rectal colonization with *C trachomatis* in infancy remains unknown. Nasopharyngeal colonization is associated with rhinitis and nasopharyngitis with nasal congestion without rhinorrhea lasting for weeks or months. Chlamydia is an uncommon cause of myocarditis and otitis media.

■ DIAGNOSIS

Diagnosis of chlamydial infection is confirmed by inoculation of McCoy cells in tissue culture with conjunctival or nasopharyngeal scrapings and by demonstration of the characteristic intracytoplasmic inclusions after several days of incubation. Conjunctivitis is diagnosed by sampling the inflamed lower conjunctiva, not the purulent drainage, because the organism resides within the epithelial cells of the conjunctiva. Diagnosis of chlamydial pneumonia is based on a typical clinical syndrome and demonstration of *C trachomatis* in specimens obtained from the nasopharynx or endotracheal aspiration. Chlamydia also may be identified in lung tissue and pleural fluid.

Rapid detection tests of chlamydial antigen in clinical specimens are available for routine use. A monoclonal antibody directed against chlamydial elementary bodies in a direct immunofluorescent stain of clinical specimens has shown a sensitivity and specificity of 100% in chlamydial conjunctivitis. In nasopharyngeal specimens, however, the sensitivity is only 85% and the specificity, 75%. A second method is an enzyme-linked immunoassay that is semiautomatic and demonstrates sensitivity of 93% and specificity of 97% in examination of conjunctival smears.

Serologic evaluation is not useful in the diagnosis of chlamydial conjunctivitis because most infants do not develop IgM antibodies, and their antichlamydia IgG is of maternal origin. When pneumonia is present, however, measurement of antichlamydia IgM titer is preferred over nasopharyngeal culture for the diagnosis of chlamydial pneumonia because it is always elevated when clinical disease is apparent.

■ TREATMENT

The recommended treatment for both chlamydial conjunctivitis and pneumonia is a 2-week course of either erythromycin estolate (10 mg/kg every 8 hours) or erythromycin ethylsuccinate (10 mg/kg every 6 hours) administered orally. The advantage of orally administered erythromycin over topical antibiotic containing ophthalmic solutions or ointments is the eradication of *C trachomatis* from the nasopharynx in infants. A shorter clinical course with lower relapse rates after oral therapy for conjunctivitis has been observed. Topical therapy in addition to oral erythromycin is not necessary because therapeutic levels of the drug are achieved in tears after oral administration. Treatment of the mother and her sexual partner with erythromycin, tetracycline, or doxycycline for 7 days is recommended at the time of diagnosis of the infant's infection. One gram of azithromycin as a single oral dose has been found effective for treatment of chlamydial infection in adults.

■ PREVENTION

Ophthalmic prophylaxis at birth with 1% silver nitrate, 0.5% erythromycin ointment, or 1% tetracycline ointment does not prevent chlamydial conjunctivitis. Identification and treatment of pregnant women colonized with *C trachomatis* and their sexual partners with erythromycin (tetracycline or doxycycline for the partner) is the most efficacious method of preventing infection and disease in neonates.

GENITAL MYCOPLASMAS

The genital mycoplasmas consist of *Mycoplasma hominis*, *Mycoplasma fermentans*, *Mycoplasma genitalium*, and *Ureaplasma urealyticum* (T-strain mycoplasma). Only *M hominis* and *U urealyticum* are clinically significant. Mycoplasmas are pleomorphic organisms that lack a cell wall. Serologic studies demonstrate 7 serotypes of *M hominis* and at least 14 serotypes of *U urealyticum*. *M hominis* and *U urealyticum* are sexually transmitted organisms accounting for female urogenital colonization rates of 20% to 30% and 60% to 80%, respectively. Although both organisms are associated with a variety of adverse pregnancy outcomes, convincing evidence exists only for their association with histologic chorioamnionitis and with postpartum fever and endometritis.

■ TRANSMISSION

The rate of vertical transmission of *U urealyticum* is 45% to 65% in full-term and 59% in preterm infants. Similar data are lacking for *M hominis*. Vertical transmission of mycoplasmas occurs in utero or during delivery. In utero transmission occurs either transplacentally or by an ascending route from a colonized maternal genital tract. Mycoplasmas have been isolated from maternal blood at the time of delivery and from amniotic fluid, endometrium, placenta, and aborted fetal tissue. Mycoplasmas also have been isolated from mucosal surfaces of newborn infants delivered by cesarean section performed before the onset of labor and rupture of amniotic membranes. More commonly, however, acquisition of mycoplasmas by newborn infants occurs at delivery through contact with a colonized birth canal. Colonization of newborn infants increases with decreasing gestational age and birth weight. Postpartum or nosocomial transmission in neonates is not well documented, but probably occurs.

■ CLINICAL MANIFESTATIONS

The role of these organisms in neonatal disease is being defined. *M hominis* and *U urealyticum* have been recovered from the lungs, brain, heart, and viscera of aborted fetuses and stillborn infants with histologic finding of bronchopneumonia present in the lungs of these fetuses. The genital mycoplasmas also have been isolated from blood, urine, CSF, and lung tissue of newborn infants with clinical signs of infection. The following clinical associations with *U urealyticum* have been made: fatal neonatal pneumonia in a term infant documented by isolation of the organism from lung at autopsy and demon-

stration of elevated serum IgG and IgM titers to *U urealyticum* in the infant; pneumonia and persistent pulmonary hypertension in five infants from whom *U urealyticum* was isolated from blood, endotracheal aspirate, pleural fluid, or lung at autopsy; afebrile pneumonitis in infants younger than 3 months of age; development of chronic lung disease in low-birth-weight infants whose respiratory tracts are colonized with *U urealyticum* in the first week of life; isolation of *U urealyticum* from lung biopsy tissue of four infants with chronic lung disease; and isolation of *U urealyticum* from CSF of both preterm and full-term infants.

Isolation of *U urealyticum* and *M hominis* from the CSF of predominantly preterm infants with suspected meningitis is associated with CSF pleocytosis consisting of a polymorphonuclear or mononuclear cellular response, hypoglycorrhachia, and elevated protein content. Sequelae of meningitis due to *U urealyticum* and *M hominis* include hemiplegia, hydrocephalus, and developmental delay. The isolation of *U urealyticum* from CSF in preterm infants is associated with severe intraventricular hemorrhage. Among full-term infants, isolation of *U urealyticum* and *M hominis* is associated with minimal, if any, CSF abnormalities.

Other manifestations of infection with *M hominis* are brain and scalp abscess, ventriculitis, submandibular adenitis, conjunctivitis, and pericardial effusion. Clinical significance of the isolation of genital mycoplasmas from urine obtained by suprapubic bladder aspiration in infants is undetermined.

■ DIAGNOSIS

Genital mycoplasmas may be isolated on special broth and solid media that are commercially available. *M hominis*, but not *U urealyticum*, may be presumptively identified on blood agar as tiny pinpoint colonies.

The diagnosis of mycoplasmal infection is made by isolation of the organism from a normally sterile body fluid or suppurative focus. Because colonization of newborn infants with mycoplasmas occurs frequently, an etiologic role for these agents cannot be supported by isolation from mucosal surfaces only. Serologic tests used to measure antibody to genital mycoplasmas include modified metabolic inhibition test, mycoplasmacidal test, indirect hemagglutination, indirect immunofluorescent test, ELISA, and immunoblotting. Use of these tests for diagnosis of mycoplasmal infection in infants is problematic and not well established.

■ TREATMENT

Mycoplasmas are not susceptible to antimicrobial agents routinely used to treat neonatal infections. Because mycoplasmas lack a cell wall, they are insensitive to penicillins, cephalosporins, polymyxins, and vancomycin. Although they may have moderate sensitivity to aminoglycosides, the minimum inhibitory concentrations of these agents for the genital mycoplasmas are usually too high for therapeutic use. The drugs of choice for treatment of infection due to *M hominis* are chloramphenicol, clindamycin, doxycycline, and tetracycline; for treatment of ureaplasmal infections, erythromycin, doxycycline, tetracycline, and chloramphenicol are the drugs of choice. *M hominis* is resistant to erythromycin. Antibiotic susceptibility testing should be performed on all clinically significant isolates because multiple-drug resistance occurs.

(Abridged from Pablo J. Sanchez and Jane D. Siegel, Congenital and Perinatal Infections, in Oski, DeAngelis, Feigin, McMillan, Warshaw: *Principles and Practice of Pediatrics, Second Edition*, J.B. Lippincott, 1994.)

Oski's Essential Pediatrics,
edited by Kevin B. Johnson and Frank A. Oski.
Lippincott–Raven Publishers,
Philadelphia © 1997

60

Rhinoviruses

Rhinoviruses (RVs) cause about 30% to 50% of all acute respiratory illness. RV infections are found in varying degrees year-round but show the greatest incidence from spring through early fall. This seasonal pattern occurs worldwide.

Schoolchildren are the most important reservoir of RVs; the highest rate of transmission occurs at home and school. Dissemination within susceptible family members averages about 50%, and within a schoolroom ranges from 0% to 50%.

■ CLINICAL MANIFESTATIONS

RV infections in any age group usually cause only mild respiratory tract illnesses (*ie,* common colds with simple coryza). Complete recovery usually occurs in a week or two. It has been shown since the discovery of the first RV serotypes, however, that these viruses can cause serious lower respiratory illness, especially in young children.

RVs are important precipitants of "wheezy bronchitis" or "infectious asthma." It appears that RVs may be the most important cause of asthma attacks in children older than 1 to 2 years, but respiratory syncytial virus (RSV) is most important in the first year of life.

RVs are implicated in cases of bronchiolitis, pneumonia, chronic bronchitis, sinusitis, and acute otitis media. Although acute otitis media is primarily a bacterial disease, it is often preceded or accompanied by a viral upper respiratory illness.

■ DIAGNOSIS

RV infections cause such a wide spectrum of respiratory illness that it is not possible to diagnose them clinically. RV infections can be isolated year-round, but there is a seasonal pattern of infection recognized internationally; many mild to moderate respiratory infections of the spring-summer-fall months are caused by RVs. Nasal specimens are superior to throat swabs for RV isolation. No methods exist for rapid diagnosis of RV infection.

■ PREVENTION AND THERAPY

Because there are 101 serotypes, a conventional vaccine seems unlikely. Several drugs, including alpha interferon, are under investigation as a preventative. Overall, there is no clear indication for any therapeutic modality (including vitamin C and zinc), although a few trials in 1987 demonstrated an improvement in signs and symptoms of patients infected with one serotype of RV.

(Abridged from Dick EC, Byers RL, Rhinoviruses, in Oski, DeAngelis, Feigin, McMillan, Warshaw: *Principles and Practice of Pediatrics, Second Edition,* J.B. Lippincott, 1994.)

Oski's Essential Pediatrics,
edited by Kevin B. Johnson and Frank A. Oski.
Lippincott–Raven Publishers,
Philadelphia © 1997

61

Adenoviruses

■ ADENOVIRAL DISORDERS

Adenoviruses are DNA viruses that cause a diverse array of diseases; serologic surveys indicate that these viruses are responsible for 10% of respiratory infections in children. Rarely, adenoviruses cause common colds. Usually, respiratory infections with adenoviruses are characterized by fever and pharyngitis. Symptoms that occur with acute adenoviral pharyngitis include malaise, headache, sore throat, cough, cervical adenopathy, abdominal pain, and rhinitis, especially in the young. Pharyngeal exudates may be thin and spotty or thick and membranous. Laryngotracheitis, bronchitis, pneumonia, and, rarely, bronchiolitis may occur concomitantly with pharyngeal disease. Illness of 5 to 7 days is common, although symptoms may persist for 2 weeks.

Pulmonary infection with adenoviruses can be severe, especially in infants, toddlers, and immunocompromised patients. High fever, dyspnea, wheezes, and rhonchi are present in these cases, and radiographs may reveal diffuse infiltrates, hyperinflation, lobar atelectasis, and, rarely, pleural effusions. Associated symptoms may include seizures, lethargy, vomiting, diarrhea, and conjunctivitis. Manifestations of extrapulmonary involvement may be present, including meningitis, encephalitis, hepatitis, myocarditis, nephritis, and exanthems. Severe infections result in bronchiectasis, bronchiolitis obliterans, and hyperlucent lung.

Pertussislike Syndrome

Adenoviral infections occasionally are associated with illness characterized by paroxysmal cough with associated post-tussive whoop, vomiting, apnea or hypoxemia, and lymphocytosis. The illness often begins with mild coryza without fever. Convalescence occurs usually in 1 to 3 months. Recent studies suggest that some of these pertussislike illnesses are *Bordetella pertussis* infections in which the adenovirus is a coinfecting agent.

Pharyngoconjunctival Fever

The constellation of acute fever, conjunctivitis, coryza, pharyngitis, and cervical adenitis occurring historically in summer epidemics, usually associated with inadequately chlorinated swimming pools, can be ascribed with some certainty to adenoviral infection. Both the bulbar and palpebral conjunctivae are involved. The palpebral conjunctiva may have a granular appearance. Initially, disease may be monocular, although the unaffected eye usually becomes involved. Bacterial superinfection of the conjunctiva is rare and resolution is complete.

Epidemic Keratoconjunctivitis

A number of adenoviruses have been found to cause epidemics of keratoconjunctivitis, commonly type 8, although more recently type 37 as well. Adenoviral kerato-conjunctivitis is nonseasonal, primarily affects adults, and is transmitted by fomites, ophthalmic instruments and solutions, and bodies of fresh water. After 4 days to 2 weeks of incubation, a follicular conjunctivitis develops with symptoms of lacrimation, photophobia, and foreign-body sensation. Hyperemia and edema of the conjunctiva are present, and preauricular adenopathy is common. About half of affected persons have rhinitis and pharyngitis. Keratitis with punctate epithelial and sometimes subepithelial lesions develop as the conjunctivitis resolves. Visual disturbances may occur and persist for several years. Similar epidemics of keratoconjunctivitis associated with respiratory and constitutional symptoms have been described in infants and young children.

Genitourinary

Hemorrhagic cystitis due to adenovirus begins acutely with dysuria and frequency; hematuria develops within 24 hours. Occasionally, there is concomitant suprapubic pain, fever, or upper respiratory tract symptoms. Resolution occurs in several days to 2 weeks and appears to be complete. This illness is not seasonal. Boys are affected more frequently than girls.

Nephritis has been reported in cases of disseminated adenoviral infections and in rare instances with respiratory infections.

Gastrointestinal

The adenoviral types commonly associated with respiratory illnesses may also cause vomiting and diarrhea. Adenoviruses types 40 and 41 along with rotavirus are thought to cause most gastroenteritis in infants and young children. Watery diarrhea usually lasts 1 to 2 weeks and in the initial days may be associated with vomiting. Mild fever and, uncommonly, respiratory symptoms may occur with enteric adenoviral infections.

Mesenteric lymphadenitis with abdominal pain, fever, and other symptoms suggestive of appendicitis is associated with adenoviral infections. Hepatitis has been reported with adenoviral infection in infants, young children, and immunocompromised patients.

■ DIAGNOSIS

Differential diagnosis for adenoviral illnesses differs with various clinical manifestations. Pharyngoconjunctival fever and keratoconjunctivitis are often recognized as adenoviral infections based on clinical findings because of their characteristic symptom complex and epidemic nature. Adenoviral pharyngitis must be differentiated from streptococcal, Epstein-Barr, influenza, parainfluenza, and enteroviral infections. Adenoviral pneumonia may be clinically difficult to distinguish from illness caused by other viral and bacterial pathogens. Eye disease must be distinguished from herpes simplex virus keratitis and, in the neonate, from conjunctivitis due to *Neisseria gonorrhoeae* and *Chlamydia* spp. Bacterial and parasitic intestinal infections sometimes produce symptoms like those of adenoviral infections. Specific diagnosis commonly is achieved by tissue culture methods, specific antigen detection, or seroconversion.

■ TREATMENT

No specific treatment exists for adenoviral infections. The patient should be discouraged from strenuous activity, and supportive care should be given. Steroid treatment is to be avoided, and immunosuppressive regimens should be reduced or suspended. Steroid preparations should be administered carefully to patients with pneumonia and wheezing. Steroids may contribute to development of severe disease and may complicate recovery. Experimental treatment of severe adenoviral infections has included administration of immunoglobulins with high titers against the specific adenovirus.

(Abridged from Cherry JD, Frenkel LM, Adenoviruses, in Oski, DeAngelis, Feigin, McMillan, Warshaw: *Principles and Practice of Pediatrics, Second Edition*, J.B. Lippincott, 1994.)

Oski's Essential Pediatrics,
edited by Kevin B. Johnson and Frank A. Oski.
Lippincott–Raven Publishers,
Philadelphia © 1997

62

Influenza Viruses

Influenza viruses cause acute respiratory infections that usually occur in outbreaks or epidemics. In contrast to other respiratory viral infections that occur in outbreaks, acute febrile illnesses occur in both adults and children. Influenza viral infections in children are associated with considerable morbidity and mortality, and the spectrum of clinical illness is broad.

Influenza viruses are orthomyxoviruses. There are three major antigenic types—A, B, and C—and multiple antigenic subtypes.

Influenza is spread from person to person via the respiratory route. The most common mechanism is inhalation of large airborne particles produced by coughing and sneezing. Spread may also occur by direct or indirect contact with fine-particle aerosols.

■ CLINICAL MANIFESTATIONS

Clinical manifestations of influenza follow a short, 2- to 3-day incubation period. Although the predominant manifestations of influenza viral infections are respiratory, systemic complaints are an integral part of the illness. In general, the manifestations of influenza in children fall into two categories based on age. In school-age children and adolescents, the illness is similar to that which occurs in adults (classic influenza). Illness onset is abrupt with fever, facial flush, chills, headache, myalgia, and malaise. Temperature varies between 39°C (102.2°F) and 41°C (105.8°F) and is generally lower in older patients. Systemic complaints, on the other hand, are generally more severe in the older patient. Initially, dry cough and coryza occur, but these symptoms are of lesser concern to the patient than the severe systemic manifestations. About half of patients complain of sore throat, which is associated with a nonexudative pharyngitis. Ocular symptoms are common and include tearing, photophobia, burning, and pain with eye movement. In uncomplicated illness, the fever lasts from 2 to 5 days. Occasionally, the temperature shows a biphasic pattern that may or may not be due to secondary bacterial complications.

The course of illness changes by day 2 to 4 of illness, when the respiratory symptoms become more prominent and the systemic complaints begin to subside. Major coughing—dry and hacking—usually persists for up to a week. Occasionally, coughing persists well after other symptoms have subsided. Influenza A and B infections are generally similar, although B viral infections may have more prominent nasal and eye complaints and fewer systemic findings such as dizziness and prostration than comparable influenza A illnesses. Although influenza C outbreaks are rarely discerned, illness due to this virus is indistinguishable from that due to A and B viral types.

The leukocyte count in uncomplicated influenza usually is normal, but frequently leukopenia (less than 4500 cells/mm^3) occurs. About one third of patients have a relative lymphopenia and one third have a relative neutropenia. In general, about 10% of older children have clinical signs and radiographic evidence of pulmonary involvement.

In younger children and infants, the manifestations of influenza viral infections frequently are similar to those of other common respiratory viral infections. Laryngotracheitis, bronchitis, bronchiolitis, and pneumonia all occur. Frequently, primary infection is an undifferentiated febrile upper respiratory illness. Temperature usually exceeds 39.5°C (103°F). Affected children appear mildly toxic and have cough, coryza, and irritability. On examination, pharyngitis is usually noted, and pulmonary involvement is common. Other findings include vomiting, diarrhea, otitis media, and fleeting erythematous or erythematous-maculopapular discrete rashes.

Acute laryngotracheitis due to influenza A virus is occasionally more severe than infection due to parainfluenza viruses. In neonates, influenza infection cannot be distinguished clinically from bacterial sepsis. Lethargy, poor feeding, petechiae, poor peripheral circulation with mottling of skin, and apneic spells all occur.

■ COMPLICATIONS

The most common complications of influenza are bacterial infections of the respiratory tract (pneumonia, otitis media, and sinusitis). Acute myositis is a particular complication of influenza B viral infections in children. It is characterized by severe pain and tenderness in the calves of both legs. Onset is sudden, and usually the affected child refuses to walk. Serum creatinine phosphokinase (CPK) and aspartate immunotransferase (SGOT) levels may be increased.

Although the pathogenesis is obscure, Reye's syndrome is a complication of both influenza A and B infections. Outbreaks of Reye's syndrome are related to epidemic activity of influenza.

Other rare complications of influenza viral infections include neurologic manifestations (encephalitis, Guillain-Barré syndrome, and transverse myelitis), pericarditis and myocarditis, and sudden death.

■ DIAGNOSIS

During outbreaks and epidemics, the clinical diagnosis of influenza can be made with some reliability. Important in the clinical diagnosis of influenza is the occurrence in the community of similar illness with fever in both adults and children.

The serologic diagnosis of influenza classically employs either complement fixation or hemagglutination-inhibition techniques. Complement fixation detects antibody against soluble nuclear protein antigens common to all strains of influenza A or B. Recently, the enzyme-linked immunosorbent assay (ELISA) has proved useful for the serologic diagnosis of influenza.

■ TREATMENT

Symptomatic treatment is the cornerstone of management and consists of rest, adequate hydration with oral fluids, control of fever and myalgia with acetaminophen, and maintenance of comfortable breathing by means of humidified air and, occasionally, nasal decongestants. Persistent irritative cough during convalescence often can be relieved with dextromethorphan or codeine.

The physician should be alert to the possibility of secondary bacterial infection. These infections are suggested by a prolonged febrile course or recrudescence of fever during early convalescence. Before antibiotic therapy is begun, the site of infection should be identified and appropriate cultures obtained. Most infections are caused by *Streptococcus pneumoniae*, *Haemophilus influenzae*, *Streptococcus pyogenes*, or, less commonly, *Staphylococcus aureus*.

The antiviral agent amantadine hydrochloride is active in vitro against influenza A viruses and has prophylactic and therapeutic benefits in adults. This drug also has a prophylactic effect in community-acquired influenza A in children, but few studies have considered its therapeutic efficacy in children. Nevertheless, it seems reasonable to administer amantadine therapeutically to severely ill, hospitalized children if the illness is likely to be caused by influenza A virus. Influenza B viruses are not susceptible to amantadine.

The broad-spectrum antiviral agent ribavirin also is effective in vitro against both influenza A and B viruses. Ribavirin given by aerosol has benefited adult patients with influenza A and B infections. Ribavirin is not approved for treatment of influenza in children.

■ PREVENTION

Inactivated influenza viral vaccines are safe and effective in preventing influenza if the antigens in the vaccine correlate with circulating influenza viruses. In general, routine immunization of normal children or adults is not recommended. Vaccine is recommended for children at high risk for complications. Specifically, this includes children with cardiovascular disorders such as rheumatic, congenital, or hypertensive heart disease; chronic bronchopulmonary disease such as tuberculosis, cystic fibrosis, asthma, and bronchiectasis; chronic metabolic diseases such as diabetes; chronic glomerulonephritis; and chronic neurologic disorders in which there is weakness or paralysis of respiratory muscles.

(Abridged from James D. Cherry, Influenza Viruses, in Oski, DeAngelis, Feigin, McMillan, Warshaw: *Principles and Practice of Pediatrics, Second Edition*, J.B. Lippincott, 1994.)

Oski's Essential Pediatrics,
edited by Kevin B. Johnson and Frank A. Oski.
Lippincott–Raven Publishers,
Philadelphia © 1997

63

Parainfluenza Viruses

Parainfluenza viruses are second only to respiratory syncytial virus as a cause of significant morbidity and mortality due to respiratory illnesses in infancy. Each of the four types of parainfluenza viruses cause specific diseases, usually during specific seasons.

■ CLINICAL MANIFESTATIONS

Clinical manifestations directly reflect the sites of infection. Type 1 parainfluenza virus causes mild upper respiratory illness but is the virus most commonly associated with croup, accounting for 20% to 40% of cases. The older child or adult experiences laryngitis. Disease due to type 2 parainfluenza virus is generally mild and confined to large airways. Type 3 parainfluenza virus causes disease that varies from symptoms of a common cold to fatal pneumonia. It ranks second to respiratory syncytial virus as a cause of bronchiolitis and bronchopneumonia in infants. Children with immunodeficiency syndromes are prone to severe, sometimes fatal, pneumonitis. Infection of the pericardium and brain also has been described.

LARYNGOTRACHEITIS

■ CLINICAL MANIFESTATIONS

Acute laryngotracheitis and laryngotracheobronchitis are the most common significant illnesses caused by the parainfluenza viruses. Laryngotracheitis accounts for about 15% of respiratory tract infections below the level of the pharynx in children. Laryngotracheitis occurs in children of all age groups and is noted throughout the year. Initial symptoms are nasal stuffiness and sore throat. Fever ranging from 37.8°C to 40°C (100°F to 104°F) follows within 24 hours, then a barking cough becomes the predominant symptom. For most patients, the illness progresses no further and symptoms abate over 3 to 5 days. Occasionally within hours, but usually more gradually, upper airway obstruction progresses in some patients and stridor appears. On examination, the child has hoarseness, coryza, and supraclavicular and substernal retractions. Position has no effect on the degree of obstruction. Examination of the pharynx discloses minimal erythema. If infection causes laryngotracheobronchitis or laryngotracheopneumonitis, the respiratory rate is elevated and the child can have a prolonged expiratory phase and wheezing in addition to inspiratory stridor. In severe disease, progressive obstruction leads to hypoxia, restlessness, and cyanosis.

Laryngotracheitis of viral etiology must be differentiated from other causes of severe upper airway compromise. These distinctions are made on clinical grounds with skillful, unobtrusive examinations and with selective roentgenographic and laboratory tests. The clinical characteristics of infectious causes of upper airway obstruction are listed in Table 63–1.

■ TREATMENT

Fewer than 10% of children with acute viral laryngotracheitis require hospitalization, fewer than 10% of these hospitalized children require tracheal intubation, and fewer than 1% of these hospitalized children die. Therapy is primarily supportive.

Nebulized racemic epinephrine has short-term beneficial effect and is used as an interim measure in hospitalized patients with severe airway obstruction. Outpatients with laryngotracheitis should not be given racemic epinephrine because of the short-lived effect and the potential for a more severe rebound effect.

TABLE 63-1. Clinical Characteristics of Infectious Causes of Upper Airway Obstruction

	Epiglottitis	Laryngotracheitis	Bacterial Tracheitis	Retropharyngeal Abscess
Peak age	2–7 yr	7–36 mo	7–36 mo	3–24 mo
Prodrome	None to nonspecific URI	Coryza, cough	Coryza, cough	Nonspecific URI
Onset of fever	Sudden, high	Gradual, variable	Variable, frequently with sudden high rise	Sudden, high
Striking feature	Stridor	Stridor/cough	Stridor	Drooling respiratory distress ± stridor
Other major symptoms:				
Hoarseness	–	+++	++	–
Cough	–	+++	++	–
Drooling	+++	–	+++	+++
Dysphagia	+++	±	±	+++
Major signs	Severe obstruction, toxicity	Obstruction, none to mild toxicity	Obstruction, toxicity	Toxicity, obstruction
Associated findings	Visibly swollen epiglottis	Rhinorrhea, mild pharyngitis	Rhinorrhea, mild pharyngitis	Rhinorrhea, bulging posterior pharynx
Preferred position	Sitting, sniffing	None	None	Hyperextension of neck

URI, *upper respiratory tract infection; ±, sometimes present; ++, frequently present; +++, hallmark of disease.*

Corticosteroid therapy is warranted in hospitalized patients with moderately severe obstruction. Valid interpretation of studies has been hampered by variabilities in populations, degree of obstruction, etiology of obstruction (*eg*, spasmodic croup), agents and dosages, and the small size of studies. Rapidly progressive viral pneumonia concurrent with steroid therapy is reported.

(Abridged from Sarah S. Long, Parainfluenza Viruses, in Oski, DeAngelis, Feigin, McMillan, Warshaw: *Principles and Practice of Pediatrics, Second Edition*, J.B. Lippincott, 1994.)

Oski's Essential Pediatrics,
edited by Kevin B. Johnson and Frank A. Oski.
Lippincott–Raven Publishers,
Philadelphia © 1997

64

Respiratory Syncytial Virus

Respiratory syncytial virus (RSV) is by far the most important lower respiratory tract pathogen of early life, accounting for the most hospitalizations for acute respiratory disease in children younger than 2 years old and for the most fatal outcomes. The annual health care costs of disease due to RSV are estimated to be close to $400 million.

Infection with RSV is an inescapable feature of infancy. In the Houston Family Study, infection rate was 69 per 100 children in the first year of life and 83 per 100 children in the second year of life. Rates of infection, severe disease manifestations, and mortality are highest at age 2 to 6 months in lower socioeconomic groups.

Epidemic disease, easily recognized as outbreaks of bronchiolitis, occurs annually in midwinter to spring peaks (December through April) with virtual absence of RSV activity from August through October.

Transmission is by infected nasal secretions. Hand transmission of secretions and fomites from infected persons to the nasal or conjunctival mucosa of the recipient is far more important than airborne transmission. The hospital, its patients, and staff are major vectors in the transmission of RSV.

■ CLINICAL MANIFESTATIONS

Clinical illnesses caused by RSV infection include nonspecific upper respiratory illness, acute otitis media, laryngotracheobronchitis, bronchiolitis, and pneumonitis. Forty percent of infected children younger than 2 years of age have involvement of the lower respiratory tract.

Bronchiolitis

Bronchiolitis is the most commonly diagnosed illness due to RSV and is almost exclusively confined to children younger than 2 years old. It is a clinical state of acute infection due to RSV (and less commonly to other viruses) in which obstruction of small airways is the predominant feature.

Clinical Presentation

The incubation period is 4 to 7 days. Rhinorrhea is the usual initial event, followed by fever in at least 50% of cases, irritability, poor feeding, and cough. Cough progresses over 3 to 5 days, wheezing occurs, and dyspnea ensues. Very young infants and premature infants are more likely to have lethargy, apnea, and increased requirements for oxygen if on ventilators. Respiratory distress is the reason for hospitalization of most infants; approximately 20% have cyanosis. Otitis media, pharyngeal hyperemia, and conjunctivitis can be present. Hyperinflation of the lungs pushes the liver and spleen into palpable positions in the abdomen.

Laboratory Findings

Abnormalities in the peripheral white blood cell (WBC) count are so variable as to be of little use. The chest radiograph universally demonstrates overaerated lungs with an increased anteroposterior diameter of the chest, flattened or everted diaphragms, a more horizontal position of the ribs, and, sometimes, a diminished heart size. Peribronchial thickening is common. Overall, hyperaerated lung with areas of atelectatic lung is the radiographic hallmark of the disease. Peripheral interstitial infiltrates are less frequent. Lobar consolidation or pleural effusion is unusual.

Hypoxemia is common and is out of proportion to that expected from the degree of clinical illness. An increasing resting rate above 60 breaths per minute correlates very well with decreasing PaO_2. Fatigue results in retention of CO_2 and acidosis.

Apnea appears to occur during RSV bronchiolitis at an increased frequency. Apnea is occasionally the reason for hospitalization; almost invariably it disappears within 48 hours of hospitalization. Premature infants, very young infants, and those with a history of episodes of apnea are more prone to this event.

Virus is present in nasal secretions for 24 hours before the onset of symptoms and persists for 4 to 21 days after hospitalization. Laboratory confirmation of specific RSV etiology is useful and is enhanced by the availability of rapid diagnostic tests. Both enzyme-linked immunosorbent assay (ELISA) and a direct fluorescent antibody technique identify about 85% of cases subsequently confirmed by virus isolation.

The course of RSV disease is occasionally severe in normal children, but is predictably severe in those with congenital heart disease, especially when pulmonary hypertension exists. Mortality from RSV bronchiolitis in these patients is as high as 30%. Children with bronchopulmonary dysplasia, certain congenital anomalies, neuromuscular disorders, malnutrition, and congenital or acquired abnormalities of immunologic function also have excessive morbidity and mortality.

■ TREATMENT

The administration of oxygen and delivery of general supportive care are the cornerstones of treatment for RSV bronchiolitis. Severity of an episode can be assessed using blood gas values or pulse oximetry if measurements are required frequently.

Ribavirin is a synthetic nucleoside analogue that is licensed for use in the treatment of RSV bronchiolitis. The spectrum of antiviral activity is broad and includes parainfluenza, influenza, and adenoviruses, as well as RSV. Aerosol is given by hood, tent, or nasotracheal tube for 12 to 20 hours out of 24 hours. Teratogenicity was noted when ribavirin was given orally to pregnant rodents for 2 weeks, but this finding has not been duplicated in primates.

In patients with bronchiolitis proved or highly suspected to be caused by RSV, the following groups should be considered for ribavirin therapy: infants with congenital heart disease, infants with bronchopulmonary dysplasia or other chronic lung disease, certain premature infants (*eg*, those of postconception age less than 34 weeks and those with a history of apnea), infants with congenital or acquired immune deficiency syndrome as well as older children with disease- or drug-associated immunosuppression, infants with severe illness (*eg*, PaO$_2$ less than 65 mm Hg, increasing PaCO$_2$, or respiratory rate above 60 breaths/minute), and very young infants (less than 6 weeks old).

Other therapy that should be considered includes humidification and oxygen, and adrenergic bronchodilators (although there is controversy about their efficacy.) Corticosteroids have not been shown to be beneficial for the treatment of bronchiolitis.

Outcome

An estimated 1% of patients hospitalized for bronchiolitis die. This relatively high mortality is a reflection of the number of infections in patients with underlying risk factors for severe disease and of the inability to provide antiviral therapy and assisted ventilation.

■ PREVENTION

The importance of contact with infected nasal or conjunctival secretions in the transmission of RSV and the importance of handwashing to interrupt transmission cannot be overstressed.

(Abridged from Sarah S. Long, Respiratory Syncytial Virus, in Oski, DeAngelis, Feigin, McMillan, Warshaw: *Principles and Practice of Pediatrics, Second Edition*, J.B. Lippincott, 1994.)

Oski's Essential Pediatrics,
edited by Kevin B. Johnson and Frank A. Oski.
Lippincott–Raven Publishers,
Philadelphia © 1997

65

Parvoviruses

Parvoviruses infect and cause disease in a great variety of insects and animals. The human parvovirus B19 was serendipitously discovered in 1975 and found to be associated with human disease in the early 1980s. B19 virus is the cause of erythema infectiosum (fifth disease) and transient red blood cell aplasia (aplastic crisis).

■ PARVOVIRAL DISORDERS

Erythema Infectiosum

Although erythema infectiosum is recognized classically by its distinct rash, recent studies in volunteers suggest a biphasic illness. Approximately 1 week after infection, there is a nonspecific febrile illness with headache, chills, malaise, and myalgia. These symptoms last 2 to 3 days, followed by an asymptomatic interlude of about 7 days, then the exanthematous phase of the illness. The exanthem occurs in three stages. The first stage is the appearance of a fiery red rash on the cheeks ("slapped-cheek" appearance) and a relative circumoral pallor. The facial appearance is suggestive of scarlet fever, an allergic reaction, or collagen vascular disease. The facial exanthem may be accentuated when the affected person moves from outdoors to a warm room.

The second stage follows the onset of facial involvement by 1 to 4 days as an erythematous maculopapular rash on the trunk and extremities. Initially, this rash is discrete, but soon it takes on a characteristic lacy or reticular pattern.

The third stage of the exanthem is characterized by changes in the intensity of the rash with periodic evanescence and recrudescence. The duration of the third stage is highly variable; fluctuations are related to environmental factors such as exposure to sunlight and temperature.

The rash is often pruritic, especially in adults, and is generally more prominent on the extensor surfaces. Occasionally, slight desquamation is noted in some patients.

Other symptoms and signs are uncommon in erythema infectiosum. Headache occurs in about one fifth of affected children and one half of affected adults. Enanthem is rare, although children occasionally have pharyngitis. Joint pain and swelling and myalgia are particularly troublesome in adults.

Arthritis

The most common complication of erythema infectiosum is arthritis. It occurs in 80% or more of affected adults but in less than 10% of children with erythema infectiosum. The illness ranges in severity from mild arthralgia to frank arthritis. Joint involvement is usually transient, lasting only a few days, but in some adults these symptoms may persist for weeks or, rarely, months. Arthritis is more common in women than in men and most often involves the knees, ankles, and proximal interpharyngeal joints; involvement is usually bilateral. The onset of arthritis usually occurs 1 to 6 days after the onset of the rash, but occasionally it has been noted before the exanthem. Many adults have arthritis without skin manifestations of infection.

Aplastic Crisis

In individuals with hemolytic anemias, the profound reticulocytopenia associated with acute B19 virus infection may result in critical depression of hemoglobin concentrations. This transitory arrest of erythrocyte production is termed *aplastic crisis* and can occur in any individual whose erythrocytes have a short lifespan. Individuals at risk for aplastic crisis with acute B19 virus infections include those with sickle cell anemia, hereditary spherocytosis, thalassemia, pyruvate kinase deficiency, and acquired hemolytic anemias.

In association with aplastic crisis, most patients have fever, malaise, and gastrointestinal symptoms; some also have respiratory symptoms. Typical erythema infectiosum is rare.

Laboratory studies in afflicted patients reveal reticulocyte counts between 0% and 1% and hemoglobin values 10% to 30% below baseline values. Occasionally, lymphocytosis, eosinophilia, and neutropenia are noted.

Intrauterine Infection

Infection in pregnancy results in fetal hydrops, fetal death, and miscarriage. Recent studies indicate that maternal B19 virus infection results in a transplacental transmission rate of 33% and a fetal death rate of 9%.

■ DIAGNOSIS

The exanthem of erythema infectiosum is characteristic, so the diagnosis is easy during epidemics. Sporadic cases can be a problem because rubella, scarlet fever, and enteroviral infections can be confused with erythema infectiosum. Other differential diagnostic considerations are collagen vascular diseases, drug reactions, and allergic responses to environmental substances.

The specific diagnosis of a B19 viral infection can be made by demonstrating B19-specific IgM antibody in the serum of ill or convalescing individuals via enzyme-linked immunosorbent assay (ELISA), radioimmunoassay, or immunofluorescence.

■ TREATMENT AND PREVENTION

There is no specific treatment for B19 viral infections. Pregnant women should, when possible, avoid contact with susceptible school-age children, because of the risk of hydrops fetalis due to parvovirus B19 infection.

(Abridged from James D. Cherry, Parvoviruses, in Oski, DeAngelis, Feigin, McMillan, Warshaw: *Principles and Practice of Pediatrics, Second Edition,* J.B. Lippincott, 1994.)

Oski's Essential Pediatrics,
edited by Kevin B. Johnson and Frank A. Oski.
Lippincott–Raven Publishers,
Philadelphia © 1997

66

Polioviruses

Polioviruses are a subgroup of the enteroviruses. They are single-stranded RNA viruses with three distinct antigenic types. Infection with a poliovirus results in lifelong immunity to the homologous virus type but confers no immunity to the other two viral types.

■ CLINICAL FINDINGS

In susceptible persons, 90% to 95% of infections are inapparent, about 4% to 8% are classified as minor illness (abortive poliomyelitis), and rarely does nonparalytic poliomyelitis (aseptic meningitis) or paralytic poliomyelitis develop. In general, older persons are more likely to have severe paralytic disease and higher mortality. Bulbar poliomyelitis may be precipitated by tonsillectomy at the time of inapparent infection; a history of tonsillectomy is also related to a higher rate of bulbar disease.

Nonparalytic Poliomyelitis (Aseptic Meningitis)

Nonparalytic poliomyelitis is similar to aseptic meningitis caused by many other enteroviruses. Initially, illness is characterized by nonspecific fever, malaise, and headache. Other complaints are anorexia, nausea, vomiting, constipation, and diarrhea. Fever is usually moderate (37.8°C to 39.5°C [100°F to 103°F]), and there is usually aching of muscles. Soon thereafter, the neck, back, and hamstrings become stiff, and sometimes there is hyperesthesia and paresthesia. Occasionally, the illness is biphasic with an initial phase (minor illness) consisting of fever and nonspecific complaints and a second phase (central nervous system [CNS] or major illness) with symptoms that indicate CNS involvement.

On physical examination, there are nuchal-spinal signs. For example, when sitting, the patient uses his hands in a tripod supporting position, indicative of spinal rigidity. Nuchal rigidity can be noted by asking the patient to flex the chin to the chest. Kernig's and Brudzinski's signs are usually positive. In nonparalytic poliomyelitis, the reflexes are usually normal. It is important to observe the reflexes over time, however, because changes may indicate impending paralysis. The white blood cell count is usually normal or slightly elevated. The cerebrospinal fluid (CSF) cell count range usually varies from 20 to 300 cells/mm³. Although the differential cell count usually has a predominance of lymphocytes, greater than 50% polymorphonuclear leukocytes may be seen early in an illness. The CSF glucose level is usually normal, and the protein concentration is normal or slightly elevated. In the usual case, recovery occurs in 3 to 10 days.

Paralytic Poliomyelitis

The initial findings in paralytic poliomyelitis are similar to those in nonparalytic poliomyelitis, except, occasionally, findings are more pronounced. Fever is likely to be higher and muscle pain is more conspicuous. Before the onset of actual muscle weakness, superficial and deep tendon reflexes diminish or disappear.

The onset of paralysis may be sudden with complete loss of function within a few hours, or it may progress gradually over 3 to 5 days. Asymmetric involvement is typical, particularly in milder cases. About 20% of affected patients have bladder paralysis, which is temporary; paralytic ileus due to bowel atony is common in severe cases. In general, lower limbs are affected more commonly than upper limbs. Sensory abnormalities usually do not occur.

In bulbar disease, the 10th cranial nerve nuclei are most commonly involved, resulting in paralysis of the pharynx, soft palate, and vocal cord. Facial paralysis is less common, and ocular palsies are unusual. There is an encephalitic form of the disease characterized by irritability, disorientation, drowsiness, and coarse tremors. Hypoxia and hypercapnea resulting from respiratory insufficiency due to inadequate ventilation can produce disorientation without true encephalitis.

■ COMPLICATIONS

The most important complication of paralytic poliomyelitis is respiratory insufficiency due to inadequate ventilation. Myocardial failure sometimes occurs, either secondary to pulmonary complications or as a direct result of acute myocarditis. Not infrequently, patients who have had paralytic poliomyelitis develop what appear to be new neuromuscular symptoms later in life. The late-onset weakness and muscle atrophy are most likely the results of routine attrition of remaining anterior horn cells associated with aging rather than persistent neural infection with polioviruses.

■ DIAGNOSIS

If poliovirus infection is suspected, specimens for viral diagnostic studies should be obtained from the throat, stool, and CSF. All diagnostic virologic laboratories have the facilities to isolate polioviruses, and hospitals unequipped for virus isolation should refer specimens to regional laboratories.

Patients infected with polioviruses regularly develop neutralizing antibody to the type-specific virus. Therefore, the cause of the illness can be confirmed by examining acute and convalescent serum antibody titers to the three polioviral types. A fourfold rise in neutralizing antibody titer is indicative of infection. In acute illness, specific IgM neutralizing antibody for a specific poliovirus type is also diagnostic.

All patients with paralytic disease should be hospitalized. Impaired ventilation must be looked for and treated early. Constipation is a common complication and should be treated early to prevent fecal impaction. Consultation with other services (orthopedics and physiotherapy) should be obtained early in an illness so fixed deformities can be prevented.

(Abridged from James D. Cherry, Polioviruses, in Oski, DeAngelis, Feigin, McMillan, Warshaw: *Principles and Practice of Pediatrics, Second Edition*, J.B. Lippincott, 1994.)

Oski's Essential Pediatrics,
edited by Kevin B. Johnson and Frank A. Oski.
Lippincott–Raven Publishers,
Philadelphia © 1997

67

Nonpolio Enteroviruses

The nonpolio enteroviruses (coxsackieviruses, echoviruses, and enteroviruses) are responsible for significant and frequent human illness with protean clinical manifestations. The enteroviruses belong to the Picornaviridae (*pico*, small; *RNA*, ribonucleic acid); they are single-stranded RNA viruses.

■ CLINICAL FINDINGS

Nonpolio enteroviral infections are exceedingly common in the United States. Virtually all children have one or more infections each summer and fall. There are few specific enteroviral diseases but rather a variety of interrelated syndromes and anatomically associated illnesses.

Asymptomatic Infection

Historically, the finding of enteroviruses in the stool of healthy children led to the assumption that the majority of enteroviral infections were asymptomatic. This reasoning was in error, because enteroviruses may be excreted in stool for months after acute infection, and the finding of an enterovirus on a particular day is no indication of what happened when the infection first occurred. Although most enterovirus infections appear to go unrecognized, it is likely that most affected persons have some symptoms, but usually the illnesses are trivial. The available data suggest that, on average, 50% or fewer of all infections are asymptomatic.

Nonspecific Febrile Illness

Nonspecific febrile illness is the most common manifestation of nonpolio enteroviral infections. This illness usually has an abrupt onset without prodrome. In young children, frequently only fever and malaise are observed. In older children, headache may be noted. Fever usually lasts days and varies between 38.3°C (101°F) and 40°C (104°F). Occasionally, the fever is biphasic. Headache, malaise, and anorexia are generally related to the degree of fever. Additional findings in nonspecific febrile illness include mild nausea, vomiting, diarrhea, and abdominal discomfort. Older patients may complain of sore throat.

In general, the findings on physical examination are benign. The usual duration of illness is 3 to 4 days with extremes of 1 to 6 days.

Respiratory Manifestations

Respiratory manifestations are common in enteroviral infections. The most common manifestation is pharyngitis; in summer, nonpolio enteroviruses are the most common cause of this illness in children. Enteroviral pharyngitis is usually abrupt in onset. Although physical examination reveals pharyngitis early in infection, the symptoms in younger children often are not particularly referable to the throat. The usual initial complaint is fever, and young children may exhibit malaise and anorexia. Older children may complain of sore throat, headache, and myalgia. Mild vomiting or diarrhea also may occur.

Herpangina is a particular specific enteroviral pharyngitis. In addition to fever, children with herpangina have a characteristic enanthem. Vesicles and ulcers 1 to 2 mm in diameter appear on the anterior tonsillar pillars, soft palate, uvula, tonsils, pharyngeal wall, and occasionally on the posterior buccal surfaces. The lesions are usually discrete and average about five per patient. Some patients have only 1 or 2 lesions; others have 14 or more. The lesions are particularly characteristic when they occur on the soft palate. Early virologic studies indicated several coxsackieviruses A as the causative agents. Subsequent study indicated that in addition to coxsackieviruses A, most coxsackieviruses B and many echoviruses also cause herpangina.

The common respiratory viral illnesses of children that involve areas below the pharynx (croup, bronchitis, bronchiolitis, infectious asthma, pneumonia) may in sporadic instances be due to enteroviral infections. Except for pneumonia, these illnesses, when caused by enteroviruses, are generally more mild than their counterparts caused by typical respiratory viral agents.

A specific enteroviral illness of the respiratory tract is pleurodynia (Bornholm disease). Historically, pleurodynia was an epidemic disease with the majority of cases occurring in older children and young adults. Today in the United States, most cases occur sporadically and outbreaks are rare. Most cases in adults are probably diagnosed incorrectly. The onset of illness is characterized by sudden occurrence of pain typically located in the chest or upper abdomen. It is muscular in origin and of variable intensity. Often, the pain is excruciatingly severe and sudden and is associated with profuse sweating. The patient may appear pale, as though in shock. The pain events occur in spasms that last from a few minutes to several hours. During spasms, patients usually have rapid shallow and grunting respirations that suggest pneumonia or pleural inflammation. In older children and adults, the pain is often described as stabbing or knifelike; in adults, the illness can be confused with a heart attack. The symptoms usually last only 1 to 2 days, but frequently the illness is biphasic, so a patient apparently recovers only to have a recurrence several days later.

Gastrointestinal Manifestations

Gastrointestinal manifestations are almost universal in nonpolio enteroviral infections. Some manifestations such as nausea, vomiting, and diarrhea are very common but usually not severe and are only a part of a more general overall illness. On the other hand, abdominal pain may be a striking specific finding of enteroviral infections in young children.

Ocular Manifestations

Mild conjunctivitis occurs frequently in many enteroviral illnesses, but in these illnesses it is usually not troublesome. A specific acute hemorrhagic conjunctivitis, however, occurs in major epidemics. This illness is caused mainly by enterovirus 70 but has also been caused by coxsackievirus A24. During epidemics, the highest attack rate is in school-age children. The illness has a sudden onset with severe eye pain, photophobia, blurred vision, lacrimation, erythema and congestion of the eye, and edematous and chemotic lids. Subconjunctival hemorrhages occur, and transient punctate epithelial keratitis, conjunctival follicles, and preauricular lymphadenopathy are noted frequently. Systemic symptoms, including fever, are rare. The illness lasts 7 to 12 days. In a few cases, a paralytic illness that is poliomyelitislike or Guillain-Barré-like follows enterovirus 70 acute hemorrhagic conjunctivitis.

Cardiovascular Manifestations

Pericarditis and myocarditis are infrequent but important severe manifestations of nonpolio enteroviruses. The Group B coxsackieviruses have been most frequently implicated. Group B coxsackieviruses are also an etiologic factor in some cases of acute myocardial infarction in young adults.

Genitourinary Manifestations

Group B coxsackieviruses are second only to mumps as causative agents of orchitis. Orchitis frequently occurs as a second phase in a biphasic illness; the initial phase is usually nonspecific febrile illness, aseptic meningitis, or pleurodynia. Other rare genitourinary findings associated with nonpolio enterovirus infections are listed in Table 67–1.

Muscle and Joint Manifestations

After intraperitoneal inoculation of suckling mice, Group A coxsackieviruses routinely cause myositis; these viruses, therefore, have been candidates for muscle infection in humans. Although myalgia is a common complaint of illness due to nonpolio enteroviruses, myositis associated with human enteroviral infections has been documented only in persons with immunologic disorders. In particular, dermatomyositis-like syndromes due to echoviral infections have been noted in children with agammaglobulinemia.

Arthritis has occasionally been reported in association with enteroviral infections.

Skin Manifestations

The nonpolio enteroviruses cause a variety of skin manifestations. Specific exanthematous manifestations by frequency of viral type are listed in Table 67–2. In summer and fall, enteroviruses are the leading cause of exanthem in children.

Echovirus 9 is the agent most commonly associated with exanthem in children. This exanthem is erythematous, maculopapular, and usually discrete. Often it is petechial and is noted in association with aseptic meningitis. The illness mimics meningococcemia. Other enteroviruses cause petechial and purpuric rashes (see Table 67–2), and these can be confused with septicemic illnesses.

The hand, foot, and mouth syndrome, which is most commonly caused by coxsackievirus A16, is a clearly recognizable enteroviral illness. The exanthem is predominantly vesicular and located on the hands, feet, and buttocks. The enanthem usually involves the anterior mouth and consists of large ulcerative lesions.

Neurologic Manifestations

Neurologic illness is common in nonpolio enteroviral infections; aseptic meningitis is the most common (see Table 67–1). The most common causes of aseptic meningitis are coxsackieviruses A9, B2, B4, and B5 and echoviruses 4, 6, 9, 30, and 33.

Paralytic illness similar to that caused by polioviruses is also an occasional manifestation of the nonpolio enteroviruses. Paralysis due to the nonpolio enteroviruses is usually less severe and causes less residual damage. Recently, there have been outbreaks of illness due to enterovirus 71.

Neonatal Infections

Nonpolio enteroviral infections in neonates result in a wide variety of clinical manifestations. Although these neonatal infections may be mild, a significant number are particularly severe, and deaths are not uncommon. In particular, the infections may be generalized with both myocarditis and meningoencephalitis. Outbreaks have occurred in newborn nurseries.

Of particular importance is a sepsislike illness that can be the manifestation of several different nonpolio enteroviruses. This illness is characterized by fever, poor feeding, abdominal distention, irritability, rash, lethargy, and hypotonia. Patients also may have diarrhea, vomiting, seizures, and apnea. Severe fatal illness is most often due to echovirus 11. In fatal cases, jaundice, hepatitis, disseminated intravascular coagulation, thrombocytopenia, and hypotension occur.

■ DIAGNOSIS

Contrary to popular belief, many common enteroviruses grow rapidly in tissue culture, so isolation of an enterovirus as a cause of a specific illness frequently takes less than a week. The identification of an isolated enterovirus is more difficult and can take much longer.

■ THERAPY

There is no specific therapy for any nonpolio enteroviral infection. It has been shown recently that commercially available immune globulins contain antibodies to most enteroviruses. In severe catastrophic enteroviral infections such as those that occur in neonates, it is reasonable to

TABLE 67-1. Clinical Manifestations of Nonpolio Enteroviruses

Clinical Categories	Virus Types		
	Coxsackieviruses A	Coxsackieviruses B	Echoviruses and Enteroviruses
Nonspecific febrile illness	All types	All types	All types
Respiratory			
Common cold	Mainly 21, 24; rarely other types	Mainly 1–5; rarely 6	Mainly 2, 20; rarely other types
Pharyngitis (pharyngitis, tonsillitis, nasopharyngitis)	Probably all types; mainly 9	Probably all types, mainly 1–5	Probably all types; mainly 2, 4, 6, 9, 11, 16, 19, 25, 30, 71
Herpangina	1–10, 16, 22	1, 5	6, 9, 16, 17, 22, 25
Lymphonodular pharyngitis	10		
Stomatitis and other lesions in the anterior mouth	5, 9, 10, 16	2, 5	9, 11, 20, 71
Parotitis	Coxsackievirus A not typed	3, 4	70
Croup	9	4, 5	4, 11, 21
Bronchitis		1, 4	8, 12–14
Bronchiolitis and asthmatic bronchitis	Many types	Many types	Many types
Pneumonia	9, 16	1–5	6, 7, 9, 11, 12, 19, 20, 30
Pleurodynia	1, 2, 4, 6, 9, 16	1–6	1–3, 6–9, 11, 12, 14, 16–19, 23–25, 30
Gastrointestinal			
Nausea and vomiting	9, 16	2–5	2, 4, 6, 9, 11, 16, 18–20, 22, 30
Diarrhea	1, 9, 16	2–5	3, 4, 6, 7, 9, 11–14, 16–22, 25, 30
Constipation	9	3–5	4, 6, 9, 11
Abdominal pain	9, 16	2–5	4, 6, 9, 11, 18, 19, 30
Pseudoappendicitis			1, 8, 14
Peritonitis		1	
Mesenteric adenitis		5	7, 9, 11
Appendicitis		2, 5	
Intussusception		3	7, 9
Hepatitis	4, 9, 10, 20, 24	1–5	1, 3, 4, 6, 7, 9, 11, 14, 20, 21, 30, 72
Reye's syndrome	2	4	14, 22
Pancreatitis	9	3–5	
Diabetes mellitus		1–5	
Acute hemorrhagic conjunctivitis	24		70
Pericarditis and myocarditis	1, 2, 4, 5, 7–10, 16	1– 5	1, 4, 6–9, 11, 14, 17, 19, 22, 25, 30
Genitourinary			
Orchitis and epididymitis		1–5	6, 9, 11
Nephritis		4	6, 9
Hemolytic-uremic syndrome	4, 9	2–5	22
Pyuria, hematuria, or proteinuria		5	1, 6, 9
Myositis and arthritis	2, 9	4	9, 18, 24
Exanthem	2–5, 7, 9, 10, 16	1–5	1–7, 9, 11, 13, 14, 16–19, 21, 22, 24, 25, 30, 32, 33, 71
Neurologic manifestations			
Aseptic meningitis	1, 14, 16–18, 21, 22, 24	1–6	1–9, 11–27, 29–33, 71
Encephalitis	2, 4–7, 9, 10, 16	1–5	1–9, 11–25, 27, 30, 33, 71
Paralysis (lower motor neuron involvement)	2, 4–7, 9–11, 14, 21	1–6	1–4, 6–9, 11, 12, 14, 16–19, 25, 27, 30, 31, 70, 71
Guillain-Barré syndrome and transverse myelitis	2, 4–6, 9, 16	1–4	6, 7, 19, 22, 70
Cerebellar ataxia	4, 7, 9	3, 4	6, 9, 16
Peripheral neuritis			9

Modified with permission from Cherry JD. Enteroviruses. In: Nelson's textbook of pediatrics. 13th ed. Philadelphia: WB Saunders; 1987:689.

TABLE 67-2. Clinical Exanthematous Manifestations of Coxsackieviruses and Echoviruses

Clinical Feature	Virus Subgroup	Associated Viral Agents and Prevalence of Manifestation		
		Common	Occasional	Rare
Macular rash	Coxsackievirus A			
	B		1, 2, 5	
	Echovirus and enterovirus		2, 4, 5, 13, 14, 17, 19, 30	18, 71
Maculopapular rash	Coxsackievirus A	9	2, 4, 5, 10, 16	6, 7
	B		1–5	
	Echovirus and enterovirus	4, 9	2, 5–7, 11, 16–19, 25, 30, 71	1, 3, 13, 14, 22, 27, 33
Vesicular rash	Coxsackievirus A	5, 16	8, 10	4, 7
	B			1–3, 5
	Echovirus and enterovirus		11	6, 9, 17, 71
Petechial or purpuric rash	Coxsackievirus A	9	4	
	B		2–5	
	Echovirus	9	4, 7	3
Urticarial rash	Coxsackievirus A	9	16	
	B		4, 5	
	Echovirus		11	
Erythema multiforme or Stevens-Johnson syndrome	Coxsackievirus A		9	10, 16
	B			4, 5
	Echovirus			6, 11
Exanthem and meningitis	Coxsackievirus A		2, 9	7
	B	1, 2, 4, 5		
	Echovirus and enterovirus	4, 9	6, 11, 17, 18, 25, 30	3, 14, 33, 71
Exanthem and pneumonia	Coxsackievirus A		9	7
	B			1
	Echovirus			9, 11
Hand, foot, and mouth syndrome	Coxsackievirus A	16	5, 10	7, 9
	B			1, 3, 5
	Echovirus and enterovirus			71
Hemangioma-like lesions	Coxsackievirus A			
	B			
	Echovirus			25, 32
Herpangina and exanthem	Coxsackievirus A		4	9
	B			2
	Echovirus		16, 17	
Roseola-like illness	Coxsackievirus A			6, 9
	B		5	1, 2, 4
	Echovirus		16, 25	9, 11, 27, 30
Anaphylactoid purpura	Coxsackievirus A			4
	B			
	Echovirus			9, 18
Zoster-like rash	Coxsackievirus A			
	B			
	Echovirus			5, 6
Pityriasis-like rash	Coxsackievirus A			
	B			
	Echovirus			6
Chronic or recurrent rash	Coxsackievirus A	16		
	B			
	Echovirus			11

Cherry JD. Enteroviruses: polioviruses (poliomyelitis), coxsackieviruses, echoviruses. In: Feigin RD, Cherry JD, eds. Textbook of pediatric infectious diseases, 3rd ed. Philadelphia: WB Saunders; 1992:1720. Used with permission.

administer intravenous immune globulin to the infant, but there is no evidence that this therapy is beneficial. Immune globulin has a limited beneficial effect in the treatment of subacute and chronic enteroviral infections in patients with immune deficiencies.

(Abridged from James D. Cherry, Nonpolio Enteroviruses, in Oski, DeAngelis, Feigin, McMillan, Warshaw: *Principles and Practice of Pediatrics, Second Edition,* J.B. Lippincott, 1994.)

68

Infectious Mononucleosis

Although there are earlier accounts, the clinical entity of infectious mononucleosis was first clearly identified in the 1920s. However, it was not until 1968 that Epstein-Barr virus (EBV), an agent discovered a few years earlier in laboratory cultures of Burkitt lymphoma cells, was first identified as the cause of classic infectious mononucleosis.

■ CLINICAL MANIFESTATIONS

Acute symptomatic primary EBV infection is not synonymous with infectious mononucleosis unless a minimum of typical clinical, hematologic, and serologic findings is present. Clinical manifestations should include fever, malaise, cervical lymphadenitis, tonsillopharyngitis, and spleen or liver enlargement. Minimal hematologic features include a relative lymphocytosis of at least 50% and a relative atypical lymphocytosis of at least 10% of all leukocytes, or at least an absolute concentration of total lymphocytes of greater than or equal to 5000/mm³ or atypical lymphocytes greater than or equal to 1000/mm³. Serologic criterion is a characteristic heterophil antibody response or development of EBV-specific antibodies.

Figure 68–1 shows the spectrum of clinical manifestations of EBV infectious mononucleosis in children. Fever commonly lasts for 1 to 2 weeks. The enlarged lymph nodes are usually nontender or minimally tender and lack overlying skin erythema. The lymphadenopathy is located predominantly and most dramatically along both sides of the neck, less frequently in the axillae or other sites. Tonsillopharyngitis, another typical feature, is commonly associated with an exudate, even in very young patients. Children, especially young children, have a greater rate of "spontaneous" rashes, abdominal pain, and upper respiratory tract infections with the infectious mononucleosis episode than young adult patients. Yet, the correlation between administration of ampicillin and subsequent development of a skin rash as reported in adult patients may not be as apparent in children. Certain uncommon manifesta-

tions appear to be unique or more closely associated with childhood EBV infectious mononucleosis: failure to thrive, early-onset otitis media, and recurrent episodes of tonsillopharyngitis before or after the acute infectious mononucleosis episode.

■ GENERAL LABORATORY FINDINGS

Although a minimal quantity of atypical lymphocytes (discussed above) is essential for the diagnosis of infectious mononucleosis, the mean relative percentage of these cells in affected children, particularly those younger than 4 years old, tends to be lower than in young adult patients. The concomitant relative neutropenia seen acutely often is severe. In one report, a segmented band form count of less than 500/mm³ was detected in 10.6% of children younger than 4 years old and in 6.1% of older children. Serum transaminase levels are moderately elevated, although not usually above 600 U/dL, in at least 50% of children during an acute infectious mononucleosis episode. Jaundice, however, is rare.

■ COMPLICATIONS

Approximately one in five children (20%) with infectious mononucleosis develops one or more significant complications involving mainly the respiratory, neurologic, and hematologic systems (Table 68–1). Complications usually develop during or shortly after the peak of clinical illness. They may also develop during early convalescence or, as is not uncommon in the case of petechial rashes and neurologic signs, during the prodrome period. The complications characteristically last only days to a few weeks and rarely produce permanent sequelae. Splenic rupture has been noted in approximately 0.2% of adult patients; the incidence in children is not known.

■ LABORATORY DIAGNOSIS

Heterophil Antibodies

Heterophil antibodies are serum antibodies of the IgM class that can agglutinate sheep and horse erythrocytes, among others. Horse erythrocytes are the most sensitive agglutination indicators and are used in laboratory tests to

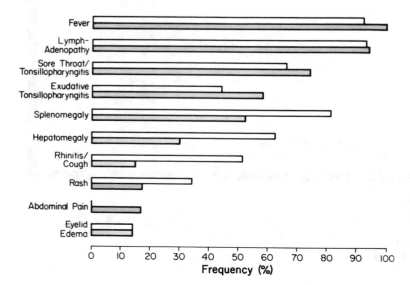

Figure 68-1. Frequency of clinical findings of infectious mononucleosis in two age groups less than 4 years old (open bars) and 4 to 16 years old (solid bars): (Sumaya CV, Ench Y. *Pediatrics* 1985;75:1003. Reproduced by permission of the American Academy of Pediatrics.)

TABLE 68-1. Complications Present in Childhood Epstein-Barr Virus Infectious Mononucleosis

Complication	No. of Children (%)
Respiratory tract	
Pneumonia	6 (5.3)
Severe airway obstruction*	4 (3.5)
Neurologic	
Seizures	4 (3.5)
Meningitis/encephalitis	2 (1.8)
Peripheral facial nerve paralysis	1 (0.9)
Guillain-Barré syndrome	1 (0.9)
Hematologic	
Thrombocytopenia with hemorrhages	4 (3.5)
Hemolytic anemia	1 (0.9)
Infectious	
Bacteremia	1 (0.9)
Recurrent tonsillopharyngitis	3 (2.7)
Liver: jaundice	2 (1.8)
Renal: glomerulonephritis	1 (0.9)
Genital: orchitis	1 (0.9)
TOTAL	31†

*Criteria consisted of nasal alar flaring, suprasternal retractions, or stridor.

†Because four children had more than one of these complications, this total is composed of 24 different children, or 21.2% of the study group.

Sumaya CV, Ench Y. Epstein-Barr virus infectious mononucleosis in children: I. Clinical and general laboratory findings. Pediatrics. 1985;75: 1003. Reproduced by permission of the American Academy of Pediatrics.

detect these antibodies. Heterophil antibodies associated with infectious mononucleosis are differentiated from heterophil antibodies associated with other illnesses by their absorption to beef red blood cells (RBCs) but not guinea pig kidney.

The rapid slide test, a qualitative test, is the most widely used method to detect serum heterophil antibodies of infectious mononucleosis.

In general, the serum heterophil antibody responses of children older than 4 years is similar to that of adults, whereas children younger than 4 years have appreciably lower rates of detectable heterophil antibody responses. In children younger than 4 years, the more sensitive quantitative Paul-Bunnel-Davidsohn test and possibly the immune adherence hemagglutination test are more reliable indicators of a heterophil antibody response than the rapid slide test.

EBV-Specific Serologic Testing

Distinct structural or viral-associated antigens—capsid antigen, early antigen, and nuclear antigen, among others—and their corresponding antibodies have been described. The pattern of these antibody responses is an important clue to the temporal onset of EBV infection and allows discrimination of acute, convalescent, or old infection.

In most cases, a single early serum sample obtained within 3 to 4 weeks, sometimes longer, after the clinical onset of the infectious mononucleosis episode reveals an IgM antibody response and other characteristic antibody responses that can be interpreted reliably to indicate an acute primary EBV infection (Table 68–2). If properly performed, detection of IgM antibody to EBV capsid antigen alone is probably sufficient to make an accurate diagnosis of an acute infection.

TABLE 68-2. Interpretation of EBV Serum Antibody Patterns

Interpretation	IgM Capsid Antigen	IgG Capsid Antigen	IgG Early Angigen D	IgG Early Angigen R	Antinuclear Antigen
Susceptible	−	−	−	−	−
Acute primary infection (IM presentation)	+	+	+	−*	−†
Acute primary infection (non-IM presentation or asymptomatic)	+	+	−	+	−†
Old, quiescent infection	−	+	−	−‡	+§
Reactivated infection	±	+	+ or +		+‖

*A few (<10%) adults and a greater number (10% to 20%) of children with acute IM develop an antibody response directed to R instead of D component.

†A low antibody titer (1.5 in our laboratory) may also be detected in acute infection.

‡Occasionally a weak, probably nonspecific, antibody response to R component is present.

§Moderate, stable titers of antibody should be present.

‖Stable levels of antibody, although in low or absent levels in immunosuppressed and immunodeficient patients, are present.

Sumaya CV, Epstein-Barr virus serologic testing: diagnostic indications and interpretations. Pediatr Infect Dis J 1986;5:337 Reproduced by permission of Williams & Wilkins Co.

In the absence of an IgM antibody response, a combination of other antibody responses (or lack thereof) may suggest, although not reliably, a recent infection. Testing a second serum sample 4 to 6 weeks after the first was collected during the acute phase of the illness is not of much diagnostic assistance. The titers of IgG antibody to EBV capsid antigen and early antigen usually peak in the early acute serum specimen. Therefore, it is too late to detect significant IgG antibody titer rises, a practice used to retrospectively diagnose recent infections by other viruses.

■ DIFFERENTIAL DIAGNOSIS

The classic presentation of infectious mononucleosis should not produce a diagnostic problem. Diagnostic difficulties may arise early in the clinical course, however, when few typical manifestations are apparent; when a principal typical feature is absent or extremely prominent; or when an organ or system that is uncommonly (or even commonly) affected shows extensive involvement.

Bacterial or viral tonsillopharyngitis is a frequently encountered differential diagnostic possibility. Group A *Streptococcus,* adenoviruses, and *Corynebacterium diphtheriae* may produce a severe tonsillopharyngitis, including an exudate, along with fever and cervical adenopathy—the clinical picture resembling that of EBV infectious mononucleosis. The absence of other typical features and the more transient course of the streptococcal (treated or untreated) or viral (non-EBV) induced tonsillopharyngitis should distinguish these entities from infectious mononucleosis.

Drug-induced hypersensitivity reactions from dilantin (phenyl-hydantoin derivatives) or isoniazid (INH), or serum sickness can produce a clinical picture similar to that of infectious mononucleosis. The lack of significant tonsillopharyngitis and an intense atypical lymphocytosis, or the pronounced migrating arthritis and eosinophilia seen in serum sickness, distinguish these disorders.

■ PROGNOSIS

Infectious mononucleosis is almost always a self-limited illness of several weeks' duration. Complications, if they occur, usually are transient and produce no permanent sequelae. Although an accurate figure for the mortality from infectious mononucleosis in either adults or children is not available, fatal cases appear to be rare.

In a few selected individuals, often with an underlying immunocompromised state, the infectious mononucleosis episode may be prolonged and lead to serious morbidity and death.

■ TREATMENT

Measures to alleviate symptoms remain the management of choice for children (and adults) with uncomplicated infectious mononucleosis. Reduction of activity and bed rest according to the tolerance of the patient usually are recommended. Contact sports should be avoided while the spleen is palpable (*ie,* clinically enlarged). Ampicillin should be avoided because of the potential development of an immunologically mediated rash, although the rash may not be as common a problem in children with infectious mononucleosis as in adults.

Life-threatening airway obstruction produced by significant tonsillopharyngeal and upper respiratory tract inflammation commonly is treated by insertion of an artificial airway rather than by emergency tonsillectomy as it was in the past. Nonoperative treatment of splenic rupture also has increased in recent years.

(Abridged from Ciro V. Sumaya, Infectious Mononucleosis, in Oski, DeAngelis, Feigin, McMillan, Warshaw: *Principles and Practice of Pediatrics, Second Edition,* J.B. Lippincott, 1994.)

Oski's Essential Pediatrics,
edited by Kevin B. Johnson and Frank A. Oski.
Lippincott–Raven Publishers,
Philadelphia © 1997

69

Postnatal Herpes Simplex Virus

■ THE VIRUS

Herpes simplex virus (HSV) is a moderately large DNA virus. Although highly infectious, HSV is not transmitted casually from person to person. Most infections do not cause significant or specific symptoms. The largest percentage of seropositive persons (although still harboring latent HSV) are unaware of having ever encountered these viruses. The spectrum of symptomatic HSV infections ranges from minor localized recurrences, usually at mucocutaneous junctions, to severe and even fatal illnesses.

■ SPECIFIC INFECTIONS

Gingivostomatitis

Gingivostomatitis is the most common form of HSV-induced primary illness seen in children. Symptomatic illness may occur in 30% or more of seropositive infants. It is usually seen in young children between 6 months and 3 years of age. Before age 6 months, the presence of residual maternal antibody probably modifies or prevents the appearance of recognizable symptoms in association with HSV infection.

The incubation period is a few days and the illness is ushered in by fretful behavior and fever. The infant usually refuses to eat and may even refuse fluids. Vesicular lesions appear on and around the lips, along the gingiva, on the anterior tongue, and on the anterior (hard) palate (Figure 69–1). Vesicles break down rapidly and lesions usually appear as 1- to 3-mm shallow gray ulcers on an erythematous base. The gums are generally mildly hypertrophic, ulcerated, and erythematous. They may appear friable and frequently bleed on contact. It is not uncommon for vesicles to extend about the lips and chin or down the neck in the immunologically normal child. The lesions bleed easily and may become covered with a black crust. Cervical and submental nodes are often swollen and tender. The process evolves for 4 to 5 days, and resolution requires at least an additional week. Autoinoculation may cause lesions on the hands (whitlow) and, less commonly, on the trunk or genital area.

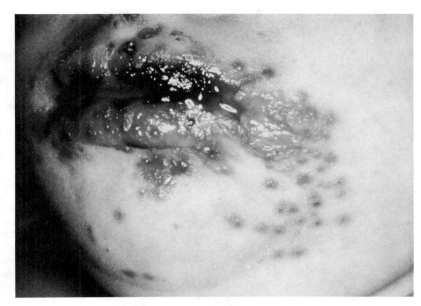

Figure 69-1. Primary herpes gingivostomatitis in a normal toddler at the ulcerative vesicular stage. (Kohl S. Postnatal herpes virus simplex infection. In: Feigin RD, Cherry JD, eds. *Textbook of pediatric infectious diseases*, 2nd ed. Philadelphia: WB Saunders, 1987:1577. Reproduced by permission.)

Herpes simplex virus gingivostomatitis is differentiated from herpangina, a manifestation of enteroviral infection, by the predominance of ulcers in the anterior and posterior portion of the oropharynx; herpangina is usually a posterior pharyngeal ulcerative condition. In addition, unlike HSV infection, herpangina often has a more acute onset, shorter duration, and seasonal occurrence.

In adolescents and especially in college-age patients, primary HSV infection often manifests as a posterior, occasionally exudative pharyngitis. The characteristic findings are shallow tonsillar ulcers with a gray exudate. In this setting, it must be differentiated from streptococcal, Epstein-Barr virus, adenovirus, and, rarely, diphtheria or tularemia-induced pharyngitis. In one study of college students of high socioeconomic status, HSV was the etiology of acute pharyngitis diagnosed most often (24%). This manifestation is most often due to HSV-1, although with the increasing frequency of oral–genital sexual practices among both heterosexual and homosexual individuals, HSV-2 pharyngitis is becoming more commonly encountered.

Vulvovaginitis

Primary herpetic vulvovaginitis may rarely occur in very young infants and children if HSV is introduced inadvertently when handling the genital area with contaminated hands. Moreover, genital herpes may reflect sexual abuse of young children. The occurrence of genital HSV in young children warrants a sensitive and careful appraisal of the family dynamics.

The incidence of genital infection in adolescents and young adults has increased markedly in the past two decades. There is a paucity of data on the incidence in children. Some 35% to 50% of patients with the first episode of genital herpes report a history of genital HSV in their contact. HSV-1 accounts for approximately 25% of primary genital HSV. The incubation period is 2 to 14 days. Primary illness is accompanied by fever, headache, malaise, and myalgias. Other systemic symptoms include an aseptic meningitis syndrome (11% to 35%). Although HSV-2 occasionally may be grown from the cerebrospinal fluid (CSF), aseptic meningitis syndrome differs from HSV-1 encephalitis in that it is generally mild, self-limited, and not associated with neurologic residua. Local genital symptoms include severe pain, itching, dysuria, vaginal or urethral discharge, and tender inguinal adenopathy. In primary illness, lesions begin as vesicles or pustules and progress to wet ulcers and then to healing ulcers with or without crusts. Crusts usually occur only on squamous epithelium. Lesions tend to last for 2 to 3 weeks before complete healing. Virus shedding occurs for a mean of 11½ days.

In addition to aseptic meningitis syndrome, complications of primary HSV genital infection include sacral autonomic nervous dysfunction manifested as poor rectal sphincter tone, constipation, sacral anesthesia, urinary retention, impotence, extragenital lesions, secondary yeast infections in women, and pharyngitis.

Beyond discomfort and embarrassment, the importance of HSV in the female genital tract relates to the potential impact of the virus on offspring, especially when a child is born to a mother with active genital lesions, particularly in connection with a primary maternal infection. In addition, although some individuals cope easily with the illness and the likelihood of recurrent disease, a sizable number exhibit profound depression, poor self-esteem, complete abstention from sexual activity, and general withdrawal. Self-help groups of individuals who have genital HSV are useful and are located in many cities of the United States.

Other Primary HSV Skin Infections

Virtually any part of the skin and mucous membranes may be involved in HSV infections. Altered skin often provides a portal of entry for HSV. Vesicular lesions spread throughout the affected skin, usually crusting and resolving in about 1 week. The illness accompanying eczema herpeticum can be severe and even fatal, although, in most cases, the infection resolves without specific therapy and leaves no sequelae (Figure 69–2). Herpetic whitlow is a painful, erythematous, swollen lesion occurring at a site of broken skin on the terminal phalanx of fingers (69%) and thumb (21%). Occasionally, the whitlow, which may persist for 7 to 10 days, initially is accompanied by a few vesicles that may give a clue to the etiology of the infection. It is important that the herpetic condition be diagnosed because

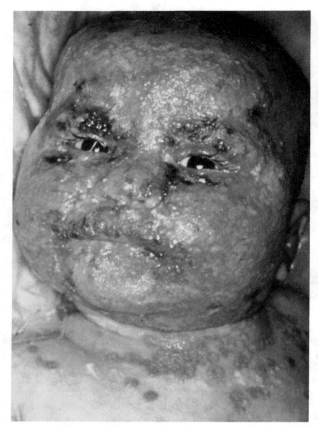

Figure 69-2. Extensive HSV infection in an infant with atopic eczema (Kaposi varicelliform eruption). (Kohl S. Postnatal herpes simplex virus infection. In: Feigin RD, Cherry JD, eds. *Textbook of pediatric infectious diseases*, 2nd ed. Philadelphia: WB Saunders, 1987:1577. Reproduced by permission.)

it usually is confused with a bacterial felon or paronychia and is incised and drained. This is not indicated in therapy of HSV whitlow. Only a needle aspiration and culture are necessary for diagnosis of herpetic whitlow. Appropriate infection control measures will lessen the spread of virus due to whitlows.

Primary HSV infection of the eye may manifest as a blepharitis or a follicular conjunctivitis, often accompanied by preauricular lymphadenopathy. If restricted to the conjunctiva, the infection, which can be accompanied by vesicular herpetic lesions elsewhere on the face or in the nose or mouth, usually resolves without sequelae. Herpetic infection of the eye may, however, progress to involve the cornea with more serious potential consequences. For this reason, an ophthalmologist should always examine and evaluate these cases.

The affected child complains of severe photophobia, blurred vision, chemosis, and lacrimation. Primary eye infection may include stromal involvement, uveitis, and rarely retinitis. Spontaneous healing, which generally requires 2 to 3 weeks, can be speeded by the use of topical therapy. Corticosteroids are contraindicated.

HSV Infections of the Central Nervous System

Herpes simplex virus is the most common identifiable cause of sporadic encephalitis and is usually very serious. It accounts for 2% to 5% of all cases of encephalitis in the

United States, but for up to 20% of all etiologic diagnoses (60% to 70% of cases of encephalitis remain without a diagnosis). The case-fatality rate associated with untreated HSV encephalitis is approximately 70%, and survivors generally exhibit considerable permanent neurologic disability. The spread of HSV-1 to the central nervous system (CNS) seems to proceed by way of neurogenic pathways. Although HSV encephalitis may involve virtually any area of the brain, it shows a striking tendency to involve the frontal and temporal lobes after the neonatal period.

It is important to differentiate the HSV-induced aseptic meningitis syndrome, usually due to HSV-2 and usually a complication of primary genital infection, from HSV encephalitis. In the former, signs of meningitis, including headache, photophobia, and stiff neck, appear shortly after genital lesions are noted. Seizures and focal CNS findings are usually absent. The CSF examination reveals a lymphocytosis (with 300 to 2600 white blood cells [WBCs] per cubic millimeter) and sometimes a low glucose level. This syndrome may recur with genital recurrences. Usually, there is complete recovery without specific therapy. HSV occasionally may be grown from the CSF.

HSV encephalitis, in contrast to meningitis, is a highly lethal disease. In 96% of cases, it is caused by HSV-1. It may be a result of primary (30%) or recurrent (70%) infection. A larger percentage of HSV encephalitis in younger individuals probably is due to primary infection. One third of cases occur in the pediatric age range. As in most manifestations of HSV infection, but unlike most other common forms of viral encephalitis (enterovirus, arbovirus), there is no seasonality to HSV encephalitis. It is an acute illness with fever, malaise, irritability, and nonspecific symptoms lasting 1 to 7 days, progressing to signs and symptoms of CNS involvement in 3 to 7 days, and finally to coma and death (Table 69–1). Fever and altered behavior in any child should evoke suspicion of encephalitis. Meningeal signs are uncommon. There is no correlation between the isolation of HSV from sites extrinsic to the CNS (such as the oropharynx or genital tract) and the diagnosis of HSV encephalitis. Thus, the presence of oral or genital lesions is of no help in the diagnosis or exclusion of HSV encephalitis. In recent studies, both identical and discordant viruses have been isolated from the brain and oral secretions.

The CSF generally reveals a pleocytosis with up to 2000 WBCs/mm^3, usually (80% of cases) greater than 50 WBCs/mm. In 90% of cases, more than 60% of cells are lymphocytes. Early in the infection, neutrophils may predominate. In 75% to 85% of cases, red blood cells (RBCs), reflecting the hemorrhagic necrosis, are seen in the CSF. Between 5% and 25% of patients have hypoglycorrhachia and 80% have elevated CSF protein levels (median, 80 mg/dL), which rise to striking levels with disease progression. The CSF is normal in 2% to 3% of patients with early HSV encephalitis. HSV almost never is grown from lumbar CSF and rarely from ventricular fluid. Thus, although the CSF examination is helpful, it is not diagnostic of HSV encephalitis unless polymerase chain reaction (PCR) is used to detect HSV DNA.

Neurodiagnostic tests are of limited use. Probably the most useful is electroencephalography (EEG). A "typical" pattern of unilateral or bilateral (poor prognosis) periodic focal spikes against a background of slow (flattened) activity (paroxysmal lateral epileptiform discharges, or PLEDs) is associated with HSV encephalitis. In 80% to 90% of patients, the EEG is not only abnormal but also localizing. Less helpful early in the illness is the brain scan or computed tomography (CT). An abnormal CT scan is a poor prognostic factor. Magnetic resonance imaging (MRI) seems to be an early sen-

TABLE 69-1. Historical and Clinical Findings in HSV Encephalitis

Historical Findings	%	Findings at Presentation	%
Alteration of consciousness	97	Fever	92
Fever	90	Personality changes	85
Personality changes	71	Dysphasia	76
Seizures	67	Autonomic dysfunction	60
Vomiting	46	Ataxia	40
Hemiparesis	33	Seizures	38
Memory loss	24	Focal	28
		Generalized	10
		Cranial nerve defects	32
		Visual field loss	14
		Papilledema	14

Kohl S. Postnatal herpes simplex infection. In: Feigin RD, Cherry JD, eds. Textbook of pediatric infectious diseases, *2nd ed. Philadelphia: WB Saunders; 1987:1577. Reproduced by permission.*

sitive test for localizing HSV encephalitis (Figure 69–3). It is probably the technique of choice for early diagnosis of HSV encephalitis. The finding of focal abnormality on EEG, MRI, CT, or radionuclide brain scan is significantly more likely to occur in HSV encephalitis than in other illnesses that are confused with it.

The clinical and laboratory data acquired by noninvasive methods are valuable only for increasing the index of suspicion for HSV encephalitis; they do not confirm the diagnosis. The differential diagnosis of this condition is relatively large and includes many treatable conditions (Table 69–2). Therefore, unless reliable HSV DNA detection by PCR is positive, a brain biopsy test is essential in patients with suspected HSV encephalitis, both to provide optimal aggressive therapy for that condition and to achieve a diagnosis for the 50% to 60% of patients without HSV infections, roughly one half of whom would benefit from other specific therapies.

The risk of brain biopsy test is low. In a national collaborative study of 182 biopsy tests, there were three complications—hemorrhage in two patients and herniation of brain tissue in a third. Roughly 3% of brain biopsies were false negative, usually due to biopsy of the wrong site.

Recurrent HSV Infections

All of the sites discussed in connection with primary HSV disease may also be involved in recurrent infections. HSV infection may occur without specific lesions. With the aid of cocultivation techniques, HSV has been recovered from dorsal root ganglia subserving the areas of skin in which individuals have experienced recurrent herpes lesions. HSV-1 has been found in trigeminal ganglia, and HSV-2 has been recovered from sacral ganglia. By in situ hybridization, HSV DNA also has been detected in ganglia. Concomitant infection of oral and genital sites by HSV is most likely to result in oral recurrences if type 1 and in genital recurrences if type 2 virus.

The most common manifestation of recurrent HSV infection is herpes labialis ("cold sores," "fever blisters"), which is estimated to occur in 25% to 50% of the general population. Most individuals experience a prodrome (pain,

burning, tingling, or itching) at the site lasting 6 hours to several days. There is then a progression from papules (lasting 12 to 36 hours) to vesicles (usually gone by 48 hours) to ulcers and crust (lasting 2 to 4 days). Most outbreaks are healed by 5 to 10 days. Most pain occurs during the vesicular stage. Virus is isolated readily from vesicles and less commonly from ulcers and crusts.

Recurrences tend to occur at the same location or closely related areas. In general, they occur on the lips, mucocutaneous junction, or other parts of the face. Recurrent lesions inside the mouth are rarely due to HSV and are more likely aphthous lesions. Intraoral HSV recurrences tend to occur on tissue adjacent to bone, such as the gums or palate, and not on the lips or buccal mucosa.

Recurrent genital HSV is probably the second most common manifestation of HSV and one of the most bothersome.

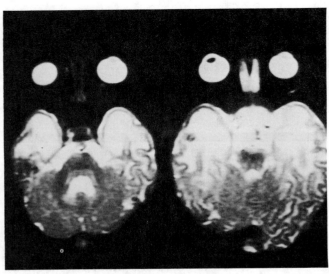

Figure 69-3. Magnetic resonance image of patient with early HSV encephalitis. Note the bilateral temporal lobe enhancement. (Kohl S. Herpes simplex encephalitis. In: New topics in pediatric infectious diseases. *Pediatr Clin North Am*, 1988;35(3):465. Reproduced by permission.)

TABLE 69-2. Differential Diagnosis of HSV Encephalopathy

INFECTIONS

Fungal
Especially *Cryptococcus*
Bacterial
Abscess, cerebritis
Listeria monocytogenes meningitis
Subdural, epidural empyema
Tuberculosis
Bacterial endocarditis
Lyme disease
Mycoplasma Rickettsial
Protozoal
Toxoplasmosis
Amoebic
Viral
Mumps virus
Coxsackievirus, echovirus
Arbovirus (especially St. Louis encephalitis)
Postinfluenza encephalitis
Reye's syndrome
Lymphocytic choriomeningitis virus
Rabies virus
Epstein-Barr virus
Rubella virus
Cytomegalovirus
Adenovirus
Tickborne encephalitis virus
Human immunodeficiency virus-1
Progressive multifocal leukoencephalopathy
Subacute sclerosing panencephalitis

NONINFECTIOUS DISORDERS

Tumor
Vascular disease
Arteriovenous malformations
Toxins
Alcoholic encephalopathy
Hematoma
Adrenal leukodystrophy

Modified with permission from Kohl S. Postnatal herpes simplex virus infection. In: Feigin RD, Cherry JD, eds. Textbook of pediatric infectious disease, 2nd ed. Philadelphia: WB Saunders; 1987:1577.

to crusting and healing by 9 to 11 days. Virus is shed for an average of 3 to 4 days. In dry areas, vesicles are seen, but in wet areas, the vesicles rapidly break down into ulcers. Symptoms are generally milder and of shorter duration than in primary genital disease.

Other cutaneous recurrences may occur at each anatomic site in which primary infection occurs. HSV may recur on the face or trunk in a typical dermatome distribution like that associated with varicella-zoster virus. Frequent repeated attacks of zosteriformlike lesions on any part of the body in a normal host suggests HSV and not varicella-zoster infection.

HSV in the Immunocompromised Host

Table 69–3 lists the states associated with unusually severe HSV infections. Other than the several cases of HSV encephalitis in patients with agammaglobulinemia (who also had concomitant infections with enterovirus), the common links in these varied groups are either skin abnormalities (eczema, burns) or immunologic defects, primarily in the cell-mediated aspects of the immune system.

■ PROGNOSIS, COMPLICATIONS, AND SEQUELAE

HSV infections occurring after the fetal and neonatal periods are annoying but usually not immediately life-threatening. The outcome of HSV encephalitis can be serious, ranging from extensive and permanent neurologic disability to death. HSV is one of the most common causes of infectious blindness in industrialized countries. In immunocompromised patients, it is a major cause of morbidity and mortality. Genital HSV may not have life-threatening potential but is a significant cause of physical and psychological morbidity.

■ THERAPY

The therapy for HSV infection in children is outlined in Table 69–4.

HSV Encephalitis

Intravenous acyclovir is the drug of choice in the treatment of HSV encephalitis. The patient's mental status at initiation of therapy markedly influences the outcome of patients with HSV encephalitis treated with acyclovir. Lethargic patients have a 15% mortality rate, whereas comatose patients have a 40% mortality rate.

Genital HSV Infection

Acyclovir (Zovirax) is the drug of choice for HSV genital infection. Specifically, intravenous acyclovir has an impressive effect on primary genital HSV infection. Used in a dose of 5 mg/kg each 8 hours for 5 days, acyclovir decreased duration of viral shedding and shortened local and systemic symptoms by 20% to 50%. Complications such as extragenital lesions and urinary retention were significantly reduced. Although intravenous acyclovir may shorten viral shedding and duration of symptoms in recurrences, it is not recommended for treatment of recurrent genital disease.

Recurrence rates are much more common after primary HSV-2 (90%) than HSV-1 (55%) infection. The mean rate of recurrence is 0.1 episode per month after primary genital HSV-1 and 0.3 episode per month after primary HSV-2 genital infection.

Only 5% to 12% of individuals with recurrent genital HSV have constitutional symptoms. Local symptoms include pain (averaging 4 to 6 days), itching, dysuria, adenopathy, and lesions lasting 4 to 5 days and progressing

TABLE 69-3. Conditions Contributing to Unusually Severe Herpes Simplex Virus Infection

Newborn period
Malnutrition
Malignancy
Immunosuppressive therapy
    Antineoplastic
    Transplantation
    Corticosteroids or ACTH
Primary immunodeficiency disease
    Agammaglobulinemia
    Common variable hypogammaglobulinemia
    Natural killer cell deficiency
    Wiskott-Aldrich syndrome
    Ataxia telangiectasia
    Severe combined immunodeficiency syndrome
    Nucleoside phosphorylase deficiency
Acquired immunodeficiency syndrome (AIDS)
Pregnancy
Burns
Trauma
Skin abnormalities
    Atopic eczema
    Bullous impetigo
    Burns
    Pemphigus
Viral infection
    Measles
Pertussis
Tuberculosis
Severe bacterial infection
    Haemophilus meningitis, pertussis
Sarcoidosis

Adapted with permission from Kohl S. Postnatal herpes simplex virus infection. In: Feigin RD, Cherry JD, eds. Textbook of pediatric infectious diseases. 2nd ed. Philadelphia: WB Saunders; 1987:1577.

TABLE 69-4. Therapy of HSV Infection in Children

GENITAL DISEASE
Primary
Oral acyclovir, 200 mg 5 times a day for 10 days (1 capsule = 200 mg)
Intravenous acyclovir, 15 mg/kg/day in 3 divided doses for 5–7 days
Recurrent
Oral acyclovir, 200 mg 5 times a day for 5 days
Suppressive
Oral acyclovir, 200 mg 3 to 5 times a day or 400 mg 2 times a day for up to 12 months
Oral dose for children should not exceed 80 mg/kg/day

ORAL DISEASE (PRIMARY)
Same as for primary genital infection. Oral dose for children should not exceed 80 mg/kg/day

ENCEPHALITIS
Intravenous acyclovir, 30 mg/kg/day in 3 divided doses for 10–14 days†

NEONATAL
Intravenous acyclovir, 30–45 mg/kg/day in 3 divided doses for 10–14 days†
Intravenous vidarabine, 30 mg/kg/day in 1 dose (12-h infusion) for 10–14 days

IMMUNOCOMPROMISED PATIENTS
Intravenous acyclovir, 15–30 mg/kg/day in 3 divided doses; duration as warranted clinically
Oral acyclovir, 200 mg 3 to 5 times a day, not to exceed 80 mg/kg/day; duration as warranted clinically*
Intravenous vidarabine, 10 mg/kg/day in 1 dose (12-h infusion)
Acyclovir Resistant Isolates
Intravenous foscarnet, 120 mg/kg/day in 3 divided doses*

OCULAR INFECTION
Trifluorothymidine (Viroptic), 1% ophthalmic solution; 1 drop every 2 h to a maximum of 9 drops, then 1 drop every 4 h (5 drops/day), do not exceed 21 days
Vidarabine (Vira-A), 3% ophthalmic ointment, 5 times a day; change to different agent if no healing in 7–9 days
Iododeoxyuridine (Stoxil), 0.1% ophthalmic solution or 0.5% ophthalmic ointment
Solution: one drop each hour during the day and every 2 h during the night
Ointment: 5 times a day every 4 h and before bedtime; change to different agent if no healing in 7–9 days

*This is an unlicensed use, and controlled trials in children have not been performed.

†The large dose has been found effective and nontoxic in these particular clinical conditions and patients.

Adapted with permission from Kohl S. Postnatal herpes simplex virus infection. In: Feigin RD, Cherry JD, eds. Textbook of pediatric infectious diseases, 2nd ed. Philadelphia: WB Saunders; 1987:1577.

Oral acyclovir has therapeutic effects on both primary and recurrent HSV infection in adults. In a dosage of 200 mg five times per day for 5 to 10 days, acyclovir significantly reduced viral shedding, lesion formation, duration of lesions, and duration and severity of symptoms in primary infection. Neither oral nor intravenous acyclovir reduces the rate of recurrence when used to treat either primary or recurrent genital infection.

■ PREVENTION

Environmental Control or Barrier Prevention

Because HSV is sensitive to heat, light, and lipid solvents, the use of antiseptics, soap and hot water, or chlorine decreases the risk of transferring the virus in settings such as the home, spas, pools, and hospitals. Wrestlers with skin lesions should be excluded from participation in practice or competition until herpes infection is ruled out. Medical and dental personnel who handle respiratory or oral secretions and administer oropharyngeal and tracheostomy care should wear gloves and wash carefully before and after working with patients and their secretions. Parents and caretakers of infants with eczema or severe diaper rash should be especially careful to avoid directly or indirectly contacting this altered skin with an active HSV lesion. Burn patients should be protected against exposure to or direct contact with personnel or visitors who have active HSV lesions. Immunosuppressed patients who develop evidence of HSV infection are usually manifesting evidence of reactivation of latent virus. Primary HSV infections in immunosuppressed individuals, as in neonates, may be especially severe, and it is important to protect these susceptible patients against exposure to HSV lesions. Hospital personnel with active cold sores or herpetic whitlow should not care for immunosuppressed patients. Although there are no human data, in vitro experiments have shown that condoms retard the passage of viable HSV.

Chemoprophylaxis

Oral acyclovir (200 mg given two to five times per day) administered long-term decreases recurrence of genital HSV by 50% to 70% in immunocompetent patients with frequent recurrences. Breakthrough recurrences are mild. When oral acyclovir is discontinued, HSV recurrences revert to pretreatment frequency. Thus, oral acyclovir suppresses recurrences without curing the latent infection. Side effects are limited to mild gastrointestinal irritation.

(Abridged from Steve Kohl, Postnatal Herpes Simplex Virus, in Oski, DeAngelis, Feigin, McMillan, Warshaw: *Principles and Practice of Pediatrics, Second Edition*, J.B. Lippincott, 1994.)

Oski's Essential Pediatrics,
edited by Kevin B. Johnson and Frank A. Oski.
Lippincott–Raven Publishers,
Philadelphia © 1997

70

Roseola and Human Herpesvirus Type 6

■ ROSEOLA CLINICAL FINDINGS

As early as 1870, the mild illness now referred to as roseola infantum or exanthem subitum was recognized and described as being distinct from other exanthematous diseases of childhood. Roseola affects infants and young children typically between the ages of 6 months and 3 years with 80% of the cases occurring before 18 months of age. Roseola characteristically is manifested by an initial fever that may have an abrupt onset. The fever may reach 40°C to 40.5°C (104°F to 105°F) and typically persists, either continuously or intermittently, for approximately 3 days. During this febrile period, the affected infant or child typically maintains near normal appetite and behavior, although there may be periods of irritability during times of increased fever.

Physical examination during this preeruptive phase yields few findings to distinguish roseola from other, more worrisome illnesses. Palpebral edema is sometimes described, and careful examination usually reveals suboccipital lymphadenopathy. Mild erythema of the pharynx may be seen in about one third of the patients. A bulging or tense fontanelle is sometimes noted in young infants with roseola. If laboratory studies are undertaken, they will be unrevealing, except that as the febrile illness begins, there may be a brief, slight elevation in the white blood cell (WBC) count with a predominance of neutrophils. During the majority of the febrile period, however, the WBC typically falls to 3000 to 5000 cells/mm³ with a relative lymphocytosis.

The rash of roseola usually coincides with the abrupt termination of the febrile period. Typically, the rash is pale pink (rose) with discrete macules or, less commonly, maculopapules, predominantly on the neck and trunk. Most often the rash persists for 1 to 2 days, but it may last only a few hours. Pruritus and desquamation are not seen.

■ COMPLICATIONS

The complication most frequently associated with roseola is febrile seizure. The rapidity of the initial temperature elevation often is cited as the reason for the frequent association between febrile seizures and roseola. Encephalitis and transient hemiparesis have been reported in young infants with a febrile illness, followed by a rash characteristic of roseola. The young age of patients with roseola, combined with their high fever and occasional bulging fontanelle, often indicates the possibility of bacterial infection, including meningitis. Laboratory investigation and hospitalization for treatment with intravenous antibiotics may result.

Human herpesvirus Type 6 (HHV-6) is now known to be a cause of roseola infantum. Serologic studies indicated that maternally derived antibody to HHV-6 is present in most infants at the time of birth and that infection with HHV-6 during the first few years of life is common.

In addition to roseola, HHV-6 infection now has been associated with a variety of clinical findings in infants and children. Isolation of HHV-6 from peripheral blood mononuclear cells concomitant with a rise in antibody against HHV-6 has been reported for 14% of the children younger than 2 years of age presenting to a pediatric emergency room with fever. Rash following defervescence occurred in the minority of these children, but many of them had otitis media. HHV-6 infection also has been documented during illness associated with rash but no fever. Other findings described in infants and children with what appears to be primary HHV-6 infection include diarrhea, pneumonia, hepatomegaly, hepatocellular dysfunction, seizures, and intussusception. Complete recovery from infection in these patients has been the rule. There is also one report of a fatal hemophagocytic syndrome in an 8-month-old infant infected with HHV-6.

HHV-6 in adults has been found in association with cervical lymphadenopathy and sore throat and with fever, sometimes in association with rash in patients who are immunosuppressed. A relationship between HHV-6 and chronic fatigue syndrome has been sought, but none has been found.

■ DIAGNOSIS AND ANTIVIRAL TREATMENT

HHV-6 can be diagnosed by isolating the virus from white blood cells. This technique is cumbersome and performed only in research laboratories. An alternative diagnostic method is polymerase chain reaction amplification of

HHV-6 DNA in lymphocytes. The simplest approach, however, is measurement of serum IgM and IgG antibody titers to HHV-6.

Most cases of HHV-6 infection are either unrecognized or only moderately symptomatic (roseola) and, therefore, need no specific antiviral treatment. Antipyretic medication (acetaminophen) may be indicated for amelioration of high fever.

(Abridged from Julia McMillan and Charles Grose, Roseola and Human Herpesvirus Type 6, in Oski, DeAngelis, Feigin, McMillan, Warshaw: *Principles and Practice of Pediatrics, Second Edition*, J.B. Lippincott, 1994.)

Oski's Essential Pediatrics,
edited by Kevin B. Johnson and Frank A. Oski.
Lippincott–Raven Publishers,
Philadelphia © 1997

71

Varicella-Zoster Virus Infections

Chickenpox is the common childhood exanthem caused by the human herpesvirus varicella-zoster virus (VZV). Most children acquire chickenpox during early school years, thereby developing lifelong immunity. About 10% of young adults, however, are susceptible to primary VZV infection because they did not contract chickenpox as children. After a person recovers from chickenpox, the virus remains in a latent state in the dorsal root ganglion cells for decades. In late adulthood, as immunity wanes, the virus occasionally reactivates and causes the dermatomal exanthem known as shingles or zoster. Zoster also occurs prematurely in children who have had chickenpox, then acquire a disease that must be treated with immunosuppressive chemotherapy and irradiation (*eg,* leukemia and lymphoma).

■ PATHOGENESIS

Varicella-zoster virus is one of the seven human herpesviruses. The other six are herpes simplex types 1 (oral) and 2 (genital), cytomegalovirus, Epstein-Barr virus, and the newly discovered human herpesvirus types 6 and 7, which reside within lymphocytes.

■ TRANSMISSION OF CHICKENPOX

Chickenpox is transmitted by virus in water droplets that are carried by air currents from an infected child to a susceptible individual. Epidemiologic observation studies document that children in the late incubation period may be infectious 1, 2, and possibly 4 days before appearance of the exanthem. They remain infectious through the first few days of the rash, but probably no longer than the sixth day.

In most communities in North America and Europe, outbreaks of chickenpox occur annually from January to May. The fewest cases occur in August and September. The periodicity of chickenpox depends on susceptible children being brought together in school every autumn.

■ CLINICAL FEATURES OF CHICKENPOX

The characteristic feature of chickenpox is the vesicle. In healthy children, the exanthem develops over 3 to 6 days, usually beginning along the hairline on the face. Each lesion begins as a macule that progresses to papule and vesicle, then to a crusted vesicle. The rash subsequently emerges in successive crops over the trunk, then the extremities. Lesions in different stages of development are present throughout the first week. The rash is more confluent wherever the skin is previously abraded, such as the diaper area.

The typical course of chickenpox is documented meticulously in American children. Usually, the prodrome is mild with malaise and low-grade fever. Once the pox appear, the temperature rises, but rarely above 38.8°C (102°F). The average number of skin lesions ranges between 200 and 300 in the index case within a family. The mortality rate for chickenpox in otherwise healthy children (ages 1 to 14 years) is about 1:50,000, whereas that for infants younger than age 1 year is 1:13,000 and that for adults is 1:1400. One subgroup at risk of fatal chickenpox is children on high-dose corticosteroid therapy for diseases such as asthma or rheumatic fever.

The most frequent complication of chickenpox in a healthy child is bacterial infection of a vesicular lesion. The most common infecting organism is Group A *Streptococcus,* although staphylococcal infections also occur. Secondary diseases range from cellulitis and erysipelas to cutaneous abscesses, impetigo, and suppurative lymphadenitis. More serious, but less common, bacterial sequelae include septic arthritis and osteomyelitis, streptococcal necrotizing fasciitis, and staphylococcal pyomyositis. The onset of bacterial disease may be rapid, sometimes within 2 days of the appearance of the exanthem. This complication is usually heralded by a sudden rise in temperature and local signs of inflammation. Diagnosis of fasciitis and myositis, once a difficult procedure, is facilitated by magnetic resonance imaging (MRI).

The viral sequelae of chickenpox involve virtually all organ systems. They include pneumonitis, hepatitis, arthritis, pericarditis, glomerulonephritis, orchitis, and involvement of the nervous system. Varicella pneumonitis is one of the most feared complications in an adult with chickenpox; pregnant women are especially prone to develop this complication. Pneumonitis usually develops late in the first week of disease in those patients who have the most florid exanthem. Mild hepatitis is another frequent complication and may account for the nausea often observed during the first few days of illness. Cases of purpuric chickenpox range from mild febrile purpura to the life-threatening condition called purpura fulminans, which is large ecchymoses that appear on the legs and occasionally progress to hemorrhagic gangrene.

Neurologic manifestations include meningoencephalitis, myelitis, and polyneuritis. In particular, the acute cerebellar syndrome is the most common VZV-induced neurologic disease in children. Symptoms include unsteady gait, vomiting, speech changes, nystagmus, vertigo, and tremor. Ataxia usually begins during the second week of the illness, but it can precede the exanthem. Cerebellar signs and symptoms often persist for several weeks but resolve with no permanent neurologic deficits. The preferred method for diagnosis of viral cerebellitis is MRI, which can detect abnormal signals within the cerebellum better than can computed tomography. Other neurologic conditions include hemiparesis, ascending and transverse myelitis, and facial palsy. Eye findings include unequal pupil size (anisocoria). Chickenpox also is associated temporally with Reye's syndrome, although the etiologic relationship is obscure.

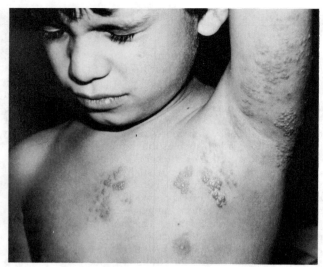

Figure 71-1. Zoster (shingles) in a child. The patient was receiving chemotherapy for treatment of leukemia when zoster was observed in the left first/second thoracic dermatome. The child had a history of chickenpox 3 years before the onset of cancer. (Grose C. Varicella-zoster virus infections: chickenpox (varicella), shingles (zoster), and varicella vaccine. In: Glaser R, ed. *Human herpesvirus infections.* New York: Marcel Dekker, in press.)

■ CHICKENPOX IN CANCER AND AIDS PATIENTS

Although chickenpox is a relatively benign condition in otherwise healthy children, VZV infection is often life-threatening when it occurs in children who are immunocompromised or immunosuppressed.

The variable outcome of chickenpox in human immunodeficiency virus (HIV) infected children depends on the immunologic status of the patient. In the HIV seropositive child without symptoms of acquired immunodeficiency syndrome (AIDS), chickenpox usually follows its typical course. In the child with very low CD4 lymphocyte counts and AIDS, chickenpox may become a progressive disease, as described in children with leukemia. Most HIV seropositive children should be considered in the higher risk category and treated with either immune globulin or acyclovir (see section on Treatment With Acyclovir).

■ ZOSTER (SHINGLES)

Zoster is the dermatomal exanthem that occurs when VZV reactivates from its site of latency and travels down a sensory nerve to the skin. Zoster is unusual in children. Estimated annual rate is about 1 case per 1000 children between ages 1 and 19 years. The younger the child at the time of chickenpox (especially younger than age 2 years), the likelier the same child will develop zoster later in childhood. Localization of zoster is also different in the young child. Rather than the lower thoracic and upper lumbar dermatomes, sites common in adults, zoster in younger children often occurs in dermatomes supplied by the cervical and sacral dermatomes. Thus, the rash frequently is seen on the arms and hands or in the groin and lower extremities.

As discussed, zoster occurs more often in immunocompromised children (Figure 71–1)

■ DIAGNOSIS

Because of the characteristic vesicular rash, diagnosis of chickenpox is usually visually apparent.

The virus infection can be identified more rapidly by antigen detection technique. For this test, cells from the base of a vesicle are dried on a glass slide before probing with a fluorescein-conjugated, VZV-specific monoclonal antibody. Cells containing virus are identified by their brilliant fluorescence.

Recent infection can be documented by obtaining acute and convalescent serum samples and demonstrating a fourfold or greater rise in VZV-specific antibody titer. Likewise, past infection can be demonstrated by persistence of anti-VZV antibody. The most reliable methods for testing VZV humoral immunity are fluorescent antibody to membrane antigen (FAMA) and enzyme-linked immunosorbent assay (ELISA).

Figure 71-2. The pathogenesis of chickenpox. Primary infection with VZV occurs when virus-laden water droplets contact the respiratory mucosa or conjunctivae of a susceptible host. The pathogenesis most likely includes a biphasic course with a primary and secondary viremia followed by typical vesicular exanthem of chickenpox. Based on this schema, varicella-zoster immune globulin must be given before primary viremia to prevent chickenpox in the exposed host. (Grose C. Varicella-zoster virus infections: chickenpox (varicella), shingles (zoster), and varicella vaccine. In: Glaser R, ed. *Human herpesvirus infections.* New York: Marcel Dekker, in press.)

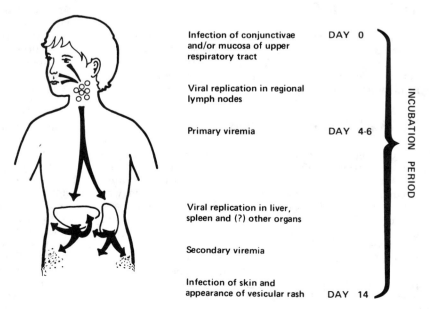

Infection of conjunctivae and/or mucosa of upper respiratory tract — DAY 0

Viral replication in regional lymph nodes

Primary viremia — DAY 4-6

Viral replication in liver, spleen and (?) other organs

Secondary viremia

Infection of skin and appearance of vesicular rash — DAY 14

INCUBATION PERIOD

■ TREATMENT MODALITIES INCLUDING VARICELLA-ZOSTER IMMUNE GLOBULIN

Chickenpox in the healthy child is rarely a serious disease. Low-grade fever can be treated with acetaminophen. Aspirin should be avoided in children with chickenpox because of its link with Reye's syndrome. For relief of itching secondary to the vesicular lesions, calamine lotion can be applied liberally to the skin. More severe pruritus, especially at night, may be ameliorated by giving Benadryl Elixir. Most children with chickenpox do not need to be seen by a physician unless they develop symptoms and signs of bacterial skin infection or one of the viral complications previously discussed. Children receiving corticosteroids for diseases such as asthma are in a high-risk category and should be seen by a physician.

The approach to the exposed child on corticosteroids or chemotherapy for cancer or AIDS is much more emergent. If the child is known to be susceptible to VZV infection, varicella-zoster immune globulin (VZIG) is the therapy of choice for passive immunization of these children at risk of developing progressive chickenpox. VZIG must be administered by intramuscular injection within 3 to 4 days after exposure to chickenpox (ie, during the early incubation period before the virus has spread throughout the body [see Figure 71–2]). The dose of VZIG is one vial (about 1.25 mL) for each 20 lb of body weight. Newly available preparations of gamma globulin for intravenous administration may be acceptable substitutes for intramuscular VZIG in the VZV-susceptible adult, but this approach has not been tested extensively.

■ TREATMENT WITH ACYCLOVIR

If the VZV-susceptible patient is beyond the fourth day post-exposure, there is no beneficial effect of passive immunization with gamma globulin. Therefore, the physician must wait until chickenpox manifests itself, then treat the patient with acyclovir (Zovirax). Acyclovir is now approved as both an intravenous and an oral formulation for treatment of chickenpox. Within 24 to 48 hours, intravenous acyclovir blocks further viral replication, thus preventing serious complications of progressive chickenpox. Because these complications (eg, pneumonitis) usually appear after the third day, the decision to administer intravenous acyclovir to high-risk children should be made on or before day 3 of the disease. The only serious side effect of acyclovir therapy is renal insufficiency. Therefore, serum creatinine levels should be monitored every 3 days.

No study shows that oral acyclovir shortens the course of chickenpox if begun on day 2 or later of the rash. Thus, the decision to prescribe this antiviral medication should be left to the discretion of physicians. Administration of oral acyclovir may not be adequate for the treatment of chickenpox in immunocompromised children. Zovirax is supplied in 200-mg capsules or as a suspension containing 200 mg per 5 mL.

■ VARICELLA VACCINATION

Alive attenuated VZV vaccine recently has been approved in the United States. The schedule for this vaccine can be found in Chapter 5.

(Abridged from Charles Grose, Varicella-Zoster Virus Infections, in Oski, DeAngelis, Feigin, McMillan, Warshaw: *Principles and Practice of Pediatrics, Second Edition*, J.B. Lippincott, 1994.)

Oski's Essential Pediatrics,
edited by Kevin B. Johnson and Frank A. Oski.
Lippincott–Raven Publishers,
Philadelphia © 1997

72

German Measles (Rubella)

Rubella is an acute infectious disease characterized by low-grade fever, erythematous maculopapular rash, and adenopathy. Rubella infection in early pregnancy may result in fetal infection with severe congenital anomalies.

■ CLINICAL MANIFESTATIONS

Incubation periods for postnatal rubella range from 14 to 21 days, usually 15 to 18 days. Inapparent infection may occur in 25% or more of infected individuals. Prodromal symptoms, usually appearing 1 to 5 days before the rash, are seen more commonly in older children and adults; they consist of low-grade fever, coryza, conjunctivitis, cough, and lymphadenopathy. A nonpathognomonic enanthem of rubella, Forschheimer spots, consists of erythematous, pinpoint or larger lesions that may be found on the soft palate in the prodromal period or on the first day of rash.

The exanthem of rubella may be the first indication of this infection in young children. It begins on the face and moves rapidly downward to the trunk and lower extremities. The exanthem lasts approximately 3 days; it may persist for 5 days or disappear within the first day. The rash of rubella is erythematous, discrete, maculopapular, and does not generally coalesce or darken as in rubeola.

Encephalitis occurs in approximately 1 in 6000 children, with the usual onset after appearance of the rash. The encephalitis usually is not fatal, and complete recovery can be expected in most cases. A mononuclear pleocytosis may occur in the cerebrospinal fluid (CSF) along with a normal or slightly elevated protein. Persistent abnormalities in the electroencephalogram have been described. Neuritis may occur during rubella infection with paresthesia being the chief complaint.

■ DIFFERENTIAL DIAGNOSIS

There are no pathognomonic findings in rubella, and with the reduced incidence of rubella, the physician must have a high index of suspicion to make the diagnosis. Helpful epidemiologic factors include age of patient, history of contact cases, documented immunization status, season of year, and incubation period.

■ DIAGNOSIS

Rubella virus may be isolated from nasopharyngeal secretions obtained from individuals with postnatal rubella, and isolation of the virus confirms the diagnosis. However, typically the diagnosis of postnatal rubella is determined by serologic testing of acute and convalescent sera obtained 10 to 14 days apart. Serologic tests now performed include enzyme immunoassay (EIA), latex agglutination, and indirect immunofluorescence.

■ TREATMENT

Treatment is largely supportive and includes use of acetaminophen for fever. Hospitalization is rarely required but may be necessary when one of the described complications occurs. Rubella arthritis usually responds to aspirin and rest of involved joints.

CONGENITAL RUBELLA

The initial report of Gregg in 1941 described a triad of congenital cataracts, heart defects, and low birth weight in infants born after maternal rubella during early pregnancy.

■ PATHOGENESIS AND EPIDEMIOLOGY

The risk of fetal infection after a maternal infection with rubella is greatest during the first month of pregnancy, with subsequent congenital anomalies seen in 30% to 60% of offspring. Risk of fetal infection apparently declines thereafter as determined by the reduced incidence of congenital anomalies, although hearing loss, ocular abnormalities, and developmental abnormalities continue to be seen. Early fetal infection results in hypoplastic organs with a subnormal number of cells.

■ CLINICAL MANIFESTATIONS

Clinical manifestations include intrauterine growth retardation (the most common manifestation and almost never an isolated finding), hepatosplenomegaly, generalized adenopathy, thrombocytopenia, hemolytic anemia, hepatitis, jaundice, meningoencephalitis (which may persist beyond the first year of life), bone lesions, large anterior fontanelle, pneumonitis, myocarditis, and nephritis.

Eye involvement is manifested by cataracts (usually noted at birth), glaucoma, retinopathy that does not interfere with visual acuity, and micro-ophthalmia, usually associated with cataracts.

Sensorineural deafness is common and may not be apparent until later in childhood. Heart defects are common; patent ductus arteriosus is most common, followed by stenosis of the pulmonary artery. More than one heart defect may coexist.

Numerous delayed manifestations with long-term implications have been described, including deafness, ocular damage, endocrinopathies (diabetes mellitus and thyroid dysfunction), progressive rubella panencephalitis, immunologic defects (particularly low levels of IgG), spastic diplegia, behavioral abnormalities, and learning disabilities.

■ DIFFERENTIAL DIAGNOSIS

Differential diagnosis includes congenital cytomegalovirus infection, syphilis, toxoplasmosis, neonatal herpes, or enteroviral infection of the newborn. Infants with congenital rubella are much more likely to be symptomatic at birth than infants with the above listed infections.

■ DIAGNOSIS

The diagnosis of congenital rubella can be made with isolation in tissue culture of the virus (throat, urine, CSF),

demonstration of rubella-specific IgM antibody that may be present until 6 to 12 months of age, or persistence of rubella antibody beyond 6 months of life. It is almost impossible to make a diagnosis of congenital rubella in those infants whose defects are identified in late infancy or childhood.

■ RUBELLA PREVENTION

Emphasis should be placed on immunization of children at an appropriate time. Adverse reactions to rubella vaccine include rash, fever, and adenopathy in a very small number of children approximately 7 to 10 days after immunization. Postvaccine arthralgias may occur 2 to 3 weeks after vaccine, are transient, and are most likely to occur in postpubertal females. Susceptible children who reside in households with pregnant women may be immunized, as well as children with minor illness. Contraindications for vaccine administration may be found in Chapter 5. For detailed recommendations or contraindications for vaccine administration, refer to the *Report of the Committee on Infectious Diseases* (Red Book).

Patients with natally acquired rubella should be considered contagious for 7 days after appearance of rash and should be isolated when necessary. Infants with congenital rubella should be considered contagious for the first year of life unless virus cultures of nasopharynx and urine prove negative, and they should be isolated (ie, hospitalized) from susceptible contacts (ie, day care, pregnant caretakers) as appropriate. Rubella is a reportable disease, and every effort should be made to diagnose all suspected cases of natally and congenitally acquired rubella and to report them to the appropriate public health agency.

(Abridged from Larry H. Taber and Gail J. Demmler, Rubella (German Measles), in Oski, DeAngelis, Feigin, McMillan, Warshaw: *Principles and Practice of Pediatrics, Second Edition*, J.B. Lippincott, 1994.)

Oski's Essential Pediatrics, edited by Kevin B. Johnson and Frank A. Oski. Lippincott–Raven Publishers, Philadelphia © 1997

73

Measles (Rubeola)

The measles virus is a highly contagious member of the family Paramyxoviridae. Infection with measles virus produces an illness characterized by a prodrome of fever, coryza, cough, conjunctivitis, an enanthem (Koplik's spots), and development of a confluent, erythematous maculopapular rash.

Transmission of the virus occurs by droplets of respiratory secretions with acquisition of infection by the nasopharyngeal route and possibly the conjunctivae. Person-to-person contact with exchange of infected secretions, particularly in young children, may lead to infection. The highest period of infectivity is the catarrhal period before appearance of the exanthem.

Measles occurs throughout the world, is essentially a winter/spring disease in temperate climates, and attacks males and females equally, although morbidity is reported to be higher in males.

■ CLINICAL MANIFESTATIONS

Persons with measles virus infection fall into four distinct groups: typical measles in the normal host; modified measles in a host with antibody; atypical measles in the host who received killed vaccine; and measles in immunocompromised persons. The clinical illness may be the same in each group but is usually different.

Typical Measles

The incubation period in typical measles is approximately 10 days, starting with a 3- to 5-day prodrome of malaise, fever, cough, coryza, and conjunctivitis. These symptoms increase over the 3- to 5-day prodrome period. Fever ranges from 39.4°C to 40.6°C (103°F to 105°F) reaching its height at the nadir of the exanthem. About 2 days before the rash, Koplik's spots (white pinpoint lesions on a bright red buccal mucosa) appear opposite the lower molars and quickly spread to involve the entire buccal and lower labial mucosa. Koplik's spots resolve by the third day of the exanthem. The exanthem of measles starts about the 14th day after exposure and appears first behind the ears and the hairline of the forehead. The rash progresses downward to the face, neck, upper extremities and trunk, and reaches the lower extremities by the third day. Initially, the rash is discrete, erythematous, and maculopapular, but it becomes confluent in the same progression as its spread. The rash eventually undergoes a brownish discoloration that does not blanch with pressure and may undergo desquamation. The exanthem lasts 6 to 7 days, and resolution of the rash begins on the third day in the same order as its appearance. In uncomplicated measles, the elevated temperature falls by either crisis or lysis; increased temperature beyond the third to fourth day of the exanthem suggests a complication.

Pharyngitis as well as generalized lymphadenopathy may be seen during the period of the exanthem. Splenomegaly is common. Diarrhea, vomiting, and abdominal pain may be prominent symptoms of measles, especially in young children. Leukopenia is a predictable finding.

Modified Measles

Modified measles occurs in children who have received immune serum globulin on exposure to measles or in young infants who still have transplacentally acquired maternal measles antibody. In addition, vaccine-modified mild measles, a form of secondary vaccine failure, can occur in individuals who were appropriately vaccinated with the live measles virus vaccine. In mild or modified measles, the prodrome period is shortened, symptoms are not as severe, and Koplik's spots do not usually occur, and, if present, they fade rapidly. The exanthem follows the progression of regular measles but does not become confluent.

Atypical Measles

Atypical measles usually occurs in persons immunized with killed measles vaccine who are exposed to natural measles. This illness may be observed in adults who received killed measles vaccine from 1963 through 1967 and were not reimmunized with live virus vaccine.

The incubation period for atypical measles is the same as for typical measles. The illness is characterized by sudden onset of fever (39.4°C to 40.6°C [103°F to 105°F]). Headache, myalgias, extreme weakness, and abdominal pain may all be present. Almost all patients have a dry, nonproductive cough. The rash of atypical measles appears first on the distal extremities and is pronounced on wrists and ankles. The rash may remain localized or may spread to involve the upper and lower extremities as well as the trunk. The palms and soles are also involved.

The rash of atypical measles may be erythematous and maculopapular (Color Figure 14); it may be vesicular, petechial, or purpuric in nature. Urticaria has been described. Edema of the hands and feet and severe hyperesthesia have also been described. Koplik's spots are rarely seen.

Pulmonary involvement occurs in almost all cases, with roentgenographic examination revealing pneumonia that frequently appears nodular. Hilar adenopathy and pleural effusion may be seen. Pulmonary involvement is accompanied by respiratory distress with tachypnea, dyspnea, and cough. Pulmonary involvement can occur without the exanthem.

Measles in Pregnancy

Measles occurring in the pregnant female may lead to increased mortality of the pregnant woman and a fetal effect of prematurity, spontaneous abortion early in pregnancy, or increased incidence of stillbirth. Perinatal measles, which has its onset in the first 10 days of life, is considered to be transplacentally acquired. Perinatal measles has a high incidence of pneumonia with resulting mortality.

■ COMPLICATIONS OF MEASLES

Complications of measles include viral pneumonia, laryngitis, laryngotracheobronchitis, and bronchiolitis. It is often difficult to differentiate between the patient who has viral pneumonia associated with measles and the patient who has a superimposed bacterial pneumonia. Therefore, when pneumonia is demonstrated by a chest roentgenogram, antimicrobial therapy should be considered. The bacteria involved include *Streptococcus pneumoniae*, *Staphylococcus aureus*, *Haemophilus influenzae*, and *Streptococcus pyogenes*. Otitis media is a common complication and is caused by the same bacterial pathogens that cause otitis media in children.

Other complications of measles include myocarditis, pericarditis, appendicitis, and corneal ulcerations as well as thrombocytopenic purpura. Hemorrhagic measles, seen frequently in former years, seldom occurs and probably was a result of disseminated intravascular coagulopathy.

Neurologic complications of measles include encephalitis, which occurs in approximately 1 in every 1000 to 2000 cases of measles. A mortality of 15% and morbidity among survivors of 25% have been observed. Encephalitis has its usual onset during the period of the exanthem, but onset may occur in the prodromal period. There is a high incidence of convulsions, cerebral edema, and other neurologic deficits in measles encephalitis. There is usually a mononuclear cell pleocytosis of the cerebrospinal fluid (CSF) and a slightly elevated protein. The electroencephalogram is abnormal in measles encephalitis but may also be abnormal in the absence of clinically diagnosed encephalitis.

Subacute sclerosing panencephalitis (SSPE) is an uncommon degenerative central nervous system (CNS) disease associated with persistent measles virus infection of the

CNS. The risk of SSPE is approximately 1 per 100,000 infections with natural measles and 1 per 1,000,000 immunizations in vaccine-associated SSPE. The incubation period is shorter in vaccine-associated SSPE than with natural measles. SSPE has an insidious onset with intellectual deterioration, myoclonic jerks, and progression to dementia and finally decorticate rigidity. The clinical picture, the typical electroencephalogram, and exceptionally high titers of measles hemagglutination-inhibition (HAI) antibody in serum and CSF are the basis for the diagnosis.

■ DIFFERENTIAL DIAGNOSIS

The differential diagnosis includes infections with those viruses that may cause erythematous maculopapular rashes: the enteroviruses, adenoviruses, rubella, erythema infectiosum, and infectious mononucleosis. Also considered in the diagnosis are infections with *Mycoplasma pneumoniae* and drug eruptions accompanied by fever. It is more likely that these illnesses would be confused with the clinical presentation of modified measles rather than typical measles. In atypical measles, the age of the patient and a history of repeated measles immunizations (killed vaccine may have been administered several times) may help confirm the diagnosis. Atypical measles has been confused with Rocky Mountain spotted fever.

■ DIAGNOSIS

Although measles virus may be isolated in tissue culture, most laboratories use the enzyme-linked immunosorbent assay (ELISA) technique to establish the diagnosis. Antibodies are usually present in a patient's serum by day 1 to 3 of the exanthem and peak some 2 to 6 weeks later. A patient with suspected measles, either in the prodromal period or with rash, should have a serum obtained immediately and a paired serum in 2 to 3 weeks. Both sera should be evaluated simultaneously in the same laboratory to determine the presence of measles antibody. A fourfold or greater rise in antibody titer in either one of the two tests or the presence of IgM antibody in either serum as determined by ELISA confirms a serologic diagnosis of measles. In atypical measles, a patient's sera may have extremely high titers of HAI antibody. This also occurs in patients with SSPE, in whom HAI antibody is found in the CSF.

■ TREATMENT

There is no specific approved therapy for measles virus infection. Fever should be controlled by acetaminophen, and room air should be humidified. Careful attention should be given to fluid intake, particularly in young infants. Antibiotics should not be given except when there are bacterial complications. Children with very serious complications of measles (eg, pneumonia, encephalitis, croup) should be hospitalized and treated. Aerosolized or intravenous ribavirin has been used on a compassionate basis to treat measles pneumonia, although its effectiveness has not been rigorously evaluated in clinical trials.

Children with measles are still considered contagious for 5 days after appearance of the rash, and measures should be undertaken to prevent their exposure to susceptible individuals. Immunocompromised persons with measles may be contagious longer.

■ MEASLES PREVENTION

General Considerations

Prevention of measles in the general population is possible by maintaining a high level of immunization among children 15 months of age or older.

There remain measles-susceptible persons of all age groups in the United States. Many parents delay immunization of children until they enter school, at which time immunization is required by law. Therefore, a number of children 15 months to 5 years of age are not immune. Children younger than 15 months of age may have no maternal antibody and, consequently, are susceptible to measles virus infections. Adults born after 1956 may never have been immunized or have had natural measles, and, thus, are susceptible to infection. Persons immunized before 1977 may have been immunized at 12 months of age or younger and may not be immune.

For detailed recommendations or contraindications for vaccine administration, refer to the *Report of the Committee on Infectious Diseases* (Red Book).

(Abridged from Larry H. Taber and Gail J. Demmler, Measles (Rubeola), in Oski, DeAngelis, Feigin, McMillan, Warshaw: *Principles and Practice of Pediatrics, Second Edition*, J.B. Lippincott, 1994.)

Oski's Essential Pediatrics, edited by Kevin B. Johnson and Frank A. Oski. Lippincott–Raven Publishers, Philadelphia © 1997

74

Mumps

Mumps is a contagious disease characterized by swelling of the salivary glands, particularly the parotid glands. Inapparent infection may occur in 40% of infected individuals. Mumps is transmitted by direct intimate contact or infected droplets from the oropharynx. Communicability is present before parotid swelling (1 to 7 days, but usually 1 to 2 days) and 7 to 9 days after onset of parotid swelling. The incubation period of mumps is approximately 18 days but may be longer. Mumps occurs in winter and spring seasons, and had its highest attack rate in 5- to 9-year-old children in the prevaccine era. Many epidemiologic features of mumps are difficult to ascertain because of the high incidence of inapparent infections.

■ CLINICAL MANIFESTATIONS

Parotitis

The classic illness of mumps is swelling of the parotid gland (ie, parotitis). Systemic symptoms include low-grade fever, headache, malaise, anorexia, and abdominal pain. Acid-containing foods may aggravate discomfort of the parotid gland. Ordinarily, the parotid gland is not palpable, but, in mumps cases, it rapidly progresses to maximum swelling over several days. Unilateral swelling usually occurs first, followed by bilateral parotid involvement. Occa-

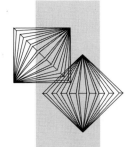

COLOR PLATES

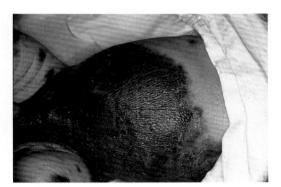

Color Figure 1

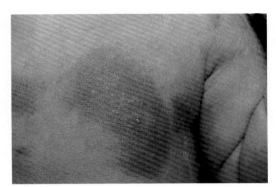

Color Figure 2

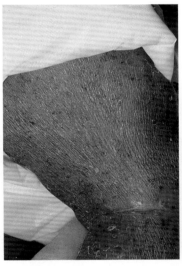

Color Figure 3

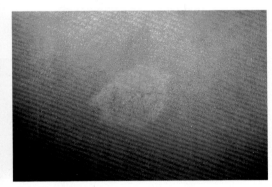

Color Figure 4

Color Figure 1. Giant congenital melanocytic nevus with atypical features, including a scalloped border, irregular pigmentation, and variable thickness.

Color Figure 2. The hallmark splotchy erythema studded with small papules and pustules of erythema toxicum.

Color Figure 3. Hyperpigmented macules of transient neonatal pustular melanosis, many of which are surrounded by a collarette of scale that is the remnant of the roof of the preceding pustule.

Color Figure 4. Incipient capillary (strawberry) hemangioma heralded by the central telangiectasia surrounded by an area of pallor.

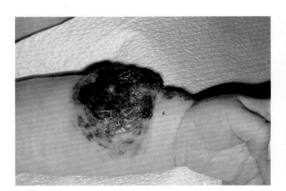

Color Figure 5

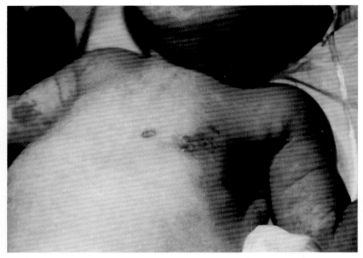

Color Figure 6

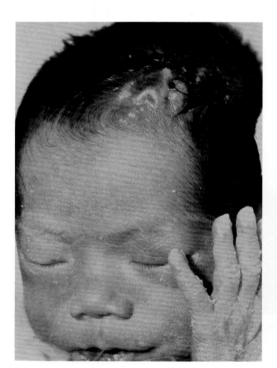

Color Figure 7

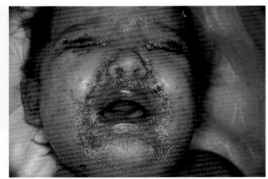

Color Figure 8

Color Figure 5. Large, mixed capillary and cavernous hemangioma on the left forearm with ulceration and crusting. The capillary component is superficial and bright red; the cavernous component is deeper and blue.

Color Figure 6. Discrete vesicles on an erythematous base in a neonate with herpes simplex virus infection.

Color Figure 7. Vesicular lesion of neonatal herpes simplex virus infection that developed at the site of a scalp electrode placed during labor for monitoring fetal heart rate. (Courtesy of Alec Wittek, MD)

Color Figure 8. Characteristic facial appearance of an infant with staphylococcal scalded skin syndrome with purulent drainage and crusting around the eyes, nose, and mouth.

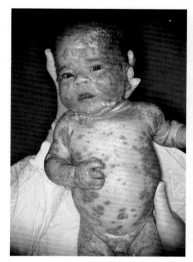

Color Figure 9

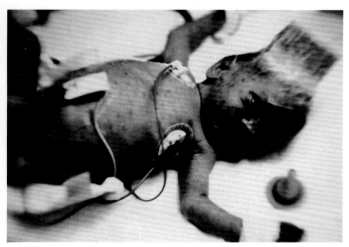

Color Figure 10

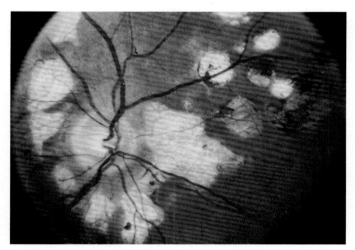

Color Figure 11

Color Figure 9. Beefy red, sharply demarcated, scaling plaques of psoriasis.

Color Figure 10. "Blueberry muffin spots." Extramedullary dermal erythropoiesis observed in the most severely affected infants with congenital cytomegalovirus infection and congenital rubella.

Color Figure 11. Patchy, yellow-white lesions of chorioretinitis seen with both congenital cytomegalovirus infection and congenital toxoplasmosis. (Courtesy of George H. McCracken, Jr, MD, Dallas, Texas)

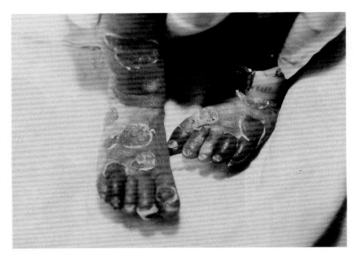

Color Figure 12

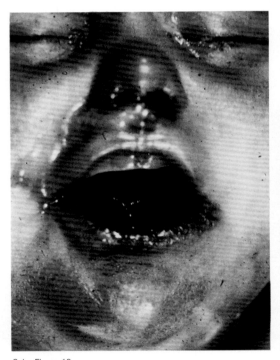

Color Figure 13

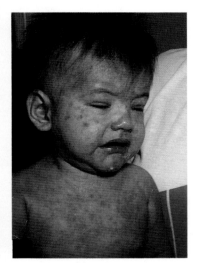

Color Figure 14

Color Figure 12. Pemphigus syphiliticus, a widely disseminated vesiculobullous eruption in an infant with early congenital syphilis. (Courtesy of Charles M. Ginsburg, MD, Dallas, Texas)

Color Figure 13. "Sniffles" or rhinitis in an infant with early congenital syphilis. This mucus discharge develops after the first week of life. (Courtesy of Charles M. Ginsburg, MD, Dallas, Texas)

Color Figure 14. Maculopapular rash in typical measles. (Courtesy of Gail Demmler, MD)

sionally, simultaneous involvement of both parotid glands occurs. Unilateral parotid disease occurs in fewer than 25% of patients. Fever subsides within 1 week and disappears before swelling of the parotid gland resolves, which may require as long as 10 days. Other salivary glands may be involved, including both submaxillary and sublingual, and orifices of the ducts may be erythematous and edematous.

Orchitis

About one third of postpubertal males develop unilateral orchitis. It usually follows parotitis but may precede parotitis or occur in the absence of parotitis. It usually appears in the first week of parotitis but can occur in the second or third week. Bilateral orchitis occurs much less frequently and, although gonadal atrophy may follow orchitis, sterility is rare even with bilateral involvement. Prepubertal males may develop orchitis, but it is uncommon in males younger than 10 years of age.

Orchitis is accompanied by high fever, severe pain, and swelling. Nausea, vomiting, and abdominal pain are not uncommon. Fever and gonadal swelling usually resolve in 1 week, but tenderness may persist.

Meningoencephalitis

Central nervous system (CNS) involvement with mumps is not uncommon and is more often a meningitis than a true encephalitis. It may precede parotitis or appear in the absence of parotitis, but it usually occurs in the first week following parotitis. Headache, fever, nausea, vomiting, and meningismus are common. Marked changes in sensorium and convulsions are not usual.

Pleocytosis of the CSF occurs in a high percentage of persons without clinical evidence of CNS involvement. In clinically diagnosed meningoencephalitis, a CSF mononuclear pleocytosis occurs as does a normal glucose, although hypoglycorrhachia has been reported. Mumps virus may be isolated from CSF early in the illness. Mumps meningoencephalitis has a good prognosis and usually an uneventful recovery.

Other clinical manifestations of mumps include pancreatitis accompanied by severe abdominal pain, chills, fever, and persistent vomiting. Thyroiditis, oophoritis, and mastitis occasionally occur.

■ COMPLICATIONS OF MUMPS

Neuritis of the auditory nerve may result in deafness. There is sudden onset of tinnitus, ataxia, and vomiting followed by permanent deafness. Other neurologic complications include facial nerve neuritis and myelitis.

More uncommon complications include arthritis, myocarditis, and hematologic complications.

■ DIFFERENTIAL DIAGNOSIS

Parotitis caused by other viruses—coxsackieviruses, influenza viruses, and parainfluenza viruses—cannot be differentiated clinically from mumps parotitis. In suppurative parotitis commonly caused by *Staphylococcus aureus* or other bacteria, the parotid gland is very tender and the overlying skin is erythematous.

Adenitis, recurrent parotitis, calculus of Stensen's duct, tumors of the parotid gland, and Mikulicz's syndrome may be considered in the differential diagnosis.

Mumps meningoencephalitis is indistinguishable from that caused by many other viruses, unless parotitis is present.

■ DIAGNOSIS

The diagnosis of mumps is usually made clinically; however, laboratory evaluation can be helpful in many caess. A serologic diagnosis of mumps may be made by testing paired sera for mumps IgG antibody obtained early in illness and 2 to 4 weeks after illness. The diagnosis of mumps also can be made from a single serum specimen if the presence of mumps IgM antibody is detected. Mumps virus also can be readily grown from saliva or swabs of material expressed directly from Stensen's duct, as well as from urine and CSF. Viral cultures are encouraged because isolation of mumps virus is timely and confirms the diagnosis.

■ TREATMENT

Treatment of mumps parotitis and other glandular involvement is largely symptomatic. Patients with orchitis may obtain relief with gentle support of the testicle and ice packs. Management of mumps meningitis is similar to that for other forms of viral meningitis. Antibiotics are not recommended. Acetaminophen can be used for fever control, but relief of pain may require a narcotic. Respiratory isolation of the hospitalized patient is advised. Patients are considered no longer contagious 9 days after onset of parotid swelling.

■ PREVENTION OF MUMPS

All children should receive measles-mumps-rubella vaccine (MMR) at 15 months of age. More than 95% of persons receiving mumps vaccine develop antibody. For detailed recommendations or contraindications for vaccine administration, refer to the *Report of the Committee on Infectious Diseases* (Red Book).

(Abridged from Larry H. Taber and Gail J. Demmler, Mumps, in Oski, DeAngelis, Feigin, McMillan, Warshaw: *Principles and Practice of Pediatrics, Second Edition*, J.B. Lippincott, 1994.)

Oski's Essential Pediatrics, edited by Kevin B. Johnson and Frank A. Oski. Lippincott–Raven Publishers, Philadelphia © 1997

75

Rotavirus

Human rotaviruses, a member of the reovirus family, were first detected in 1973 by electron microscopy in duodenal biopsy samples of children with acute gastroenteritis. Because the circular outline of the outer capsid of the viruses resembled a double-rimmed wheel, they were named rotavirus from the Latin *rota*, which means wheel. They are a major cause of diarrhea in infants and young children in developed countries and can cause severe morbidity and mortality in children in developing countries. Rotavirus gastroenteritis severe enough to require hospitalization occurs most frequently in infants younger than 1 year of age.

Rotavirus disease has been termed "winter gastroenteritis" because, in temperate climates, it occurs more often in January and February. In tropical climates, it is endemic and may be a cause of traveler's diarrhea. Rotaviruses are also frequent causes of nosocomial infection in hospital nurseries and pediatric wards. Transmission within families and day care centers often occurs as well.

The virus is shed in large quantities in the feces for 3 to 5 days and probably is spread by contact with virus-infected stool. Waterborne transmission may also occur in community swimming pools because the virus is resistant to chlorination. Many children have a concomitant rhinorrhea, so transmission may also occur by the respiratory route.

■ CLINICAL MANIFESTATIONS

Rotavirus infection usually produces clinical illness in children aged 6 months to 2 years. The illness begins with fever, upper respiratory symptoms, and vomiting, followed by a profuse, watery diarrhea that does not characteristically contain blood or fecal leukocytes. The diarrhea can last 3 to 5 days and often causes isotonic dehydration and a metabolic acidosis. Death can occur, especially in malnourished children in developing countries, due to dehydration, electrolyte imbalance, seizures, or aspiration of vomitus.

Rotavirus-induced diarrhea is usually associated with a transient disaccharidase deficiency, although chronic or recurrent diarrhea may produce villous atrophy and monosaccharide intolerance. Rotavirus can produce a chronic, symptomatic, even fatal infection in immunosuppressed patients.

■ DIAGNOSIS

The diagnosis of rotavirus disease should be considered when a young child presents with vomiting and watery diarrhea, especially if the illness occurs during winter. The presence of rotavirus particles in the stool can be confirmed by direct examination of the stool by electron microscopy or immune electron microscopy. Rotaviruses are shed in large quantities and their appearance is characteristic, making this test both sensitive and specific. A simpler, more available method is detection of rotavirus antigen by enzyme-linked immunosorbent assay (ELISA) or latex agglutination. These antigen detection tests are available commercially, do not require expensive equipment, and can be performed reliably and easily in most clinical laboratories. False-positive ELISA results can occur, especially in stool specimens collected from neonates.

■ TREATMENT

The treatment of rotavirus-associated gastroenteritis is restoration of fluid and electrolyte balance. Oral therapy with a glucose-electrolyte solution corrects mild to moderate dehydration and has been lifesaving in developing countries. Intravenous rehydration may be necessary in infants with severe dehydration, shock, or protracted vomiting. Antibiotics and antidiarrheal medications that alter intestinal motility are not indicated.

Good hygiene, handwashing, and disinfection are important to prevent spread of rotavirus in families, day care centers, and hospitals. Improved nutrition and hygiene will help decrease the severe mortality associated with this disease in developing countries.

Immunoprophylaxis using an experimental rotavirus vaccine recently has been shown to induce protective antibody and may be an important step in reducing the worldwide morbidity and mortality associated with this disease.

(Abridged from Gail J. Demmler, Rotavirus, in Oski, DeAngelis, Feigin, McMillan, Warshaw: *Principles and Practice of Pediatrics, Second Edition*, J.B. Lippincott, 1994.)

Oski's Essential Pediatrics,
edited by Kevin B. Johnson and Frank A. Oski.
Lippincott–Raven Publishers,
Philadelphia © 1997

76

Viral Gastroenteritis

Acute viral gastroenteritis is a common illness that occurs in both endemic and epidemic forms worldwide. Four categories of viruses are recognized as medically important causes of human gastroenteritis: rotavirus (which is discussed in Chapter 75); enteric adenovirus; calicivirus and calici-like virus, including Norwalk virus; and astrovirus.

ENTERIC ADENOVIRUSES

Adenoviruses are 70 to 80 nm in diameter, are nonenveloped, and contain a double-stranded DNA viral genome. By measuring antibodies induced by distinct antigenic determinants, 47 serotypes of human adenoviruses have been identified. The enteric adenoviruses are members of group F and are designated as serotypes 40 and 41. Unlike other serotypes of adenovirus, enteric adenoviruses do not grow well in conventional cell cultures and require special cell lines for replication. Enteric adenoviruses can be identified by electron microscopy. After rotavirus, enteric adenovirus is the second most common cause of viral gastroenteritis in infants and children.

Most episodes of gastroenteritis due to enteric adenoviruses occur in children younger than 2 years of age. Diarrhea is the most prominent symptom, lasting from 4 to 23 days (mean, 7 days). Symptoms are indistinguishable from those associated with rotavirus infection, although generally less severe. Blood and mucus are not present in stools. Dehydration is mild and isotonic, and death is rare. Apparent lactose intolerance occurs in some children with enteric adenovirus infection.

No specific agent for treating children with enteric adenovirus infection is available. Treatment is aimed at replacing fluid and correcting electrolyte abnormalities. Isolation of patients with gastroenteritis in hospitals, day care centers, and other institutions is the major means of interrupting spread.

CALICIVIRUSES AND CALICI-LIKE VIRUSES

Caliciviruses and calici-like viruses are nonenveloped RNA viruses 27 to 40 nm in diameter. The most extensive information is available for the Norwalk virus, which lacks typical calicivirus morphology but has been shown to be a calicivirus based on the sequence of its genome. Norwalk virus was identified first in 1972 when immune electron microscopy was applied to samples collected from an outbreak of gastroenteritis in a secondary school in Norwalk, Ohio. It was the first gastroenteritis virus discovered.

Caliciviruses have a worldwide distribution and are a common cause of waterborne and foodborne outbreaks of acute, nonbacterial gastroenteritis. Caliciviruses cause illness more frequently among infants and children, and Norwalk virus causes illness among adults.

Calicivirus outbreaks tend to occur in closed populations and have a high attack rate. Typical calicivirus infections seem common in day care centers. Common-source outbreaks occur in association with ingestion of contaminated water and food, particularly shellfish and salads. Secondary transmission presumably is person to person and fecal–oral. Symptoms generally are mild and, especially in adults, of short duration. In children, symptoms are indistinguishable from those of rotavirus gastroenteritis. Excretion lasts 5 to 7 days after the onset of symptoms in half the infected patients and can extend to 13 days. Virus excretion may continue 4 days after symptoms cease. Persistent excretion may occur in immunocompromised hosts. Asymptomatic, persistent virus excretion has been detected for months after primary calicivirus infections in animals.

Hepatitis E causes epidemics of hepatitis in Asia and Africa. Outbreaks of hepatitis E virus infection have been identified in Mexico, and imported cases have occurred in the United States.

■ DIAGNOSIS AND TREATMENT

Electron microscopy is the most widely available diagnostic tool for detection of caliciviruses in stool specimens, but it is fairly insensitive for this virus family. For Norwalk virus and certain other strains, specific diagnostic tests are available in some reference laboratories. Samples submitted for virus detection should be collected early after infection, should be stored at 4°C (39.2°F), and should not be frozen. Paired serum samples may help establish the diagnosis of infection.

As for the other viral agents, treatment is supportive. Hospitalized patients should be isolated, and infected individuals attending day care centers or similar institutions should be cohorted. Virus may be inactivated with a 1-minute exposure to 0.1% sodium hypochlorite.

ASTROVIRUSES

Astroviruses, first described in 1975, are nonenveloped RNA viruses 28 to 30 nm in diameter with a characteristic starlike appearance when visualized by direct electron microscopy. The absence of a central hollow distinguishes astrovirus stars from typical calicivirus stars in direct electron microscopy. Known astroviruses include at least five antigenic types. Human astroviruses are antigenically distinct from animal astroviruses. Initial genetic studies indicate that astroviruses are a unique virus family, distinct from caliciviruses and picornaviruses.

Symptoms generally are mild and indistinguishable from those caused by rotavirus. The incubation period is 1 to 2 days. Excretion lasts 5 days after onset of symptoms in half the infected cases. The duration of asymptomatic excretion

after onset of illness is uncertain. Persistent excretion may occur in immunocompromised hosts. Asymptomatic infections also occur.

■ DIAGNOSIS AND TREATMENT

Astroviruses are difficult to diagnose using existing laboratory tools. Electron microscopy is the most widely available diagnostic tool for detection of astroviruses in stool specimens, but it also is fairly insensitive for this family of viruses. Treatment is supportive. Enteric precautions are recommended, and control measures are the same as those for rotavirus.

(Abridged from David O. Matson, Lamia Elerian, and Larry K. Pickering, Viral Gastroenteritis, in Oski, DeAngelis, Feigin, McMillan, Warshaw: *Principles and Practice of Pediatrics, Second Edition,* J.B. Lippincott, 1994.)

Oski's Essential Pediatrics,
edited by Kevin B. Johnson and Frank A. Oski.
Lippincott–Raven Publishers,
Philadelphia © 1997

77

Mycoplasma Infections

Mycoplasmas are classified as bacteria, but are unique because they lack a rigid cell wall. For this reason, their morphology depends on the environment in which they grow, they do not take usual bacterial stains, and they are not susceptible to antibiotics that act on the cell wall, such as the penicillins. Other members of the family include *M hominis* and *Ureaplasma urealyticum*. Because *M pneumoniae* is the most common agent affecting children, it will be discussed below.

MYCOPLASMA PNEUMONIAE

■ EPIDEMIOLOGY

M pneumoniae is the most common cause of pneumonia and tracheobronchitis in school-age children and young adults treated in the outpatient setting. The average annual rate is about 5:1000 school-age children. It is an uncommon cause of lower respiratory tract disease in infants and young children, and usually does not result in hospitalization of children without chronic conditions. College students and military recruits may be confined to bed with *M pneumoniae* pneumonia.

■ CLINICAL FEATURES

The main clinical features of *M pneumoniae* disease are fever, malaise, sore throat, and a dry, hacking cough. The onset usually is gradual over several days. The affected schoolchild may not appear particularly ill, and the examiner may be surprised when chest auscultation reveals rales and rhonchi. The chest roentgenogram may show peribronchial thickening and infiltration of one or both lower lobes, with some subsegmental atelectasis. Pleural effusion is not a prominent finding. The peripheral white blood cell (WBC) count usually is in the normal range. The severity of the illness may be exaggerated in children with sickle-cell disease. These children appear toxic and require hospitalization, with prolonged high fever and peripheral WBC counts greater than 25,000/mm³. The chest roentgenogram may reveal dense infiltrates involving more than one lobe and prominent pleural effusion.

The progress of the infection may be aborted in some children who have fever and pharyngitis. A larger proportion of children have a prominent cough and rhonchi in the larger airways on auscultation; in these children, a diagnosis of tracheobronchitis is warranted.

Some children not known to wheeze previously may have expiratory wheezing on examination. A nondescript rash may accompany the infection. A few children present with acute otitis media or bullous myringitis. The total course of the illness with or without treatment may encompass 2 weeks, with a bothersome night cough persisting even longer.

■ COMPLICATIONS

A wide variety of extrapulmonary complications has been attributed to *M pneumoniae* infection, incuding Stevens-Johnson syndrome, hemolytic anemia with or without renal failure, and a plethora of neurologic syndromes, including meningoencephalitis, Guillain-Barré syndrome, transverse myelitis, and cerebral infarction.

■ DIAGNOSIS

The diagnosis of *M pneumoniae* infection can be suspected in a child who has the typical clinical picture described above. The clinical impression can be reinforced by the presence of cold agglutinins in the serum at a titer of 1:64 or greater. Cold agglutinins are IgM antibodies that may appear early in the course of the infection—probably because the organism has an antigen similar to the I antigen on the red blood cell (RBC) membrane. Cold agglutinins are not specific for *M pneumoniae* infection and are present in only about 50% of affected persons, but this finding in a child with no chronic underlying condition is helpful, because the likelihood of finding a titer of 1:64 or greater increases with the severity of the illness.

A specific diagnosis can be made by isolating the organism. Serologic diagnosis usually is accomplished by documenting a fourfold or greater rise in the level of CF antibodies between serum obtained when a patient is in the acute phase of the disease and that obtained when the patient is convalescent.

■ TREATMENT

The treatment of choice for children with *M pneumoniae* infection is erythromycin. Therapy should be started early for optimal response, which may not be dramatic under even the best of circumstances. Controlled clinical trials have shown that either erythromycin or tetracycline will shorten the clinical course and hasten improvement of the chest x-ray findings. Treatment may not eradicate the organism; it often is possible to recover *M pneumoniae* from respiratory secretions after therapy is discontinued.

(Abridged from W. Paul Glezen, *Mycoplasma* Infections, in Oski, DeAngelis, Feigin, McMillan, Warshaw: *Principles and Practice of Pediatrics, Second Edition,* J.B. Lippincott, 1994.)

Oski's Essential Pediatrics,
edited by Kevin B. Johnson and Frank A. Oski.
Lippincott–Raven Publishers,
Philadelphia © 1997

78

Rickettsial Diseases

The rickettsial diseases are caused by microorganisms that have characteristics common to both bacteria and viruses.

All rickettsial diseases are characterized clinically by fever, headache, and rash, with the exception of Q fever, which has no rash, and ehrlichiosis, which frequently has no rash. In the early stages of rickettsial diseases, all infections are susceptible to a number of broad-spectrum antibiotics. Rickettsial organisms all occur under natural conditions in insects such as lice and fleas or arachnids such as ticks and mites. These arthropods serve as vectors for the transmission of all rickettsial diseases to humans, with the exception of Q fever.

Another general characteristic is that arthropods and mammals serve as natural hosts for rickettsiae. Infection also can occur by an airborne route, however, when infectious microorganisms acquire access to respiratory surfaces or the conjunctivae.

The spotted fevers are a group of infectious diseases caused predominantly by *Rickettsia rickettsii*. Because most are transmitted by ticks, they are called tick typhuses.

ROCKY MOUNTAIN SPOTTED FEVER

Rocky Mountain spotted fever is a disease caused by *R rickettsii*, which first was recognized in areas of Idaho and Montana. Its occurrence is not limited to the Rocky Mountain area, however; the disease actually is most prevalent in the eastern United States. Nearly two thirds of all patients with Rocky Mountain spotted fever are 15 years old or younger.

Despite the use of chloramphenicol or tetracyclines, Rocky Mountain spotted fever has an overall case fatality rate of 3.9%. A considerable number of the deaths can be attributed to failure to consider and establish the diagnosis early enough for appropriate therapy to be beneficial.

The wood tick (*Dermacentor andersoni*) in the West, the Lone Star tick (*Amblyomma americanum*) in the Southwest, and the dog tick (*Dermacentor variabilis*) in the East all are carriers and vectors of this disease. Rocky Mountain spotted fever rickettsiae do not kill the arthropod host but can be passed from generation to generation of ticks transovarially.

The principal pathologic lesion of Rocky Mountain spotted fever is a vasculitis that follows the bite of an infected tick. Vascular lesions account for the more prominent clinical features noted, including rash, mental confusion, headache, heart failure, and shock. Pneumonia can be acquired by laboratory inhalation.

Changes in nitrogen balance are extreme. Early in this infection, large amounts of nitrogen may be excreted in the urine. Subsequently, nitrogen imbalances are related to insufficient protein intake. The serum albumin concentration is depressed as the result of protein losses, hepatic dysfunction related to the disease process, and protein leakage through the damaged endothelium of blood vessels.

Hyponatremia may be profound. Reported causes of the hyponatremia include a loss of sodium by the urine, a shift in water from the intracellular to the extracellular space, and an exchange of sodium for potassium at the cellular level. The intracellular sodium level increases slightly. The destruction of cells results in an increase in the serum concentration of potassium and in enormous losses of potassium in the urine. Plasma concentrations of antidiuretic hormone and aldosterone have been increased in some individuals with this disease.

■ CLINICAL MANIFESTATIONS

Fever, headache, and rash are the hallmarks of Rocky Mountain spotted fever as well as of other rickettsial diseases, although the complete triad may be present in only 45% to 62% of all cases. Mental confusion and myalgia are common features of Rocky Mountain spotted fever. The onset of disease in children usually occurs 2 to 8 days after a bite is sustained from an infected tick. The onset of clinical manifestations may be gradual or abrupt. Body temperature rises rapidly to 40°C (104°F) with a pattern characterized by persistence, although many patients do have temperature oscillations over a period of several hours.

The rash associated with Rocky Mountain spotted fever is one of the more pathognomonic features of this disease. It generally appears by the second or third day of illness, although it may be delayed for a week. Initially, the lesions are erythematous macules that can blanch on pressure. The lesions rapidly become petechial and, in untreated patients, even hemorrhagic. Sometimes skin necrosis occurs. The rash appears peripherally on the wrists and ankles, spreading within hours up the extremities and onto the trunk. The rash also appears frequently on the palms and soles. The absence of rash, however, does not exclude a diagnosis of Rocky Mountain spotted fever.

Headache in older children and adults is a characteristic finding. The headache is persistent night and day, and is intractable. Young children, however, may not complain of this symptom. Signs of meningoencephalitis are common and may be appreciated because the patient is irritable, apprehensive, restless, or exhibits signs of mental confusion or delirium. Occasionally, children may become comatose. Meningismus may be present but is not accompanied always by abnormalities in the cerebrospinal fluid. In fact, the cerebrospinal fluid generally is clear, with minor elevations seen in the lymphocyte count (less than 10 cells/mm^3). Seizures (grand mal or focal) have been observed. Central deafness (persistent or transient) and cortical blindness have been described. Other reported neurologic involvement includes sixth nerve paralysis, spastic paralysis, and ataxia. Rocky Mountain spotted fever also seems to exert a consistent effect on intellectual function, and several investigators have suggested that a higher probability of learning disability and difficulty in school performance exists in children who have had this disease.

Cardiac involvement is frequent and requires evaluation of each patient with clinically defined illness by electrocardiography, echocardiography, and other techniques if necessary. Congestive heart failure and arrhythmias are common.

Muscle tenderness is a common feature of Rocky Mountain spotted fever. Characteristically, the patient complains when the calf or thigh muscles are squeezed.

Pulmonary involvement occurs in 10% to 40% of reported cases and may be associated with abnormal chest radiograph results and abnormal arterial blood gas measurements. The chest radiograph may reveal cardiomegaly, focal infiltrates, or pulmonary edema.

Generalized edema of the face and extremities usually occurs and, in occasional cases, nuchal rigidity and conjunctival suffusion are seen. Acute tubular necrosis and glomerulonephritis can occur. Enlargement of the liver and spleen develops but is infrequent. Other gastrointestinal symptoms and signs, including nausea, vomiting, abdominal pain, and diarrhea, arise frequently during the early course of Rocky Mountain spotted fever. Icterus has been reported but is relatively rare, except in severe cases.

■ DIAGNOSIS

Specific treatment should be initiated promptly because, in most cases, laboratory evaluations do not permit a specific cause to be identified before therapy must be instituted. *R rickettsii,* however, can be identified by immunofluorescent techniques in skin specimens obtained by biopsy on days 4 through 8 of the illness. A negative immunofluorescent test result never excludes the diagnosis of Rocky Mountain spotted fever.

Specific serologic results usually are not positive before day 10 or 12 of the illness. At this time, the majority of the 20% of patients who will die if they are not treated already are moribund or dead; therefore, the provision of appropriate therapy can never await a definitive diagnosis.

■ DIFFERENTIAL DIAGNOSIS

Meningococcemia and measles are the disorders most frequently confused with Rocky Mountain spotted fever. A petechial rash involving the palms and soles that spreads in a centripetal manner suggests a diagnosis of Rocky Mountain spotted fever, although the atypical measles syndrome can produce a similar rash. The inability to differentiate meningococcemia from Rocky Mountain spotted fever does not justify delaying antimicrobial therapy, because both diseases potentially are fatal. Treatment should be initiated promptly with chloramphenicol and penicillin G if the diagnosis of either disease is entertained and neither can be excluded immediately. When the appropriate diagnosis is certain, the inappropriate drug can be discontinued.

■ TREATMENT

Chloramphenicol and the tetracyclines are highly effective when they are given early in the course of the disease and in an appropriate dosage. It is appropriate to monitor serum chloramphenicol concentrations during the course of this disease. Tetracycline may be given orally or intravenously. Treatment can be terminated 3 to 4 days after the patient's temperature has returned to normal for a full 24-hour period. The duration of therapy usually is 7 to 10 days.

Thrombocytopenia and disseminated intravascular coagulation may develop in the course of Rocky Mountain spotted fever. Adequate antimicrobial therapy is essential to prevent this complication.

The need for supportive care cannot be overemphasized. Careful evaluation of serum and urine electrolyte levels, body weight, and renal function is important to guide fluid therapy. Hyponatremia is treated best by providing maintenance fluids or, in the case of severe hyponatremia, by instituting modest fluid restriction. The administration of sodium-rich fluids precipitates cardiac decompensation and pulmonary edema in critically ill patients with Rocky Mountain spotted fever without raising the serum sodium concentration substantially. Patients who have concomitant hypotension and hypoalbuminemia may be given albumin (1 g/kg immediately). When the clotting time is prolonged in patients without disseminated intravascular coagulation, the administration of vitamin K (2 mg intramuscularly immediately) has been helpful. Anemia of a severe degree may require blood transfusion. Several investigators have suggested that steroid therapy has been helpful in shortening the febrile period. When steroids are given in sufficient doses to any febrile patient, the febrile period should be diminished, but other specific therapeutic benefits related to this course of action in Rocky Mountain spotted fever have not been proven.

■ PROGNOSIS

The mortality from Rocky Mountain spotted fever was about 25% before appropriate antimicrobial therapy became available. If appropriate antibiotics are provided before the end of the first week of illness, recovery generally is the rule. The overall mortality rate remains 5% to 7%, however, principally because diagnosis and therapy are delayed in many patients until the second week of illness. The case fatality rate in 1990 was 2.4% for persons less than 20 years of age and 6.8% for those greater than 20 years of age. When death occurs, it usually is the result of heart failure, vascular collapse, renal failure, or thrombocytopenia, either alone or in combination. Central nervous system involvement and disseminated intravascular coagulation are common.

Complications are less common in patients who receive appropriate therapy early. Bronchopneumonia may develop in critically ill patients, and the infusion of sodium-rich parenteral fluids may precipitate both cardiac failure and pulmonary edema.

Q FEVER

Q fever is a rickettsial disease that occurs worldwide. It is characterized by fever, headache, and pneumonia in more than 50% of cases. It is unique among the human rickettsial infections in that it is primarily a disease of animals that is transmitted to humans by inhalation rather than by an arthropod bite, although it can be transmitted to humans by ticks.

Rickettsiae that cause Q fever are known as *Coxiella burnetii*. Q fever is primarily a zoonosis infecting cattle, goats, sheep, and rodents on a worldwide basis, and marsupials in Australia. Humans acquire the disease when they come in contact with infected animals and materials contaminated by these animals.

■ CLINICAL MANIFESTATIONS

After an incubation period of 9 to 20 days, the disease begins with chills, high fever, general malaise, myalgias, chest pain, and an intractable headache, similar to that seen with other rickettsial diseases. This particular rickettsial disorder, however, is not accompanied by a rash.

Physical findings in the chest generally are minimal and a radiograph may be necessary to appreciate the pulmonary pathology. In about 50% of patients, multiple round segmental opacities may be seen on the chest radiograph. Other, less common findings include linear atelectasis, lobar consolidation, or pleural effusion.

Although pneumonitis is a primary characteristic of Q fever, it should be noted that Q fever is a systemic disorder, as are the other rickettsioses. Hepatosplenomegaly occurs frequently, and gastroenteritis and hemolytic anemia have been reported.

The disease usually is mild and self-limited, lasting 1 to 2 weeks, with a mortality rate of 1% or less. Patients in whom Q fever and endocarditis or chronic Q fever develop, however, have a mortality rate between 30% and 60%. Other reported complications include myocarditis, pericarditis, meningoencephalitis, hepatitis, inappropriate secretion of antidiuretic hormone, and glomerulonephritis.

■ DIAGNOSIS

Complement-fixation or immunofluorescence tests that measure anti-phase I and anti-phase II antibody are effective in diagnosing Q fever. Specific IgM to *C burnetii* can be measured by ELISA, or by complement-fixation or immunofluorescence tests. Anti-phase II antibody is present early in primary disease. Anti-phase I antibody is present in patients with chronic disease or those who have granulomatous hepatitis or endocarditis. A polymerase chain reaction test is available that has the ability to detect as few as 1 to 10 organisms.

■ TREATMENT

Q fever responds promptly to tetracyclines or chloramphenicol, and relapses are rare. Primary disease should be treated with chloramphenicol in children less than 8 years of age and with tetracycline in those 8 years of age or older. The most appropriate drug and the duration of therapy necessary for patients with endocarditis resulting from Q fever remain unclear. Combination therapy that includes quinolones recently has been shown to be effective. Tetracycline, chloramphenicol, rifampin, lincomycin, co-trimoxazole, and trimethoprim-sulfamethoxazole all have been used, with differing degrees of success.

■ PROGNOSIS

Mortality from uncomplicated Q fever is 1% or less. Most patients recover completely within 30 to 60 days, with or without antimicrobial therapy. Antibiotics shorten the course of infection. When myocarditis, pericarditis, or endocarditis occurs, permanent disability and fatality are reported in 30% to 60% of patients.

EHRLICHIOSIS

Ehrlichia canis has been recognized as a canine pathogen for many years. Human ehrlichiosis is a febrile illness characterized by headache, anorexia, and myalgias, with associated leukopenia or pancytopenia. Most patients have experienced tick attachment or bite within weeks before the onset of illness.

■ CLINICAL MANIFESTATIONS

The estimated incubation period for human ehrlichiosis is 12 to 14 days. Similar to Rocky Mountain spotted fever, ehrlichiosis is an acute febrile illness that causes fever, headache, anorexia with or without vomiting, and myalgias. Rash, which may be macular, maculopapular, or petechial, rarely occurs in adults. Among the small number of pediatric infections reported, rash has occurred commonly, with a distribution that often includes both the trunk and the extremities.

Meningitis as a manifestation of ehrlichiosis has been reported in two children, with symptoms ranging from irritability and meningismus to obtundation with response only to painful stimuli. Initial examination of the cerebrospinal fluid revealed pleocytosis ranging from about 50 to 1000 white blood cells, with a predominance of either neutrophils or lymphocytes; between 5 and 40 red blood cells; mildly elevated protein levels; and a normal to slightly low glucose value. Each of the two children recovered fully.

One half to two thirds of affected adults have mild leukopenia and thrombocytopenia. Although the numbers are small, these features also occur with similar frequency in children. One child has had a documented decline in the white blood cell count from 13,000 to 1600 over a period of several hours. Usually, thrombocytopenia is not associated with clinical bleeding; however, disseminated intravascular coagulopathy has been reported. Elevations of aspartate aminotransferase, which usually are modest, peak at about 1 week into the illness, with values ranging from twice normal to several thousand. Other uncommon manifestations of illness include elevation of renal function test results (occasionally of sufficient severity to require dialysis), hyponatremia, and hypoalbuminemia. These manifestations presumably are a consequence of the generalized vasculitis that accompanies the infection.

■ DIAGNOSIS AND DIFFERENTIAL DIAGNOSIS

The diagnosis of human ehrlichiosis is established by documenting a fourfold rise or fall in titer by an indirect fluorescent antibody test that is available through the Centers for Disease Control and Prevention. The minimum titer required by this method is 80, with a technique in which *E chaffeensis* is used as the source of antigen. Sera should be collected at the time of diagnosis and then 2 to 4 weeks after the onset of illness for serologic analysis.

■ TREATMENT

In adults, the drug of choice for ehrlichiosis is tetracycline. Because this antibiotic is not approved for use in children less than 12 years of age, the optimal therapy for children is unclear. Several children have received treatment with chloramphenicol with apparent improvement, but the experience to date is too limited to advocate chloramphenicol as the treatment of choice for pediatric ehrlichiosis. Doxycycline is an alternative regimen for children more than 12 years of age. Mild clinical illness is self-limited, and recovery without specific antimicrobial treatment has been described, although fever may be protracted.

(Abridged from Ralph D. Feigin and Marc L. Boom, Rickettsial Diseases, in Oski, DeAngelis, Feigin, McMillan, Warshaw: *Principles and Practice of Pediatrics, Second Edition,* J.B. Lippincott, 1994.)

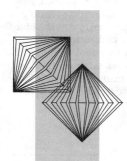

SECTION 4
Parasitic Diseases

Oski's Essential Pediatrics,
edited by Kevin B. Johnson and Frank A. Oski.
Lippincott–Raven Publishers,
Philadelphia © 1997

79

Protozoan Parasites

ENTAMOEBA HISTOLYTICA

Amebiasis is defined as infection with *Entamoeba histolytica,* with or without overt clinical symptoms. The disease is worldwide in distribution, affecting as much as 10% of the population. The highest prevalence is seen in underdeveloped areas and tropical regions. It has been estimated that about 1% to 5% of Americans who have never traveled outside the United States have amebiasis; most of these are asymptomatic carriers. Severe disease, such as ulcerative amebic colitis or liver abscess, is relatively rare.

Infection with pathogenic trophozoites is not a major clinical problem in this country, despite prevalence rates ranging from 0.1% to 50% in regional and institutional surveys. Overall, prevalence rates approach 4%. The invasive trophozoites cause diarrhea and dysentery in 2% to 8% of infected patients. Trophozoites that enter the bloodstream may pass to the liver or other organs and cause abscesses.

Humans are the natural host and reservoir for *E histolytica.* Fecal–oral transmission occurs frequently through contaminated water or foods such as vegetables.

■ CLINICAL FEATURES

Most infections are asymptomatic (luminal colonization) and elimination of the parasite from the gut occurs within 12 months. The incubation period for the illness varies but usually is 2 to 4 weeks. The severity of illness may vary from very mild symptoms to severe fulminating disease with mucosal inflammation, ulceration, and even perforation. Most patients with invasive amebiasis describe a gradual onset of cramping, abdominal pain, malaise, tenesmus (with rectal involvement), and frequent stools. Stools usually are blood-stained and mucoid. Diarrhea may persist for weeks but can wax and wane with alternating periods of constipation. In some patients, the onset of symptoms may be acute, with fever, profuse bloody mucoid diarrhea, dehydration, and electrolyte abnormalities. This fulminant picture may mimic that seen in toxic megacolon, acute inflammatory bowel disease, and bacillary dysentery. More serious disease is associated with youth, pregnancy, malnutrition, corticosteroid therapy, and underlying systemic disease. Possible complications include intestinal perforation, hemorrhage, stricture, inflammation, peritonitis, and a local inflammatory mass or ameboma. On physical examination, tenderness usually is present throughout the lower abdomen.

Hepatic amebiasis and abscess are characterized by fever, right upper quadrant abdominal pain, pleuritic pain, respiratory distress, and hepatomegaly. Patients frequently give no history of significant gastrointestinal symptoms. The most common finding on physical examination is a large, tender liver. Icterus occurs infrequently, and its presence is a ominous sign. Examination of the chest may reveal rales, decreased breath sounds, and a friction rub. Complications involve the pleural cavity or intra-abdominal extension of the abscess.

■ DIAGNOSIS

Because medical therapy is highly effective in all forms of amebiasis, the diagnosis should be made as early as possible. It is crucial to distinguish amebiasis from inflammatory bowel disease. The symptoms, findings on colonoscopy, and histologic findings on examination of biopsy material can mimic the findings in ulcerative colitis. Steroids, which frequently are prescribed for ulcerative colitis, may complicate the course of amebiasis and increase the mortality.

Microscopic examination of repeated stool specimens is the definitive diagnostic test. When the test is done correctly, the results of more than 90% of stool examinations are positive in infected patients.

■ TREATMENT

The specific therapy recommended for infection with *E histolytica* depends on the site of involvement (luminal, intramural, or systemic) and is beyond the scope of this text.

Prophylaxis for travelers to endemic areas is not recommended. The best prophylaxis is exercising caution in unsanitary conditions and endemic environments.

Acquired cellular immunity to invasive amebiasis seems to occur. Work is underway using a number of strategies to develop a subunit amebiasis vaccine. Vaccination would be the most cost-effective approach to prevention.

(Abridged from Bradley Howard Kessler and William J. Klish, Protozoan Parasites, in Oski, DeAngelis, Feigin, McMillan, Warshaw: *Principles and Practice of Pediatrics, Second Edition*, J.B. Lippincott, 1994.)

Oski's Essential Pediatrics,
edited by Kevin B. Johnson and Frank A. Oski.
Lippincott–Raven Publishers,
Philadelphia © 1997

80

Giardia lamblia

Giardia lamblia is a cosmopolitan parasite of worldwide distribution and an important cause of traveler's diarrhea. Attack rates are particularly high in travelers to Russia, especially St. Petersburg. *Giardia* also is prevalent in the mountainous western United States, where infection can be contracted by drinking water from mountain streams that have been contaminated by feces from humans, dogs, and other species susceptible to *G lamblia*. The beaver acts as a reservoir for the organism during the summer months by becoming infected (presumably from humans) and then defecating directly into the streams. Boiling water for 10 minutes kills all organisms.

Giardia also can be spread by close person-to-person contact in which fecal contamination may occur, such as in day care centers and residential institutions. In addition, contaminated food may act as a vector for this parasite.

■ CLINICAL FEATURES OF GIARDIASIS

Acute symptoms of giardiasis include watery diarrhea, nausea, bloating, belching (described as "sulfurous"), cramping, abdominal pain, and weight loss; these symptoms usually occur 1 to 2 weeks after the ingestion of cysts. The illness usually is self-limited, lasting 2 to 6 weeks, but may recur intermittently or become chronic. Chronic symptoms can include fatigue, nervousness, weight loss, growth retardation, steatorrhea, lactose intolerance, and, rarely, protein-losing enteropathy. Chronic giardiasis frequently is associated with immune deficiency syndromes such as IgA and IgM deficiencies and the acquired immunodeficiency syndrome. People who are carrying the disease chronically may be asymptomatic.

■ DIAGNOSIS

Routine laboratory values such as blood cell counts and electrolyte levels are normal in most patients. Nonspecific radiographic abnormalities that may be seen on barium contrast studies of the upper intestinal tract include thickening of the mucosal folds, hypersecretion with dilution of the barium column, and hypermotility.

Direct examination of feces for the presence of *G lamblia* cysts or trophozoites remains the hallmark for diagnosis. If the diagnosis is suspected strongly, at least three stools should be collected on different days. If both a direct smear and a concentration test are done on each stool, the chance of diagnosis is 75% from one stool, 90% from two stools, and 97% from three stools.

The diagnosis is made readily by examining the upper small intestine directly, either by mucosal biopsy or through the collection of jejunal contents. Diagnosis of giardiasis using both enzyme-linked immunosorbent assay (ELISA) and counterimmunoelectrophoresis of either stool or serum is available and has a high sensitivity and specificity.

■ TREATMENT

Treatment is indicated whenever *Giardia* is found to cause acute diarrhea, chronic intermittent disease, subclinical symptoms, or infection in others. Children with nondiarrheal giardiasis, however, who exhibit other gastrointestinal symptoms or have evidence of malabsorption should be considered for therapy. The treatment of choice in both asymptomatic and symptomatic patients is metronidazole. Alternative drugs include quinacrine and furazolidone.

(Abridged from William J. Klish, *Giardia lamblia*, in Oski, DeAngelis, Feigin, McMillan, Warshaw: *Principles and Practice of Pediatrics, Second Edition*, J.B. Lippincott, 1994.)

Oski's Essential Pediatrics, edited by Kevin B. Johnson and Frank A. Oski. Lippincott–Raven Publishers, Philadelphia © 1997

81

Malaria

Although rarely seen in the United States, malaria is the most common infectious cause of morbidity in tropical and semitropical regions of the world. An estimated 2 to 3 million deaths annually, mostly of young children, are attributed to the disease. The illness, caused by one of the four species of *Plasmodium* parasite that are specific for humans, is characterized by recurrent paroxysms of high fever, splenomegaly, and anemia.

■ THE ORGANISMS

The parasites responsible for malaria are obligate intracellular protozoa. *Plasmodium falciparum, Plasmodium vivax, Plasmodium malariae,* and *Plasmodium ovale* all are similar in their pattern of reproduction. The sexual portion of their life cycle begins when a female *Anopheles* mosquito feeds on an infected human. Malarial gametocytes ingested as part of this blood meal form zygotes in the midgut of the insect. These zygotes mature and migrate to the mosquito's salivary gland, where they reside as sporozoites until the mosquito's next feeding, at which time they are inoculated into the next human victim.

Leaving the bloodstream almost immediately, the sporozoites invade human hepatocytes. There, nestled in parenchymal tissue, the parasite undergoes multiple asexual divisions to form a cystic structure called a schizont. One to 3 weeks after the initial inoculation, the schizont ruptures, releasing thousands of infective units (merozoites) into the bloodstream. It is at this stage that important species diversity exists: with infection by *P falciparum* or *P malariae,* all the schizonts rupture, effectively ending this exoerythrocytic (ie, intrahepatic) phase. In *P vivax* and *P ovale* infections, however, some of the schizonts remain dormant in the liver, only to rupture months to years later. These dormant forms (hypnozoites) are responsible for the clinical phenomenon of malarial relapse.

On release from the hepatic schizonts, the merozoites initiate the erythrocytic phase by attaching to and invading circulating red blood cells. Once inside the erythrocyte, the protozoan, now known as a trophozoite, appears as the characteristic blue "signet ring" against the pink cytoplasm of the blood cell. The organism ingests the host cell cytoplasm and hemoglobin, developing asexually from the ring form to the mature trophozoite. Nuclear division begins, creating schizonts; these ultimately will contain 6 to 24 merozoites, depending on the species. After this process of schizogony occurs (which takes about 72 hours for *P malariae* and 48 hours for the other species), the erythrocyte ruptures. This releases the merozoites, which enter uninfected red cells to start the erythrocytic cycle again. A small percentage of the merozoites diverge from this pattern, differentiating into the sexual gametocytes. These forms circulate in the bloodstream until they are ingested in the next mosquito feeding, thereby completing the life cycle.

■ TRANSMISSION AND EPIDEMIOLOGY

Malaria is found primarily in Mexico, parts of the Caribbean, Central and South America, sub-Saharan Africa, the Middle East, the Indian subcontinent, southern Asia and Indochina, and certain islands of the South Pacific. Standing water and warm climate (each of which is required for mosquito propagation) favor endemicity. Prerequisites for spread of the disease include the presence of a suitable anopheline vector along with infected and susceptible hosts.

■ CLINICAL MANIFESTATIONS

The clinical picture in malaria may vary considerably, depending on the species involved and on the patient's age and immune status. *P falciparum* produces the most severe symptoms; this probably correlates with the degree of parasitemia (up to 500,000 parasites per cubic millimeter of blood in severe cases). The other three species produce milder symptoms and may be considered as a group. In endemic areas, very young infants are relatively protected by virtue of their high concentration of hemoglobin F and their passive acquisition of maternal antibody. Older infants and young children (and their immunologic equivalent, previously unexposed adults) are the most susceptible to severe infection. Individuals who have attained immunity by virtue of repeated exposure to malaria generally have mild symptoms, even in the face of heavy parasitemia.

Aquiescent period, corresponding to the exoerythrocytic phase of the parasite, follows the initial inoculation. During the first few cycles of erythrocytic infection, the nonimmune patient exhibits vague influenza-like symptoms of headache, malaise, irritability, anorexia, gastrointestinal complaints, and fever that may be continuous. After a number of infectious cycles, the symptoms often take on the classic "cold–hot–wet" pattern of the periodic fever paroxysm. Coinciding with erythrocytic rupture, the paroxysm consists of a brief episode of chills followed by several hours of sudden high fever, headache, nausea, vomiting, and myalgia, sometimes accompanied by delirium. Abdominal pain is prominent if rapid splenic enlargement has occurred. The patient may be prostrate and, because the ensuing defervescence is accompanied by marked diaphoresis, frequently suffers from dehydration. After a period of hours, the paroxysm ceases rather abruptly; the patient usually is fatigued and may rest soundly. With many species of *Plasmodium*, the paroxysms return in 48 to 72 hours.

When it can be observed, the malarial paroxysm is the most characteristic of clinical findings. In its absence, splenomegaly usually is the most striking feature. The spleen may be massively enlarged, and care must be taken in its palpation because the potential for rupture poses a significant danger. Tender hepatomegaly frequently occurs. Other common physical findings include orthostatic hypotension or other signs of dehydration, herpes labialis, icterus, and the pallor associated with anemia.

Laboratory data in malaria reflect hemolysis, with a normochromic, normocytic anemia, hyperbilirubinemia, and a direct Coombs' test result that frequently is positive. The leukocyte count and differential are unpredictable; an increased proportion of monocytes is common, but eosinophilia usually is not seen. Thrombocytopenia is common. The prothrombin time may be prolonged. Proteinuria often is evident. Hypoglycemia is common in patients with severe *P falciparum* malaria.

■ DIAGNOSIS

In malaria-endemic regions, diagnosis of the disease is not difficult and usually is made on clinical grounds. For individuals outside these areas, however, the key is remembering the disease as part of the differential diagnosis. Travel to endemic areas (even years earlier) and adherence to chemoprophylaxis guidelines are important clues. A history of recurrent high fevers also is helpful, if present. The triad of fever, splenomegaly, and anemia always should suggest the diagnosis. A fever paroxysm is impressive when it is witnessed firsthand by observers who are unfamiliar with the disease.

Examination of Giemsa-stained peripheral blood smears continues to be the primary method of diagnosis for malaria. Because of generally low levels of parasitemia (less than 1% of erythrocytes are infected in cases caused by species other than *P falciparum*), a thick smear is done first for screening. Multiple thick smears performed at 12-hour intervals optimize detection of the parasite. If infected red cells are found, a review of a thin smear by an experienced examiner usually will allow species identification based on the morphology of the intracellular trophozoites. Other diagnostic techniques, such as specific antibody detection and DNA probing, generally are reserved for research and epidemiologic studies.

■ TREATMENT

Once the diagnosis of malaria has been made, treatment should be initiated immediately. With severely ill patients for whom the index of suspicion is high, some authorities recommend treating presumptively before laboratory confirmation is available. Delay in treatment may affect prognosis adversely in *P falciparum* infection.

In addition to quinine, antimalarial drugs include the other arylaminoalcohols, synthetic aminoquinolines, and folate antagonists. Doxycycline and clindamycin also are chosen occasionally for prophylaxis or therapy, although their use in malaria is considered to be experimental.

Key issues in deciding on drug(s) of choice for malaria treatment include: species identity (*P falciparum* versus another species); the possibility that the strain is chloroquine-resistant if the infection is with *P falciparum*; and the ability of the patient to take medication orally. Infections with species other than *P falciparum* and those with sensitive strains of *P falciparum* are treated in the same manner in patients with acute infection (*ie*, with chloroquine [Aralen] orally or quinidine gluconate parenterally). If the history does not clearly suggest the source of a *P falciparum* infection, chloroquine resistance must be assumed and the patient treated accordingly. Oral therapy is standard, but a patient who is comatose, or one who has significant emesis or parasitemia of more than 5% will require parenteral therapy until clinical improvement allows a change to oral medication. Quinine was the parenteral drug of choice for years, but this has been supplanted in the United States by quinidine gluconate, which is more readily available and at least as efficacious.

Supportive care is an important adjunct to antimalarial chemotherapy. Volume depletion should be corrected rapidly, but with care. Analgesics and antipyretics will make the patient more comfortable. If parenteral quinidine is used, an intensive care setting with continuous cardiac monitoring and close attention to fluid status (central hemodynamic monitoring in severe cases) is recommended; frequent determinations of the QT interval (a sensitive indicator of quinidine concentration) and blood glucose level should be made. Some experts advocate the use of exchange transfusion in patients with severe or complicated malaria, as a means of rapidly reducing the level of parasitemia and possibly removing plasmodia-related toxic factors. The total volume of exchange should be based on reaching a parasitemia of less than 1%. The use of corticosteroids in cerebral malaria probably is unwarranted because they may increase complication rates and the duration of coma.

■ PREVENTION

The most successful preventive regimens combine personal environmental protection with chemoprophylaxis during exposure in endemic regions. Given the nocturnal feeding behavior of the *Anopheles* mosquito, environmental protection—avoiding mosquito bites—is most important from dusk to dawn. Recommended measures include wearing long clothing, covering exposed areas of the body sparingly with insect repellent (preparations containing N,N diethylmetatoluamide, or DEET, are most effective), remaining in screened-in areas as much as possible, and using fine mesh mosquito netting around beds. Permethrin also may be applied to clothing for extra protection. A flying-insect spray containing pyrethrum also may be useful for living quarters during the evening and nighttime.

The use of drugs to prevent malaria is recommended highly for travelers to regions where the disease is endemic. The risk of exposure generally is higher in rural areas than in cities, and the travel itinerary should be reviewed carefully to ascertain the need for chemoprophylaxis. Unless otherwise noted below, the drug should be taken once weekly, starting 1 to 2 weeks before departure, continuing throughout the trip, and ending 4 weeks after leaving the endemic area. Chloroquine in a dose of 5 mg base per kilogram orally (maximum 300 mg base or 500 mg salt) is the drug of choice for travel to areas that do not have chloroquine resistance. If this drug is not tolerated, one alternative is hydroxychloroquine (Plaquenil), at 5 mg base per kilogram (maximum 310 mg base) weekly.

(Abridged from Lori E. R. Patterson, Malaria, in Oski, DeAngelis, Feigin, McMillan, Warshaw: *Principles and Practice of Pediatrics, Second Edition*, J.B. Lippincott, 1994.)

Oski's Essential Pediatrics,
edited by Kevin B. Johnson and Frank A. Oski.
Lippincott–Raven Publishers,
Philadelphia © 1997

82

Visceral Larva Migrans

Human infection with the larval stage of the common dog roundworm, *Toxocara canis,* is the principal cause of two distinct clinical syndromes: visceral larva migrans (VLM) and ocular toxocariasis or ocular larva migrans (OLM). Because of its relative infrequency, however, OLM will not be discussed here. The majority of *Toxocara* infections occur in young children, and although most result in mild or inapparent disease, serious complications may occur. Humans do not act as a definitive host for these nematodes, but the larvae migrate throughout the tissues and provoke an eosinophilic inflammatory response that may result in striking symptoms and laboratory findings.

■ CLINICAL FEATURES

The classic manifestations of VLM reflected the fact that only clinical diagnosis of *T canis* infection was possible; fever, hepatomegaly, eosinophilic leukocytosis, and hypergammaglobulinemia defined the syndrome. Many of these patients also had pulmonary involvement (rales or wheezes) and rashes (often pruritic). Seizures were reported in more than 25% of patients in one early series. It is now agreed that the majority of *T canis* infections in children are asymptomatic, and that only a small number of these infections result in the full-blown VLM syndrome. The use of improved serologic tests should define better the clinical characteristics of less severe cases of VLM.

Hepatomegaly remains a common sign in VLM, but the most common symptoms are pulmonary and may mimic those of asthma or pneumonia. Chest radiographs reveal infiltrates in half the patients with pulmonary symptoms, but severe lung disease is uncommon. Fever, adenopathy, rash, and weight loss may occur. Ocular disease is unusual in association with VLM but may occur in severe cases. Leukocyte counts of 30,000 to 100,000/mm³ with a pronounced eosinophilia are common. The percentage of eosinophils usually is greater than 20% in acute cases of VLM and may reach 90%; eosinophilia often persists for months or years after symptoms resolve. Hypergammaglobulinemia often is present, with elevations of IgE, IgM, and IgG. Isohemagglutinin titers (anti-A, anti-B) often are elevated because the *T canis* larva expresses surface antigens that cross-react with epitopes of the blood group antigens.

The prognosis in most cases of VLM is excellent, with complete recovery the rule. Severe and even fatal cases have been reported, however. Myocardial involvement is rare, but has been reported in several fatal cases and as an incidental finding at the time of open heart surgery in two patients. *T canis* may cause eosinophilic meningitis; larvae have been found in the brain at autopsy in children with fatal infection and as an incidental finding in children with unrelated causes of death. Although seizures may occur as a complication of VLM, this appears to be a much less frequent complication than early reports suggested. The effects of asymptomatic and mild infection are largely unknown. Both a large cohort study and a large case-control study found small deficits in performance on neuropsychiatric tests in seropositive children as compared with seronegative controls. In the cohort study, confounding variables appeared to explain these differences; in the case-control study, small differences between seropositive and seronegative children remained after careful adjustment for potential confounding factors. Considering the frequency of *T canis* infection in children in the United States, more careful study of the neurologic consequences of *Toxocara* infections is merited.

■ DIFFERENTIAL DIAGNOSIS

The differential diagnosis of VLM caused by *T canis* includes infection by the larval forms of other helminths that have a tissue migratory phase to their life cycle: these include other *Toxocara* species, *Ascaris lumbricoides, Strongyloides stercoralis, Trichinella,* hookworms, and schistosomes. Eosinophilic leukemia may be considered in some patients with severe eosinophilia. The eosinophilia associated with *T canis* infection may persist for months or years, and it occurs in asymptomatic infected patients. Thus, silent or preceding *T canis* infection should be considered in the differential diagnosis of unexplained persistent eosinophilia.

Laboratory Diagnosis

Although a presumptive diagnosis of VLM can be supported by abnormalities on a variety of laboratory tests (eosinophilia, hypergammaglobulinemia, elevated isohemagglutinin levels), these tests are nonspecific and usually are normal in cases of ocular disease. A variety of immunologic tests have been developed over the years but have been largely unsuccessful, presumably because they used antigen prepared from adult worms.

Recently, an enzyme-linked immunosorbent assay (ELISA) test using antigen from larval *T canis* has been developed. The *Toxocara* Excretory–Secretory (TES) ELISA uses an excretory or secretory antigen from the supernatants of *T canis* larvae maintained in vitro. The TES ELISA has proved to be a sensitive and specific test in the diagnosis of VLM, and it appears to be useful in the diagnosis of ocular toxocariasis as well.

■ THERAPY

Discussion of potential therapy of VLM must begin with consideration of the prognosis of untreated disease. The overall prognosis of VLM is excellent. Even in more severe cases, removal of the patient from the source of exposure usually is adequate to effect satisfactory recovery. Pharmacologic treatment of VLM should be considered only when severe symptoms occur (*eg,* severe respiratory distress) or involvement of critical organs (myocardium, brain) is noted. In these situations, the use of corticosteroids may be indicated and has been reported to result in dramatic improvement of symptoms. There is no convincing evidence that antihelminthic agents such as thiabendazole or diethylcarbamazine are effective against larval forms in tissues, and these drugs have not been shown to be of clear value in the treatment of any human *Toxocara* infection.

■ PREVENTION

Newborn puppies are the principal source of infection in young children. All newborn puppies should be wormed before they reach 2 to 3 weeks of age, and worming should be repeated every 2 weeks until the puppy is 4 months old. Thereafter, fecal examinations should be performed twice yearly, with treatment as indicated. Scoop laws are of some benefit because eggs that have not undergone embryonation require 2 weeks or more to become infective. Pica should be discouraged and good hygiene practiced. In young children with persistent pica, close supervision is recommended when they play outdoors in parks, backyards, or sandboxes. Once soil is contaminated with *T canis* eggs, it cannot be decontaminated.

(Abridged from B. Keith English, Toxocariasis, in Oski, DeAngelis, Feigin, McMillan, Warshaw: *Principles and Practice of Pediatrics, Second Edition*, J.B. Lippincott, 1994.)

Oski's Essential Pediatrics,
edited by Kevin B. Johnson and Frank A. Oski.
Lippincott–Raven Publishers,
Philadelphia © 1997

83

Arthropoda

■ TICKS AND MITES

Ticks are macroscopic arthropods that may cause local disease after a bite but, more important, can transmit to humans one of several potentially serious infectious diseases (Table 83–1). Mites are microscopic arthropods that also may cause local skin irritation or transmit such diseases as rickettsialpox or scrub typhus.

Some pregnant female ticks secrete a neurotoxin associated with tick paralysis, a neurologic syndrome characterized by an ascending flaccid paralysis. Diminished nerve conduction velocity suggesting peripheral nerve dysfunction has been detected in some children. One to 2 days after the tick attaches, ataxia and areflexia develop in the patient. Subsequently, the syndrome progresses to a gradual ascending flaccid paralysis that ultimately may involve the trunk, upper extremities, pharynx, and tongue. Death may result from respiratory compromise.

Tick paralysis can be diagnosed only by neurologic improvement occurring in a patient with typical features once the tick is removed. Therapy otherwise is supportive, particularly for respiratory function.

In contrast to tick bites, most reactions to mites occur within minutes to hours of the bite. This local reaction is thought to be the result of hypersensitivity to toxins secreted during feeding, which generally takes place at night. Contact with mites in their natural habitat occurs during such activities as hiking and camping. Domestic animals such as dogs and cats as well as wild birds and rodents may harbor mites. Mite bites are treated symptomatically to reduce the pruritus and prevent secondary infections.

■ SPIDERS

In the United States, the two spiders that cause severe cutaneous and systemic reactions to envenomation are *Loxosceles reclusa,* the brown recluse spider, and *Lactrodectus mactans*, the black widow spider.

Brown Recluse Spiders

Brown recluse spiders have a characteristic fiddle-shaped marking on the dorsal cephalothorax. This spider lives mainly in the south central United States, especially the Midwest, but can be found in many other areas. It prefers dark, secluded places and often is found in closets, storage boxes, barns, garages, and other little-used areas of the home.

Shortly after sustaining a brown recluse spider bite, the patient may experience itching and tingling; the local area becomes swollen, red, and tender. The lesion may develop central necrosis and blebs. Lymphangitis and regional lymphadenopathy may occur secondarily. Systemic symptoms such as fever, chills, nausea, vomiting, and myalgias may occur 12 to 24 hours after the bite. More severe envenomation may be complicated by thrombocytopenia, disseminated intravascular coagulation, hematuria, hemoglobinuria, renal failure, and shock. In young children especially, a purplish or blanched lesion indicates ischemia, and, in these patients, the complete blood cell count, platelet count, and urinalysis should be monitored carefully.

The treatment of uncomplicated cutaneous lesions from a brown recluse spider bite is best approached conservatively. Immobilization of the affected extremity is useful. Frequent cleaning and tetanus prophylaxis, if indicated, are recommended. Administering an antipruritic drug such as diphenhydramine and covering the wound may help prevent further trauma to the area and the development of a secondary infection. Early surgical excision and corticosteroids have not proved beneficial for severe bites. Dapsone, a leukocyte inhibitor, has been shown to reduce surgical complications as well as the time required for the wound to heal. Further studies with this agent are necessary before its general use can be considered in children. Another experimental approach involves a specific antivenin.

TABLE 83-1. Infectious Diseases of Humans Transmitted by Ticks

Agent	Disease
Arbovirus	Encephalitis
Babesia microti	Babesiosis
Borrelia burgdorferi	Lyme disease
Borrelia duttonii	Relapsing fever
Coxiella burnetii	Q fever
Ehrlichia chaffeensis	Ehrlichiosis
Francisella tularensis	Tularemia
Orbivirus	Colorado tick fever
Rickettsia conorii	Fievre boutonneuse
Rickettsia rickettsii	Rocky Mountain spotted fever
Other rickettsiae	Tick typhus

Black Widow Spiders

The black widow spider bite is associated with an immediate sharp pain, followed by burning, swelling, and inflammation of the bite site. Systemic symptoms that may develop shortly include weakness, dizziness, hypotension, tremors, and abdominal muscle cramps. Hemoglobinuria and nephritis have occurred in young children.

Rest and immobilization of the involved extremity are recommended. Pain medication and muscle relaxants are used as necessary. An antivenin (manufactured by Merck, Sharp & Dohme) also can be administered, provided the patient does not have a hypersensitivity reaction to skin testing of this material.

(Abridged from Sheldon L. Kaplan, Arthropoda, in Oski, DeAngelis, Feigin, McMillan, Warshaw: *Principles and Practice of Pediatrics, Second Edition*, J.B. Lippincott, 1994.)

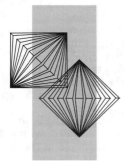

SECTION 5
Kawasaki Disease

Oski's Essential Pediatrics,
edited by Kevin B. Johnson and Frank A. Oski.
Lippincott–Raven Publishers,
Philadelphia © 1997

84

Kawasaki Disease

Kawasaki disease is an acute, febrile, multisystem syndrome of unknown etiology that predominantly afflicts children less than 9 years of age. The disease also is referred to as mucocutaneous lymph node syndrome. The diagnosis is based entirely on clinical features because there are no pathognomonic laboratory findings.

The disease first was recognized by Tomisaku Kawasaki in 1961. Subsequently, numerous cases of the disease have been recognized throughout the world in all racial groups. Kawasaki disease is one of the most common causes of acquired heart disease and inflammatory arthritis in North America.

■ EPIDEMIOLOGY

Cases reported to the Centers for Disease Control and prevention (CDC) indicate that the yearly incidence per 100,000 children aged 8 years or younger is three times higher in Asian-American than in African-American children and more than six times higher in Asian-American than in white children. The ratio of affected males to females is 1.5:1 in virtually all countries.

Kawasaki disease has been seen almost exclusively in children. In several adult cases, the disease reported seems more likely to have been caused by toxic shock syndrome than by Kawasaki disease. The syndrome has not been detected in newborn infants, but the incidence increases steadily to peak at about 13 to 24 months of age and then falls off in almost linear fashion until 12 years of age after which Kawasaki disease is most unusual.

This particular incidence pattern, which has been noted with other infectious diseases, suggests that transplacental antibody may offer some protection in young infants and that, when maternal IgG levels begin to decline and infants no longer are immune, a cohort of susceptible children is produced. As individuals either have clinical disease or acquire immunity to an as yet unknown agent, the incidence may decline toward zero. The incidence pattern described above, however, cannot be accepted as proof of an infectious cause for Kawasaki disease.

■ ETIOLOGY

The cause of Kawasaki disease is unknown. Most investigators have favored the possibility of an infectious agent or an immune response to an infectious agent or agents. Kawasaki disease has not been associated consistently with exposure to environmental pesticides, chemicals, heavy metals, toxins, or pollutants. However, one outbreak of Kawasaki disease in Denver was felt to be associated with the use of rug shampoo. There is also some evidence to suggest that Kawasaki disease may be an allergic phenomenon, given a higher incidence of allergies in children with Kawasaki disease or in members of their families than there is in control patients.

■ PATHOLOGY

Grossly, cardiac hypertrophy is common. Multiple or single beadlike or fusiform aneurysms of the coronary arteries and their branches usually are found in fatal cases. During the various clinical stages, specific pathologic findings are noted, and during days 0 to 9, the coronary arteries have perivasculitis and endarteritis, but medial sparing. Pericarditis, myocarditis, endocarditis, valvulitis, and conduction system inflammation are observed, with polymorphonuclear infiltrates. During days 12 to 25, coronary artery panvasculitis and aneurysm formation occur, with inflammation and necrosis of the media resulting in "true" aneurysms. By the second week, the inflammatory infiltrate has evolved into a lymphocytic and plasma cell dominance. Resolution of the coronary inflammation occurs near day 30, with subsequent granulation formation. Coronary artery scarring, stenosis, and endocardial fibroelastosis are described after day 40. Aneurysms of other arteries, such as the renal, iliac, and brachial arteries, may be found. Phlebitis is common, with vascular inflammation that affects larger musculoelastic arteries in their extraparenchymal portions most often and most severely. Sites of arteritis include the lung, pancreas, spleen, kidney, testis, mesentery, adrenal gland, and gastrointestinal tract.

■ CLINICAL MANIFESTATIONS

The clinical manifestations of Kawasaki disease in accordance with the CDC diagnostic criteria are given in Table 84–1.

Kawasaki disease occurs in four discrete phases. In the first phase, the previously healthy child becomes febrile and irritable. Fever is relentless, and the temperature frequently exceeds 40.6°C (105.8°F) in 40% of the patients at some time. Nonsuppurative cervical lymphadenopathy, usually in the anterior triangle and frequently bilateral, may be present, but may disappear rapidly. Within several days, rash and bilateral conjunctival injection appear. It usually is at the end of this phase that the physician first is consulted.

The second phase begins about the fourth day of illness and is characterized by continuing high, spiking fever that is unresponsive to standard antipyretic regimens or to antibiotics. The mean duration of fever is 12 days if the patient is not treated with aspirin or gamma globulin. The child is febrile and irritable, and often appears quite ill. Cervical lymphadenitis usually is present. Bilateral injection of the conjunctivae, primarily bulbar, is impressive, and unilateral subconjunctival hemorrhage may occur. Anterior uveitis may be found in 80% of all patients evaluated by slit-lamp

---

TABLE 84-1. Diagnostic Criteria for Kawasaki Disease

I. Fever of 5 or more days' duration associated with at least four of the five following changes*:

1. Bilateral conjuctival infection

2. One or more changes of the mucous membranes of the upper respiratory tract, including pharyngeal injection, dry fissured lips, injected lips, and "strawberry" tongue

3. One or more changes of the extremities, including peripheral erythema, peripheral edema, periungual desquamation, and generalized desquamation

4. Rash, primarily truncal

5. Cervical lymphadenopathy

II. The disease cannot be explained by some other known disease process.

*A diagnosis of Kawasaki disease can be made if fever and any of the changes below are present in conjunction with coronary artery disease documented by two-dimensional echocardiography or coronary angiography.

Modified from previously published diagnostic criteria from the Centers for Disease Control for Kawasaki disease and the American Heart Association Committee on Rheumatic Fever, Endocarditis, and Kawasaki Disease.

---

examination. The anterior uveitis is self-limited, and the prognosis is good. Other ocular symptoms may include vitreous opacities, punctate keratitis, and papilledema. Chorioretinal and vitreous inflammation have been noted. Purulent conjunctivitis and blepharitis may occur. Photophobia may be apparent.

The lips are bright red, dry, and cracked. A strawberry tongue may be apparent, and the oral mucosa generally is hyperemic.

A rash that is particularly prominent over the trunk consists of maculopapular, ill-defined erythematous plaques of variable size. At times, coalescent areas suggest the possibility of scarlet fever. Vesicles and sterile pustules are seen occasionally. Petechiae, pinpoint rashes, and erythema multiforme have been described in selected cases. The rash also has been noted in the diaper area and on the face.

Hepatomegaly and splenomegaly are detected occasionally but usually resolve quickly. Diarrhea may occur in the early phases of the illness. Severe abdominal pain, paralytic ileus, and icterus are common. As the second phase progresses, erythema of the palms and soles may develop (Figure 84–1). The hands and feet become edematous, and arthralgia and arthritis of large joints may be noted.

Children with this type of illness usually must be hospitalized. The white blood cell (WBC) count is elevated, with a left shift. Counts in excess of 30,000/mm^3 are noted in about 15% of patients, and counts in excess of 20,000/mm^3 are observed in about 50% of patients. A peripheral smear reveals an increased percentage of toxic neutrophils characterized by cytoplasmic swelling, vacuolation, and toxic granulation, especially with coronary lesions. Toxic granulation and Döhle bodies are seen. The erythrocyte sedimentation rate, C-reactive protein titer, A$_2$-globulin value, and A$_1$-antitrypsin level all are elevated, but normalize by 8 to 12 weeks. An elevated sedimentation rate and C-reactive protein level usually are not present with viral exanthems, hypersensitivity reactions, and measles. Mild anemia may be noted. Severe hemolytic anemia has been described but is unusual. There often is an acute rise and convalescent fall in the levels of all classes of immunoglobulins. The elevation in the IgG level is predominantly in subclasses IgG1 and IgG3. The serum complement value is normal or high. Transaminase levels may be elevated but usually are not more than three times the upper limit of normal. Hypoalbuminemia, hyponatremia, and hypophosphatemia have been described. Urinalysis may reveal proteinuria and moderate pyuria, usually reflecting urethritis. In males, meatitis may be visible. Vulvitis has been described.

Meningeal findings are rare, although nuchal rigidity and lethargy have been reported. In patients who have had lumbar punctures performed, 10 to 50 WBCs/mm^3, predominantly mononuclear, have been noted, but the cerebrospinal protein and glucose levels have been normal.

Electrocardiograms are abnormal in 77% of patients with Kawasaki disease and in all those who have pancarditis. The most common abnormalities in order of their frequency are flattened T waves initially, followed by peaked T waves in convalescence; first-degree heart block; ST segment elevation or depression; and QT interval prolongation. Auscultation may reveal sinus tachycardia, a gallop rhythm, distant heart sounds, or a frictional rub. Chest radiographs may reveal infiltrates in selected patients and some cardiomegaly. Disappearance of the rash and resolution of the adenopathy herald the end of the second phase of illness.

About day 12 of the illness, the third phase occurs and is dominated by desquamation. Desquamation sometimes can be seen several days before the fever abates, which occurs at a mean of 10 days after the onset of the illness. Desquamation is a constant feature of Kawasaki disease. It usually is noted first

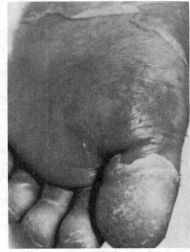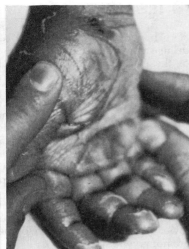

Figure 84-1. Erythema and edema of the feet and hands, characteristic of the second phase of Kawasaki disease.

in the periungual region, although other parts of the body may be involved. Desquamation may be particularly prominent in the diaper area. During the period of desquamation, arthralgias and arthritis may be noted, even though they were not present earlier. The large weight-bearing joints are involved most often. Thrombocytosis is another constant feature of the third phase of illness, with platelet counts ranging from 500,000 to 3 million/mm³. Thrombocytosis is seen rarely in the first week of illness. It usually appears in the second week, peaks in the third week, and returns gradually to normal about a month after onset in uncomplicated cases.

Bone marrow examination has revealed normal number and morphology of megakaryocytes. Increased fibrinogen levels and prolongation of the partial thromboplastin time have been noted. The third phase of illness is characterized by a gradual return of the patient toward normal. Beau's lines (transverse depressions in the fingernails and toenails) and alopecia may be seen in the weeks and months after recovery.

The fourth phase of illness is recognized in only a minority of cases. This phase is characterized by ongoing inflammation, subacute vasculitis, and an increased incidence of death from cardiac involvement.

■ COMPLICATIONS

Cardiovascular

The most serious complications of Kawasaki disease are cardiovascular and include aneurysms of the coronary arteries and other large arteries, aneurysmal rupture, hemopericardium, myocarditis, coronary thrombosis, pericardial effusions, cardiac tamponade, mitral valve disease, and arrhythmias. Aneurysms of the aorta and the cerebral, vertebral, subclavian, axillary, internal, common and external iliac, hepatic, and renal arteries have been described. In most cases, peripheral aneurysms have been associated with coronary artery aneurysms.

Other Complications

Acalculous cholecystitis has been noted repeatedly during the second phase of Kawasaki disease. Children with hydrops of the gallbladder usually have abdominal pain, a soft palpable mass in the right upper quadrant, and abdominal distention. The diagnosis can be made by ultrasonography. Most cases resolve spontaneously.

Other complications that have been described include sterile purulent otitis media, mastoiditis, retropharyngeal mass, necrotic pharyngitis, pleural effusion, myositis, renal infarcts, nephritis and nephrosis, gangrene of the fingers and toes, encephalopathy, facial nerve paralysis, hemiparesis, ataxia, and evidence of cerebral aneurysms, cerebral embolus, subarachnoid hemorrhage, and sensorineural hearing loss.

■ DIAGNOSIS AND DIFFERENTIAL DIAGNOSIS

The diagnosis of Kawasaki disease is made clinically by exclusion. Children who meet the CDC criteria should be strongly considered to have Kawasaki disease. Unfortunately, infants are less likely to have a classic presentation than are older children. In fact, children younger than 6 months of age may have coronary involvement, even though they do not fulfill the diagnostic criteria. The most common conditions that mimic Kawasaki disease are measles and group A β-hemolytic streptococcal infection. Other disorders with which Kawasaki disease can be confused are listed in Table 84–2.

TABLE 84-2. Disorders With Which Kawasaki Disease Is Confused

Roseola infantum
Meningococcemia
Rocky Mountain spotted fever
Leptospirosis
Rubella
Infectious mononucleosis
Enteroviruses
Rat-bite fever
Toxoplasmosis
Acrodynia
Collagen vascular disease
Reiter's syndrome
Behçet's syndrome
Toxic shock syndrome
Drug reactions
Gianotti syndrome

■ TREATMENT

The goals of therapy for Kawasaki disease are to decrease the inflammatory response and reduce the severity of the cardiovascular complications. The combination of intravenous gamma globulin and aspirin effectively meets these goals.

Corticosteroids appear to be contraindicated. Several investigators have reported a higher incidence of coronary artery aneurysms in patients treated with steroids than in those who received antibiotics or salicylate therapy.

Aspirin appears to be a particularly important therapeutic modality. Although it does not have an immediate antipyretic effect, aspirin can help reduce the height and duration of fever and may serve as an important antithrombotic agent. Experience with patients who receive high-dose aspirin early in the course of disease has demonstrated a lower rate of aneurysm development than in patients who are not given aspirin.

The presence of coronary aneurysms predisposes an individual to platelet deposition, embolic phenomena, and progressive intimal fibrosis with luminal obstruction. This may lead to decreased coronary artery blood flow, with resultant angina and myocardial infarction. Fibrinolytic agents, such as streptokinase, urokinase, or tissue plasminogen activator, may be used to treat myocardial infarction. If coronary artery bypass grafting is indicated, internal mammary artery grafts are the best choice, compared to saphenous vein grafts, because of their long-term patency and good growth potential.

■ PROGNOSIS

Kawasaki disease normally is acute and self-limited, although cardiac damage sustained when the disease is active may be progressive. Coronary artery aneurysms are detectable by angiography or two-dimensional echocardiography in 20% of those patients who are not treated with intravenous gamma globulin, as opposed to 3% of those who receive gamma globulin within the first 10 days of illness. These abnormalities occur usually between days 7 and 28 of the illness. For infants less than 1 year of age, however, the risk of coronary abnormalities at 8 weeks still is 15%, even with gamma globulin treatment.

Japanese surveys between 1982 and 1988 of patients with Kawasaki disease suggest an average case-fatality rate of 0.3%. US surveillance data suggest a 2.8% case-fatality rate in this country, but most investigators believe that this number is inflated artificially as a result of the selective reporting of deaths caused by this disease. It may be assumed, however, that deaths can be expected to occur in about 1% of affected American children. The case-fatality ratio for all infants may exceed 4%; for all patients 1 year of age or older, it probably is less than 1%. Nearly 90% of the infant fatalities occur in males. Most deaths related to Kawasaki disease result from coronary artery thrombosis.

(Abridged from Ralph D. Feigin, Frank Cecchin, and Guy Randolph, Kawasaki Disease, in Oski, DeAngelis, Feigin, McMillan, Warshaw: *Principles and Practice of Pediatrics, Second Edition*, J.B. Lippincott, 1994.)

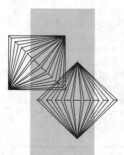

SECTION 6
Respiratory Diseases

Oski's Essential Pediatrics, edited by Kevin B. Johnson and Frank A. Oski. Lippincott–Raven Publishers, Philadelphia © 1997

85

Physiologic Considerations

■ THE ONSET OF AIR BREATHING AT BIRTH

Successful transition of the respiratory and pulmonary circulatory system from the fetal to the neonatal state determines the survival of the neonate. The fetal lung undergoes anatomic, physiologic, and biochemical development throughout gestation, so that, at term, the full complement of the airways (but not of the alveoli) is developed and the lungs are filled with fetal pulmonary fluid (30 mL/kg body weight), which includes surfactant. Whereas the fetus makes breathing movements (30% of the time in the near-term fetus), gas exchange is accomplished by the placenta.

Thus, the following major changes must occur promptly at birth so as to render the lung suitable for its lifelong air-exchanging function: (1) the onset of continuous ventilation; (2) the absorption of fetal pulmonary fluid; (3) the establishment of an air-filled, compliant lung at functional residual capacity; (4) the establishment of an intra-alveolar film of surfactant-enriched material that lowers the surface tension of the lung; and (5) dilation of the pulmonary vasculature, as well as redirection of and increase in pulmonary blood flow to ensure adequate gas exchange across the alveolar-capillary barrier.

The first breath, which is crucial to the success of this transition, is deep and is accompanied by large transpulmonary pressures that overcome surface and viscous forces; the first expiration is long and is accompanied by positive airway pressure brought about by laryngeal adduction and expiratory muscle activation. Some air already is retained in the lungs after the first breath—the beginning of the establishment of gaseous functional residual capacity.

After the first breath and over the next few hours, lung function changes progressively. Functional residual capacity increases gradually as fetal pulmonary fluid is absorbed. As the fluid is absorbed, breathing frequency decreases. After the initial deep breaths, tidal volume decreases. Lung compliance increases gradually, and total pulmonary resistance falls. Gas exchange adapts gradually to the postnatal state, as expressed by the decline in $PaCO_2$ and the rise in PaO_2. Although the time course of these changes varies depending on factors such as the mode of delivery, stable respiratory function usually is attained by the end of the first postnatal day.

■ RESPIRATORY REGULATION AND REFLEXES IN THE NEONATE

Inasmuch as neonatal respiration is a continuation of fetal breathing, consideration of the latter is important to the understanding of normal and abnormal respiratory control in the newborn.

The episodic breathing of the normal fetus is linked to its behavioral state: in the near-term human fetus (32 to 40 weeks' gestation), it has been shown by ultrasonographic techniques that breathing is least associated with the state of quiescence and most often associated with periods of body and eye movement as well as heart rate variability. Somatosensory stimuli also excite respiratory activity in the fetus. The most powerful of these is cooling, which produces vigorous fetal breathing and wakefulness.

Thus, it seems that some type of arousal is important for the sustenance of breathing activity. In fact, the "onset" of breathing at birth, which actually is the transition from discontinuous to continuous breathing, is associated with a barrage of stimuli that have an effect on arousal or a direct effect on respiratory reflexes. The former include cooling, light, sound, touch, and pressure. It also appears that the respiratory responses to the chemical stimuli CO_2 and O_2 change abruptly at birth; the response to CO_2, which involves carotid and aortic, but mainly ventral medullary chemoreception, is heightened, although it does not attain an adultlike sensitivity until several days postnatally. The response to hypoxia becomes biphasic (ie, an initial hyperventilation by peripheral chemosensory mechanisms is followed by respiratory attenuation or even apnea).

The behavior of other respiratory reflexes also differs in the perinatal period from that in later life. For example, the response of upper airway muscles to local changes in pressure, the coordination between the upper airway and the main respiratory muscles, and the intercostal–phrenic inhibitory reflex are all less developed in the newborn. Intrapulmonary reflexes are also less developed, including the slowly adapting (stretch), rapidly adapting (irritant), and C fiber (J receptor) vagal reflexes. A striking difference in behavior is shown by the laryngeal/pharyngeal chemoreflex: whereas stimulation of its chemoreceptors by materials perceived as foreign elicits a cough in the adult, it elicits apnea in the newborn. This apnea can be profound and irreversible in very young animals; its length is inversely proportional to postnatal age.

Among the brain processes that undergo postnatal development, sleep–wake states have a special importance because they reflect the maturation of neuronal networks that coordinate and integrate many somatic and autonomic systems and are linked tightly to respiration. The young neonate spends most of its time asleep, predominantly in active sleep. With time, the total time spent in sleep decreases, and quiet sleep becomes increasingly more pronounced. Furthermore, the length of sleep–wake cycles lengthens gradually, from 30 to 70 minutes in newborns to 75 to 90 minutes in children and adults. Even in normal neonates, and particularly in preterm infants, breathing pattern and respiratory reflexes depend on behavioral state. Periodic breathing and apnea are characteristic of premature infants during sleep, and are but a continuation into postnatal life of fetal patterns of breathing. The fact that these patterns exist during sleep and disappear with arousal (either natural or induced) underscores the importance of arousal in the maintenance of regular breathing. Sleep–wake states also play a role in the chemical respiratory reflexes because these are relatively diminished in sleep, particularly in active sleep. Furthermore, the chemical respiratory stimuli, especially CO_2, produce wakefulness at the same time that they stimulate ventilation. Indeed, it is thought that deficient arousal mechanisms might account for a portion of near-miss sudden death or for crib death itself.

(Abridged from Immanuela R. Moss, Physiologic Considerations, in Oski, DeAngelis, Feigin, McMillan, Warshaw: *Principles and Practice of Pediatrics, Second Edition,* J.B. Lippincott, 1994.)

Oski's Essential Pediatrics,
edited by Kevin B. Johnson and Frank A. Oski.
Lippincott–Raven Publishers,
Philadelphia © 1997

86

Causes of Respiratory Distress in the Newborn

Respiratory distress is a common presentation of disease in the newborn infant. The term is used to describe a constellation of easily observable physical signs, including rapid breathing (more than 60 breaths per minute), cyanosis, retractions (sucking in of the skin between the ribs, under the ribs, or above the sternum), flaring of the nostrils, and a grunting sound on expiration. There are many causes for these signs, and their presence is an indication that further observation or investigation is necessary. The causes of respiratory distress in the newborn include the following:

1. Airway obstruction
   a. Choanal atresia
   b. Congenital stridor (this may be caused by congenital defects such as laryngomalacia, tracheomalacia, laryngeal webs, or aberrant vessels compressing the airways)
2. Pulmonary disorders
   a. Respiratory distress syndrome (hyaline membrane disease)
   b. Transient tachypnea
   c. Pneumonia
   d. Aspiration syndromes
   e. Persistent pulmonary hypertension
   f. Air leak caused by interstitial emphysema, pneumothorax, or pneumomediastinum

g. Congenital malformations caused by diaphragmatic hernia, pulmonary hypoplasia, tracheoesophageal fistula, or congenital lobar emphysema
h. Atelectasis
i. Chronic lung disease as a result of bronchopulmonary dysplasia or Wilson-Mikity syndrome
j. Pulmonary hemorrhage

3. Nonpulmonary causes

a. Cardiac disease
b. Metabolic acidosis
c. Central nervous system disorders
d. Hypothermia or hyperthermia.

■ APPROACH TO THE NEWBORN WITH RESPIRATORY DISTRESS

Because there are many causes of respiratory distress and they cannot be differentiated by clinical examination alone, a chest radiograph is indicated in any infant who has significant respiratory distress. A sudden deterioration in respiratory status also is an indication for obtaining a chest radiograph to rule out conditions that require urgent treatment, such as pneumothorax. Very early chest films (in the first 2 to 4 hours after birth) often are not helpful in differentiating the various forms of parenchymal lung disease because the presence of lung fluid tends to produce a hazy appearance or diffuse fine infiltrates. Early radiographs are useful, however, for excluding surgical conditions such as diaphragmatic hernia and air leaks.

If there is no clear-cut pulmonary cause for the respiratory distress, it also will be necessary to exclude the presence of cardiac disease. This usually can be done by chest radiograph, electrocardiogram, and echocardiogram. The availability of echocardiography has diminished the need for cardiac catheterization and other potentially dangerous tests such as inspiration of 100% oxygen. In the presence of lung disease, the arterial PO_2 should increase after the inhalation of high concentrations of inspired oxygen, whereas with a fixed cardiac right-to-left shunt, there will be little increase in PO_2. This procedure carries the risk of causing closure of a patent ductus arteriosus in a ductal-dependent cardiac lesion. In some respiratory conditions (ie, persistent pulmonary hypertension), the echocardiogram not only is useful for excluding heart disease, but also plays a role in the diagnosis and management of the pulmonary disorder.

(Abridged from Ian Gross, Causes of Respiratory Distress in the Newborn, in Oski, DeAngelis, Feigin, McMillan, Warshaw: *Principles and Practice of Pediatrics, Second Edition*, J.B. Lippincott, 1994.)

Oski's Essential Pediatrics, edited by Kevin B. Johnson and Frank A. Oski. Lippincott–Raven Publishers, Philadelphia © 1997

87

Respiratory Distress Syndrome

Respiratory distress syndrome of the newborn (RDS, or hyaline membrane disease) is one of the most important causes of illness and death in the premature infant in developed countries. It is the result of immaturity of the lungs at birth and, therefore, with rare exceptions, is seen only in premature infants. Although alveoli first appear at 28 weeks' gestation, lung maturation usually is not adequate to sustain extrauterine life without some form of respiratory support until 32 to 34 weeks' gestation. Babies born earlier than this may have inadequate surfactant and decreased compliance of the lung. Other factors that contribute to lung compliance, such as tissue elasticity, also are believed to be abnormal in these infants. In addition, the anatomic structure of the lung is not suited as well to gas exchange as that of a full-term infant because there are smaller alveoli with larger amounts of interstitial tissue between them. The net result is a lung that is stiff and less well adapted for gas exchange.

■ INCIDENCE

In general, the incidence of RDS in infants born before 30 weeks' gestation is about 60% in those who have not been exposed to antenatal glucocorticoids and about 35% in those who have received an adequate course of glucocorticoid therapy. Between 30 and 34 weeks' gestation, the incidence is about 25% in untreated or inadequately treated infants, and about 10% in those who have received full steroid treatment. In premature infants of greater than 34 weeks' gestational age, the incidence is about 5%. RDS is rare in full-term infants. The factors associated with an increased risk of RDS include prematurity, maternal diabetes (classes A to C), delivery by cesarean section without antecedent labor, perinatal asphyxia, second twin, and history of a previous infant with RDS.

There also are conditions that appear to decrease the incidence of RDS, such as long-term maternal stress (*eg*, toxemia, hypertension), intrauterine growth retardation, maternal infection, maternal heroin exposure, and glucocorticoid treatment. Chronic low-grade maternal stress, as opposed to acute asphyxia, appears to accelerate lung maturation by a mechanism that is not entirely clear. It is possible that hormones such as glucocorticoids and catecholamines are involved.

■ PATHOGENESIS

Current concepts of the pathogenesis of RDS are illustrated in Figure 87–1. The basic deficit is immaturity of surfactant production and lung structure. This results in a lung that is stiff and prone to atelectasis.

■ CLINICAL FEATURES

The clinical course of uncomplicated RDS usually follows a fairly consistent pattern. The infant demonstrates

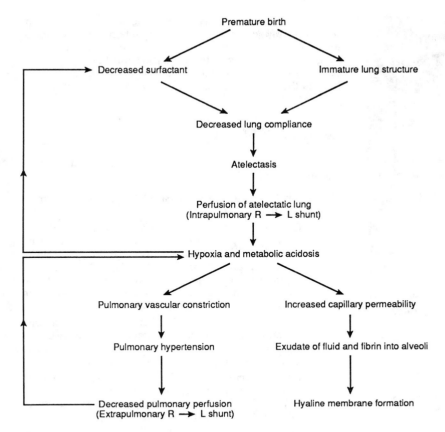

Figure 87-1. The pathogenesis of respiratory distress syndrome of the newborn.

signs of respiratory distress that become worse during the first few hours after birth. In some infants, especially those who are extremely immature, the respiratory distress may be severe from the start. The disease then progresses for 48 to 72 hours, reaches a peak, and starts to improve. The onset of recovery often is associated with diuresis. This classic course may not occur, however, in infants with very low birth weights or those who are very sick. With the use of ventilators and high oxygen concentrations, oxidant or mechanical injury may induce secondary lung damage and a prolonged respiratory illness may ensue.

Infants with RDS initially have the classic features of respiratory distress in the newborn (ie, tachypnea, flaring of the nose, retractions of the chest, cyanosis, and grunting). Radiographs taken at about 6 hours after birth reveal evidence of diffuse atelectasis and loss of lung volume (Figure 87–2). The lung fields, which are relatively opaque, have been described as resembling "ground glass" or being "reticulogranular." Because the lung fields now are relatively radiodense, the heart border may be obscured. In addition, air within the bronchi stands out in contrast to the lung fields as "air bronchograms." The air bronchograms may extend down to the diaphragm. This radiographic picture, although characteristic of RDS, also may be seen in neonatal pneumonia in premature infants, and it may be impossible to distinguish RDS and pneumonia on radiographic grounds.

If the infant dies, the characteristic features at postmortem examination are disrupted alveoli and the presence of eosinophilic hyaline membranes within the alveolar spaces. Although these proteinaceous deposits give this syndrome its name, the presence of hyaline membranes is not pathognomonic of "hyaline membrane disease." They also are seen in pneumonia, cardiac failure, and other neonatal conditions that are characterized by lung injury.

The differential diagnosis of RDS includes other causes of respiratory distress in the premature infant. The condition with which it is most likely to be confused is group B streptococcal pneumonia, which may mimic it in almost every respect. At times, it may be possible to differentiate these two disorders only retrospectively, by reviewing the course and pattern of the illness.

■ MANAGEMENT OF RESPIRATORY DISTRESS SYNDROME OF THE NEWBORN

Respiratory Care

Much of the work of neonatal intensive care units is concerned with providing respiratory care to infants with RDS. The level of intervention required depends on the severity of the respiratory distress. This is determined primarily by the arterial blood gas levels and by the amount of supplemental oxygen the infant needs to maintain an adequate arterial oxygen tension (PaO_2). The goal of therapy is to keep the PaO_2 in the range of 45 to 70 mm Hg, and the $PaCO_2$ between 35 and 45 mm Hg. Although these PaO_2 values are less than those observed in healthy full-term infants, they are used because premature infants are susceptible to oxygen injury to their eyes and it is felt that the range of 45 to 70 mm Hg is generally safe. PaO_2 levels lower than 35 mm Hg can result in tissue hypoxia and metabolic acidosis. Thus, the range used is a compromise designed to avoid hypoxia at the lower end and oxygen injury to the eyes at the high end. Management may include respiratory support, using continuous positive airway pressure (CPAP), or intubation and ventilation, using an endotracheal tube.

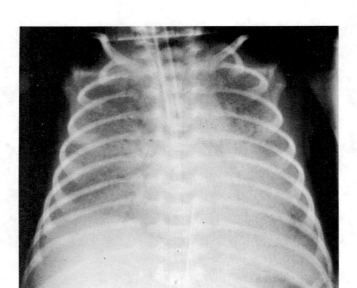

Figure 87-2. X-ray of the chest of an infant with respiratory distress syndrome. Note the diffusely opaque lung fields and the indistinct cardiac outline. Radiolucent "air bronchograms" also can be seen.

Monitoring

In addition to routine monitoring of temperature and heart rate, assessment of the respiratory status of infants with RDS by means of arterial blood gas determinations is essential. This usually is done by inserting a catheter through the umbilical artery into the aorta, or by radial artery catheterization. The catheter can be used to draw arterial samples to determine PaO_2, $PaCO_2$, and pH levels, and to record arterial blood pressure continuously by way of a transducer. Instruments for monitoring oxygenation by noninvasive methods also have been developed. The first such devices were transcutaneous oxygen sensors. Although these are useful for reflecting trends, they do not always report accurately the actual PaO_2 values. A more reliable instrument is the pulse oximeter, which records the oxygen saturation of the blood continuously by means of a probe attached to an extremity, such as a fingertip. This device is easy to use and safe, and has found widespread application. In mild cases of RDS, it may be possible to follow oxygenation by means of a pulse oximeter alone and to avoid arterial catheterization. Capillary blood specimens (*eg,* a heelstick) can be used for determination of pH and PCO_2 levels; PO_2 values obtained in this manner will be unreliable, however.

Surfactant Therapy

The successful use of pulmonary surfactant preparations for the prevention or amelioration of RDS represents one of the major advances made in neonatal care during the past decade. Surfactant preparations generally are administered as liquid suspensions that are instilled into the lungs by way of an endotracheal tube. For this reason, surfactant therapy is confined to infants who are intubated and ventilated. Two approaches to surfactant therapy have evolved. "Prevention" therapy refers to the administration of surfactant to premature infants who are at risk for having RDS immediately after birth in the delivery area. "Rescue" therapy refers to the administration of surfactant to infants with diagnosed RDS, usually within 8 hours of birth.

Large, multicenter studies have confirmed the effectiveness of modified natural and artificial surfactants for the prevention or treatment of RDS.

Surfactant therapy has been associated with few complications. There is no significant impact on the incidence of infection, patent ductus arteriosus, intraventricular hemorrhage, or necrotizing enterocolitis. In addition, there is no evidence of the development of antibodies to surfactant proteins in the serum of infants who have received natural surfactant therapy.

■ COMPLICATIONS

The major complications of RDS are related to therapy and include the following:

1. Air leak caused by increased airway pressure from ventilation or CPAP.
2. Chronic lung disease (bronchopulmonary dysplasia). This is believed to result from injury to the lungs by oxygen and ventilator pressure. The fragile lung of the extremely premature infant is particularly susceptible to this injury, and the incidence of bronchopulmonary dysplasia is increased greatly in infants with birth weights of less than 1250 g.
3. Catheter complications. The insertion of a catheter into the aorta can result in complications such as necrotizing enterocolitis, hypertension caused by renal arterial thrombosis, and infarction of other organs.
4. Intraventricular hemorrhage. There is an increased incidence of intraventricular hemorrhage in infants with RDS. The mechanism may be related to intravascular pressure swings.
5. Retinopathy of prematurity. Because RDS occurs in premature infants who are treated with oxygen, they are at particular risk for retinopathy of prematurity. Like bronchopulmonary dysplasia, this complication occurs mainly in infants with birth weights below 1500 g.

(Abridged from Ian Gross, Respiratory Distress Syndrome, in Oski, DeAngelis, Feigin, McMillan, Warshaw: *Principles and Practice of Pediatrics, Second Edition,* J.B. Lippincott, 1994.)

Oski's Essential Pediatrics,
edited by Kevin B. Johnson and Frank A. Oski.
Lippincott–Raven Publishers,
Philadelphia © 1997

88

Transient Tachypnea of the Newborn

Transient tachypnea of the newborn (also called retained fetal lung fluid, wet lung, or respiratory distress syndrome type II) is a benign, self-limited condition seen primarily in full-term infants. It is believed to result from delay in the reabsorption of fetal pulmonary fluid. There is an association between delivery by cesarean section and the development of this condition, possibly because of the compression of the chest during vaginal delivery and the mechanical "wringing out" of fetal lung fluid. These infants have respiratory distress shortly after birth. The features are tachypnea, mild retractions, and, sometimes, cyanosis. The clinical course usually is transient and mild, with resolution of the problem in 24 to 48 hours. In some infants, the condition is more severe and may persist for 72 hours or longer.

The diagnosis is made by radiography. The classic appearance is that of a well-aerated lung with streaky markings radiating out from the hilum ("star-burst" appearance) and small amounts of fluid in the fissures, particularly the right middle fissure. The major condition from which transient tachypnea must be differentiated is pneumonia. Differentiation sometimes can be difficult in prolonged cases of transient tachypnea, although resolution usually is more rapid than with pneumonia.

Treatment essentially is symptomatic. Blood gas levels or oxygen saturation are monitored, and oxygen is administered to maintain a PaO_2 of 60 to 90 mm Hg. Occasionally, a brief period of mechanical ventilation may be necessary and, if the diagnosis of pneumonia cannot be excluded, antibiotics are given, although transient tachypnea does not require antibacterial treatment. This condition is not associated with long-term sequelae such as bronchopulmonary dysplasia, and the prognosis is excellent.

(Abridged from Ian Gross, Transient Tachypnea of the Newborn, in Oski, DeAngelis, Feigin, McMillan, Warshaw: *Principles and Practice of Pediatrics, Second Edition,* J.B. Lippincott, 1994.)

Oski's Essential Pediatrics,
edited by Kevin B. Johnson and Frank A. Oski.
Lippincott–Raven Publishers,
Philadelphia © 199

89

Pneumonia in the Newborn

Pneumonia in the newborn period may arise in the first 2 to 3 days after birth (early onset) or after the first week (late onset). It may occur as an isolated infection or in association with septicemia. Pneumonia that develops shortly after birth probably is acquired in utero or intrapartum by hematogenous spread from the mother, from ascending infection from the vagina and cervix, or by aspiration of contaminated secretions immediately after birth. Late-onset pneumonia, similar to other nosocomial infections in the newborn unit, can be transmitted by the infant's caretakers. The most common pathogens are the group B streptococci and gram-negative organisms such as *Escherichia coli* and *Klebsiella*, but a wide variety of organisms may be involved. During the 1970s, group B streptococci emerged as a major cause of pneumonia and septicemia in newborns. Although group B streptococcal infection still is prevalent, it occurs now with about the same frequency as does infection with gram-negative enteric organisms.

■ CLINICAL FEATURES

Infants with early onset pneumonia usually have respiratory distress during the first few hours after birth. If they are premature, their symptoms may be indistinguishable from those of respiratory distress syndrome (RDS). Features that suggest pneumonia rather than RDS include prolonged rupture of the membranes, less rapidly progressive course, early onset of apnea, poor perfusion and shock, and other signs consistent with sepsis. The amniotic fluid lecithin:sphingomyelin ratio, if available, also is useful in differentiating pneumonia from RDS (a "mature" ratio rules out RDS).

■ RADIOGRAPHIC APPEARANCE

A variety of radiographic appearances have been described in newborn infants with pneumonia, ranging from lobar consolidation (Figure 89–1) to patchy or coarse infiltrates, to an RDS-like pattern (Figure 89–2).

■ TREATMENT

The improvement that has occurred in the survival of infants with serious neonatal infections over the past 20 years is related to advances in supportive techniques as well as antibiotic therapy.

Because a precise bacterial diagnosis usually is not available, broad-spectrum coverage, for example, with a penicillin and an aminoglycoside, usually is instituted for 7 to 10 days. If gentamicin is used, peak and trough levels of this antibiotic in the blood should be determined to ensure that the dose and frequency of administration are appropriate.

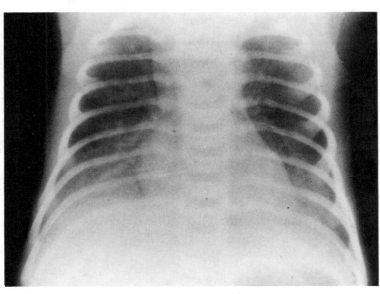

Figure 89-1. Bilateral lobar consolidation in an infant with pneumonia.

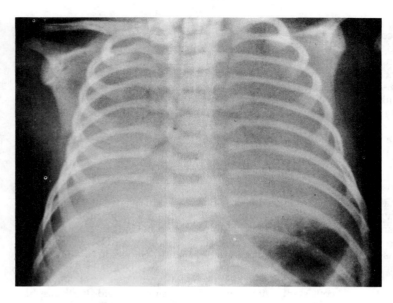

Figure 89-2. "RDS-like" pattern in a premature infant with pneumonia. The radiodensity of the lungs is greatly increased, resulting in an opacified appearance.

In those infants who demonstrate evidence of pulmonary hypertension and right-to-left shunting, a trial of tolazoline may be indicated, particularly if the PaO_2 is extremely low despite ventilation with high oxygen concentrations. If there is a favorable response to a test dose of tolazoline, a continuous infusion should be started and maintained as long as there is evidence of shunting. In some infants, the pulmonary hypertension is so severe and intractable that institution of extracorporeal membrane oxygenation (ECMO) is indicated. Tolazoline and ECMO therapy are discussed in the chapter on pulmonary hypertension.

Most infants with pneumonia do well and survive without long-term sequelae. Patients who require prolonged ventilation with high peak inspiratory pressures and high oxygen concentrations may have chronic lung disease.

(Abridged from Ian Gross, Pneumonia, in Oski, DeAngelis, Feigin, McMillan, Warshaw: *Principles and Practice of Pediatrics, Second Edition*, J.B. Lippincott, 1994.)

Oski's Essential Pediatrics,
edited by Kevin B. Johnson and Frank A. Oski.
Lippincott–Raven Publishers,
Philadelphia © 1997

90

Meconium Aspiration Syndrome

Meconium is passed into the amniotic fluid in about 10% of all births. Although meconium passage may be associated with intrauterine fetal hypoxia, it also occurs in normal deliveries in the absence of asphyxia. Meconium aspiration is not seen in premature infants of less than 34 weeks' gestation; these infants rarely demonstrate meconium-stained amniotic fluid. It is more common in postmature babies.

It is important that infants who are born covered with thick meconium and who have not yet cried vigorously have adequate aspiration of the meconium from their pharynx and trachea. It has been shown that tracheal suctioning in the delivery room before respiration is established is of benefit.

Meconium that has not been cleared from the trachea migrates peripherally and obstructs the smaller airways. Partial occlusion may result in a one-way valve effect, with distal hyperinflation. Alternatively, the small airways may be blocked completely, leading to atelectasis. In some infants, persistent pulmonary hypertension develops, and this considerably complicates their management. The management of persistent pulmonary hypertension is discussed in Chapter 91.

Infants with meconium aspiration present clinically with respiratory distress and an overdistended chest. Coarse rales may be heard. The chest radiograph reveals hyperinflation of the lungs with patchy infiltrates. Because of the air-trapping effect of meconium in the airways, pneumothorax is common, occurring in 20% to 50% of cases.

Management of these patients is symptomatic. They require oxygen supplementation and, frequently, ventilator therapy. The diffuse small-airway obstruction often necessitates the use of high peak inspiratory pressures to maintain adequate ventilation. The use of antibiotics is controversial; some neonatologists do not use antibiotics in uncomplicated cases of meconium aspiration, whereas others do because of concern for secondary infection.

(Abridged from Ian Gross, Meconium Aspiration Syndrome, in Oski, DeAngelis, Feigin, McMillan, Warshaw: *Principles and Practice of Pediatrics, Second Edition*, J.B. Lippincott, 1994.)

Oski's Essential Pediatrics,
edited by Kevin B. Johnson and Frank A. Oski.
Lippincott–Raven Publishers,
Philadelphia © 1997

91

Persistent Pulmonary Hypertension

During fetal life, there is increased tone in the pulmonary vasculature and the pressure on the right side of the heart is greater than that on the left. Consequently, blood is shunted from the right to the left side of the heart through the foramen ovale and the ductus arteriosus (Figure 91–1). The blood that enters the right atrium by way of the superior vena cava tends to flow into the right ventricle, whereas that which enters the right atrium from the inferior vena cava tends to be shunted across the foramen ovale to the left atrium. Much of the flow from the right ventricle then is shunted to the aorta through the ductus arteriosus. After birth, pressure in the pulmonary circulation decreases and there is functional closure of the foramen ovale, followed by anatomic closure of the ductus arteriosus. In some infants, pulmonary hypertension develops again after birth. This results in reestablishment of right-to-left shunting through the foramen ovale or ductus arteriosus; for this reason, this condition sometimes is referred to as "persistent fetal circulation."

Pulmonary hypertension also is associated with pulmonary hypoplasia, particularly that which results from diaphragmatic hernia. In this condition, there is not only pulmonary vasospasm, but also a smaller pulmonary vascular bed in association with the hypoplastic lung. The hypoxia in these infants may be particularly severe and resistant to therapy.

■ DIAGNOSIS

The diagnosis of persistent pulmonary hypertension (PPH) is suggested by the triad of cyanosis, absence of heart disease, and clear lung fields or meconium aspiration. The usual presentation is that of a full-term or postmature infant who may have a history of asphyxia or meconium aspiration. The baby initially may appear to be well, but, within the first 24 hours after birth, there is progressive cyanosis and tachypnea. A chest radiograph taken at this stage will reveal clear lungs or scattered infiltrates in the case of meconium aspiration. The lungs may have decreased vascular markings, consistent with diminished pulmonary blood flow. The cyanosis, if untreated, will continue to progress until, eventually, it becomes profound. Shock with decreased peripheral perfusion and hypotension also may become apparent.

The combination of severe cyanosis with clear lung fields or small infiltrates should raise the suspicion of PPH; the clue is cyanosis that is disproportionate to the underlying lung disease. The diagnosis cannot be made, however, and the infant should not be treated for pulmonary hypertension, until heart disease has been ruled out, preferably by an echocardiogram. Infants with transposition of the great vessels or other causes of cyanotic heart disease initially may exhibit very similar symptoms. The echocardiogram will exclude anatomic heart disease and confirm the diagnosis of pulmonary hypertension and right-to-left shunting. It may reveal tricuspid regurgitation resulting from the high right-sided pressure. The echocardiogram also is useful for assessing right ventricular filling and myocardial contractility, and it can be used as a guide for determining intravenous fluid requirements.

■ MANAGEMENT

Infants with PPH present perhaps the most difficult medical management problem in the newborn intensive care unit, and their care draws on all the resources available to modern neonatology. They should be managed by physicians who are experienced with this problem and in an environment where the appropriate support is available. Management includes careful monitoring of oxygen and carbon dioxide concentration in blood perfusion, fluid status, and blood pressure.

Ventilation

The ventilatory management of infants with PPH is controversial. Over the past 10 years, treatment of this disorder by hyperventilation has become common. Hyperoxia and

Figure 91-1. (A) and **(B)** Comparison of mature and fetal circulations. In fetal life, blood is shunted from the right to left side of the heart across the foramen ovale and the ductus arteriosus because of the increased pressure in the pulmonary circulation. If arterial pressure in the pulmonary circulation rises again after birth, the shunting recurs. *SVC,* superior vena cava; *RA,* right atrium; *LA,* left atrium; *RV,* right ventricle; *LV,* left ventricle; *IVC,* inferior vena cava; *PA,* pulmonary artery; *AO,* aorta; *FO,* foramen ovale; *DA,* ductus arteriosus.

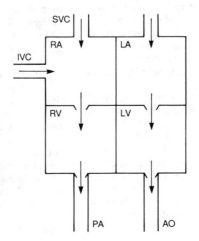

A. Mature Circulation

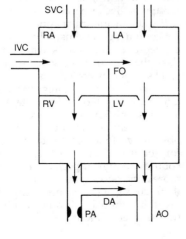

B. Fetal Circulation

alkalosis are pulmonary vasodilators. The goal of hyperventilation is to reduce the $PaCO_2$ to 20 to 25 mm Hg, so that a respiratory alkalosis develops, and to increase the PaO_2.

Oxygen and alkalosis are potent pulmonary vasodilators, as discussed above. No specific pulmonary vasodilator drugs are available. A variety of agents with limited effectiveness are used for this purpose, however. The most widely used and probably the most effective agent is tolazoline, a histamine releaser and α-adrenergic blocker. In about one third of infants with PPH, tolazoline is successful in dilating the pulmonary vasculature and improving the PaO_2. Recent preliminary reports suggest that endothelium-derived relaxing factor, which actually is nitric oxide, is a potent pulmonary vasodilator in adults and infants. Studies to evaluate the effectiveness of inhaled nitric oxide in the management of PPH are in progress.

A type of pulmonary bypass, extracorporeal membrane oxygenation (ECMO) is being used increasingly for the treatment of severe cases of PPH. In this procedure, blood is diverted from the jugular vein, anticoagulated, pumped through a membrane oxygenator, and then returned to the baby by way of the carotid artery. The use of ECMO has been justified on the grounds that, if it were not used for the sickest infants, they would have a very high rate of mortality. Although the use of ECMO for infants with PPH has not been subjected to large-scale, randomized, controlled clinical trials, it does appear to be an effective rescue therapy for selected infants with severe irreversible hypoxia who are not responding to conventional medical therapy. Because the procedure involves ligating the carotid artery and heparinizing the blood, there have been concerns about bleeding and neurologic side effects, but follow-up studies of survivors have reported encouragingly good outcomes.

■ PROGNOSIS

Although the rate of survival for infants with pulmonary hypertension was 50% or less in 1980, survival rates of 80% or better have been reported recently by a number of centers in association with advances in conventional supportive therapy. Similar survival rates also have been attained in severely ill infants with the use of ECMO. Those infants who survive appear to do fairly well. Some have residual lung disease resulting from prolonged ventilation and oxygen administration. Significant neurologic problems have been reported in about one fifth of the survivors, whether treated with conventional therapy or ECMO.

(Abridged from Ian Gross, Persistent Pulmonary Hypertension, in Oski, DeAngelis, Feigin, McMillan, Warshaw: *Principles and Practice of Pediatrics, Second Edition*, J.B. Lippincott, 1994.)

Oski's Essential Pediatrics,
edited by Kevin B. Johnson and Frank A. Oski.
Lippincott–Raven Publishers,
Philadelphia © 1997

92

Apnea

Apnea is defined as a respiratory pause of 20 seconds or longer, or a shorter pause associated with cyanosis, abrupt pallor or hypotonia, or bradycardia. Apnea is an extremely common finding in premature infants. The incidence increases with decreasing gestational age. About 50% of infants weighing less than 1500 g at birth, and almost all infants weighing less than 1000 g, will require intervention for apnea. Because most cases of apnea are related to prematurity, the incidence of apnea decreases with increasing postconceptual age, and usually resolves by 35 to 36 weeks' postconceptual age. Infants with extremely low birth weights (less than 1000 g) may have persistent apnea beyond 40 weeks' postconceptual age.

Apnea can be categorized into three types. Central apnea is characterized by a total lack of chest wall movement and nasal airflow; obstructive apnea is associated with chest wall movement, without nasal airflow; and mixed apnea is obstructive followed by central apnea. The latter accounts for about 50% of apneic episodes in premature infants. In contrast to apnea, periodic breathing is defined as three or more respiratory pauses of more than 3 seconds with less than 20 seconds of breathing between pauses. Periodic breathing probably is a normal breathing pattern in premature and term infants.

■ MANAGEMENT

Apnea is a symptom or sign of an underlying disorder; however, the most common cause of apnea in premature infants is related to immaturity of the ventilatory control mechanism. All infants at risk for apnea of prematurity (*ie*, those of less than 34 weeks' gestation) require cardiac or cardiac/thoracic impedance monitoring when they are admitted to the nursery. Apnea of prematurity is a diagnosis of exclusion, and before this diagnosis can be made, the other causes of apnea must be considered (Table 92–1). A careful history and physical examination will direct further evaluation. An investigation for sepsis/meningitis should be performed in infants who have other signs and symptoms of sepsis, in those with apnea beyond 34 weeks' gestation, in those with a sudden onset of apnea after being asymptomatic, and in those with severe apnea requiring bag mask ventilation. Management of apnea of prematurity is determined by the frequency and severity of the episodes. If these are mild and are not associated with cyanosis or bradycardia, they may be treated with gentle stimulation, clearance of secretions from the airway, and avoidance of neck flexion. If the infant continues to have significant apnea, the next step is to treat with methylxanthines. These agents are effective against central and obstructive apnea. Proposed mechanisms of action of methylxanthines for apnea include increased sensitivity of the medullary respiratory center to CO_2, increased afferent nerve traffic to the brain stem, and improved skeletal and diaphragmatic muscle contraction. Theophylline is the most commonly used agent. Caffeine, which is given orally and has a longer half-life and a wider therapeutic range, may be used as an alternative to theophylline. Theophylline is metabolized in part to caffeine in premature infants.

Persistent apnea despite methylxanthine therapy is an indication for nasal continuous positive airway pressure

TABLE 92-1. Causes of Apnea

Apnea of prematurity
Central nervous system disorders
    Intraventricular/periventricular hemorrhage
    Subarachnoid hemorrhage
    Infarction
Cardiorespiratory disorders
    Respiratory distress syndrome
    Bronchopulmonary dysplasia
    Patent ductus arteriosus
Metabolic disorders
    Hypoglycemia
    Hypocalcemia
    Electrolyte imbalance
Hematologic
    Anemia
Infection
    Sepsis/meningitis
Gastrointestinal
    Necrotizing enterocolitis
    Gastroesophageal reflux
Medications
    Phenobarbital
    General anesthesia
Temperature
    Rapid warming
Obstruction
    Secretions
    Neck flexion
    Congenital airway anomalies
Stimulation of inhibitory reflexes

(CPAP), which is effective against obstructive and mixed apnea spells. The proposed mechanism of action for CPAP involves stabilization of the upper airway and chest wall, as well as reduction in inhibitory respiratory reflexes.

Intubation and mechanical ventilation are indicated if significant apnea persists despite the above measures. Severe apnea may be associated with a decrease in cerebral blood flow resulting in neurologic injury.

Infants with apnea of prematurity may be discharged home if they are more than 35 to 36 weeks' postconceptual age and remain free of apnea for 7 to 10 days. Although the incidence of sudden infant death syndrome (SIDS) increases with decreasing birth weight, parents should be reassured that apnea of prematurity is not an independent risk factor for SIDS. Home monitoring may be used to shorten the hospitalization of premature infants with persistent apnea beyond 36 weeks' postconceptual age. The home monitor may be discontinued if the infant has no significant episodes for 2 or 3 months. No evidence exists, however, that home monitoring prevents SIDS. Apnea of prematurity that has resolved is not in itself an indication for home monitoring.

(Abridged from Robert Herzlinger, Apnea, in Oski, DeAngelis, Feigin, McMillan, Warshaw: *Principles and Practice of Pediatrics, Second Edition*, J.B. Lippincott, 1994.).

Oski's Essential Pediatrics, edited by Kevin B. Johnson and Frank A. Oski. Lippincott–Raven Publishers, Philadelphia © 1997

93

Bronchopulmonary Dysplasia

Most neonates with acute lung disease recover completely within the first week of life. Some of these infants, however, have chronic respiratory disease characterized by tachypnea, dyspnea, hypoxemia, and hypercarbia. In children who survive hyaline membrane disease, one sees the typical clinical, radiologic, and pathologic manifestations of *bronchopulmonary dysplasia* (BPD).

■ DIAGNOSIS

The diagnosis of BPD is suspected when a neonate with acute lung disease fails to follow the anticipated course of resolution or has a gradual increase in oxygen and ventilator requirements during the first month of life. The disease was characterized in 1979 as tachypnea, retractions, and supplemental oxygen requirement for more than 28 days in infants who had received positive-pressure ventilation for at least 3 days in the first week of life. Associated chest radiograph findings included strandlike densities in both lung fields alternating with areas of normal or increased lucency. The diagnosis must be made on the basis of both clinical and radiographic characteristics. There are no specific tests that can be used to confirm the diagnosis. The distinction between unresolved acute lung disease and chronic lung disease at 28 days of age is an arbitrary one, based in part on the likelihood that pulmonary dysfunction that persists for at least 4 weeks will be associated with increased long-term morbidity and mortality. The distinction can be problematic when considering therapeutic modalities begun at 1 to 3 weeks of age in infants with pulmonary dysfunction or when classifying deaths from respiratory failure at 1 to 4 weeks of age. More recently, a more stringent diagnostic criterion, oxygen therapy at 36 weeks' corrected postnatal gestational age, has been recommended. This recommendation was based on the observation that this definition is a more specific predictor of long-term pulmonary morbidity.

Other diseases commonly associated with pulmonary insufficiency in neonates are Wilson-Mikity syndrome, cystic fibrosis, α_1-antitrypsin deficiency, viral pneumonia, and patent ductus arteriosus.

■ COMPLICATIONS

Pulmonary hypertension and cor pulmonale can result from many forms of chronic lung disease, including BPD. Mortality is very high in infants with severe BPD and cor pulmonale, so therapeutic endeavors should be directed toward preventing the development of cor pulmonale. Pulmonary arterial pressure can be decreased by increased oxygen administration in infants with BPD.

Congestive heart failure with pulmonary and systemic venous congestion frequently complicates the treatment of infants with BPD. Infants with BPD have an increased susceptibility to severe bacterial and viral pneumonia. Respiratory syncytial virus and pertussis infections can be fatal in infants with BPD.

■ PREVENTION

The management of acute lung disease in premature infants should be directed toward the prevention of BPD. As discussed above, BPD results from the complex interaction of many factors. Limited exposure to mechanical ventilation and oxygen therapy, judicious fluid administration, prompt management of the patent ductus arteriosus, and attention to optimal nutrition may reduce the risk of BPD in susceptible infants. Surfactant replacement has not significantly reduced the incidence of BPD. Short-term steroid treatment has been shown to be beneficial for ventilator-dependent infants at 3 to 6 weeks of age; however, the long-term benefits are less clear, and there are serious risks associated with steroid therapy.

■ MANAGEMENT

Although exposure to high concentrations of oxygen is thought to be a contributing factor in the pathogenesis of BPD, chronic administration of oxygen is one of the most important aspects in the management of chronic lung disease in infants. Maintaining a PaO_2 greater than 60 mm Hg or an O_2 saturation greater than 90% should reduce the risk of cor pulmonale from chronic hypoxemia. Many infants have decreased oxygenation during sleep and feedings, and may require additional oxygen therapy during these times.

Although diuretic therapy is used commonly in infants with BPD, the diuretic and nondiuretic cardiopulmonary effects of chronic diuretic therapy in these infants have not been explored fully. Diuretic therapy may allow for increased fluid administration, and diuretic agents have been shown to improve pulmonary mechanics in infants with BPD. The efficacy of furosemide versus thiazide diuretics in infants with BPD is unknown, and careful attention must be given to electrolyte balance when diuretics are used in these infants. Replacement of potassium and chloride may be necessary to prevent metabolic alkalosis and hypoventilation during diuretic therapy. Sodium supplementation enhances fluid retention and defeats the purpose of diuretic therapy. Many infants with BPD also are at risk for osteopenia of prematurity, and thiazide diuretics may have the advantage of decreasing urinary calcium excretion.

Infants with BPD have increased airway resistance and increased work of breathing compared to age-matched control infants. Some of these infants have bronchial hyperreactivity that responds favorably to bronchodilator therapy with theophylline or β-adrenergic agonists. Response to bronchodilator therapy has been demonstrated in infants as young as 2 weeks' postnatal age.

Adequate nutrition is necessary for lung growth and repair, but meeting nutritional needs often is a challenge in infants with BPD. Infants with BPD have tachypnea and increased respiratory effort, and they may require more calories for adequate growth than do infants without respiratory disease. The caloric needs of an individual infant should be determined by the intake required to achieve a sustained weight gain of at least 10 g/kg/day. Some infants may require as much as 150 kcal/kg/day. If oral or naso-gastric feedings are not tolerated, prolonged peripheral parenteral nutrition rarely provides adequate calories and central total parenteral nutrition should be considered.

■ PROGNOSIS

In a study of 179 infants with BPD born between 1975 and 1982, the predischarge mortality rate was 14%. Those infants who survived until discharge from the hospital had a postdischarge death rate of 11%. Survivors had an increased incidence of neurodevelopmental abnormalities, visual and hearing deficits, and rehospitalization for respiratory illness in the first year of life when compared to premature infants without BPD. Pulmonary function improves over the first several years of life in infants with BPD, and most survivors have normal exercise tolerance by school age. With formal pulmonary function testing, however, some evidence of increased airway reactivity persists into early adulthood.

With carefully monitored long-term oxygen therapy to reduce the risk of cor pulmonale and aggressive management of respiratory infections, the prognosis for infants with BPD may continue to improve. The long-term outlook for infants in whom BPD develops is impossible to determine. Encouraging information about 20-year-old survivors of HMD who had a different disease spectrum may not apply to the infants treated today.

(Abridged from Kathleen A. Kennedy and Joseph B. Warshaw, Bronchopulmonary Dysplasia, in Oski, DeAngelis, Feigin, McMillan, Warshaw: *Principles and Practice of Pediatrics, Second Edition*, J.B. Lippincott, 1994.)

Oski's Essential Pediatrics,
edited by Kevin B. Johnson and Frank A. Oski.
Lippincott–Raven Publishers,
Philadelphia © 1997

94

Acute and Chronic Bronchitis

The term *bronchitis* describes inflammation of the large airways, namely, the trachea and bronchi. Bronchitis can occur throughout the year but is more likely to be seen in the winter months and in association with viral and bacterial infections.

ACUTE BRONCHITIS

Acute bronchitis is encountered commonly in children. Most clinicians describe acute bronchitis as a febrile illness with cough, rhonchi, and referred breath sounds. Causative agents are many, predominantly adenovirus, influenza viruses, and respiratory syncytial virus. Influenza viruses A and B have been implicated in epidemics of bronchitis; influenza A is associated with a severe respiratory illness in very young children. Bacterial infections identified include *Bordetella pertussis* and *Haemophilus influenzae* (Table 94–1). Additionally, *Mycoplasma pneumoniae* is a common cause of acute bronchitis in children, especially after 6 years of age.

■ CLINICAL PRESENTATION

By definition, fever and cough are associated with acute bronchitis, almost invariably in connection with upper respiratory congestion (predominantly nasal). The patient's temperature can range from 37°C to 39°C (100°F to 103°F). Cough usually is dry and harsh without sputum production in young infants. Coughing can be accompanied by gagging and vomiting, leading to poor oral intake and dehydration.

TABLE 94-1. Infectious Agents Associated With Acute Bronchitis

Agent	Importance in Causation*
VIRUSES	+++
Adenoviruses types 1–7, 12	
Enteroviruses	+
Coxsackieviruses B	+
Echoviruses 8, 12, 14	+
Polioviruses	+
Herpes simplex	+
Influenza	+++
A	++
B	++
C	+
Measles	+
Mumps	+
Parainfluenza	+++
1	+
2	++
3	+++
4	+
Respiratory syncytial virus	+++
Rhinoviruses	++
BACTERIA	
Bordetella pertussis	+
Bordetella parapertussis	±
Haemophilus influenzae	+
Streptococcus pneumoniae	±
Streptococcus pyogenes	±
OTHER	
Chlamydia psittaci	+
Mycoplasma pneumoniae	+++

*+++, very common; ++, common; +, rare; ±, of questionable etiologic significance.

Modified from Cherry JD. Lower respiratory tract infections: Acute bronchitis. In: Feigin RD, Cherry JD, eds. Textbook of pediatric infectious disease. 2nd ed. Philadelphia: WB Saunders, 1987:272.

Older children with persistent cough occasionally will produce sputum and may complain of chest wall pain. The clinical illness usually is preceded by 24 to 48 hours of lassitude or malaise. Subsequently, fever and cough develop; these findings may persist for as long as 1 week. A relatively slow recovery phase, spanning 1 to 2 weeks, with persistent cough is characteristic. Secondary bacterial infection can complicate the recovery period, causing exacerbation of fever and other clinical findings.

On physical examination, lung auscultation reveals rhonchi and referred upper airway breath sounds. Rhinitis usually is present and may be mucopurulent. Chest radiographs typically are normal unless secondary bacterial infection has occurred. Laboratory data are of limited value, usually suggesting a viral process (ie, the white blood cell count is elevated mildly and only a third of all cases are associated with an increased neutrophil count).

■ DIFFERENTIAL DIAGNOSIS

Acute bronchitis should be distinguished from chronic bronchitis, infectious asthma, and asthmatic bronchitis and sinusitis. More serious illnesses associated with recurrent acute upper respiratory tract infections (*eg,* immunodeficiency states, immotile cilia syndrome, and cystic fibrosis) should be distinguished from acute bronchitis. Acute bronchitis is a self-limited illness, and one bout of clinical disease does not warrant additional investigation.

An epidemiologic history often is helpful in identifying a possible causative agent; pandemics of respiratory viral illnesses occur characteristically during the winter months, and spread of respiratory viruses occurs easily in day care settings. *M pneumoniae* is more common in school-age children.

■ TREATMENT AND COMPLICATIONS

Acute bronchitis usually is a benign illness unless secondary infection occurs. When specific respiratory viruses are isolated from nasopharyngeal secretions and the infection is severe enough to warrant hospitalization, then therapy with antiviral agents such as aerosolized ribavirin or amantadine can be considered.

Persistent coughing with gagging and vomiting can precipitate dehydration and serum metabolic changes. Monitoring of these parameters in the severely affected host and reconstitution of deficits by oral or parenteral rehydration are indicated.

When secondary bacterial infection is suggested by exacerbation of fever or by evidence of pneumonia on a chest radiograph, broad-spectrum antibiotic therapy may be indicated. Specific antimicrobial therapy can be provided when *H influenzae* or *Streptococcus pneumoniae* is isolated.

Recurrent acute bronchitis has been associated with reactive airway disease or asthma. Complications of acute bronchitis are few; in the majority of cases, the outcome is excellent, with resolution of disease and return to baseline health.

CHRONIC BRONCHITIS

Chronic bronchitis, which is described widely in the literature on adults, is ill-defined in children and is described less frequently in this population. The prevalence of childhood bronchitis is variable, ranging from 2% to 40% in selected series.

■ CLINICAL PRESENTATION AND DIFFERENTIAL DIAGNOSIS

Clinically, chronic bronchitis is characterized by excessive mucus production and by cough that is present on most days for a minimum of 3 months per year. Fever can accompany the cough, and the temperature can range from 37°C to 39°C (100°F to 103°F). Chronic bronchitis can be a clinical manifestation of a number of disorders, some of which are listed in Table 94–2.

■ PATHOGENESIS AND PATHOPHYSIOLOGY

Many viral infections have been implicated in the etiology of chronic bronchitis (see Table 94–1). These include rhinoviruses, respiratory syncytial virus, parainfluenza viruses, influenza viruses A and B, adenoviruses, and enteroviruses. Bacterial agents are implicated more commonly in chronic bronchitis. The predominant pathogens isolated from sputum in a group of 40 pediatric patients with chronic bronchitis are shown in Table 94–3. Treatment of exacerbations of chronic bronchitis with antibiotic therapy usually is effective in reducing sputum volume and purulence, but shows no parallel elimination of the cultured microorganisms.

TABLE 94-2. Conditions Associated With Chronic Cough (3 Months or Longer) or Lower Respiratory Tract Illness

ASTHMA

RECURRENT EPISODES OF BRONCHITIS

INFECTIONS—CHLAMYDIA, PERTUSSIS, MYCOBACTERIUM

CYSTIC FIBROSIS

PRIMARY CILIARY DYSKINESIA

Kartagener's syndrome

Immotile cilia syndrome

IMMUNODEFICIENCY

Selective IgA deficiency

Subclass of IgG deficiency

Hypogammaglobulinemia (primary and secondary)

Ataxia-telangiectasia

Graft-versus-host disease after bone marrow transplant

ANATOMIC LESIONS

Foreign body

Previous esophageal atresia repair

Mediastinal tumors

Congenital heart disease

IRRITANTS

Milk aspiration (gastroesophageal reflux, tracheoesophageal fistula)

Tobacco smoke

Pollution

Occupational exposure

Modified from Morgan WT, Taussig LM. The chronic bronchitis complex in childhood. In: The pediatric airway. Pediatr Clin North Am. 1984;31:853.

TABLE 94-3. Dominant Pathogens in Washed Sputum From Patients With Chronic Bronchitis (40 Cases)

Pathogen	Number of Cases (%)
HAEMOPHILUS INFLUENZAE AND STREPTOCOCCUS	21 (52.5)
H INFLUENZAE	17 (42.5)
STAPHYLOCOCCUS AUREUS	2 (5.0)
SUPERINFECTION WITH GRAM-NEGATIVE RODS	
PSEUDOMONAS AERUGINOSA	4
Klebsiella pneumoniae	2
Escherichia coli	1
Enterobacter cloacae	1

Kubo AS, Funabashi S, Uehara S, et al. Clinical aspects of "asthmatic bronchitis" and chronic bronchitis in infants and children. J Asthma Res. 1978;15:99.

■ TREATMENT

When a specific diagnosis can be identified with chronic cough or wheezing, therapy is directed toward the primary disease entity in addition to the clinical presentation. Hence, bronchodilators (theophylline preparations, β-adrenergic agents, cromolyn sodium, corticosteroids) are used when deemed appropriate in the treatment of chronic cough associated with asthma.

Antimicrobial therapy in chronic bronchitis is reserved for patients with severe illness in whom the likelihood of secondary bacterial infection is great. In these instances, therapy usually consists of ampicillin, erythromycin, or, in adolescents and adults, tetracycline. Sequential monitoring of pulmonary function studies is important. The prognosis for the chronic bronchitis complex is varied and depends on the specific diagnosis.

(Abridged from I. Celine Hanson and William T. Shearer, Acute and Chronic Bronchitis, in Oski, DeAngelis, Feigin, McMillan, Warshaw: *Principles and Practice of Pediatrics, Second Edition*, J.B. Lippincott, 1994.)

Oski's Essential Pediatrics,
edited by Kevin B. Johnson and Frank A. Oski.
Lippincott–Raven Publishers,
Philadelphia © 1997

95

Nonbacterial Pneumonia

Nonbacterial pneumonias are the most common pulmonary infections encountered in pediatrics. The varied causes of these conditions, excluding bacteria and fungi, cover a broad taxonomic spectrum. With improvement in microbiologic techniques, the number of known causative agents continues to increase. Although most nonbacterial pneumonias have a good prognosis, they occasionally are life-threatening. In Table 95–1, the major agents causing disease in various age groups are presented according to their

TABLE 95-1. Etiologic Agents in Nonbacterial Pneumonia

Etiologic Agents	Frequency*			Usual Degree of Severity†			Mode of Access to Lung
	0–3 mo	4 mo–5 y	6–16 y	0–3 mo	4 mo–5 y	6–16 y	
VIRUSES							
Respiratory syncytial virus	+++	++++	+	++	++	+	Respiratory
Parainfluenza viruses							
Type 1	+	++	+	++	++	+	Respiratory
Type 2	+	+	+	++	++	+	Respiratory
Type 3	++	+++	++	++	++	+	Respiratory
Influenza viruses							
Type A	++	+++	+++	++	++	+	Respiratory
Type B	++	++	+	++	++	+	Respiratory
Adenoviruses‡	+	++	++	+++	++	+	Respiratory
Rhinoviruses§	+	+	+	−	++	+	Respiratory
Enteroviruses¶	+	+	+	++	++	+	Respiratory (hematogenous)
Coronaviruses	−	+	+	−	++	+	Respiratory
Measles virus	+	++	++	+++	++	++	Respiratory (hematogenous)
Rubella virus	+	−	−	++	−	−	Hematogenous
Human immunodeficiency virus	+	++	+	++	++	++	Hematogenous
Varicella-zoster virus	+	+	+	+++	+++	+++	Hematogenous (respiratory)
Cytomegalovirus	++	+	+	++	+++	+++	Hematogenous (respiratory)
Epstein-Barr virus	−	+	++	−	++	+	Hematogenous (respiratory)
Herpes simplex viruses	++	+	+	++++	+++	+++	Hematogenous (respiratory)
MYCOPLASMAS							
Mycoplasma pneumoniae	−	+	++++	−	++	+	Respiratory
Mycoplasma hominis	?	−	−	?	−	−	Respiratory
Ureaplasma urealyticum	?	−	−	?	−	−	Respiratory
CHLAMYDIAE							
Chlamydia pneumoniae	?	?	+++	?	?	+	Respiratory
Chlamydia psittaci	−	+	+	−	++	++	Respiratory
Chlamydia trachomatis	++++	−	−	++	−	−	Respiratory
RICKETTSIAE							
Coxiella burnetii	−	+	+	−	++	++	Respiratory (hematogenous)
PROTOZOA							
Pneumocystis carinii	+	+	+	+++	+++	+++	Respiratory

*++++, most frequent; +++, frequent; ++, infrequent; +, rare; −, no reported cases; ?, uncertain.

†++++, often fatal; +++, severe; ++, usually hospitalized; +, home management; −, no reported cases; ?, uncertain.

‡Types 1, 2, 3, 4, 5, 7, 14, 21, and 35.

§Ninety or more types known.

¶Coxsackieviruses A9, A16, B1, B4, and B5; echoviruses 9, 11, 19, 20, and 22.

Modified from Boyer KM, Cherry JD. Nonbacterial pneumonia In: Feigin RD, Cherry JD, eds. Textbook of pediatric infectious disease. 3rd ed. Philadelphia: WB Saunders, 1992:256.

overall frequency, their typical degree of severity, and their usual mode of access to the lung.

■ EPIDEMIOLOGY

The rates of childhood pneumonia show a rough inverse correlation with age, ranging from 40:1000 in children younger than 5 years to 7:1000 in adolescents 12 to 15 years. Respiratory syncytial virus (RSV) is the most common causative agent in children less than 5 years of age; *Mycoplasma pneumoniae* is most common in older children.

In children, congenital heart disease and bronchopulmonary dysplasia are associated with viral pneumonia of greater severity, particularly that caused by RSV. Pulmonary deterioration in patients with cystic fibrosis has been shown to be associated with respiratory viral infection. Surprisingly, common respiratory viruses have only moderately greater impact in patients with hematologic malignancy and immunosuppressed states than they have in normal hosts.

■ CLINICAL PRESENTATION

Acute nonbacterial pneumonia in the infant or young child generally follows 1 or 2 days of coryza, decreased appetite, and low-grade fever. The onset generally is gradual, with increasing fretfulness, respiratory congestion, vomiting, cough, and fever. In the very young infant, fever may be minimal and apneic spells ("near-miss" sudden infant death syndrome [SIDS] or "apparent life-threatening events") the most prominent (and frightening) presenting complaint. The most reliable physical findings of pneumonia are those of respiratory distress: tachypnea, tachycardia, nasal flaring, and retractions, but without the stridor that is characteristic of upper airway obstruction. In the patient with diminished functional residual capacity, grunting may be present. Cyanosis generally accompanies apneic spells or coughing attacks, but it may be present at rest if significant ventilation–perfusion mismatch has developed.

Other physical findings are variable and may be normal. Wheezing is present in infants with bronchiolitis. Hyperresonance may be noted if significant air trapping is present. Diminished local percussion or breath sounds may indicate lobar consolidation or atelectasis. In patients with interstitial pneumonia, fine crackling rales may be present diffusely or locally. Also important in the initial assessment is an evaluation of the young child's state of hydration, because increased insensible losses from fever and hyperventilation, coupled with anorexia, can result in significant fluid deficits.

The afebrile pneumonitis syndrome of young infants, in contrast to the usual acute viral pneumonias affecting this age group, is subacute to chronic in its development and is nonseasonal. Characteristic features include the absence of fever, a "staccato" cough pattern, and diffuse rales on auscultation. Radiographic findings usually consist of interstitial infiltrates with subsegmental atelectasis. Hypergammaglobulinemia and mild eosinophilia are common laboratory abnormalities.

Nonbacterial pneumonia in the older child and adolescent occurs clinically more nearly like that in an adult. Premonitory complaints generally include such systemic symptoms as malaise, myalgia, and anorexia in addition to upper respiratory tract symptoms. "Chilliness" may occur, but rigors generally are absent. Cough usually is irritative and nonproductive. A temperature above 39°C (102.2°F) is unusual. Although tachypnea, flaring, and retractions generally are present, they may be less apparent than in the infant or young child. Findings on examination of the chest are more reliable than in infancy and may include local percussion dullness or diminished breath sounds and local or diffuse fine rales. Because apnea is rare in older patients, cyanosis is an ominous sign of impairment of gas exchange. Although mild dehydration often is present, it generally is not evident on examination.

Radiologic findings in nonbacterial pneumonias vary according to the patient's age and the infecting agent. In the infant and young child, bilateral air trapping and perihilar infiltrates are the most frequent findings. Patchy areas of consolidation may represent lobular atelectasis or alveolar pneumonia. In the older child and the adolescent, lobar involvement can be defined more often, but the affected areas typically are not consolidated completely. Although lobar consolidation may occur in patients with nonbacterial pneumonia, this finding should be distinguished from atelectasis and is more consistent with a bacterial cause of disease. Similarly, although small pleural effusions may be detected in decubitus films in patients with nonbacterial pneumonias, effusions are much more suggestive of bacterial infection.

Peripheral leukocyte counts are variable but tend to be less than 15,000/mm³ in patients with nonbacterial pneumonia. Gram stains of sputum or tracheal secretions tend to show epithelial cells as the predominant cell type, with a mixed bacterial population representing normal pharyngeal flora. Dominance of polymorphonuclear leukocytes and a uniform bacterial population are more consistent with bacterial infection.

■ DIFFERENTIAL DIAGNOSIS

In the differential diagnosis of nonbacterial pneumonias, the following factors must be considered: the status of the host (normal or compromised); the environment (family or school exposure); the age of the patient; and the season of the year. In certain epidemiologic settings, the specific cause of nonbacterial pneumonia may be guessed with relative certainty. Often, however, this category of pulmonary infection is a diagnosis of exclusion. The major conditions to be differentiated include noninfectious pulmonary diseases, bacterial pneumonias that are amenable to conventional antibiotics, and the more unusual bacterial, fungal, or parasitic infections that may require specialized forms of therapy.

Noninfectious conditions that may simulate nonbacterial pneumonia are summarized in Table 95–2. The demarcation between infectious and noninfectious conditions is not always sharp. In a child with sickle cell anemia, for example, pulmonary vascular occlusive crisis presents with fever, leukocytosis, and patchy pulmonary infiltrates. Differentiation from pneumococcal, *Haemophilus*, or *Mycoplasma* pneumonia, to which the child with sickle cell is susceptible, can be difficult.

■ THERAPY

Therapy for nonbacterial pneumonia is primarily expectant and supportive. The course of uncomplicated viral pneumonia is not influenced by the administration of antibiotics. In the vast majority of cases in which pulmonary involvement is uncovered, however, antibiotic therapy is used because bacterial disease cannot be ruled out with certainty. In all but the most mild cases, this approach is both reasonable and practical. It is important, though, that antibiotic therapy in routine cases be appropriate for the most common bacterial pathogens (*S pneumoniae* and *H influenzae*). In the immunocompromised host or when secondary infection is a possibility, *Staphylococcus aureus* and other hospital-associated and opportunistic pathogens must be considered.

In certain fulminant viral pneumonias, such as varicella in a compromised host, antiviral chemotherapy with acyclovir may be lifesaving, but it should be recalled that as many as half of all patients with this condition have complicating bacterial sepsis that is amenable to antibiotic therapy. The treatment of pneumonia caused by cytomegalovirus (CMV) in an immunocompromised host now consists of the combination of ganciclovir and intravenous hyperimmune globulin. Inhalational administration of the antiviral compound ribavirin appears to shorten the course of viral pneumonias caused by RSV and influenza. This drug is recommended particularly for the treatment of RSV infection in infants with underlying cardiopulmonary disease. Other infants with proven or suspected RSV disease for whom ribavirin has been recommended include those with severe disease and impending respiratory failure, and those with initially milder disease, but risk factors such as prematurity, young age (<6 weeks), and neuromuscular compromise. Crystallization in ventilator valves is a technical difficulty associated with the administration of ribavirin to patients on mechanical ventilation. With protective filtration devices in

TABLE 95-2. Noninfectious Conditions That May Simulate or Underlie Pneumonia in Children

TECHNICAL	ATELECTASIS
Poor inspiratory chest radiograph	Cardiomegaly
Underpenetrated chest radiograph	Mucus plug
PHYSIOLOGIC	Foreign body
Prominent thymus	**DAMAGE BY PHYSICAL AGENTS**
Breast shadows	
CHRONIC PULMONARY DISEASE	Bronchopulmonary dysplasia
	Lipoid pneumonia
Asthma	Petroleum distillate ingestion
Cystic fibrosis	Near drowning
Bronchiectasis	Smoke inhalation
Bronchiolitis obliterans	**IATROGENIC PULMONARY DAMAGE**
Pulmonary sequestration	
Congenital lobar emphysema	Fluid overload
Pulmonary hemosiderosis	Drugs (nitrofurantoin, bleomycin)
Desquamative interstitial pneumonitis	Radiation pneumonitis
	Graft-versus-host disease
RECURRENT ASPIRATION	**PULMONARY INFARCTION**
Gastroesophageal reflux	Sickle vaso-occlusive crisis
Tracheoesophageal fistula	Fat embolism
Craniofacial defect	**MISCELLANEOUS**
Neuromuscular disorders	
Familial dysautonomia	Systemic lupus erythematosus
PULMONARY EDEMA	Sarcoidosis
Congestive heart failure	Neoplasms (lymphoma, teratoma, neuroblastoma)
Adult respiratory distress	Pleural effusion or reaction
Syndrome	Bronchogenic cyst
Total anomalous pulmonary Venous return	Vascular ring
	Histiocytosis
ALLERGIC ALVEOLITIS	
Dusts (farmer's lung)	
Molds (allergic aspergillosis)	
Excreta (pigeon-breeder's lung)	

Modified from Boyer KM. Pneumonia. In Dershewitz RA, ed. Ambulatory pediatric care. 2nd ed. Philadelphia: JB Lippincott; 1992:621.

Because of ventilation–perfusion abnormalities and alveolocapillary block, most children with nonbacterial pneumonia have some degree of hypoxemia. In a child with respiratory distress, provision of supplemental oxygen reduces anxiety and ventilation rates. Increases in inspired oxygen to about 30% are provided easily in mist tent environments, which are the most convenient means of administering oxygen. More severe respiratory distress or cyanosis requires documentation of the patient's respiratory status by means of arterial blood gas determinations and more exact regulation of inspired oxygen administered by nasal prongs, hood, or face mask. Oximetry, capnography, or transcutaneous monitoring can reduce the need for frequent blood gas sampling and insertion of arterial lines. In patients with respiratory failure, mechanical ventilation is required to maintain oxygenation and control CO_2 retention.

Apnea and bradycardia occur commonly in young infants with pneumonia that is caused by RSV, parainfluenza viruses, and influenza viruses, and are particularly frequent complications in those with a history of premature birth. Although the mechanism for these episodes is unclear, continuous monitoring for apnea is prudent in a young infant with viral pneumonia.

■ PROGNOSIS

The child with pneumonia should be reevaluated clinically 2 to 3 weeks after the condition was diagnosed. If the child is asymptomatic, has returned to normal activities, and has benign results on physical examination, a follow-up radiograph is not required. Repeated chest radiographs are indicated in children with complicated clinical courses, underlying cardiopulmonary disease, or prior episodes of pneumonia, or if signs or symptoms of respiratory difficulty persist at the time of follow-up. It should be recognized that about 20% of patients with uncomplicated cases of pneumonia have persistent radiographic abnormalities 3 to 4 weeks after diagnosis, but a selective approach to follow-up films permits the early recognition of atelectasis or chronic disease.

(Abridged from Kenneth M. Boyer, Nonbacterial Pneumonia, in Oski, DeAngelis, Feigin, McMillan, Warshaw: *Principles and Practice of Pediatrics, Second Edition,* J.B. Lippincott, 1994.)

Oski's Essential Pediatrics,
edited by Kevin B. Johnson and Frank A. Oski.
Lippincott–Raven Publishers,
Philadelphia © 1997

the circuitry, however, ribavirin has proven to be safe and effective in patients with critical RSV illness.

Specific antimicrobial therapy for mycoplasmal, chlamydial, and rickettsial pneumonias with erythromycin or tetracycline shortens the course of the illness, but generally has a less dramatic therapeutic effect than does specific antibiotic therapy for bacterial infections. The drug of choice for *Pneumocystis* pneumonia is trimethoprim-sulfamethoxazole.

The elements of supportive therapy include adequate hydration, high humidity, maintenance of oxygenation, and mobilization of lower respiratory tract secretions. Because of increased insensible fluid losses as a result of fever, hyperventilation, and anorexia, mild dehydration frequently is observed initially, and continuing losses usually occur during the acute phase of illness. Thus, restoration of deficits and adequate maintenance of fluid intake are desirable. With regard to the latter, it should be remembered that fluid requirements increase by about 12% per °C of fever, and that hyperventilation increases fluid requirements by an additional 15%.

96

Hypersensitivity Pneumonitis

The term *hypersensitivity pneumonitis* defines a spectrum of pulmonary disorders that includes granulomatous, interstitial, and alveolar filling diseases. These respiratory disorders are associated causally with intense and frequently prolonged exposure to inhaled organic antigens. The range of vegetable and animal antigens implicated is broad. Table 96–1 lists some of the most common offenders.

TABLE 96-1. Causative Agents in Hypersensitivity Pneumonitis

Antigen	Antigen Source	Name of Disorder
ACTINOMYCETE AND FUNGAL-LADEN VEGETABLE PRODUCTS		
Thermophilic actinomycetes (*Micropolyspora faeni, Thermoactinomyces vulgaris*), *Aspergillus species*	Moldy hay	Farmer's lung disease
Thermophilic actinomycetes (*Thermoactinomyces sacchari, T vulgaris*)	Moldy pressed sugarcane (bagasse)	Bagassosis
Thermophilic actinomycetes (*M faeni, T vulgaris*)	Moldy compost	Mushroom worker's disease
Penicillium species	Moldy cork	Suberosis
Aspergillus clavatus	Contaminated barley	Malt worker's lung
Cryptostroma corticale	Contaminated maple logs	Sequoiosis
Alternaria species	Contaminated wood pulp	Wood-pulp worker's disease
Thermophilic actinomycetes (*Thermoactinomyces candidus, T vulgaris*), *Penicillium* species, *Cephalosporium* species, amebae	Contaminated humidifiers, dehumidifiers, air conditioners	Humidifier lung
Bacillus subtilis	Contaminated wood dust in walls	Familial hypersensitivity pneumonitis
Penicillium species	Cheese casings	Cheese washer's disease
Rhizopus species, *Mucor* species	Contaminated wood trimmings	Wood trimmer's disease
Saccharomonospora viridis	Dried grasses and leaves	Thatched roof disease
Streptomyces albus	Contaminated fertilizer	*Streptomyces*-hypersensitivity pneumonia
Cephalosporium	Contaminated basement (sewage) pneumonitis	*Cephalosporium* hypersensitivity
Pullularia species	Sauna water	Sauna taker's disease
B subtilis enzymes	Detergent	Detergent worker's disease
Mucor-stolonifer	Paprika dust	Paprika splitter's lung
ANIMAL PRODUCTS		
Pigeon-serum proteins	Pigeon droppings	Pigeon breeder's disease
Duck proteins	Feathers	Duck fever
Turkey proteins	Turkey products	Turkey handler's disease
Parrot-serum proteins	Parrot droppings	Budgerigar fancier's disease
Chicken proteins	Chicken droppings	Feather plucker's disease
Bovine and porcine proteins	Pituitary snuff	Pituitary-snuff taker's lung
Rat-serum protein	Rat urine and droppings	Rat lung
INSECT PRODUCTS		
Ascaris siro (mite)	Dust	
Sitophilus granarius (wheat weevil)	Contaminated grain	Miller's lung
REACTIVE SIMPLE CHEMICALS		
Altered proteins (neoantigens) or hapten protein conjugates	Toluene diisocyanate	TDI*-hypersensitivity pneumonitis
		TMA†-hypersensitivity pneumonitis
	Tremetallic anhydride	
Hapten protein conjugates	Diphenylmethane diisocyanate	MDI‡-hypersensitivity pneumonitis
Hapten protein conjugates	Heated epoxy resin	Epoxy-resin lung

*TDI, *toluene diisocyanate.*
†TMA, *tremetallic anhydride.*
‡MDI, *diphenylmethane diisocyanate.*
Salvaggio JE. Hypersensitivity pneumonitis. *J Allergy Clin Immunol. 1987;79:558.*

■ CLINICAL PRESENTATION

The clinical presentation of hypersensitivity pneumonitis is variable and traditionally is separated into three somewhat distinct clinical entities: acute, subacute, and chronic. The acute form of hypersensitivity pneumonitis frequently is related to intermittent, intense inhalation of the offending antigen, with symptoms precipitated 4 to 6 hours after antigen contact. Typical clinical symptoms include elevated temperature in the range of 38.3°C to 40.0°C (101°F to 104°F), dry cough, dyspnea, and malaise. Constitutional symptoms can persist for weeks after exposure, but usually resolve within 24 hours. The patient appears ill on physical examination, and lung auscultation typically documents bilateral bibasilar rales. Wheezing or evidence of reversible reactive airway disease is uncommon and provides evidence against the diagnosis of hypersensitivity pneumonitis.

Characteristic laboratory findings in patients with an acute episode of hypersensitivity pneumonitis (which can be reproduced by antigen inhalation challenge also) include leukocytosis, with white blood cell counts as high as 25,000/mm³; eosinophilia (in about 10% of patients); polyclonal elevation of serum immunoglobulin levels; and nonspecific reactive rheumatoid factor results. Positive evidence of antigen-specific serum precipitins is documented well in both symptomatic and asymptomatic exposed individuals, so using this measure solely to diagnose hypersensitivity pneumonitis is not always valid.

The subacute presentation of hypersensitivity pneumonitis lacks the characteristic findings of fever, malaise, and dyspnea that are noted in the acute form of the disorder. Clinically, the patient may complain of persistent anorexia or weight loss and malaise. Pulmonary symptoms such as progressive shortness of breath or insidious onset of dyspnea on exertion may be late. The chronic form of hypersensitivity pneumonitis usually is related to long-term, low-dose antigen exposure. Clinical findings include a normal physical examination, with the exception of pulmonary rales detected on auscultation of the chest. Wheezing rarely accompanies chronic hypersensitivity pneumonitis. Lung disease related to the chronic form of the disorder usually is poorly responsive to traditional therapeutic intervention. Initial pulmonary findings include the following: severe restrictive impairment (coupled with a diffusion defect); pulmonary fibrosis (determined radiographically and histologically, with noncaseating granulomas noted); and progressive nonreversible obstructive disease that is characterized by hyperinflation and sometimes is associated histologically with evidence of obliterative bronchiolitis and emphysema.

Chest radiographs of patients with acute hypersensitivity pneumonitis may reveal bibasilar interstitial infiltrates or multibasilar nodular densities. In chronic disease forms, pulmonary fibrosis can be seen, with evidence of contracted lung tissue. When progressive obstructive lung disease complicates hypersensitivity pneumonitis, hyperinflation may be noted radiographically.

■ TREATMENT AND COMPLICATIONS

The therapy of choice for patients with hypersensitivity pneumonitis is avoidance of the offending agent, if it can be identified. Because causative agents often are related to a person's occupation, however, patients frequently are reluctant to limit their exposure to the offending antigen. For children, this usually is not a difficult problem. For acute and subacute forms of the disease, avoidance alone often is not sufficient to cause clinical improvement. In these instances, corticosteroid therapy has proven useful in controlling pulmonary exacerbations and reversing some restrictive lung components. Antihistamines and bronchodilators are ineffective therapeutic modalities in patients with acute and subacute hypersensitivity pneumonitis.

With chronic lung disease (interstitial fibrosis, obliterative bronchiolitis), steroid therapy usually is not effective in reversing pulmonary function deficits or improving clinical symptoms. Patients with chronic lung disease occasionally have evidence of obstructive lung disease and sometimes benefit from bronchodilator therapy. Given appropriate clinical suspicion and astute and pertinent historical data collection, these affected individuals should be identified before irreversible lung disease ensues.

(Abridged from I. Celine Hanson and William T. Shearer, Hypersensitivity Pneumonitis, in Oski, DeAngelis, Feigin, McMillan, Warshaw: *Principles and Practice of Pediatrics, Second Edition,* J.B. Lippincott, 1994.)

Oski's Essential Pediatrics,
edited by Kevin B. Johnson and Frank A. Oski.
Lippincott–Raven Publishers,
Philadelphia © 1997

97

Pneumocystis carinii Pneumonia

Pneumocystis carinii pneumonia is an opportunistic infection of increasing importance to pediatricians. A marked increase in the prevalence of this disorder in the United States over the past 2 decades has paralleled therapeutic advances in the management of immunologic and neoplastic diseases, resulting in longer survival of children with these underlying disorders. Most important, *P carinii* pneumonia is currently occurring in epidemic proportions in association with the acquired immunodeficiency syndrome (AIDS).

The dramatic nature of *P carinii* pneumonia tends to obscure the fact that its severity is the result of the susceptibility of the host rather than the virulence of the parasite. During the past 2 decades, pneumocystic pneumonia has occurred almost exclusively in patients with primary or acquired immunologic disorders or in those receiving immunosuppressive treatment of oncologic disease or organ transplantation.

Pneumocystis carinii pneumonia is unique in that the pathologic findings, with rare exceptions, are limited to the lungs, even in fatal cases. In the infantile "epidemic" form of the disease, essentially all alveoli contain large numbers of organisms.

The natural course of *P carinii* infections in children is highly variable and depends primarily on the status of host defenses in individual patients. Infantile epidemic pneumocystosis is typified in premature, debilitated, or marasmic infants between the ages of 2 and 6 months. These patients often have chronic diarrhea and weight loss before the development of respiratory symptoms. Characteristically, the onset is insidious, with progression of cough, tachypnea, and respiratory distress over a 1- to 4-week interval. Fever is either absent or low-grade in most cases. Symptoms in immunosuppressed children or adults may be more abrupt in onset and more rapidly progressive than in infantile epidemic cases; in these older patients, the severity and duration of disease before diagnosis are highly variable, but the mortality rate is about 100% if treatment is not provided. Unlike in infantile cases, fever generally is present and high-grade, and it often precedes the onset of a nonproductive cough, tachypnea, and severe dyspnea or the appearance of pulmonary infiltrates on radiography. The onset of clinical disease in high-risk patients is unpredictable, but it often has been observed to occur after the discontinuation of corticosteroid therapy or reduction in drug dosage. Observations suggest that the development of clinical disease depends in part on whether inflammatory responses are normal or are impaired somewhat as a result of the patient's underlying disease, therapeutic regimen, or both.

Physical examination at the time of initial presentation may reveal tachypnea, nasal flaring, and intercostal, subcostal, or supracostal retractions. An ashen color or cyanosis may be present or may develop rapidly. Auscultation of the chest frequently is characterized by a conspicuous absence of adventitious sounds despite rapid (80 to 100 per minute), shallow respirations. Scattered rales, rhonchi, or wheezes usually are detected later in the clinical course as resolution occurs. Aside from variable temperature elevation, few physical abnormalities are noted except those that are referable to pulmonary disease or secondary to the patient's underlying disease or treatment.

Various radiographic abnormalities have been observed in documented cases of isolated *P carinii* pneumonia. These variations, in part, are a result of observations being made at different stages in the course of the disease. Bilateral diffuse parenchymal infiltrates are seen most commonly, but no pattern is specific enough either to exclude or to confirm a consideration of *P carinii* disease. Although it initially is a reticulogranular interstitial process, *Pneumocystis* pneumonitis progresses to a predominantly alveolar process, with coalescence and air bronchogram formation. Late in the course of the disease, complete opacification of the lung fields may occur. Hilar adenopathy and pleural effusion are not characteristic of the disease unless they are a result of an underlying disorder.

A variety of techniques have been used to obtain suitable materials for diagnostic purposes. Bronchoalveolar lavage, endobronchial brush biopsy, and transbronchial lung biopsy have been used successfully to establish a diagnosis of *P carinii* pneumonia in adult patients. Bronchoalveolar lavage has been shown to be safe and effective, especially in patients with AIDS. These techniques have been employed successfully in infants as young as 2 months of age. Their routine use in children is not justified, however, given the limited experience and significant morbidity associated with these procedures in pediatric patients. Invasive techniques, including open lung biopsy, closed needle biopsy, and percutaneous needle aspiration, are the most reliable methods of confirming a diagnosis. Open lung biopsy provides the most reliable specimen for identification of both the organism and the extent of the infection; its chief disadvantage is that it requires general anesthesia. Percutaneous needle aspiration has proved to be a reliable and safe procedure in some centers.

Before the availability of specific therapeutic agents, the overall prognosis of patients with *P carinii* pneumonia was poor. Pentamidine became available to investigators in the United States in 1967, with dramatic results. Although pentamidine was effective in treatment of this disorder, the high incidence of toxicity emphasized the need for an alternative therapeutic agent. At present, trimethoprim-sulfamethoxazole appears to be the drug of choice for the treatment and prevention of *P carinii* pneumonia. In addition to antimicrobial agents, the administration of corticosteroids early in the course of moderately severe pneumonitis reduces the occurrence of respiratory failure and improves oxygenation among adult patients with AIDS.

P carinii pneumonitis can be prevented effectively by providing chemoprophylaxis with co-trimoxazole. Use of this medication can prevent this infection in as many as 95% of high-risk patients.

(Abridged from Donald C. Anderson, *Pneumocystis carinii* Pneumonia, in Oski, DeAngelis, Feigin, McMillan, Warshaw: *Principles and Practice of Pediatrics, Second Edition*, J.B. Lippincott, 1994.)

Oski's Essential Pediatrics,
edited by Kevin B. Johnson and Frank A. Oski.
Lippincott–Raven Publishers,
Philadelphia © 1997

98

Bacterial Pneumonia

In the United States, recognized infection of the lower respiratory tract occurs annually in 15 to 20 per 1000 infants less than 1 year of age and in 30 to 40 per 1000 children 1 to 5 years of age. Although the respiratory viruses and *Mycoplasma pneumoniae* are the most common agents of lower respiratory tract disease in children and young adults, pyogenic bacteria cause a substantial minority of cases of pneumonia; a recent study found that bacteria were responsible for 19% of pneumonia cases among ambulatory children. Bacterial pneumonia is observed most often in the winter and early spring, and occurs almost twice as frequently in males as in females.

Diseases involving the airways, such as bronchopulmonary dysplasia, cystic fibrosis, and bronchiectasis, and anatomic defects, such as cleft palate or tracheoesophageal fistula, predispose to the development of bacterial pneumonia. Pneumonia and lung abscess are common infections in children with severe cognitive neurologic disorders or diminished levels of consciousness. Children with hemoglobinopathies, especially sickle-cell disease, have higher rates of bacterial pneumonia. Children who are immunodeficient on the basis of inherited or acquired disease, or because they are receiving immunosuppressive therapy have an increased risk of pneumonia from a wide spectrum of bacteria in addition to viruses, fungi, protozoa, and parasites.

In practice, bacterial pneumonia may be difficult to distinguish from other forms of pneumonia. Young children do not produce adequate sputum for Gram stain and culture, and more invasive procedures are not warranted except in a few patients who are severely ill or have underlying immunodeficiency.

■ ETIOLOGY

The age of the child and the presence or absence of underlying disease are the two most important patient characteristics determining the cause of bacterial pneumonia. Bacterial pneumonia presenting in the first 2 days of life is caused by the same organisms that are responsible for generalized neonatal sepsis (ie, group B streptococci, *Listeria monocytogenes*, *Haemophilus influenzae*, and gram-negative enteric bacilli). After the neonatal period, *Streptococcus pneumoniae*, *H influenzae*, type b, *Staphylococcus aureus*, and group A streptococci are responsible for virtually all cases of bacterial pneumonia in otherwise healthy children. In patients older than 4 or 5 years, the spectrum of bacteria causing pneumonia narrows, with *S pneumoniae* and *M pneumoniae* predominating. *Mycoplasma* infections are unusual in young children but are common after the age of 5 years.

■ CLINICAL FEATURES

The signs and symptoms of bacterial pneumonia vary with the age of the child, the infecting organism, and the presence or absence of underlying disease. Older children and adolescents characteristically have fever, chills, headache, dyspnea, productive cough, chest pain, abdominal pain, and nausea or vomiting. Young infants, however, are likely to have the largely nonspecific symptoms of fever, lethargy, poor feeding, vomiting, or diarrhea. Tachypnea may be overlooked by the parents, and cough, if present, often is not a prominent finding in very young infants. Similarly, the findings on physical examination of young infants with pneumonia are less definitive; percussion and auscultation usually do not elicit the characteristic dullness to percussion and decreased breath sounds that are found in older children and adults with pneumonia, and rales may be difficult to distinguish from the sounds produced by a congested upper respiratory tract.

■ DIAGNOSIS

In practice, the diagnosis of pneumonia is made with the demonstration of infiltrates on anteroposterior and lateral chest radiographs. (Keep in mind that many noninfectious diseases of the lung may mimic the radiographic appearance of pneumonia, including malignancy, collagen vascular disease, congestive heart failure, pulmonary embolus, allergic alveolitis, pulmonary hemorrhage, and hemosiderosis.) A pattern of peribronchial or "patchy" infiltrates (bronchopneumonia) does not distinguish viral or mycoplasmal pneumonia from bacterial pneumonia, but demonstration of hyperinflation is most consistent with viral infection. Resolution of the pulmonary infiltrates will lag behind clinical improvement of the patient. Routine follow-up radiographs contribute little to the treatment of a child with an uncomplicated course of pneumonia.

A white blood cell (WBC) count and differential, and an erythrocyte sedimentation rate test are performed routinely on all pediatric patients with suspected pneumonia. An attempt to determine the cause of the infection should be made in all cases of suspected bacterial pneumonia in hospitalized children. Cultures of blood and pleural fluid, if the latter is present, usually are obtained from children who require hospitalization. Gram stain of expectorated sputum may be of considerable value in the diagnosis of pneumonia in a school-age child or adolescent, especially when a single organism is seen in association with polymorphonuclear leukocytes, and culture of an adequate sputum specimen usually yields the pathogenic organism. Infants and young children are incapable of producing a spontaneous sputum specimen, however, and efforts to induce sputum in younger children generally are unsuccessful. Cultures of the nasopharynx and throat are not useful and should not be attempted because of the risk of producing misleading information. Invasive procedures such as bronchoalveolar lavage or open lung biopsy are justified in cases of pneumonia that are severe or complicated by underlying disease. Direct transthoracic needle aspiration of the lung has proven to be useful in cases in which recovery of an organism is critical for treatment.

■ TREATMENT

The treatment of pneumonia depends on the severity of the illness and the presence or absence of underlying chronic disease. In practice, children with mild to moderate pneumonia often are treated as outpatients. Some physicians choose to withhold antibiotic therapy for cases that, in their judgment, are more likely to have a viral cause. Other physicians prefer to "cover" with an oral antibiotic that is effective against the most likely bacterial pathogens. Oral penicillin V or erythromycin often is used for outpatient treatment of older children and adolescents with pneumonia. Erythromycin often is considered the drug of choice for this age group because of its activity against *M pneumoniae*, but as many as 5% to 20% of group A streptococci and clinical isolates of *S pneumoniae* may be resistant. For children less than 5 years of age, amoxicillin-clavulanate (Augmentin) is an excellent choice for oral therapy. Although ampicillin and amoxicillin are used widely in oral therapy for pneumonia in young children, they are ineffective against 10% to 30% of the strains of *H influenzae*, type b and β-lactamase–producing strains of *S aureus*. For hospitalized children with more serious disease, antibiotics and maintenance of adequate oxygenation are the mainstays of treatment of bacterial pneumonia; chest physical therapy and intermittent positive-pressure treatments are of little additional benefit. Antibiotics should be chosen that are effective against the major bacterial pathogens expected, given the child's age. Initial therapy can be guided by the results of a sputum Gram stain and can be modified, if necessary, once the results of cultures of blood, sputum, or pleural fluid are reported. A variety of options are available for parenteral antibiotic treatment of the infant or young child with suspected bacterial pneumonia, including ampicillin-sulbactam (Unasyn), cefuroxime, a third-generation cephalosporin, or the combination of oxacillin and chloramphenicol.

■ PNEUMONIA CAUSED BY SPECIFIC BACTERIAL PATHOGENS

S pneumoniae is a common cause of pneumonia in patients of all ages. Serotypes 1, 3, 6, 7, 14, 18, 19, and 23 are the most common of the 84 serotypes found in children, differing slightly from the distribution of serotypes that cause bacteremia pneumonia in adults. Pleural effusion occurs in a minority of cases, but frank empyema is unusual, and pneumatocele formation is rare. About 30% of children with pneumococcal pneumonia have positive blood culture results when they are first seen, a finding associated with more severe disease. Rapid resolution of fever and dyspnea with appropriate antibiotic therapy is the rule, but prolonged courses occur, especially with extensive lung involvement and with empyema. The mortality rate in children is about 10%, and there is little or no residual impairment of lung function. Rare complications include pericarditis, meningitis, endocarditis, arthritis, and bursitis.

H influenzae, type b pneumonia is indistinguishable clinically and radiographically from pneumococcal pneumonia and is nearly as common in children less than 2 years of age. Seventy-five percent to 90% of children with *H influenzae* pneumonia have positive blood culture results, however, and 40% to 75% have accompanying pleural effusions. Importantly, 10% to 30% of children with *H influenzae* pneumonia also have meningitis, epiglottitis, or another serious pyogenic infection. The mortality rate is 5% to 10%.

S aureus pneumonia appears to be less common now than it was in the past, but it remains an important cause of serious pneumonia, especially in infants younger than 6 months. Staphylococcal pneumonia presents initially similar to pneumonia of other causes but progresses characteristically to pneumatocele formation and empyema, even in the presence of appropriate antibiotic therapy. Although recovery of staphylococci from the blood occurs in only 10% of affected infants, organisms usually are present in large numbers in a Gram-stained tracheal aspirate. Mortality resulting from staphylococcal pneumonia is 20% to 30%, and recovery in survivors may take weeks.

(Abridged from John F. Modlin, Bacterial Pneumonia, in Oski, DeAngelis, Feigin, McMillan, Warshaw: *Principles and Practice of Pediatrics, Second Edition,* J.B. Lippincott, 1994.)

Oski's Essential Pediatrics,
edited by Kevin B. Johnson and Frank A. Oski.
Lippincott–Raven Publishers,
Philadelphia

99

Foreign Bodies

Foreign bodies in the respiratory tract are a common and important pediatric problem. From the nose to the distal airways, the respiratory tree has been the recipient of a wide range of unnatural, exogenous materials. Aspiration of foreign bodies remains a major cause of morbidity and mortality in children.

■ NOSE

Nasal foreign bodies usually are more of an annoyance than a threat to life. The majority are inserted by toddlers or preschoolers, more often mischievously than truly accidentally. Occasionally, a piece of tissue inserted to stop a nosebleed miraculously will avoid dislodgment and stay in place for days to weeks. The classic finding is a persistent, unilateral, purulent nasal discharge that may be blood-tinged. Foul odor is common. Although they generally are not considered to be very dangerous, nasal foreign bodies have dislodged posteriorly and been aspirated, either spontaneously or during an attempt at removal. Although the diagnosis should be readily apparent, the foreign body occasionally is obscured by copious or dried secretions. Alternatively, the foreign object may be misinterpreted as a nasal polyp.

Removal of most nasal foreign bodies is accomplished readily in the office without general anesthesia. Sedation may be required, but even this usually is not necessary.

Soft or irregularly shaped objects that can be grasped easily by forceps are best removed in this way. Removal of a round, hard object, such as a bead, is accomplished best by insertion of an ear curet past the foreign body and then application of gentle forward pressure.

■ UPPER AIRWAY (LARYNX AND TRACHEA)

Aspiration of foreign material into the larynx and trachea occurs frequently and, not uncommonly, proves lethal. It has been estimated that aspiration of foreign bodies into the upper airway is the second leading cause of accidental death in the home among children younger than 5 years. In most cases, the diagnosis is immediately evident. Sometimes, however, a child may aspirate while asleep or alone and may be seen either as a sudden, unexpected death or with the sudden onset of severe respiratory distress. Although the aspirated material usually is a piece of food or candy, a variety of other objects have been recovered from the larynx and trachea. The plastic cap of a water pistol, a fragment of balloon, and a piece of bubble gum are examples of objects that have been recovered at autopsy.

Very small foreign objects in the trachea generally are not life-threatening. Although one would imagine that such objects would promptly be coughed out or aspirated more deeply, in reality, this is not always the case; they may remain in the trachea for days or even weeks, often becoming embedded in granulation tissue. Although the predominant clinical feature is inspiratory stridor, associated expiratory wheezing is present in about 25% to 50% of cases. Cases have been misdiagnosed as croup or tumors. Eggshell, plastic toys or parts of toys, and watermelon seeds are examples of objects that have remained in the trachea for extended periods.

Signs and symptoms of an upper airway foreign body may be mimicked by a foreign body in the esophagus that is pressing on the posterior trachea. Remarkably, in some cases, such foreign bodies cause stridor or wheezing without any dysphasia or difficulty in swallowing.

It is not surprising that the treatment of acute, life-threatening upper airway obstruction due to a foreign body is controversial. The great majority of patients with this catastrophic event are treated in the field, usually by someone who is not a physician. By the very nature of the condition, few patients requiring urgent treatment survive to reach the hospital without intervention.

To perform the abdominal thrust (Heimlich maneuver) with the victim sitting or standing, the rescuer stands behind the patient with his or her arms wrapped around the victim's abdomen and one fist grabbed by the other hand, slightly above the navel and well below the xiphoid process. The rescuer then forces the fist into the abdomen with a quick upward thrust. If the patient is supine, the rescuer places the heel of one hand, with the other hand on top, on the abdomen in the location described above and then exerts a sudden upward pressure in the midline. Back blows are applied with the heel of the hand high between the scapulae. Chest thrusts are similar to external cardiac compression, delivered smartly as four thrusts.

■ LOWER AIRWAY (BRONCHI)

The majority of aspirated foreign bodies either are coughed out promptly or lodge beyond the carina, in a major bronchus or more distal airway. The peak incidence of pulmonary aspiration of foreign bodies in children is between the first and second birthdays. More than 90% of foreign body aspiration occurs before the fifth birthday. The variety of foreign bodies that have been aspirated is impressive. Unfortunately, most aspirated foreign bodies are radiolucent.

In the classic case (which, of course, is seen only occasionally), a previously well toddler suddenly starts to choke and cough, often while eating, playing with a toy, or crawling on a carpet. The coughing and choking subside, only to be followed by wheezing. Often, however, there is no history to suggest a discrete episode of aspiration, or the episode is recalled only in retrospect when the foreign body has been removed and identified. The onset of symptoms may be gradual. Occasionally, the onset may coincide fortuitously with an upper respiratory tract infection and fever, making diagnosis especially difficult.

Although wheezing is one of the most common signs associated with a pulmonary foreign body, it is far from invariably present. In a 1980 study of children with bronchial foreign bodies, wheezing was exhibited in only 60% and stridor in only 13%.

To a large extent, the clinical picture, especially the physical and roentgenographic findings, is dictated by whether the foreign body causes partial or total obstruction of the bronchus in which it resides. Partial obstruction results in wheezing that is predominantly expiratory and may be either unilateral (on the side of the foreign body) or bilateral. In some cases of bilateral wheezing, the expiratory wheeze is clearly louder over the ipsilateral hemithorax. It is not clear whether the contralateral wheezing in these cases represents a generalized reflex bronchoconstriction or merely transmission of the wheezing sound. Partial obstruction results in a check-valve mechanism in the airway, with progressive air trapping in the involved lung, lobe, or segment. On physical examination, breath sounds may be decreased over the involved lung, and the trachea and cardiac impulse are shifted *away* from the involved lung. Tachypnea and retractions are common. Cyanosis generally is seen only in severe cases, usually when the foreign body is obstructing a major bronchus. Radiographically, obstructive emphysema involving a lung, lobe, or segment is the hallmark of a foreign body that is partially occluding an airway. In some cases, the over-expansion of the involved lung is mild and not discernible on an ordinary roentgenogram of the chest. In such situations, fluoroscopy, inspiratory and expiratory roentgenograms, or right and left decubitus films may show an apparent shift of the mediastinum away from the involved lung during expiration. This results from the fact that the uninvolved lung is able to empty and, therefore, gets smaller during expiration, whereas the involved lung is obstructed and remains hyperinflated. Visually, this appears as if the mediastinum were moving away from the involved lung.

When the foreign body occludes the involved airway completely, the result is atelectasis rather than hyperaeration. Clinically, this is evident by decreased breath sounds, with or without rales. Although the trachea and cardiac impulse usually are unchanged, in severe cases, they may be shifted *toward* the involved lung. Chest roentgenography will reveal atelectasis of the affected area.

Fever, rales, purulent sputum, and radiographic evidence of pneumonia can occur with either partial or complete occlusion. Pneumonia may be noted in 15% to 20% of cases.

The mainstay of management of foreign bodies in the lower airways is endoscopic removal. If the presence of a foreign body is unclear, endoscopy can be diagnostic as well as therapeutic. Although, for a time, postural drainage was recommended as a less invasive approach to pulmonary foreign bodies, it quickly was recognized that this form of therapy is fraught with considerable danger. The obstructing foreign body can be dislodged into the opposite main stem bronchus, obstructing that bronchus while the original lung is unable to recover instantly from the insult. Edema of the airway, as well as parenchymal changes in the lung from which the foreign body was just dislodged, may take hours to days to subside. Such instances can be catastrophic.

The gold standard for therapy is endoscopy, usually under general anesthesia with rigid endoscopic equipment. The procedure should be performed in the operating room, and the endoscopist should be familiar with, and comfortable in caring for, the pediatric patient. State-of-the-art endoscopic equipment should be available. Optimal treatment includes assessment by an anesthetist who is skilled in the care of young children and in treating patients during endoscopic procedures. These ideal conditions often are not available, and, if the patient's condition is stable, it may be best to transfer the child to a facility where skillful pediatric endoscopic treatment is available. If endoscopy is unsuccessful because the object is too small, or if the object fragments on attempted removal, then a course of postural drainage is reasonably safe and should be undertaken.

With proper treatment, the mortality rate for aspiration of foreign bodies into the lower airways should be exceedingly low.

(Abridged from Martin I. Lorin, Foreign Bodies, in Oski, DeAngelis, Feigin, McMillan, Warshaw: *Principles and Practice of Pediatrics, Second Edition*, J.B. Lippincott, 1994.)

Oski's Essential Pediatrics, edited by Kevin B. Johnson and Frank A. Oski. Lippincott–Raven Publishers, Philadelphia © 1997

100

Laryngeal Disorders

■ CONGENITAL SUBGLOTTIC STENOSIS

Congenital stenosis is an anatomic defect in the larynx resulting in a narrowed airway. Stenosis at the subglottic level is secondary most often to a cartilaginous abnormality—the cricoid typically is smaller in circumference than normal and somewhat flattened in shape. Another common finding is telescoping of the first tracheal ring within the cricoid cartilage and, as a consequence, narrowing of the airway. Soft-tissue airway compromise occurs when either an increased amount of connective tissue or hyperplastic dilated mucous glands encroach on the subglottic lumen.

Minimal stenosis rarely causes problems except in association with upper respiratory tract infections. In contrast, marked subglottic stenosis produces nearly constant biphasic stridor and sternal retractions. Pulmonary secretions are cleared ineffectively, and a barking cough and recurrent pulmonary infections are common.

Fortunately, most neonates with congenital subglottic stenosis respond to conservative therapy and can be treated with antibiotics and steroids during episodes of upper respi-

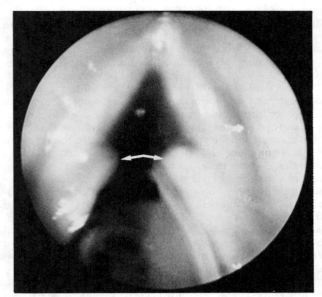

Figure 100-1. Intubation granulomas hugging the endotracheal tube, which can be seen inferiorly

ratory tract infection and increased respiratory stridor. Fewer than 50% require a tracheotomy, and this frequently can be removed as airway cross-sectional area increases with growth and development. A weight increase from 2 to 10 kg is associated with an increase in the area of the airway at the cricoid from 20 to 60 mm². This tripling results in a ninefold decrease in airway resistance and, in many instances, obviates the need for major surgery.

More commonly, glottic and subglottic stenosis are the sequelae of prolonged intubation. The mucosa of the larynx is highly reactive and vulnerable to injury, and an inappropriately large tube or repeated or traumatic attempts at intubation cause extensive tissue damage. Mucosal changes occur almost immediately. In the first few hours after intubation, edema develops in the laryngeal mucosa. Within days, the epithelium becomes eroded and mucosal necrosis occurs. At the sites of injury, granulation tissue forms and often can be seen around the endotracheal tube if a direct

laryngoscopy is done (Figure 100–1). Attempted extubation at this time often is unsuccessful, as the granulation tissue further narrows an already compromised airway.

The reported incidence of subglottic stenosis as a complication of intubation ranges from 0.23% to 8.0%. In many instances, surgery is required before extubation is possible. Treatment possibilities that must be considered in the face of failed attempts to remove the endotracheal tube range from endoscopic laser surgery to cricoid-splitting procedures. If these therapeutic techniques are unsuccessful, a tracheotomy is required. In most instances, the stenosis is so severe that conservative treatment will not permit decannulation for several years, if at all.

■ SUBGLOTTIC HEMANGIOMA

Hemangiomas are hamartomatous collections of endothelial cells similar to those from which the vascular system is derived. Capillary loops, sinusoidal spaces, or arteriovenous fistulas predominate, and hemangiomas are subclassified accordingly. They are the most common benign tumor of the head and neck in children, with an estimated prevalence of 10% to 12% in whites. This figure increases to 22% in preterm babies weighing less than 1000 g. The female:male preponderance is 3:1.

Most commonly, hemangiomas appear in the skin, usually as a single tumor, although multiple cutaneous lesions occur occasionally, often with involvement of other organ systems. If the hemangioma is present in the subglottic area, the lesion potentially can be life-threatening. Subglottic hemangiomas usually are capillary, submucosal, and unencapsulated; in contrast, the rarer supraglottic hemangioma is more likely to be cavernous. Similar to hemangiomas in general, subglottic hemangiomas are more common in females and, in 50% of affected children, are associated with concomitant cutaneous hemangiomas. The site of predilection for these associated hemangiomas is in the head and neck.

Subglottic hemangiomas are present at birth, but typically go unnoticed until several weeks to months have passed. The natural history is one of progressive enlargement of the hemangioma during the first 12 months of life, followed by autogenous embolization in the ensuing years. Varying degrees of airway distress develop, bringing these infants to the attention of their pediatrician.

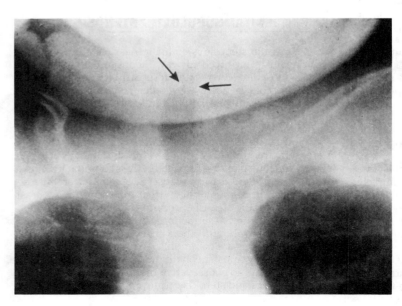

Figure 100-2. Soft-tissue roentgenogram of the airway, showing encroachment of the tracheal air column by a right-sided subglottic hemangioma.

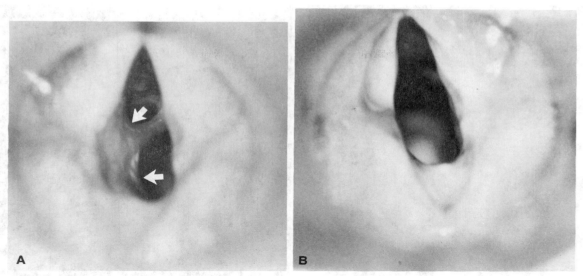

Figure 100-3. Endoscopic view of a left posterolateral subglottic hemangioma, before (**A**) and after (**B**) laser therapy.

Plain roentgenograms of the neck can reveal an asymmetric subglottic mass, and supplemental studies such as a cine-esophagram can show the extent of invasion of the common tracheoesophageal wall (Figure 100–2). The definitive diagnosis is made under controlled conditions by direct laryngoscopy. A biopsy is not required because the appearance of the pink to bluish compressible mass in the lateral or posterolateral subglottic space is pathognomonic (Figure 100–3).

Small subglottic hemangiomas do not cause airway compromise and may require no treatment; with larger, life-threatening hemangiomas, however, a tracheotomy often is essential. Although this secures the airway, the high mortality rate makes further intervention essential. Local compression is believed to hasten the regression of hemangiomas, and some lesions respond to a 10- to 14-day period of intubation. Systemic steroids may be administered concomitantly, although proof of their efficacy is lacking and their mechanism of action on hemangiomas is not clear. Presumably, steroids enhance the sensitivity of endothelial cells to endogenous circulating vasoconstrictors. Unfortunately, when used alone, they usually are unsuccessful at relieving obstruction and afford only a transient improvement in the airway condition.

Surgical treatment options include the injection of sclerosants, cryotherapy, laser therapy, and excisional surgery. Of the choices, the precision that is possible and the discrete area of tissue damage that is produced make the CO_2 laser especially applicable to endolaryngeal surgery. A beam of coherent light of 10.6 μm in wavelength is generated. The radiant energy produced by the CO_2 laser is absorbed strongly by homogenous water, and the extinction length in soft tissue is only 0.03 mm. Reflection and scattering are negligible. For these reasons, only a small area of tissue destruction results, and the exposed cells absorb energy and are vaporized immediately. Hemangiomas usually must be treated several times before enough scarring and fibrosis form to restore the airway to an adequate size (see Figure 100–3).

■ LARYNGEAL PAPILLOMA

The most common benign tumor of the larynx is the papilloma. It accounts for more than 80% of laryngeal growths and, although benign, tends to recur, can be difficult to cure, and can cause fatal airway obstruction. These char-

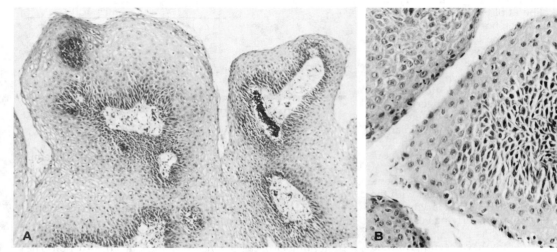

Figure 100-4. Histologic appearance of a papilloma, showing (**A**) fibrovascular cores and acanthosis, and (**B**) additionally, under higher power, focal koilocystosis.

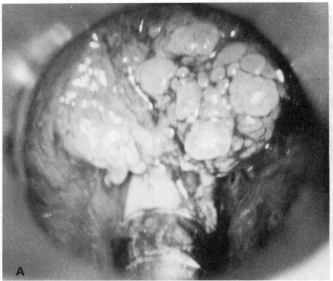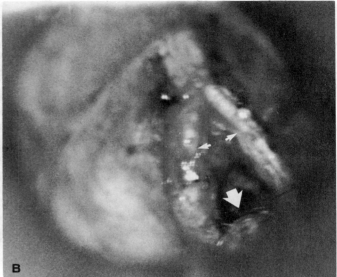

Figure 100-5. Marked laryngeal papillomatosis, before (**A**) and after (**B**) laser therapy. *Small arrows*, vocal cords; *large arrow*, endotracheal tube.

acteristics are reflected in its common name, recurrent respiratory papillomatosis (RRP). RRP is induced virally, most frequently by human papillomavirus subtypes 6 and 11. The majority of affected individuals are children less than 7 years of age, although papillomas do occur in people of all ages.

Juvenile laryngeal papillomas can be extremely aggressive and resistant to treatment. Most frequently, the anterior portion of the true vocal cords, the false vocal cords, and the laryngeal surface of the epiglottis are involved. Exuberant growth can cover normal anatomy and spread to contiguous areas, which can lead to involvement of the vallecula and hypopharynx, esophagus, trachea, and bronchi. Treatment is extremely frustrating because recurrences are common even after apparently complete removal. Additionally, the clinical course is unpredictable, with spontaneous regression seen occasionally at puberty.

The most common presenting symptoms reflect vocal cord disease and airway compromise. Hoarseness or stridor, a voice change or complete aphonia, a weak cry, and respiratory distress may occur. Occasionally, the degree of papillomatosis is so severe that a tracheotomy is necessary. Tracheotomy increases the likelihood of tracheal and bronchial spread, however, and should not be undertaken without serious reflection. Involvement of the lower airways is the harbinger of a particularly bleak prognosis.

The diagnosis of papilloma is made easily by visual examination of the larynx, using either a laryngeal mirror or a flexible fiberoptic laryngoscope. The histologic picture is pathognomonic. Papillary lesions with long, fingerlike projections of connective tissue abound. These are covered with acanthotic and hypoplastic ingrowing epithelium. Enlarged stromal vessels lie contiguous to hypoplastic epithelium immediately adjacent to the basement membrane, without apparent intervening stroma (Figure 100–4).

In most cases, surgery is the favored form of treatment. CO_2 laser vaporization of papillomas is performed with the patient under general anesthesia using a direct laryngoscope and a surgical microscope. The small underlying vessels also can be cauterized easily (Figure 100–5).

Large trials of interferon therapy have been performed in several centers, and dramatic results have been seen occasionally.

Optimal treatment requires serial laser laryngoscopy with the use of interferon in selected cases. The unpredictable course of papilloma makes several procedures the rule, without a guarantee of cure. Recent advances in molecular biology have demonstrated the presence of the viral genome in normal-appearing mucosa in children with laryngeal papilloma. This suggests that the infection is more widespread than is clinically apparent. Advances in medical rather than surgical therapy will be necessary to cure this disorder permanently. Especially promising are the host of antiviral agents being developed.

(Abridged from Nancy M. Bauman and Richard J.H. Smith, Laryngeal Disorders, in Oski, DeAngelis, Feigin, McMillan, Warshaw: *Principles and Practice of Pediatrics, Second Edition,* J.B. Lippincott, 1994.)

Oski's Essential Pediatrics,
edited by Kevin B. Johnson and Frank A. Oski.
Lippincott–Raven Publishers,
Philadelphia © 1997

101

Cystic Fibrosis

Cystic fibrosis (CF) is the most common lethal or semilethal genetic disease affecting whites. The triad of chronic obstructive pulmonary disease, pancreatic exocrine deficiency, and abnormally high sweat electrolyte concentration is present in most patients. CF is the major cause of chronic debilitating pulmonary disease and pancreatic exocrine deficiency in the first 3 decades of life and accounts for a significant number of cases of neonatal intestinal obstruction. The name of the disease is derived from the characteristic histologic changes seen in the pancreas.

■ GENETICS

Estimates of the incidence of CF vary according to the population studied, but a reasonable figure for whites is 1 in 2500. The incidence of CF in American blacks is 1 in 17,000. The CF gene is rare in African blacks and Asians. Transmission is autosomal recessive. Based on incidence figures, 4% of whites in the United States are estimated to be carriers (heterozygous) of the CF gene.

Gene Defect

The gene responsible for CF has been localized to 250,000 base pairs of genomic DNA located on the long arm of chromosome 7. It encodes a protein of 1480 amino acids called the cystic fibrosis transmembrane conductance regulator (CFTR). A 3-base deletion removing a phenylalanine residue at position 508 of CFTR (Δ F508 mutation) is present on about 70% of CF chromosomes.

■ PATHOPHYSIOLOGY

Most clinical manifestations can be related to abnormal secretions that result in obstruction of organ passages and to abnormal function of the eccrine sweat glands. Glands are affected in varying distribution and degrees of severity and fall into three types: those obstructed by viscid or solid eosinophilic material in the lumen (pancreas, intestinal glands, intrahepatic bile ducts, gallbladder, submaxillary glands), those that produce an excess of histologically normal secretions (tracheobronchial and Brunner's glands), and those that are histologically normal but secrete excessive electrolytes (sweat, parotid, and small salivary glands). The high concentration of electrolytes in sweat is due to decreased transductal reabsorption of chloride and sodium.

■ CLINICAL FEATURES

Table 101–1 is a summary of clinical manifestations of CF. Some of the more significant manifestations are described below.

Pulmonary

The respiratory tract is invariably involved, and pulmonary complications usually dominate the clinical picture. Manifestations may not appear, however, until weeks, months, or even years after birth. Autopsy studies suggest that the lungs are normal at birth. The initial pulmonary lesion is obstruction of the small airways by abnormally thick mucus secretions. Secondary to obstruction, there is bronchiolitis and mucopurulent plugging of the airways. Bronchial changes are more common than parenchymal changes. Bronchiectasis is present in almost all patients older than age 18 months. It progresses with age and is especially striking in older patients. Emphysema is not common. Figure 101–1 shows a proposed mechanism for pulmonary manifestations seen in patients with CF.

Infection

Secondary bacterial infection, first due to *Staphylococcus aureus* then to *Pseudomonas aeruginosa*, initiates a cycle of chronic infection, tissue damage, and obstruction. More than 80% of patients with advanced disease consistently harbor

TABLE 101-1. Summary of Clinical Manifestations of Cystic Fibrosis

UPPER RESPIRATORY TRACT	NUTRITIONAL/METABOLIC
Nasal polyposis	Diabetes
Sinusitis	Hypokalemic alkalosis
PULMONARY	Hypoprothrombinemia
Allergic bronchopulmonary aspergillosis	Iron deficiency anemia
	Salt depletion syndrome
Atelectasis	Protein–calorie malnutrition
Bronchiectasis	Vitamin A deficiency
Bronchiolitis	Vitamin E deficiency
Bronchitis	**MISCELLANEOUS**
Cor pulmonale	Arthritis/arthropathy
Hemoptysis	Absent vas deferens
Pneumothorax	Aspermia
Pneumonia	Decreased female fertility
Reactive airway disease	Delayed puberty
Respiratory failure	Digital clubbing
HEPATOBILIARY	Erythema nodosum
Cholecystitis	Failure to thrive
Cholelithiasis	Growth retardation
Cholestasis	Malnutrition
Cirrhosis/portal hypertension	
GASTROINTESTINAL	
Gastroesophageal reflux	
Intussusception	
Meconium ileus	
Meconium ileus equivalent	
Meconium plug syndrome	
Pancreatic exocrine deficiency	
Pancreatitis	
Peptic ulcer disease	
Rectal prolapse	

strains of *P aeruginosa*, most of which are heavy slime producers known as mucoid variants. Once established, *Pseudomonas* is virtually impossible to eradicate. Systemic defense mechanisms appear to be intact, and infection tends to be localized to the respiratory tract. Septicemia and extrapulmonary infections are rare.

Signs and Symptoms

Half of patients present with pulmonary manifestations, usually consisting of chronic cough and wheezing along with recurrent or chronic infections. Young infants can present with atelectasis, often involving the right upper lobe, or a severe bronchiolitic syndrome. The most prominent and constant feature of pulmonary involvement is chronic cough. At first, the cough may be dry, but with progression it becomes paroxysmal and productive. Older patients expectorate mucopurulent sputum, particularly in association with pulmonary exacerbations. Wheezing is often a prominent feature, especially in association with pulmonary exacerbations, but it is unclear if this reflects inflammation and bronchial obstruction or coincidental atopy. A few patients develop allergic bronchopulmonary aspergillosis. Physical findings include a barrel-chest deformity, use of accessory muscles of respiration, growth retardation, digital clubbing, pulmonary hypertrophic osteoarthropathy, and cyanosis.

Radiographic Changes

Chest x-ray findings can help in the diagnosis of CF. Hyperinflation and bronchial wall thickening are the earliest findings (Figure 101–2). Subsequent changes include areas of infiltrate, atelectasis, and hilar adenopathy. With advanced disease, segmental or lobar atelectasis, bleb formation, bronchiectasis, and pulmonary artery and right ventricular enlargement are seen. Characteristic branching, fingerlike opacifications represent mucoid impaction of dilated bronchi.

Pulmonary Function

Airway obstruction, air trapping, and ventilation–perfusion inequalities are the most important functional changes in CF. Ventilation–perfusion scans usually demonstrate focal areas of inequality. Pulmonary function tests reveal hypoxemia; reduction in forced vital capacity (FVC), in forced expiratory volume in 1 second (FEV$_1$), and in FEV$_1$ to FVC ratio; and an increase in residual volume and in the

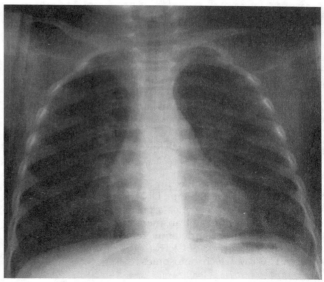

Figure 101-2. Chest radiograph from a 6-year-old patient showing increased lung markings and focal areas of peribronchial thickening.

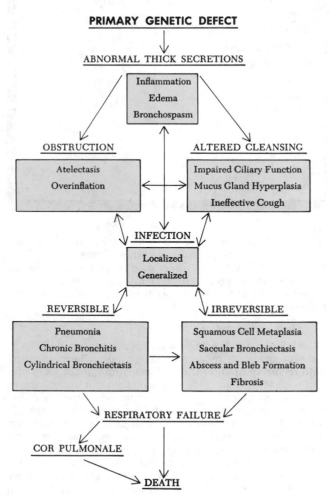

Figure 101-1. Proposed mechanism for the pulmonary manifestations seen in patients with CF. (With permission from *Guide to Diagnosis and Management of Cystic Fibrosis*. Bethesda, MD: Cystic Fibrosis Foundation; 1979:8.)

ratio of residual volume to total lung capacity. Airway reactivity is present in 50% of patients and may be associated with accelerated progression of pulmonary disease. The response to bronchodilators is unpredictable and varies with time and changes in underlying pulmonary status.

Pneumothorax

In patients with advanced lung disease, pneumothorax, hemoptysis, and cor pulmonale are frequent complications. Pneumothorax occurs secondary to rupture of apical subpleural blebs. The overall incidence is 2% to 10% and, in adults, may be as high as 16%. Patients typically present with acute onset of chest pain and shortness of breath. After a pneumothorax on one side, there is a 50% incidence on the contralateral side within 6 to 12 months.

Hemoptysis

Patients often experience blood streaking of their sputum. Bleeding is due to erosion of bronchial arteries into a bronchus, often in association with an exacerbation of the underlying pulmonary infection. Massive hemoptysis is a serious complication associated with significant mortality, a high recurrence rate, and a poor prognosis. The site of bleeding may be localized by bronchoscopy.

Cor Pulmonale

Cor pulmonale, manifested by hypertrophy of the right ventricle, is seen in 70% of patients dying with CF and occurs in 50% of patients surviving past age 15 years. Chronic alveolar hypoxia and hypoxemia serve as a stimulus to reflex vasoconstriction and medial hypertrophy of the pulmonary arteries. Severe cor pulmonale has been consistently associated with PaO$_2$ values of less than 50 mm Hg. Clinically, cor pulmonale may be difficult to recognize. Peripheral edema is present in only two thirds of cases and is often a late manifestation. Liver tenderness may be an early clue. The electrocardiogram does not correlate consistently with the presence of right ventricular hypertrophy. Echocardiography is probably the most practical and reliable way of documenting cor pulmonale and following its course.

Course

The pulmonary course is characterized by chronic suppurative bronchitis with recurrent pulmonary exacerbations, often following viral respiratory infections. Infection with respiratory syncytial virus may be an important cause of significant respiratory morbidity in young infants. By age 10 years, 90% of patients have intermittent sputum production; by age 15 years, 90% of patients have daily sputum production. There is progressive shortness of breath and exercise intolerance. Pulmonary involvement advances at a variable rate, usually faster in females than males, but eventually leads to respiratory failure, cardiac failure, or both.

Upper Respiratory Tract

The upper respiratory tract is usually affected secondary to the hyperactive mucus-secreting glands and the hyperplasia and edema of mucous membranes. Chronic nasal congestion and rhinitis are common. Radiographic evidence of opacification of the paranasal sinuses is present in almost all patients and may be helpful diagnostically in patients with equivocal sweat test results.

Nasal polyps occur in 6% to 24% of patients. Clinical manifestations include obstruction to nasal airflow, mouth breathing, localized infection, epistaxis, rhinorrhea, and widening of the nasal bridge. Polyps occur at a much younger age in patients with CF as compared with those with underlying atopy, can be differentiated histologically, and tend to recur.

Gastrointestinal

Pancreatic Exocrine Deficiency

The most common gastrointestinal manifestations result from loss of pancreatic enzyme activity and consequent intestinal malabsorption of fats, proteins, and, to a lesser extent, carbohydrates. Complete loss of pancreatic activity is seen in 85% to 90% of patients. Loss of function may be progressive. Clinical manifestations include poor or no weight gain, abdominal distention, deficiency of subcutaneous fat and muscle tissue, rectal prolapse, and frequent passage of pale, bulky, foul-smelling, often oily stools. Steatorrhea and azotorrhea are pronounced. Secondary to pancreatic insufficiency, patients have low serum lipid levels and may be deficient in linoleic acid. Although infants may appear to have a voracious appetite, caloric intake is often deficient. In adolescent patients, there may be absence of a pubertal growth spurt and delayed maturation. In general, growth retardation correlates more closely with the degree of pulmonary involvement. Adolescents and young adults with residual pancreatic function may have recurrent episodes of pancreatitis, sometimes as the presenting manifestation. Patients with residual pancreatic function tend to have lower sweat chloride values, less severe pulmonary involvement, and better survival. Tests of fat absorption, including 72-hour fecal fat excretion, provide indirect assessment of pancreatic exocrine function.

Carbohydrate Intolerance

In addition to pancreatic exocrine dysfunction, up to 40% of patients show carbohydrate intolerance that progresses to frank diabetes in 2% to 5% of cases. The incidence of carbohydrate intolerance increases with age, but diabetes has been seen at age 6 months.

Meconium Ileus

Meconium ileus, in which there is obstruction of the distal ileum by inspissated, tenacious meconium, occurs in 10% to 15% of newborn infants with CF. With rare exception, meconium ileus is always associated with CF. Clinically, infants present with evidence of intestinal obstruction. Abdominal films show distended bowel loops with a "bubbly" pattern of inspissated meconium in the terminal ileum. Contrast enema shows a microcolon from disuse secondary to intrauterine obstruction. Associated intestinal complications, including small-bowel atresia, volvulus, and perforation/peritonitis are present in 40% to 50% of cases. Meconium ileus tends to recur in the same family. A delay in the passage of meconium and distal colonic obstruction secondary to the meconium plug syndrome also may be presenting manifestations of CF and are indications for a sweat test.

Late Intestinal Complications

The intestinal contents tend to be abnormally thick and puttylike as a result of abnormal behavior of intestinal gland secretions, decreased chloride secretion across the colonic epithelium, deficiency of pancreatic enzymes, and prolonged intestinal transit time. This may lead to a variety of late intestinal complications. There may be recurrent episodes of partial or complete obstruction of the small or large bowel, often preceded or accompanied by colicky abdominal pain and a palpable firm mass in the right lower quadrant. This symptom complex is referred to as meconium ileus equivalent or the distal intestinal obstruction syndrome and occurs in as many as 20% of patients. These episodes may be precipitated by decreased fluid intake, change in diet, or cessation of pancreatic enzyme supplements. Precipitated by the abnormal intestinal contents, there may be episodes of small-bowel volvulus or intussusception. The latter complication occurs in 1% of older patients and may be the presenting manifestation. Episodes tend to recur and may be associated with chronic symptoms.

Upper Gastrointestinal Complications

Patients with CF have an increased incidence of gastroesophageal reflux, probably related to chest hyperinflation along with increased abdominal pressure due to coughing. It may be manifested by vomiting and failure to thrive in infants and by abdominal pain, esophageal ulcerations, stricture formation, and blood loss in older patients.

Nutritional/Metabolic

Vitamin and Mineral Deficiencies

Secondary to pancreatic achylia, there is malabsorption of fat-soluble vitamins. Low serum vitamin A levels are due to steatorrhea and a depression of retinol-carrier protein and retinol-binding protein. Xerophthalmia and night blindness occur rarely, usually in association with hepatic involvement. A bulging fontanelle, secondary to vitamin A deficiency, may be the presenting manifestation in infants. Overt rickets is rare, but a significant reduction in vitamin D biologic activity with associated secondary hyperparathyroidism, reduced bone mineral content, and delayed bone maturation is common. Significant demineralization is present in half of all patients. Severe bleeding in association with hypoprothrombinemia and deficiency of clotting factors II, VII, IX, and X may occur in infants secondary to vitamin K deficiency.

Edema and Hypoproteinemia

The syndrome of edema and hypoproteinemia, secondary to pancreatic enzyme deficiency, may be the presenting manifestation in as many as 8% of patients with CF. It is seen most often in infants 1 to 6 months of age who are breast-fed or receive soy-based formula. Associated findings include hepatomegaly, elevation of liver enzymes, skin rash, and anemia. False-negative sweat test results can be seen in the presence of edema.

Hepatobiliary

Liver

The liver is extensively involved in CF. Focal biliary cirrhosis—characterized by the inspissation of amorphous, eosinophilic material in the intrahepatic bile ducts, bile duct proliferation, inflammatory reaction, a variable degree of fibrosis, and focal distribution—is pathognomonic of CF. Hypoalbuminemia in infancy may predispose to later liver complications. Portal hypertension, which is manifested by hepatomegaly, esophageal varices, and hypersplenism, develops in 2% to 3% of all patients and in 5% of adults. Liver failure is rare, and liver function tests may show only mild transaminase elevation until late in the course of disease. Fatty infiltration of the liver secondary to protein–calorie malnutrition may present clinically as massive hepatomegaly. In some patients, liver complications may be the predominant and, at times, presenting features. Liver complications are seen only in those patients with pancreatic insufficiency; there may be a familial pattern to their occurrence.

Reproductive System

Male

Aspermia and infertility are seen in 98% of adult males. Histologically, the testes show active but decreased spermatogenesis. There is mechanical obstruction of sperm transport, however, secondary to absence or atresia of the vas deferens, along with associated abnormalities of the epididymis and seminal vesicle. The prostate is normal. All postpubescent males should have their semen analyzed for purposes of counseling.

Female

Although fertility is decreased, many women with CF bear children. Histologically, there is excessive cytoplasmic and extracellular mucus, and there is often plugging of the cervical os by tenacious, dehydrated mucus. This probably acts as a barrier to sperm penetration. The ovaries and endometrium are normal. Among women who become pregnant, there may be deterioration of pulmonary status and there is an increased incidence of spontaneous abortion, prematurity, and stillbirth, possibly related to maternal hypoxemia.

Back Pain and Spinal Deformity

Back pain that is not associated with trauma is present in most patients. It usually affects the mid and lower back, may be exacerbated by coughing, and often interferes with exercise, coughing, daily activities, and physiotherapy. Associated features include decreased range of motion and muscle strength, a "hunched over" posture, and a high incidence of vertebral wedging. Treatment consists of exercise and postural counseling.

Psychosocial

Impact on Family

Cystic fibrosis is accompanied by a series of psychological crises from the time of diagnosis to the patient's death. Initially, parents may be frustrated and angry by medical delays in making the diagnosis of CF. After the diagnosis is confirmed, there is shock and disbelief, accompanied by the guilt associated with the transmission of a genetic disease. Eventually, there is acceptance of the diagnosis, but denial is used as the overriding defense mechanism. If adaptive, denial enables families to cope; if maladaptive, it can lead to serious problems resulting in denial of the diagnosis by the patient as well as noncompliance with the treatment program. Impact on family functioning is usually significant. Hardest to accept by families is the concept of intensive, long-term care carried out with no guarantee of success. There is often a breakdown in intrafamilial communication and withdrawal from the community. Psychosomatic complaints and depression are common. Siblings often resent the extra care and time required by the patient with CF, but generally function quite well. The occupational goals of the parents may have to be modified, and the financial burden can be considerable.

Impact on Patient

The reaction of the patient to the diagnosis of CF varies with age and parental response. There is often denial of symptoms. There may be maladaptive use of fantasy, repression, and regression. Feelings of anxiety and depression can lead to psychosomatic complaints and problems with discipline and academic work at school. The well-adjusted child is not embarrassed about having CF, discusses it openly with friends, and readily takes medications and treatments in front of others. Adolescence is a critical period for patients, and psychological problems are prominent. Patients are dissatisfied with their appearance and have to cope with a delay in physical development and maturation. They may be forced to realistically compromise their academic and vocational goals. The extended dependency caused by CF interferes with the normal process of separation from parents. Conflicts during adolescence are often manifested by social withdrawal, noncompliance with medical regimens, and risk-taking behavior.

■ DIAGNOSIS

Clinical Presentation

The physician should remain vigilant for CF and consider this diagnosis in a wide range of clinical situations. Although two thirds of cases are diagnosed by age 1 year, 10% of cases escape detection until adolescence or adulthood. In most patients, the diagnosis is suggested because of pulmonary manifestations or steatorrhea, often associated with failure to thrive, a positive family history, or a variety of miscellaneous manifestations related to salt depletion or deficiencies of vitamins, protein, minerals, or calories. The spectrum of clinical features is so varied and symptoms may be so minimal that one cannot exclude the possibility of CF even with a normal growth pattern, absence of pulmonary disease, or normal pancreatic exocrine function. A patient should never be deprived of an evaluation because of "looking too well to have CF."

Sweat Testing

The diagnosis of CF should always be confirmed by documentation of an elevated sweat electrolyte concentration. Indications for a sweat test are outlined in Table 101–2.

Newborn Screening

Screening of newborns for CF is possible. Newborns with CF have elevated blood levels of immunoreactive trypsin (IRT), presumably due to a secretory obstructive defect in the pancreas in utero. Mass newborn screening programs are not yet recommended for the United States, however, pending results of cost–benefit analysis. The IRT test also may be helpful in evaluating neonates with a positive family history for CF. In such cases, it may yield information 2 to 3 weeks earlier than the age at which an adequate sweat sample can be obtained. In no case should the IRT test be used as a substitute for the sweat test or as the basis of a definitive diagnosis. False-negative IRT results occur in as many as 25% of newborns with intestinal obstruction.

■ MANAGEMENT

Because of multisystem involvement, frequency of complications, psychosocial burden, and uncertain prognosis, a comprehensive, intensive therapy program is essential. Patients should be followed at intervals of 2 to 3 months by an experienced, available physician, as well as by nursing, nutrition, physical–respiratory therapy, and counseling personnel. The Cystic Fibrosis Foundation, Bethesda, MD, supports a nationwide network of centers involved in patient care, teaching, and clinical and basic research. Services provided by the centers include sweat testing and confirmation of diagnosis; evaluation and provision of a therapeutic plan; continuity of outpatient and inpatient services; patient and family education; nutrition counseling; instruction in physical and respiratory therapy; psychosocial support, including individual counseling and education/support groups for patients, parents, and siblings; financial counseling; genetic counseling; subspecialty consultative services; and opportunity to participate in clinical research projects. Vocational, educational, financial, and premarital counseling can help the increasing number of adult patients make a smooth transition to independent living. Optimal patient management involves coordination of services between the CF center and the primary care provider who can provide ongoing psychosocial support, offer general medical care, coordinate home, community, and educational services, and interpret the significance of medical developments. Goals of therapy include maintaining adequate nutrition and normal growth, preventing or providing aggressive therapy for pulmonary complications, encouraging appropriate physical activity, and providing psychosocial support.

Pulmonary

Antibiotic Therapy

Treatment of pulmonary manifestations of CF is directed at clearing excess mucus from the tracheobronchial tree and providing aggressive antimicrobial therapy. Except in the case of acute respiratory illness, guidelines for the use of antibiotics in these patients are not well established. Patients with CF may require high doses of aminoglycosides to achieve acceptable serum concentrations.

Improved methods for providing stable venous access have made home intravenous antibiotic therapy an attractive alternative to hospitalization. This type of therapy is cost-effective, is associated with few complications, and does not interfere with normal activity.

Physical and Respiratory Therapy

Chest physiotherapy, consisting of postural drainage, manual or mechanical percussion, vibration, and assisted coughing, enhances the removal of bronchial secretions and usually is recommended at the first indication of pulmonary involvement.

Aerosol Therapy

Although a variety of aerosolized agents have been used in CF therapy, evidence to support their use is largely anecdotal. Bronchodilators, administered either orally or by nebulization, may be useful in selected patients. The response of CF patients to these agents is highly variable, and they should be used only after observing an obvious clinical response or documenting a beneficial response by pulmonary function testing.

Immunotherapy

Evidence supports a role for glucocorticoid therapy in patients with CF. Use of glucocorticoids in the treatment of

---

TABLE 101-2. Indications for Sweat Testing

PULMONARY/UPPER RESPIRATORY	METABOLIC/OTHER
Atelectasis (especially right upper lobe)	Acrodermatitis enteropathica
Bronchiectasis	Aspermia/absent vas deferens
Chronic cough	Edema and hypoproteinemia
Digital clubbing	Failure to thrive
Hemoptysis	Hypoprothrombinemia
Mucoid *Pseudomonas* colonization	Metabolic alkalosis
Nasal polyps	Positive family history
Pansinusitis	Salt depletion syndrome
Recurrent/chronic pneumonia	Salty taste/salt crystals
Tachypnea/retractions	Vitamin A deficiency (bulging fontanelle)
Wheezing and hyperinflation	
GASTROINTESTINAL	
Cirrhosis and portal hypertension	
Intestinal atresia	
Meconium ileus	
Meconium plug syndrome	
Mucoid-impacted appendix	
Prolonged neonatal jaundice	
Recurrent intussusception	
Recurrent pancreatitis	
Rectal prolapse	
Steatorrhea	

CF probably should be limited to patients with severe bronchiolitic syndrome, significant airway obstruction that is not responsive to conventional bronchodilators, allergic bronchopulmonary aspergillosis, and evidence of hypersensitivity characterized by recurrent episodes of fever, rash, and joint pain. Patients on long-term glucocorticoid therapy need to be carefully monitored for development of carbohydrate abnormalities, cataracts, and growth retardation.

Hemoptysis Management

Heavy blood streaking of sputum and episodes of hemoptysis usually reflect increased pulmonary infection. The site of bleeding may be localized by bronchoscopy. In patients with heavy blood streaking, intensive antibiotic therapy alone may be sufficient. With massive hemoptysis (more than 300 mL/24 h) or with protracted or recurrent episodes of moderate bleeding, percutaneous catheter embolization of the involved bronchial arteries is the procedure of choice. Bleeding immediately ceases in more than 80% of patients. After the procedure, however, repeat bleeding is common, and one third to one half of patients require repeat embolization.

Cor Pulmonale Management

The management of right-sided failure includes therapy of the underlying pulmonary obstruction and infection along with diuretics, salt restriction, and oxygen. Digitalis is not generally useful. Overall, results have not been favorable. In adults with chronic obstructive pulmonary disease, pulmonary hypertension may be reversed by long-term continuous oxygen therapy. This has not been demonstrated in CF cases, however, and the role of oxygen therapy remains poorly defined. It is usually prescribed to relieve symptomatic hypoxemia (ie, headaches and dyspnea) and to improve exercise tolerance.

Gastrointestinal

Pancreatic Exocrine Deficiency

Pancreatic enzyme supplements, derived from hog pancreas, constitute the primary therapy of the pancreatic enzyme defect. The most effective preparations consist of capsules containing pancrelipase in pH-sensitive enteric-coated microspheres. The enteric coating prevents gastric acid inactivation of the enzyme. Enzyme supplements are given with all meals and snacks; the dosage is determined by the frequency and character of the stools along with the patient's growth pattern.

Nutrition

The goal of nutrition therapy is to promote normal growth. Because of incomplete correction of steatorrhea and increased metabolic demands, it is recommended that patients receive 50% more calories than usual daily allowances. Supplements with medium chain triglyceride (MCT) oil and polycose can boost caloric intake. In patients who have poor growth and inadequate caloric intake, despite nutritional counseling and attempts at oral supplementation, enteral supplementation may be useful. This is accomplished by nightly infusion of high-calorie elemental formulas by way of a nasogastric, gastrostomy, or jejunostomy tube.

Vitamin deficiencies can be prevented by daily administration of a water-miscible vitamin preparation. Additional dietary salt should be provided at times of thermal stress, including increased activity in hot weather. Supplementation with salt tablets is not usually indicated.

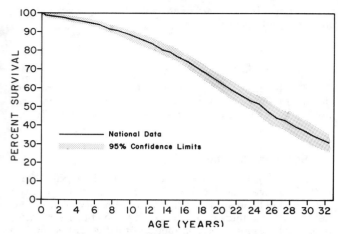

Figure 101-3. Survival curve for patients seen in CF centers in the United States in 1990. (Courtesy of Cystic Fibrosis Foundation, Bethesda, MD.)

Meconium Ileus Equivalent

In cases of meconium ileus equivalent in which there is no evidence of intestinal obstruction, oral administration of a cleansing electrolyte solution (Golytely) is the treatment of choice. If there is evidence of intestinal obstruction, enemas with hyperosmolar contrast material may be diagnostic as well as therapeutic.

■ COURSE AND PROGNOSIS

The course of disease varies from patient to patient, possibly related to genetic heterogeneity and environmental factors. Prognosis is largely determined by degree of pulmonary involvement. Some patients retain near-normal lung function over 5 to 7 years but, in general, there is an exponential decline in pulmonary function of about 2% to 3% per year. Early colonization with *Pseudomonas* may be associated with a more severe course. Passive exposure to cigarette smoke is associated with a more rapid decline in clinical status and should be avoided. Patients with clinically intact pancreatic function have milder pulmonary disease and better survival. Improved prognosis is related to early diagnosis and institution of a comprehensive treatment program before irreversible pulmonary changes are established. Evidence shows that survival may correlate with intensity of the treatment regimen, particularly with antibiotic usage. Clinical scoring systems are available for longitudinal assessment of patients for prognosis counseling and for classifying patients for clinical studies.

There has been steady improvement in prognosis over the past four decades. In 1950, survival past infancy was unusual. By 1990, the median age at time of death was 28 years (Figure 101–3). About one fourth of all patients under care at specialized CF centers are older than 18 years of age. There is a trend toward poorer early survival but better late survival among black patients. For reasons that are not clear, survival of male patients at every age appears better than that of female patients, but in recent years the gap has narrowed.

(Abridged from Beryl J. Rosenstein, Cystic Fibrosis, in Oski, DeAngelis, Feigin, McMillan, Warshaw: *Principles and Practice of Pediatrics, Second Edition,* J.B. Lippincott, 1994.)

Oski's Essential Pediatrics,
edited by Kevin B. Johnson and Frank A. Oski.
Lippincott–Raven Publishers,
Philadelphia © 1997

102

Idiopathic Diffuse Interstitial Lung Disease in Children

■ DESCRIPTION

The term *interstitial pneumonia* describes a variety of pathologic states characterized by a diffuse inflammatory process that involves the interstitium or supporting structures of the lung as opposed to the alveolar spaces. Interstitial pneumonia is a nonspecific reaction to injury that can be a manifestation of infection, drugs, toxic inhalants, collagen vascular diseases, or a variety of genetic, metabolic, or inflammatory disorders. It may present clinically ranging from an acute fulminant to a chronic indolent form. Interstitial pneumonia is generally subdivided, based on histologic pattern, into four groups: usual interstitial pneumonia (UIP), desquamative interstitial pneumonia (DIP), lymphoid interstitial pneumonia (LIP), and giant-cell interstitial pneumonia (GIP). A rapidly progressive form of interstitial pneumonia with a characteristic histologic picture has variously been called acute interstitial pneumonia, rapidly progressive interstitial pneumonia, and Hamman-Rich syndrome. These diseases are unusual in both adults and children, except in individuals with collagen vascular disease or acquired immunodeficiency syndrome (AIDS).

The most common pattern of interstitial lung disease seen in children is a cellular interstitial pneumonia without the specific histologic features of the better known interstitial pneumonias, which are more common in adults. Most children with chronic interstitial lung disease have a nonspecific picture of more uniform alveolar epithelial cell hyperplasia and patchy interstitial mononuclear cell infiltration without the features of coexistent hyaline membranes and fibrosis seen in UIP, which suggests both chronicity and activity. This pattern has an unpredictable course. Steroid therapy is the usual treatment. Some patients with this disease pattern do well, whereas others progress to pulmonary fibrosis.

■ USUAL INTERSTITIAL PNEUMONIA

Usual interstitial pneumonia, the most common of these conditions in adults, is a patchy interstitial process with variable microscopic features reflecting progressive infiltration and scarring of the lung parenchyma. These features include the coexistence in the same biopsy specimen of both active lesions with hyaline membranes and cellular infiltration and regions of scarring with collagen deposition. This pathologic picture is described under various names, including fibrosing alveolitis and Hamman-Rich syndrome. The latter term is better reserved for the rapidly progressive variant of interstitial pneumonia, which differs clinically from UIP by its rapid fulminant course and differs histologically by the marked fibroplasia without collagen deposition and the relative paucity of inflammatory cells. The histologic picture of Hamman-Rich syndrome does not show the variability of UIP; its lesions are all of the same age and progression. In UIP, the major signs and symptoms include tachypnea, dyspnea, hypoxia, cough, and failure to thrive. Respiratory and cardiac failure, pulmonary hypertension, and spontaneous pneumothorax are the most common reported major complications. Clinical signs in infancy and childhood are similar to those in adults, but the clinical course is often more rapid in childhood, and fatal if untreated. UIP has been seen in children with rheumatoid arthritis, chronic active hepatitis, ulcerative colitis, thyroid disease, and systemic lupus erythematosus. There are a few familial cases, both children and adults, which suggests an autosomal dominant mode of inheritance. Current treatment is high-dose steroid therapy with a starting dosage of about 2 mg/kg/day, continued for a minimum of 4 to 8 weeks and sometimes for as long as 1 to 2 years. Immunosuppressant therapy has been tried on a limited number of children with mixed results. Those patients with onset of disease before 1 year of age have a shorter mean survival than older patients who may survive for 5 to 10 years. The mortality rate, even with good treatment, may be as high as 50%.

■ LYMPHOID INTERSTITIAL PNEUMONIA

Lymphoid interstitial pneumonia was a rare disease in children. With the increase in the number of children with human immunodeficiency virus (HIV) infection, LIP is more prevalent. The incidence of LIP in pediatric AIDS patients is estimated at about 25%. Although LIP was initially grouped with the interstitial pneumonias, it is a manifestation of lymphoproliferative disease involving the lung. LIP is characterized histologically by a prominent interstitial infiltrate of mature lymphocytes with a variable admixture of plasma cells and other lymphoreticular elements; it may be either diffuse or patchy. Many presenting signs and symptoms are similar to those seen in UIP and DIP. LIP is associated with a variety of immunologic disorders including hypergammaglobulinemia or hypogammaglobulinemia, rheumatoid diseases, Sjögren's syndrome, and, more recently, AIDS in the pediatric age group, for which it is an indicator disease. Familial LIP has been reported. The usual treatment is steroids. Cytotoxic drugs are used when response to steroids is poor.

(Abridged from Iley Browning and Claire Langston, Idiopathic Diffuse Interstitial Lung Disease in Children, in Oski, DeAngelis, Feigin, McMillan, Warshaw: *Principles and Practice of Pediatrics, Second Edition*, J.B. Lippincott, 1994.)

Oski's Essential Pediatrics,
edited by Kevin B. Johnson and Frank A. Oski.
Lippincott–Raven Publishers,
Philadelphia © 1997

103

Recurrent or Persistent Lower Respiratory Tract Symptoms

Recurrent cough and wheeze are common symptoms in children. They raise parental and physician concern that an underlying chronic lung disease is present. When confronted with this situation, the physician needs to distinguish between multiple acute unrelated respiratory infections and a significant chronic pulmonary disease. The history and physical examination are extremely important in making this distinction and cannot be overemphasized.

■ DETERMINING DISEASE SEVERITY

Although chronic cough and wheeze commonly are found in children with serious pulmonary problems, they are also manifestations of acute self-limited illness. Therefore, the presence of other signs and symptoms is useful in identifying children with an underlying chronic disorder.

Table 103–1 lists signs and symptoms that suggest chronic pulmonary disease. If acute infection is present, it usually is accompanied by fever, purulent secretions, and an overall toxic appearance of the child. Fever accompanied by grunting often represents a pneumonic process with frequent pleural involvement. Noisy breathing or snoring during sleep is often associated with enlarged adenoids, nasal

TABLE 103-1. History and Physical Findings Suggesting Chronic Lung Disease

HISTORY
Chronic cough
Recurrent wheeze
Decreased activity
Malabsorption symptoms
Fever for longer than 3 weeks
Weight loss
Recurrent pneumonia
Chronic sputum production
Multiple serious bacterial infections

PHYSICAL
Poor growth and nutritional status
Tachypnea
Cyanosis
Deviated trachea
Increased anteroposterior diameter of chest
Wheezing, crackles
Clubbing
Neurologic delay

TABLE 103-2. Differential Diagnosis for Chronic Cough in Children

INFANT
Aspiration
   Congenital malformations
   Tracheoesophageal fistula
   Vascular ring
   Neuromuscular weakness or pharyngeal incoordination
   Gastroesophageal reflux
Infections
   Congenital
      Cytomegalovirus
      Rubella
   Acquired
      Respiratory syncytial virus
      Adenoviruses
      Influenza and parainfluenza virus
Other
   Bordetella pertussis
   Chlamydia trachomatis
   Mycobacterium tuberculosis
Cystic fibrosis
Asthma
Congenital heart disease with congestive failure
Acquired immunodeficiency syndrome (AIDS)
Environmental irritants

PRESCHOOL-AGE CHILD
Aspiration
   Neuromuscular weakness or pharyngeal incoordination
Infection
   Viral
      Adenoviruses
      Influenza and parainfluenza virus
Other
   M tuberculosis
Cystic fibrosis
Foreign-body aspiration
Chronic sinusitis
Asthma
Congenital heart disease with congestive failure
AIDS
Environmental irritants

SCHOOL-AGE ADOLESCENT
Infections
Other
   M tuberculosis
   Histoplasmosis
   Mycotic infections
   Mycoplasma pneumoniae
Cystic fibrosis
Chronic sinusitis
Smoking
Psychogenic cough
Hypersensitivity pneumonitis
Kartagener's syndrome
Sarcoidosis

TABLE 103-3. Differential Diagnosis for Wheezing in Children

INFANT	TODDLER/PRESCHOOL-AGE CHILD	SCHOOL-AGE ADOLESCENT
Congenital malformation	Aspiration (less common)	Infection
Tracheobronchial anomalies	Infection	Viral
Lung cyst	Viral	Adenoviruses
Vascular ring	Adenoviruses	Influenza
Mediastinal lesions	Parainfluenza, influenza viruses	Other
Aspiration	Other	Tuberculosis
Pharyngeal incoordination	Tuberculosis	Histoplasmosis
Gastroesophageal reflux	Histoplasmosis	Mycotic infections
Tracheoesophageal fistula	Mycotic infections	Tumor
Laryngotracheoesophageal cleft	Parasitic	Leukemia
Infections	Visceral larva migrans	Lymphoma
Viral	Tumor	Lymphosarcoma
Respiratory syncytial virus	Leukemia	Asthma
Adenoviruses	Lymphoma	Cystic fibrosis
Parainfluenza, influenza viruses	Foreign-body aspiration	Kartagener's syndrome
Other	Asthma	Hypersensitivity pneumonitis
Tuberculosis	Congenital heart disease with left-to-right shunt	
Histoplasmosis	Cystic fibrosis	
Mycotic infections	Pulmonary hemosiderosis	
Asthma	AIDS	
Congenital heart disease with large left-to-right shunt		
Bronchopulmonary dysplasia		
Cystic fibrosis		
AIDS		

polyposis, choanal narrowing, nasal foreign body, or Pierre Robin syndrome.

The physical examination can help confirm the presence of underlying lung disease, but normal findings in the examination do not exclude the possibility of significant abnormalities. The child's recent health can be assessed by evaluating the overall nutritional status. The physical examination should determine the pattern of respiration, adequacy of gas exchange, and location of disease. Head-bobbing can be seen in a sleeping infant and is a sign of dyspnea. Flaring of the alae nasi, use of accessory muscles of respiration, wheezing, grunting, and retractions are all signs of dyspnea and indicators of respiratory disease in a child.

To establish the location of disease, the head, neck, chest, and extremities should be closely inspected. Allergic shiners under the eyes, nasal mucosal swelling, or a crease across the bridge of the nose are commonly observed in children with allergic disease. An increase in the anteroposterior diameter of the chest is consistent with severe obstructive lung disease. Auscultation of the chest can reveal crackles, wheezes, or suppression of breath sounds. Clubbing of the extremities is an uncommon finding in children and rarely occurs in asthmatic individuals. If present, an extensive evaluation should be undertaken to rule out chronic liver, heart, and gastrointestinal disease. Clubbing can be familial. If a pulmonary disorder is suspected, however, diseases such as bronchiectasis, cystic fibrosis, immotile cilia syndrome, and disorders causing interstitial fibrosis should be sought.

If a serious respiratory disorder is suspected after the history and physical examination, evaluation should proceed based on an age-dependent differential diagnosis.

■ CHRONIC OR RECURRENT COUGH

A chronic cough is defined as a persistent cough lasting for 3 weeks or longer. Table 103–2 lists potential etiologies of cough by age group.

■ DIFFERENTIAL DIAGNOSTIC FEATURES OF WHEEZING BY AGE

A wheeze is a high-pitched musical sound produced by rapid vibration of a large bronchial wall. It indicates airflow obstruction from isolated or multiple sites of airway narrowing. Table 103–3 lists potential etiologies of wheezing by different age groups.

(Abridged from Peter W. Hiatt, Recurrent or Persistent Lower Respiratory Tract Symptoms, in Oski, DeAngelis, Feigin, McMillan, Warshaw: *Principles and Practice of Pediatrics, Second Edition*, J.B. Lippincott, 1994.)

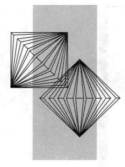

SECTION 7

Cardiovascular Diseases

Oski's Essential Pediatrics,
edited by Kevin B. Johnson and Frank A. Oski.
Lippincott–Raven Publishers,
Philadelphia © 1997

104

Epidemiology of Congenital Heart Disease

Congenital heart disease (CHD) is a leading cause of death during the first year of life. Malformations of the heart occur in about 8:1000 liveborn infants, resulting in up to 36,000 cases per year in the United States. Children with CHD use between 25% and 30% of the beds in most pediatric intensive care units and, therefore, consume a large fraction of pediatric health care resources. Because the majority of severe cases now are being managed successfully by surgery, most of these patients are surviving into their reproductive years. Recent studies have shown that the offspring of women with CHD are at much greater risk of having cardiac malformations. In the next decade, the prevalence of CHD may increase as a result of longer survival and the increase in incidence of heart defects in the offspring of survivors. Pediatric health care providers need to be informed of the incidence of CHD, the familial risk of CHD recurrence, and risk factors for CHD.

■ PREVALENCE AND FAMILIAL RISK OF RECURRENCE OF CONGENITAL HEART DISEASE

The frequency of occurrence of various types of CHD among liveborn infants is shown in Table 104–1.After the diagnosis of CHD has been made, parents want to know the chance of recurrence. In some cases, the affected offspring exhibits manifestations of a recognizable syndrome that has specific known genetic risks. CHD in about 8% of children may be explained on the basis of a primary genetic defect. In the majority of cases, however, a specific genetic defect is not recognized. It has been postulated that genetic predisposition interacting with an environmental trigger causes the cardiovascular malformation. In families having a child with CHD, the genetic predisposition already has been expressed, and subsequent pregnancies are associated with a higher risk of cardiac maldevelopment. The recurrence risk when one offspring has been born with CHD varies with the specific lesion, as shown in Table 104–2 Ranges of risk in the table are listed to indicate differences among studies. When a second case does occur, the infant frequently has a form of CHD that differs from that of the first child. It often is useful to present the information in a positive fashion (*eg,* in a family having a child with an atrial septal defect, the likelihood of the next infant having a normal heart is about 97%).

Over the past decade, more information has become available regarding the risk that a parent with a congenital

TABLE 104-1. Frequency of Specific Defects in Live Births With Congenital Heart Disease

Lesion	Percentage (%)
Ventricular septal defect	30.3
Patent ductus arteriosus (full-term)	8.6
Pulmonary stenosis	7.4
Atrial septal defect (secundum)	6.7
Aortic coarctation	5.7
Aortic stenosis	5.2
Tetralogy of Fallot	5.1
Transposition	4.7
Endocardial cushion defects	3.2
Hypoplastic right heart	2.2
Hypoplastic left heart	1.3
Total anomalous pulmonary veins	1.1
Truncus arteriosus	1.0

TABLE 104-2. Estimated Risk of Congenital Heart Disease (CHD) Recurrence: One Offspring With CHD

Lesion	Recurrence Risk (%)
Ventricular septal defect	3–6
Patent ductus arteriosus	3–8
Atrial septal defect	3
Tetralogy of Fallot	3
Pulmonic stenosis	2–9
Coarctation	2–8
Aortic stenosis	2
Transposition	2
Endocardial cushion defect	2
Endocardial fibroelastosis	4
Tricuspid atresia	1
Hypoplastic left heart	2–10
Truncus arteriosus	1
Ebstein's malformation	1

TABLE 104-3. Estimated Risk of Occurrence in Offspring: Parent With Congenital Heart Disease (CHD)

Lesion	CHD in Father (%)	CHD in Mother (%)
Aortic stenosis	3–8	13–18
Atrial septal defect	1–7	4–14
Atrioventricular canal	1	14
Coarctation	2–8	4–6
Patent ductus arteriosus	2.5	4–9
Pulmonic stenosis	2	6–15
Tetralogy of Fallot	1.5	2.5
Ventricular septal defect	2	6–17

heart defect will have a child with a heart defect (Table 104–3). The risk of recurrence is greater when the heart disease is in the mother. Estimating the risk for mothers with cyanotic CHD is confounded by their higher rates of spontaneous abortion and interrupted pregnancy. Ranges of risk are shown in Table 104–3 because important discrepancies are found among different studies. Because it has not been feasible for any center to follow all patients with CHD through childbearing age, sampling biases may have occurred that result in underestimates or overestimates of risk. In addition, recent studies have reported higher risks of recurrence than those previously reported for families having left-heart obstructive lesions such as coarctation, aortic stenosis, and hypoplastic left-heart syndrome.

(Abridged from David E. Fixler and Norman S. Talner, Epidemiology of Congenital Heart Disease, in Oski, DeAngelis, Feigin, McMillan, Warshaw: *Principles and Practice of Pediatrics, Second Edition*, J.B. Lippincott, 1994.)

Oski's Essential Pediatrics,
edited by Kevin B. Johnson and Frank A. Oski.
Lippincott–Raven Publishers,
Philadelphia © 1997

105

Cyanotic Congenital Heart Disease

■ TRANSPOSITION OF THE GREAT ARTERIES

Transposition of the great arteries, or complete transposition, is a common form of cardiac abnormality found in about 5% of all patients with congenital heart disease. The distinguishing anatomic feature of transposition is the discordant ventriculoarterial connection of the great arteries whereby the aorta originates from the morphologic right ventricle and the pulmonary artery from the morphologic left ventricle. The consequence of this anatomic arrangement is that unoxygenated systemic venous blood returning to the heart passes through the right atrium and right ventricle and

is ejected into the aorta. Similarly, oxygenated pulmonary venous blood reaches the left side of the heart and is returned to the pulmonary artery. The clinical situation that results from this cardiac anomaly is characterized by severe, life-threatening hypoxemia early in life. The presence or absence of associated cardiac abnormalities dictates the presentation, clinical course, and surgical approach to the management of the three main categories of patients with transposition:

1. Transposition with an intact interventricular septum (complete transposition). These patients may or may not have left ventricular outflow tract obstruction (subpulmonary stenosis).

2. Transposition with ventricular septal defect, which is complete transposition and an interventricular communication, but without narrowing in the left ventricular outflow tract.

3. Complex transposition, which is complete transposition, ventricular septal defect, and varying degrees of left ventricular outflow tract obstruction. These patients usually have significant subpulmonic stenosis and equal right and left ventricular pressures. This category includes patients with pulmonary atresia.

■ DIAGNOSIS

Cyanosis, with or without associated heart murmur, is the most common presenting manifestation of transposition of the great arteries. As previously stated, associated lesions temporarily may provide adequate blood mixing, so the infant may be only mildly cyanotic or have significant cyanosis only during exercise (feeding or crying). In patients with transposition and an intact interventricular septum, there is often no murmur; other than cyanosis, the only abnormalities on physical examination may be a loud, single second heart sound and a prominent right ventricular impulse.

The electrocardiogram shows right axis deviation and right ventricular hypertrophy, which is a normal pattern in a newborn. Although the classic "egg-on-a-string" radiographic pattern may be seen in about one third of patients, usually the chest roentgenogram is normal in the first few days of life.

Cross-sectional echocardiography has had a dramatic impact on the noninvasive diagnosis of transposition of the great arteries. With this technique, it is possible to demonstrate reliably the atrioventricular and ventriculoarterial connections, thus enabling the diagnosis of transposition of the great arteries. All of the echocardiographic modalities—cross-sectional, M-mode, and Doppler—are important in demonstrating the associated lesions and physiologic derangements that occur in these patients.

■ MANAGEMENT

Balloon atrial septostomy was the first interventional procedure used in the cardiac catheterization laboratory. It was extremely effective in providing immediate palliation for the patient with transposition of the great arteries. By the early 1970s, successful initial palliation was achieved in more than 85% of patients with transposition. Effective long-term palliation for as long as 2 to 3 years was possible for 65% to 75% of patients who underwent balloon atrial septostomy during infancy. Until development of blade atrial septostomy by Park in 1975, no other nonsurgical option was available for the approximately 25% of patients in whom balloon atrial septostomy was not effective either initially or subsequently during infancy. In an extensive collaborative study reported in 1982, about 80% of these patients who required additional palliation by blade septostomy during infancy and childhood had an adequate result.

Many types of partial and complete atrial redirection operations, including the Senning operation, were suggested but had little success before the description of the atrial baffle repair by Mustard in 1964. Subsequently, this technique was the only procedure used by most centers to repair transposition until the early 1980s when it became popular to use the Senning operation. The goal of both the Mustard and Senning atrial baffle procedures is to redirect the venous inflow to the heart so systemic venous drainage is channeled to the mitral valve, then into the pulmonary circulation, whereas the pulmonary venous drainage is channeled to the tricuspid valve and, eventually, out into the aorta.

Concerns about long-term systemic ventricular function, along with problems of atrial baffle obstruction and electrophysiologic abnormalities that are present with both types of atrial baffle repair, led surgeons to consider arterial switch repair. A variety of procedures for switching aorta and pulmonary arteries, and connecting one or both coronary arteries to the reconnected aorta has been suggested or attempted. All procedures were unsuccessful until the report by Jatene and associates of survival following an arterial switch repair that included transplantation of both coronary arteries into the reconnected aorta. Although this procedure was associated with high mortality during its initial use, the recent mortality is at more acceptable levels and this anatomic repair is now a worldwide standard.

■ LATE RESULTS

Although most patients have good functional results, a number of long-term problems have been identified in patients who have undergone atrial baffle procedures. About 10% to 20% of patients who underwent a Mustard operation developed systemic venous obstruction postoperatively.

Atrial arrhythmias (atrial flutter, supraventricular tachycardia, and sick-sinus syndrome) are important problems in patients who underwent a Mustard operation. The percentage of atrial arrhythmias continues to increase in frequency with increasing length of postoperative follow-up. Modifications of operative technique to avoid injury to the sinoatrial node or its artery have been successful in reducing the incidence of early postoperative rhythm disturbances.

These problems, which are present with both types of atrial baffle repair, led to development of the arterial switch procedure. Because this operation results in an anatomic as well as physiologic correction, it is theorized that this procedure will provide a better functional result over many years. Long-term results of patients who underwent an arterial switch repair for transposition of the great arteries are still unknown. A number of questions may yet be answered by studying survivors of arterial switch procedure. Maintenance of normal coronary artery blood flow is of major importance, and long-term effects related to growth are unknown. Another concern is the site of anastomosis for reconnection of the great arteries. Stenosis at the site of anastomosis of the great arteries (particularly the pulmonary artery) is fairly common, and some patients have required reoperation to correct this problem. Despite the lack of long-term follow-up to decide questions such as the

growth of anastomotic sites and the fate of transplanted coronary arteries, the arterial switch repair is the preferred procedure for surgical management of the patient with transposition of the great arteries.

(Abridged from William H. Neches, Sang C. Park, and Jose A. Ettedgui, Cyanotic Congenital Heart Disease, in Oski, DeAngelis, Feigin, McMillan, Warshaw: *Principles and Practice of Pediatrics, Second Edition*, J.B. Lippincott, 1994.)

Oski's Essential Pediatrics,
edited by Kevin B. Johnson and Frank A. Oski.
Lippincott–Raven Publishers,
Philadelphia © 1997

106
Tricuspid Atresia

Tricuspid atresia, the third most common form of cyanotic congenital heart disease, consists of complete agenesis of the tricuspid valve and absence of direct communication between the right atrium and the right ventricle. The prevalence of tricuspid atresia in clinical series of patients with congenital heart disease ranges from 0.3% to 3.7%. The prevalence rate in autopsy series is 2.9%. Tricuspid atresia occurs in 1:17,857 to 1:10,000 live births.

An opening in the atrial septum allows egress of blood from the right atrium. The interatrial communication can be or can become restrictive. Additional cardiovascular abnormalities occur in 18% of patients with normally related great arteries and in 63% of patients with transposed great arteries. These include coarctation of the aorta, patent ductus arteriosus, and right aortic arch. Extracardiac anomalies occur in 20% of cases.

■ HEMODYNAMICS

In tricuspid atresia, hemodynamics depend on presence or absence of pulmonary atresia, degree of pulmonary stenosis, presence of normally related or transposed great arteries, and presence or absence of subpulmonary or subaortic stenosis. Because all systemic venous return (blood oxygen saturation low) and pulmonary venous return (blood oxygen saturation high) mix in the left atrium, the level of blood oxygen saturation reaching the left ventricle, and subsequently the aorta, depends on the relative volumes of pulmonary venous return and systemic venous return.

■ CLINICAL FINDINGS

History

Because of the presence of cyanosis, congestive heart failure, or growth failure, tricuspid atresia usually is detected in infancy. Cyanosis is the prominent feature in patients whose pulmonary blood flow is limited by pulmonary atresia or pulmonary stenosis. Symptoms of pulmonary edema and congestive heart failure predominate in patients with unobstructed pulmonary blood flow; cyanosis also can be apparent. If pulmonary blood flow depends on the patency of the ductus arteriosus, the degree of cyanosis and arterial hypoxemia may increase dramatically if the ductus arteriosus closes. If pulmonary atresia is present, closure of the ductus can produce profound hypoxemia, acidosis, and death. For patients with unobstructed pulmonary blood flow, as pulmonary vascular resistance decreases and pulmonary blood flow increases, signs and symptoms of congestive heart failure and pulmonary edema can increase.

Without surgical intervention, significant pulmonary vascular obstructive disease occurs in patients with unrestricted pulmonary blood flow. Pulmonary vascular obstructive disease is much less common in patients with tricuspid atresia and normally related great arteries than it is in patients with transposed great arteries. This is because most patients with normally related great arteries have or will have (at about 1 year of age) pulmonary or subpulmonary stenosis.

Bacterial endocarditis and brain abscess are relatively common complications of tricuspid atresia. Neurologic complications also can result from cerebrovascular accidents secondary to polycythemia or to intravascular thrombosis or embolic phenomena.

Physical Examination

Cyanosis is the most common clinical feature of tricuspid atresia. Infants with tricuspid atresia and normally related great arteries may have excessive pulmonary blood flow and little cyanosis, but the degree of cyanosis may increase as the ventricular septal defect becomes progressively restrictive, causing subpulmonary stenosis and decreasing blood flow.

Cardiac murmurs are present in 80% of patients with tricuspid atresia. A low-frequency holosystolic or, at times, a crescendo–decrescendo murmur is produced by the flow of blood through the ventricular septal defect. A systolic mid-frequency crescendo–decrescendo murmur is present in patients with pulmonary stenosis. Patients with pulmonary atresia and a systemic-to-pulmonary collateral blood supply, as well as patients who have had a surgical systemic arterial-to-pulmonary arterial anastomosis, have a continuous murmur. A diastolic mitral murmur may be audible in patients who have excessive pulmonary blood flow.

Electrocardiogram

First-degree atrioventricular block occurs in 15% of cases and presumably is due to prolonged atrial conduction, because atrioventricular node function usually is normal. Because of early origin of the left bundle from the common bundle, the frontal plane QRS axis usually is leftward or superior and the frontal plane electrocardiographic loop is counterclockwise. Rarely, the frontal plane QRS axis is normal, which suggests the presence of transposed great arteries. The right ventricular electrocardiographic forces are diminished, and there is evidence of left ventricular hypertrophy and, frequently, of discordant QRS and T waves.

Chest Radiograph

The heart usually is enlarged. The right heart border may be prominent, reflecting enlargement of the right atrium. The pulmonary vascular markings are increased when the pulmonary blood flow is excessive. In 80% of patients with tricuspid atresia, however, the pulmonary blood flow is diminished and the pulmonary vascular markings are decreased.

Echocardiogram

Basic anatomy, size of the atrial septal defect, size of ventricular septal defect, ventricular function, great artery relationships, and valvular function can be ascertained by using M-mode, two-dimensional, and color flow imaging echocardiography.

Cardiac Catheterization

In infants, the major use of cardiac catheterization is to determine sources and reliability of pulmonary blood flow. Administration of prostaglandin E_1 to maintain ductal patency has improved the safety of cardiac catheterization for babies with decreased or ductal-dependent pulmonary blood flow. Cardiac catheterization may be necessary in infants (2 to 6 months of age) to measure pulmonary artery pressure and resistance as a guide to the need for pulmonary artery banding to prevent development of pulmonary vascular obstructive disease.

■ CLINICAL MANAGEMENT

Three major considerations should guide the management of infants with tricuspid atresia:

1. The need for manipulating the amount of pulmonary blood flow, either to decrease hypoxemia and polycythemia by increasing pulmonary blood flow or to decrease symptoms of congestive heart failure by decreasing pulmonary blood flow

2. The need to preserve myocardial function, pulmonary vascular integrity, and the pulmonary vascular bed to optimize conditions for future Fontan operation

3. The need to reduce risks of associated cardiovascular complications such as bacterial endocarditis and thromboembolism.

Babies with severe hypoxemia and acidosis should be treated promptly with an infusion of prostaglandin E_1 to maintain patency of the ductus arteriosus, thus improving pulmonary perfusion. Cardiac catheterization and angiography establish sources of pulmonary blood flow and help plan for type of surgical systemic-to-pulmonary artery anastomosis.

Infants with transposed great arteries and unrestricted pulmonary blood flow have signs and symptoms of pulmonary edema and congestive heart failure. They benefit from treatment with digitalis and diuretics. Classically, these patients have had a pulmonary artery band surgically placed to decrease pulmonary blood flow. Some investigators suggest, however, that pulmonary artery banding might accelerate ventricular septal defect closure. In tricuspid atresia with transposed great arteries, this would create subaortic obstruction and lead to marked ventricular hypertrophy. Because marked ventricular hypertrophy is an adverse risk for subsequent successful Fontan operation, surgical procedures to reduce pulmonary blood flow and to bypass potential areas of subaortic obstruction have been recommended.

Advantages of these more complicated and riskier palliative procedures have not been established.

In 1971, Fontan and associates described a unique procedure to separate the systemic and pulmonary venous return to eliminate the right-to-left intracardiac shunt and reduce the volume of ventricular overload. They constructed a Glenn anastomosis to direct superior vena caval systemic venous return to the right lung, directed inferior vena caval systemic venous return to the pulmonary artery with a valve-containing conduit connecting the right atrium and the pulmonary artery, inserted a valve into the inferior vena cava, closed the interatrial communication, and obliterated the connection between the pulmonary artery and the ventricle. Since its original description, the procedure has been modified considerably, but the concept of directing systemic venous return directly to the pulmonary artery retains the eponym "modified Fontan procedure."

(Abridged from David J. Driscoll, Tricuspid Atresia, in Oski, DeAngelis, Feigin, McMillan, Warshaw: *Principles and Practice of Pediatrics, Second Edition*, J.B. Lippincott, 1994.)

Oski's Essential Pediatrics,
edited by Kevin B. Johnson and Frank A. Oski.
Lippincott–Raven Publishers,
Philadelphia © 1997

107

Tetralogy of Fallot

■ DEFINITION

Tetralogy of Fallot refers to a spectrum of anatomic abnormalities that have in common a large, unrestrictive ventricular septal defect and right ventricular outflow tract obstruction—two features of the tetralogy. Clinical presentation varies from the asymptomatic acyanotic child with a heart murmur to the severely hypoxic newborn infant. Severity of presentation largely depends on the nature and degree of the outflow obstruction. The anatomic hallmark of tetralogy of Fallot is the anterocephalad deviation of the outlet portion of the interventricular septum. Apart from producing infundibular pulmonary stenosis, this also accounts for the ventricular septal defect and the third feature of the tetralogy—aortic override (Figure 107–1). The fourth feature of the tetralogy, hypertrophy of the right ventricle, is the result of the underlying anatomic and hemodynamic abnormalities. The severity of the infundibular stenosis ranges from mild to severe pulmonary stenosis and to pulmonary atresia. Further obstruction to pulmonary blood flow often occurs at other levels. Pulmonary valve stenosis is common, and stenoses are also often found in the supravalvar region at the bifurcation of the pulmonary artery branches or in the distal pulmonary arteries.

The typical ventricular septal defect in tetralogy of Fallot is large and unrestrictive and is due to malalignment of the outlet portion with the rest of the interventricular septum. Muscular ventricular septal defects, an inlet defect, or a complete atrioventricular septal defect also may be present.

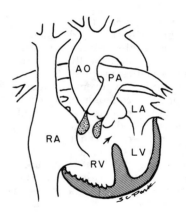

Figure 107-1. Anatomic abnormalities in tetralogy of Fallot. *Ao*, aorta; *LA*, left atrium; *LV*, left ventricle; *PA*, pulmonary artery; *RA*, right atrium; *RV*, right ventricle. Note the ventricular septal defect (*arrow*), the infundibular pulmonary stenosis (*stippled area*), and the overriding aorta.

Other possible associated abnormalities include an atrial septal defect (so-called pentalogy of Fallot) or coronary artery abnormalities. About 25% of patients with tetralogy of Fallot have a right-sided aortic arch, an important consideration if a patient undergoes systemic to pulmonary artery anastomosis.

Tetralogy of Fallot occurs in about 6% of infants born with congenital heart disease. The etiology is obscure. Although tetralogy of Fallot and most other forms of congenital heart disease generally occur as isolated abnormalities, children with tetralogy of Fallot are afflicted with additional major extracardiac malformations significantly more often (15.7%) than are patients with other congenital heart defects (6.8%). In addition, the extracardiac malformations may be more serious in patients with tetralogy of Fallot and include cleft lip and palate, hypospadias, and skeletal malformations. Although tetralogy of Fallot is not commonly part of specific hereditary malformation syndromes or chromosomal abnormalities, it is often found in a number of malformation associations, including cardiofacial, VACTERL, and CHARGE associations as well as DeLange, Goldenhar, and Klippel-Feil syndromes. These syndromes are outlined in the Pediatrician's Companion, later in this book.

■ PHYSIOLOGY AND HEMODYNAMICS

The presenting symptoms and severity of clinical manifestations in patients with tetralogy of Fallot depend on the relation between the resistances to systemic and pulmonary outflow. If the total right ventricular outflow obstruction is such that pulmonary outflow resistance is less than systemic resistance, there is a net left-to-right shunt, and clinical manifestations are similar to those of patients with a small to moderate size ventricular septal defect. If pulmonary and systemic resistances are similar, there is a balanced shunt with nearly equal pulmonary and systemic blood flows at rest. Lastly, when resistance to pulmonary outflow exceeds systemic resistance, there is a net right-to-left shunt, and systemic flow is greater than pulmonary flow.

Cyanosis may be mild or undetectable at rest in patients with tetralogy of Fallot but usually becomes apparent or increases with physical activity. With exercise, increased cardiac output and decreased systemic arteriolar resistance result in a considerable increase in the degree of right-to-left shunting. Although effective cardiac output is maintained, right-to-left shunting produces a rapid decrease in systemic arterial oxygen saturation and results in exertional dyspnea and decreased exercise tolerance. In contrast to episodes of paroxysmal hypoxemia (tetralogy spells), the systemic desaturation is limited by the duration of exercise and improves as soon as activity ceases.

Squatting is a common posture in patients with tetralogy of Fallot, particularly in young children who easily assume the more comfortable knee–chest position. Squatting is often seen in children after exercise. They also are frequently seen to assume this position while playing quiet games with their peers who are sitting. It is likely that squatting results in an increase in systemic arterial resistance due to kinking and compression of the major arterial circulation to the lower extremities. This increase in peripheral resistance, in the presence of relatively fixed pulmonary outflow resistance, decreases the degree of right-to-left shunting and increases pulmonary blood flow. The result is an immediate increase in systemic arterial oxygen saturation.

Episodes of paroxysmal hypoxemia, also called hypercyanotic or tetralogy spells, often are seen in infants and children with tetralogy of Fallot and other cardiac malformations with similar physiology. These spells are usually self-limited and last less than 15 to 30 minutes, although they may be longer. The spells are seen more often in the morning but may occur during the day and may be precipitated by activity, a sudden fright, or injury or may occur spontaneously without any apparent cause. The spell is characterized by increasing cyanosis and an increased rate and depth of respiration. The physiologic change that produces a hypoxemic spell is an increase in right-to-left shunting and concomitant decrease in pulmonary blood flow. The exact mechanism by which this occurs is unknown.

■ DIAGNOSIS

The presentation of patients with tetralogy of Fallot ranges from the small infant with severe hypoxemia to the asymptomatic child with "pink tetralogy." The severity of symptoms is related to the degree of pulmonary stenosis. Cyanosis usually is present in the neonate with severe tetralogy of Fallot or with associated pulmonary atresia. Another relatively common presentation is the asymptomatic infant with a heart murmur. These patients may seem to have only a ventricular septal defect because the murmur of the right ventricular outflow obstruction in the infant with tetralogy of Fallot may be indistinguishable from that of an isolated ventricular septal defect. The presence of significant right ventricular hypertrophy on the electrocardiogram may be a clue to the nature of the underlying abnormality.

Cyanosis and clubbing may be present on physical examination of the child with tetralogy of Fallot. There may be an increased left parasternal impulse, indicating right ventricular hypertrophy. The first heart sound is usually normal, whereas the second sound is single because the pulmonary closure sound is very soft. An ejection systolic murmur is heard at the mid-upper left sternal border and may radiate toward the back. Loudness of the murmur depends on the volume of blood crossing the right ventricular outflow tract. As infundibular stenosis becomes more severe, less blood flows through the right ventricular outflow, and the murmur becomes softer and shorter. In the child having a hypoxemic spell, there is much less antegrade flow into the pulmonary arteries and the murmur disappears.

The chest radiograph in older children with tetralogy of Fallot exhibits the classically described "boot-shaped" heart. This is caused by mild enlargement of the right ventricle and concavity of the upper left heart border caused by absence of the main pulmonary artery segment. In infants, the chest radiograph may be normal or may only show decreased pulmonary vascular markings.

The anatomic features of tetralogy of Fallot are identified by echocardiography. Doppler echocardiography demonstrates an increased velocity of blood flow in the main pulmonary artery and is useful in estimating the gradient across the right ventricular outflow tract.

Cardiac catheterization and angiocardiography are important in the evaluation of the patient with tetralogy of Fallot. In the preoperative patient, it is important to define the levels and severity of stenosis in the right ventricular outflow tract and pulmonary artery and to predict whether the repair is likely to be successful. Associated abnormalities such as multiple ventricular septal defects or coronary artery abnormalities that might adversely affect the success of surgical repair also can be demonstrated. In the postoperative patient with residual defects, cardiac catheterization provides an assessment of the hemodynamic result, ventricular function, severity of residual anatomic abnormalities, and electrophysiologic status.

■ MEDICAL MANAGEMENT

Although many patients with tetralogy of Fallot are acyanotic in early infancy, the subpulmonary stenosis tends to be progressive and usually results in the appearance of cyanosis during infancy or early childhood. Before the development of systemic to pulmonary artery anastomoses in the mid-1940s, about 50% of patients with tetralogy of Fallot died in the first year of life, and it was unusual for a patient to survive past the third decade.

Treatment of significant resting hypoxia or hypercyanotic spells is surgical. Medical management in patients with tetralogy of Fallot, therefore, is directed toward treating associated noncardiac abnormalities, avoiding problems associated with anemia or polycythemia, preventing infectious complications such as bacterial endocarditis or brain abscess, and acutely managing paroxysmal hypoxemic spells. Hypoxemic spells usually are self-limited and last less than 15 to 30 minutes, but can be prolonged. In addition to comforting the patient during one of these episodes, the physician should have the patient assume the knee–chest position. Squatting, or assuming the knee–chest position, may cause increased peripheral resistance in the lower extremities, which, in turn, promotes increased pulmonary blood flow. In a hospital situation, oxygen is administered by face mask during a hypoxemic spell. When combined with the above physical maneuvers, this is often sufficient management for a short spell. If this is not successful and the patient's hypoxemic episode does not appear to resolve, morphine sulfate can be administered either intramuscularly, subcutaneously, or intravenously. The effectiveness of morphine sulfate in treating hypoxemic spells has been known for many years, but its exact mechanism of action is unclear. Because this drug can be administered intramuscularly, it is valuable to use morphine for initial management of a hypoxemic spell when an intravenous route is unavailable. Once an intravenous line is placed, the dose of morphine sulfate can be repeated. Because metabolic acidosis appears quickly after the onset of a hypoxemic spell, sodium bicarbonate can be given empirically as soon as intravenous access is available. If these measures are unsuccessful, a beta-adrenergic blocking agent such as propranolol is valuable in managing a hypoxemic spell. The total calculated dose should be diluted with 10 mL of fluid in a syringe, and no more than half of the calculated dose should be given initially as an intravenous bolus. The remainder can be given slowly over the next 5 to 10 minutes if necessary. Propranolol also has been used in the long-term nonoperative management of paroxysmal hypoxemic spells. It is administered orally in a dose of 1 to 4 mg/kg of body weight per day in four divided doses.

■ SURGICAL MANAGEMENT

Surgical palliation became possible in the 1940s with the development of the Blalock-Taussig shunt, an end-to-side anastomosis between the subclavian artery and the pulmonary artery. Currently, a modified Blalock-Taussig or "H type" shunt is popular. This consists of interposition of a synthetic tube between the subclavian artery and the pulmonary artery, thus preserving blood flow to the arm.

Total correction is preferred, if possible, and consists of patch closure of the ventricular septal defect and relief of the right ventricular outflow tract obstruction. Occasionally, infundibular resection alone relieves the subpulmonary stenosis, but placement of a patch of synthetic material to further widen the right ventricular outflow tract is generally necessary.

■ LATE RESULTS

In most centers, more than 90% of patients who undergo complete repair of tetralogy of Fallot will survive to adulthood and have a good functional long-term result.

Arrhythmias, particularly ventricular ectopy, are of concern in patients who have undergone repair of tetralogy of Fallot. Sudden unexpected death occurs in a small percentage of postoperative patients and may be caused by a ventricular arrhythmia. The combination of ventricular ectopy and hemodynamic abnormalities, especially residual pulmonary stenosis with high right ventricular pressure and right or left ventricular dysfunction, is especially worrisome and is treated in most centers.

After complete repair, patients with tetralogy of Fallot are still at risk of subacute bacterial endocarditis and should receive appropriate antibiotic prophylaxis. Preservation of good right and left ventricular function and the possible effects of coronary artery disease in a heart with a repaired congenital defect are potential long-term problems.

(Abridged from William H. Neches and Jose A. Ettedgui, Tetralogy of Fallot, in Oski, DeAngelis, Feigin, McMillan, Warshaw: *Principles and Practice of Pediatrics, Second Edition*, J.B. Lippincott, 1994.)

Oski's Essential Pediatrics, edited by Kevin B. Johnson and Frank A. Oski. Lippincott–Raven Publishers, Philadelphia © 1997

108

Hypoplastic Left Heart Syndrome

The term *hypoplastic left heart syndrome* describes a spectrum of congenital cardiac anomalies in which there is an underdeveloped left ventricle and ascending aorta. Severe mitral stenosis, mitral hypoplasia, or mitral atresia is seen in 84% of cases; common atrioventricular canal with the atrioventricular valve malaligned to the right with respect to the muscular ventricular septum accounts for the remaining 16%.

■ EPIDEMIOLOGY

The frequency of hypoplastic left heart syndrome is about 0.36 per 1000 live births, and, before surgical palliation was possible, it was responsible for 23% of neonatal deaths due to congenital heart disease. As with other left-sided obstructive lesions, there is a male predominance, with about 60% of cases occurring in males. When hypoplastic left heart syndrome occurs in females, Turner's syndrome should be considered.

■ PHYSIOLOGY

Patients with hypoplastic left heart syndrome have complex preoperative physiology. Because of the hypoplasia of the left ventricle and ascending aorta, the right ventricle must maintain both systemic and pulmonary output. This requires both left-to-right shunting of pulmonary venous return and right-to-left shunting of right ventricular output. If the pulmonary veins return normally to the left atrium, as is the usual case, the left-to-right shunt must occur through either a stretched foramen ovale or a true atrial septal defect. The right-to-left shunt must occur through the ductus arteriosus. The carotid, subclavian, and coronary arteries are perfused retrograde by way of the ductus arteriosus. With the aorta and pulmonary arteries connected in parallel, the percentage of right ventricular stroke volume that goes to the systemic and pulmonary circuits depends on the relative resistances of each of these circuits. Because fetal circulation involves a patent ductus arteriosus with low systemic resistance, high pulmonary resistance, and oxygenation in the placenta, the infant with hypoplastic left heart syndrome develops normally in utero. After birth, lungs are the source of oxygenation. Patency of the ductus arteriosus is required for adequate systemic blood flow. Usually, systemic and pulmonary perfusion remain adequate in the presence of a nonrestrictive ductus. Occasionally, excessive pulmonary blood flow develops when the pulmonary to systemic resistance ratio falls rapidly. In these cases, arterial oxygen saturation increases secondary to the high pulmonary blood flow, but metabolic acidosis ensues because of marginal systemic perfusion. In less than 5% of cases, inadequate pulmonary blood flow and severe cyanosis result from a congenitally small foramen ovale. Metabolic acidosis ensues in these patients because of inadequate oxygen delivery.

■ CLINICAL FEATURES

History

Because systemic perfusion and oxygenation are normal in utero, the infant frequently appears normal at birth and has normal Apgar scores. When hypoplastic left heart syndrome presents with marked cyanosis on the first day of life, severe obstruction to blood flow at the interatrial level (congenitally small or absent foramen ovale) usually is present.

More typically, on day 2 or 3 of life, the patient with hypoplastic left heart syndrome develops cyanosis, tachypnea, and respiratory distress. As the ductus arteriosus closes, systemic perfusion is compromised and acidosis develops. If the ductus arteriosus remains patent, however, the onset of cyanosis and respiratory distress could be delayed for weeks.

Physical Examination

On physical examination, the child with hypoplastic left heart syndrome usually is mildly cyanotic, tachypneic, and tachycardiac. Peripheral pulses are normal to absent depending on the degree of ductal closure at the time of evaluation. Although rales occasionally may be heard, breath sounds are usually normal. The right ventricular impulse is dominant with a diminished left ventricular (apical) impulse. Auscultation usually reveals a normal S1 and a single S2 that is increased in intensity. A nonspecific soft grade I/VI systolic murmur, reflecting relative pulmonic stenosis, is commonly heard at the left sternal border. In rare cases with a dysplastic pulmonary valve, an early systolic ejection click may be heard.

Electrocardiogram

The underlying pathology is reflected in the electrocardiogram. About 30% to 40% of patients have right atrial enlargement and about 80% to 90% have right ventricular hypertrophy with a qR, rSR', or pure R wave pattern in lead V_1. Q waves usually are absent in the lateral precordial leads, and 30% to 40% of patients have diminished left ventricular forces. A leftward superior axis usually is present in patients with malaligned common atrioventricular canal.

Chest Radiograph

Cardiomegaly and increased pulmonary vascular markings typically are seen in the chest x-ray of patients with hypoplastic left heart syndrome. A reticular pattern similar to that seen in obstructed total anomalous pulmonary venous connection may be seen in patients with a severely restrictive atrial septal defect.

Two-Dimensional and Doppler Echocardiography

The diagnosis of hypoplastic left heart syndrome is made by two-dimensional echocardiography (Figure 108–1).

■ THERAPY

Because patients with hypoplastic left heart syndrome are ductal dependent, therapy consists of preoperative stabilization followed by surgical treatment.

Operative Management

Two major surgical approaches exist for this lesion. In one operation, the patient's own cardiovascular tissues are reconstructed to provide for hemodynamics compatible with life until a Fontan procedure can be performed; in the second operation, a cardiac transplantation replaces the hypoplastic

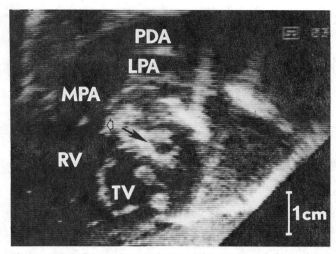

Figure 108-1. Echocardiogram demonstrating a subcostal short axis cut in a child with hypoplastic left heart syndrome. *PDA*, patent ductus arteriosus; *LPA*, left pulmonary artery; *MPA*, main pulmonary artery; *RV*, right ventricle; *TV*, tricuspid valve orifice. The solid black arrow points to the hypoplastic left ventricle and the hollow black arrow points to the pulmonary valve.

heart. The patient's own tissues are used in the reconstructive approach, which eliminates the need for immunosuppression; whereas, a two-ventricular repair is achieved in the transplantation approach. The reconstructive approach typically involves three stages. In the first stage, the main pulmonary artery is transected and the proximal portion is anastomosed to the hypoplastic ascending aorta. This allows the right ventricle to continue functioning as the systemic ventricle. The remainder of the aortic arch is then augmented with pulmonary homograph. The ductus arteriosus is ligated, and a 4-mm polytetrafluoroethylene shunt is placed between the systemic and pulmonary arterial circuits. This shunt provides for pulmonary blood flow. Potential complications of the first stage reconstruction include development of a restrictive atrial septal defect, neoaortic arch obstruction, pulmonary artery hypoplasia or distortion, and ventricular dysfunction. Long-term survival for the first stage of the reconstructive approach is 70%. At 6 to 12 months of age, the patient undergoes a bidirectional cavopulmonary shunt or "hemi-Fontan." In this operation, the superior vena cava is directly anastomosed to the pulmonary artery and excluded from the right atrium. The shunt is removed, and the pulmonary arteries are augmented. This prevents the rapid diminution in end-diastolic volume that can occur with removal of the systemic to pulmonary artery shunt during the Fontan operation. About 6 months after the "hemi-Fontan," the Fontan procedure is completed by channeling the inferior vena cava to the pulmonary arteries. There is a 6% mortality from the "hemi-Fontan" and a 7% mortality from the completion of the Fontan procedure. Some patients, because of deterioration in the function of the right ventricle, are not good candidates for a Fontan operation. These patients can be managed successfully by cardiac transplantation. Cardiac transplantation has been adopted by several centers as the treatment of choice for children with hypoplastic left heart syndrome. Children with hypoplastic left heart syndrome account for 38% of heart transplantations for congenital heart disease. Because the hypoplastic heart is replaced in the transplantation approach, the surgical technique is the same as that for any other cardiac transplantation. Complications of transplantation in this age group include rejection (about 1.5 rejection episodes per patient), infection (about 1 episode per patient), and seizures (about 4% of patients). There is a 13% early and an 8% late mortality for neonatal cardiac transplantation. True long-term results from either the reconstructive approach or cardiac transplantation approach remain to be seen, but, with the 60% to 80% intermediate survival, hypoplastic left heart syndrome should no longer be considered a hopeless condition.

(Abridged from Gerald Barber, Hypoplastic Left Heart Syndrome, in Oski, DeAngelis, Feigin, McMillan, Warshaw: *Principles and Practice of Pediatrics, Second Edition,* J.B. Lippincott, 1994.)

Oski's Essential Pediatrics,
edited by Kevin B. Johnson and Frank A. Oski.
Lippincott–Raven Publishers,
Philadelphia © 1997

109

Defects of the Atrial Septum Including the Atrioventricular Canal

Congenital defects of the atrial septum are common. They may be located in different anatomic portions of the atrial septum, and the location of the defect generally reflects the abnormality of embryogenesis that led to the anomaly (Figure 109–1). An atrial septal defect (ASD) may be isolated or may be associated with other congenital cardiac abnormalities. Sizes of ASDs vary greatly. Functional consequences of defects of the atrial septum, then, are related to the anatomic location of the defect, size of the defect, and presence or absence of other cardiac anomalies.

ISOLATED ATRIAL SEPTAL DEFECTS

■ DEFECTS OF SMALL SIZE

Small ASDs are defined as those with a pulmonary-to-systemic flow ratio (Qp:Qs) of less than 2:1 in the absence of significant associated cardiovascular anomalies. Presence of a small atrial septal defect does not cause major changes in cardiac hemodynamics.

■ DEFECTS OF MODERATE AND LARGE SIZE

Moderate and large ASDs are defined as those associated with a Qp:Qs of greater than 2:1 in the absence of significant associated cardiovascular anomalies. As a result of the ASD, shunting of blood across the atrial septum occurs, but the direction of the atrial shunt is determined by the relative pressures in the right and left atria. Because atrial pressures are principally determined by the resistances to filling of the respective ventricles, the volume of the shunting is most dependent on the relative compliances of the right and left ventricles.

■ NATURAL HISTORY

Isolated secundum ASDs do not cause major symptoms in most cases during infancy and childhood. Exercise intolerance may develop in some patients as early as the second decade of life. Others may remain asymptomatic for several more decades. The two most common complications of unrecognized ASDs are congestive heart failure secondary to increasing left-to-right shunting, and atrial arrhythmias, such as atrial flutter, secondary to stretching of the atria from large shunts.

■ DIAGNOSTIC EXAMINATION: PHYSICAL EXAMINATION

The height and weight of patients with ASDs are often below normal, although usually not substantially so. The presence of a hypoplastic thumb, radius, or phocomelia should cause suspicion that the patient has the Holt-Oram syndrome, an autosomal dominant disorder in which an upper limb deformity is found with congenital heart disease, most often an ASD in association with prolonged atrioventricular (AV) conduction. Cyanosis may be present in infants, particularly in those with right ventricular outflow obstruction of any form.

The arterial pulse is normal at rest in patients with uncomplicated ASDs. However, when a Valsalva's maneuver is employed, patients without cardiac anomalies show a decrease in cardiac output secondary to a decrease in systemic venous return, whereas patients with ASDs and relatively large left-to-right shunts are able to maintain ventricular output due to the large volume of blood pooled in the lungs.

Auscultation

In patients with ASDs, the first heart sound, best heard at the apex and lower left sternal edge, often is split and the second component is increased in intensity. ASDs with moderate to large left-to-right shunts are associated with a pulmonary systolic murmur that begins shortly after the first heart sound, peaks in early systole to midsystole, and ends before the second heart sound. Rapid flow through the peripheral pulmonary arteries may cause systolic crescendo–decrescendo murmurs that are most prominent at locations in the chest other than the second intercostal space.

The characteristic auscultatory finding in ASD is the wide, fixed splitting of the second sound. This finding is present in patients with large left-to-right shunts and normal pulmonary artery pressure.

The diastolic murmur most often associated with ASD is a mid-diastolic murmur resulting from the high flow across the tricuspid valve. This murmur becomes apparent when the left-to-right shunt is greater than 2:1. The murmur is of low to medium frequency and does not increase with inspiration. Another diastolic murmur sometimes associated with ASD is a low-pitched murmur of pulmonic regurgitation, probably a consequence of dilatation of the pulmonary artery.

Electrocardiogram

Sinus rhythm is customary in young patients with uncomplicated secundum ASDs. Prolongation of the PR interval is common and sometimes has a familial association. Beyond the third decade of life, patients with ASD have a

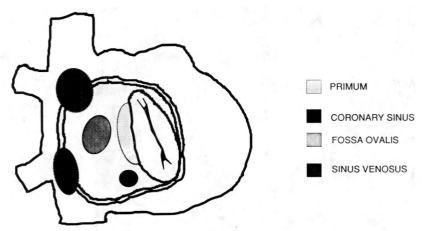

PRIMUM

CORONARY SINUS

FOSSA OVALIS

SINUS VENOSUS

Figure 109-1. Atrial septal defects. Only defects within the fossa ovalis region are true defects of the interatrial septum, although all of the defects permit interatrial shunting.

high frequency of atrial arrhythmias, particularly atrial fibrillation but also including atrial flutter and supraventricular tachycardia.

Chest Radiograph

The chest radiograph in patients with secundum ASD and sizable left-to-right shunts generally shows cardiac enlargement and increased pulmonary vascularity (Figure 109–2). Increased pulmonary vascularity typically extends to the periphery of the lung fields, with a dilated pulmonary trunk and central branches. Right atrial and right ventricular enlargement usually are seen, but left atrial and left ventricular sizes usually are normal.

Echocardiogram

Two-dimensional echocardiography enables direct, noninvasive visualization of all types of ASDs (Figure 109–3). In addition to direct visualization of the ASD, two-dimensional echocardiography also may demonstrate enlargement of the right atrium, right ventricle, and pulmonary arteries, and often shows paradoxical motion of the

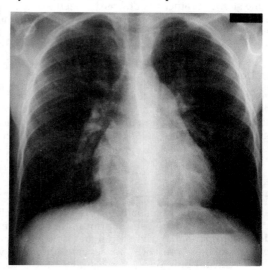

Figure 109-2. Chest x-ray of a patient with a secundum atrial septal defect. Note the cardiomegaly and increased pulmonary vascular markings. The main pulmonary artery is enlarged, and the aortic knob is small.

ventricular septum in a two-dimensional format. In many cases, the pulmonary and systemic venous connections also can be demonstrated.

Continuous wave Doppler echocardiography can be of assistance in the evaluation of patients with ASD. It is particularly useful in evaluating the gradient across the atrial septum in patients with left atrial hypertension and restrictive ASDs and in evaluating patients for obstruction to pulmonary venous return.

Transesophageal echocardiography often is helpful in these patients. Two-dimensional anatomic visualization of the atrial septum from the transesophageal approach generally is excellent.

■ TREATMENT AND PROGNOSIS

Isolated secundum ASDs associated with a large left-to-right shunt and either symptoms or significant cardiomegaly should be electively closed in childhood.

Surgical results in uncomplicated secundum ASD are good. Mortality is less than 2% in many large series. Mortality and morbidity are increased with advanced age or congestive heart failure. After the operation, the left-to-right shunt and its consequent cardiac volume overload are eliminated in nearly all patients. Without closure, patients with moderate and large secundum ASDs generally do well until the third decade of life, after which they tend to become progressively more symptomatic with a substantially higher mortality than that for the general population.

PERSISTENT COMMON ATRIOVENTRICULAR CANAL DEFECTS

AV canal defects include a range of malformations, a central feature of which is usually an ASD of the primum type, and which also involve the ventricular septum and one or both AV valves. A number of terms have been applied to these malformations, including endocardial cushion defect, AV septal defects, and persistent common AV canal.

■ NATURAL HISTORY

The natural history of AV canal defect primarily depends on the pathologic anatomy of the malformation. In

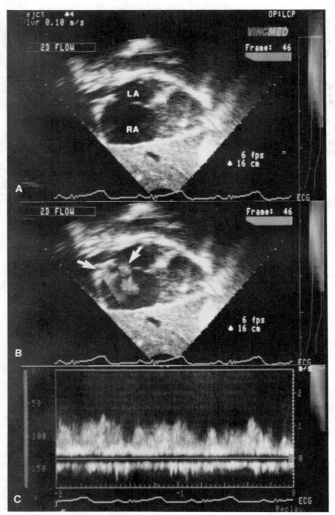

Figure 109-3. Two-dimensional echocardiogram demonstrating a fossa ovalis atrial septal defect. (**A**) Note the opening in the fossa ovalis region of the septum between the left atrium (LA) and the right atrium (RA). (**B**) Color Doppler study demonstrating flow across the atrial septum from left to right through the secundum atrial septal defect. (**C**) Pulsed Doppler study demonstrating low-velocity flow from left to right across the defect.

those patients with only an ostium primum ASD and minimal insufficiency of the left AV valve, the clinical course is similar to that of patients with a large secundum ASD. Generally, these patients do well without treatment during infancy, childhood, and adolescence. During adulthood, they have an increasing tendency to develop congestive heart failure, particularly as atrial arrhythmias develop and with the increasing mitral regurgitation that occurs with time.

Those patients with ostium primum ASDs and moderate-to-severe left AV valve insufficiency develop congestive heart failure in early life with a consequent high morbidity and mortality that relates primarily to the severity of the AV valve insufficiency.

Patients with complete AV canal defects generally develop severe symptoms of congestive heart failure in early infancy. They have frequent respiratory infections and poor weight gain. If they survive infancy untreated, they generally develop pulmonary vascular disease with fixed pulmonary hypertension as an additional major deleterious factor.

■ DIAGNOSTIC EXAMINATION: PHYSICAL EXAMINATION

Patients with partial AV canal defects and minimal mitral insufficiency usually appear normal in infancy and childhood. More severely affected children may manifest growth failure and other signs of chronic congestive heart failure. If there are no signs of chronic congestive heart failure in a patient with known complete common AV canal defect, pulmonary stenosis or pulmonary vascular obstructive disease should be suspected.

The patient with Down's syndrome, which frequently is associated with endocardial cushion defects, has a characteristic physical appearance. When Down's syndrome is seen in conjunction with physical signs of chronic congestive heart failure, the coexistence of complete common AV canal should be suspected. Other types of congenital heart disease also occur in Down's syndrome.

In partial endocardial cushion defect, mitral regurgitation sometimes is associated with a water-hammer pulse that is caused by rapid ejection of a large left ventricular stroke volume. When a large left-to-right shunt is present, a palpable impulse in the second and third left intercostal spaces often is found, reflecting the presence of a dilated, pulsatile, pulmonary artery trunk. Sometimes, the pulmonic component of the second heart sound is palpable. The right ventricular volume and pressure overload associated with complete AV canal defects cause a prominent systolic impulse or heave at the left sternal border and in the subxiphoid area.

Auscultation

Complete AV canal defects may be associated with a variety of auscultatory manifestations, depending on the nature of the underlying pathologic physiology. Because one common AV valve is present, the first heart sound is usually single. The second sound usually manifests a fixed split. A murmur of AV valve incompetence frequently is present. This murmur usually is maximal at the left ventricular apex and often radiates toward the sternum rather than toward the left axilla, reflecting the predominance of left ventricular to right atrial shunting over left ventricular to left atrial shunting.

Electrocardiogram

The most characteristic electrocardiogram abnormality of AV canal defect is a superiorly oriented QRS frontal plane axis with a counterclockwise depolarization pattern. Electrocardiographic manifestations of right ventricular hypertrophy also may be present.

Chest Radiograph

Cardiac enlargement usually is present in the chest radiograph in patients with ostium primum or complete AV canal defects. In particular, right atrial and right ventricular enlargement often are present. With severe pulmonary vascular disease, distal pulmonary vessels may have a lucent, pruned appearance. Severe enlargement of the pulmonary trunk and left atrium may compress the left main stem bronchus and cause atelectasis of parts of the left lung.

Echocardiogram

The two-dimensional echocardiogram is highly reliable in identifying AV canal defects. The hallmark of the diagnosis is the demonstration of an absent AV septum. In ostium primum ASDs, the AV valve leaflets appear to originate from the crest of the ventricular septum. In complete AV canal defects, the bridging leaflets of the common AV valve cross the ventricular septum. Doppler echocardiography also can contribute substantially to the evaluation of AV canal defects.

■ TREATMENT

Medical

When heart failure and associated pulmonary congestion are present, anticongestive measures such as diuretics and digoxin are indicated. Long periods of fluid restriction generally are counterproductive because the patients in distress are usually small infants and such restriction deprives them of calories needed for growth. Most cardiologists do not favor prolonged medical therapy in these patients if their symptoms are refractory, but rather refer them for surgical treatment.

Surgical

Recommendations for surgical treatment depend on the anatomic characteristics of the defect and associated anomalies. Patients with an osium primum ASD, separate AV valves, no ventricular defect, and minimal AV valve insufficiency generally are asymptomatic during infancy and childhood. Because repair of ostium primum ASD is associated with a substantially greater morbidity and mortality than repair of a secundum ASD, many cardiologists do not recommend surgery at any age if cardiomegaly is absent, which usually is the case when AV valve insufficiency is mild and pulmonary-to-systemic flow ratio is less than 2:1. Infants with partial AV canal defects that are symptomatic almost invariably have severe AV valve regurgitation. Pulmonary artery banding generally does not help these patients. Therefore, corrective surgery with mitral valvuloplasty and ASD closure usually is recommended. Asymptomatic patients with ostium primum ASDs that do exhibit substantial cardiomegaly usually are referred for elective surgical repair when they are near school age.

For patients with uncomplicated complete AV canal defects, most centers advocate corrective surgery in early infancy. Palliative procedures such as pulmonary artery banding, however, may be more appropriate in patients who have AV canal defects in association with other anomalies such as hypoplasia of the left ventricle. When pulmonary pressures are near systemic, as they generally are in patients with complete AV canal defects who do not have associated right ventricular outflow obstruction, pulmonary vascular disease usually develops after the first year of life. Therefore, either corrective surgery or a palliative procedure to protect the pulmonary circulation during infancy is recommended in these patients.

■ PROGNOSIS

Long-term results of surgical therapy depend greatly on the degree of preoperative pulmonary vascular disease and on the extent of residual left AV valve regurgitation. In many cases, the left AV valve regurgitation is reduced substantially and the left-to-right shunt is abolished or reduced to minimal levels by corrective surgery. When pulmonary vascular disease is present preoperatively, however, hospital morbidity and mortality are high, and little improvement is seen in the late follow-up period for those patients who survive the operation. Postoperative arrhythmias can occur, including complete heart block, and may increase in frequency as patients grow older. With advancing age, patients may require mitral valve replacement.

(Abridged from G. Wesley Vick III and Jack L. Titus, Defects of the Atrial Septum Including the Atrioventricular Canal, in Oski, DeAngelis, Feigin, McMillan, Warshaw: *Principles and Practice of Pediatrics, Second Edition*, J.B. Lippincott, 1994.)

Oski's Essential Pediatrics, edited by Kevin B. Johnson and Frank A. Oski. Lippincott–Raven Publishers, Philadelphia © 1997

110
Ventricular Septal Defect

Ventricular septal defect (VSD) is the most common cardiac malformation in children. The incidence is estimated at 1.5 to 2.5 per 1000 live births, although this figure varies depending on the method used to identify the defect. VSD accounts for about 20% of patients followed by pediatric cardiologists in the United States.

■ ANATOMY

The ventricular septum is a curvilinear, spiraling structure that separates the left ventricle from the right ventricle and, to a small extent, from the right atrium. The ventricular septum consists of a membranous and a muscular portion, and is subdivided into inflow, trabecular, and outflow regions. Defects in the septum may occur in each region. They range in size from "pinhole" defects of 1 mm or less to virtual absence of the septum.

The location of a defect within the ventricular septum is not of great hemodynamic consequence, but is a critical surgical consideration and an important determinant of natural history. The majority of defects are bounded by both a portion of the membranous septum and a portion of muscular septum. The margin of a perimembranous defect, then, is partially membrane and partially muscle. Less common are true muscular defects, which are bounded entirely by muscle. These tend to be multiple and are more difficult to repair. They also have a greater frequency of spontaneous closure.

■ CLINICAL MANIFESTATIONS

Small VSDs seldom cause significant symptoms and usually come to the attention of a physician because of the associated heart murmur. Although the murmur is not present in the immediate newborn period, it may be audible as early as the second day of life and usually is heard at the routine 2-week checkup. It is characteristically a high-pitched, harsh, holosystolic murmur, well localized along the left sternal border. A small VSD may produce a murmur of lower pitch, but a high-pitched murmur strongly suggests that the defect is not large. The precordium is quiet, but a localized thrill may be palpable. The first and second heart sounds are normal, and there is seldom a diastolic murmur. Except finding mild tachypnea in small infants, other physical findings are normal. Small defects, sometimes called maladie de Roger, do not interfere with normal growth. A significant number, estimated from 30% to 70%, undergo spontaneous closure, usually in the first 2 years of life. Small defects that do not close rarely require treatment. Their chief importance lies in their distinction from other anomalies (in young infants, this includes distinction from larger defects) and the risk for developing bacterial endocarditis. Certain types of defects, regardless of size, may predispose to development of secondary conditions, especially secondary aortic regurgitation and left ventricular outflow tract obstruction. For this reason, children older than 2 years of age with physical findings of a small VSD should have an echocardiographic examination to confirm the diagnosis and localize the defect.

Large defects may come to the attention of a physician later than small defects because elevated pulmonary vascular resistance may delay the appearance of a murmur. When present, symptoms are those of congestive heart failure. They include irritability, increased respiratory effort, poor feeding, and poor weight gain. Recurrent respiratory infections are common, and pneumonia is often the preliminary diagnosis.

Signs of congestive heart failure include tachycardia, tachypnea, increased work of breathing, pallor, diaphoresis, and failure to thrive. Pulmonary rales are a late finding. The precordium is hyperactive, and a thrill is often palpable. The second heart sound is single or narrowly split. When audible, it is usually accentuated, but often it is obscured by a loud, low-pitched, harsh, holosystolic murmur. The murmur is loudest along the left sternal border, but is much less well localized than is the murmur of a small VSD. It may radiate to the right of the sternum, but radiates poorly to the back. A diastolic murmur or rumble heard at the lower left sternal border is related to increased mitral flow. Its presence implies a pulmonary-to-systemic flow ratio exceeding 2:1. Pulses may be diminished with severe congestive heart failure but are symmetric in the absence of aortic coarctation. The liver and sometimes the spleen are enlarged.

Moderately sized defects may produce physical findings suggestive of small defects, although rarely a murmur of high pitch. There is usually some degree of tachypnea and increased respiratory effort. Because of increased volume load of the left ventricle, the precordial impulse is hyperactive and there is often a thrill. When associated with low pulmonary vascular resistance and high pulmonary blood flow, a moderate-sized defect may produce findings similar to a large defect, including those of congestive heart failure.

Large defects with high resistance, and, thus, little increase in pulmonary blood flow, may cause no symptoms or growth failure in the small child. Although the precordial impulse is hyperactive and the pulmonic closure sound is accentuated, an absent or subtle murmur may allow this effect to pass undetected. Older children with more advanced pulmonary vascular occlusive disease (PVOD) have resting cyanosis, exercise intolerance, and nailbed clubbing. A murmur of VSD flow usually is not heard, but a systolic murmur of tricuspid regurgitation or a diastolic murmur of pulmonic regurgitation may be present.

■ NONINVASIVE AND INVASIVE STUDIES

Radiographic findings generally reflect the size of the left-to-right shunt. Small defects may produce mild cardiac enlargement on a plain chest roentgenogram, but usually the chest radiograph is normal. Moderately sized defects are associated with cardiomegaly, usually of a predominant left ventricular type. The left atrium may be enlarged on the lateral projection. Pulmonary blood flow is increased. Large defects produce a more diffuse cardiomegaly, increased pulmonary vascular markings, and often signs of pulmonary edema. In patients with large VSD and PVOD, only mild cardiomegaly is shown on the chest roentgenogram. The main pulmonary artery segment usually is prominent, and central vascular markings are normal or diminished.

Electrocardiographic changes with small VSD are minimal. Moderately sized defects usually produce some degree of left ventricular hypertrophy. Large defects commonly produce combined ventricular hypertrophy on electrocardiogram. Large defects with PVOD may show more right ventricular hypertrophy than left.

Echocardiography and Doppler echocardiography are the primary modality for anatomic and physiologic assessment of VSD. Real-time two-dimensional echocardiographic imaging in the standard views discloses the presence, location, and size of nearly all defects (Figure 110–1) as well as the presence of associated lesions. Color flow Doppler investigation increases the sensitivity of standard imaging, particularly for small or multiple defects. Pulsed and continuous wave Doppler studies facilitate assessment of right ventricular pressure and pressure gradients between ventricles. Systemic and pulmonary blood flows can be estimated indirectly by measuring semilunar valve diameter and recording flow velocity.

■ MANAGEMENT

Infants and children with small VSD seldom require treatment. Young infants should be evaluated periodically in the first 6 months of life, when pulmonary vascular resistance is expected to decline. Physical examination and noninvasive studies should be used to ascertain the expected minimal increase in pulmonary blood flow and absence of pulmonary hypertension. Many small defects close spontaneously. Older children with persistent defects should be evaluated periodically, both to screen for acquired lesions (aortic regurgitation, subaortic membrane, right ventricular muscle bundle) and to reemphasize the need for endocarditis prophylaxis.

Infants with moderate-sized and large defects generally have symptoms caused by increased pulmonary blood flow. Most infants with congestive heart failure due to isolated VSD can be treated successfully with conservative therapy. This usually begins with diuretic therapy. Digoxin is a conventional component of therapy for these children.

Afterload-reduction therapy—hydralazine, captopril, or enalapril—may help patients whose response to diuretic therapy and digoxin is limited. A decrease in systemic vascular resistance can favorably affect relative systemic-to-pulmonary blood flow ratio, especially in patients with low pulmonary vascular resistance.

Even with aggressive medical treatment, infants with excessive pulmonary blood flow may gain weight poorly. Goals of medical therapy are relief of symptoms and adequate growth. When these cannot be achieved, early surgical repair should be considered. Children with normal pulmonary artery pressure and persistent significant left-to-

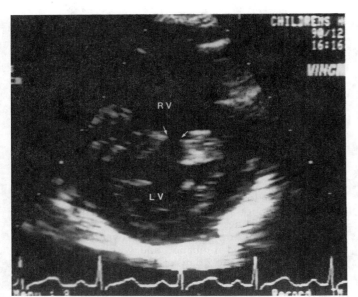

Figure 110-1. Short-axis two-dimensional echocardiographic view of a large muscular VSD. Arrows point to margins of the defect. *RV*, right ventricle; *LV*, left ventricle.

right shunt (pulmonary-to-systemic flow ratio greater than 2:1) may undergo elective repair in late infancy or in childhood. Surgery generally is not advocated if pulmonary-to-systemic flow ratio is less than 2:1.

(Abridged from Carl H. Gumbiner, Ventricular Septal Defect, in Oski, DeAngelis, Feigin, McMillan, Warshaw: *Principles and Practice of Pediatrics, Second Edition,* J.B. Lippincott, 1994.)

Oski's Essential Pediatrics,
edited by Kevin B. Johnson and Frank A. Oski.
Lippincott–Raven Publishers,
Philadelphia © 199

111

Patent Ductus Arteriosus

■ DESCRIPTION

The patent ductus arteriosus is a normally occurring essential structure in the fetus and becomes abnormal only when it persists after birth. In the term infant, the persistent ductus probably represents a structural abnormality in the ductus tissues present at birth. Persistent patent ductus arteriosus is the second most common congenital heart defect, accounting for about 10% of all congenital heart defects in full-term infants.

All factors resulting in persistent patency of the ductus are not understood. Factors such as high altitude or severe pulmonary disease that cause persistent hypoxia predispose to persistent patency of the ductus. Continued high

prostaglandin levels, in the presence of a compromised or inefficient pulmonary clearing function (found in premature infants or in marked decrease pulmonary flow occurring in some pulmonary atresia patients), contribute to the persistent patency of the ductus. Rubella (and possibly other viral infections) during the first trimester of pregnancy frequently results in patency of the ductus. Some evidence shows that a lower socioeconomic status, probably resulting in inadequate perinatal nutrition, may predispose to persistent patency of the ductus.

When the ductus remains open and, with normal lungs, pulmonary resistance drops, blood flows from the aorta through the ductus into the pulmonary arteries. Eventual flow to the lungs from the ductus depends on size and shape of the ductus and on how close to normal levels the pulmonary vascular resistance drops. With normal pulmonary resistance, the flow through the ductus begins during midsystole to late systole and continues through diastole. This flow pattern corresponds to the timing of the maximal pressure gradient between the aorta and the pulmonary artery during the various phases of the cardiac cycle.

The uncomplicated patent ductus places a pure volume workload on the left heart with little or no effect on the right heart. The blood from the aorta flows through the ductus into the pulmonary arteries, through the pulmonary vascular bed into the left atrium, into the left ventricle, and back into the aorta. The total additional workload on the left ventricle depends directly on the size of the persistent ductus arteriosus and the resultant flow through the ductus. The additional blood from the ductus mixes with the blood ejected from the right ventricle into the pulmonary artery; however, in the absence of increased pulmonary resistance, the extra blood does not add significantly to the work of the right ventricle. As a result, in the absence of increased pulmonary resistance, there is little or no additional volume or pressure work placed on the right ventricle and no physical or clinical laboratory signs suggesting right-sided involvement.

■ CLINICAL FINDINGS AND DIAGNOSIS

Clinical histories of patients with persistent patent ductus range from florid heart failure in the young infant to incidental murmur in an otherwise perfectly healthy child or, occasionally, adult. The patient with a patent ductus may present as early as the newborn period and anytime thereafter, including late adulthood. The most common presentation of the patient with a persistent patent ductus is a heart murmur discovered incidentally in an asymptomatic young child being examined for some other reason. The infant or child with a moderate-to-large patent ductus may be prone to, or more susceptible to, secondary involvement in the lower respiratory tract or even infections after initial upper respiratory infection. This probably is due to the decreased compliance of the lungs associated with significantly increased pulmonary blood flow.

The murmur and associated clinical finding of a patent ductus usually are characteristic and often pathognomonic of the defect. The typical murmur of a patent ductus is continuous (sounding like machinery) and is maximum in the first and second left intercostal spaces in the left midclavicular line. Peripheral pulses are bounding in quality as a result of both the increased left ventricular stroke volume and the diastolic runoff into the lungs.

The electrocardiogram in the uncomplicated ductus is normal or, in the larger ductus, shows left ventricular hypertrophy and left atrial enlargement. The chest radiograph shows cardiomegaly proportionate to the flow through the ductus with a prominent main pulmonary artery segment, large ascending aorta and arch, increased pulmonary vascular markings, and a "left ventricular" contour to the heart shadow, with possible left atrial enlargement.

The diagnosis can be supported further by the echocardiogram. The ductus usually can be seen on two-dimensional echocardiogram. Turbulent flow by Doppler interrogation in the main pulmonary artery support the echocardiogram. Even the very tiny ductus that is too small to be audible or visualized by echocardiogram can be detected by continuous wave Doppler, or the flow can be seen using color Doppler.

When all clinical findings of the ductus are assimilated and are absolutely characteristic, the diagnosis is established without further study. If there is even one atypical feature in any part of the clinical assessment, then the diagnosis should be established by cardiac catheterization.

■ THERAPY

Therapy for patent ductus can be supportive or definitive. Supportive therapy is treatment of symptoms resulting from the patent ductus. Patients with a large persistent ductus have signs and symptoms of pulmonary overcirculation with shortness of breath, dyspnea, even overt pulmonary edema. Symptoms can be treated with digoxin and vigorous diuretic therapy. Occasionally, the young infant with a large patent ductus needs intubation and ventilation with end-expiratory positive pressure to control pulmonary overcirculation. These medical measures help control symptoms but do not treat the underlying anatomic defect.

Definitive therapy for the ductus is complete interruption of blood flow through the ductus. Heretofore, the established definitive therapy for the persistent ductus was surgical ligation and division of the ductus. Definitive therapy is indicated when supportive therapy does not allow normal growth, development, and activity of the infant or child. When no supportive therapy is necessary or when supportive therapy is required and satisfactorily maintains the patient, then elective surgical repair is considered for the patient anytime after 2 to 3 years of age, but usually before the child enters school. The only urgency for repair of the asymptomatic ductus is the anxiety of the child's physician, which often is relayed to the parents.

Surgical repair of the ductus requires a thoracotomy; however, it does not require cardiopulmonary bypass and is a "minor" cardiac surgical procedure. Nevertheless, it is a surgical procedure with the inherent discomfort and morbidity of a surgical procedure. The thoracic surgical patient requires general anesthesia, intubation, and a thoracotomy. There is a 1- to 2-day stay in the recovery ward with a period of continued intubation and with a chest tube in place, followed by 5 to 7 days of hospitalized recovery. The patient has a further 4- to 8-week convalescence before returning to full normal physical activity. In addition to the acute risks of surgery and recovery, there are rare but possible permanent complications. These include vocal cord or diaphragmatic paralysis from intrathoracic nerve injury or even ligation of the wrong vessel or structure within the chest. In addition to the morbidity of the surgery, there is a small, finite mortality associated with surgical repair of the patent ductus.

(Abridged from Charles E. Mullins, Patent Ductus Arteriosus, in Oski, DeAngelis, Feigin, McMillan, Warshaw: *Principles and Practice of Pediatrics, Second Edition,* J.B. Lippincott, 1994.)

Oski's Essential Pediatrics,
edited by Kevin B. Johnson and Frank A. Oski.
Lippincott–Raven Publishers,
Philadelphia © 199

112

Pulmonary Stenosis

Obstruction of pulmonary blood flow may occur within the right ventricle, at the valve, or anywhere in the pulmonary arterial system. In general terms, pulmonary stenosis occurs in about 20% to 30% of all patients with congenital heart disease. In about half of these cases, the ventricular septum is intact.

■ PULMONARY VALVE STENOSIS

Pulmonary valve stenosis constitutes about 7% to 12% of all congenital heart disease and up to 80% to 90% of all lesions causing obstruction of right ventricular output.

Clinically, pulmonary valve stenosis with intact ventricular septum is described best as either mild, moderate, or severe. Mild stenosis is defined here as a systolic transvalvular gradient of less than 40 mm Hg or right ventricular pressure of less than half of left ventricular pressure.

Moderate obstruction is considered present when the systolic gradient across the pulmonary valve is greater than 40 mm Hg or right ventricular pressure of greater than half of, but less than, the left ventricular pressure. Severe stenosis is classified as a systolic gradient of more than 80 mm Hg or the presence of suprasystemic right ventricular pressure.

Patients with mild stenosis are asymptomatic with normal growth and development and no cyanosis. The jugular venous pulse is normal, and there is no sign of congestive heart failure. Children with moderate stenosis and intact ventricular septum may develop mild dyspnea with exertion but are frequently asymptomatic. Cyanosis with exertion may be noted occasionally if an atrial septal defect is present. Individuals with severe valvular stenosis usually demonstrate symptoms, although as many as 25% of these patients are asymptomatic. Frequently, dyspnea and fatigue with only a moderate amount of exertion are present. Central cyanosis is one of the most important signs in patients with an atrial communication; it may be present at rest or with minimal exercise. Some evidence shows the degree of cyanosis increases with age.

A high-pitched ejection sound or systolic click usually is audible along the left upper sternal border. The click probably originates from the sudden opening and doming of the thickened pulmonary valve leaflets. As the severity of obstruction increases, the systolic ejection click occurs earlier, until, in severe stenosis, it may be indistinguishable from the first heart sound. The second heart sound usually is

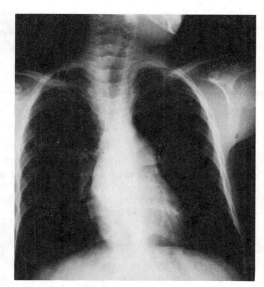

Figure 112-1. Chest roentgenogram from an 8-year-old boy with mild stenosis of the pulmonary valve. Heart size is usually normal. Pulmonary vascular markings are unremarkable. The most distinctive radiographic feature of this disease is poststenotic dilation of the pulmonary turnk, as depicted in this chest film. The degree of dilatation is unrelated to the severity of stenosis.

split and of normal intensity in mild stenosis. The degree of splitting is directly proportional to the severity of obstruction. There also appears to be an inverse relationship between the severity of stenosis and the intensity of the pulmonary component of the second heart sound. In severe stenosis, therefore, there is wide splitting of the second heart sound, with a very soft pulmonary component that is often heard as a single second sound.

The most consistent and distinctive radiographic feature is prominence in the main pulmonary artery segment secondary to poststenotic dilatation of the pulmonary trunk and the proximal left pulmonary artery (Figure 112–1). This finding is present in as many as 90% of patients but does not cor-

relate with the severity of obstruction. In severe stenosis, the cardiac apex may be tilted upward with generalized cardiomegaly and right atrial prominence, especially if right-sided failure is present. The aortic arch is usually left-sided. Presence of a right arch should lead the physician to consider the diagnosis of tetralogy of Fallot.

The noninvasive evaluation of abnormalities of the pulmonary valve by M-mode and two-dimensional echocardiography has been less than satisfactory. With recent advances of Doppler echocardiography and color flow mapping techniques, however, both the sensitivity and specificity of diagnosis of pulmonary valve stenosis have improved.

The natural history of mild pulmonary valve stenosis is benign. There is little improvement in severe obstruction, however, and often the transvalvular gradient increases with age. There is a definite risk of right-sided congestive heart failure, myocardial fibrosis, and sudden death in these patients. The clinical course of and prognosis for moderate pulmonary valve stenosis is under debate, but recent exercise studies demonstrating right ventricular dysfunction in adults are alarming. The risk of infective endocarditis in patients with pulmonary valve stenosis is low, but all individuals, regardless of the severity of stenosis or whether intervention has taken place, should receive selected antibiotics for infective endocarditis prophylaxis during dental or surgical procedures.

Medical treatment of children with pulmonary valve stenosis usually is confined to neonates with critical obstruction. They present with cyanosis, right-sided congestive failure, and cardiomegaly. Because adequate pulmonary blood flow in these neonates depends on patency of the ductus arteriosus, prostaglandin E$_1$ intravenous infusion is life-saving. Anticongestive medications (*eg*, digoxin, furosemide, dopamine) also may be necessary. The treatment of choice in these neonates, as well as in children with moderate to severe stenosis, however, is balloon pulmonary valvuloplasty performed in the cardiac catheterization laboratory.

Since its initial description in 1982, balloon-dilation valvuloplasty for pulmonary valve stenosis has evolved into a fairly standard treatment performed by the pediatric cardiologist with special training. After hemodynamics and angiograms are obtained, a proper-sized balloon is chosen

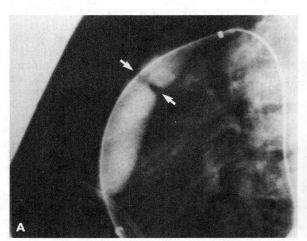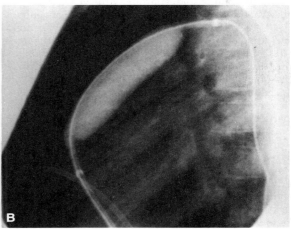

Figure 112-2. Proper postioning of the balloon catheter for pulmonary valvuloplasty using the lateral view under fluoroscopy. (**A**) A guidewire passes through the catheter from the right ventricular outflow tract into the left pulmonary artery. The balloon is inflated with diluted contrast (20%) until a "waist" is seen that corresponds to the stenotic valve leaflets (*arrows*). Attempts to maintain the waist at the midportion of the balloon should be made while the catheter is positioned. In this case, the waist is toward the distal third of the balloon. (**B**) The balloon is repositioned more distally and is completely inflated, using a hand-held manometer. Note that the hourglass waist has disappeared.

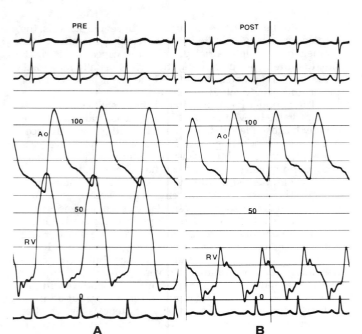

Figure 112-3. Pressure recordings obtained at cardiac catheterization before and after balloon valvuloplasty for moderate pulmonary valve stenosis. (**A**) The right ventricular (RV) systolic pressure is somewhat greater than 70 mm Hg before balloon valvuloplasty. Note the triangular appearance of the RV pressure curve indicative of significant stenosis. (**B**) The RV systolic pressure decreases to 30 mm Hg with a completely normal pressure curve. Aortic (Ao) pressure remained unchanged during the procedure.

(1.3 times the size of the angio-measured annulus or equal to the echo-measured annulus). After positioning the balloon catheter over a guidewire through the stenotic pulmonary valve, the balloon is inflated to 4 to 6 atmospheres of pressure using a hand-held gauge (Figure 112–2). Occasionally, two balloon catheters are required in large children and adults with a pulmonary valve annulus larger than 20 mm in diameter. Immediate relief of the transvalvular gradient is seen frequently (Figure 112–3). Balloon valvuloplasty produces relief of obstruction by commissural splitting of the valve. According to the Valvuloplasty and Angioplasty of Congenital Anomalies (VACA) Registry, the risk of a major complication is 0.6%, including death (0.2%), cardiac perforation with tamponade (0.1%), and severe tricuspid insufficiency (0.2%). Minor complications occur in 1.3% of patients, whereas 2.6% experience an incident defined as arrhythmia, hypoxemia, or venous bleeding. The incidence of complications and incidents is inversely related to age. It is substantially higher in infants, particularly in neonates.

Although surgical pulmonary valvotomy is a relatively low-risk procedure (3% to 4% mortality rate), it is seldom necessary because balloon-dilation valvuloplasty is available. When surgery is required, inflow occlusion with transarterial valvotomy or "open" valvotomy using cardiopulmonary bypass is the method usually employed. The incidence of pulmonary insufficiency after surgery varies from 57% to 90%, whereas an incidence of 13% to 20% has been reported after balloon valvuloplasty.

(Abridged from John P. Cheatham, Pulmonary Stenosis, in Oski, DeAngelis, Feigin, McMillan, Warshaw: *Principles and Practice of Pediatrics, Second Edition,* J.B. Lippincott, 1994.)

Oski's Essential Pediatrics,
edited by Kevin B. Johnson and Frank A. Oski.
Lippincott–Raven Publishers,
Philadelphia © 1997

113

Coarctation of the Aorta

Coarctation of the aorta is a congenital malformation characterized by a constriction of a segment of the aorta. Usually, an abrupt narrowing of the lumen of the vessel occurs in the thoracic descending aorta, producing obstruction to blood flow (Figure 113–1).

■ OCCURRENCE

Coarctation of the aorta is a common congenital defect occurring in frequency just after ventricular septal defect and patent ductus arteriosus in most series. It has a striking male-to-female preponderance in excess of 2:1. Patients with the full XO Turner's syndrome with ovarian agenesis and short stature have a high incidence of coarctation in 20% of cases. A more extreme anomaly with complete interruption of the aortic arch in a slightly different location just proximal to the origin of the left subclavian artery has a high association with DiGeorge's anomaly and is functionally analogous to severe coarctation with a reverse ductus arteriosus.

■ CLINICAL FEATURES

Coarctation Beyond Infancy

Coarctation of the aorta beyond infancy is recognized clinically when blood pressure recordings are obtained from all four extremities; its hallmark is hypertension in the upper extremities and decreased blood pressure in the lower extremities. It is the discrepancy in blood pressure rather than an absolute level of proximal blood pressure elevation that is most striking; however, evaluation of any patient with hypertension should exclude coarctation as a cause. Most individuals with isolated coarctation have no cardiac symptoms, although minor complaints of cold feet, leg cramps, and nose bleeds are volunteered often. Unilateral headaches, particularly of unusual severity, rarely point to an associated cerebral aneurysm, but may be worrisome enough to prompt a full neurologic evaluation. On physical examination, there is striking inequality in the strength of pulses from vessels arising proximal to the obstruction compared to those distal to the obstruction. Simultaneous palpation of brachial and femoral pulses is recommended; in the presence of well-developed collateral vessels, femoral pulses can be felt easily despite coarctation, and it is the discrepancy in timing and pulse volume that should be sought. Auscultation should be performed systematically in an attempt to explain the auscultatory findings rather than with a prejudice that a particular murmur is always found with coarctation. A systolic murmur generated from the coarctation site may be heard best in the left infraclavicular area, in the axilla, or over the left posterior chest. The murmur may seem to originate after the first heart sound, accentuates in later systole, and extends into diastole. The murmur reflects an apparent lag between cardiac systole and flow through the coarctation site as well as the persistence of a coarctation gradient in early diastole.

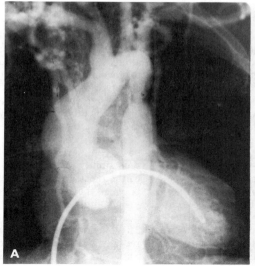
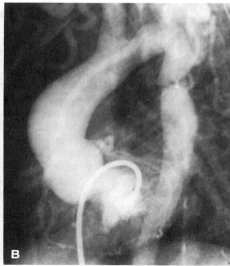

Figure 113-1. (**A**) AP and (**B**) lateral frames from left ventricular angiogram. Discrete coarctation is seen in the descending thoracic aorta. Well-developed collateral vessels are evident.

True continuous murmurs may be generated by collateral vessels. Presence of an aortic ejection click and an ejection murmur in the aortic area may raise suspicion of an additional bicuspid aortic valve, which is found with high frequency in as many as 85% of patients with aortic coarctation. A thrill at the right upper sternal border or suprasternal notch may accompany significant aortic stenosis but can also be found with coarctation alone due to rapid ejection into the dilated proximal aorta.

Despite significant aortic coarctation, the electrocardiogram may be normal in older children. When changes occur, they are manifested chiefly by voltage criteria for left ventricular hypertrophy. The rare patient with severe coarctation and left ventricular dysfunction additionally may have ST-T wave changes indicative of ischemia.

The typical radiologic examination of an older child reveals normal heart size, with less common findings of mild enlargement and left ventricular contour. There may be dilatation of the ascending aorta. In some patients, radiographic evidence of the prestenotic and poststenotic dilatation resulting from coarctation appears along the left paramediastinal shadow and is referred to as the 3 sign. Reversed 3 sign, or E sign, refers to the mirror-image prestenotic and poststenotic dilatation impinging on a barium-filled esophagus. Rib notching, if present, is pathognomonic of coarctation of the aorta but is related to age, because erosion of the inferior portion of the ribs caused by dilated intercostal collateral vessels is a slow process, rarely seen before a patient reaches school age (Figure 113–2). The principal values of echocardiography are that associated defects can be assessed, left ventricular function and hypertrophy can be quantitated, and, if visualization of the coarctation site is possible, a more confident recommendation can be made to the surgeon that a typical coarctation is present. Pulsed Doppler echocardiography does reveal patterns of flow thought to be additionally confirmatory of coarctation of the aorta.

Magnetic resonance imaging has a newer application in prospective identification and follow-up of patients with coarctation of the aorta, and testing of this method's contribution is ongoing.

Coarctation in Infancy

Coarctation syndrome in infancy is characterized by a high association with other defects that results in systemic

right ventricle, reversed flow from right to left through the ductus arteriosus, and more severe hypoplasia of a greater portion of the aortic arch, although discrete coarctation may be present. Infants with coarctation can appear to be well at birth, but cardiac failure, respiratory distress, and cardiogenic shock may appear rapidly as the ductus constricts. Because of the severe impairment of cardiac output, a murmur may not be detected until the infant is stabilized and treated. The pulse discrepancy may not be apparent in the infant because the widely patent ductus serves as a route for flow to the descending aorta, so coarctation is not excluded even if normal pulses are felt on a routine newborn examination. There is potential for differential cyanosis, with shunting of the blood with a lower saturation to the lower body from the pulmonary artery by way of the ductus; however, the high frequency of associated defects, particularly left-to-right shunts, may allow pulmonary saturations to be only slightly lower than aortic saturations, masking this difference clinically. Marked benefit can be obtained by dilating the ductus arteriosus with prostaglandin infusion, thus enabling improved renal perfusion and reversal of acidosis and cardiogenic shock.

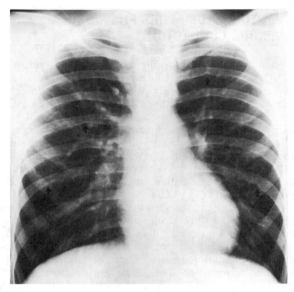

Figure 113-2. Posteroanterior chest film with rib notching and "3 sign" identified in a 7-year-old child.

■ TREATMENT

Surgical

Coarctation of the aorta has been considered a congenital defect amenable to surgical repair since the mid-1940s. The expected result is complete relief of the obstruction so flow to the distal aorta remains unobstructed. Best results are obtained by elective resection and end-to-end anastomosis in a school-age child, with the single operation providing immediate and long-term relief of hypertension without the need for reoperation. Because of the high rate of restenosis when resection and end-to-end procedures were used in infants, with a reoperation rate of up to 60%, a repair using a flap of the subclavian artery was popularized. This vascular flap enables bridging of a long-segment hypoplasia, with the presumption that growth will be permitted. Patch angioplasty and interposition grafts are techniques that can be used when more complex anatomy dictates the need. Complications of surgery include injury to the recurrent laryngeal nerve with resulting hoarseness, diaphragmatic injury from phrenic nerve trauma, bleeding from high-pressure suture lines, chylothorax, and, rarely, spinal cord injury, which is less likely when a well-developed collateral circulation is present.

■ NATURAL HISTORY AND FOLLOW-UP

The former natural history of coarctation of the aorta with an estimated 75% rate of mortality by midadult years has been altered by surgical treatment. Endocarditis with the potential for mycotic aneurysm formation is a lifelong threat, and endocarditis prophylaxis should be observed by all patients both preoperatively and postoperatively. The reversibility of hypertension is thought to be favored by repair in early childhood, avoiding longstanding preoperative hypertension as well as permitting complete relief of obstruction. Considerations based on normal growth of the aorta and concern about reversibility of preoperative hypertension have led pediatric cardiologists to recommend elective repair of aortic coarctation between the ages of 3 years and 9 years.

A high incidence of congenital berry aneurysms is described, estimated at up to 10% of patients with coarctation. The likelihood of intracranial hemorrhage is thought to be reduced by successful coarctation repair. Follow-up of patients with coarctation for restenosis, recurrent or residual hypertension, endocarditis, and surveillance of aneurysm formation at sites of repaired coarctation continue to be appropriate.

(Abridged from Mary J.H. Morriss and Dan G.McNamara, Coarctation of the Aorta, in Oski, DeAngelis, Feigin, McMillan, Warshaw: *Principles and Practice of Pediatrics, Second Edition*, J.B. Lippincott, 1994.)

Oski's Essential Pediatrics, edited by Kevin B. Johnson and Frank A. Oski. Lippincott–Raven Publishers, Philadelphia © 1997

114

Anomalous Pulmonary Venous Connections

■ PARTIAL ANOMALOUS PULMONARY VENOUS CONNECTION

Partial anomalous pulmonary venous connection (PAPVC) occurs when one or more, but not all, pulmonary veins connect anomalously to the right atrium, either directly or through a systemic venous tributary. PAPVC, which often is found in association with an atrial septal defect, demonstrates hemodynamic findings of an acyanotic cardiac lesion with increased pulmonary blood flow similar to that observed in an atrial septal defect (ASD) alone.

When all pulmonary veins connect anomalously to the systemic venous circulation, total anomalous pulmonary venous connection (TAPVC) is defined. TAPVC is associated with total mixing of pulmonary and systemic venous blood at the level of the right atrium and, as such, is defined as a cyanotic form of cardiac disease that may demonstrate increased or decreased pulmonary blood flow. Increased pulmonary blood flow is usual. Decreased pulmonary blood flow may occur when there is severe obstruction in the anomalous pulmonary venous channel. In addition, TAPVC always is associated with an interatrial communication, usually a patent foramen ovale.

■ TOTAL ANOMALOUS PULMONARY VENOUS CONNECTION

Total anomalous pulmonary venous connection (TAPVC) affects 2% to 5% of all patients with congenital heart disease. In all cases, systemic blood flow is maintained by way of right-to-left shunting through an interatrial communication, usually a patent foramen ovale. The male-to-female ratio is equal in most types of TAPVC, except there is a strong male predominance (3:1) in infants with TAPVC of the infradiaphragmatic type. In the group of patients with this abnormality, about one third have other significant major cardiac malformations, including single ventricle, atrioventricular canal defect, hypoplastic left heart, patent ductus arteriosus, and transposition of the great vessels. Many patients in this group have been found to have abnormalities of atrial and visceral situs associated with the heterotaxy syndromes (asplenia and polysplenia). Most cases of TAPVC are sporadic and are not associated with syndromes or chromosomal abnormalities.

Anatomy

TAPVC can be classified according to the site of insertion of the anomalous channel. The four types and their frequency of occurrence are type I, supracardiac connection (55%); type 2, cardiac connection (30%); type 3, infracardiac (infradiaphragmatic) connection (13%); and type 4, mixed connection (2%; Figure 114–1).

Obstruction of pulmonary venous return may occur at many sites along the anomalous venous pathway. Obstruction occurs less often in supracardiac and cardiac TAPVC but is almost universal in connection of the infracardiac type because pulmonary venous blood returning through the portal venous system must traverse the hepatic sinusoids.

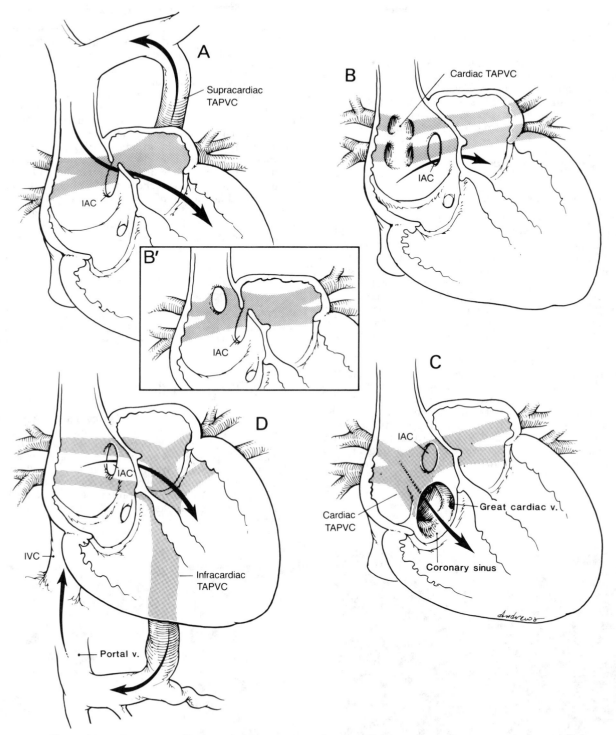

Figure 114-1. Types of total anomalous pulmonary venous connection. (**A**) Supracardiac connection to left innominate vein. (**B**) Cardiac connection via four separate veins. (**B**) Cardiac connection via single common orifice. (**C**) Cardiac connection to coronary sinus. (**D**) Infracardiac (subdiaphragmatic) connection to portal system. *IAC*, interatrial communication. (Adapted with permission from Reardon, et al. Total anomalous pulmonary venous return: report of 201 patients treated surgically. Texas Heart Institute Journal, 1985.)

Hemodynamics

The primary physiologic derangement in patients with TAPVC is a pretricuspid left-to-right shunt with mixing of both pulmonary venous and systemic venous blood in the right atrium, resulting in cyanosis of a variable degree. Factors that determine blood flow distribution in the systemic and pulmonary venous circuits, thus the predominant clinical symptoms, include the presence and severity of obstruction in the extracardiac pulmonary venous channels and the relative size of the interatrial communication.

When obstruction occurs in the pulmonary venous channels, pulmonary venous pressures become elevated, leading to pulmonary edema, reflex pulmonary vasoconstriction, and pulmonary hypertension. Pulmonary blood flow diminishes due to right-to-left shunting through the foramen ovale and ductus arteriosus. Progressive systemic hypoxemia leads to metabolic acidosis, multisystem organ failure, and death within a few days if the obstruction is not relieved.

■ CLINICAL FEATURES

TAPVC With Obstruction

Infants born with obstruction in the anomalous pulmonary venous channels develop symptoms shortly after birth and demonstrate severe cyanosis and respiratory distress. Physical examination reveals a prominent right ventricular impulse, accentuation of the second heart sound, and, at times, a gallop rhythm over the left lower sternal border. Murmurs are infrequent. Hepatomegaly usually is present and often is dramatic in anomalous pulmonary venous connection to the portal venous system. The electrocardiogram may demonstrate right ventricular hypertrophy and a paucity of left ventricular forces.

The chest radiograph at times is diagnostic in TAPVC with obstruction. The cardiac size usually is normal. Pulmonary vascular markings are striking, characterized by a diffuse, linear reticular pattern radiating from the hilar regions (Figure 114–2). Overt pulmonary edema with Kerley B lines may be present. Hyperinflation of the lungs may be seen, which should differentiate this cardiac anomaly from early hyaline membrane disease. Increased pulmonary vascularity helps distinguish this entity from persistent fetal circulation syndrome.

TAPVC With a Restrictive Interatrial Communication

Infants born with a restrictive interatrial communication are usually asymptomatic at birth and during the first few weeks of life; then, they develop respiratory distress, feeding difficulties, and poor weight gain. Physical examination reveals tachypnea with perioral duskiness, a hyperdynamic precordium, and hepatomegaly. Auscultation demonstrates a pulmonary systolic murmur, fixed splitting of the second heart sound, and, often, a diastolic murmur over the left lower sternal border. Occasionally, a continuous venous hum may be detected in an area overlying the anomalous venous connection. The electrocardiogram demonstrates right axis deviation, right atrial enlargement, and right ventricular hypertrophy. The chest roentgenogram reveals cardiomegaly, dilatation of the pulmonary artery, and increased pulmonary vascularity. Distinctive radiographic features may be observed, reflecting the course of the anomalous pulmonary venous channel (Figure 114–3).

TAPVC With a Nonrestrictive Interatrial Communication

Infants with a large ASD or who have undergone an atrial septostomy may have minimal symptoms in the first year of life. These patients often can be operated on electively after 1 year of age, with a low mortality rate.

■ DIAGNOSTIC STUDIES

Echocardiography and cardiac catheterization are the diagnostic procedures of choice in patients with TAPVC. Although surgery may be performed based on two-dimensional and Doppler echocardiography alone, catheterization and selective angiography are often required to delineate the anatomy in patients with complex cardiac defects or in mixed-type TAPVC. In addition, atrial septostomy can be performed during catheterization if surgery is to be delayed until the patient is older.

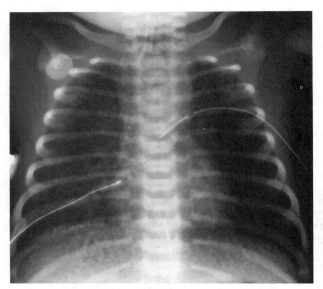

Figure 114-2. TAPVC with obstruction. Heart size is normal and lungs are hyperinflated. Pulmonary vascularity demonstrates a diffuse, linear reticular pattern radiating from the hilum, representing a pulmonary venous engorgement.

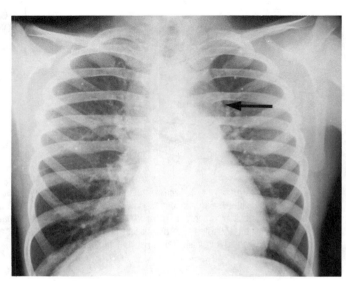

Figure 114-3. Supracardiac TAPVC. Chest radiograph in a child with connection to the left innominate vein demonstrating figure-of-eight or "snowman" appearance. Arrow points to anomalous vertical vein. (Courtesy of Teresa Stacy, MD.)

■ TREATMENT

In infants with TAPVC who present with marked cyanosis, respiratory distress, and cardiovascular collapse in the first few days of life, severe obstruction in the extracardiac pulmonary venous channels must be assumed. Surgery must be undertaken immediately after diagnostic studies are performed. Prostaglandin E₁ has been used before surgery to dilate the ductus venosus to enhance pulmonary venous return to the portal venous system in patients with TAPVC. Operative mortality rates can be as high as 36% in these patients.

Infants without obstruction are treated somewhat differently. Some cardiac centers prefer to operate soon after the diagnosis is established, whereas others elect to use medical therapy after an adequate atrial septostomy to delay surgery until the second year of life. The two approaches are equally successful, resulting in operative mortality rates of less than 10%. The surgical technique involves anastomosis of the pulmonary venous confluence to the left atrium with ligation of the anomalous channel.

The long-term outlook after surgery is excellent, although a few patients may require reoperation for obstruction due to inadequate growth of the pulmonary venous confluence–left atrial anastomosis.

(Abridged from Kent E. Ward, Anomalous Pulmonary Venous Connections, in Oski, DeAngelis, Feigin, McMillan, Warshaw: *Principles and Practice of Pediatrics, Second Edition*, J.B. Lippincott, 1994.)

Oski's Essential Pediatrics,
edited by Kevin B. Johnson and Frank A. Oski.
Lippincott–Raven Publishers,
Philadelphia © 1997

115

Mitral Valve Prolapse

Mitral valve prolapse is the most common cardiac diagnosis of childhood, with prevalence estimates of 0.5% to 35%. The overall prevalence in the general population is 4% to 8%. Since Barlow's first report on midsystolic clicks with late systolic murmur in 1963, several reports have documented the syndrome in children.

■ DIAGNOSIS

The diagnosis of mitral valve prolapse may be made by auscultatory, echocardiographic, angiocardiographic, and pathologic criteria. Criteria vary according to the examiner and method used. Mitral valve prolapse is divided into normal mitral valve prolapse and pathologic mitral valve prolapse. Normal mitral valve prolapse may have superior systolic motion into the left atrium, which may produce a click. Pathologic mitral valve prolapse has an abnormal valve function and failure of leaflet edge apposition, causing mitral regurgitation.

Specific clinical criteria have been proposed for the diagnosis of mitral valve prolapse. The midsystolic click and the late systolic murmur are diagnostic auscultatory criteria of pathologic mitral valve prolapse. Two-dimensional echocardiogram showing marked superior systolic displacement of the mitral leaflets with failure of leaflet edge apposition, or mild to moderate superior systolic displacement of the mitral leaflets with chordal rupture, Doppler mitral regurgitation, and annular dilatation are echocardiographic diagnostic criteria. The diagnosis may not be made based on symptoms, physical appearance, electrocardiographic abnormalities, chest radiograph abnormalities, or nonspecific echocardiographic abnormalities.

■ ASSOCIATED CONDITIONS

Mitral valve prolapse may be seen in as many as 40% of patients with an isolated secundum atrial septal defect. This high incidence does not persist after surgical repair of the secundum atrial septal defect. This association probably is based on left ventricular size and geometry, which is changed with correction of the atrial septal defect. Mitral valve prolapse may be a primary condition or secondary to several disorders.

■ CLINICAL FEATURES

Most children with mitral valve prolapse are asymptomatic and initially are referred for cardiac evaluation because of a click or a murmur detected during a routine examination. A number of studies report a high incidence of symptoms with mitral valve prolapse, but these are due to selection bias. Small subgroups of patients may be highly symptomatic.

Symptoms may include chest pain, easy fatigability, weakness, palpitations, dyspnea, dizziness, syncope, anxiety, and orthostatic hypotension.

Abnormalities on physical examination include thoracic and skeletal abnormalities such as a tall slender habitus, pectus excavatum, pectus carinatum, scoliosis, or kyphosis. A high arched palate, increased joint laxity, or abnormal dermatoglyphics patterns may be present.

Mitral valve prolapse is characterized by a midsystolic click or a late systolic murmur. The click and murmur vary depending on the patient's position and may vary in auscultatory findings at different times in different patients. The change in the click and murmur is due to alterations in left ventricular geometry. Maneuvers such as moving from a sitting to a supine position, from a standing to a squatting position, passive leg raising, and maximal isometric exercise increase left ventricle volume and decrease the degree of mitral valve prolapse and mitral regurgitation. The click and murmur move toward the second heart sound, and the murmur is shorter.

Administration of amyl nitrate, Valsalva's maneuver, sudden change from a supine to a sitting position, from a sitting to a standing position, from a squatting to a standing position and inspiration, decrease left ventricular size and left ventricular volume. Mitral valve prolapse and mitral valve regurgitation increase, thus the click and murmur move toward the first heart sound, and the murmur becomes longer. Because of the changing intensity or timing with different body positions, auscultation should be carried out with the patient in many positions.

The high-pitched, low-intensity, nonejection midsystolic click is heard best at the apex of the heart. It may occur from just after the first heart sound to just before the second heart sound. Multiple clicks may be present in certain patients. The crescendo, late systolic murmur of mitral valve prolapse, is usually preceded by a click and is best heard at the apex. Occasionally, the murmur is described as having a honking or whooping quality and may be heard without a stethoscope.

The chest radiograph and electrocardiogram are usually normal, unless associated cardiac defects are present. If routine chest roentgenogram shows thoracic spine and chest wall abnormalities, then a deliberate search for mitral valve prolapse is indicated.

The apical four-chamber view in two-dimensional echocardiography is sensitive but not specific for the diagnosis of mitral valve prolapse. Many patients who have a normal auscultatory examination may have mitral valve prolapse as documented by the apical four-chamber view. The mitral valve annulus is not flat but has a saddle shape. The four-chamber view may show superior displacement of the mitral valve leaflets, but this may not be true mitral valve prolapse. The long axis view seems to be the most specific view to determine presence or absence of mitral valve prolapse.

■ COMPLICATIONS

The prognosis of mitral valve prolapse in children is excellent. Complications such as endocarditis, significant arrhythmias, sudden death, progressive mitral regurgitation, and cerebral ischemia occur infrequently. Other complications of mitral valve prolapse are chest pain, infective endocarditis, thromboembolism, arrhythmias, and mitral regurgitation.

■ MANAGEMENT

Evaluation of a patient for presence of mitral valve prolapse is first done by a thorough physical examination that includes maneuvers to elicit the click and murmur, a two-dimensional echocardiogram, and a Doppler study.

A resting electrocardiogram is recommended in all patients to look for evidence of ST-T wave changes, a long QT interval, or an arrhythmia. If coexisting cardiac defects are not present, a chest roentgenogram is not needed in patients with isolated mitral valve prolapse. A 24-hour Holter monitor or exercise treadmill is indicated in patients with palpitations, lightheadedness, dizziness, syncope, arrhythmias on resting electrocardiogram, family history of sudden death, complaints of chest pain, and a long QT interval on resting electrocardiogram. Angiography may be indicated if other cardiac defects coexist.

An asymptomatic patient with an isolated midsystolic click, no evidence of mitral regurgitation, or dysplastic mitral valve should be reassured of the benign nature of mitral valve prolapse and followed up every few years.

Indications for mitral valve replacement are severe mitral regurgitation, severe life-threatening arrhythmias, and uncontrollable chest pain, all unresponsive to medical management.

Prophylactic treatment of patients for cerebral ischemia is not indicated. Patients with mitral valve prolapse who have transient ischemic attacks should receive prophylaxis with antithrombotic and antiplatelet therapy.

Patients with mitral valve prolapse should not participate in competitive athletics if there is a history of syncope or near syncope, a history of disabling chest pain, complex ventricular arrhythmias, significant mitral regurgitation or left ventricular enlargement or dysfunction, prolongation of the QT interval, Marfan's syndrome, or a family history of sudden death. Patients who are asymptomatic and found to have isolated uniform premature ventricular contractions (PVCs) may participate in competitive athletics if there is no history of exercise-induced syncope or increase in ectopic beats with exercise.

(Abridged from Victoria E. Judd, Mitral Valve Prolapse, in Oski, DeAngelis, Feigin, McMillan, Warshaw: *Principles and Practice of Pediatrics, Second Edition*, J.B. Lippincott, 1994.)

Oski's Essential Pediatrics,
edited by Kevin B. Johnson and Frank A. Oski.
Lippincott–Raven Publishers,
Philadelphia © 1997

116
Myocarditis

The term *myocarditis* refers to inflammation of the muscular walls of the heart. Myocarditis may be secondary to many of the common infectious illnesses that affect children and infants (Table 116–1) or may occur as a manifestation of hypersensitivity or as a toxic reaction to drug administration. Myocarditis is a relatively uncommon finding in children. Not all cases of myocarditis are recognized by the clinician, however, and a much higher incidence is noted in autopsy series.

In a significant number of cases of myocarditis, manifestations may be subclinical and recognized either through other findings (*eg,* electrocardiogram changes) or, perhaps, not at all. Myocarditis also may be only one component of a generalized disease and, if the cardiac dysfunction is mild, may be completely overlooked. This could explain the discrepancy between the clinical and the autopsy series.

■ EPIDEMIOLOGY

Myocarditis generally is a sporadic disease, although epidemics have been reported. Coxsackievirus B is the most frequently reported cause of epidemics in children. Although much less common, coxsackievirus A and echoviruses, herpes simplex viruses, and prenatally acquired rubella virus are also suspected etiologies.

■ CLINICAL PRESENTATION

The clinical presentation of myocarditis varies in response to host factors, including age and immunocompetence. Although the majority of cases probably are unnoticed with no apparent clinical illness, a rapidly fatal illness may occur. Newborn infants are susceptible to infection with coxsackievirus B, which may result in the severe form of myocarditis. Infections with rubella, herpes simplex, and toxoplasmosis also may result in a severe form of illness in infants.

Myocarditis may be merely one component of a more severe generalized illness, with coexisting hepatitis or encephalitis. Myocardial involvement may be only a mild clinical disturbance in these cases. In a review of 25 infants with myocarditis due to coxsackievirus B, symptoms of lethargy and anorexia heralded the onset of severe disease. Fever was recorded in more than 50% of the cases, although hypothermia was also noted. Cyanosis, respiratory distress or tachycardia, cardiomegaly, or electrocardiogram changes were present in 19 of 23 infants; vomiting was noted in 4. Initial symptoms in infants include irritability and periodic episodes of pallor, which may precede sudden onset of cardiorespiratory symptoms.

Clinical manifestations of myocarditis generally are less severe in older infants and children than in newborns. Rapidly fatal illness has been reported in association with myocarditis of unknown etiology, enteroviruses, adenoviruses, mumps, varicella, cytomegalovirus, and diphtheria. The usual clinical picture is either an acute or a subacute

TABLE 116-1. Etiologic Agents of Myocarditis

VIRAL	BACTERIAL	FUNGI AND YEASTS	HYPERSENSITIVITY/ AUTOIMMUNE
Coxsackievirus A	Meningococcus	Actinomycosis	Rheumatoid arthritis
Coxsackievirus B	*Klebsiella*	Coccidiomycosis	Rheumatic fever
Echoviruses	*Leptospira*	Histoplasmosis	Ulcerative colitis
Rubella virus	Diphtheria	*Candida*	Systemic lupus erythematosus
Measles virus	*Salmonella*		
Adenoviruses	Clostridia	**TOXIC**	**OTHER**
Polio viruses	Tuberculosis	Scorpion (diphtheria)	Sarcoidosis
Baccinia virus	*Brucella*		Scleroderma
Mumps virus	*Legionella pneumophilia*	**DRUGS**	Idiopathic
Herpes-simplex virus	*Streptococcus*	Sulfonamides	Cornstarch
Epstein-Barr virus		Phenylbutazone	
Cytomegalovirus	**PROTOZOAL**	Cyclophosphamide	
Rhinoviruses	*Trypanosoma cruzi*	Neomercazole	
Hepatitis viruses	Toxoplasmosis	Acetazolamide	
Arboviruses	Amebiasis	Amphotericin B	
Influenza viruses		Indomethacin	
Varicella virus	**OTHER PARASITES**	Tetracycline	
	Toxocara canis	Isoniazid	
RICKETSII	Shistosomiasis	Methyldopa	
Rickettsia ricketsii	Heterophyiasis	Phenytoin	
Rickettsia tsutsugamushi	Cysticercosis	Penicillin	
	Echinococcus		
	Visceral larva migrans		

illness, often beginning with a mild respiratory infection and low-grade fever.

Physical examination usually shows the child to be anxious and apprehensive, although some children appear apathetic and listless. Pallor and mild cyanosis may be present, with the skin cool to the touch and mottled in appearance. Respirations usually are rapid and sometimes labored; grunting may be prominent. The pulse is thready, although blood pressure may be normal or slightly reduced unless the patient is in shock. Palpation of the chest demonstrates a quiet precordium. Tachycardia usually is present. Heart sounds may be muffled, especially in the presence of pericarditis, and a gallop rhythm is heard frequently. With severe ventricular dysfunction, mitral regurgitation with a pansystolic murmur at the apex may be heard. Auscultation of the lungs reveals scattered rhonchi and fine crepitations in the lung bases. Peripheral edema is rare, but hepatomegaly is found almost uniformly. Some infants may have only mild congestive heart failure without evidence of peripheral circulatory compromise, whereas others have such a mild illness that the only abnormal finding may be a conduction disturbance visible on surface electrocardiogram.

■ DIAGNOSIS

The diagnosis of myocarditis often is difficult to establish but should be suspected in any infant or child who presents with unexplained congestive heart failure. Fever is a common occurrence in children, and the frequency of viral illness may be so high as to invalidate the causal relationship in the history of recent illness in the child who presents with congestive heart failure. If this relationship is found, however, it should be documented for epidemiologic purposes.

A sinus tachycardia out of proportion to the level of fever and in association with a quiet precordium and a gallop rhythm should strongly suggest the diagnosis. A third heart sound, which is a common finding in healthy children, usually is associated with a relatively hyperdynamic precordium with heart sounds that are increased or crisp. When a prominent third heart sound exists without these findings, a significant disturbance in ventricular compliance usually is present and deserves further investigation by chest radiograph, electrocardiogram, and echocardiogram. Children with myocarditis and congestive heart failure usually show cardiomegaly and pulmonary edema on chest radiograph.

When an arrhythmia occurs after a febrile illness, the clinician should suspect the diagnosis and look for other signs of disease. One study found significant arrhythmias in five infants with isolated myocarditis. Four of the five infants died, and three of them had paroxysmal atrial tachycardia. Paroxysmal atrial tachycardia also has been reported in patients with viral myocarditis.

The electrocardiographic pattern classically described in myocarditis is that of low-voltage QRS complexes (less than 5 mm of total amplitude in all limb leads), with low-amplitude or slightly inverted T waves and a small or absent Q wave in leads V_5 and V_6. The low voltage also may be present in the precordial leads.

The echocardiogram is essential in establishing the diagnosis. Pericardial effusion, as a cause of cardiomegaly, can be determined using either single-crystal or two-dimensional techniques. Depressed ventricular function with dilatation of one or more chambers in the absence of any structural abnormality helps establish the diagnosis.

Nuclear imaging has been used recently as a screening test to help establish the diagnosis of myocarditis. Screening of patients with dilated cardiomyopathy using gallium 67 may help in selecting a subgroup of patients who could benefit from endomyocardial biopsy. This technique has not been used in children but may prove to be a relatively safe and effective method of helping select children for biopsy testing.

Endomyocardial biopsy helps to establish the diagnosis of myocarditis and possibly to classify the phase of disease (acute, healed, chronic).

Laboratory Tests

Although rarely successful, an attempt should be made to identify the offending organism for each child with the suspected diagnosis of myocarditis. Early in the course of illness, it is possible to isolate the virus from the stool, throat washings, or, rarely, blood. Active infection is diagnosed when a fourfold increase is found in antibody titer to the isolated virus.

Even when a diagnosis of myocarditis is likely, blood cultures should be obtained in any infant with fever and signs of compromised cardiovascular function. A complete blood count should be ordered; a leukemoid reaction may be noted. The erythrocyte sedimentation rate usually is elevated during acute myocarditis, although a normal value does not exclude the diagnosis. Elevated levels of serum glutamic-oxaloacetic and glutamic-pyruvic transaminase can occur as the result of a generalized viral infection, although they may also be seen during episodes of diphtheritic myocarditis. Creatine phosphokinase and lactate dehydrogenase enzymes should also be measured. One study found elevation of isozyme 1 of lactate dehydrogenase was a specific finding in patients with idiopathic myocarditis.

■ DIFFERENTIAL DIAGNOSIS

Any cause of acute circulatory failure may mimic the presentation of acute myocarditis. Hypoxia, hypoglycemia, and hypocalcemia in newborns may be seen with heart failure. Circulatory collapse with shock frequently occurs in cases of overwhelming sepsis in this age group. Anomalous left coronary artery arising from the pulmonary artery should be investigated by echocardiography and angiography. Type II glycogen storage disease (Pompe's disease), medial necrosis of the coronary arteries, and left atrial myxoma are among the many diseases that can present a clinical picture similar to that of myocarditis.

Pericarditis, which may be secondary to viral illness, usually occurs in children rather than infants. The clinical history may be similar to that in patients with myocarditis. Cardiovascular function, however, is usually less severely compromised for the degree of apparent cardiomegaly because of the amount of pericardial effusion. Cardiac tamponade may occur in severe cases and present with circulatory collapse. When pericarditis and myocarditis coexist, "perimyocarditis" results, and a clinical picture consistent with both diseases may be found. Perimyocarditis may be seen with rheumatic fever, collagen vascular disease, other autoimmune diseases, and coxsackievirus B disease. Myocarditis also has been described with rheumatoid arthritis, systemic lupus erythematosus, and ulcerative colitis.

■ TREATMENT

Although no specific therapy aimed at reversing myocardial injury is recommended widely, maintenance of cardiac output at levels that supply adequate tissue perfusion and prevent metabolic disturbance is essential. In cases of congestive heart failure, digitalis may be used and has effected dramatic improvement in some instances. Diuretics frequently are administered in conjunction with digitalis.

When these measures fail to reestablish an adequate cardiac output, a positive inotropic agent is administered. Dopamine in doses of 2 to 10 µg/kg/min is recommended to support blood pressure and effect some degree of dilatation of the renal vasculature. When chronic oral therapy is possible, an afterload-reducing drug such as captopril, an angiotensin-converting enzyme inhibitor, may be used with digitalis and diuretics.

Arrhythmias should be treated vigorously. Supraventricular tachyarrhythmias often are suppressed with digitalis, which usually has been administered previously for the treatment of congestive heart failure. Ventricular arrhythmias usually are responsive to lidocaine.

The use of immunosuppressive agents in suspected or proven viral myocarditis is controversial. A tabulation of results from most studies showing the effects of immunosuppressive therapy revealed that 60% of 82 biopsy-proven cases of myocarditis improved with therapy. Patients who had lower grade changes apparently did better than those with greater involvement. Complications of immunosuppressive therapy, including opportunistic infections and a cushingoid state, should be considered before administration of these drugs. Controlled studies are underway in the adult population to address the usefulness of immunosuppressive therapy, including use of cyclosporine; a similar study in children should be undertaken before firm recommendations can be given to clinicians.

The prognosis for acute myocarditis in newborns is poor. A 75% mortality rate was found in 25 infants with suspected coxsackievirus B myocarditis. The highest rate of mortality occurred in the first week of illness. For the six infants who survived, there were no apparent sequelae, although long-term follow-up was not reported. Older infants and children have a better prognosis, with a mortality rate between 10% and 25% in clinically recognizable cases. Adult patients who recover may be asymptomatic at rest or with light exertion but may demonstrate a reduced working capacity with exercise stress testing.

The etiology of the disease may affect prognosis. Patients who develop conduction abnormalities or arrhythmias with diphtheritic myocarditis have a poor prognosis. Some investigators report a 100% rate of mortality in the patients with conduction disturbances or supraventricular tachycardia.

(Abridged from Richard A. Friedman, Myocarditis, in Oski, DeAngelis, Feigin, McMillan, Warshaw: *Principles and Practice of Pediatrics, Second Edition*, J.B. Lippincott, 1994.)

Oski's Essential Pediatrics,
edited by Kevin B. Johnson and Frank A. Oski.
Lippincott–Raven Publishers,
Philadelphia © 1997

117

Cardiomyopathy

The term *cardiomyopathy* refers to any structural or functional abnormality of the ventricular myocardium that is not associated with disease of the coronary arteries, high blood pressure, valvular or congenital heart disease, or pulmonary vascular disease. It can be divided into two categories: primary or "heart muscle disease of known cause associated with disorders of other systems" and secondary (Table 117–1).

TABLE 117-1. Classification of Cardiomyopathy in Children

PRIMARY

Dilated
    Idiopathic dilated
    Cardiomyopathy
    Endocardial fibroelastosis
Hypertrophic
    Obstructive
    Nonobstructive
Restrictive
    Endomyocardial fibrosis
    Löffler eosinophilic endomyocardial disease
    Hemochromatosis
    Fabry's disease
    Pseudoxanthoma elasticum
Arrhythmogenic
    Arrhythmogenic right ventricular dysplasia
    Oncocytic cardiomyopathy

SECONDARY

Infection
Metabolic
General system disease
Heredofamilial
Sensitivity and toxic reactions

There are four types of primary cardiomyopathies: dilated (which will be discussed in this chapter), hypertrophic, restrictive, and arrhythmogenic. The most common causes of secondary cardiomyopathy in childhood are listed in Table 117–2.

■ DILATED CARDIOMYOPATHY

Dilated cardiomyopathy is characterized by dilatation of the left ventricle (or both ventricles), with resultant cardiomegaly. Dilatation is accompanied by some hypertrophy. Functionally, it impairs systolic function, and the clinical picture is one of congestive heart failure.

Idiopathic Dilated Cardiomyopathy

Idiopathic dilated cardiomyopathy (IDC) is a disease of infancy. More than 50% of patients present before 2 years of age. Incidence is equal in both sexes. Etiology is unknown. Familial incidence is 600 to 700 times that of the general population, and, in some cases, a hereditary basis has been documented. Over the past 5 years, numerous reports have described various cardiovascular abnormalities, including dilated cardiomyopathy, in children infected with the human immunodeficiency virus (HIV). The pathologic process usually involves the myocardium of both ventricles in a uniform fashion, producing generalized cardiac dilatation. The myocardium is pale, and the endocardium is thin and translucent. Microscopic examination shows interstitial fibrosis, myofiber hypertrophy, degeneration, and necrosis.

■ CLINICAL FINDINGS

In one third to one half of reported cases, the initial presentation is preceded by a respiratory or gastrointestinal illness. Symptoms of congestive heart failure—tachypnea, fatigue during feedings, excessive perspiration, and, occasionally, failure to thrive—are usually dominant at the initial presentation. Some patients initially present with ventricular or supraventricular arrhythmias.

Physical examination usually reveals an ill-looking child in moderate to severe respiratory distress. Cyanosis is unusual, but pallor of the skin is common. Peripheral pulses are often weak, blood pressure is low with a narrowed pulse pressure, and *pulsus alternans* is a common finding. Murmurs often are absent at the time of initial presentation, but the soft apical pansystolic murmur of mitral regurgitation often appears after a few days, once the cardiac function improves. The liver edge is usually palpable well below the right costal margin, and it is rounded as a result of passive congestion. Neck vein distention and peripheral edema are rarely found in infants but are not unusual in older children and young adults.

■ LABORATORY FINDINGS

The chest radiograph shows cardiomegaly secondary to dilatation of the left atrium and left ventricle, as well as evidence of pulmonary venous congestion that can progress to frank pulmonary edema (Figure 117–1). The electrocardiogram shows sinus tachycardia with ST-T wave abnormalities and left ventricular hypertrophy in most patients (Figure 117–2). The echocardiographic features include dilatation of the left atrium and dilatation of the left ventricle with reduction of the shortening fraction.

■ TREATMENT

During the acute phase of illness, treatment is directed at controlling congestive heart failure and includes bed rest, fluid restriction, and use of agents that decrease the cardiac load or improve myocardial contractility.

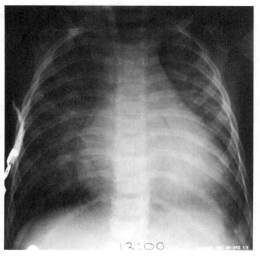

Figure 117-1. This chest radiograph of a 12-month-old boy with idiopathic dilated cardiomyopathy shows cardiomegaly and pulmonary venous congestion.

TABLE 117-2. Secondary Cardiomyopathies

INFECTIONS

Viral
Coxsackie B
Echovirus
Mumps
Rubella
Rubeola
HIV
Bacterial
Diphtheria
Meningococcal
Pneumococcal
Gonococcal
Fungal
Candidiasis
Aspergillosis
Protozoal
American trypanosomiasis (Chagas' disease) toxoplasmosis
Rickettsial
Rocky Mountain spotted fever
Spirochetal
Lyme disease

METABOLIC CONDITIONS

Endocrine
Thyrotoxicosis
Hypothyroidism
Diabetes mellitus:
Infant of diabetic mother
Diabetic cardiomyopathy
Hypoglycemia
Pheochromocytoma/neuroblastoma:
Catecholamine
Cardiomyopathy
Familial Storage Disease
Glycogen storage disease
    Pompe's disease (type II)
    Cori's disease (type III)
    Andersen's disease (type IV)
    McArdle's disease (type V)
    Hers' disease (type VI)
Mucopolysaccharidoses
    Hurler's syndrome
    Hunter's syndrome
    Morquio's syndrome
    Scheie's syndrome
    Maroteaux-Lamy syndrome
Sphingolipidoses
    Niemann-Pick disease
    Farber's disease
    Fabry's disease
    Gaucher's disease
    Tay-Sachs disease
    Sandhoff's disease
    GM, gangliosidosis
    Refsum's disease

NUTRITIONAL DEFICIENCY

Protein: kwashiorkor
Thiamine: beriberi
Vitamin E and selenium (Keshan's disease)
Phosphate
Others
Carnitine deficiency
    Primary
    Secondary: diphtheritic cardiomyopathy
B-ketothiolase deficiency
Hypertaurinuria

GENERAL SYSTEM DISEASES

Connective Tissue Disorders
Systemic lupus erythematosus
Juvenile rheumatoid arthritis
Polyarteritis nodosa
Kawasaki disease
Pseudoxanthoma elasticum
Infiltrations and Granulomas
Leukemia
Sarcoidosis (not in children)
Amyloidosis (not in children)
Others
Hemolytic-uremic syndrome
Mitochondrial cytopathy
Reye's syndrome
Peripartum cardiomyopathy
Osteogenesis imperfecta
Noonan's syndrome

HEREDOFAMILIAL CONDITIONS

Muscular Dystrophies and Myopathies
Juvenile progressive (Duchenne's disease)
Myotonic dystrophy (Steinert's disease)
Limp-girdle (Erb's disease)
Juvenile progressive spinal muscular atrophy (Kugelberg-Welander disease)
Chronic progressive external ophthalmoplegia (Kearns)
Nemaline myopathy
Myotubular myopathy
Neuromuscular Disorders
Friedreich's ataxia
Multiple lentiginosis

SENSITIVITY AND TOXIC REACTIONS

Sulphonamides
Penicillin
Anthracyclines
Iron (hemochromatosis)
Chloramphenicol
Dexamethasone

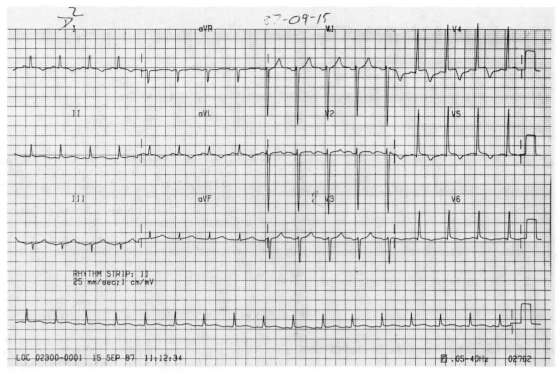

Figure 117-2. This 12-lead ECG from a 12-month-old boy with idiopathic dilated cardiomyopathy shows LVH and diffuse ST-T wave abnormalities.

The role of afterload-reducing agents in the treatment of patients with IDC is well established. Although significant atrial or ventricular arrhythmias should be treated according to accepted principles, the question of such arrhythmias representing an independent prognostic factor remains unanswered.

The role of corticosteroids and other immunosuppressive agents such as azathioprine is unclear and controversial in the treatment of children with IDC. Because of the high risk of serious side effects such as growth retardation, bone narrow suppression, and infection, use of corticosteroids and immunosuppressive agents should be restricted to those patients in whom myocardial inflammation is documented by endomyocardial biopsy.

Patients who fail to respond to medical therapy and whose condition deteriorates rapidly are candidates for cardiac transplantation. Indications for cardiac transplantation are New York Heart Association class IV symptomatology and a life expectancy of less than 6 months. It is suggested that patients who present after age 2 years and those who present before 2 years but have persistent cardiomegaly or develop significant atrial or ventricular arrhythmias during follow-up are candidates for transplantation.

■ **PROGNOSIS**

The prognosis for infants with IDC is poor, with mortality rates ranging from 35% to 63%. Other factors suggestive of poor outcome include persistent congestive heart failure or cardiomegaly and development of significant arrhythmias (ie, atrial fibrillation or flutter, or complex ventricular ectopy) during follow-up. The most common cause of death is intractable congestive heart failure, followed by sudden death secondary to an arrhythmia. About half of the survivors recover completely, whereas the other half continue to present clinical or echocardiographic evidence of myocardial dysfunction.

(Abridged from Marc Paquet and Brian D. Hanna, Cardiomyopathy, in Oski, DeAngelis, Feigin, McMillan, Warshaw: *Principles and Practice of Pediatrics, Second Edition,* J.B. Lippincott, 1994.)

Oski's Essential Pediatrics,
edited by Kevin B. Johnson and Frank A. Oski.
Lippincott–Raven Publishers,
Philadelphia © 1997

118

Infective Endocarditis

Infective endocarditis (IE) refers to a condition in which an organism or organisms infect the endocardium, valves, or related structures. These structures have been previously injured by surgery, trauma, or prior disease. The infecting organism may be bacterial, fungal, chlamydial, rickettsial, or viral. In the first half of the 20th century, many patients with IE had had prior rheumatic heart disease. In the latter part of the century, most children with IE have complex congenital heart defects.

■ **CLINICAL MANIFESTATIONS**

The clinical manifestations of IE depend on the underlying pathophysiologic processes of the disease. The extent of local involvement of the myocardium or valves, emboliza-

TABLE 118-1. Symptoms and Physical Findings in Infective Endocarditis

Symptom/Finding	Incidence (%)
Fever	56–100
Anorexia/weight loss	8–83
Malaise	40–79
Arthralgias	16–38
Gastrointestinal problems	9–36
Chest pain	5–20
Heart failure	9–47
Splenomegaly	36–67
Petechiae	10–50
Embolic events	14–50
New/changing murmur	9–44
Clubbing	2–42
Osler's nodes	7–8
Roth's spots	0–6
Janeway's lesions	0–10
Splinter hemorrhages	0–10

tion from vegetations, and activation of immunologic mechanisms play essential roles in clinical expression. Patients with acute IE may present in shock and with a clinical picture consistent with overwhelming sepsis. In some cases, confirmation of endocarditis may be found only at autopsy. The subacute form of the disease may follow an indolent course, and a diagnosis may not be established for weeks or months. Because endocarditis frequently occurs in children with underlying heart disease, subtle changes in their physical examination may be missed unless the examiner is discerning and alert. Table 118–1 lists the major clinical manifestations of IE and their relative frequency of occurrence in children.

The most common finding in IE is fever, although approximately 10% of patients have no fever. It usually is low grade and shows no specific pattern, especially in the subacute form. Other nonspecific complaints include malaise, anorexia, weight loss, fatigue, and sleep disturbances. Involvement of the large joints, with arthralgias or arthritis, occurs in 24% of patients. Nausea, vomiting, and nonspecific abdominal pains are found in 16% of patients. Chest pains, which usually are related to myalgias but are sometimes secondary to pulmonary embolism, especially with tricuspid valve involvement, occur in as many as 10% of older children.

Heart murmurs in patients with infective endocarditis have been accepted as a classic finding. They occur in as many as 90% of affected children, but most of these patients have underlying congenital defects and initially presented with murmurs specific for their lesions. A new or changing murmur occurs in approximately 25% of children. Congestive heart failure (CHF) may affect as many as 30% of children with IE, and it is especially common in patients who develop a new murmur of valvular insufficiency. Exacerbation of CHF in children with rheumatic or congenital lesions should alert the clinician to consider the diagnosis of IE for patients who previously had been controlled well on medical therapy for their chronic condition.

Signs and symptoms of neurologic involvement are seen in about 20% of children with IE. The sudden develop-

ment of a clinical picture consistent with cerebral infarction in a child with an underlying heart defect should suggest the diagnosis. Acute hemiplegia, seizures, ataxia, aphasia, focal neurologic defects, sensory loss, and changing mental status may occur as presenting features or even years after the disease process has been treated.

Splenomegaly occurs in about 55% of children with IE, usually in those with subacute disease and activated immune systems. On palpation, the spleen is not tender. Hepatomegaly also is observed in many patients. Infarction of the spleen or abscess formation should be suspected in patients with left upper quadrant pain and tenderness that radiates to the shoulder area. A pleural friction rub or pleural effusion may be observed.

Specific skin lesions associated with IE are more common in adults than in children. Petechiae are seen in about a third of the children, especially in those with a more chronic course. Common sites of involvement are the mucous membranes of the mouth, the conjunctivae, and the extremities. Petechiae are the most common skin manifestation in IE, occurring in as many as 40% of patients; purpura is rare. Osler's nodes, which also have been described in systemic lupus erythematosus and in extremities distal to the sites of prolonged arterial catheterization, are exquisitely tender lesions. They are found most commonly on the pads of the fingers and toes, the thenar and hypothenar eminences, the sides of the fingers, and the skin on the lower part of the arm. Janeway's lesions are nontender, hemorrhagic plaques that occur frequently on the palms and the soles and represent septic emboli with bacteria, neutrophils, and subsequent necrosis with subcutaneous hemorrhage. Roth's spots are small, pale retinal lesions with areas of hemorrhage that are usually located near the optic disc. Osler's nodes, Janeway's lesions, splinter hemorrhages, and Roth's spots occur in only 5% to 7% of children with endocarditis.

The tricuspid valve is the site most commonly affected, and these patients often have pulmonary complications, including infarction, abscess formation, and signs and symptoms of pleural effusion. Tricuspid insufficiency with findings of a murmur of tricuspid regurgitation, a pulsatile liver, and a gallop rhythm are found in 33% of patients.

■ DIAGNOSIS

Laboratory Investigation

Table 118–2 summarizes the most common laboratory findings in children with IE. Blood cultures are the single most important diagnostic tool for establishing the diagnosis of IE. Because bacteremia usually is continuous and low grade, the timing and site of collection do not affect the yield. Blood cultures may be negative in 10% to 15% of cases of suspected endocarditis.

TABLE 118-2. Laboratory Findings

Finding	Incidence (%)
Elevated erythrocyte sedimentation rate	71–94
Positive rheumatoid fever	25–55
Anemia	19–79
Positive blood culture	68–98
Hematuria	28–47

Echocardiography

The role of echocardiography in helping to establish the diagnosis of IE has grown considerably since the introduction of two-dimensional echocardiography. The sensitivity of echocardiography in detecting vegetative lesions in suspected endocarditis in adults ranges from 13% to 83%, with a greater sensitivity exhibited in the more recently published series using the two-dimensional technique. Several studies have concluded that patients with a "positive echo" were twice as likely to develop serious complications (usually emboli, more commonly cerebral than peripheral) and that patients were at higher risk for death or severe CHF if the vegetation was larger than 1 cm². However, the risk of embolization does not appear to correlate with vegetation size.

The use of transesophageal echocardiography (TEE) to evaluate the patient for vegetations has become important. TEE takes advantage of the proximity of the heart, especially the left atrium, to the esophagus. This technique also eliminates the inability to image transthoracically in some patients who do not have good "echo windows" from that approach. The quality of the image is better, making diagnosis more certain.

A negative echocardiographic study does not rule out the presence of vegetations. The limit of resolution on most equipment limits the detection of vegetations to those larger than 2 to 3 mm. Poor technique also may hinder evaluation. Rheumatic heart disease with preexisting valve disease, mitral valve prolapse with thickened leaflets, marantic vegetations, Löffler's endocarditis, Chiari's networks in the right atrium, and valve ring abscesses pose interpretive problems to the echocardiographer.

Electrocardiography

Numerous electrocardiographic abnormalities may be found throughout the course of IE. Ventricular ectopy in patients with hemodynamic compromise may be life threatening. Atrial fibrillation in adults and children may be secondary to atrioventricular valve regurgitation. Extension of abscess formation or an inflammatory response may cause direct injury to the conduction system. Complete right bundle branch block, left anterior or posterior fascicular block, and complete atrioventricular block have been reported. Abscess formation in the perivalvular aortic region may cause direct injury to the atrioventricular node because of its proximity to that structure. This may result in sudden death unless temporary and eventually permanent pacing is instituted.

■ PROPHYLAXIS

The use of antibiotics before and during any procedure that induces a transient bacteremia has become standard medical practice for the prevention of IE. The Committee on Rheumatic Fever and Bacterial Endocarditis of the Council on Cardiovascular Diseases in the Young of the American Heart Association published recommendations in 1985 (Table 118–3).

■ MICROBIOLOGY

Many different organisms have been associated with infective endocarditis in humans. Table 118–4 lists the most common causative agents responsible for the development

TABLE 118-3. Recommended Antibiotic Regimens for Endocarditis Prophylaxis in Children

For Dental/Respiratory Tract Procedures			For Gastrointestinal/Genitourinary Procedures		
Regimen	Condition	Dosage	Regimen	Condition	Dosage
Standard	For dental procedures that cause gingival bleeding and oral/respiratory tract surgery	Amoxicillin 50 mg/kg PO (up to 3 gm) 1 h before the procedure, then ½ initial dose 6 h later G (1–2 million U IV or IM 30–60 min before, and 0.5–1.0 million units 6 h later)	Standard	For genitourinary/gastrointestinal tract procedures indicated	Ampicillin (50 mg/kg IM or IV) plus gentamicin (2.0 mg/kg IM or IV) given 30 min to 1 h before procedure; one follow-up dose may be given 8 h later
Special	Parenteral regimen for use when maximal protection is desired (eg, for patients with prosthetic valves)	Ampicillin (50 mg/kg IM or IV) plus gentamicin (2.0 mg/kg IM or IV) 0.5 h before the procedure, followed by Amoxicillin 25 6 h later; alternatively, parenteral regimen may be repeated once 8 h later	Special	Oral regimen for minor or repetitive procedures in low-risk patients	Amoxicillin (50 mg/kg orally 1 h before procedure and 25 mg/kg 6 h later)
	Oral regimen for penicillin-allergic patients and those on rheumatic fever prophylaxis	Erythromycin (20 mg/kg orally 2 h before, then 10 mg/kg 6 h later)		Penicillin-allergic patients	Vancomycin (15–20 mg/kg IV) plus gentamicin (2 mg/kg IM or IV) 1 h before procedure; may be repeated once 8 h later
	Parenteral regimen for penicillin-allergic patients and those on rheumatic fever prophylaxis	Clindamycin 10 mg/kg (max 300 mg) IV: 0.5 h before; then 5 mg/kg IV 6 h later			

From Committee on Rheumatic Fever, Endocarditis, and Kawasaki Disease of the Council on Cardiovascular Disease in the Young, the American Heart Association, JAMA 264:2919, 1990.

TABLE 118-4. Causative Agents in Pediatric Infective Endocarditis

Organism	Incidence (%)
Streptococci	
Viridans	17–72
Enterococci	0–12
Pneumococci	0–21
β-Hemolytic	0–8
Staphylococci	
S aureus	5–40
S epidermidis	0–15
Gram-negative aerobic bacilli	0–15
Fungi	0–12
Miscellaneous	0–10
Culture negative	2–32

of infective endocarditis. Gram-positive cocci are the etiologic agents of 90% of cases in which an organism is isolated. Streptococci, especially of the viridans group, remain the bacteria isolated most frequently. Because of the increasing role of surgery and prosthetic material in the correction and palliation of congenital heart disease, the percentage of cases caused by staphylococci, gram-negative bacilli, and fungi have increased. Identification of the causative agent is the single most important procedure involved in confirming the diagnosis, directing therapy, and predicting outcome and possible complications.

■ TREATMENT

Several general principles provide the basis for treatment of IE. The preferable route of antibiotic administration is intravenous. Oral antibiotics may be absorbed poorly or erratically, especially in infants, which may result in treatment failure. A course of at least 4 and up to 6 weeks or longer is required to sterilize vegetations and prevent relapse. Bacteriostatic agents are contraindicated and may lead to failure or relapse if employed. Synergism between certain agents may produce a rapid bactericidal effect and allow smaller doses of each drug to be administered, thereby reducing possible toxic side effects. Certain drug combinations, however, such as penicillin and chloramphenicol, may be antagonistic.

After initiation of therapy, daily blood cultures should be obtained. Although negative blood cultures may not necessarily correlate with a therapeutic success, continued positive blood cultures usually indicate a need for investigation of the serum concentration of the drug in the patient, for the addition of another agent, or for a change in therapy. If the patient has not responded clinically to initial antibiotic therapy within several days, more blood cultures should be obtained. In addition, attention to the patient's clinical course is essential. Patients usually begin to improve within a few days of the initiation of appropriate therapy, although persistent fever may occur occasionally in patients who eventually have a good outcome.

■ PROGNOSIS

The course and prognosis of patients depend on many underlying factors, including the severity of the primary car-

diac lesion, the presence of prosthetic material, the infecting organism, the duration of illness before diagnosis and initiation of appropriate therapy, and the clinical condition at the time of diagnosis (eg, degree of respiratory, neurologic, and cardiovascular or renal compromise).

Patients who survive will always be at risk for future development of IE. After an apparently successful course of therapy, the disease may recur early (within 3 months of completion of therapy) or late (3 to 6 months after completion of therapy), and it should be suspected if fever or other symptoms recur shortly after antibiotics are discontinued. The organism found at relapse may be identical to or different from the organism identified initially.

(Abridged from Richard A. Friedman, Starke JR, Infective Endocarditis, in Oski, DeAngelis, Feigin, McMillan, Warshaw: *Principles and Practice of Pediatrics, Second Edition*, J.B. Lippincott, 1994.)

Oski's Essential Pediatrics, edited by Kevin B. Johnson and Frank A. Oski. Lippincott–Raven Publishers, Philadelphia © 1997

119

Rheumatic Fever

Rheumatic fever (RF) is a delayed, nonsuppurative sequela to upper respiratory infection with group A β-hemolytic streptococci. It is a diffuse inflammatory disease of the connective tissue that involves principally the heart, blood vessels, joints, central nervous system, and subcutaneous tissues.

The term *acute rheumatic fever* is a misnomer, because it may not be acute, rheumatic, or febrile. Although the term emphasizes involvement of the joints, the disease owes its importance to involvement of the heart. As early as 1884, Lasegue described this feature: "Rheumatic fever is a disease that licks the joints but bites the heart."

Rheumatic fever occurs more commonly in the winter and spring, a seasonal variation similar to that of streptococcal pharyngitis. Recurrent streptococcal infections are the most important predisposing factor in the occurrence and recurrence of RF. About 1% to 5% of streptococcal throat infections are followed by RF. The most important factors that may be related to the attack rate of RF after streptococcal pharyngitis are the magnitude of the immune response to the antecedent infections and the duration of convalescent carriage of the organisms. Skin infections are unlikely to produce the disease.

■ CLINICAL MANIFESTATIONS

Antecedent Streptococcal Infection

The interval between the onset of pharyngitis and the symptoms of RF is 1 to 5 weeks (average, 3 weeks). However, clinical evidence for a preceding streptococcal infection may be lacking. About one third of patients have had no apparent illness during the preceding month.

Polyarthritis

Inflammation affects the large joints and moves from one to another. The affected joint is hot, red, tender, and swollen. The arthritis characteristically leaves the joints without any sequelae and responds almost immediately to salicylates. The severity of joint involvement is inversely proportional to the severity of cardiac involvement.

Carditis

In contrast to the seriousness of its prognosis, rheumatic carditis, unless it causes heart failure or pericarditis, produces no symptoms of its own and is usually diagnosed during examination of a patient with arthritis or chorea.

The development of an apical systolic murmur that is propagated to the axilla and is accompanied by a muffled first sound and a third sound indicates the development of mitral insufficiency. A systolic murmur over the apex without these characteristics may be caused by fever and not by mitral valvulitis.

The occurrence of a mid-diastolic murmur over the apex is a definite sign of mitral valvulitis. The diastolic apical murmur is caused by narrowing of the mitral orifice by the thickened, edematous cusps. The murmur may persist, indicating permanent damage, but it frequently disappears for a variable period, followed later by the appearance of the diastolic murmur of stenosis caused by the development of adhesions between the valve cusps.

The occurrence of a high-pitched, early-diastolic murmur over the base indicates aortic valvulitis. As in mitral valvulitis, the occurrence of a systolic murmur over the base may be caused by fever or by aortic valvulitis.

The murmurs of mitral and aortic valvulitis may disappear or may be followed by the establishment of valve regurgitation, stenosis, or both, according to the pathologic process occurring in the valve. Regurgitation, the result of damage, takes a short time to develop, but stenosis, the result of union between mobile cusps, takes years to decades to occur.

Myocarditis usually is accompanied by valvulitis and leads to tachycardia (especially if it persists during sleep) that is disproportionate to the patient's fever and can lead to gallop rhythm, rapid cardiac enlargement, and heart failure. Pericarditis accompanies valvulitis in approximately 5% to 10% of patients. The degree of effusion in pericarditis varies from none to moderate.

Electrocardiographic changes characteristically include prolongation of the PR and QT intervals. Second-degree or a complete AV block may occur in response to inflammation of the conduction system. There may be ST wave and T wave changes of pericarditis or myocarditis. Echocardiographic changes can detect valvular and myocardial involvement or pericardial effusion.

Chorea

Rheumatic or Sydenham's chorea, which is a late manifestation of RF, is more common among female than male patients. Chorea may last from 1 week to more than 2 years. Chorea is never seen simultaneously with arthritis, but it may coexist with carditis. If there is no carditis, the sedimentation rate is not elevated. In such cases, the ASO and other streptococcal antibody titers may not be increased, probably because chorea appears only after a latent period as long as 6 months after the streptococcal infection, and, by that time, the acute-phase reactants and the streptococcal antibody titer may have returned to normal.

There are involuntary, incoordinate, jerky movements accompanied by hypotonia and emotional disturbances, with abrupt alterations between laughter and tears. Flexion at the wrist and dorsiflexion of the fingers occur in the outstretched hands. Objects often fall from the hands. The patient, after protruding the tongue for inspection, may withdraw it rapidly, snapping the jaws over it.

Subcutaneous Nodules

Rarely seen in recent years, subcutaneous nodules usually indicate severe carditis. The nodules are attached to the tendon sheaths and occur on the extensor surfaces and bony prominences of the arms and legs and on the scapula and the mastoid processes. Histologically, they consist of collections of Aschoff bodies.

Erythema Marginatum

The rash of erythema marginatum generally appears as an area of erythema. The margins progress as the center clears. The rash occurs chiefly over the trunk and the proximal parts of the limbs (Figure 119–1).

Signs of Inflammation

Pallor, epistaxis, elevated temperature, tachycardia, anorexia, and loss of weight are signs of inflammation. They indicate rheumatic activity in a patient already diagnosed as having rheumatic fever. Pleurisy, pneumonia, and abdominal pain (simulating appendicitis) due to vasculitis have the same significance.

■ DIAGNOSIS

Laboratory tests typically show a high erythrocyte sedimentation rate, anemia, leukocytosis, and C-reactive protein. The ASO antibody is elevated abnormally in 70% to 85% of patients with RF. A single value of 500 units indicates recent streptococcal infection, and a value of 333 units is of borderline significance. If the ASO titer is 333 units or less, additional antistreptococcal antibody assays should be obtained. ASO and anti-DNase are most often used for diagnosis, and antihyaluronidase is a third choice.

The diagnosis of RF is important because serious cardiac disease can be prevented or minimized by long-term antistreptococcal therapy. There is no single diagnostic test for RF. The laboratory tests indicate recent streptococcal infection, but diagnosis of RF rests on the ability to satisfy the Duckett Jones criteria (Table 119–1). It is mandatory to demonstrate recent streptococcal infection (usually by elevation of ASO titer) and to find one major and two minor criteria or to identify two major criteria. The minor manifestations are less specific for the illness.

RF should be differentiated from juvenile rheumatoid arthritis, innocent murmur with a febrile illness, bacterial arthritis, systemic lupus erythematosus, Schönlein-Henoch purpura, acute leukemia, sickle-cell anemia, and mucocutaneous lymph node syndrome.

■ COURSE AND PROGNOSIS

RF usually follows a characteristic clinical course. The latent period is short for disease complicated with arthritis

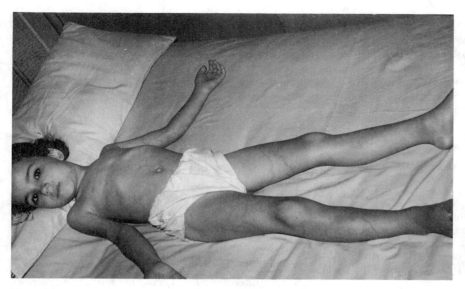

Figure 119-1. A 6-year-old girl with erythema marginatum has acute rheumatic fever with severe carditis. (Courtesy of Samir Kassem, MD, Alexandria Medical School.)

and erythema marginatum, longest for RF with chorea, and midlength for RF with carditis and subcutaneous nodules. The duration of active disease is usually less than 3 months. Fewer than 5% of patients with RF have disease that remains active for more than 6 months, a condition known as chronic active carditis. The prognosis is excellent for the patient who does not develop carditis during the initial attack. The prognosis becomes poorer with increasing severity of initial carditis.

■ TREATMENT

Prophylactic Therapy

Prevention of RF is achieved by improving socioeconomic circumstances and sanitation.

The aim of primary prophylaxis is to prevent initial attacks of RF by prompt and accurate recognition and treatment of streptococcal pharyngitis or by antibiotic prophylaxis using benzathine penicillin intramuscularly for members of a susceptible population. Modern outbreaks in the United States were blamed in part on diminished adherence to conventional recommendations for penicillin, which is highly effective in preventing RF due to pharyngeal infections.

Secondary prophylaxis is the prevention of recurrences of RF by continuous chemoprophylaxis. The most effective method is a single monthly intramuscular injection of ben-

zathine penicillin. The duration of secondary prophylaxis depends on the variables that influence the recurrence rate and the degree to which the heart has been affected. The risk of recurrence declines with age and with an increased free RF interval from the last rheumatic attack after 10 years.

No vaccine is available, but purification and immunologic study of streptococcal M proteins hold the promise of a streptococcal vaccine in the near future.

Curative Therapy

Bed rest is required until the signs and symptoms of acute inflammation disappear. Salt is restricted if signs of heart failure are observed.

A course of antibiotics should be initiated after a throat culture has been obtained. Antibiotics should be administered even in the absence of positive throat cultures. One intramuscular injection of benzathine penicillin (600,000 to 1,200,000 U) or a 10-day course of oral penicillin G (500 to 1000 mg, four times daily) is recommended.

Acetylsalicylic acid (aspirin) is analgesic and antipyretic and reduces malaise. It causes such dramatic improvement of the arthritis that it can be given as a therapeutic test, but it has no effect on carditis. Aspirin is given to patients with or without mild carditis, if there are side effects or contraindications to corticosteroids, and during and after withdrawal from corticosteroids. Side effects include tinnitus, gastric irri-

TABLE 119-1. Duckett Jones Criteria for the Diagnosis of Rheumatic Fever

Requirements for Diagnosis	Major Criteria	Minor Criteria
Two major criteria,	Carditis	Previous rheumatic fever
or	Arthritis	Arthralgia
One major plus two minor,	Chorea	Fever
plus	Erythema marginatum	Raised erythrocyte sedimentation rate
Evidence of previous streptococcal infection: (eg, elevated ASO titer)	Subcutaneous nodules	Elevated leukocyte count
		Prolonged PR interval
		C reactive protein

tation, bleeding due to inhibition of platelet function, metabolic acidosis, hyperventilation that may lead to respiratory alkalosis, and hypoglycemia. The dosage is 60 to 120 mg/kg/day, given in six divided doses and administered until a satisfactory clinical response is obtained. The dosage is then reduced by one third and continued until all laboratory findings return to normal, which usually requires 6 to 9 weeks. The dosage is decreased gradually to avoid the rebound that occurs if the drug is stopped abruptly.

Corticosteroids do not markedly shorten the course of illness or diminish the likelihood of cardiac damage. Steroids do produce prompt control of the subcutaneous nodules, erythema marginatum, fever, and arthritis. Corticosteroids are indicated for patients with severe carditis. The dosage of prednisone or prednisolone is 2 mg/kg/day (not to exceed 60 mg/day) for 3 to 4 weeks. Shortly before or at the time steroid therapy is discontinued, aspirin (90 to 120 mg/kg/day) should be given, and it should be continued for 1.5 to 6 months, probably until active inflammation subsides.

(Abridged from Galal M. El-Said, Rheumatic Fever, in Oski, DeAngelis, Feigin, McMillan, Warshaw: *Principles and Practice of Pediatrics, Second Edition,* J.B. Lippincott, 1994.)

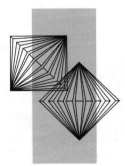

SECTION 8

Diseases of the Blood

Oski's Essential Pediatrics,
edited by Kevin B. Johnson and Frank A. Oski.
Lippincott–Raven Publishers,
Philadelphia © 1997

120

The Nutritional Anemias

The important nutritional anemias result from dietary deficiencies of iron, folic acid, or vitamin B_{12}. Deficiencies of other nutrients such as vitamins B_6 and E may be associated with anemia, but they are unusual in pediatric practice.

IRON DEFICIENCY ANEMIA

Anemia due to iron deficiency is the most common hematologic disease of infancy and childhood. The body of the newborn infant contains 0.3 to 0.5 g of iron; the adult's iron content is estimated at 5 g. To make up the 4.5-g difference, an average of 0.8 mg of iron must be absorbed each day during the first 15 years of life. In addition to this requirement for growth, a small amount of iron is necessary to balance normal losses, estimated at 0.5 to 1 mg/day. To maintain a positive iron balance during childhood, 0.8 to 1.5 mg of iron must be absorbed each day from the diet. Because less than 10% of dietary iron is absorbed from the average mixed diet, 8 to 15 mg of iron daily is necessary for optimal nutrition. During the first years of life, when relatively small quantities of iron-rich foods are ingested, it is difficult to attain these amounts. The infant's diet should include iron-fortified foods, such as cereals or iron-supplemented formulas, by no later than 6 months of age.

■ PATHOPHYSIOLOGY

Anemia due solely to inadequate dietary iron is unusual during the first 4 to 6 months of life, but it becomes common from 9 to 24 months of age. The usual dietary pattern of infants with iron deficiency anemia is the consumption of large amounts of milk and carbohydrates not supplemented with iron. Blood loss must also be considered in the genesis of iron deficiency anemia. Chronic iron deficiency anemia from occult bleeding may be caused by a peptic ulcer, Meckel's diverticulum, polyp, or hemangioma. As many as one third of the infants with severe iron deficiency in the United States have chronic intestinal blood loss induced by ingestion of a heat-labile protein in whole cow's milk. This can be prevented by reducing the quantity of whole cow's milk or by using a milk substitute. This gastrointestinal reaction is not related to lactase deficiency or to milk allergy.

■ CLINICAL PRESENTATION

Pallor is the most frequent sign of iron deficiency anemia. In mild to moderate deficiency (ie, hemoglobin level of 7 to 10 g/dL), few symptoms of anemia are seen, but irritability and anorexia may be prominent. As the anemia progresses, tachycardia, cardiac dilation, and systolic murmurs occur.

The spleen is palpable in 10% to 15% of patients, and some chronic cases of anemia are associated with widening of the marrow cavity of the skull. The child with iron deficiency anemia may be obese or underweight with other evidence of undernutrition.

Some children have pica. This and the characteristic irritability may reflect a deficiency in tissue iron-containing enzymes. With iron therapy, striking symptomatic improvement occurs before significant hematologic improvement. In the past, the intracellular enzyme iron compartment was believed to be maintained even in the face of severe deficiency, but this view is no longer supported. Iron deficiency anemia and even iron deficiency without significant anemia may adversely affect the attention span, behavior, and performance of the affected infants.

■ LABORATORY FINDINGS

A sequence of biochemical and hematologic changes of iron deficiency have been described. First, the iron stores (ie, liver and bone marrow hemosiderin) disappear. Serum ferritin levels less than 10 ng/mL indicate iron deficiency. As the serum iron levels decrease to less than 30 g/dL, the iron-binding capacity of the serum increases, resulting in serum transferrin saturation values of less than 15%. As deficiency progresses, the erythrocytes become smaller than normal with decreased hemoglobin content. The reticulocyte count is normal or minimally elevated, and leukocyte counts are normal. Elevated platelet counts (>600,000/mm^3) are often seen. The bone marrow is hypercellular, with erythroid hyperplasia. The normoblasts have scanty cytoplasm, with poor hemoglobinization.

Iron deficiency must be differentiated from other hypochromic, microcytic anemias. In lead poisoning, the erythrocytes are morphologically similar, but coarse basophilic stippling of the erythrocytes is prominent. Tests reveal elevations of blood lead and marked elevation of free erythrocyte protoporphyrins. Many cases of lead poisoning have concomitant iron deficiency. β-Thalassemia trait resembles iron deficiency, but there are characteristic elevations in the level of hemoglobin A$_2$. α-Thalassemia trait occurs in about 3% of blacks and in many Southeast Asian peoples, but it is difficult to prove after the neonatal period. Thalassemia major with its organomegaly, erythroblastosis, and hemolytic component is usually obvious. The erythrocyte morphology of chronic inflammatory or infectious conditions may be microcytic. In these conditions, the serum iron and iron-binding capacity are reduced, and serum ferritin levels are normal or elevated.

■ TREATMENT

The response of iron deficiency anemia to adequate amounts of iron is an important diagnostic and therapeutic feature. Oral administration of simple ferrous salts is satisfactory therapy. Four to 6 mg/kg of elemental iron in three divided doses is optimal; larger doses do not result in a more rapid hematologic response. Medicinal iron should be administered between meals to ensure good absorption. Parenteral iron therapy is almost never indicated unless compliance is poor.

Within 4 days after administration of iron, peripheral reticulocytosis is seen, with the magnitude of the reticulocytic response proportional to the severity of the anemia. The hemoglobin level rises to normal. Iron medication should be continued for 4 to 6 weeks. Iron therapy fails if the child does not receive the prescribed medication or if there is unrecognized continuing blood loss. An incorrect diagnosis of iron deficiency anemia may also be revealed by therapeutic failure.

MEGALOBLASTIC ANEMIASF

The megaloblastic anemias are uncommon disorders characterized by abnormal erythrocyte morphology and maturation. The erythrocytes are larger than normal. The nucleated erythrocytes have an open, finely dispersed arrangement of chromatin and asynchronous maturation of nucleus and cytoplasm. Megaloblastic anemias are a consequence of disordered syntheses of DNA, and megaloblastic cells have increased amounts of RNA relative to DNA.

The rare megaloblastic anemia of infancy is caused by a deficient intake or malabsorption of folic acid often aggravated by infection. Goat's milk and powdered cow's milk are poor sources of folic acid, and vitamin C deficiency impairs folate absorption. Megaloblastic anemia has a peak incidence at 4 to 7 months of age. In addition to showing pallor, affected infants are irritable, fail to gain weight, and often have chronic diarrhea.

■ LABORATORY FINDINGS

Megaloblastic anemia is macrocytic (ie, mean corpuscular volume >95 fL). The reticulocyte count is low, but nucleated erythrocytes demonstrating megaloblastic morphology may be seen in the blood. Advanced cases have thrombocytopenia and neutropenia, and many of the neutrophils are hypersegmented (ie, two lobes or more). Serum folate levels are usually reduced, but low levels of erythrocyte folate are a better indication of chronic deficiency. Serum lactate dehydrogenase activity is markedly elevated. The bone marrow is hypercellular because of erythroid hyperplasia and shows prominent megaloblastic changes. Large, abnormal neutrophilic forms (ie, giant metamyelocytes) with cytoplasmic vacuolization are also seen.

FOLIC ACID DEFICIENCY

Because folic acid is absorbed throughout the small intestine, diffuse inflammatory or degenerative disease of the intestine may impair its absorption. Celiac disease, chronic infectious enteritis, and enteroenteric fistulas may lead to folic acid deficiency. Folic acid supplements are indicated in these states.

Many patients have low serum levels of folic acid during therapy with anticonvulsant drugs. Malabsorption of folic acid appears to be induced by these drugs. These patients usually have no anemia or symptoms. However, if anemia develops, it is responsive to folic acid therapy even if administration of the drug is continued. Megaloblastic anemia has been seen in users of oral contraceptives. Drugs such as methotrexate prevent the utilization of folic acid by inhibiting reduction to its active coenzymatic forms.

VITAMIN B$_{12}$ DEFICIENCY

To be absorbed, dietary vitamin B$_{12}$ must combine with a glycoprotein (ie, intrinsic factor) secreted by the parietal cells of the gastric fundus. The B$_{12}$–intrinsic factor complex passes to the terminal ileum, where specific absorptive receptors exist. Vitamin B$_{12}$ deficiency can result from inadequate dietary intake, lack of secretion of intrinsic factor, disruption of the B$_{12}$–intrinsic factor complex, or abnormalities or absence of the receptor sites in the terminal ileum.

Vitamin B$_{12}$ is present in many foods, and pure dietary deficiency is rare. Deficiency may be seen in patients (ie, vegans) subsisting on extreme diets that contain no milk, eggs, or animal products. It has also been reported in breast-fed infants whose mothers were B_{12}-deficient because of diet or pernicious anemia. Because the vitamin occurs in so many foods, most cases of B_{12} deficiency are a consequence of failure to absorb the vitamin.

■ THERAPY

Initially, folic acid should be administered parenterally in a dosage of 2 to 5 mg every 24 hours and treatment should be continued for 3 to 4 weeks. Antibiotic therapy should be used for superimposed bacterial infection.

Therapy with folic acid should not be started in a patient with megaloblastic anemia until a diagnosis of folate deficiency has been established. Folic acid therapy is contraindicated in vitamin B_{12} deficiency.

(Abridged from Paul L. Martin and Howard A. Pearson, The Nutritional Anemias, in Oski, DeAngelis, Feigin, McMillan, Warshaw: *Principles and Practice of Pediatrics, Second Edition*, J.B. Lippincott, 1994.)

Oski's Essential Pediatrics,
edited by Kevin B. Johnson and Frank A. Oski.
Lippincott–Raven Publishers,
Philadelphia © 1997

121

The Hemoglobinopathies and Thalassemias

The genetic, molecular, and biochemical characteristics of human hemoglobin are well known. The genes for the polypeptide chains of hemoglobin are located on chromosomes 11 and 16, and their DNA sequences have been determined. Each of the α and β chains of adult hemoglobin consist of about 150 amino acids. It is possible to identify and locate the single amino acid substitution in these chains that causes each abnormal hemoglobin syndrome. Although more than 400 types of abnormal human hemoglobin have been characterized, only a few of them are prevalent.

Hemoglobin variants are identified by hemoglobin electrophoresis, a technique that usually permits a specific genotypic diagnosis. The thalassemias are associated with decreased production of the normal polypeptide chains of hemoglobin. The thalassemias are quantitative rather than qualitative abnormalities of hemoglobin.

SICKLE-CELL DISEASE AND TRAIT

The gene for sickle-cell hemoglobin (Hb S) is not exclusively African, although there is a broad periequatorial sickle-cell belt in Africa. From Africa, the sickle gene was introduced into the Western hemisphere by the 16th through 18th century slave trade. In the United States, sickling disorders are particularly prevalent in the South and in the urban North, reflecting the demography of African Americans. In Latin America, relatively high frequencies are seen in the Caribbean, Panama, Guyana, and Brazil, but not in Mexico and most of South America. A high incidence of sickle genes, apparently resulting from independent mutational events, is found in Italy, Greece, the Middle East, and India.

■ PATHOPHYSIOLOGY

In Hb S, a valine residue is substituted for the usual glutamic acid in the β chains of the hemoglobin molecule. When Hb S becomes deoxygenated, polymerization occurs with the formation of long, crystalline tactoids. These ultimately form elongated, sickled erythrocytes. Sickled erythrocytes have markedly shortened survival, and they can obstruct small blood vessels and cause distal tissue ischemia and necrosis.

Heterozygosity for a sickle gene has a benign clinical course. About 8% of African Americans have the trait. The sickle gene is thought to confer a degree of resistance in areas endemic for falciparum malaria in infancy. The erythrocytes in sickle trait contain only 30% to 40% Hb S, and sickling does not occur under physiologic conditions. Rarely, hypoxia resulting from shock or from flying at high altitudes in unpressurized aircraft may produce vaso-occlusive phenomena. Unexpected death has also been observed in military recruits during the extreme exertion of basic training. Spontaneous hematuria, usually from the left kidney, and mild hyposthenuria also occur. Anemia or hemolysis should not be attributed to the sickle trait.

In persons homozygous for the sickle gene, sickle-cell anemia is a severe, chronic hemolytic anemia. The clinical course is marked by episodes of pain caused by occlusion of small blood vessels by the spontaneously sickled erythrocytes. These events have traditionally been called crises.

■ CLINICAL MANIFESTATIONS

Manifestations of sickle-cell disease do not usually appear until the second 6 months of life, coincident with the postnatal decrease in fetal hemoglobin (Hb F) and increase in Hb S. The hemolytic process is evident by 6 months of age.

The painful or vaso-occlusive crises are the most frequent clinical symptoms. Symmetric, painful swelling of the hands and feet (ie, hand–foot syndrome) caused by infarction of the small bones of the hands and feet may be the initial manifestation of sickle-cell anemia in infancy. Older patients may have painful involvement of the larger bones and joints and severe abdominal pain resembling acute surgical conditions. Strokes may leave permanent paralysis. Extensive pulmonary consolidation occurs, and it is difficult to differentiate infarction from pneumonia. Vaso-occlusive crises are not usually associated with changes in the usual hematologic picture.

A second type of crisis, seen only in young infants and children, is called the sequestration crisis. Large amounts of blood become pooled in the abdominal organs. The spleen becomes massively enlarged, and signs of circulatory collapse develop rapidly. If volume replacement is given, much of the sequestered blood is remobilized. The sequestration crisis is an important cause of death in infants with sickle-cell disease.

The third well-characterized type of crisis is the aplastic crisis (see Chapter 123).

In addition to these acute crises, a variety of clinical signs and symptoms result from chronic severe hemolytic anemia and vaso-occlusive disease. Impairment of liver function contributes to the jaundice of these patients. Gallstones can occur in children as young as 3 years of age. Renal function is progressively impaired by diffuse glomerular and tubular fibrosis, resulting in hyposthenuria and polyuria.

As many as 30% of children with sickle-cell anemia develop pneumococcal sepsis during the first 5 years of life.

The increased risk is a result of functional hyposplenia and low levels of specific serum antibodies. Increased susceptibility to *Salmonella* osteomyelitis is also a feature of sickle-cell disease.

By midchildhood, most patients are underweight, and puberty is delayed, particularly in boys. Chronic leg ulcers are common in adolescence and early adult life.

■ LABORATORY FINDINGS

Table 121–1 outlines typical laboratory findings in patients with sickle-cell disease. Diagnostic studies to demonstrate Hb S include the sickle-cell preparation and hemoglobin solubility studies. However, hemoglobin electrophoresis is more conclusive and is necessary for a precise diagnosis. After infancy, the erythrocytes of patients with sickle-cell anemia contain approximately 90% Hb S, 2% to 10% Hb F, and a normal amount of Hb A$_2$; they do not contain Hb A.

■ TREATMENT

No antisickling pharmacologic agent has proved safe or of consistent value. For mild or moderately painful crises, analgesics are indicated. Parenteral narcotics are often necessary for severe pain. Dehydration and acidosis should be corrected. Bacterial infections require appropriate antibiotic therapy. The risk of sepsis from encapsulated organisms is high enough to justify the use of prophylactic penicillin in all sickle-cell patients from 6 months to at least 6 years of age. The value of prophylaxis after 6 years of age is being studied. Blood transfusions are unnecessary for the usual painful crises but are indicated for prolonged or extreme pain, for extensive involvement of lungs or central nervous system, and as preparation for general anesthesia. When the homozygous patient's circulating Hb SS erythrocytes can be diluted to less than 40% by transfusions of normal blood, vaso-occlusive symptoms usually abate. Partial exchange transfusion can be done to rapidly lower the percentage of Hb SS erythrocytes.

Newborn screening for sickle hemoglobinopathies is mandated in 38 states. Medical counseling of affected families and initiation of prophylactic penicillin for affected infants have been effective in decreasing early mortality from sickle-cell disease.

OTHER HEMOGLOBINOPATHIES

■ HEMOGLOBIN SC

When the genes for Hb S and Hb C occur in the same person, a moderately severe anemia with splenomegaly results. Vaso-occlusive episodes are usually less frequent

TABLE 121-1. Laboratory Findings in Patients With Sickle-cell Disease

Diagnosis	Frequency	Clinical Severity	HGB (gm/dl)	HCT (%)	MCV (µ³)	% RETIC	RBC Morphology	Solubility Test	Electro-phoresis	Distribution HbF
SS	1:625	Moderate-Severe	7.5 (6–10)	22 (18–30)	93	11 (4–30)	Many ISCs, target cells, nucleated red cells	Positive	80–90%S 2–20%F <3.6%A$_2$	Uneven
SC	1:833	Mild-Moderate	10 (9–14)	30 26–40	80	3 (1.5–6)	Many target cells, rare ISCs	Positive	45–55%S 45–55%C 0.2–8%F	Uneven
S/B° Thal		Moderate-Severe	8.1 (7–12)	25 (20–36)	69	8 (3–18)	Marked hypochromia, microcytosis and target cells, variable ISCs	Positive	50–85%S 2–30%F >3.8%A$_2$	Uneven
S/B⁺ Thal	1:1667	Mild-Moderate	11 (8–13)	32 (25–40)	76	3 (1.5–6)	Mild microcytosis, hypochromia, rare ISCs	Positive	55–75%S 15–30%A 1–20%F >3.6%A$_2$	Uneven
S/HPFH	1:25,000	Asymptomatic	14 (11–15)	40 (32–48)	84	1.5 (0.5–3)	No ISCs, occasional target cells, and mild hypochromia	Positive	60–80%S 16–36%F 1–3%A$_2$	Even
AS	1:17	Asymptomatic	Normal	Normal	Normal	Normal	Normal	Positive	38–45%S 50–55%A 1–3%A$_2$	Uneven
ASα Thal	1:300	Asymptomatic	Low/Normal	Low/Normal	70	Normal	Microcytic	Positive	29–35%S 71–75%A	Uneven

SS = Homozygous sickle cell disease.
S = Sickle trait.
C = C hemoglobin.
B°, B⁺ = β-Thalassemias.
HPFH = Hereditary persistence of fetal hemoglobin.
ISC = Irreversible sickle cells.
Reference: Lubin, B., Kleman, K., and Pennathur-Das, R.: Lab. Management, 18:38, 1980.

and milder than in sickle-cell disease. Aseptic necrosis of the femoral head is an occasional complication, and severe retinal damage also occurs.

Hb SC disease does not usually affect growth and is compatible with extended survival. The hemoglobin concentration averages 9 to 10 g/dL. Target cells are seen in large numbers on blood smears. Hemoglobin electrophoresis reveals an almost equal mixture of Hb S and Hb C, with a slight elevation of Hb F.

THALASSEMIAS

The thalassemias are a group of hereditary hypochromic anemias associated with defective synthesis of one of the polypeptide chains of hemoglobin. In the United States, they chiefly affect persons of Mediterranean and Southeast Asian ethnic backgrounds. In the heterozygous state, thalassemia genes produce mild anemia. In the homozygous form, they are associated with severe hematologic disease.

■ CLINICAL PRESENTATIONS

Heterozygous thalassemia of the β-chain variety (ie, thalassemia minor) is a mild familial hypochronic microcytic anemia. Hemoglobin levels are 2 to 3 g/dL below age-appropriate normal values. The mean corpuscular volume averages 68 fL (range, 58 to 75 fL). The erythrocytes are hypochromic and microcytic, with target cells, ovalocytes, and basophilic stippling. Elevation of Hb A_2 levels (>3.5%) establishes the diagnosis. No therapy is effective or necessary.

Homozygous β-thalassemia (ie, thalassemia major, Cooley's anemia) usually becomes symptomatic in the first year of life. The anemia is so profound that regular blood transfusions are necessary to sustain life; untreated, the life expectancy is only a few years. However, about 10% of homozygous patients are able to maintain hemoglobin levels of 6 to 8 g/dL without regular transfusions (ie, thalassemia intermedia). In the untransfused or poorly transfused patient, massive splenomegaly and progressive bone changes become evident during the first few years of life.

■ LABORATORY FINDINGS

The erythrocyte changes of thalassemia major are extreme. In addition to severe hypochromia and microcytosis, there are many poikilocytes and target cells. Large numbers of nucleated erythrocytes circulate, especially after splenectomy. Typically, the hemoglobin level falls progressively to less than 5 g/dL unless transfusions are given. The unconjugated serum bilirubin level is elevated. The serum iron level is high, with increasing saturation of iron-binding capacity. Lactate dehydrogenase activities are very high, reflecting ineffective erythropoiesis. Large amounts of fetal hemoglobin are contained in the erythrocytes. The level of Hb F exceeds 70% during the early years of life but tends to decline with increasing age.

■ TREATMENT

Transfusions of packed erythrocytes are given to maintain the hemoglobin level above 10 g/dL. This hypertransfusion has striking clinical benefit: it permits normal activity with comfort and prevents progressive marrow expansion and its attendant cosmetic problems and osteoporosis. Transfusions are necessary every 4 to 5 weeks.

Hemosiderosis is an inevitable and fatal consequence of prolonged transfusion therapy, because each 200 mL of erythrocytes contains about 200 mg of iron that cannot be physiologically excreted. The iron burden can be reduced with iron-chelating agents, especially desferoxamine. This must be given parenterally, administered subcutaneously at night over 8 to 12 hours using a battery-driven pump. In many patients, negative iron balance is possible. A chronic chelation program can reverse the poor prognosis of this disease if patient compliance with the demanding regimen can be obtained. Iron-chelating drugs, especially those that can be taken orally, are undergoing clinical testing. If efficacious and safe, these new drugs will improve compliance with chelation therapy and significantly reduce the incidence of hemosiderosis in chronically transfused patients.

Splenectomy is often necessary because of the size of the organ or because of secondary hypersplenism, but it has no effect on the basic hematologic disease. Immunization with pneumococcal polysaccharide vaccine is indicated, and prophylactic penicillin therapy is advocated by some authorities.

Bone marrow transplantation from HLA-identical and partly mismatched siblings has been performed in over 400 children with thalassemia. Early death from toxicity and graft-versus-host disease is low (<10%) in young patients without hepatic dysfunction. The risk of death is considerably higher for older patients, especially if liver function is already compromised by hemosiderosis. If an HLA-matched, healthy sibling is available, bone marrow transplantation should be considered, especially in a patient without symptoms of hemosiderosis. Introduction of a normal β-globin gene using gene therapy remains an area of active research.

OTHER THALASSEMIAS

■ ALPHA THALASSEMIAS

A group of diseases especially prevalent in Southeast Asians results from genetic deletions of α-chain genes. There are normally four α-chain genes. Five percent of African Americans have α-thalassemia trait associated with deletion of two α-chain genes. Clinically, it is characterized by microcytic anemia that is unresponsive to iron. Three and four α-chain deletions are rare among African Americans. The diagnosis is made by excluding other causes of anemia. Hemoglobin electrophoresis is not helpful after the immediate postnatal period. In the newborn period, hemoglobin electrophoresis shows 3% to 6% Hb Barts. Patients are asymptomatic but should be counseled so they may prevent well-meaning health care providers from prescribing iron for presumed iron deficiency or from performing a workup for anemia.

In Asians, the four distinct α-thalassemia syndromes are the silent carrier state, α-thalassemia trait, Hb H disease, and fetal hydrops syndrome. These result from increasing numbers of α-thalassemia gene deletions, from one to four. Deletion of four α-thalassemia genes produces the clinical picture of hydrops fetalis in utero. The predominant hemoglobin is Barts (γ_4). This variant has abnormal oxygen dissociation properties that make oxygen unavailable to the tissues, causing fetal death.

Deletion of three α-thalassemia genes causes the less severe Hb H disease. This is a moderately severe anemia that resembles thalassemia major or intermedia. It is characterized by 5% to 10% of unstable Hb H (β_4).

■ HEREDITARY PERSISTENCE OF HIGH FETAL HEMOGLOBIN

Hereditary persistence of high fetal hemoglobin (HPFH) is associated with high levels of normal fetal hemoglobin but few hematologic abnormalities. It occurs predominantly in black and Mediterranean people. The erythrocytes contain 15% to 30% Hb F. There is an even distribution of Hb F in the erythrocyte population, in contrast to the thalassemias, in which Hb F content varies from cell to cell. The HPFH homozygote has 100% Hb F but no significant anemia. If HPFH and a sickle gene affect the same person, only Hb S and Hb F are found. However, the even distribution of Hb F in the erythrocyte population prevents sickling, and hematologic and clinical symptoms are minimal.

(Abridged from Paul L. Martin and Howard A. Pearson, The Hemoglobinopathies and Thalassemias, in Oski, DeAngelis, Feigin, McMillan, Warshaw: *Principles and Practice of Pediatrics, Second Edition,* J.B. Lippincott, 1994.)

Oski's Essential Pediatrics,
edited by Kevin B. Johnson and Frank A. Oski.
Lippincott–Raven Publishers,
Philadelphia © 1997

122

The Hemolytic Anemias

INTRINSIC HEMOLYTIC ANEMIAS

■ HEREDITARY SPHEROCYTOSIS

Hereditary spherocytosis (HS; congenital hemolytic anemia, congenital acholuric jaundice) occurs predominantly in persons of North European ancestry, although it has been found in patients of many ethnic groups. The typical features are a familial hemolytic anemia of various degrees of severity, splenomegaly, and spherical erythrocytes found on the blood smear.

In about three quarters of patients, pedigree analysis indicates an autosomal dominant transmission. Sporadic dominant mutations have been invoked, and autosomal recessive transmission is suggested in some cases. The gene for HS is located on chromosome 8.

Pathophysiology

A deficiency or abnormality of the erythrocyte membrane structural protein spectrin appears to affect most patients with HS. This deficiency is associated with an accelerated loss of the erythrocyte membrane, which reduces the erythrocyte surface area. Because there is no concomitant loss of cellular volume, the erythrocytes assume a spherical shape. Increased membrane cation flux can be demonstrated.

The spleen is intrinsically involved in the hemolytic process. The splenic circulation imposes a metabolic stress on spherocytic cells. The spherocyte is relatively rigid and passes with difficulty through the splenic cords and sinuses. This results in their sequestration and destruction. The hemolytic process regresses after splenectomy, although biochemical and morphologic abnormalities persist.

Clinical Presentation

The disease may present in the neonatal period with anemia and hyperbilirubinemia that may require phototherapy or exchange transfusion. The anemia varies considerably in severity but tends to be similar within the same family. The patient usually has slight jaundice. Expansion of the marrow cavities occurs to a lesser extent than in thalassemia. The spleen is almost always palpably enlarged after 2 or 3 years of age. Pigmentary gallstones have occurred as early as 4 years of age. Aplastic crises associated with parvovirus infections are the most serious complications during childhood (see Chapter 123).

Laboratory Findings

The hemoglobin level ranges from 6 to 10 g/dL, and the reticulocyte count ranges from 5% to 20% (average, 10%). The spherocytic erythrocytes are smaller than normal erythrocytes and lack the central pallor of the biconcave disk, but only a relatively small proportion of the cells are spherocytic. There is erythroid hyperplasia in the marrow, but erythrocyte precursors are not spherocytic.

Abnormality of the erythrocyte can be demonstrated by osmotic fragility studies. When erythrocytes are placed in hypotonic saline solutions, water enters the cells, causing them to swell. The normal biconcave erythrocyte can increase its volume, but the spherical cell already has maximal volume for its surface area and hemolyzes at a higher saline concentration (ie, increased osmotic fragility) than normal. In 10% to 20% of HS cases, the osmotic abnormality can be demonstrated only if the blood is incubated at 37°C (98.6°F) for 24 hours.

HS must be differentiated from other congenital hemolytic states. Family history, blood smear, and osmotic fragility studies offer the most diagnostic value. Acquired spherocytosis of the erythrocytes is seen in autoimmune hemolytic anemias, in which the spherocytosis is often more pronounced than in HS, and the direct Coombs' test result is positive. It may be difficult to differentiate HS from hemolytic disease because of ABO incompatibility in the newborn infant. A period of observation may be necessary to clarify the diagnosis.

Therapy

Splenectomy almost invariably produces a clinical cure, although in a few instances of severe HS with recessive transmission, the operation was not curative. Splenectomy should be deferred if possible until the patient is at least 5 or 6 years of age. If anemia is severe enough to impair growth or normal activity, the operation can be considered earlier after a period of observation. Splenectomy prevents gallstones and eliminates the threat of aplastic crises.

After splenectomy, jaundice and reticulocytosis disappear. The hemoglobin level becomes normal, although the spherocytosis and osmotic fragility abnormalities become more pronounced. Overwhelming sepsis after splenectomy occurs infrequently if the surgery is delayed until the child is 5 or 6 years of age, but the febrile child must be carefully evaluated for sepsis. Polyvalent pneumococcal vaccine should be given before splenectomy. Prophylactic penicillin therapy after splenectomy is advocated by some authorities and is definitely indicated if the operation is done before the child is 6 years of age.

■ HEREDITARY ELLIPTOCYTOSIS

Some oval or elliptical erythrocytes may be seen in a number of conditions, especially thalassemia and iron deficiency; however, they occur in much larger numbers as a dominantly inherited trait in hereditary elliptocytosis (HE; hereditary ovalocytosis). Fifteen percent to 50% of the circulating erythrocytes of these persons are elongated. In most patients, there is no associated hemolysis, and the hematologic values, including reticulocyte counts, are normal. However, in about 10% of patients with elliptical cells, there is evidence of hemolysis, with hemoglobin levels averaging 8 to 10 g/dL and reticulocytes comprising 5% to 15% of the cells.

Pathophysiology

A structural abnormality of spectrin has been described in erythrocytes from some HE patients with or without hemolysis. The bases for hemolytic HE and HE without hemolysis are unclear. In most family studies of hemolytic HE, one parent has elliptical erythrocytes without hemolysis, and the other parent is hematologically normal.

Clinical Presentation

HE with hemolysis may be associated with neonatal jaundice, but characteristic elliptocytosis may not be evident at birth. The blood smear instead shows bizarre poikilocytes and pyknocytes. The usual features of chronic hemolytic process, including anemia, jaundice, splenomegaly, and osseous changes, may be seen later. Cholelithiasis occurs in later childhood, and aplastic crises have been reported.

Laboratory Findings

The morphology of the erythrocytes is the most important diagnostic feature. Elliptical cells characterized by a length more than 1.5 times the diameter account for 15% to 70% of the erythrocytes. The reticulocyte count is increased. Erythroid hyperplasia is evident in the bone marrow, but the erythrocyte precursors are not elliptical. Increased erythrocyte osmotic fragility and increased thermal instability occur in hemolytic HE. This has sometimes led to designating cases of hemolytic HE as pyropoikilocytosis.

Therapy

If there is significant hemolysis, splenectomy is usually beneficial. Erythrocyte morphology is not changed after the operation, and it may become even more abnormal.

■ PYRUVATE KINASE DEFICIENCY

An inherited deficiency of pyruvate kinase (PK) is the most frequent of the erythrocyte glycolytic enzyme deficiencies. PK activity, measured in the erythrocytes, is markedly reduced, but the enzyme activity in other blood cells and tissues is normal.

Pathophysiology

The disease is caused by homozygosity for an autosomal recessive gene, which results in markedly decreased production of a mutant PK isoenzyme. The PK-deficient erythrocytes are ATP depleted, and their survival is compromised. Levels of glycolytic intermediates, especially 2,3-diphosphoglycerate (2,3-DPG), are greatly increased. The increase in 2,3-DPG causes a right shift of the oxygen dissociation curve, which may reduce symptoms of anemia. Heterozygotes for PK deficiency have intermediate enzyme levels.

Clinical Presentation

In PK-deficient homozygotes, there is a broad spectrum of clinical and hematologic findings, ranging from a mild, completely compensated hemolytic state to severe anemia. Anemia and hyperbilirubinemia may occur in the neonatal period. In the older patient, pallor, scleral icterus, and splenomegaly are usual findings.

Laboratory Findings

The blood smear shows polychromatophilic erythrocytes, indicating an elevated reticulocyte count. A few small, spiculated erythrocytes are seen, but no spherocytes are found. Osmotic fragility is normal.

Treatment

Hyperbilirubinemia in the neonatal period may require exchange transfusion. Severe disease may require repeated transfusions for anemia during infancy. Splenectomy, although not curative, often improves the anemia and should be considered in patients with severe disease. Marked reticulocytosis occurs after splenectomy.

■ GLUCOSE-6-PHOSPHATE DEHYDROGENASE DEFICIENCY SYNDROMES

Glucose-6-phosphate dehydrogenase (G6PD) deficiency results in two kinds of hematologic problems: a common, acute condition manifested by hemolytic episodes induced by infection or certain drugs and a rare, chronic, nonspherocytic hemolytic anemia.

The G6PD gene is on the X chromosome. In the hemizygous affected male, the condition results from inheritance of one abnormal G6PD gene. In the affected homozygous female, two abnormal genes are inherited. The normal G6PD enzyme found in most Caucasian populations is designated, G6PD B$^+$. A normal isozyme designated G6PD A$^+$ is common in blacks. More than 100 distinct enzyme variants of G6PD have been documented.

Pathophysiology

Thirteen percent of African-American males and 2% of African-American females have a mutant enzyme called G6PD A$^-$, which is unstable and associated with reduced erythrocyte enzyme activity (5% to 15% of normal). Affected persons of Mediterranean, Arabic, and Asian ethnic groups have relatively high frequencies of G6PD deficiency because of a variant designated G6PD B$^-$. The enzyme activity of the homozygous female or the hemizygous male is less than 5% of normal.

G6PD, the rate-limiting enzyme of the pentose phosphate pathway, is crucial for protection of the erythrocytes from oxidant stress. In G6PD deficiency, oxidant metabolites of a number of drugs produce denaturation and precipitation of hemoglobin, causing erythrocyte injury and rapid hemolysis. Hemolysis occurs only if the patient is exposed to oxidant drugs, such as antipyretics, sulfonamides, antimalarials, and naphthaquinolones, or to the fava bean. The degree of hemolysis varies with the drug, the amount ingested, and the severity of the enzyme deficiency in the patient.

Laboratory Findings

Hemoglobinemia and hemoglobinuria occur 24 to 48 hours after the ingestion of an oxidant substance. The hemoglobin level may fall as low as 2 to 5 g/dL. Heinz bodies are not visible on stained blood smears. They can be initially demonstrated on supravital preparations, but they disappear after 3 or 4 days. Spontaneous recovery is usual and is heralded by reticulocytosis and an increase in hemoglobin concentration, starting 4 or 5 days after the acute hemolytic episode.

Diagnosis depends on direct or indirect demonstration of reduced G6PD activity in erythrocytes. By direct measurement, enzyme activity in affected persons is less than 15% of normal. The reduction of enzyme activity is more extreme in Caucasians and Asians than in G6PD-deficient blacks. Immediately after a hemolytic event, G6PD activity may be normal. A repeat examination several weeks later may be necessary to prove the diagnosis.

Therapy

Prevention of hemolysis by avoiding oxidant drugs is important. Males belonging to ethnic groups in which there is a significant incidence of G6PD deficiency should be tested for the defect before drugs that are known to be potent oxidants are given. After hemolysis has occurred, supportive therapy is indicated, including blood transfusions if the anemia is severe and the patient is symptomatic.

■ CHRONIC NONSPHEROCYTIC HEMOLYTIC ANEMIA ASSOCIATED WITH GLUCOSE-6-PHOSPHATE DEHYDROGENASE DEFICIENCY

Instances of chronic hemolytic anemias not associated with oxidant drug ingestion have been associated with profound deficiencies of G6PD due to several enzyme variants. These have occurred predominantly in persons of North European ancestry. For this X-linked disease, splenectomy has been of minimal value.

EXTRINSIC HEMOLYTIC ANEMIAS

Agents that damage erythrocytes may lead to their premature destruction. The most clearly defined of these agents are the antibodies associated with immune hemolysis. Antibodies directed against specific intrinsic membrane antigens damage the erythrocytes and produce hemolysis. The most important feature of these diseases is the positive Coombs'

test, which detects immunoglobulins or components of complement on the erythrocyte surface.

■ AUTOIMMUNE HEMOLYTIC ANEMIAS

In the autoimmune hemolytic anemias (AIHAs), the patient's antibodies are directed against the erythrocytes. The factors evoking such an autoimmune response are unknown, but they include viral infections and occasionally specific drugs.

Pathophysiology

AIHAs associated with an underlying disease process such as lymphoma, lupus erythematosus, or immunodeficiency are said to be secondary. In idiopathic AIHA, there is no such underlying disease. Drugs such as penicillin cephalosporins and α-methyldopa evoke the formation of antibodies in some patients.

Clinical Manifestations

AIHAs occur in two clinical patterns. The first type, a fulminant variety that occurs in infants and young children, is frequently preceded by a respiratory infection. The onset is acute, with pallor, jaundice, and hemoglobinuria. The spleen is enlarged. A consistent response to corticosteroid therapy, low mortality rate, and complete recovery are characteristic. No underlying disease is found. A second type of AIHA has a prolonged course and a significant mortality rate. Underlying diseases are frequently found.

Laboratory Findings

The anemia may be severe, with hemoglobin levels less than 6 g/dL. Spherocytosis and polychromasia are prominent. Reticulocytosis and nucleated erythrocytes are found, and leukocytosis is common. The platelet count is usually normal; occasionally, there is concomitant immune thrombocytopenic purpura (ie, Evans syndrome).

The direct and indirect Coombs' test results are positive, indicating the presence of antibodies attached to the erythrocytes or free in the serum. These antibodies belong to the IgG class. They are often nonspecific panagglutinins, but they may have specificity for common antigens of the Rh system (eg, LW). Because of spontaneous erythrocyte agglutination, the patient may be mistakenly typed as blood group AB, Rh positive. In acute transient cases, only complement is found on the erythrocytes, chiefly the C3 and C4 components. In chronic AIHA, a pure IgG Coombs' test result is often found.

Treatment

Transfusion may be required, but it offers only transient benefit. It is difficult to find compatible blood, and it is often necessary to give blood that is "incompatible" as judged by the crossmatch. Prednisone should be administered in a dosage of 2 to 4 mg/kg every 24 hours. Treatment should be continued until hemolysis decreases. The dose can then be gradually reduced. The acute form of disease usually remits spontaneously within a few weeks or months, but the Coombs' test may remain positive for an extended period.

Splenectomy may be beneficial in severe refractory cases. Immunosuppressive agents have been used in patients refractory to conventional therapy. In AIHA secondary to lymphoma or lupus erythematosus, the disease tends to be chronic, and the course of the underlying disease determines ultimate prognosis.

(Abridged from Paul L. Martin and Howard A. Pearson, The Hemolytic Anemias, in Oski, DeAngelis, Feigin, McMillan, Warshaw: *Principles and Practice of Pediatrics, Second Edition*, J.B. Lippincott, 1994.)

Oski's Essential Pediatrics, edited by Kevin B. Johnson and Frank A. Oski. Lippincott–Raven Publishers, Philadelphia © 1997

123

The Hypoplastic and Aplastic Anemias

HYPOPLASTIC ANEMIAS

The hypoplastic anemias (*ie,* pure erythrocyte anemias, aregenerative anemias) constitute an uncommon group of congenital or acquired blood disorders characterized by anemia, reticulocytopenia, and a paucity of erythroid precursors in otherwise normally cellular bone marrow. Unlike the aplastic anemias (*ie,* pancytopenias), the other formed elements of the blood are usually present in normal or increased numbers.

■ CONGENITAL HYPOPLASTIC ANEMIA

At the 1938 meeting of the American Pediatric Society, Diamond and Blackfan described four children with severe aregenerative anemia that developed during the first year of life and required regular transfusions for survival. Only about 300 cases of congenital hypoplastic anemia (CHA) have been described in the literature, but many more cases have been recognized.

A familial recurrence in some families suggests that genetic factors may occasionally be operative, but in most cases, no inherited pattern is evident. About 25% of the patients have physical abnormalities of various kinds, including short stature and facial, cardiac, and renal abnormalities. A subset of patients have thumbs with three rather than the usual two phalanges (*ie,* Wranne syndrome).

Clinical Presentation

Anemia at or shortly after birth is the presenting manifestation of CHA. About a quarter of the patients are pale at birth. Sixty-five percent are anemic by 6 months of age, and almost all are anemic by 1 year of age. CHA described in older infants, particularly those reported before 1970,

must be viewed with some skepticism, because the cases may have represented transient erythroblastopenia of childhood.

Laboratory Findings

At the time of diagnosis, the hemoglobin levels may be as low as 2.5 g/dL. The erythrocytes are macrocytic and have biochemical properties of fetal erythrocyte (*ie,* increased levels of Hb F for the patient's age, presence of the i erythrocyte antigen, and increased levels of age-dependent erythrocyte enzymes such as glucose-6-phosphate dehydrogenase). These findings may be of limited diagnostic value in early infancy when fetal cells are still present.

The reticulocyte count is characteristically very low, even in the presence of severe anemia. The remainder of the peripheral blood count is usually normal, although elevated platelet counts and modest neutropenia have occasionally been found.

Serum bilirubin levels are normal. Serum iron levels are usually elevated with increased transferrin saturation. Plasma and urinary levels of erythropoietin (EPO) are elevated.

The most important diagnostic features are found in the bone marrow. The marrow in patients with CHA is normally cellular with normal numbers of megakaryocytes, lymphocytes, and myeloid precursors. However, erythrocyte precursors at every level of development are absent or markedly reduced. The proportion of myeloid to erythroid precursors in the bone marrow (M:E ratio), normally 3:1, is markedly increased (10:1 to 200:1). In some patients, a few primitive pronormoblasts can be recognized, but no more mature erythroid precursors are seen. Bone marrow erythroid cultures consistently have few BFU-E and CFU-E.

Therapy

The degree of anemia is often so profound at presentation that erythrocyte transfusions are necessary. About 10% to 20% of patients are refractory to therapy and continue to require regular transfusions. Transfusions with packed, leukocyte-poor erythrocytes are given to maintain a hemoglobin level compatible with normal activity and comfort, usually above 8.0 g/dL.

When chronic transfusion therapy is necessary, transfusional hemosiderosis inevitably occurs. Serum ferritin levels should be monitored periodically, and chelation therapy should be begun when there is evidence of tissue iron overload.

The use of adrenocorticotropic hormone and corticosteroids in CHA was suggested as early as 1949, but it was not until 1961 that a relatively large number of steroid-treated patients were reported. Between 60% and 70% of patients respond to corticosteroid therapy. The mechanism of steroid action may involve an enhancement of the effect of EPO on CFU-E proliferation and maturation. Corticosteroids, such as prednisone, are administered. Response is heralded by the appearance of erythropoietic precursors in the bone marrow within 1 to 2 weeks, followed by reticulocytosis and an increase in the hemoglobin level. The full dose of prednisone is continued until the hemoglobin attains a normal level. The dose can then be gradually decreased until a minimal effective dose is attained. In many instances, it is possible to administer corticosteroids on alternate-day schedules that further decrease steroid side effects. Some patients do not respond to the usual dose of steroids and should be given a trial with larger doses. About 20% to 30%

of these children are nonresponsive to steroids and require regular blood transfusions.

Children refractory to steroids have usually not responded to other forms of therapy including androgenic and immunosuppressive agents. Bone marrow transplantation has been effective for a few patients.

■ TRANSIENT ERYTHROBLASTIC ANEMIA OF CHILDHOOD

Transient erythroblastic anemia of childhood (TEC) is a striking syndrome of temporary failure of erythropoiesis, which is increasingly encountered in clinical practice. It is characterized by moderate to severe aregenerative anemia in an otherwise healthy child. The condition is self-limited and usually does not recur.

Clinical Presentation

The condition occurs in children older than 1 year of age, but it has been seen as early as 4 months of age. Pallor and symptoms of anemia are the usual presenting manifestations. Because the anemia reflects a complete cessation of erythropoiesis without increased hemolysis, the anemia develops very slowly.

If a patient has a hemoglobin level of 5 g/dL on presentation, it can be assumed that erythrocyte production has been minimal for at least 2 months. Because the anemia develops insidiously, pallor or symptoms may not be noticed by the parents. Except for the features of anemia, the remainder of the physical examination is normal.

Laboratory Findings

The degree of anemia may be severe, as low as 2.5 g/dL, with a low reticulocyte count. The leukocyte count is normal. The platelet count is usually normal but may be elevated. Other laboratory findings include a high serum iron level reflecting decreased use. The bone marrow shows a paucity of erythrocyte precursors with a high M:E ratio. The other marrow elements are normal.

Recovery occurs spontaneously within a few weeks and is accompanied by a brisk reticulocytosis and rapid increase in hemoglobin level.

The major differential diagnosis of TEC is CHA, particularly in the infant younger than 1 year of age. In contrast to CHA, in TEC the erythrocyte population at presentation has age-appropriate characteristics; a mean corpuscular volume of 70 to 80 fL; Hb F less than 2% to 5%; normal levels of erythrocyte age-dependent enzymes (G6PD); and the usual adult I erythrocyte antigen. Erythrocyte adenosine deaminase levels are not elevated.

A patient first seen in the recovery state of TEC may be erroneously considered to have a hemolytic process because of the concomitant low hemoglobin and high reticulocyte count. Observation can clarify the diagnosis.

Therapy

No specific therapy is necessary. Corticosteroid therapy is not indicated. If the anemia is severe, a small erythrocyte transfusion may be considered to sustain the child until recovery occurs. Most children have no recurrence of this disease.

■ APLASTIC CRISIS OF HEMOLYTIC ANEMIAS ASSOCIATED WITH PARVOVIRUS INFECTION

Episodes of exaggerated anemia and reticulocytopenia in patients with various kinds of hemolytic anemias have been recognized for many years. Such episodes usually occur in the wake of viral infections and often affect several family members.

A correlation between aplastic crises patients in sickle-cell disease and infection by the parvovirus was established in 1981 by the demonstration of virus particles in the blood of these patients. It is likely that most severe aplastic crises in patients with hemolytic anemias are caused by the parvovirus, an organism that also has been established as the cause of erythema infectiosum (ie, fifth disease). Intrauterine parvovirus infection has been invoked as a possible cause of severe anemia and nonimmunologic hydrops fetalis.

Clinical Presentation

During aplastic crises, the degree of anemia worsens and jaundice decreases. There is profound reticulocytopenia and no erythrocyte precursors in the bone marrow. Early in the aplastic crisis, parvovirus particles can be found in the serum by electron microscopic examination. Later evidence of infection can be documented by changes in antibody titers in acute and convalescent sera.

Treatment

Supportive blood transfusions are indicated if the degree of anemia is severe or if the patient is symptomatic. Because parvovirus infections evoke protective levels of circulating antibodies, aplastic crises do not recur in the same patient.

APLASTIC ANEMIAS

The aplastic anemias have diverse causes whose common features are varying degrees of peripheral pancytopenia accompanied by marked hypocellularity of the bone marrow.

■ ACQUIRED APLASTIC ANEMIA

Pathophysiology

In many instances, aplastic anemia is believed to be a result of destruction or dysfunction of the pluripotential stem cell (CFU-S) that is the progenitor of erythrocytes, platelets, monocytes, and granulocytes. An environmental toxin or agent is believed to cause the stem cell damage, but in as many as a third of patients, aplastic anemia appears to be an autoimmune disorder mediated through an inhibitory process involving T lymphocytes. Other mechanisms, such as an abnormal microenvironment for bone marrow proliferation, have been postulated.

Many drugs, infections, and environmental factors have been associated with the development of aplastic anemia. Some of these agents are directly toxic to the bone marrow and regularly produce marrow hypoplasia in a dose-dependent manner. Such obligate marrow suppressors include ionizing radiation, a variety of chemicals, and many antineoplastic agents.

Another group of drugs produces marrow hypoplasia in only a small proportion of patients who receive them, so that the disease is considered to represent an idiosyncratic reaction. These include a variety of antibiotics, anti-inflammatory agents, and anticonvulsants. Chloramphenicol has been the drug most frequently associated with aplastic anemia. It has been estimated that only about 1 of 20,000 to 50,000 persons taking chloramphenicol develops aplastic anemia, but in as many as 50% of the cases of drug-related aplastic anemia, chloramphenicol has been implicated. A particularly serious form of aplastic anemia occurs in the wake of viral hepatitis. In about half of these patients, no causative factor can be implicated, and their disease is designated idiopathic, although an environmental factor cannot be excluded.

Clinical Presentation

The signs and symptoms of aplastic anemia reflect the degree of pancytopenia at presentation. The most common initial manifestations are petechiae and bruising as a consequence of thrombocytopenia. Pallor and bacterial infections develop as anemia and neutropenia ensue. The spleen, liver, and lymph nodes are not enlarged.

Laboratory Findings

A variable degree of pancytopenia is found at diagnosis. Platelet counts are moderately to severely reduced (5000 to 50,000/mm³). A moderate to severe, usually macrocytic anemia (Hb of 3 to 10 g/dL; mean corpuscular volume >90 fL) with low reticulocyte counts (<0.1%) and neutropenia (absolute neutrophil count <1500/mm³) are observed at the time of diagnosis or develop within a few months.

Diagnosis is established by examination of the bone marrow by aspiration and biopsy. The marrow is hypocellular due to a loss of hematopoietic elements. Megakaryocytes are reduced, and fat is increased. Bone marrow cultures reveal a marked reduction of progenitor cells of erythroid, granulocytic, and megakaryocytic lines.

The disease is classified as severe if two of the following three peripheral blood value abnormalities occur in combination with severe hypocellularity of the marrow biopsy: neutrophil count of less than 950/mm³, platelet count of less than 20,000/mm³, and a corrected reticulocyte count of less than 1%.

Therapy

Anemia and thrombocytopenia may require transfusions of erythrocytes and platelets. These should be used sparingly to prevent isoimmunization that could compromise future bone marrow transplantation. If an HLA-compatible sibling is available, bone marrow transplantation is the preferred treatment. The survival rate after bone marrow transplantation for young, untransfused patients with aplastic anemia is between 85% and 95%. Because the patient is already aplastic, reduction in the conditioning before bone marrow transplantation has allowed most patients to avoid serious long-term side effects, including infertility. Clinical trials with various hematopoietic colony-stimulating factors have been unsuccessful. The use of HLA-incompatible mar-

row transplantation has been attempted with success in a few patients.

In patients who do not have an HLA-compatible sibling as a donor, various forms of immunosuppressive therapy have been employed, including injections of horse or sheep anti-thymocyte or anti-lymphocyte globulin, high-dose methylprednisone, and cyclophosphamide. Response rates as high as 50% to 60% have been reported. Androgens have been ineffective in severe aplastic anemia but may produce a degree of hematologic improvement in patients with moderate disease.

■ CONGENITAL APLASTIC ANEMIA

Congenital aplastic anemia (CAA; Fanconi syndrome, constitutional aplastic anemia) was first described by Professor Fanconi in Switzerland in 1927. More than 600 cases have been reported in many ethnic groups. Although CAA is genetically determined and transmitted as an autosomal recessive disorder, it is not usually hematologically evident during infancy and early childhood. Clinical CAA is characterized by severe pancytopenia, hypoplasia of the bone marrow, and a constellation of physical abnormalities. Some patients do not have obvious physical anomalies.

Pathophysiology

CAA is believed to be caused by an ill-defined defect in DNA that renders the patient's cells susceptible to damage by environmental agents. This sensitivity may predispose the patient to bone marrow failure.

The cells of these patients demonstrate abnormal mitotic divisions in tissue culture. This is evident in phytohemagglutinin-stimulated lymphocyte cultures. Structural abnormalities include chromatid breaks, exchanges, and gaps and endoreduplication. These occur in more than 10% of metaphases. Other cell culture lines from these patients, including skin fibroblasts, show similar changes, and this has made prenatal diagnosis possible.

Clinical Presentation

Short stature and generalized hyperpigmentation affect most patients. About half of the patients with CAA have congenital skeletal anomalies. The most striking of these include bilateral absence or hypoplasia of the thumb, sometimes accompanied by abnormalities of the radii. About one third of patients have renal abnormalities, including unilateral aplasia and horseshoe kidney. About 50% of patients have no gross anatomic abnormalities.

The onset of progressive bone marrow failure is initially manifested by petechiae and ecchymosis secondary to thrombocytopenia between 2 and 22 years of age (mean age, 7). Anemia and neutropenia develop somewhat later than thrombocytopenia.

Laboratory Findings

Disordered erythropoiesis is manifested by macrocytosis (mean corpuscular volume >90 fL) and elevated levels of Hb F before the onset of marrow failure. Ultimately, severe pancytopenia develops. Serial bone marrow examinations show progressive hypocellularity and ultimately frank aplasia. The peripheral blood lymphocytes, when cultured in the presence of diepoxybutane, an alkylating agent, consistently show chromosomal abnormalities. This is a useful test when the physical stigmata of Fanconi anemia are absent.

Treatment

Supportive therapy, including transfusions of erythrocytes and platelets, offers only temporary benefit. In the past, about three quarters of these patients died within 2 years of the onset of marrow failure.

Therapy with pharmacologic doses of androgenic hormones produces a hematologic improvement in more than two thirds of patients. The response to these agents may be sustained for several years, but maintenance therapy is usually necessary. Complications of androgen therapy, including masculinization and liver dysfunction, are common. Ultimately, most patients become refractory to androgens and again require transfusions. Bone marrow transplantation using HLA-compatible siblings who do not themselves have CAA has been successful in many patients.

Long-term complications of the disease and its therapy include androgen-associated hepatic disease and tumors and an increased risk of acute myeloid leukemia and other malignancies.

(Abridged from Paul L. Martin and Howard A. Pearson, The Hypoplastic and Aplastic Anemias, in Oski, DeAngelis, Feigin, McMillan, Warshaw: *Principles and Practice of Pediatrics, Second Edition*, J.B. Lippincott, 1994.)

Oski's Essential Pediatrics,
edited by Kevin B. Johnson and Frank A. Oski.
Lippincott–Raven Publishers,
Philadelphia © 1997

124

The Spleen and Lymph Nodes

The spleen and lymph nodes are the major components of the mononuclear-phagocyte system (MPS), which serves as a filter, delivers antigens to the immune system, and removes damaged cells and particulate matter. Originally called the reticuloendothelial system, the MPS consists of fixed phagocytic cells in different organs: macrophages in lymph nodes and the spleen, Kupffer cells in the liver, and histiocytes in connective tissue. These cells all share a common derivation from circulating blood monocytes. Functionally, these phagocytes interact locally with lymphocytes and play an essential role in the recognition and interaction of immunocompetent cells with antigens. The MPS constitutes a crucial component of our immunologic defense mechanisms.

■ SPLENOMEGALY

Splenomegaly is the most frequent and important clinical problem involving the spleen. The most important causes of splenic enlargement are listed in Table 124–1.

■ HYPERSPLENISM

Hypersplenism is a clinical syndrome in which normal splenic function becomes excessive as the spleen and its MPS tissues enlarge. The more formal definition includes the following criteria: splenomegaly, a deficiency of at least one or more of the peripheral blood cell lines, normal or increased levels of bone marrow precursors, and an expectation that splenectomy will resolve the cytopenias.

As the spleen enlarges, its minimal erythrocyte reservoir can greatly expand to sequester up to 45% of the total erythro-

TABLE 124-1. Causes of Spenomegaly in Children

HYPERPLASIA OF THE MONOCYTE-PHAGOCYTE SYSTEM

Excessive antigenic stimulation
  Viral infections
    Infectious mononucleosis
    Cytomegalovirus
    Acquired immunodeficiency syndrome
  Bacterial infections
    Septicemia
    Endocarditis
    Salmonella
  Protozoal infections
    Toxoplasmosis
    Malaria
  Fungal infections
    Histoplasmosis
Disorders of immunoregulation
    Juvenile rheumatoid arthritis
    Systemic lupus erythematosus
    Serum sickness
Excessive destruction of blood cells
    Hereditary spherocytosis
    Sickle-cell anemia
    Neonatal Rh or ABO incompatibility

NEOPLASTIC INFILTRATION

Acute leukemias
Hodgkin's disease
Non-Hodgkin's lymphoma
Neuroblastoma
Histiocytosis X

DISORDERED SPLENIC BLOOD FLOW

Cavernous transformation of the portal vein
Hepatic cirrhosis
Congestive heart failure

INFILTRATION WITH ABNORMAL MATERIAL

Gaucher's disease
Niemann-Pick disease

SPACE-OCCUPYING LESIONS

Hematomas
Pseudocysts
Congenital cysts

EXTRAMEDULLARY HEMATOPOIESIS

Thalassemia major
Osteopetrosis

cyte mass. The sequestered cells are not destroyed; they exchange slowly with circulating blood. As plasma volume expands to preserve circulating blood volume, the dilutional effect decreases the hemoglobin concentration in peripheral blood. However, erythrocyte mass remains normal or increases. The anemia is, in large part, dilutional. There may be excessive erythrocyte destruction by splenic macrophages, but it is limited. Erythrocyte survival is only slightly decreased, and overt hemolysis is rare. The sequestration of leukocytes and platelets may be more severe than that of erythrocytes.

The most common cause of hypersplenism is venous obstruction. Because of the absence of valves in the portal venous system, an increase in portal pressure is reflected immediately in the splenic venous sinuses. This impairs blood flow out of the cords and results in splenic sequestration and hypersplenism.

Hypersplenism in children often is caused by portal hypertension due to extrahepatic venous obstruction, often secondary to thrombosis of the portal vein due to umbilical venous catheterization, septic omphalitis, or thrombosis due to dehydration or shock. Less common causes of extrahepatic obstruction include congenital stenosis, atresia, or aneurysms of the splenic or hepatic portal venous system. Intrahepatic obstructions include cirrhosis due most commonly to hepatitis, cystic fibrosis of the pancreas, galactosemia, Wilson's disease, and alpha₁-antitrypsin deficiency. Schistosomiasis and malaria are important causes in endemic areas.

Children with hypersplenism can present with simple fatigue, pallor, and irritability or with unexplained splenomegaly. When the vascular obstruction is beyond the splenic vein, portal hypertension causes increased flow through minor collateral vessels between the portal and systemic circulation. Increased flow through the superficial abdominal and hemorrhoidal veins can cause clinically recognizable dilatation of the superficial veins on the abdominal wall and hemorrhoids, respectively. Dilatation of the short gastric and esophageal veins can result in esophageal varices, which may present with sudden and catastrophic gastrointestinal hemorrhage. Laboratory studies reveal neutropenia, thrombocytopenia, and anemia, singly or in combination, with evidence of active hematopoiesis in the bone marrow. Hepatocellular disease may be evident. Esophagoscopy is the most accurate means for confirming esophageal varices. Angiography, measurements of portal venous pressure, and scans using radioactively labeled blood cells can be used to evaluate the vascular obstruction.

Therapy depends on the site and nature of the vascular obstruction. Splenectomy cures the pancytopenia, but it is usually not indicated. The leukopenia and thrombocytopenia are rarely severe enough to cause sufficient infection or bleeding to justify any therapy. Splenectomy carries significant risks and may limit the potential for subsequent shunting procedures by removing the splenic vein. To prevent esophageal variceal hemorrhage, surgical procedures that relieve the pressure may be helpful by shunting blood from the obstructed hepatic portal system directly to the systemic circulation. In the young child, direct anastomosis between the portal vein and the inferior vena cavae (ie, portacaval shunt) is preferred to shunts between the splenic and renal veins.

Hypersplenism occurs less frequently as a result of splenomegaly in the absence of venous obstruction. Specific causes include infections such as malaria and storage diseases such as Gaucher's disease.

The splenic sequestration crisis is a distinct form of acute hypersplenism in young children with sickle-cell anemia, and it is an important cause of death. Even after functional hyposplenism develops, young children with sickle-cell disease may develop sudden and massive splenic enlargement with sequestration of large portions of blood volume. These children manifest sudden weakness, dyspnea, left-sided abdominal pain, and increasing splenomegaly. So much blood can be trapped within the spleen that death due to hypovolemia can rapidly result. Treatment consists of restoration of blood volume and transfusion. To prevent recurrences, splenectomy is performed after one or two episodes of sequestration.

■ LYMPHADENOPATHY

By adult standards, almost all children have lymphadenopathy. Absence of palpable cervical or inguinal nodes in children is unusual and even may provide a clinical clue to an underlying immune deficiency. Common viral or bacterial illnesses of childhood often result in additional lymph node enlargement that can be dramatic. These factors explain the difficulty in determining whether enlarged lymph nodes in children represent a normal finding, transient hyperplasia in response to a simple viral illness, or more serious underlying pathology. This decision is based on clinical experience and judgment, but general guidelines are useful. Normal nodes usually do not exceed 2.5 cm in diameter and demonstrate neither warmth, tenderness, fluctuance, overlying erythema, nor any tendency to mat together into less well-defined masses. The groups of nodes involved are important. Palpable cervical, axillary, and

TABLE 124-2. Causes of Generalized Lymphadenopathy in Children

INFECTIONS
Viral
    Common upper respiratory infections
    Infectious mononucleosis
    Cytomegalovirus
    Acquired immunodeficiency syndrome
    Rubella
    Varicella
    Measles
Bacterial
    Septicemia
    Typhoid fever
    Tuberculosis
Protozoal
    Toxoplasmosis
Fungal
    Coccidioidomycosis

AUTOIMMUNE DISORDERS AND HYPERSENSITIVITY STATES
Juvenile rheumatoid arthritis
Systemic lupus erythematosus
Serum sickness
Drug reactions (eg, phenytoin, allopurinol, isoniazid)

ABNORMAL PROLIFERATION OF CELLS
Acute leukemias
Non-Hodgkin's lymphoma
Hodgkin's lymphoma
Neuroblastoma
Histiocytosis X

STORAGE DISEASES
Gaucher's disease
Niemann-Pick disease

inguinal nodes are expected; however, supraclavicular nodes, if noticed at all, should be no greater than 1 to 2 mm.

Lymphadenopathy can be caused by an increase in the number of normal lymphocytes and macrophages during a response to an antigen (eg, viral illness such as mononucleosis), nodal infiltration by inflammatory cells in response to an infection localized to the nodes themselves (eg, lymphadenitis), proliferation of neoplastic lymphocytes or macrophages (eg, lymphoma), or infiltration of nodes by metabolite-laden macrophages in storage diseases (eg, Gaucher's disease).

The following sections provide an overview of lymphadenopathy, the most common clinical problem related to lymph nodes and one of the more frequent diagnostic problems in pediatrics. The differential diagnosis of lymphadenopathy has much in common with that of splenomegaly, which is not surprising in view of the common MPS functions of the two organs. Most children with lymphadenopathy have benign disorders, but, in a few children, serious and even life-threatening problems will be identified.

Generalized Lymphadenopathy

Lymphadenopathy is considered to be generalized when it involves enlargement of two or more noncontiguous lymph node regions. Disorders causing generalized lymphadenopathy are usually associated with other findings in the history, physical examination, and laboratory data that usually make it relatively easy to establish a diagnosis. Hepatosplenomegaly often is an associated finding. A careful search for any significant clinical or laboratory abnormalities is essential (Table 124–2). Common causes of lymphadenopathy are discussed below.

Infection

Viral infections are the most common cause of generalized lymphadenopathy. The nodal enlargement is most often the result of transient responses to common viral upper respiratory infections. Other specific viral infections associated with adenopathy include infectious mononucleosis and cytomegalovirus. Rubella, varicella, and measles are causes readily recognized on the basis of their exanthems. Acquired immunodeficiency syndrome (AIDS) is becoming an increasingly important cause of lymphadenopathy. Viral infections are usually associated with soft and minimally tender nodes. Bacterial infections are associated with more tender, warm, and sometimes fluctuant nodes with overlying erythema. In some cases, the bacterial infection is acute and associated with toxic symptoms, as with septicemia and typhoid fever. In other instances, such as tuberculosis, systemic symptoms are much less severe. Other infectious causes include *Chlamydia*, protozoa (eg, toxoplasmosis) and fungi (eg, coccidioidomycosis).

Abnormal Proliferation of Cells in Lymph Nodes

Although malignancies are not a frequent cause of lymphadenopathy in children, they always must be considered because of the importance of rapidly establishing a diagnosis and instituting therapy. Lymph nodes enlarged because of malignant disease are usually nontender and are not associated with overlying erythema; the nodes may have a rubbery texture, and groups of nodes may become matted together, losing their individual character. Acute lymphoblastic leukemia, the most common childhood malignancy, is associated with lymphadenopathy in as many as 70% of these patients, but this is usually an incidental finding and not the presenting complaint. Lymphadenopathy is a frequent finding at presentation of the acute nonlymphoblastic leukemias.

Non-Hodgkin's lymphoma is often associated with bilateral adenopathy, and Hodgkin's disease more often presents with unilateral involvement. Occasionally, lymphadenopathy is the presenting sign of neuroblastoma.

Histiocytic infiltration of nodes occurs in a number of disorders, of which histiocytosis X is the most common. In its systemic form, it is frequently associated with lymphadenopathy and hepatosplenomegaly, although these are not usually the presenting manifestations.

■ LYMPH VESSELS

The lymphatic vessels collect lymph from almost all tissues except the central nervous system, striated muscle, and nonvascular structures, such as cartilage and the cornea. The lymph is essentially colorless extracellular fluid containing large numbers of lymphocytes and material too large to be absorbed into blood capillaries. This fluid and its contents are delivered into blind lymph capillaries and then carried by thin-walled transparent lymph vessels to regional nodes. The lymph enters the nodes by afferent lymphatics, and, within the node, the fluid is filtered, and immunologic material is phagocytized and undergoes immunologic processing. The nodes act as protective barriers to prevent the spread of local infections and to facilitate immunologic responses that are effective locally and systemically. Large numbers of lymphocytes are added to the lymph, which exits the nodes through efferent lymphatics and eventually reaches the thoracic duct and the right lymphatic duct. At this point in the base of the neck, the lymph enters the great venous system.

Acute Lymphangitis

During a local bacterial infection, the lymphatics act as a protective drain that delivers bacteria to regional nodes for clearance and immunologic response. When the infection is not contained locally, it may involve the lymphatic vessels in an acute lymphangitis. Erythematous streaks that are a few millimeters to several centimeters wide may be seen extending from the primary site of infection to regional nodes. Painful swelling of regional nodes usually occurs soon thereafter. Peripheral edema may occur as a result of lymphatic obstruction. Bacteremia may follow as soon as 24 to 48 hours from the onset of the initial lesion. Acute lymphangitis is generally caused by group A streptococci. Rapid institution of penicillin is indicated for local control and to prevent complicating bacteremia.

Lymphedema

Lymphedema is a diffuse, pitting edema that results from obstruction of the lymphatic flow. It most commonly involves the lower extremities and may be complicated by verrucous hypertrophy of the skin and recurrent infections. Congenital lymphedema occurs in Milroy disease, in which there are multiple congenital obstructions within the lymphatic system, and as part of the syndrome of gonadal dysgenesis. Acquired lymphedema can be the result of inflammatory processes or of surgical or radiologic obliteration of lymphatic channels; it may have no identifiable cause. Treatment is ineffective.

(Abridged from Richard H. Sills, The Spleen and Lymph Nodes, in Oski, DeAngelis, Feigin, McMillan, Warshaw: *Principles and Practice of Pediatrics, Second Edition*, J.B. Lippincott, 1994.)

Oski's Essential Pediatrics,
edited by Kevin B. Johnson and Frank A. Oski.
Lippincott–Raven Publishers,
Philadelphia © 1997

125

Disorders of Coagulation

Abnormalities of the hemostatic system are commonly encountered in hospitalized children, because primary diseases of hemostasis often require hospitalization and systemic diseases severe enough to require hospitalization often produce abnormalities of hemostasis. In addition, pediatricians are frequently called on to evaluate coagulation abnormalities before or after surgery.

Coagulation disorders can be divided into conditions with abnormal bleeding (*ie,* hypocoagulable states) and those associated with the development of thromboses (*ie,* hypercoagulable states). Current knowledge of factors necessary for normal clotting to occur and for maintaining blood in a fluid state is sufficiently complex that a full understanding of all the mechanisms involved is a challenge even for an experienced hematologist. New information is being acquired rapidly, especially in the area of hypercoagulability. Despite this surge of new information, most abnormalities of hemostasis can still be approached in an orderly fashion, beginning with a detailed history and physical examination, the evaluation of readily available laboratory tests, and a general overview of hemostatic mechanisms.

■ HISTORY AND PHYSICAL EXAMINATION

Although the search for a possible bleeding disorder is often initiated by an abnormal laboratory test result, the history and physical examination remain the most useful approaches for defining the presence and type of hemorrhagic diathesis. For example, purpura and mucosal bleeding are common presentations of platelet disorders. Abnormalities of the plasma clotting factors are much more likely to present with deep soft-tissue bleeding or hemarthrosis. The history may indicate that the coagulation abnormality is a secondary phenomenon and lead to the recognition of an underlying systemic illness.

In obtaining a history of abnormal bleeding, the clinician should ask specific rather than general questions. The question, "Do you or your child bruise easily?" is answered affirmatively by so many parents that a positive answer is often of little value. The examiner should use specific questions, using recognizable childhood events as a trigger for the parent's memory, such as "Was separation of the cord or circumcision associated with abnormal bleeding?". Approximately one half of hemophiliacs have a history of bleeding in the neonatal period, a fact that is often overlooked or unsolicited in the history. Patients with factor XIII deficiency may experience delayed bleeding after cord separation. Did the child bleed at the sites of immunization? Did the child bleed during eruption of teeth or after minor trauma to the mouth (*eg,* from falling into furniture)? Prolonged bleeding from a torn frenulum suggests factor VIII deficiency. Does the child bleed after minor trauma, such as falling from playground equipment? How frequent are epistaxis, and how long do they last? These questions are useful in gaining positive and negative information. For example, the complaint of frequent nosebleeds often raises concern about a possible coagulation disorder, but

nosebleeds that predictably stop within minutes are rarely encountered in patients with significant bleeding disorders. How long does the child bleed from minor cuts? Did the wound heal normally? It is useful to find a scar, which often jogs the parent's memory about a forgotten laceration.

Previous surgical procedures are an extremely important source of information about potential coagulation abnormalities. The child who has had a tonsillectomy or dental extractions without unusual bleeding is less likely to have a serious coagulopathy. In questioning parents about dental procedures, it should be remembered that bleeding for 24 to 48 hours after dental extractions may occur even in normal persons and should not cause undue alarm.

A detailed history of drug administration is essential. Many substances (*eg,* aspirin, antihistamines) are available in over-the-counter prescriptions and are not reported by parents unless specifically mentioned by the examiner. A history of prolonged antibiotic administration or use of drugs that antagonize or interfere with the absorption of vitamin K (*eg,* anticonvulsants, antibiotics) may prompt a diagnosis of vitamin K deficiency. Ingestions of rodent poisons containing coumarins may cause coagulopathy.

A careful family history often provides important information. The finding of a sex-linked pattern of transmission of a bleeding tendency may be the first clue to deficiencies of factor VIII (*ie,* classic hemophilia A) or factor IX (*ie,* classic hemophilia B). The discovery of an autosomal dominant mode of transmission is characteristic of von Willebrand's disease. Idiopathic thrombocytopenic purpura is commonly encountered in families in which other immunoregulatory abnormalities, such as lupus and thyroid disease, are prevalent.

The physical examination can provide important diagnostic clues. Petechiae, easily overlooked, are an important indication of reduced platelet number or function. Bruises with firm nodular or indurated centers are commonly seen in hemophilia and may be the first sign of a congenital factor deficiency. Poorly healed scars may be seen in patients with factor XIII deficiency. The finding of an enlarged liver may be an indication of a systemic illness or that a coagulation disturbance is secondary to a primary hepatic disorder. An enlarged spleen may reflect significant portal hypertension with consequent hypersplenism and thrombocytopenia. The finding of characteristic angiomatous skin and mucous membrane lesions in a child with gastrointestinal bleeding may lead to a diagnosis of hereditary hemorrhagic telangiectasia. Patients with the stigmata of Ehlers-Danlos syndrome may also manifest purpura.

■ LABORATORY EVALUATION

Excellent screening procedures and tests for specific abnormalities are available for evaluating the patient with a possible coagulation disorder. The physician should first consider whether any laboratory testing is required.

Appropriate laboratory testing (or no laboratory testing) can then be obtained. A tabulation of all of the available tests of coagulation is beyond the scope of this chapter, but some of the commonly used screening procedures are outlined in Table 125–1. Coulter counter technology is readily available. Numeration and sizing of platelets by this method are routine and inexpensive.

■ DISORDERS OF PLATELETS

Abnormalities of platelets may be quantitative (*ie,* due to reduced platelet number) or qualitative (*ie,* due to an intrinsic defect that diminishes function).

Quantitative Congenital Abnormalities of the Platelets

Thrombocytopenia–Absent Radius Syndrome

The thrombocytopenia–absent radius syndrome is perhaps the most striking and most easily recognized of the congenital thrombocytopenias. Clinical recognition of the disorder occurs soon after birth in the infant with purpura and characteristic limb deformities. Although absence of the radius is the most consistent finding in this condition, cardiac, renal, or other skeletal malformations (eg, complete or partial agenesis of other bones or joints, bony synostoses) may also occur. Leukoerythroblastic responses, often associated with severe diarrhea, are often observed in the neonatal period and infancy. The inheritance pattern appears to be autosomal recessive. Bone marrow specimens exhibit reduced numbers of megakaryocytes, which often appear dysplastic. Transfused platelets survive normally, and with the use of HLA-matched platelets, many patients can be maintained on weekly platelet transfusions for long periods. The thrombocytopenia tends to remit spontaneously in the second and third year of life.

Quantitative Acquired Abnormalities of Platelets

Idiopathic (Immune) Thrombocytopenic Purpura

Idiopathic thrombocytopenic purpura, sometimes referred to as immune or autoimmune thrombocytopenic purpura (ITP or ATP), is perhaps the most commonly encountered acquired platelet disorder of childhood.

Etiology and Pathogenesis. Although mounting evidence indicates an immunologic basis for this disease, in most cases the cause of the immunologic aberration is not clear, and the term *idiopathic* is preferred. Clinically, the disease is recognized in acute and chronic forms, and a multitude of pathogenetic mechanisms are probably involved. The immunologic basis of the disease has been suggested by classic experiments demonstrating that homologous and autologously transfused platelets are rapidly removed from the circulation; that the illness in adults can be passively transmitted from one person to another by administration of serum from an affected patient; that platelets from patients with ITP typically show increased amounts of IgG associated with the platelet membrane in several in vitro tests; that, in some cases, specific antiplatelet antibodies can be demonstrated by Western-blotting techniques and other assays; and that the disease can be produced in infants by passive transplacental transfer of antiplatelet antibodies from the

mother to the fetus. The reticuloendothelial system of the spleen is the major site of destruction of platelets in ITP, with a less important contribution from the reticuloendothelial system of the liver, bone marrow, and lungs.

Although the concept that there is an immunologic basis for ITP is well accepted, the inciting cause for antibody production often remains obscure. Acute ITP in childhood is often preceded by a viral illness, and it has been postulated that viral antigens may trigger the production of antibodies that cross-react with the platelet membrane. The most convincing evidence for this hypothesis is the finding that postinfectious sera from some patients with varicella contain an antibody that cross-reacts with specific platelet membrane glycoproteins. Specific antiglycoprotein IIb/IIIa antibodies have been demonstrated in the chronic forms of ITP, which often occurs in the setting of other known autoimmune illnesses. However, the exact significance of the autoantibodies demonstrated in ITP remains the subject of debate. Recent studies suggest that much of the platelet-associated IgG (PAIgG) in ITP is not directed against specific platelet antigens. Other serum proteins are associated with platelet membranes in increased amounts, possibly as a nonspecific response to platelet injury. Studies have shown decreased production of platelets in otherwise classic cases of ITP, suggesting that the thrombocytopenia may be the consequence of decreased production and increased destruction in some cases.

Clinical and Laboratory Features. Acute and chronic ITP tend to vary considerably in their initial presentations. In acute ITP, the onset of purpuric symptoms is typically abrupt, so much so that parents can often recount the exact hour that they became aware of the problem. In chronic ITP, the onset of purpura is often much more insidious. Acute ITP most often presents in previously healthy children, whereas chronic ITP is more common in patients with other underlying immunoregulatory abnormalities, such as systemic lupus erythematosus, IgA deficiency, autoimmune endocrinopathy, common variable immunodeficiency, or autoimmune hemolytic anemia (ie, Evans' syndrome). Acute ITP tends to occur equally in both sexes, whereas chronic ITP is more common in females. Acute ITP is predominately a disease of early childhood. Chronic ITP is much more common in children older than 10 years of age.

In acute and chronic ITP, purpura and mucosal bleeding are the most prominent symptoms. The fact that the children generally appear well except for the purpuric lesions is helpful in excluding other illnesses associated with severe thrombocytopenia. Gastrointestinal and renal hemorrhage sometimes occurs. Central nervous system bleeding is the most feared complication of ITP, but it occurs in fewer than 1% of

TABLE 125-1. Normal Values for Screening Coagulation Tests

Assay	Normal Adult	Term	32–36 Weeks of Gestation	<31 Weeks of Gestation	Age at Which Adult Values Are Reached
Platelet count ($10^3/mm^3$)	300 ± 50*	310 ± 68	290 ± 70	275 ± 60	
aPTT (sec)	44	55 ± 10	70	108†	2–9 mo
PT (sec)	13 (12–14)	16 (13–20)	17 (12–21)	23	1 wk
Bleeding time	4 ± 1.5	4 ± 1.5	4 ± 1.5	NA	

*Means ± 1 S.D. or range when available are given.

†Indicates upper limit of normal for cord blood.

these patients, usually early in the course of the illness. Such hemorrhages are often fatal. Platelet counts vary from normal (in a compensated phase) to undetectable, but they tend to be lower in acute ITP than in chronic ITP. Bone marrow aspirates should exhibit normal to increased numbers of megakaryocytes. PAIgG on the platelet surface (*ie*, the direct test) is usually positive if sufficient platelets can be obtained for study, but the patient's serum may or may not increase the amount of IgG on the surface of control platelets (*ie*, the indirect test). The PT and aPTT should be normal.

The resolution of symptoms and the thrombocytopenia occur in a variety of patterns, from abrupt to slow with frequent relapses. ITP is generally not considered chronic unless symptoms persist for more than 6 months. Relapses are common in chronic ITP. Acute ITP tends not to recur, but relapses have been reported. Improvement of symptoms often precedes a detectable rise in the platelet count.

Treatment. Because the spontaneous remission rate for acute ITP is extremely high, a waiting period is usually warranted before attempting therapy if the disease is mild (*ie*, platelet count >20,000/mm^3, no bleeding other than purpura). Platelet counts less than 20,000/mm^3 and extensive mucosal hemorrhage indicate a higher risk for internal hemorrhage, and treatment should be considered. If serious complications are present or suspected or if a protective environment cannot be guaranteed, treatment should be initiated. Historically, steroid administration has been the most commonly used therapy. The effectiveness of steroids in this disease is still debated.

Intravenous γ-globulin is a relatively new but useful modality in the treatment of ITP. The mechanism of action of this agent is not clear, but the best evidence to date suggests that it may act by causing a reticuloendothelial blockade, as evidenced by the reduced splenic clearance of sensitized erythrocytes after administration. Anti-idiotypic or anti-Fc receptor antibodies may be involved. Modulation of T- or B-cell function has been postulated, and it has also been speculated that the clearance of infection or antigenemia may play a role in the process.

Platelet transfusions are generally eschewed in ITP because of the shortened survival of transfused platelets. However, platelet transfusions may be effective in immediately reducing serious bleeding. Splenectomy is effective in resolving the thrombocytopenia in approximately two thirds of patients, but is generally used only in emergencies or in extremely resistant cases. Other therapeutic approaches, such as vinca-loaded platelets or vincristine infusions, other immunosuppressive agents, or danazol, have been used in chronic ITP. In general, these therapies should be used after more conventional modes of therapy have failed.

Thrombocytosis

Thrombocytosis occurs commonly in children. In most instances, the elevation of the platelet count is attributable to an underlying disorder associated with thrombocytosis. Common causes of thrombocytosis include acute and chronic bleeding, inflammatory or infectious processes, iron or vitamin E deficiency, hemolytic anemia, and asplenia. Thrombocytosis may occur as a result of neoplastic processes, drug administration (*eg*, vinca alkaloids, epinephrine), nephrotic syndrome, graft-versus-host disease, or during treatment of megaloblastic anemias. Kawasaki disease is frequently associated with extremely high platelet counts. Rarely, thrombocytosis is the result of a primary hematologic disease, essential thrombocythemia. In this condition, platelet production occurs autonomously, with the loss of the normal control mechanisms for thrombopoiesis. Ironically, primary thrombo-

cythemia is associated with bleeding rather than thrombosis. Thrombocytosis may be seen as part of polycythemia vera and chronic myelogenous or megakaryocytic leukemia.

Although an underlying disease causing an elevation of the platelet count frequently requires attention, treatment for the thrombocytosis is rarely required. Symptomatic thromboses in children due to elevated platelet counts appear to be rare. Although aspirin and dipyridamole are sometimes prescribed for extreme thrombocytosis, their efficacy in preventing thrombotic complications in children has not been demonstrated. The natural history of thrombocythemia is poorly understood, and the value of treatment of this disorder with chemotherapeutic agents has not been documented.

■ DISORDERS OF COAGULATION FACTORS

Congenital Abnormalities of Coagulation Factors

Abnormalities of the Factor VIII Complex

Classically, two major congenital disorders have been attributed to abnormalities of the factor VIII molecule: hemophilia A, also referred to as factor VIII deficiency, and von Willebrand's disease. Hemophilia A represents a defect in factor VIII procoagulant activity in which platelet function is normal, whereas von Willebrand's disease involves a defect in platelet function associated with a variable abnormality of factor VIII procoagulant activity. The abnormality of platelet function in von Willebrand's disease is caused by decreased or defective von Willebrand's factor, a substance necessary for platelet adhesion to blood vessel walls and maintenance of a normal bleeding time.

In the past, the relation of factor VIII procoagulant activity to the von Willebrand's factor was poorly understood. Advances in the molecular biology and protein biochemistry of factor VIII have demonstrated that circulating factor VIII is a complex of two different proteins: the factor VIII procoagulant protein (*ie*, factor VIII:C) and the von Willebrand's factor (*ie*, factor VIIIR:vWF or vWF). These proteins are products of separate genes, and each has unique antigenic sites. The von Willebrand's factor is a macromolecular structure (*ie*, multimer) composed of multiple smaller subunits and appears to act as a carrier protein for the factor VIII procoagulant molecule. Factor VIII procoagulant activity is likely to be reduced when the von Willebrand's factor is not present in sufficient quantities. The designation factor vWF:Ag refers to the major antigen on vWF that is recognized by heterologous antisera against the factor VIII complex; the designation factor VIIIR:C.F. (*ie*, ristocetin cofactor) indicates the activity of the von Willebrand's factor in vitro, which is the ability of the molecule to support ristocetin-induced agglutination of platelets. An appreciation of these relationships is essential to understanding the clinical disease states.

Factor VIII Deficiency

Etiology and Pathogenesis. Factor VIII deficiency (*ie*, hemophilia A) is a sex-linked disorder, occurring in about 1 of 10,000 Caucasian male births. The disease results from a deficient or abnormal factor VIII procoagulant molecule. Clinical severity of the disease varies with the degree of deficiency of factor VIII activity and tends to breed true among affected males in a given kindred.

Clinical and Laboratory Features. Factor VIII deficiency is characterized by a lifelong tendency toward serious and often life-threatening hemorrhage. Although surface bleeding and purpura can occur, deep soft-tissue bleeding and hemarthrosis are the hallmarks of the disease. Hemophiliacs can be divided into three groups based on clinical severity and the level of factor VIII activity: severe (<1% factor VIII activity), moderate (1% to 5% factor VIII activity), and mild (5% to 25% factor VIII activity). Severe hemophiliacs are subject to spontaneous bleeding into joints or soft-tissue sites. Moderate hemophiliacs classically develop severe bleeding only after trauma, but mild hemophiliacs may be symptomatic only after surgery or major trauma. Life-threatening bleeding can occur in all groups. Severe hemophiliacs may not bleed excessively immediately after small lacerations or venipunctures due to lack of impairment of platelet function. However, delayed bleeding at such sites is common, particularly if sutures have been placed.

The symptoms tend to vary with age. Approximately 50% of hemophiliacs escape detection in the neonatal period, even if circumcisions are performed. Mucous membrane bleeds in the mouth and bruises, particularly palpable subcutaneous hematomas, are much more common in infancy than later life. The frequency of hemarthrosis tends to increase as the child becomes ambulatory.

Although bleeding may occur at virtually any anatomical site, the most common bleeds encountered in hemophiliacs are hemarthroses, with knees, elbows, and ankles representing the most commonly affected joints; shoulders, wrists, and hips are less frequently involved. The onset of hemarthrosis is often marked by development of pain without other objective findings, followed by acute swelling, warmth, and tenderness of the joint, sometimes accompanied by erythema or discoloration. Bleeding into soft tissues and bursae around the joint may occur. Repeated bleeding into the same joint results in synovial damage and hypertrophy, producing secondary cartilaginous and bony abnormalities. The development of muscular atrophy and contraction of ligamentous structures around such "target" joints is common. The combination of soft-tissue, bony, and cartilaginous abnormalities results in an anatomically abnormal joint that is more susceptible to successive bleeds. Disruption of the epiphyseal structures may result in growth abnormalities. The development of bony cysts represents a late complication of hemarthrosis. Rarely, erosive "pseudotumors" of bone may be seen.

Central nervous system bleeding is one of the most feared complications of hemophilia. It is usually the result of trauma. Symptoms may be minimal immediately after the traumatic event, and the seriousness of the bleeding may not become evident until several days after the initial incident. Even minor episodes of head trauma may be followed by intracranial bleeding, and spontaneous intracranial hemorrhage may occur.

Hemorrhage with dental procedures can be severe. Lip or tongue lacerations occur frequently in toddlers and younger children and can be troublesome, possibly because of the high level of fibrinolytic activity of saliva. Excessive bleeding from a torn frenulum can indicate hemophilia, as does the development of a large fleshy clot. Other gastrointestinal bleeding can occur and is usually associated with some type of structural abnormality. Bleeding into retroperitoneal spaces occurs with some frequency and can sometimes be mistaken for an intra-abdominal process. Hematuria is relatively common and can be persistent. Bleeding into muscles or soft tissue can occur at any site. The seriousness of these bleeds is usually dictated by their anatomical location. Entrapment of nerves or blood vessels can be particularly problematic. Bleeding in the area of the airway should be managed as a life-threatening event. Severe hemorrhage may be experienced after surgery if adequate replacement therapy is not administered.

The diagnosis of hemophilia A requires the demonstration of low factor VIII:C activity in the presence of a normal von Willebrand's factor assay. The PTT usually is prolonged, and the PT is normal. However, in some mild forms of factor VIII deficiency, the PTT may be normal. Tests of platelet function are usually normal, although abnormal template bleeding times have been observed in some hemophiliacs. A family history may reveal a sex-linked pattern of inheritance. However, the family history may be negative because of a predominance of females in successive generations or the high rate of spontaneous mutations.

Treatment. Prevention of bleeding should be a major goal of treatment, with care taken to avoid an environment of overprotection. Infants should be provided with padded cribs and playpens. Contact sports should be prohibited, but nontraumatic sports such as swimming should be encouraged. Platelet-inhibitory substances such as aspirin should be avoided. Immunizations should be administered after replacement with factor VIII or be given intradermally rather than intramuscularly to avoid hemorrhagic complications. Immunization against hepatitis B should be given as early as possible. Prophylactic dental treatment should be encouraged. Invasive procedures such as lumbar puncture should be performed only under coverage with factor VIII.

Replacement therapy with factor VIII remains the most important part of the care of the hemophiliac. Home therapy has gained widespread acceptance and offers the opportunity for earlier treatment of bleeding episodes and increased autonomy for the hemophiliac. Such programs require close physician supervision.

Von Willebrand's Disease. The term *von Willebrand's disease* encompasses a heterogeneous group of disorders involving primary defects or deficiencies in the vWF portion of the factor VIII complex, with variable deficiencies of factor VIII:C, the procoagulant component of the factor VIII molecule. The abnormalities of vWF result in decreased platelet adhesiveness, impairment of agglutination of platelets in the presence of ristocetin, and prolongation of the bleeding time. Abnormalities of factor VIII procoagulant activity contribute to the coagulation disturbance. Unlike hemophilia A, von Willebrand's disease is usually transmitted as an autosomal dominant trait. Compound heterozygotes have been described. In rare instances, transmission may be autosomal recessive. Studies suggest that 0.8% to 1.6% of the general population show biochemical abnormalities consistent with von Willebrand's disease, making von Willebrand's disease the most common of the inherited coagulation disorders.

Several classifications of von Willebrand's disease have been suggested. All of these schemes recognize that there are two major forms: those due to quantitative abnormalities of vWF and those due to qualitative abnormalities. Mild quantitative deficiencies of vWF and factor VIII:C are referred to as type I or classic von Willebrand's disease. Qualitative abnormalities are classified as type II, and severe quantitative deficiencies as type III. Type II abnormalities can be subcategorized on the basis of abnormalities of vWF subunit and multimer structure, as demonstrated by immunoelectrophoretic techniques and decreased or increased responsiveness to ristocetin in platelet aggregation studies. Quantitative deficiencies of vWF and factor VIII:C may or may not be found in type II disorders. In types I and III, the level of factor VIII:C activity correlates with the amount of vWF. Type III patients are thought to be homozygotes or compound heterozygotes.

Most patients with von Willebrand's disease have a mild to moderate bleeding tendency, usually involving mucocutaneous surfaces. Epistaxis, increased bruisability, and hemorrhage after dental extraction are common manifestations. Melena and menorrhagia may occur. Excessive bleeding after trauma or surgery can develop. Hemarthroses are unusual, except in type III disease, or after significant trauma. Many persons with biochemical abnormalities consistent with von Willebrand's disease report no bleeding symptoms.

The diagnosis of von Willebrand's disease is complicated by the fact that results of laboratory testing sometimes vary, not only within families, but for the same person on repeated determinations. Bleeding times are abnormal at some time for most persons. The PTT may be abnormal, depending on the level of VIII:C activity. Types I and II can usually be differentiated by measuring antigenic vWF (vWF:Ag) and factor VIII:C in conjunction with crossed-immunoelectrophoresis or multimer analysis. Both vWF:Ag and factor VIII:C should be reduced in type I disease, with normal crossed-immunoelectrophoresis or size distribution on multimer analysis. In type II disease, vWF:Ag and or VIII:C may or may not be reduced, but crossed-immuno-electrophoresis or multimer analysis should show abnormal variants or lack of high-molecular-weight multimers of vWF. Assessment of platelet aggregation in response to ristocetin in vitro should define the persons with qualitative abnormalities who show hyper-responsiveness to low doses of ristocetin and are, therefore, at risk for in vivo platelet aggregation and thrombocytopenia. In type III von Willebrand's disease, vWF:Ag and factor VIII:C are markedly reduced.

Cryoprecipitate contains intact vWF of all molecular weights and appears to be effective in treating most subtypes. The bleeding time is corrected for only a few hours after administration of cryoprecipitate, despite the prolonged increase in factor VIII:C. Factor VIII concentrates may lack the high-molecular-weight forms of vWF and are not consistently effective in correcting the bleeding time in von Willebrand's disease. The treatment of choice for mild to moderate bleeding episodes in type I von Willebrand's disease is 1-desamino-8-D-arginine vasopressin (DDAVP) because of the infectious risks of cryoprecipitate. This therapy is often sufficient for surgical procedures, but adjunctive therapy with plasma products may be required for extensive surgery or serious hemorrhagic episodes. DDAVP should not be given to patients who show increased responsiveness to ristocetin in platelet aggregation studies, because they may be at risk for thrombocytopenia. It may lack effectiveness in some type II patients. The effect of DDAVP on the bleeding time is transient, approximately 3 to 4 hours, and tachyphylaxis may occur. Patients should be tested for efficacy before it is used as a therapeutic agent. In very mild cases of von Willebrand's disease, specific treatment is often not required.

Acquired Abnormalities of Coagulation Factors

Vitamin K Deficiency

Vitamin K is an essential substrate for the synthesis of procoagulant and anticoagulant proteins, including factors II, VII, IX, X, protein C, and protein S. Identical clinical states can be produced by absence of vitamin K or interference with its action by pharmacologic means. Dietary vitamin K consists mainly of vitamin K_1, a fat-soluble naphthaquinone found in leafy vegetables. Intestinal bacteria also synthesize vitamin K compounds. Therapeutically and physiologically, the fat-soluble forms of vitamin K appear to be most useful, and toxicity has resulted from the administration of water-soluble analogues. True dietary deficiency of vitamin K appears to be unusual, except in early infancy or in the setting of prolonged intravenous feedings without supplemental administration of vitamin K. Most cases of apparent dietary insufficiency in older children are caused by malab-

sorptive syndromes, such as pancreatic insufficiency, biliary obstruction, prolonged diarrhea affecting absorption of vitamin K in the upper small intestine, or the administration of drugs. Drugs that antagonize or interfere with the metabolism of vitamin K include phenobarbital, diphenylhydantoin, some cephalosporins, rifampin, isoniazid, and coumarin. Vitamin K deficiency due to antibiotic suppression of intestinal flora appears to be unusual without a dietary deficiency of vitamin K.

Uncomplicated vitamin K deficiency is characterized by bleeding symptoms (eg, bruising, oozing from puncture sites of the skin, visceral hemorrhage) with an acquired prolongation of the PT and aPTT and a normal fibrinogen. Other clotting factors that are produced in the liver but are not vitamin K dependent (eg, factors V, XI, XII, VIII) are normal. However, the clinical and laboratory picture is often affected by a primary disorder that produces liver disease and malabsorption or decreased utilization of vitamin K, such as biliary atresia, cystic fibrosis, hemolytic anemia with obstructive jaundice, hepatitis, α_1-antitrypsin deficiency, or a beta-lipoproteinemia. In the absence of severe hepatic disease or antagonists, the response to vitamin K is rapid, usually occurring within 6 hours. Anaphylactoid reactions may occur with parenteral administration of vitamin K, but they are unusual. Infusion of plasma is effective in emergent situations.

Disseminated Intravascular Coagulation

Disseminated intravascular coagulation (DIC) describes a constellation of clinical and laboratory abnormalities indicative of a combination of accelerated fibrinogenesis and fibrinolysis. Rather than being considered a disease in and of itself, DIC should be thought of as a secondary phenomenon that occurs in response to a variety of stimuli. DIC may be triggered by local or systemic factors. Examples of local problems that can result in systemic DIC include hemangiomas (ie, Kasabach-Merritt syndrome), in which a localized vascular lesion results in consumption of fibrinogen and platelets and in which elevations of fibrin degradation products can be massive, and brain injury, in which release of thromboplastic substances may initiate systemic clotting. Abruptio placenta and massive pulmonary emboli may also produce systemic signs of DIC. Systemic causes of DIC include sepsis, shock of any cause, transfusion of incompatible blood, and injection of snake venom. DIC is encountered in toxemia of pregnancy, respiratory distress syndrome, malignancies, burns, hypothermia, heat stroke, postoperative states, and any situation in which massive tissue damage is encountered. The severity of DIC varies widely, from transient and insignificant to overwhelming. Patients with DIC manifest purpura, and oozing from incisions or venipuncture sites is common. Circulatory collapse may occur.

Purpura fulminans represents a special systemic form of DIC. This rare disorder is characterized at its onset by purpura and DIC, usually in association with viral (eg, varicella), bacterial (eg, meningococcal, streptococcal) or rickettsial infections or severe hypernatremia. Pathologically, this disease is characterized by widespread microthrombi in the vascular bed of a variety of organs. Renal failure is common. The purpuric lesions are often symmetric and show sharply demarcated borders with a surrounding inflammatory reaction. Scarring of the skin and loss of extremities are common, and the fatality rate is high. Rarely, purpura fulminans may be seen as a manifestation of protein C deficiency, which was discussed previously.

Laboratory findings in DIC include thrombocytopenia, prolongation of the PT and aPTT, and a reduction of clotting factors, particularly fibrinogen and factors II, V, and VIII.

Protein C levels are reduced. Microangiopathic changes in the erythrocytes may be seen in the peripheral blood smear. Plasma levels of fibrin degradation products are usually elevated and may play a pathogenetic role by inhibiting clotting and platelet function. Measurement of fibrinopeptide A, a cleavage product of fibrinogen, and fibrinogen turnover studies increase the diagnostic sensitivity, but these assays are not routinely available.

Treatment of DIC should be aimed primarily at correcting the inciting cause. Concern has been raised about the possibility of "feeding the fire" by administering clotting factors and platelet concentrates. However, the risk of allowing severe thrombocytopenia or hypofibrinogenemia to develop is not warranted on the basis of what are mostly theoretical concerns, and replacement therapy should be given if the consumption has been severe. Heparin may be helpful in some cases if the underlying defect cannot be corrected, but its usefulness is still a matter of debate. Some authors think that heparin is particularly effective in purpura fulminans if initiated early in the illness. Epsilon-aminocaproic acid may be helpful in cases of DIC with low levels of α_2-antiplasmin due to hypergranular promyelocytic leukemia, but it is not considered useful in other forms of DIC.

(Abridged from James F. Casella, Disorders of Coagulation, in Oski, DeAngelis, Feigin, McMillan, Warshaw: *Principles and Practice of Pediatrics, Second Edition*, J.B. Lippincott, 1994.)

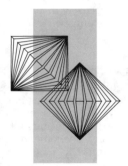

SECTION 9

Neoplastic Diseases

Oski's Essential Pediatrics,
edited by Kevin B. Johnson and Frank A. Oski.
Lippincott–Raven Publishers,
Philadelphia © 1997

126

Acute Lymphoblastic Leukemia in Childhood

In the past 25 years, there has been dramatic improvement in the treatment of children with acute lymphoblastic leukemia (ALL). ALL once was considered an incurable disease, but approximately 65% of the children newly diagnosed with ALL now survive in complete continuous remission for more than 5 years and remain free of disease.

■ ETIOLOGY

Acute leukemia is the most common malignancy diagnosed in children. Based on mortality statistics, the overall incidence is estimated at 40 per one million children younger than 15 years of age. In the United States, childhood ALL has a peak incidence between 2 and 6 years of age in white populations but not in blacks. The reason for this difference is unexplained. Childhood ALL occurs more frequently in boys than in girls, and the difference increases with age. Geographic variation in incidence, rates, and subtype of leukemia (ie, leukemic clusters) has been reported in the United States and worldwide. For example, in Turkey, acute myelomonocytic leukemia accounts for approximately 35% of the cases, and in Shanghai, China, almost one half of the children with a diagnosis of leukemia have acute nonlymphocytic leukemia.

An unusual susceptibility to leukemia has been associated with certain heritable diseases, chromosomal disorders, and constitutional syndromes. Children with trisomy 21 (ie, Down's syndrome) have at least a 10-fold to 15-fold increased risk for developing leukemia compared with normal children.

Several immunodeficiency states have an associated increased risk for lymphoma and leukemia. These conditions include the syndromes of Wiskott-Aldrich, X-linked agammaglobulinemia, severe combined immune deficiency, and ataxia telangiectasia.

■ CLINICAL PRESENTATION

In ALL, an uncontrolled proliferation of immature lymphoid cells produces bone marrow failure and may be associated with extramedullary infiltration. The presenting signs and symptoms are a reflection of these events (Table 126–1). The most common presenting symptoms are fever, pallor, purpura, and pain. The onset may be abrupt or insidious. The evolution of symptoms may proceed over a few days, weeks, or months. At first, symptoms may be nonspecific and may mimic other nonmalignant conditions. Fever, although a nonspecific complaint, is a significant symptom in the child with ALL. Fever, particularly if coupled with

TABLE 126-1. Frequency of Presenting Complaints in Childhood ALL

Symptoms	Frequency (%)
Fever	43–61
Pallor	39–55
Bleeding	24–55
Bone/joint pain	31–38
Abdominal pain	9–19
Anorexia	17–33
Fatigue	30

other nonspecific complaints, may mimic more common pediatric illnesses. Of the first 400 children with ALL treated at Texas Children's Hospital, 6% presented with fever of unknown origin and no other clinical or laboratory evidence for leukemia. The diagnosis was established by bone marrow examination. Because many of these children have absolute neutropenia (neutrophil count <500/mm3) secondary to bone marrow failure, they are at extreme risk for bacterial sepsis.

Anemia occurs in 76% of patients. It is gradual in onset, normocytic, and rarely associated with significant symptoms. In some patients, tachycardia, air hunger, apprehension, and restlessness may signal acute blood loss with impending hypovolemic shock.

Petechiae and bruising are frequently noticed on physical examination and are related to the high incidence (71%) of thrombocytopenia. Epistaxis is not uncommon, especially when thrombocytopenia is severe (platelets <20,000/mm3). Under such conditions, the child may swallow blood, experience gastrointestinal irritation, nausea, and vomiting with hematemesis, followed by melena or bloody diarrhea. All of these symptoms have a profound psychological effect on the child, parents, and unsuspecting physician.

Symptoms of anorexia and vague abdominal pains are common. Children may present with bone, hip, or joint pain. Arthralgias and refusal to walk may reflect leukemic infiltrations of the bony cortex or the joint compartment. Lymphadenopathy is common, and some degree of hepatosplenomegaly occurs in more than half of the patients. Massive infiltrations can occur but are uncommon.

■ INITIAL LABORATORY FINDINGS

Clinical laboratory data often reveal a broad spectrum of abnormal findings. In addition to anemia and thrombocytopenia, the leukocyte counts and morphology may be abnormal. Approximately 20% of children present with leukocyte counts greater than 50,000/mm³ (range, 100 to 1,000,000/mm³). About 44% of children have leukocyte counts less than 10,000/mm³. Occasionally, hypereosinophilia has been observed and is thought to be a reactive phenomena. Leukemic blasts may or may not be seen on peripheral smears.

■ DIAGNOSIS

The diagnosis of leukemia cannot be established from peripheral blood examination alone. Osteopetrosis, myelofibrosis, granulomatous infections, sarcoid, Epstein-Barr virus (EBV) infection in the very young, other acute viral infec-

tions, and metastatic tumor are conditions that can result in the release of immature-appearing blasts into the circulation.

The diagnosis of ALL is established by bone marrow examination. In children, the bone marrow specimen is usually obtained from the posterior iliac crest rather than by sternal or pretibial puncture. Diagnostic aspirations may be technically difficult to perform because of the density of blast forms or the presence of marrow fibrosis or necrosis.

The normal bone marrow contains less than 5% blasts. A minimum of 25% lymphoblasts on differential examination of the bone marrow aspirate is necessary for the diagnosis of ALL. Most children with ALL have hypercellular marrow with 60% to 100% of the cells as blasts. The presenting characteristics of childhood ALL are outlined in Table 126–2.

■ DIFFERENTIAL DIAGNOSIS

Because children with ALL present with a variety of nonspecific symptoms, several pediatric nonmalignant conditions may be confused with leukemia. Idiopathic thrombocytopenic purpura is a common cause of bruising and petechiae in children. Anemia, leukocyte disturbances, and significant hepatosplenomegaly are not typical findings. Bone marrow examinations reveal normal or increased num-

TABLE 126-2. Presenting Characteristics of Children With ALL

Characteristic	Frequency (%)*
Age (yr) <1.5	6–8
>1.5–10	72–80
>10	15–22
Sex (male)	54–57
Race (white)	80–89
Leukocyte count <10,000/mm³	44
10,000–50,000/mm³	34
>50,000/mm³	22
Platelets <20,000/mm³	20
20,000–100,000/mm³	51
>100,000/mm³	29
Hemoglobin <7.5 g/dL	46
<7.5–10 g/dL	30
>10 g/dL	24
Hepatomegaly (below umbilicus)	8–13
Splenomegaly (below umbilicus)	11–14
Lymphadenopathy	
None/minimal	73
Moderate/marked	28
Mediastinal mass	8
CNS symptoms	4
Immunoglobulin abnormalities (1 or more)	9
FAB L1	82
L2	17
L3	1
Karyotype abnormality	45

*Percentages are estimates based on accumulated data from large numbers of patients treated by the Pediatric Oncology Group and the Children's Cancer Study Group.

bers of megakaryocytes and no increase in blast forms in children with thrombocytopenic purpura. Children with infectious mononucleosis (*ie*, EBV) or other acute viral illnesses may present with fever, malaise, adenopathy, splenomegaly, rash, and lymphocytosis. In the young child with EBV, lymphocytosis may be extreme (80 to 100,000/mm³), and thrombocytopenia and immunohemolytic anemia may further confuse the diagnosis. The atypical lymphocytes characteristic of these diseases are larger and pleomorphic, have more abundant pale blue cytoplasm, and may resemble the leukemic lymphoblast. Specific viral serologies can establish the diagnosis, but a bone marrow examination sometimes is necessary.

Leukemoid reactions may be observed in bacterial sepsis, acute hemolysis, granulomatous diseases, vasculitis, and metastatic tumor to the bone marrow. In these circumstances, underlying clinical events may offer some clues to the differential diagnosis. A bone marrow aspirate usually reveals myeloid hyperplasia. The leukemoid reaction resolves as the underlying disease is successfully managed. Isolated neutropenia may also be observed in asymptomatic infants after the use of certain medications for overwhelming bacterial sepsis. In this case, the bone marrow examination may reveal a maturational arrest of the granulocytic precursors, but increased blast forms are not usually seen.

Children with ALL presenting with fever, arthralgias, arthritis, or a limp may frequently be confused with juvenile rheumatoid arthritis (JRA). Anemia, leukocytosis, and mild splenomegaly, all of which may be observed in JRA, can be misleading. Of the first 400 children with ALL treated at Texas Children's Hospital, 4.5% presented with a diagnosis of osteomyelitis or JRA. Several of these patients were receiving anti-inflammatory agents for several weeks before the diagnosis of ALL. Until a reliable positive test for JRA becomes available, a bone marrow examination to exclude ALL should be strongly considered as part of the diagnostic evaluation of patients with atypical presentations of JRA.

Pancytopenia and fever are presenting symptoms for aplastic anemia and ALL in children, but lymphadenopathy and hepatosplenomegaly are unusual findings in aplastic anemia. The bone marrow aspirate and biopsy usually clarify the diagnosis. Patients with aplastic anemia have a hypocellular marrow with cellularity usually less than 10%, no normal marrow precursors, and only small lymphocytes seen on smears. Occasionally, the bone marrow in children with ALL is initially hypocellular, and multiple aspirates and biopsies from additional sites are necessary to establish the diagnosis. Myeloproliferative syndromes and preleukemic conditions are rare in childhood but must be considered in the differential diagnosis whenever a disturbed or dysmyelopoietic bone marrow examination is observed.

Leukemia is a small blue cell malignancy. Other small blue cell malignancies can present in childhood and may produce bone marrow invasion, with the resulting signs and symptoms of fever, pain, petechiae, bruising, and pancytopenia. Neuroblastoma is the most common pediatric solid tumor that is associated with a high frequency (70%) of bone marrow invasion in children older than 2 years of age at diagnosis. The pattern of bone marrow infiltration, including discrete clumps or rosettes, the usual presence of a retroperitoneal mass, and elevated urinary catecholamines help to differentiate this disease from ALL. Other small blue cell tumors that may produce bone marrow infiltration include rhabdomyosarcoma, non-Hodgkin's lymphoma, retinoblastoma, medulloblastoma, and Ewing's sarcoma. Other significant clinical abnormalities characteristic of these diseases help to establish the correct diagnosis.

■ PROGNOSTIC FACTORS

For childhood ALL, the patient's age at diagnosis and the initial leukocyte count have been the two most reliable indicators for response to therapy. The very young or older child does less well with current therapy. Infants younger than 1 year of age at diagnosis have a particularly poor prognosis. Patients with high leukocyte counts (>50,000/mm³) are thought to have a greater leukemic burden, an increased risk for emergence of resistant clones, and a greater risk for relapse with standard therapy. Selected leukemic karyotypic abnormalities have been associated with poor prognosis. The commonly recognized prognostic factors for childhood ALL are listed in Table 126–3. Prognostic factors will continue to be defined and redefined as therapeutic interventions improve.

■ TREATMENT

The treatment of childhood ALL has become progressively complex. Curative therapy for ALL has not been established, and investigational therapy is the treatment of choice. These therapeutic programs recognize that ALL is a heterogeneous disease, that certain risk factors may have importance for response to therapy, that optimal scheduling and delivery of effective chemotherapeutic agents have not been defined, that factors leading to relapse are unknown, and that answers to these and other questions can be obtained only through carefully conducted and critically evaluated cooperative clinical trials. Consequently, the best therapy for the child newly diagnosed with ALL is offered by pediatric cancer centers participating in ongoing clinical therapeutic trials.

Combination chemotherapy is the principal therapeutic modality for childhood ALL. The therapy can be divided into four phases:

TABLE 126–3. Prognostic Factors for Childhood ALL at Diagnosis

Factor	Favorable	Unfavorable
Cell type	Lymphoid	Nonlymphoid
Leukocyte count	<10,000/mm³	>50,000/mm³
Age	3–5 yr	<2 or >10 yr
Ploidy	>1.16	<1.16
Karyotype	Hyperdiploid (>53 chromosomes)	Pseudodiploid
		Hypodiploid
		Translocation
Cell lineage	CD10 positive	CD10 negative
	Early Pre-B cell	B > T > Pre-B cell
Race	Caucasian	Black
Sex	Female	Male
Central nervous system involvement	−	+
Organomegaly	−	+
Mediastinal mass	−	+

Symbols: +, present; −, absent.

Remission induction and consolidation (*ie*, intensification)

Presymptomatic central nervous system (CNS) therapy (*ie*, prophylaxis)

Maintenance

Elective discontinuation of therapy and long-term, late-effects follow-up

Induction and Consolidation Therapy

The objectives of remission induction are to eliminate as many leukemic cells as biologically tolerable and to reestablish a normal clinical and hematologic state for the patient. Most pediatric cancer centers use at least three drugs to achieve remission: vincristine, prednisone, L-asparaginase with or without doxorubicin or daunorubicin.

The assessment of prognostic factors at diagnosis becomes useful at this point. Patients with high-risk leukemia (*ie*, patients with high leukocyte counts, unfavorable immunophenotypes such as T-ALL, or unfavorable cytogenetic characteristics such as the Philadelphia translocation) are assigned to more intensive treatment regimens at diagnosis. The morbidity of therapy is counterbalanced by the need for more intensive cytoreductive therapies for biologically more aggressive leukemias.

The concept of intensification of therapy was extended to the period immediately after achievement of hematologic remission. This consolidation phase of treatment was designed to deliver multiple chemotherapeutic agents in a relatively short period. The objective of treatment was to further reduce residual leukemia and minimize the development of cross-resistance. The BFM West German study group employed an intensive eight-drug induction and consolidation program (*ie*, BFM 76/79) followed by a late reinforcement schedule and achieved an overall disease-free survival rate of 68% at 5.5 years. The Memorial Sloan-Kettering group developed two aggressive chemotherapy regimens (*ie*, L-2, L-10) for childhood ALL. The overall survival for all patients on the L-2 protocol was 57% at greater than 7 years' median follow-up. The Children's Cancer Study Group (CCSG) is investigating modifications of the BFM and L-10 protocols for children with high-risk ALL. The estimated EFS for both studies is greater than 60%. However, toxic effects, particularly life-threatening infectious complications, have been a major concern in the early developmental phases of these protocols. The Dana Farber Cancer Institute has reported an overall 72% EFS at 7 years for childhood ALL using a schedule of intensive asparaginase during consolidation. Pediatric Oncology Group (POG) studies using intensive courses of intravenous methotrexate and 6-mercaptopurine in children with lower-risk ALL (*ie*, POG 8399) report a 4-year EFS rate of greater than 90%. Overall, patients with low-risk prognostic features at diagnosis are experiencing a superior response to these forms of intensive therapy and have a better chance for long-term survival.

Central Nervous System Therapy

Presymptomatic CNS prophylaxis therapy is an integral component of ALL therapy. Effective CNS treatment programs have decreased the incidence of CNS leukemia as a primary site of relapse from 50% to between 6% and 10%. Several regimens have been investigated and include intrathecal methotrexate and cranial irradiation (2400 cGy); intrathecal triple therapy with methotrexate, hydrocortisone, and ara-C; and intrathecal methotrexate coupled with high-dose intravenous methotrexate.

Cessation of Therapy

The minimal duration for effective chemotherapy has not been established, partially because of an inability to recognize minimal residual disease. The standard duration of therapy is 2 to 3 years. Improved disease-free survival has not been clearly established for therapy schedules extending beyond 3 years in remission. Historically, 20% to 25% of the children with ALL discontinuing therapy after 3 years relapsed. The risk of relapse was greatest within the first year off therapy, with virtually no relapses occurring 4 years after cessation. Unfortunately, isolated cases of relapsed leukemia have been reported as late as 10 to 15 years after cessation of therapy.

For children who remain in continuous complete remission for 2 to 3 years on therapy, it has been the practice to discontinue therapy and to observe closely during the first 1 to 2 years off therapy for evidence of relapse. Because of the risk for late recurrence, these children require periodic monitoring indefinitely. Whether children will continue to experience this rate of relapse after discontinuation of current protocols remains to be determined.

Complications of Therapy and Supportive Care

At diagnosis, the critical issues of management relate directly to complications of the leukemic burden. Patients with high leukocyte counts at diagnosis, massive organomegaly, or immunophenotypes such as T- or B-ALL are at greatest risk for these complications (Table 126–4).

Bone Marrow and Extramedullary Relapse and Transplantation

The most serious complication of ALL treatment is bone marrow relapse. Although reinduction of remission is possible, most patients will relapse again and eventually succumb to their disease. Patients who relapse while receiving continuation therapy have the worst prognosis. This event usually signals the emergence of resistant leukemic clones. Remission duration after successful reinduction is usually less than 1 year. In this group of patients, ablative chemotherapy and allogeneic bone marrow transplantation may offer the only hope for long-term survival. The reported experience for the Seattle Transplant Service in this group of patients is a 40% disease-free survival rate with a plateau from 2.5 to 10 years in follow-up.

Transplantation remains a form of investigational therapy. Treatment schedules, bone marrow processing, and post-transplant support measures are undergoing continual refinement. The procedure is risky, with an estimated 15% to 25% mortality rate from all causes during the first 100 days after transplantation. Acute and chronic graft-versus-host disease, interstitial pneumonitis, and relapse of leukemia are some of the many significant complications that may follow the transplantation procedure.

Patients who relapse more than 6 to 12 months after cessation of therapy may have a somewhat better prognosis. Reinduction of remission is usually successful, and long durations of remission have been achieved, with some patients actually discontinuing therapy for a second time.

The CNS and the testes are the most common sites of extramedullary relapse. However, these isolated events

TABLE 126-4. Potential Complications of Childhood ALL and Its Therapy

Metabolic complications

    Hyperuricemia

    Hyperkalemia

    Hyperphosphatemia

    SIADH

    Hyponatremia

Hemorrhage (platelets <20,000/mm³)

    Skin: mucous membranes; occasional GI, CNS

Hyperleukocytosis (WBC >100, 000/mm³)

    Infarction: pulmonary, CNS hemorrhage

Infection

    Agranulocytic: bacterial (staph, enteric organisms)

    Lymphopenic: *Pneumocystis,* fungal, viral (HSV, CMV, varicella)

Extravasation burns: vincristine, doxorubicin, daunorubucin

Anaphylaxis: L-asparaginase, VP-16, VM-26

Myelosuppression: doxorubicin, daunorubicin, cyclophosphamide, cytosine arabinoside, 6-mercaptopurine, methotrexate, etoposide, nitrogen mustard, procarbazine, dactinomycin

Emetic: High-dose methotrexate, cytosine arabinoside, cyclophosphamide, doxorubicin, daunorubicin, VP-16, VM-26

Dysuria: cyclophosphamide

Mucositis: High-dose methotrexate, cytosine arabinoside, doxorubicin

Hypertension: prednisone

Hepatic dysfunction: methotrexate 6-mercaptopurine, cytosine arabinoside

Pancreatic dysfunction: L-asparaginase, cytosine arabinoside

should be considered as localized manifestations of recurrent systemic disease; aggressive systemic chemotherapy is an essential part of the management.

Other sites of extramedullary infiltration with ALL have been observed in children. Renal infiltrates are found in 40% of the children at diagnosis and may contribute to metabolic complications and hypertension during induction therapy. Isolated ovarian involvement has been reported occasionally and may extend to the fallopian tubes, uterus, and pelvic nodes. Radiographic changes in the skeleton, with or without associated symptoms, may be seen in as many as 30% of the patients at diagnosis. Leukemic infiltrates have been observed in the lower gastrointestinal tract, oral and gingival regions, retina and iris, heart, lungs, and skin.

■ LONG-TERM SURVIVAL, LATE EFFECTS, AND THERAPEUTIC DIRECTIONS

As with all children with cancer, the management of the child with ALL requires a team approach. Pediatric nurse specialists, psychologists, play therapists, dietitians, and other hospital and clinic personnel play an important role in the total care of these patients. The stresses that frequently are faced by families with a child with ALL include concerns about the discomfort or disfigurement (especially alopecia) associated with chemotherapy, the financial pressures of medical care or disruption of family employment schedules, school performance and peer relationships, particularly for the older child, communication about fears and apprehensions among parents, patient, and siblings, and anxiety preceding the elective cessation of therapy.

With prolonged survival, monitoring for late effects of antileukemic therapy assumes increasing importance. The areas of interest include monitoring for specific organ dysfunction, impaired genetic or immunologic mechanisms, and second malignancies. Several long-term problems have been associated with CNS prophylaxis. These may include a 50% incidence of cranial CT scan abnormalities for children treated with cranial irradiation and intrathecal methotrexate,

seizures, neuropsychological deficits that result in school problems, and endocrine disturbances (*eg,* growth hormone deficiency). These problems are remediable and are insufficient reasons for altering a successful treatment program. Current leukemia protocols are seeking to obviate some of these complications by the use of high-dose systemic chemotherapy and intrathecal therapy without irradiation. The success of these programs remains to be established.

Delayed sexual maturation may be observed in children receiving irradiation to gonadal tissue, such as boys with testicular leukemia. Male adolescents may be at risk for spermatogenic dysfunction after cyclophosphamide therapy. Successful parenthood in long-term survivors has been reported, but the progeny of survivors of childhood leukemia are few. The data from cooperative late effects studies do not indicate an excess of congenital abnormalities or cancer in the offspring.

Clinical and laboratory-based research for childhood ALL probably will proceed along two principal lines. First, an increased understanding of the molecular and genetic events that regulate normal cellular proliferation and differentiation is essential. By recognizing normal regulatory events in bone marrow and lymphoreticular tissues, it should be possible to identify abnormal regulatory mechanisms and devise strategies for treatment. An increased understanding of the genetic mechanisms that offer the leukemic cell specific and nonspecific resistance advantages against antileukemic therapy will be necessary before we can solve the problem of leukemic relapse. Second, refinements in antileukemic therapy should proceed along more pharmacologically oriented schedules. Early antileukemic therapy was principally based on empiric data. Advances in the technologies of drug pharmacology, immunology, and cell kinetics will contribute to more effective treatment combinations that target specific mechanisms of leukemic proliferation or differentiation and increase the patient's chance for long-term survival.

(Abridged from Donald H. Mahoney Jr., Acute Lymphoblastic Leukemia in Childhood, in Oski, DeAngelis, Feigin, McMillan, Warshaw: *Principles and Practice of Pediatrics, Second Edition,* J.B. Lippincott, 1994.)

Oski's Essential Pediatrics,
edited by Kevin B. Johnson and Frank A. Oski.
Lippincott–Raven Publishers,
Philadelphia © 1997

127

Acute Myeloid Leukemia

■ EPIDEMIOLOGY

Between 350 and 500 new cases of acute myeloid leukemia (AML) are diagnosed in children annually in the United States. The incidence is one fifth to one sixth that of acute lymphocytic leukemia (ALL) in the same age group. The therapy for childhood AML has not reached the degree of success achieved for childhood ALL.

■ PRESENTING FEATURES AND DIAGNOSIS

As with ALL, children with AML manifest symptoms of bone marrow infiltration and failure. Pallor, bone pain, fever, and bleeding are the most common complaints at diagnosis. There is no sex predominance, and the age-adjusted incidence is constant. Enlargement of the liver and spleen affects approximately half of the children. Lymphadenopathy is not usually a prominent feature. Testicular involvement at any stage of disease is infrequent. Chloromas or granulocytic sarcomas, particularly of the orbit and skin, may occur in a small percentage of patients. Gingival hyperplasia develops most commonly in children whose disease has a monocytic component.

Cerebrospinal fluid (CSF) studies demonstrate leukemic involvement in 10% of patients at diagnosis. This is higher than for children with ALL. These CSF findings are usually unaccompanied by symptoms. If detected at diagnosis, central nervous system (CNS) leukemia in childhood AML is responsive to specific therapy and does not adversely affect treatment outcome, although, as systemic therapy improves, this observation may change. An exception is the infant (<2 years of age) with monocytic leukemia and CNS disease at diagnosis. These patients do not respond well to therapy. In childhood AML, the initial leukocyte count is usually less than 50,000/mm³, but extreme leukocytosis (≥100,000/mm)³ is recorded in one of five AML patients and is considered an adverse prognostic factor.

Coagulation studies may indicate a consumptive coagulopathy, particularly in patients with acute promyelocytic leukemia (APL). In contrast to adult APL patients, heparinization may not be necessary to prevent bleeding complications in children with APL. Most respond to transfusion support and early aggressive chemotherapy.

There has not been universal agreement about the prognostic factors in childhood AML because of the generally poor outcome of all subgroups. It has been suggested that extreme leukocytosis, particularly in children younger than 2 years of age at diagnosis and the monocytic subgroup are adverse indicators. However, there are considerable data that fail to confirm the importance of these factors in various studies, and the impact of therapy rather than disease as the prognostic factor determinant should not be underestimated.

Studies of leukemic bone marrow growth patterns in various culture systems have been performed in an effort to define the disease and prognosis on the basis of colony and cluster patterns and ratios. The results of these studies were contradictory, and the utility of these observations is questionable. There are ongoing efforts to relate drug sensitivities in culture systems with the results observed in clinical trials.

■ THERAPY

For AML patients, successful induction of remission requires regimens more toxic than those used in ALL. It is necessary to create transient marrow aplasia to achieve a complete remission in AML. The therapeutic index for such regimens is narrow, and early death rates are 5% to 15%, although in the past they have been as high as 30%. Complete remissions in childhood AML are being obtained in 70% to 85% of newly diagnosed patients.

Approximately 50% of the responders are expected to remain in remission. The median disease-free survival for all patients in most pediatric AML series is 12 to 18 months. An interesting subgroup is patients with Down's syndrome and AML. The increased incidence of AML associated with trisomy 21 is well established. The response of these patients to therapy appears to be exceptionally good.

Improved therapy for childhood AML depends on several factors: a better understanding of the molecular basis of disease, an appreciation of the interactions of malignant cell growth characteristics with the effects of chemotherapeutic agents, and the development of effective new agents or approaches.

(Abridged from C. Philip Steuber, Acute Myeloid Leukemia, in Oski, DeAngelis, Feigin, McMillan, Warshaw: *Principles and Practice of Pediatrics, Second Edition,* J.B. Lippincott, 1994.)

Oski's Essential Pediatrics,
edited by Kevin B. Johnson and Frank A. Oski.
Lippincott–Raven Publishers,
Philadelphia © 1997

128

Bone Marrow Transplantation for Childhood Leukemia

Bone marrow transplantation is the process of replacing a patient's diseased, defective, or damaged marrow elements with healthy donor marrow cells. In malignancies, marrow grafts offer an opportunity to circumvent the therapeutic dosage limitations imposed by myelosuppressive toxicities and to further intensify therapy.

With improvements in histocompatibility testing, immunosuppressive therapies, and supportive care during the last two decades, bone marrow transplantation is increasingly the therapy chosen for a variety of otherwise fatal conditions. Most marrow transplantations have been performed for patients with leukemia.

The first marrow transplants for leukemia were syngeneic or allogeneic and were given to patients with advanced refractory disease to rescue them from myeloablative therapies. The few successes (5% to 10%) observed at that time outnumbered those seen with other therapies and led investigators to explore the indications for and optimal applications of the transplant procedure.

Current guidelines for considering the use of bone marrow transplantation for childhood leukemia include the following diagnoses:

Acute myelogenous leukemia (AML) in first remission

Selected high-risk acute lymphocytic leukemia (ALL) in first remission (eg, Ph¹-positive ALL)

Adult and juvenile forms of chronic myelogenous leukemia during the chronic phase

Recurrent or refractory leukemia of any type

Most marrow transplantations done for leukemia through 1987 have used HLA/MLC-compatible donor–recipient pairs. These pairs are identical at the A, B, and D loci. The restricted availability of matched, related allogeneic donors reduces the number of patients eligible for transplant by 67%. In an attempt to increase the donor pool for patients without matched siblings, efforts have been directed toward the use of partially matched family members, such as parents (ie, haploidentical). Bone marrow donor registries have been established to catalog unrelated histocompatible persons. Preliminary data suggest that the use of HLA-matched nonrelated donors may result in less graft-versus-host disease (GVHD) than is seen using partially matched related donors.

To reduce the anticipated increase in the incidence and severity of GVHD under such disparate conditions, methods are used to purge the donor marrow of immunocompetent T cells. Most T-cell depletion procedures involve monoclonal antibodies directed at T cells. These purging methods are effective in reducing the GVHD-related problems, but the incidence of graft rejection and of recurrent leukemia increases. These observations underscore the contribution of immunocompetent donor T cells to engraftment and to disease control.

There are several obstacles to the ultimate success of bone marrow transplantation: acute and chronic GVHD, recurrent disease, fatal infection (particularly in patients with GVHD), lethal toxicity from the conditioning regimen, and failure to engraft, although engraftment rarely fails with the current preparative regimens.

GVHD is a process in which donor T lymphocytes produce injury in host tissue, particularly the skin, liver, and gastrointestinal tract. The severity of GVHD correlates to some extent with measures of histocompatibility, but it occurs even in complete A-, B-, and D-loci matches, reflecting the limitations of current histocompatibility assessment. Acute GVHD usually occurs within 3 months of grafting. It develops in approximately half of patients receiving allografts. All bone marrow transplant patients receive some form of immunosuppressive therapy in an effort to abrogate or ameliorate the appearance of GVHD. Methotrexate, prednisone, and cyclosporine are the agents most often used in various combinations for GVHD prophylaxis. Attempts can be made to deplete donor marrows of T cells before infusion to reduce the incidence and severity of GVHD, but this process introduces other undesirable complications. Successful, aggressive GVHD prophylaxis may contribute to a greater incidence of relapse.

Despite these complicating factors and unsettled issues, the successes of bone marrow transplant are substantial. For children with AML in first remission, the disease-free survival rate is approximately 60% to 65% after allogeneic transplants. These figures are markedly reduced if the grafting takes place in second or subsequent remission or at the time of overt relapse. In patients transplanted for AML, most failures are caused by transplant-related causes, and the relapse rate appears to be less than 15%. However, recent advances in drug treatment for childhood AML may require a reevaluation of the timing of bone marrow transplantation for those patients.

The responses of children with ALL to transplant have been somewhat less gratifying. Because more than half of the newly diagnosed patients with ALL respond to chemotherapy regimens, bone marrow transplantation usually is reserved for ALL patients who fail initial therapy and are in second remission. Under such circumstances, long-term, disease-free survivals have been of the magnitude of 30% to 35%, with relapse accounting for the largest number of failures (30% to 50%). Selected patients with ALL in first remission who are considered to be at high risk for chemotherapy failure are considered for transplantation. A widely accepted high-risk feature is the presence of the Philadelphia chromosome (Ph¹). Relapse after transplantation reflects the inadequacy of the conditioning regimen. Improved preparative programs use agents more specific for lymphoproliferative disorders and appear to have increased the projected disease-free survival rates to 50%, but the data are preliminary. The use of autologous marrow for leukemia patients in remission who do not have matched donors provides another approach to leukemia therapy. Autografting allows for higher-dose chemoradiotherapy without the limitations imposed by marrow-suppressive toxicity, and it enables hematopoietic recovery without the risk of GVHD seen in allografts. There are disadvantages of autografting. If the remission marrow being reinfused remains contaminated with leukemic cells, the disease may recur as a result of the reinfused malignant cells. The therapy regimens used to treat the patient are similar to those used in allogeneic transplants, but autografts do not have the added benefit of the GVHD effect. There is no accurate method of determining if relapse under these circumstances reflects reinfusion of disease or inadequate systemic conditioning therapy.

Marrow autografting is being used to treat increasing numbers of patients with refractory solid tumors. Children with lymphomas, neuroblastoma, sarcomas, and even brain tumors have responded to aggressive myeloablative therapies followed by "rescue" with their own previously cryopreserved marrows. For solid tumors with a proclivity for marrow involvement, the questions of marrow contamination with malignant cells and of the indications and methods for purging remain unsettled.

(Abridged from C. Philip Steuber, Bone Marrow Transplantation for Childhood Leukemia, in Oski, DeAngelis, Feigin, McMillan, Warshaw: *Principles and Practice of Pediatrics, Second Edition*, J.B. Lippincott, 1994.)

Oski's Essential Pediatrics, edited by Kevin B. Johnson and Frank A. Oski. Lippincott–Raven Publishers, Philadelphia © 1997

129

Hodgkin's Disease

Lymphomas comprise the third largest group of childhood malignancies, accounting for about 14% in whites and 11.3% in blacks. The actual incidence is 6.2 cases of Hodgkin's disease (HD) per million Caucasian children per year and 6.9 cases of non-Hodgkin's lymphoma. White children have about half again as many cases of lymphomas as blacks, with an incidence of 16.2 per million whites and 10.2

per million blacks. The differences are most striking in the non-Hodgkin's lymphomas (NHL); the incidence is twice as high for white children as for black children.

■ EPIDEMIOLOGY

Hodgkin's disease is a malignancy of the interdigitating, antigen-processing cells, which are found in the paracortical regions of the lymph nodes or spleen. The neoplastic counterpart, known as the Reed-Sternberg cell, can also be found in bone, bone marrow, liver, lung, and in skin and brain in the late stages of disease.

HD occurs rarely in children younger than 7 years of age and is diagnosed equally in boys and girls. The incidence increases until age 25 and then decreases until the midthirties.

There has been significant controversy about the possible association of tonsillectomy and incidence of HD. The relative incidence varied from 0.7 to 3.6 in 12 studies seeking to answer the question of an association. The incidence varied with sibship size, and there are probably several confounding variables involved. For example, compared with the general population, more HD patients are single children, although this group is only 12.5% of patients.

■ CLINICAL FEATURES AND DIAGNOSIS

Presenting Signs and Symptoms

Most children present with painless lymphadenopathy, usually of the cervical, supraclavicular, axillary, or inguinal nodes. Splenic or hepatic enlargement is infrequently found in early stages of HD. Fewer than 20% of patients have the classic fever and night sweats that adults with HD demonstrate. These initial signs could be caused by a variety of diseases.

A mediastinal mass is seen on chest x-ray films in 17% to 40% of patients and is found more often in children over 12 years of age. It is almost always found when low cervical or supraclavicular nodes are enlarged. Most of the older children have masses less than one third the diameter of the chest, but 30% have mediastinal masses greater than one third of the diameter, which may cause dysphagia, dyspnea, cough, or the superior vena cava syndrome.

Staging

The routine evaluation of a patient with suspected HD should include a complete history with emphasis on constitutional symptoms such as fever and weight loss, previous infections, family exposures to toxins and parental occupational hazards, and evidence for underlying immune deficiencies and familial cancer. A complete physical examination means assessment of general health, height and weight, size and location of lymphadenopathy, liver and spleen size, skin infiltrations, pulmonary findings, and neurologic signs. Laboratory evaluation should include a complete blood count, bilateral bone marrow biopsies and aspirates, erythrocyte sedimentation rate, renal and liver function tests (including lactate dehydrogenase levels), urinalysis, anteroposterior and lateral chest x-ray films, and computerized

tomography (CT) scans of the abdomen and chest with oral and intravenous contrast.

There are two aspects to staging: clinical and pathologic. Clinical staging refers to an assessment of the disease extent based on history, physical examination, and radiologic tests. Pathologic staging is accomplished by histologic examination of tissues removed at a staging laparotomy and by the bone marrow biopsy. Table 129–1 outlines the Ann Arbor staging system for Hodgkin's disease in children or adults.

■ TREATMENT

Patients with pathologically staged I through IIA disease have, until recently, been treated primarily with irradiation to involved areas plus an extended field to contiguous regions that are frequently sites of relapse. For a child with a cervical node involvement, this means the neck, supraclavicular, and axillary ("mini-mantle") regions must be treated. If there is a mediastinal mass, it may require a special boost of radiation if the mass is greater than one third of the chest diameter. Historically, this approach has provided disease-free survival rates of more than 80% for stage I and II HD. Some centers have routinely added extended-field irradiation to para-aortic nodes and to splenic or hepatic regions, even for limited supradiaphragmatic disease. This helped improve survival when B symptoms or extensive mediastinal disease suggested a worse prognosis, but the price paid for this extra therapy was toxicity in the form of musculoskeletal growth problems.

(Abridged from Kenneth L. McClain, Hodgkin's Disease, in Oski, DeAngelis, Feigin, McMillan, Warshaw: *Principles and Practice of Pediatrics, Second Edition,* J.B. Lippincott, 1994.)

TABLE 129-1. Ann Arbor System for Staging of Hodgkin's Disease

Stage I	Involvement of a single lymph node region (I) or a single extralymphatic organ or site (I_E)
Stage II	Involvement of two or more lymph node regions on the same side of the diaphragm II, or extension to an extralymphatic site and one or more lymph node regions on the same side of the diaphragm (II_E)
Stage III	Involvement of lymph node regions on both sides of the diaphragm (III), localized involvement by extension to an extralymphatic organ or site (III_E), or involvement of the spleen
Stage IV	Diffuse or disseminated involvement of one or more extralymphatic organs or tissues with or without associated lymph node enlargement.

All stages are further classified as A or B to indicate the absence or presence, respectively, of systemic symptoms: (1) unexplained fever, (2) night sweats, or (3) weight loss greater than 10% of normal body weight. If laparotomy and histologic review show that disease is limited to spleen, splenic, celiac, or portal nodes, the classification is substage IIIA1. Involvement of the lower abdominal nodes, such as para-aortic, iliac, and inguinal nodes, designates substage IIIA2.

From Carbone PP, Kaplan HS. Report of the committee on Hodgkin's disease staging classification. Cancer Res. *197;31:1860.*

Oski's Essential Pediatrics,
edited by Kevin B. Johnson and Frank A. Oski.
Lippincott–Raven Publishers,
Philadelphia © 1997

130

Non-Hodgkin's Lymphoma

Non-Hodgkin's lymphomas (NHLs) represent 10% of all tumors in the pediatric age group. The peak incidence occurs among children 7 to 11 years of age, and there is a male predominance. There are three major histologic varieties: Burkitt's lymphoma, which is the subject of this chapter, and the less common lymphoblastic and large cell, or histiocytic, lymphomas.

■ BURKITT'S LYMPHOMA

Burkitt's lymphoma is the most common (39%) type of NHL in childhood. The children usually present with an abdominal mass that may originate in the bowel, kidneys, or gonads and be accompanied by massive ascites. Striking enlargement of the tonsils or thyroid gland and CNS disease may be evident. Bone marrow involvement may show the L3 variety of lymphoblast containing vacuoles staining with oil red O.

Burkitt's lymphoma is a particularly dangerous form of childhood cancer because it frequently masquerades as an apparently "benign" tonsillitis or intussusception from a leading enlargement of cecal, ileal, or mesenteric nodes. Surface marker studies show a mature B cell with surface immunoglobulin. The B lymphoblast is the fastest growing human tumor cell, with doubling times of less than 24 hours. The disease can change from a barely palpable node to massive tumor in a matter of days.

Although the cell of origin and clinical behavior are similar to the African variety originally named after Dr. Denis Burkitt, the association with Epstein-Barr virus is lacking and the source of chronic antigenic stimulation (*eg*, malaria, parasites) is less obvious in western countries. There is a histologic variation of this tumor that causes some confusion; pathologists may report "nonBurkitt's, Burkitt's lymphoma." This designation reflects the heterogeneity of cell size and has little clinical relevance.

■ PATIENT EVALUATION AND DIAGNOSIS

Initial evaluation of NHL patients should include a thorough history and physical examination. Laboratory investigations should include a complete blood count, urinalysis, chest x-ray film, spinal tap, and bone marrow biopsy and aspirate, with samples sent for chromosome and cell marker analysis. Requisite blood chemistry evaluation includes serum electrolytes, including calcium and phosphate; liver function tests and blood urea nitrogen; and creatinine, uric acid, and serum lactate dehydrogenase (LDH) levels. The renal tests are especially important because of frequent kidney involvement in lymphoblastic and Burkitt's lymphomas.

Because of the rapid turnover of these cells and tumor lysis from chemotherapy, the physician must know if cell breakdown has resulted in dangerous levels of uric acid, cal-

TABLE 130-1. Staging of Childhood Non-Hodgkin's Lymphoma

Stage I	Single tumor in a node or extralymphatic site, excluding the mediastinum or abdomen
Stage II	Single extranodal tumor with one regional node positive Two or more nodal areas on the same side of the diaphragm; two extranodal tumors on the same side of the diaphragm regardless of nodal involvement; or primary gastrointestinal tract tumor plus or minus associated mesenteric nodes, grossly completely excised
Stage III	Two single extranodal tumors on opposite sides of the diaphragm; two or more nodal areas above and below the diaphragm; all tumors originating in mediastinum, pleura, or thymus; or all extensive primary intra-abdominal disease (usually many implants, not totally resectable), often with ascites
Stage IV	Any of the above with initial central nervous system or bone marrow involvement

From Murphy SB. Childhood non-Hodgkin's lymphoma. N Engl J Med. 1978;299:1446.

cium, or phosphate, which may precipitate in the kidney. This complication is usually preventable by vigorous hydration, alkalinization, and use of allopurinol before the treatment is begun.

The serum LDH is an important marker for following the progress of disease and has prognostic importance. If the LDH level is over 1000, there is a high probability of massive disease and a poor outcome. Chest x-ray and abdominal computed tomography examinations are necessary for determining the extent of intracavitary disease. Lymphangiograms are not helpful.

Removal of abdominal or tonsilar masses or biopsy of mediastinal nodes is required to make the diagnosis. Tissue samples should be sent for cell surface marker studies, chromosome analysis, and special molecular studies for further understanding of the tumor biology. A staging laparotomy as is done for Hodgkin's disease is unnecessary for NHL. The clinical staging categories are listed in Table 130–1.

■ TREATMENT

Stage I and II Burkitt's lymphoma patients have been treated with vincristine, doxorubicin, cyclophosphamide, prednisone, and intrathecal medications as induction and consolidation therapy. Some patients continue with maintenance for 33 weeks of mercaptopurine and methotrexate like acute lymphoblastic leukemia patients. A 94% complete remission rate has been reported. Stage III or IV patients had only a 10% chance of survival until the advent of very aggressive chemotherapy treatments. It is now possible to cure 80% of stage III and 50% of stage IV patients. These patients represent an especially challenging group because the high metabolic turnover of their tumor puts them at risk for renal and electrolyte complications (*ie*, tumor lysis syndrome) before and during induction therapy. Generous prehydration, alkalinization, and allopurinol treatment are necessary. The total time of treatment ranges from 3 to 5 months.

(Abridged from Kenneth L. McClain, Non-Hodgkin's Lymphoma, in Oski, DeAngelis, Feigin, McMillan, Warshaw: *Principles and Practice of Pediatrics, Second Edition,* J.B. Lippincott, 1994.)

Oski's Essential Pediatrics,
edited by Kevin B. Johnson and Frank A. Oski.
Lippincott–Raven Publishers,
Philadelphia © 1997

131

Malignant Brain Tumors in Children

Primary brain tumors are the second most common type of cancer reported in children and adolescents. In the United States, the annual incidence of primary brain tumors in children younger than 15 years of age is 24 per million persons in the general population or approximately 1200 new cases each year. Unfortunately, progress in the field of pediatric neuro-oncology has been slow compared with that in other childhood malignancies.

■ SYMPTOMS ON PRESENTATION

Early symptoms of central nervous system (CNS) tumors are frequently nonspecific. In infants with open sutures, these may consist of increased head circumference, irritability, head tilt, and loss of developmental milestones. Older children may present with headache. This symptom usually increases in frequency, becomes more severe in the morning, and is typically followed by vomiting. Approximately 85% of the children with malignant brain tumors have abnormal findings on neurologic or ocular examinations within 2 to 4 months of the onset of headaches.

Children who report an unchanging pattern of headaches without focal neurologic findings for more than 12 months have a low probability for CNS tumors. Specific neurologic symptoms, such as ataxia, somnolence, hemiparesis, seizures, head tilt, cranial nerve palsies, diencephalic

syndrome, and diabetes insipidus, may occur later in the illness and may suggest localization of the CNS tumor.

The differential diagnosis for CNS tumors in children is extensive and includes brain abscesses, hemorrhage, nonneoplastic hydrocephalus of any cause, arteriovenous malformations or aneurysm, and indolent virus infections.

■ CLASSIFICATION

Traditionally, CNS tumors of childhood have been classified on the basis of location (*eg,* infratentorial versus supratentorial) and histology. In children between the ages of 4 and 11 years, infratentorial (posterior fossa) tumors predominate. These include cerebellar tumors and brain stem tumors. Supratentorial tumors occur more frequently during the first years of life and during late adolescence and young adulthood. Approximately 45% of the childhood brain tumors arise in the cerebellum. Cerebellar astrocytomas and medulloblastomas are the tumors diagnosed most frequently in this region. Ependymomas that arise in and around the fourth ventricle represent between 3% and 14% of all childhood tumors and have been included as cerebellar tumors by some authorities.

The cerebrum is the next most common site of involvement in children, accounting for 20% to 27% of all brain tumors. The most frequent tumors include astrocytomas, glioblastomas, and ependymomas. Brain stem neoplasms account for 9% to 15% of all intracranial neoplasms. Approximately 75% of all brain stem tumors occur in children younger than 10 years of age. Midline tumors, which include a mix of germ cell tumors, craniopharyngiomas, pinealomas, optic gliomas, and pituitary adenomas, account for another 10%.

■ DIAGNOSTIC EVALUATIONS

Computed tomography (CT) scanning, with and without contrast enhancement, has been the standard noninvasive diagnostic tool for more than a decade. The unenhanced CT

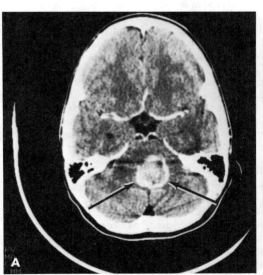
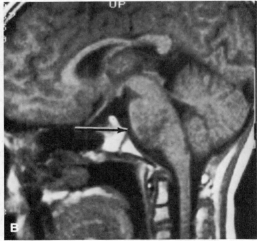
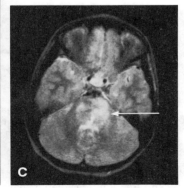

Figure 131-1. CT scan and MRI study of a brain-stem glioma. (**A**) CT scan demonstrating a ringlike enhancing mass (*arrows*) involving the mid pons. (**B**) Six months after the diagnosis and radiotherapy, the MRI sagittal view (T1 weighted) reveals an enlarging mass in the mid pons (*arrows*). (**C**) The axial T2-weighted scan reveals abnormal signal intensity (*arrow*) extending into the left brachium pontis.

scan can suggest whether a lesion is cystic or solid and whether there are calcifications, hemorrhage, edema, and hydrocephalus. After intravenous contrast, enhancement of the tumor occurs because of a disruption of the blood–brain barrier. This improves detection of small tumors, definition of isodense or hypodense regions within the tumor, and differentiation of areas of edema surrounding the tumor mass. Subarachnoid and leptomeningeal seeding of tumor may also be detected with enhanced scans. Cranial CT scans have a sensitivity of greater than 94% for primary brain tumors, but certain limitations of resolution must be recognized. Small lesions within the posterior fossa, especially within the brain stem, and small midline cystic structures near the base of the skull occasionally escape detection.

Magnetic resonance imaging (MRI) with gadolinium enhancement is a sensitive neuroimaging technology for the diagnosis of CNS tumors and is becoming more widely available. MRI scans are potentially superior to CT scans in the detection and definition of low-grade glial tumors and of lesions at the vertex, within the posterior fossa (especially within the brain stem), near the wall of the middle fossa, and at the base of the skull (Figure 131–1). MRI myelography with gadolinium enhancement is the best method for detecting spinal cord tumors or delineating leptomeningeal tumor invasion. Limitations include increased cost, longer scan times, an inability to detect calcifications, and limited access to the patient during the actual scan time.

■ TREATMENT

Published treatment results for various childhood malignant brain tumors vary widely and should be interpreted with caution. The number of patients with specific tumor histologies available for clinical investigations is small, and studies may report results from trials with limited patient entries. Despite this caveat, progress has been made in the treatment of several pediatric CNS tumors. Continued efforts must be made to enroll these patients in prospective, multimodal, cooperative treatment studies and accelerate the development of more effective therapeutic strategies.

(Abridged from Donald H. Mahoney Jr., Malignant Brain Tumors in Children, in Oski, DeAngelis, Feigin, McMillan, Warshaw: *Principles and Practice of Pediatrics, Second Edition*, J.B. Lippincott, 1994.)

Oski's Essential Pediatrics,
edited by Kevin B. Johnson and Frank A. Oski.
Lippincott–Raven Publishers,
Philadelphia © 1997

132

Wilms' Tumor

Wilms' tumor is a malignant embryonal neoplasm of the kidney of mixed cellular histology. The incidence remains remarkably constant, with 7.8 cases per million children younger than 15 years of age reported annually. It is diagnosed only slightly less often than neuroblastoma, and, like neuroblastoma, it is a tumor of young children: 77% occur in children younger than 5 years of age, and 90% occur in children younger than 7 years of age. The incidence peaks in children between the ages 1 and 3 years (median, 3.5 years). The tumors associated with cytogenic aberrations occur at a slightly earlier age. Girls are more frequently affected than boys (2:1), and they may present at a slightly older age.

■ CLINICAL AND DIAGNOSTIC FEATURES

The classic Wilms' tumor appears as a silent mass in the abdomen in almost two thirds of the patients. The tumor is often detected accidentally by the parents or incidentally during the course of a physical examination performed for other medical reasons. Abdominal pain occurs in approximately one third of the patients. The mass is usually hard, smooth, and confined to the flank or one side of the abdomen. Occasionally, a patient with Wilms' tumor experiences a sudden hemorrhage into the tumor and presents with rapid abdominal enlargement and anemia. Hematuria has been observed in 12% to 25% of the patients, and hypertension has been reported for as many as 63%. Nonspecific symptoms such as fever, malaise, constipation, and anorexia may be reported, but weight loss is an uncommon association.

The diagnosis of Wilms' tumor must be suspected in any child who has an abdominal mass. The evaluation includes complete blood counts, liver and kidney function studies, a skeletal survey, a chest radiograph, ultrasonography, and a computed tomography (CT) scan of the abdomen. If the abdominal CT scan fails to substantiate a renal lesion, a bone marrow examination is indicated before surgical intervention. A CT scan of the lungs may identify metastasis not seen on routine chest films.

The differential diagnosis includes neuroblastoma, rhabdomyosarcoma, leiomyosarcoma, renal cell sarcoma, fibrosarcoma, hypernephroma, polycystic kidneys, adrenal hemorrhage, renal vein thrombosis, dysplastic kidney, and renal carbuncle—almost anything that can cause a mass in the upper abdomen.

The final diagnosis depends on a biopsy or a complete excision of the tumor and subsequent histologic examination.

Rarely, syndromes of polycythemia, acquired von Willebrand's disease, and hypercalcemia have been associated with Wilms' tumor. Wilms' tumor occurs rarely in adults, who have a much poorer prognosis than the pediatric patients.

■ TREATMENT

Wilms' tumor is sensitive to chemotherapy and radiation therapy. Nevertheless, the first line of therapy is complete surgical excision of the tumor whenever possible.

An aggressive approach to metastatic disease has resulted in the salvage of many patients. Pulmonary irradiation plus chemotherapy with multiple agents has achieved survival rates of 40% to 50%. Many institutions excise liver or lung metastases if the lesions are surgically accessible and then administer chemotherapy or combined chemoradiotherapy. The prognosis is poorer for metastatic lesions that develop during the initial therapy, but it is reasonably good for patients off chemotherapy who develop metastatic disease.

The late effects of therapy can be very significant. The most prominent effects are bone and muscle changes secondary to radiation therapy. Significant among these are degrees of muscle atrophy and impairment of vertebral bone growth, which result in a high incidence of scoliosis. The younger the patient, the more profound is the subsequent damage, and many of these children have required corrective surgery, back braces, and long-term physiotherapy. Irradiation to the chest can damage mammary tissue in young patients. The incidence of second malignancies is low, but second tumors, benign and malignant, have been described in a few patients. These include exostoses, osteochondromas, mesotheliomas, and leukemia.

(Abridged from C. Philip Steuber and Donald J. Fernbach, Wilms' Tumor, in Oski, DeAngelis, Feigin, McMillan, Warshaw: *Principles and Practice of Pediatrics, Second Edition*, J.B. Lippincott, 1994.)

Oski's Essential Pediatrics,
edited by Kevin B. Johnson and Frank A. Oski.
Lippincott–Raven Publishers,
Philadelphia © 1997

133

Neuroblastoma

Neuroblastoma, ganglioneuroblastoma, and ganglioneuroma are tumors that develop from neural crest tissue and may arise from a number of widely separated anatomical sites along the craniospinal axis. After brain tumors, neuroblastoma is the most common solid tumor in childhood, with an incidence of approximately 10 per million white children per year and 7 per million black children per year. It is slightly more common in boys than in girls. Over half of the tumors occur in children younger than 2 years of age, and 75% are diagnosed during the first 4 years of life.

The actual incidence is probably much greater if based on random sections at autopsy of the adrenal glands of infants younger than 3 months of age, in which the incidence of neuroblastoma in situ has been reported to be as high as 1 in 39. These findings and the propensity for this tumor to regress spontaneously during the first year of life have important implications. Infants appear to possess an innate mechanism to cause regression of active tumor, eliminating a large percentage of the in situ tumors, or there is a biologic difference of the tumors of infants.

■ ETIOLOGY

The cause of neuroblastoma is unknown. No seasonal variation has been confirmed, but almost all services and surveys report significant variations in the annual incidence of this tumor. It is rare to find more than one case in a family, but there are reports of tumors occurring in siblings or successive generations. The concomitant occurrence of neuroblastoma with congenital anomalies of other organ systems has been described, but no specific defect exceeds the normal expectation of incidence. The findings of increased catecholamine excretion in the siblings of children with neuroblastoma supports the contention that all members of the family should be examined.

■ CLINICAL FEATURES

In almost 70% of the children with neuroblastoma, metastasis has occurred before the diagnosis is made, and the first clinical manifestations may be the result of metastatic disease. Commonly, however, the tumor appears as a large, "silent," intra-abdominal mass, and the signs and symptoms are attributable to compression of other tissues by the primary tumor or by the metastatic deposits. About 55% of the primary tumors are found in the abdomen, and about 33% arise from the adrenal gland. The abdominal mass is usually firm, irregular, nontender, and crosses the midline. Extrinsic pressure by the tumor on the genitourinary structures may result in increased urinary frequency or a partial obstruction to the flow of urine. The primary abdominal tumor may cause intracranial hypertension and other bizarre neurologic abnormalities.

Thoracic tumors may displace the chest organs and can compromise the airway or cause superior vena caval obstruction. Unexplained fever is a common presenting complaint. Bone pain may occur in the absence of visible skeletal lesions but may be absent in the presence of widespread, destructive lesions. Unfortunately, this tumor has a predilection for involvement of the skull and facial bones, which may result in bilateral proptosis. This can cause severe deformity later. In association with proptosis, ecchymoses of the upper eyelids are a clue that this symptom is more likely to be caused by infiltrative disease than by trauma.

Skin nodules, which are seen commonly in infants, have a bluish cast and have been given the sobriquet "blueberry muffin." Signs and symptoms occasionally result from the catecholamine production of the tumor and may include flushing, increased perspiration, hypertension, headaches, and tachycardia. Diarrhea unresponsive to medical therapy is rare, as is failure to thrive, but both have been described in association with this type of metabolic activity. Another rare complaint is acute cerebellar ataxia associated with oculogyric crisis (*ie*, opsomyoclonus). These signs and symptoms, including paraplegia, are all potentially reversible after removal or destruction of the tumor.

■ DIAGNOSTIC FEATURES

Peripheral hematologic studies often reveal anemia and reticulocytopenia, which are usually a reflection of metastatic disease involving the bone marrow. A bone marrow examination should be performed in every case of suspected neuroblastoma. Over half of all the children with neuroblastoma have tumor cells in the bone marrow. The tumor cells are seen easily on the bone marrow smears but are difficult to differentiate from other small round cell tumors of childhood such as lymphoma, leukemia, rhabdomyosarcoma, or Ewing's sarcoma. Electron microscopic examination may reveal the neurosecretory granules, which are diagnostic of neuroblastoma.

With the establishment of the relation between neuroblastoma and elevated urinary catecholamine excretion, neuroblastoma became one of a number of malignant neoplasms that have a fairly specific tumor marker. Increased amounts of vanillylmandelic acid or homovanillic acid are detected in the urine in more than 75% of these patients. These tests now can be done on a few milliliters of urine and with much greater accuracy than with the outdated 24-hour urine collection. The newer techniques measure all of the metabolic by-products of dopamine, norepinephrine, and epinephrine. Urinary metabolites now can be found in the urine of more than 90% of the children with neuroblastoma, with the exception of those with tumors arising from the spinal routes and ganglia, which are nonsecretors of catecholamines. Each laboratory must establish its own range of normal values. The level of catecholamine excretion has little prognostic significance, but the appearance or reappearance of elevated levels in children known to have had neuroblastoma indicates recurrent disease and a poor prognosis.

The complete evaluation of a child suspected of having neuroblastoma should include a total skeletal survey, including the skull. In the skull, osteolytic radiographic lesions and separation of the sutures are practically pathognomonic of neuroblastoma. Lytic lesions of the long bones and pelvis are common, but metastases from neuroblastoma are not easily distinguishable from Ewing's sarcoma, leukemia, or osteomyelitis. Chest radiographs may expose mediastinal or cervical tumors by delineating a mass and displacement of the mediastinal structures. The lateral chest x-ray film may help to reveal tumors in the left chest, where the heart may obscure lesions on routine anteroposterior films. Abdominal tumors may be seen on flat films of the abdomen and may show calcium deposits in many cases. An intravenous pyelogram may help differentiate an extrarenal from an intrarenal tumor.

The computed tomography scan and magnetic resonance imaging (MRI) are particularly useful for examining the abdomen. MRI has replaced standard myelography for the detection of intraspinal tumors and is useful in determining bone disease. Ultrasound examination is a useful tool for diagnosing intra-abdominal tumors and can also demonstrate calcifications. As a noninvasive imaging tool, sonography is particularly useful in serial follow-up evaluations. Arteriography, myelography, and lymphangiography have almost been replaced by the newer techniques but still may have a role in selected cases. Liver scans may show defects in the liver as an indication of metastatic disease. Regardless of all other findings, the diagnosis must always be confirmed by histologic examination.

■ DIFFERENTIAL DIAGNOSIS

Because of the metabolically active products and the propensity for this tumor to metastasize early, the symptoms may be quite variable. Lesions of the skull may resemble those of Langerhans' histiocytosis. Abdominal masses may suggest other diagnoses, including Wilms' tumor, lymphoma, mesenteric cysts, hydronephrosis, and splenomegaly. Occasionally, a mediastinal neuroblastoma may be confused with thymoma. Bone pain may resemble rheumatoid arthritis, osteomyelitis, and leukemia. All things considered, unless the tumor is very undifferentiated, it is usually not a difficult diagnosis to make after a proper biopsy specimen is obtained.

■ TREATMENT

Almost all treatment programs offer experimental therapy. The prognosis is related to the age of the patient, stage of the disease, and, in many cases, the biologic characteristics at the time of diagnosis. Patients younger than 1 year of age with stage I (stage A) disease have an excellent prognosis, and almost 100% of these children survive. If the tumor is localized (stage I or stage A) at any age, complete surgical excision is the treatment of choice. For metastatic disease, value of surgical excision of the presumed primary lesion is unclear, but second-look surgery is being used more frequently, particularly after initial intensive chemotherapy. The second-look procedure is useful in planning future therapy by identifying residual disease.

Radiation therapy plays an important role in the management of high-risk stage C disease in patients older than 1 year of age. Chemotherapy is an important component of therapy for low-risk or highly aggressive disease.

Allogeneic and autologous forms of bone marrow transplantation have been explored as therapeutic options. Transplantation allows dose intensification for highly resistant and relapsed disease. Allogeneic transplantation appears to offer no advantage over autologous transplantation. The use of autologous transplantation avoids the risk of graft-versus-host disease associated with allogeneic transplantation. The results of autologous bone marrow transplantation for patients with neuroblastoma vary widely. Progression-free survival rates at 2 years are in the range of 20% to 50%. Controversy continues about the utility of marrow purging, the need for total-body irradiation, and the appropriate preparative technique. A large, randomized trial may be necessary to answer the questions raised by transplantation. All investigators agree that intensified therapy is essential in the management of patients with high-risk neuroblastoma. Unfortunately, it is not clear which therapy offers the best opportunity to maximize outcome.

■ PROGNOSIS

Age and stage remain important prognostic variables, and biologic markers are becoming increasingly indispensable as additional predictors of outcome. After 1 year of age, the outcome becomes markedly worse, especially for children with stage II, III, or IV disease. Children who develop neuroblastoma after the age of 8 seem to have an improved survival (almost 50%). Patients younger than 1 year of age who have stage III or IV disease have a much more favorable response than those between the ages of 1 and 8. Infants with Evans stage IVs disease probably do as well without chemotherapy but may benefit from chemotherapy if the tumor is rapidly progressive, has unfavorable biologic characteristics, or appears to be acutely threatening the life of the patient. Spontaneous remissions are high in this group of children.

(Abridged from ZoAnn E. Dreyer and Donald J. Fernbach, Neuroblastoma, in Oski, DeAngelis, Feigin, McMillan, Warshaw: *Principles and Practice of Pediatrics, Second Edition*, J.B. Lippincott, 1994.)

Oski's Essential Pediatrics, edited by Kevin B. Johnson and Frank A. Oski. Lippincott–Raven Publishers, Philadelphia © 1997

134

Rhabdomyosarcoma

The soft tissue sarcomas form a diverse group of malignant neoplasms that arise from embryonal mesenchyma. As a group, these tumors are rare in children, and most of the information known about these diseases is derived from treating adults. The exception is rhabdomyosarcoma, a tumor of embryonal mesenchyma that gives rise to striated skeletal muscle. This malignancy is the most common soft tissue sarcoma of children and accounts for 5% to 15% of all malignant solid tumors in patients younger than 15 years of age.

■ INCIDENCE AND EPIDEMIOLOGY

Rhabdomyosarcoma is the most common of the soft tissue sarcomas in children, accounting for 4% to 8% of all malignant diseases in children younger than 15 years of age. It is the seventh most common malignant tumor in children. The annual incidence is estimated to be 4.4 per million white children and 1.3 per million black children. The ratio of males to females is 1.4:1. Low socioeconomic status has been associated with this disease, implying an environmental role in its pathogenesis.

Relatives of children with rhabdomyosarcoma have a high frequency of carcinoma of the breast and of brain tumors. Rhabdomyosarcoma is a recognized complication of neurofibromatosis and has been associated with other congenital abnormalities as well. Bone sarcoma has been reported as a second malignancy in patients with rhabdomyosarcoma.

■ CLINICAL MANIFESTATIONS

Rhabdomyosarcoma can occur anywhere in the body. The percentage of cases presenting at each anatomical location is depicted in Table 134–1. The head and neck (including the orbit) are the most common sites of primary occurrence, with 38% of the cases presenting in this region. The orbit accounts for 10% of the total presentations. The genitourinary tract is next in order of frequency, followed by the trunk, extremities, retroperitoneum, and other sites.

Approximately 70% of the tumors occur in children younger than 10 years of age, with a peak incidence between the ages of 2 and 5. The signs and symptoms relate to the primary site of the tumor or the metastases. Usually a painless, enlarging mass is noticed.

Tumors in the orbit can produce proptosis, chemosis, and ocular paralysis. These tumors can begin as a mass in the conjunctiva or eyelid. Tumors in the nasopharynx can cause a nasal voice, dysphagia, airway obstruction, epistaxis, or pain. Tumors in the paranasal sinuses cause swelling, pain, discharge, sinusitis, obstruction, or epistaxis. Laryngeal tumors cause hoarseness. Tumors in the middle ear are associated with a polypoid tumor in the external auditory canal that can cause pain, chronic otitis media, and a facial nerve palsy. Rhabdomyosarcoma may present as a painless facial or parotid mass. Neck masses may present with hoarseness or dysphagia. Parameningeal tumors may extend into the central nervous system, resulting in meningeal symptoms, cranial nerve palsies, or respiratory paralysis.

Tumors arising from the trunk, extremities, or paratesticular region usually occur as painless masses that are noticed by the child or parents. Tumors in the retroperitoneum usually are asymptomatic or are found as large masses that may cause gastrointestinal or urinary tract symptoms. Bladder and prostate tumors usually produce urinary tract symptoms. Tumors from the perineum may involve the bowel or bladder. Botryoid tumors appear as grapelike clusters of clear tissue protruding from the uterus or cervix.

The tumor characteristically grows with indistinct margins along fascial planes and infiltrates into surrounding tissues. Metastases spread hematogenously and by lymphatics to the lung, bone, bone marrow, lymph nodes, central nervous system, heart, and breast.

■ DIFFERENTIAL DIAGNOSIS

The differential diagnosis of rhabdomyosarcoma reflects the presenting complaint. With orbital tumors, it includes infection (*ie,* orbital cellulitis), proptosis secondary to hyperthyroidism, hemangioma, metastatic neuroblastoma, optic nerve glioma, retinoblastoma, granuloma, lymphoma, granulocytic sarcoma, fibrous dysplasia of bone, and Langerhans' histiocytosis.

Other tumors that can arise in the nasopharynx and paranasal sinus include inflammatory granulomas, lymphoma, other soft tissue sarcomas, carcinomas, and juvenile nasopharyngeal angiofibroma. Tumors in the neck must be differentiated from inflammatory lesions, branchial cleft cyst, lymphoma, carcinoma, sinus histiocytosis, and Langerhans' histiocytosis.

An intra-abdominal mass must be differentiated from a mesenteric cyst, intestinal duplication, Wilms' tumor, neuroblastoma, hepatoma, hemangioma, lymphoma, teratoma, carcinoma, and other soft tissue sarcomas. A paratesticular mass could be a benign tumor, including a varicocele or hydrocele, a seminoma, teratoma, embryonal carcinoma, lymphoma, or a rare tumor of the spermatic cord. In the bladder, neurofibroma, hemangioma, and transitional cell carcinoma or leiomyosarcoma should be considered. In the vagina, rhabdomyoma, a benign lesion, must be excluded.

Other soft tissue sarcomas can occur on the trunk. Bone tumors and neurogenic sarcoma should be considered in the differential diagnosis of tumors of an extremity.

■ DIAGNOSTIC EVALUATION

Open biopsy of the tumor is the definitive diagnostic procedure for an unexplained mass. Certain tests are performed before the surgical procedure to assess the extent of the disease for staging and therapeutic purposes.

Preoperative assessment should include a complete blood count, urinalysis, measurement of electrolytes (including calcium and phosphorus), liver and renal function tests, and a uric acid determination. Computed tomography (CT) or magnetic resonance imaging (MRI) of the primary tumor

TABLE 134-1. Primary Sites of Rhabdomyosarcoma

Site	Frequency (%)
Orbit	10
Head and neck	28
Trunk	7
Extremities	18
Genitourinary tract	21
Intrathoracic tissues	3
Gastrointestinal and hepatic systems	3
Perineum and anus	2
Retroperineum	7
Other sites	1

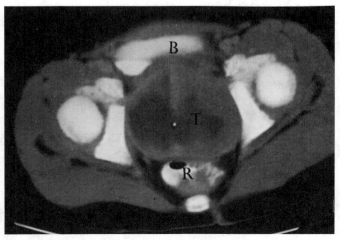

Figure 134-1. In the CT scan of a patient with a pelvic mass that was shown to be rhabdomyosarcoma after a surgical biopsy, the large pelvic tumor (*T*) is possibly associated with prostate, displacing the rectum (*R*) posteriorly, the bladder (*B*) anteriorly, and extending to the side walls bilaterally. Notice the Foley catheter in the center of the tumor and the central area of necrosis depicted by the darker region of the mass.

TABLE 134-2. Proposed Staging Criteria
for Rhabdomyosarcoma

Stage I	Primary tumors found at sites considered to be of favorable prognosis without distant metastases
Stage II	All other primary tumors less than 5 cm in diameter without metastases
Stage III	1. All other tumors greater than 5 cm in diameter 2. All other tumors with adjacent nodal involvement
Stage IV	All tumors with distant metastases at diagnosis

should be performed to delineate the involvement of adjacent structures and to aid in the surgical management of the patient. A CT scan of the chest, bone marrow examination, bone scan or skeletal survey, and liver scan should be performed to look for metastases. Patients with cranial parameningeal tumors should also have a CT or MRI scan of the head and an examination of the cerebrospinal fluid (CSF) to look for evidence of meningeal seeding with CSF pleocytosis, elevation in protein, and reduction of glucose. A CT scan may be employed to assess retroperitoneal lymph node involvement in patients with lower extremity and genitourinary tumors. Figure 134–1 demonstrates a solid tumor in the pelvis that was shown to be rhabdomyosarcoma after surgical biopsy.

■ TREATMENT

The therapy for rhabdomyosarcoma consists of a coordinated approach using surgery, radiation therapy, and chemotherapy. The surgeon provides tissue for diagnosis and attempts a total resection of the primary tumor, if possible without radical extirpative procedures. A reduction in tumor burden is achieved if total resection is not possible. Current surgical management includes second-look surgery to assess treatment response and the control of complications due to tumor regrowth and metastases. Aggressive excision surgery is not indicated in treating these children.

■ PROGNOSIS

Staging and 5-year survival rates are shown in Tables 134–2 and 134–3. The differences in survival between patients in group I and group II are not statistically significant and have led to discussion about changing the staging system. Preliminary analysis of patients treated on the IRS III study suggests that disease-free survival in the group III

TABLE 134-3. Five-Year Survival Rates
for Rhabdomyosarcoma*

Clinical Group	Five-Year Survival (%)
All	62
I	82
II	78
III	64
IV	27

*Based on data accumulated in IRS II.

children may be significantly improved from that reported in IRS II. These patients received more intensive therapy. It is clear from this table that the discovery of metastatic disease is an ominous finding. Tumors arising from the orbit, head and neck, and the genitourinary tract have been found to have a significantly better prognosis than do tumors arising from other sites (94% versus 65% 3-year survival rate). Local or distal recurrence carries a grave prognosis. Occasionally, a prolonged remission can be attained, especially if the tumor recurs after the completion of chemotherapy in a site amenable to surgery. Relapses, when they do occur, usually are seen within 2 years of institution of therapy, although a relatively small risk of late recurrences has been reported.

(Abridged from Richard L. Hurwitz, Soft Tissue Sarcomas, in Oski, DeAngelis, Feigin, McMillan, Warshaw: *Principles and Practice of Pediatrics, Second Edition,* J.B. Lippincott, 1994.)

Oski's Essential Pediatrics,
edited by Kevin B. Johnson and Frank A. Oski.
Lippincott–Raven Publishers,
Philadelphia © 1997

135

Retinoblastoma

■ INCIDENCE, LATERALITY, AND MORTALITY

Retinoblastoma is a rare, highly malignant tumor of the retina of young children. It is the seventh most common pediatric malignancy in the United States. The worldwide incidence of retinoblastoma is relatively stable at one case per 18,000 to 30,000 live births. There is no significant difference in incidence between sexes or among races. The average age at presentation ranges between 13 and 18 months; more than 90% of the cases are diagnosed before age 5 years. Retinoblastoma is a relatively slow-growing tumor that usually remains confined to the eye for months or even years. With early diagnosis, the overall 5-year survival rate exceeds 90%. However, when disease extends beyond the eye, mortality approaches 100%.

Retinoblastoma occurs unilaterally in 20% to 35% of cases. In more than 70% of cases, the tumor originates from a single focus and, when clinically detected, involves more than half the retina, with extension into the vitreous chamber. Multifocal involvement may be observed with unilateral retinoblastoma but is more common with bilateral disease. Although multiple tumor foci usually present simultaneously, in as many as 25% of cases new foci may develop within weeks to months after the original diagnosis. The potential for metachronous occurrence of retinoblastoma warrants careful follow-up examination, even of the previously unaffected retina. Bilateral disease is detected at an earlier age (median, 13 months) than unilateral disease (median, 24 months). The outlook for bilateral disease is significantly worse than for unilateral disease because of an increased incidence of second, nonocular malignant tumors in bilaterally affected cases.

■ GENETICS

Retinoblastoma occurs in both hereditary and nonhereditary forms. Knudson has postulated a "two-hit" mutational event as necessary for the development of disease. The retinoblastoma gene locus resides on human chromosome 13 at band q14. This retinoblastoma gene has been further characterized, mapped, and cloned and is the prototype for a class of recessive human cancer genes (tumor suppressor genes) in which a loss of activity of both normal alleles is thought to be associated with tumor genesis. Retinoblastoma gene mutations also have been found in some osteosarcomas, soft-tissue sarcomas, breast carcinomas, small-cell carcinomas of the lung, and prostatic carcinomas.

More than 90% of the patients have no family history of retinoblastoma and represent the first mutational event within the family. All patients with bilateral retinoblastoma and about 15% of the patients with unilateral retinoblastoma harbor a germinal mutation and have a hereditary form of the disease. According to Knudson's hypothesis, a somatic mutation following the germinal mutation is necessary to form the disease. About 85% of sporadic unilateral cases are nonhereditary; according to Knudson's hypothesis, two somatic mutations are required to produce the disease in these patients. When patients with either bilateral or unilateral retinoblastoma have the germinal mutation, 50% of their offspring will be affected by the disease, and one out of 100 will harbor a gene but not express the disease. Using DNA sequence polymorphism for recognizing the retinoblastoma locus, it is possible to predict familial predisposition to retinoblastoma in families with two or more affected members. Diagnosis of the hereditary form may be possible using direct DNA sequence analysis.

■ SIGNS AND SYMPTOMS

In the United States, the most common presenting sign is a white pupillary reflex called leukokoria (Figure 135–1). This abnormal reflex, present in 60% of the patients, is the result of a centrally located tumor at the posterior pole. Replacement of the vitreous with tumor or retinal detachment may also be noted.

The second most common sign is strabismus, present in 20% of the patients. In children under age 4, strabismus is usually the result of esotropia. With retinoblastoma, both esotropia and exotropia may occur and usually indicate tumor involvement of the macular area. Other signs include a red, painful eye with glaucoma (7%), poor vision (5%), unilateral dilated pupil, heterochromia (different-colored irises), or nystagmus. Children with advanced stages of disease may present with signs of lethargy, anorexia, failure to thrive, neurologic defects, orbital mass, proptosis, or blindness.

■ DIAGNOSIS AND DIFFERENTIAL DIAGNOSIS

The diagnosis of retinoblastoma is made by visual examination alone. The examination is best done by an experienced ophthalmologist using an indirect ophthalmoscope. The patient should be sedated or under general anesthesia, and the pupils should be dilated. Any child presenting with the above signs and symptoms requires prompt attention, with these examinations at a minimum.

The differential diagnosis for retinoblastoma depends on whether the tumor presents as a solitary mass or underlies an area of retinal detachment. When the tumor presents as a mass, there are two principal considerations: astrocytic hamartomas and granulomas of *Toxocara canis*. If the eye contains a retinal detachment, there are three diagnoses to consider: Coats' disease, retrolental fibroplasia, and persistent hyperplastic primary vitreous. The patient's age, past medical history (*ie*, oxygen exposure for retrolental fibroplasia, tuberous sclerosis for astrocytic hamartomas), and presentation will help the experienced ophthalmologist distinguish among these disorders.

■ TREATMENT

The priorities in treatment for retinoblastoma are to preserve life, to retain the eye, to retain vision, and to ensure favorable cosmetic results. Modalities in current use are enucleation, radiation (external beam and localized radioactive plaques), photocoagulation, cryotherapy, and systemic chemotherapy.

The following indications have been proposed for enucleation: unilateral group V eyes, most bilateral group V eyes, any blind eye with active tumor, any eye with glaucoma from invasive tumor, any eye that has failed all other forms of treatment, and patients who may not be available for future follow-up. At surgery, care must be taken to avoid rupture at tumor insertions, and attempts must be made to remove a long stump of optic nerve.

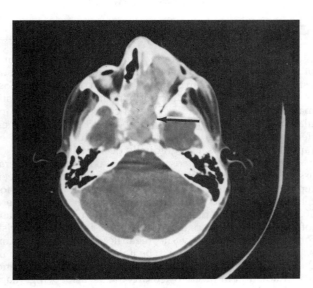

Figure 135-2. CT scan of face, sinuses, and orbits of a 14-year-old with bilateral retinoblastoma, treated 12 years prior. Note the large destructive osteosarcoma involving the left ethmoid and sphenoid area.

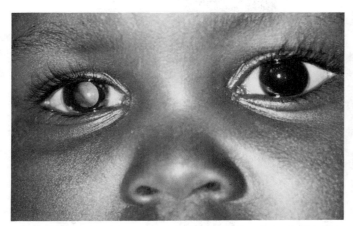

Figure 135-1. Abnormal white reflex, leukokoria, in a 7-month-old child with unilateral retinoblastoma.

■ SECOND TUMORS

Patients who have the germinal mutation for retinoblastoma and who survive the ocular tumor have a high risk for developing other malignancies. Tumors appear both within and outside the field of radiation. Tumors within the field include osteogenic sarcoma, fibrosarcoma, soft-tissue sarcoma, neuroblastoma, and meningioma. Osteosarcoma of the skull occurs 2000 times more frequently in survivors of bilateral retinoblastoma than in the general population (Figure 135–2). Patients with primitive neuroectodermal tumors involving the pineal region have been described as having "trilateral" retinoblastoma. The most common tumor outside the radiation field is osteosarcoma.

More than 90% of the patients with the germinal mutation who survive retinoblastoma develop a second malignancy within 32 years after treatment. The reason for this extraordinarily high incidence is linked to the retinoblastoma gene, which has been identified in several of these nonocular tumors. The mortality associated with second malignancies is high.

(Abridged from Donald H. Mahoney Jr., Retinoblastoma, in Oski, DeAngelis, Feigin, McMillan, Warshaw: *Principles and Practice of Pediatrics, Second Edition*, J.B. Lippincott, 1994.)

Oski's Essential Pediatrics,
edited by Kevin B. Johnson and Frank A. Oski.
Lippincott–Raven Publishers,
Philadelphia © 1997

136

Malignant Bone Tumors in Children

OSTEOGENIC SARCOMA

■ INCIDENCE AND EPIDEMIOLOGY

Osteogenic sarcoma is a malignant spindle-cell sarcoma of bone in which the tumor cells directly form neoplastic osteoid. Osteogenic sarcoma, or osteosarcoma, is the most common primary malignancy of bone in children. The estimated incidence in adolescence is 11 cases per 1 million population. The male/female ratio is about 1.5:1. The peak incidence occurs within the second decade, during periods of rapid growth spurts, and gradually declines thereafter.

The etiology of osteosarcoma is unknown, but several associations with underlying medical conditions have been reported. Patients who have the germinal mutation for retinoblastoma and who survive the ocular tumor have a 2000-fold increased risk for osteosarcoma in irradiated craniofacial bones. These patients have a 500-fold increased risk for osteosarcoma at any site regardless of prior radiation exposure. This risk appears to be linked to the expression of the retinoblastoma gene, located on chromosome 13, band q14. Radiation-induced osteosarcoma is also being diagnosed with increased frequency in long-term survivors of childhood cancer. Pediatric cancer groups studying late effects estimate a 40-fold risk for bone cancer in survivors

who have received more than 6000 rad to the bone. The median time to onset is 10 years. There is also an increased risk associated with alkylating agents, proportional to cumulative doses. In older patients with Paget's disease, there is an increased risk for osteosarcoma involving the affected bone. Occasional cases also have been reported in association with chondroma, osteochondromatosis, and nonossifying fibroma.

■ SIGNS, SYMPTOMS, AND DIAGNOSTIC STUDIES

The metaphyseal portion of the long bone is the site of predilection. Almost half of all new cases present with involvement in the region of the knee. In order of presentation, the most common sites are the distal femur, proximal tibia, and proximal humerus. However, any membranous bone may be involved, and even cases of extraosseous osteosarcoma have been reported.

Pain, which initially may be intermittent, and swelling of the extremity, which may evolve over several weeks, are the cardinal symptoms. Because these symptoms are nonspecific, adolescents presenting with pain in the area of the knee without a history for trauma should undergo a radiographic examination. Pathologic fractures are uncommon. However, minor trauma with disproportional symptoms of pain may cause these patients to present for evaluation and lead to the recognition of a preexisting pathologic lesion.

The diagnosis of osteosarcoma may be suspected from good-quality radiographs; tumors may appear as lytic, sclerotic, or mixed lesions. Irregular periosteal new bone formation in the metaphyseal region may be an initial observation. In more advanced cases, cortical destruction, sclerosis, a sunburst pattern of periosteal new bone formation, and contiguous, calcified soft-tissue extensions may be noted (Figure 136–1). Submicroscopic extension along the diaphysis can produce "skip" metastases some distance from the primary lesion.

The diagnosis is best made by incisional biopsy and permanent section. A carefully performed needle biopsy also may provide material sufficient for diagnosis. Extreme care

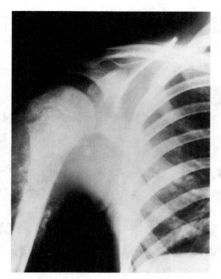

Figure 136-1. A large permeative lesion of the proximal right humerus, representing osteosarcoma beginning at the metaphyseal plate, with soft-tissue extension and calcifications due to osteosarcoma.

must be taken in the biopsy of these lesions, because an incorrectly directed biopsy may produce an inadequate or misleading diagnosis or may leave a tract that will complicate possible consideration for limb salvage therapy. Ultimately, the biopsy tract must be excised en bloc with the tumor at the time of definitive surgery. In view of the rarity of these tumors and because of recent developments in the multimodal management of these patients, referral to a pediatric cancer center for definitive biopsy and diagnosis is in the patient's best interest.

Patients considered for limb preservation require computed tomography (CT) or magnetic resonance imaging (MRI) examinations of the tumor-bearing bone and occasionally angiography. MRI scans are very accurate in the assessment of intraosseous extension of tumor and are the preferred examination for patients undergoing limb salvage procedures.

■ TREATMENT

Before the 1970s, the prognosis for children with osteosarcoma of the extremity was dismal. Despite control of the primary tumor with amputation, distant metastases developed in most patients, and survival was about 20% at 5 years from diagnosis. Current multimodal treatment strategies for osteosarcoma have reversed this trend, and about 60% to 65% of patients with nonmetastatic disease of the extremities are surviving their disease. Both surgery and high-dose chemotherapy play a significant part in achieving this result.

Surgery has an established role in the treatment of osteosarcoma. Ablative procedures usually involve amputation through the bone above the affected bone. It is generally accepted that the amputation should be 7 cm beyond the most proximal limits of the lesion to minimize the risk for local recurrence. Large lesions involving the proximal femur or humerus occasionally require a disarticulation procedure.

With the availability of more effective chemotherapy programs, limb salvage surgery, after en bloc tumor excision and endoprosthetic replacement, has become a viable alternative for many patients. Candidates considered eligible for the limb salvage procedure are generally selected on the basis of the following criteria:

- Attainment of complete or nearly complete physical growth for patients with lesions of the lower extremities
- Anatomical site of the lesion such that no sacrifice of major arteries or nerves is involved
- Absence of metastases at diagnosis, or isolated metastasis that responded to preoperative treatment
- Full understanding by the patient and parents of the nature of the procedure, reasonable expectations for functional outcome, and estimated risks for complications, local recurrence, and possible failure of procedure.

Limb salvage may be performed by immediate en bloc resection or may follow a brief course of chemotherapy. The potential advantages of preoperative chemotherapy are that it allows for planning and acquisition of a custom prosthesis, it may allow some definition of the antitumor efficacy of the chemotherapy regimen to be used as postoperative adjuvant therapy, and the antitumor effects may enhance the safety of the surgical procedure. Several pediatric cancer centers have extended the process of preoperative treatment to all osteosarcoma patients, but the value of this approach remains to be established.

Pulmonary metastases remain the major obstacle for cure for patients with osteosarcoma. The number and time of presentation of metastases may have clinical significance: early-appearing, multiple lesions may be associated with drug-resistant disease and poor prognosis. Aggressive surgical treatment, including multiple and occasionally bilateral thoracotomies, coupled with intensive chemotherapy, may salvage 25% to 50% of these patients. Complete removal of all metastatic tumor at the time of the initial thoracotomy may have the greatest importance for long-term survival. Refinement of limb salvage techniques in the future will increase the number of children who might enjoy a more functionally and cosmetically satisfying result from the primary surgical treatment.

EWING'S SARCOMA

■ INCIDENCE AND EPIDEMIOLOGY

Ewing's sarcoma is an uncommon primary sarcoma of nonosseous origin that usually arises in children or adolescents. James Ewing is credited with the first description of this tumor in 1921. Ewing's sarcoma represents about 1% of all cancers reported in children but about 30% of all bone tumors in this age group. The estimated incidence is two per 1 million population in the United States for Caucasians under age 20; it is rare in the nonwhite population. The male:female ratio is 1.54:1.

The etiology for Ewing's sarcoma is unknown. Unlike osteosarcoma, ionizing radiation exposure does not represent a significant risk factor.

■ CLINICAL PRESENTATION AND DIAGNOSTIC EVALUATION

Pain is the most common first symptom in Ewing's sarcoma, occurring in more than half of the patients. Swelling associated with a soft-tissue mass may become evident weeks to months thereafter. Fever and an elevated erythrocyte sedimentation rate (ESR) may develop in time and may confound the diagnosis. Pathologic fractures are uncommon.

The femur is the bone most commonly involved, but any bone of the body may be involved (Figures 136–2 and 136–3). The classic radiographic feature is a diffuse, mottled, lytic lesion affecting the medullary cavity and cortical bone. There may be regions of increased density associated with new bone formation. Tumor that penetrates the cortex and extends into the periosteum may produce elevations characterized by multiple layers of reactive new bone formation, creating an "onion-skin" appearance on radiographic examination. The tumor may expand the affected bone and resemble a cystic malformation. A soft-tissue mass, rarely including calcifications, may be associated with the primary bone tumor. Although these radiographic features have been clearly described with Ewing's tumors, several conditions can produce similar features, including acute and chronic osteomyelitis, eosinophilic granuloma, osteosarcoma, metastatic sarcomas, and lymphoma. An MRI scan of the affected bone gives the best assessment of intramedullary tumor extension.

An open biopsy is the procedure of choice to establish the diagnosis of Ewing's sarcoma. In general, needle biopsies do not provide sufficient material for interpretation and have, on occasion, produced confusing information. The two conditions most often mistaken for Ewing's sarcoma are

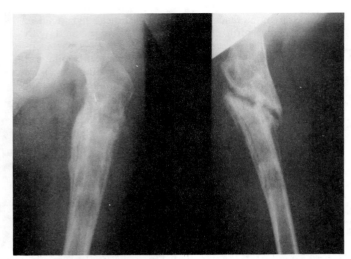

Figure 136-2. Two radiographic views of the left femur demonstrating a diffuse, destructive process due to Ewing's sarcoma, involving the intertrochanteric region and extending to the mid-shaft. There is a pathologic fracture.

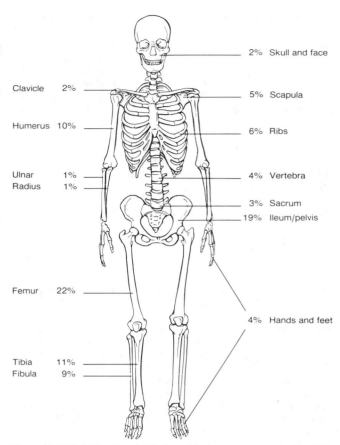

Figure 136-3. Anatomical distribution of Ewing's sarcoma, based on 836 cases. (After Sutow WW, Fernbach DJ, Vietta TJ, eds. *Clinical pediatric oncology*, St Louis: CV Mosby; 1984:chap 29.)

eosinophilic granuloma and osteomyelitis. The presence of necrosis or inflammatory cells within the tumor can be misleading if the biopsy material is inadequate. Biopsy of cortical lesions should be as small and round as possible, avoiding the tension side of the bone if possible, and should include touch preparations and material for electron microscopy. If a malignant bone tumor is suspected in a child or adolescent, referral to a pediatric cancer center for the definitive diagnosis will ensure the most experienced surgical assessment and optimum biopsy for these patients.

Once the diagnosis of Ewing's sarcoma is established, clinical staging is essential, including chest radiographs, a CT scan of the chest, an MRI scan of the bone, a radionuclide bone scan, and bone marrow aspiration and biopsy. These investigations are pursued because the lungs and bones are the most common sites of metastases (90% of the cases). Other baseline studies are also recommended, including serum lactate dehydrogenase, alkaline phosphatase, and ESR. These tests may reflect the extent of tumor activity. Urinary catecholamines may be helpful to rule out neuroblastoma in the younger patient.

■ TREATMENT AND PROGNOSIS

Ewing's sarcoma is a highly malignant tumor with a great propensity for metastatic spread before diagnosis. Before the 1960s, surgery and radiotherapy were the mainstays of therapy. Local control was adequate, but long-term disease-free survival (DFS) was only 9%. A multidisciplinary approach is now the recognized treatment of choice.

There is a renewed interest in surgical management of the primary tumor, due to the improved survival in patients with complete removal, the increased risk of orthopedic complications after chemoradiotherapy, the difficulty in confirming that the primary site has been sterilized, and the concern that residual microscopic disease might produce distant metastases. The exact role for surgery in the treatment of Ewing's sarcoma is yet to be determined. Possible applications include aggressive surgery for lesions in expendable bones, in which resulting disability is acceptable (*ie*, lesions in the foot, fibula, rib, forearm bone, clavicle, or scapula). Amputation may be recommended for extremity lesions in which there are huge destructive components, pathologic

fractures, or involvement of distal femoral epiphysis in children under age 6. Debulking of large pelvic primaries following initial tumor reduction with chemotherapy may also increase the chances for long-term survival.

The presence of metastatic disease at diagnosis has been reported in 14% to 35% of patients and is associated with a poor prognosis. Historically, the median DFS for patients with metastatic disease at diagnosis has been 75 weeks. Patients developing distant metastases while receiving therapy have resistant disease and an expected median survival of 37 weeks.

For survivors of Ewing's sarcoma, several late consequences of treatment may have a significant impact. Pathologic fractures may occur at primary tumor sites involving lower extremities at periods of 6 months to 3 years from diagnosis. This complication may be related to impaired bone remodeling following radiation and chemotherapy. Demineralization and radiation-associated delayed healing may aggravate this situation by causing nonunion of the fracture site. Other potential complications of radiation therapy include retarded bone growth, limb-length discrepancy, fibrosis, sclerosis, and functional limitations. The combination of radiation and chemotherapy has carcinogenic potential. The estimated rate for second cancers is 72 times the expected value in the normal population. Other potential complications include sterility associated with prolonged use of cyclophosphamide, and cardiotoxicity associated with doxorubicin.

(Abridged from Donald H. Mahoney Jr., Malignant Bone Tumors in Children, in Oski, DeAngelis, Feigin, McMillan, Warshaw: *Principles and Practice of Pediatrics, Second Edition,* J.B. Lippincott, 1994.)

Oski's Essential Pediatrics,
edited by Kevin B. Johnson and Frank A. Oski.
Lippincott–Raven Publishers,
Philadelphia © 1997

137

Langerhans Cell Histiocytosis

The terminology for histiocytic proliferative disorders is in the process of changing. Experts in the field have suggested that the original terminology for the various syndromes in the "histiocytosis-X" category (Letterer-Siwe disease, Hand-Schüller-Christian syndrome, and eosinophilic granuloma) should be replaced by the term *Langerhans cell histiocytosis* (LCH) because the proliferative cell that causes these entities is known. The cell is the dendritic histiocyte, also called the Langerhans' cell, which contains characteristic pentalaminar Birbeck granules seen by electron microscopy (Figure 137–1). To establish the diagnosis of Langerhans histiocytosis, positive electron microscope identification of Birbeck granules is necessary, and additional data are helpful.

The Langerhans cell diseases are not malignancies, but manifestations of complex immune dysregulation. The proliferation of these "normal" cells causes destruction or impairment of other organ systems. The Langerhans cell is a distinct member of the antigen-processing cells such as monocytes or histiocytes in the bone marrow. Like other antigen-processing cells, it produces a stimulating factor for T lymphocytes (a lymphokine, interleukin-1) that is necessary for the activation and response of T cells. They, in turn, make interleukin-2, which stimulates other T cells. Feedback stimulation on Langerhans cells (or other histiocytes) results from production of gamma-interferon and prostaglandin E_2 by the T cells. Somewhere in the interactive cycle, a regulatory element is lost such that the histiocytes proliferate locally or diffusely.

There is abundant evidence of immunologic abnormalities in LCH patients. Elevation of at least one type of immunoglobulin is found in 75% of patients, with most having high IgM. Although the mitogenic response is normal in most patients' lymphocytes, the number of suppressor T cells is often low. Circulating lymphocytes that were spontaneously cytotoxic to cultured human fibroblasts have been reported.

■ CLINICAL SYNDROMES

Clinical syndromes of LCH should now be identified according to the degree or number of organ systems involved, such as LCH, solitary skull lesion, instead of eosinophilic granuloma.

Solitary Lesions

This is the most benign form of LCH and frequently presents as one or more well-circumscribed lesions in the skull. The patient presents with pain or swelling in the region. Often the defects are easy to palpate. Any bone in the body can be involved, but the other most common sites are the femur, pelvis, vertebra, and mandible. Orbital lesions causing proptosis have been reported. Most children present between 1 and 9 years of age.

Treatments used include curettage or low-dose radiotherapy for resolution of pain, deformity, or danger of pathologic fractures. Some centers treat patients with prednisone or vinblastine sulfate instead of radiotherapy until there is some resolution of the radiographic findings. Most patients show sclerosis of the margins or more than 75% filling of the defect by 5 months after beginning therapy. Complete healing may take years.

Multiple Lesions

Multiorgan involvement is more prevalent in children under 5 years of age. Prognosis depends on the age of presentation and whether any organ system function is impaired. A good-risk patient is one older than 2 years with no organ dysfunction; this implies a chance of survival of more than 80%. Those younger than 2 years at diagnosis are

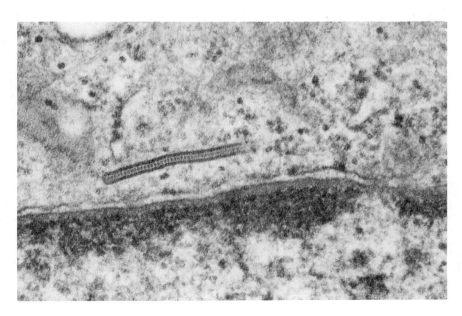

Figure 137-1. Electron micrograph of a Langerhans histiocytosis cell showing the striated, multilaminar granule (Birbeck granule) diagnostic of the Langerhans histiocytoses (magnification x141,831). (Courtesy of Dr. H.K. Hawkins, Department of Pathology, Texas Children's Hospital, Houston.)

by age alone in an intermediate group and have only a 60% to 70% chance of survival. The poorest-risk group includes very young children with multisystem disease, but can include any age with organ dysfunction; this group has an overall survival of less than 50%.

In these contexts, organ dysfunction includes evidence of hepatic failure by total protein less than 5.5 g/dL, albumin less than 2.5 g/dL, total bilirubin over 1.5 mg/dL, edema, and ascites. Hematologic dysfunction includes hemoglobin less than 10 g/dL, leukocyte count less than 4000/mm^3, neutrophils less than 1500/mm^3, and platelets 100,000/mm^3. Pulmonary dysfunction includes tachypnea, dyspnea, cyanosis, cough, pneumothorax, and pleural effusion.

Many of these children will present with a seborrheic rash of the scalp and periauricular regions that mimics "cradle cap" or eczema. The chronic draining ears at first appear to be a chronic otitis externa. Hepatosplenomegaly, anemia, thrombocytopenia, and pulmonary disease make the diagnosis more obvious clinically, but the diagnostic cell type must be confirmed by the methods previously mentioned. Other clinical findings that accompany the various forms of LCH include diabetes insipidus, growth retardation, hyperprolactinemia, hypogonadism, panhypopituitarism, and hyperosmolar syndrome secondary to pituitary involvement. Infiltration of the thyroid and pancreas with resultant organ deficiencies has been reported. Occasionally skull x-rays show evidence of "floating" teeth when the mandible is involved. Gingivitis is also seen.

Of the children presenting with generalized LCH, involvement of various organ systems are found in bone (100%), skin (88%), liver (71%), lung (54%), lymph nodes (42%), spleen (25%), pituitary (25%), bone marrow (18%), and central nervous system (CNS; 16%).

The evaluation should include a complete history and physical examination with complete blood count, bone marrow aspirate and biopsy when an abnormal blood count is found, radiographic survey of the complete skeleton and chest, bone scan, lumbar puncture when CNS symptoms are present, careful monitoring of intake and output, serum and urine osmolality, and biopsy of an affected site for confirmatory histologic diagnosis. The biopsy material should be sent for electron microscopy to look for Birbeck granules. The S-100 and T6 stains should be performed as additional confirmatory data.

■ TREATMENT AND LONG-TERM OUTLOOK

Standard therapy for disseminated LCH has included prednisone 40 to 60 mg/m^2/day orally and vinblastine sulfate 6 mg/m^2 (0.1 mg/kg) intravenously weekly. The duration of therapy and need for escalation depend on the patient's response.

LCH is a chronic disease with a waxing and waning nature that tries the patience of all involved. When the disease is active for more than 5 years, many patients will have diabetes insipidus, growth failure, intellectual impairment, neurologic deficit, emotional or orthopedic problems, chronic lung disease, or hearing deficits.

(Abridged from Kenneth L. McClain, Histocytic Proliferative Diseases, in Oski, DeAngelis, Feigin, McMillan, Warshaw: *Principles and Practice of Pediatrics, Second Edition*, J.B. Lippincott, 1994.)

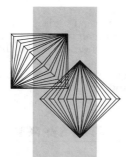

SECTION 10

Genitourinary Disorders

Oski's Essential Pediatrics,
edited by Kevin B. Johnson and Frank A. Oski.
Lippincott–Raven Publishers,
Philadelphia © 1997

138

Disorders of Renal Development and Anomalies of the Collecting System, Bladder, Penis, and Scrotum

■ DISORDERS OF RENAL DEVELOPMENT

Anomalies of Position

Simple Ectopia

Simple renal ectopia is a condition in which a kidney is located in an abnormal position but remains on its own side of the midline. Often there is associated incomplete rotation of the renal unit. The most common position is in the true pelvis; less common locations are the thorax or iliac fossa. Ectopia occurs in one in 500 to 1200 live births and is more common on the left.

An ectopic kidney is associated with other anomalies in many patients. The most common are other urologic abnormalities and musculoskeletal, cardiovascular, gastrointestinal (GI), and otolaryngologic anomalies. Treatment, if any, should address pathologic factors (primarily ureteral obstruction) rather than the position of the renal unit.

Fusion Anomalies

In patients with fusion anomalies, the two renal units are connected. Horseshoe kidneys are the most common fusion anomalies, accounting for about 90% of these abnormalities. They often are discovered incidentally during evaluation of associated anomalies or urinary infection or at autopsy. The kidneys are positioned lower than normal, with their lower poles joined by an isthmus of tissue. They are incompletely rotated and their axes are more vertical than normal, a consistent and characteristic sign on intravenous urography. The isthmus usually crosses the midline anterior to the great vessels below the inferior mesenteric artery, which blocked further ascent of the kidneys during fetal development. The ureters may be somewhat dilated above the location where they cross in front of the isthmus; however, the need for surgical repair is unusual. Associated anomalies are common but usually are less serious than

those related to crossed renal ectopia. Urologic evaluation should include a voiding cystourethrogram because reflux is a common finding. Treatment decisions are based on the same criteria as for a normal kidney (Figure 138–1).

Anomalies of Renal Parenchyma

Agenesis

Unilateral renal agenesis is present in one in 450 to 1800 live births. Its etiology is related to maldevelopment of the metanephric duct (primitive ureter) and renal blastema. Often the ipsilateral ureter and vas deferens are absent because their embryologic origins are intertwined. Compensatory hypertrophy of the solitary kidney is common but not pathognomonic for this lesion. Diagnosis often is made during investigation of other anomalies (cardiovascular, GI, musculoskeletal). No treatment is needed, but the child and parents should be cautioned that only a single kidney is present so that they may avoid activities that might put the kidney at undue risk of injury (*eg*, organized football, riding motorcycles).

Polycystic Kidney

Polycystic kidney disease is an inherited disorder, either autosomal recessive (infantile polycystic disease) or autosomal dominant (adult polycystic disease). The two entities are distinct and should not be confused. The recessive form is found in homozygotes, the dominant form in heterozygotes. Other organs are involved, especially the liver; in the dominant form, cerebral aneurysms are common.

In the recessive form, the kidneys retain their reniform configuration but are enlarged. The parenchyma is filled with dilated renal collecting tubules that appear as small radial cysts. The collecting system (renal pelvis and ureter) is normal, as is the renal pedicle. All children with recessive polycystic kidney disease have involvement of the liver consisting of bile duct dilation and proliferation with varying amounts of periportal fibrosis. Areas of uninvolved parenchyma are interspersed among these involved segments. The degree of renal and hepatic involvement appears to be inversely related, with younger children having more renal but less hepatic involvement. Children who are older when they present usually have more severe hepatic impairment with marked periportal fibrosis. Prognosis is related to age at diagnosis, those children discovered at birth having the worst outcome. Those in whom the disease is found late in childhood do better, but most die before reaching adulthood, often of hepatic complications.

The disease in infants usually is discovered as part of an evaluation for palpable renal masses noted on routine examination. An ultrasound will show enlarged kidneys with increased, diffuse echogenicity. Intravenous urography will show typical radial streaking of the dilated collecting

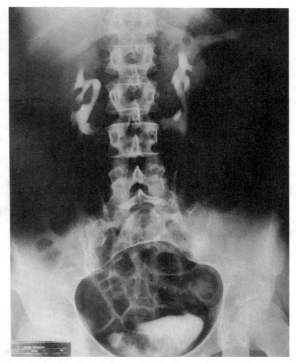

Figure 138-1. IVP of a horseshoe kidney. Note the axis deviation and incomplete rotation of the kidneys.

tubules. Although the kidneys function, they do so poorly; without delayed films, visualization of dye in the renal pelvis, ureter, or bladder is unusual (Figure 138–2).

The dominant form is usually noted in adults and is a completely different disease. It too is slowly progressive and ultimately results in renal insufficiency in most cases. The cysts are of various sizes and may be large. The kidneys may

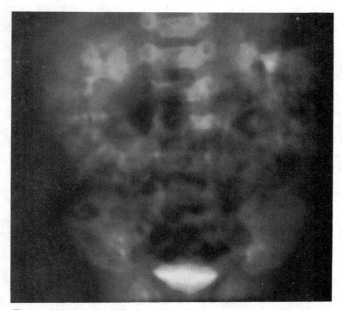

Figure 138-2. In this IVP of a child with recessive polycystic kidney disease, note the massive enlargement of the kidneys, good excretion and linear streaking of the contrast material. (Gonzales ET Jr. Genitourinary disorders in the neonate. In: Whitaker RH, Woodard JR, eds. *Paediatric urology.* London: Butterworth's; 1985.)

be huge and fill almost the entire abdomen. Treatment is usually limited to controlling hypertension and any infections that occur and intervention with dialysis or transplantation when necessary. A complete and thorough family history for the past several generations is imperative to identify other affected family members and to assist in the diagnosis. Appropriate genetic counseling should be done.

■ ANOMALIES OF THE COLLECTING SYSTEM

Ureteropelvic Junction Obstruction

Obstruction at the ureteropelvic junction (UPJ) is the most common cause of hydronephrosis in childhood and one of the two most common etiologies for a renal mass in neonates (the other is a multicystic kidney). The obstruction is often caused by an intrinsic fibrosis at the junction of the renal pelvis and ureter that disrupts the peristaltic wave across that region. Less common etiologies include a crossing renal vessel, kinking of the ureter, stenosis of the junction, and adhesions or extrinsic fibrosis at the UPJ. The obstruction leads to increased intrapelvic pressure, which causes dilation of the pelvis and calyces. This obstruction predisposes to urinary stasis, infection, hematuria, pain, and gradual destruction of renal parenchyma.

The diagnosis is often suggested by prenatal ultrasound and confirmed by postnatal studies. Other signs and symptoms include urinary tract infection (UTI), pyelonephritis, abdominal or flank pain, sepsis, palpable masses, nausea, failure to thrive, or an incidental finding during the evaluation of associated congenital anomalies. Investigations should include a renal ultrasound, intravenous pyelogram (IVP), or renal scan. These studies should demonstrate pyelocaliectasis and late emptying of the renal pelvis. Because the IVP often shows poor excretion, delayed films out to 24 hours may be necessary. The renal scan can help estimate the relative contribution of the obstructed kidney to overall renal function, and the addition of diuresis (with furosemide) may show a prolonged washout period that suggests obstruction. A voiding cystourethrogram is necessary because high-grade vesicoureteral reflux can mimic a UPJ obstruction or cause a secondary UPJ obstruction as a result of the large volume of refluxed urine. In both of these cases, control of the reflux will resolve the upper tract difficulties (Figure 138–3).

A pyeloplasty is the surgical repair of a UPJ obstruction. Its goal is to provide a funneled and dependent pelvis leading to the ureter. Reduction of pelvic size may be necessary to facilitate renal emptying. Significant improvement in radiographic appearance and renal function is usual after relief of obstruction, especially in infants. Therefore, efforts should be made to repair even those kidneys with poor function. There is a trend toward earlier exploration and repair of kidneys; some advocate surgery within the first several weeks of life. Neonates tolerate the surgery well, and, with the use of optical magnification, the procedure is technically feasible in even the youngest children. Long-term follow-up is necessary both for confirmation of an adequate postoperative anatomical result and for final assessment of renal function.

Ureteral Duplication and Ectopia

Complete Duplication

Ureteral duplication is the most common congenital urologic anomaly; it affects about one in 150 individuals. Etiologically it can be traced to two ureteral buds arising from

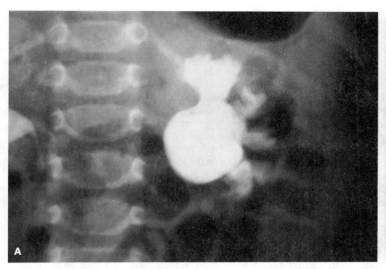
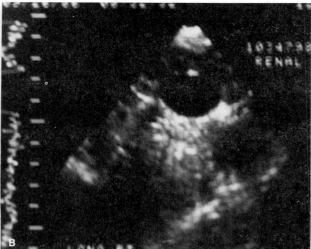

Figure 138-3. Ureteropelvic junction obstruction demonstrated by (**A**) IVP and (**B**) renal ultrasound.

a single Wolffian duct. Both buds reach the developing metanephros and stimulate renal differentiation. The ureter to the lower segment is absorbed into the developing bladder earlier and, therefore, travels further along the trigone, finally resting lateral and cephalad to the upper pole ureter, which lies medial and caudal. This relationship is known as the Weigert-Meyer law. The lower pole ureter is prone to

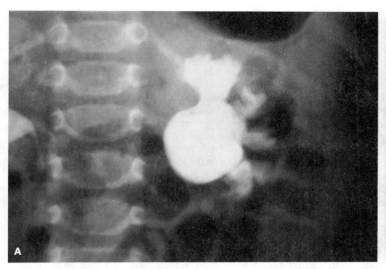

Figure 138-4. IVP of a neonate with a right duplication anomaly. There is nonvisualization of the right upper pole with the "drooping lily" deformity of the lower pole moiety. (Gonzales ET Jr. Genitourinary disorders in the neonate. In: Whitaker RH, Woodard JR, eds. *Paediatric urology.* London: Butterworth's; 1985.)

reflux, whereas the upper pole ureter (medial and inferior) is more often associated with obstruction from either ectopia or an ectopic ureterocele.

A full spectrum of renal involvement has been observed, ranging from the child with severe bilateral lower pole reflux and bilateral obstructing ureteroceles to the asymptomatic adult in whom duplication anomalies are discovered serendipitously. In the severe case, the diagnosis may be made on the basis of prenatal ultrasound, but more often the diagnosis is made during the workup of a UTI. An IVP may show a nonfunctioning upper pole moiety depressing the functioning lower pole collecting system and pushing it laterally (the so-called drooping lily deformity) (Figure 138–4). A renal ultrasound will show similar findings: a hydronephrotic upper pole "cap" of tissue depressing a normal lower pole segment. The bladder may demonstrate a negative filling defect caused by nonopacification of a large ureterocele. A renal scan can estimate the functional capacity of each segment, and a voiding cystourethrogram is required for assessment of possible lower pole reflux.

Treatment is as varied as the presentation. Often when the upper pole has no function, an upper pole partial nephroureterectomy is done. If, on the other hand, there is good function in that segment, a ureteropyelostomy connecting the upper pole ureter to the lower pole renal pelvis is done in conjunction with partial resection of the distal upper pole ureter. If lower pole reflux is present with an upper pole ureterocele, some surgeons reimplant the ureters at the same sitting. Other surgeons delay any bladder surgery for several months or years in the hope that the reflux may resolve once the ureterocele, which has been distorting the bladder, has been decompressed. When reflux to the lower pole is present without upper pole obstruction, a common sheath ureteroneocystostomy may be all that is required.

The prognosis depends on the degree of renal damage present at the time of intervention. However, renal function is generally adequate, and further problems are unusual.

■ VESICOURETERAL REFLUX

Vesicoureteral reflux is the retrograde regurgitation of urine from the bladder toward the kidney. Reflux is either primary or acquired; in children, primary reflux is more prevalent. Its etiology is embryologically related to a malpositioning of the ureteral bud on the Wolffian duct. This location causes the ureteral orifice to be lateral and cephalad on the trigone, thus foreshortening the submucosal tunnel. The tunnel provides the valvelike mechanism against urinary reflux, and, if it is deficient, reflux can occur. The degree of reflux may range from very mild (when urine enters the ureter but does not reach the kidney) to very severe (when the ureters are widely dilated and tortuous with gross pyelocaliectasis). An objective system using well-described criteria for grading reflux is used throughout the world and is based on the voiding cystourethrogram.

The diagnosis of reflux is best made with a voiding cystogram (Figure 138–5). Initially, a radiologic study is done because it provides reproducible quantification of the reflux, defines anatomical anomalies at the ureteral insertion area (paraureteral diverticula, ectopia), and also visualizes the urethra, which is imperative in boys to rule out the presence of urethral obstruction causing reflux. In subsequent follow-up studies, a nuclear cystogram may be substituted for the voiding cystourethrogram. The main advantage of the nuclear cystogram is that radiation exposure is lower compared with standard contrast cystography.

Quantification of the reflux is important for prognosis because the lower grades of reflux tend to resolve spontaneously. Higher grades of reflux resolve less often and are more likely to lead to renal injury and scarring.

The basis of treatment for reflux is the premise that sterile reflux is not harmful to the kidney. Therefore, children who have reflux can be treated with a daily low-dose prophylactic antibiotic, generally nitrofurantoin or trimethoprim-sulfamethoxazole, to prevent infection and allow the kidney to grow normally. As the bladder matures, the reflux may spontaneously resolve. While the child is receiving prophylactic treatment, urinalysis and cultures should be done every 3 to 4 months and whenever clinically indicated to monitor for possible infection. Cystography should be repeated at regular intervals so that, if resolution of the reflux occurs, the medications can be stopped and the child observed. Normal renal growth and development should follow.

The other treatment option is ureteral reimplantation (ureteroneocystostomy). In uncomplicated cases, the success rate exceeds 98%. After surgery, antibiotics can be discontinued and the child watched. The decision for either medical or surgical treatment is usually made by parents with information and guidance from their physicians. The only absolute indication for surgery is a breakthrough infection, a UTI while the child is receiving appropriate chemoprophylactics.

Several other factors, including age, sex, family situation, and presence of renal scarring, may play a role in determining treatment. Location of the ureteral orifices as determined by cystoscopy may predict the likelihood of spontaneous resolution of reflux and can be taken into account when treatment decisions are made. Because of an increased incidence (30%) of reflux in siblings of a refluxer, they also should be investigated. The most accurate screening test is cystography, but, in the older asymptomatic child with no history of urinary infection, a renal ultrasound may be adequate. If significant reflux is present, the renal ultrasound will uncover upper tract dilation or scarring. If low-grade reflux is present and missed by ultrasound, the older child is thought to be beyond the age when most renal damage secondary to reflux occurs, and treatment may not be needed. If identified, such a child should receive the same treatment as anyone else with documented reflux.

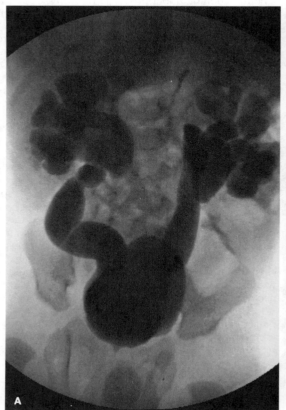
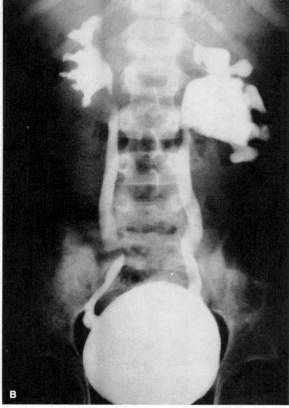

Figure 138-5. (A) Severe high-grade reflux. (Gonzales ET Jr. Genitourinary disorders in the neonate. In: Whitaker RH, Woodard JR, eds. *Paediatric urology.* London: Butterworth's; 1985.) **(B)** More moderate reflux.

■ BLADDER AND URETHRAL ANOMALIES

Posterior Urethral Valves

Posterior urethral valves are rare congenital obstructing leaflets in the region of the verumontanum in the prostatic urethra. There is no analogous structure or pathology in the female. Their etiology is unclear, but they are thought to be related to anomalous development of the urethrovaginal folds. Their pathophysiology stems from their narrowing of the bladder outlet, proximal to the external urethral sphincter. The obstruction they cause increases voiding pressure with dilation of the prostatic urethra, hypertrophy of the bladder neck, bladder trabeculation, and saccule formation. Renal dysplasia is common and often associated with vesicoureteral reflux.

Clinical presentation is varied and often unique. Recently, with the advent of prenatal ultrasonic monitoring, children with these problems have been diagnosed before birth with typical findings of bilateral hydroureteronephrosis, a thickened bladder, and occasionally a widened and elongated prostatic urethra. Neonatal discovery may be prompted by the findings of a distended bladder, palpable kidney, UTI, renal insufficiency, and a poor or dribbling urinary stream. Constitutional symptoms such as failure to thrive, abdominal distention, and vomiting may signal the presence of posterior urethral valves. In older boys, voiding problems may predominate and may be obvious. They vary from the expected (poor stream, urinary retention, and bladder distention) to subtle (hematuria, enuresis, and hesitancy). The diagnosis is best made on a voiding cystourethrogram (Figure 138–6).

Treatment is directed toward relief of the obstruction. Initial therapy, especially in the neonate, is placement of a transurethral catheter, hemodynamic stabilization, normalization of electrolytes, and treatment of any existing infection. If the renal function is normal or near normal,

transurethral ablation of the valves is done within a few days. In neonates with rising creatinine, uncontrollable infection, or a urethra too small to accept an infant cystoscope, a temporary vesicostomy or supravesical diversion is appropriate. The older boy can almost always undergo transurethral surgery because size is not a problem and severe renal insufficiency is rare.

Traditionally, the younger the child is at diagnosis, the poorer the prognosis. This, however, has been modified by prenatal ultrasound, because even mild cases may be discovered before birth. The best predictor of prognosis is the nadir serum creatinine after treatment. Those in whom the creatinine drops below 1.0 tend to do well, but, if the creatinine stays above 1.0, the boys are more apt to have difficulties with renal function as they grow. Renal failure with resultant dialysis and transplant is common in the latter group of patients.

Long-range difficulties are associated with both renal and bladder function. The bladder problems include vesicoureteral reflux, which may require surgery, and voiding dysfunction caused by the effects of the high intravesical pressures produced by the obstructing valves during prenatal development and infancy. The difficulties with renal function have been noted above.

■ ANOMALIES OF THE PENIS

Hypospadias

Hypospadias is a congenital penile deformity resulting from incomplete development of the distal or anterior urethra. The urethral meatus may be located at any point along the ventral shaft of the penis, midline of the scrotum, or perineum. The more proximal the urethral meatus, the more likely the penis is to be curved because of inelasticity of the dysplastic urethral plate and a foreshortening of the ventral aspect of the paired corpora cavernosa. This curvature is termed *chordee* and may preclude intercourse if severe. The prepuce in these patients is incompletely formed. The ventral foreskin is absent, but there is usually abundant dorsal skin that drapes over the glans as a dorsal "hood."

Hypospadias is the most common congenital anomaly of the penis, affecting about 3.5 boys out of 1000 births. Etiology is thought to be secondary to an in utero disorder of virilization, possibly a temporary deficiency or insensitivity to testosterone. Associated anomalies consist mainly of inguinal pathology, either hernias or undescended testes. Upper tract abnormalities are uncommon unless other organ systems are involved, in which case upper tract screening, by either IVP or renal ultrasound, is appropriate. For boys with bilateral cryptorchidism associated with hypospadias, consideration must be given to an intersex abnormality and appropriate testing should be done. Furthermore, patients with severe hypospadias may have a large utriculus masculinas or vaginal remnant, which can sequester urine and lead to a UTI. In such instances, cystoscopy and cystography may be warranted.

There is a definite familial tendency toward hypospadias. If a boy has hypospadias, his brother has a 14% chance of having hypospadias; if two brothers have hypospadias, the chances of a third brother having the same defect increase to 21%. If a boy has hypospadias, there is an 8% chance that his father is similarly affected. It seems that a multifactorial inheritance pattern is the most consistent explanation for the incidence of hypospadias.

In the initial evaluation of a boy with hypospadias, the position of the urethral meatus (glandular, coronal, distal shaft, midshaft, proximal shaft, penoscrotal, scrotal, per-

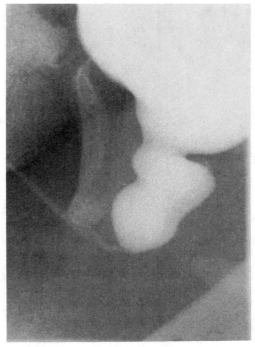

Figure 138-6. A newborn boy with typical x-ray findings of posterior urethral valves. (Gonzales ET Jr. Genitourinary disorders in the neonate. In: Whitaker RH, Woodard JR, eds. *Paediatric urology.* London: Butterworth's; 1985.)

ineal) should be noted so the degree of required surgical repair can be estimated. Because almost every hypospadias repair uses preputial skin, documentation of its position and amount is important, and neonatal circumcision is contraindicated. Slight perineal pressure on the corpora cavernosa will mimic an erection by obstructing venous outflow. This erection should help the clinician to assess the degree (mild, moderate, severe) and location (glandular, distal shaft, midshaft, or proximal shaft) of chordee. In cases of severe hypospadias, there may be an element of penoscrotal transposition; the scrotal folds envelop or wrap around the proximal penile shaft. This abnormality can be addressed at the same time as the hypospadias and chordee to improve the patient's appearance (Figure 138–7).

The objectives of surgical repair in patients with hypospadias are threefold. The first is to provide a straight penis that is adequate for intercourse. The second is to extend the urethral meatus to the tip of the glans penis, and the third is to make the appearance of the penis that of a normal circumcised phallus. Most pediatric urologists suggest that surgery be performed at age 6 to 18 months. Sexual identification is not complete at this age, and the surgical procedure will not be remembered. A single surgical procedure is used to correct all but the most severe problems. In instances of penoscrotal or perineal defects, a two-stage procedure remains a reasonable option.

Generally, cosmetic results after hypospadias surgery are excellent, but there is still a significant (15% to 40%) complication rate for patients with proximal defects. These problems consist mainly of fistulas, urethral strictures, and recurrent chordee. Any of these could require a second procedure for revision of the hypospadias repair. Unfortunately, despite our best efforts, some patients will undergo multiple procedures before an acceptable result is achieved.

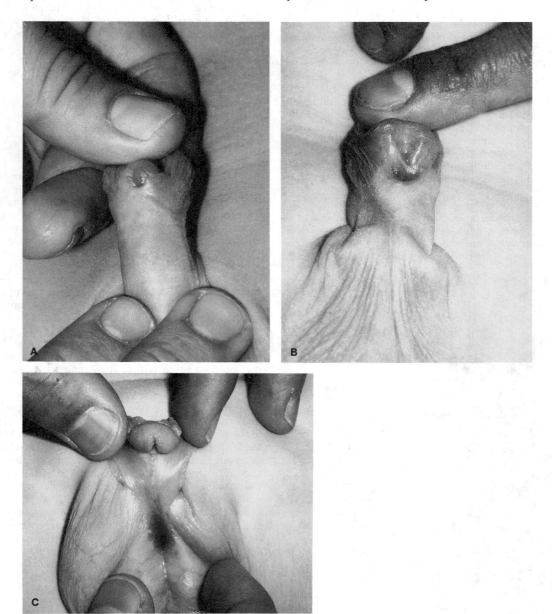

Figure 138-7. Three cases of hypospadias with varying degrees of involvement. (**A**) A distal meatus without evidence of concomitant chordee. (**B**) A more severe case in which there is severe chordee and deficiency of the ventral penile skin. (**C**) A perineal hypospadias with severe chordee.

Difficulties With the Prepuce

Phimosis

Phimosis is a condition in which scarring or narrowing of the preputial opening precludes its retraction over the glans penis. In the newborn, the preputial space is not completely developed and there are normal adhesions between the inner aspect of the prepuce and the glans penis. Therefore, in neonates, the foreskin normally is difficult to retract. With normal erections and development, these adhesions will separate to allow retraction of the prepuce. By age 3, the preputial opening should be large enough to allow easy retraction of the prepuce. Boys older than 3 years who have a persistent narrowing of the preputial opening, either congenital or from scarring, are candidates for circumcision. Attempts at blunt retraction and stretching of this opening may lead to tearing, bleeding, and edema, and should be discouraged.

Paraphimosis

Occurrence of paraphimosis, as distinguished from phimosis, is an emergency that can require surgical reduction. Paraphimosis is a condition in which the prepuce is incarcerated behind the glans penis, producing edema and swelling of the prepuce. Local discomfort is universal, and prompt reduction is mandatory. Usually, pressure around the prepuce to reduce edema, followed by direct pressure to the glans in conjunction with counteraction on the prepuce, will resolve the situation. If not, incision of the restricting band or circumcision is required.

Infection

Balanitis is a fairly common infection of the prepuce (incidence 6%). It usually responds to oral and topical antibiotics and warm baths. If simple measures are unsuccessful, parenteral antibiotics or circumcision may be required. Most often, mixed flora or organisms are cultured from the exudate. There have been reports of both Group A beta-hemolytic streptococcus and Group B streptococcus causing balanitis. In sexually active teenagers, trichomonal balanitis and candidal infections are possibilities and, if present, should prompt investigation of sexual partners.

The first episode of balanitis may not be the last. Repeated episodes of balanitis can lead to preputial scarring and phimosis. Therefore, once an episode of balanitis has occurred, circumcision should be considered as an option for further management.

Several studies report greater frequency of UTIs in infant boys who have not undergone circumcision (1.8%) than in circumcised boys (0.2%). Generally, the infections were not severe, but they did require hospitalization and parenteral antibiotics when they occurred in neonates.

Complications of Circumcision

Neonatal circumcision is safe when done by an experienced practitioner within the first several weeks of life. Reported complications include hemorrhage (1%), infection (0.4%), dehiscence (0.16%), denudation of shaft (0.05%), glandular injury (0.02%), and urinary retention (0.02%). There is no medical indication for the procedure. Most pediatric urologists suggest circumcision only for boys who have had difficulties with their foreskin (phimosis, paraphimosis, balanitis) or whose parents desire the surgery for personal reasons.

■ TESTICULAR AND SCROTAL ANOMALIES

Cryptorchidism

Testicular descent occurs late in fetal life and is regulated by many factors, including intra-abdominal pressure, hormonal influence, and gubernacular presence. The absence of any one of these elements may contribute to testicular maldescent. The incidence of maldescent depends on fetal age, with up to 30% of premature boys having either one or both testes undescended. In boys born normally at term, the incidence is between 3% and 4%. During the first several months of life, a transient increase in serum gonadotropin and testosterone is responsible for a spontaneous descent in more than half of boys with cryptorchidism at birth. After 1 year of life, testicles have descended in all but about 1% of boys. After that age, descent is rare; the incidence of cryptorchidism in untreated adults is about 1%.

True cryptorchidism must be distinguished from retractile testes, which are believed to be normal testes temporarily drawn into the inguinal canal by a hyperactive cremasteric muscle. With manipulation, these can be brought into the deep scrotum. No treatment is needed for these, because, given time, the testes will spontaneously descend, remain in the scrotum, and function normally. Therefore, one must accurately differentiate the retractile from the truly undescended testis.

The examination should take place in a relaxed, warm, and nonthreatening environment. The examiner should ensure that his or her hands are warm and should try to make the patient feel at ease. Repeated examinations with the patient in multiple positions (supine, sitting cross-legged, and squatting) may be beneficial. The history is also important, as a parent may remark that the testes are down during baths or diaper changes. The examination should be performed with two hands. One hand should start from the lateral area of the anterior superior iliac spine and sweep caudally along the inguinal canal, thereby "trapping" a testis so that it does not ascend into the abdomen. The second hand should palpate the lower groin and scrotum to identify the gonad.

There is some enthusiasm for the "ascending testis," a gonad that at birth appears well descended in the scrotum, but subsequently is found in the inguinal region, often in the superficial inguinal pouch. It is unclear whether these testes were truly descended or were inguinal testes that could be manipulated into the scrotum during infancy.

The position of the testis should be documented as either palpable (80%) or nonpalpable (20%). Palpable testes should be further described as inguinal, low inguinal, high scrotal, or ectopic. Even if the testes are not felt, it is often possible to identify testicular membranes on the spermatic cord; these should be documented for help in planning further therapy.

Treatment is suggested for several reasons. It has been established that progressive injury to the testis occurs as long as the testis remains in an extrascrotal position. Ultrastructural changes have been documented as early as 2 years of age, and it has been reported that after age 6 sperm production is impaired. After puberty, hormonal production has been impaired in a cryptorchid testis, and orchiectomy is often more appropriate than orchiopexy. Fifty percent of adults with a history of unilateral cryptorchidism have oligospermia, but paternity rates approach normal. On the other hand, bilateral cryptorchidism is associated with both oligospermia (80%) and infertility. It is difficult to show, however, that treatment at any age improves ultimate testicular function and fertility.

A second reason for relocating the testes in the scrotum is the increased incidence of malignant degeneration in testes with a history of maldescent. Testicular cancer, which is rare before puberty, affects about 3 of 100,000 men. In males with a history of cryptorchidism, the incidence is from 4 to 40 times higher. Yet there is no evidence that an orchiopexy will provide protection against future malignancy. Ideally, a neoplasm in an orthotopic testis will be discovered and treated earlier than one in an inguinal or abdominal position and thus increase the chance of survival, because early, small-volume testicular cancer has a cure rate of better than 95%.

The last reason for medical intervention is to improve the patient's self-image so that he, like his friends, will have two intrascrotal testes.

Most pediatric urologists suggest treatment of cryptorchidism before the child is 2 years old, preferably when he is between 6 and 18 months. The modalities available are surgical or hormonal. Surgery usually is done on an outpatient basis, and the results generally are excellent. An absent gonad is noted in about 20% of nonpalpable testes and can be confirmed by finding a blind-ending vas deferens and testicular vessels, either at exploration or in some cases by laparoscopy. Laparoscopy has been suggested for evaluation of nonpalpable testes, both to document anorchia and to help plan the surgical approach.

Usually an orchiopexy can relocate the cryptorchid testis into the scrotum without problem; however, when the testis is intra-abdominal or in a high inguinal position, division of the testicular artery and vein may be required so the testis can reach the scrotum. In such an instance, the blood supply depends on the vasal artery and its supporting mesentery. The success rate in such a procedure drops from 98% to 70% or 80%. Its main complications are that of any orchiopexy—atrophy and retraction. A patent processus vaginalis (pediatric hernia) occurs in association with 90% of cryptorchid testes and should be repaired at the same time.

The other treatment modality is hormonal manipulation, based on the observation that increased testosterone may encourage testicular descent. In the United States, intramuscular human chorionic gonadotropin (HCG) is given in a series of injections at varying doses. Success rates with HCG are lower than those with an orchiopexy and at best reach 30%. In Europe, there is a growing trend toward the use of intranasal gonadotropin-releasing hormone (GnRH), given twice daily for a month. Success has been claimed in 80% of the patients, although these data have been questioned, with studies in the United States showing only 20% success. No long-term side effects have been observed in association with this short-term hormonal therapy. However, for some patients, orchiopexy is often preferable to repeated injections and hormonal treatment.

When neither testicle is palpable, the question arises as to whether any testicular tissue is present and whether surgical intervention is necessary. Certain observations based on genital appearance and endocrinologic findings can assist in this decision. The presence of adequate levels of fetal testosterone during the first trimester is necessary for normal penile formation. During the last two trimesters, fetal testosterone promotes phallic growth. If the boy has a normal-sized penis, one can deduce that he had functioning testicular tissue until late in gestation; however, the presence of hypospadias or micropenis raises further questions regarding testicular function and development.

Endocrine evaluation of bilateral anorchia consists of measuring serum luteinizing hormone (LH), follicle-stimulating hormone (FSH), and testosterone before gonadotropin stimulation and serum testosterone after HCG administra-tion. To ensure adequate stimulation, HCG should be given over a 2-week period. In the absence of testicular tissue (the penis must be normally developed), one will find an increased FSH but normal LH in young boys and increased FSH and LH in older boys. Serum testosterone levels will be prepubertal before and after HCG administration. When these rigid criteria are adhered to, it is safe to make the diagnosis of bilateral anorchia in this limited subgroup of patients without significant exploration.

Torsion

Spermatic Cord and Testes

Torsion of the testicle is one of the few true emergencies in pediatric urology. It is the most common intrascrotal disorder in boys and requires prompt surgical intervention to avoid testicular necrosis. Testicular torsion must be differentiated from epididymitis and torsion of a testicular appendage, because neither of these requires surgery.

Testicular torsion occurs within the tunica albuginea (intravaginal) or includes the tunica albuginea (extravaginal). Intravaginal torsion is more common and occurs most frequently in early adolescence. It is thought to result from the absence of posterior attachments between the tunica vaginalis and testis that normally stabilize the gonad within the scrotum. Signs of testicular torsion consist of the acute onset of severe hemiscrotal pain, nausea, and vomiting. The attacks may be intermittent. Examination reveals an enlarged tender testis and frequently some degree of scrotal edema. The testis may be noted to have an unusual lateral lie. As time goes on, the intrascrotal elements become confluent, and torsion may be difficult to differentiate from acute or chronic epididymitis. Additional investigations that may be beneficial include a nuclear technetium scan of the testes or Doppler examination of the scrotum to assess testicular blood flow.

Prompt surgical exploration and detorsion are mandatory, because irreversible changes in the testis may occur within 4 hours. If treatment is not prompt, orchiectomy may be required. Because the abnormality (absence of posterior testicular attachment) is often bilateral, a contralateral scrotal orchiopexy should be done whenever an intravaginal torsion is diagnosed.

Torsion of a Testicular Appendage

Torsion of a testicular appendage must be distinguished from testicular torsion. Unless the diagnosis can be made with confidence, one must pursue a more thorough evaluation or surgically explore the acute scrotum. Often the symptoms of a torsed appendage are less severe than those of a testicular torsion. At times, the appendage is palpable in the upper aspect of the scrotum, and, if infarcted, a pathognomonic blue dot may be visible. Appropriate treatment consists of bed rest; the natural course is slow, steady improvement.

Hydrocele and Hernia

In children, a hernia represents the persistent patency of the processus vaginalis, which normally obliterates before birth. This allows communication of fluid between the scrotum and peritoneum, accounting for both variation in scrotal size and the characteristic inguinal swelling (Figure 138–8). A noncommunicating hydrocele, which is rare in children, represents partial obliteration of the processus vaginalis, leaving a sac of fluid about the testicle but no communication with the peritoneum. A communicating hydro-

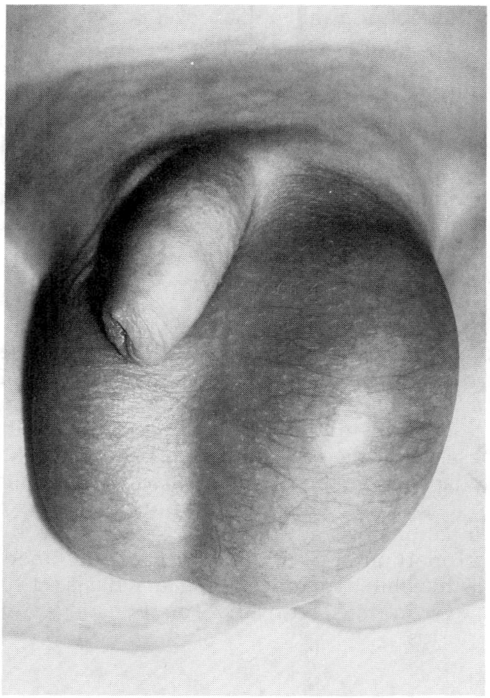

Figure 138-8. A large, tense hydrocele.

cele is equivalent to a hernia and should be repaired promptly so incarceration of bowel does not occur. Simple hydroceles, on the other hand, do not need emergency attention; because they tend to resolve spontaneously before age 1, intervention is usually delayed until that time. Reactive hydroceles secondary to infection, trauma, and torsion of an appendage resolve spontaneously and do not need separate attention. In general, the surgical approach to scrotal pathology is through the groin unless an obvious diagnosis of a torsion of the testis or an appendage is made.

Epididymitis

Epididymitis is an unusual finding in a preadolescent boy, but its recognition is important because symptoms resemble those of testicular torsion. The treatment for the former is antibiotics and bed rest; for the latter, prompt surgical exploration is mandatory. The physical findings may be similar for the two entities—scrotal erythema, swelling, and pain. Laboratory data such as fever, leukocytosis, pyuria, and a positive urine culture suggest a diagnosis of epididymitis. Often, because the diagnosis remains in question, a scrotal exploration is done.

Once epididymitis is confirmed in a prepubertal child, an IVP or renal ultrasound and voiding cystourethrogram should be obtained to identify any congenital anomalies. Positive findings—ureteral and vasal abnormalities predominate—can be expected in more than one third of the children. In these cases, correction of the problem often requires surgery.

(Abridged from David R. Roth and Edmond T. Gonzales Jr., Disorders of Renal Development and Anomalies of the Collecting System, Bladder, Penis, and Scrotum, in Oski, DeAngelis, Feigin, McMillan, Warshaw: *Principles and Practice of Pediatrics, Second Edition*, J.B. Lippincott, 1994.)

Oski's Essential Pediatrics,
edited by Kevin B. Johnson and Frank A. Oski.
Lippincott–Raven Publishers,
Philadelphia © 1997

139

Urinary Tract Infection

The urinary tract ranks second only to the upper respiratory tract as a source of morbidity from bacterial infection in childhood. The neonatal period is the only time that the incidence of male urinary tract infection (UTI) exceeds that of the female. A boy has about a 1% chance of developing an infection during childhood. In male neonates, the incidence of asymptomatic bacilluria is 1.5%, but it decreases to 0.2% by the time boys are of school age. In newborns, the incidence of UTI in uncircumcised boys is about 10 times that of boys who have been circumcised. Still, this is not thought to be an indication for routine circumcision in the newborn, because complications from circumcision potentially negate the benefit of reduced infections. The presence of a foreskin is not thought to increase the risk of UTI in older boys. A girl's chance of developing an infection during childhood is close to 3%. Random screening of preschool and school-age girls has shown an incidence of asymptomatic bacilluria in 1%. The incidence peaks between age 2 and 3 years, a time that coincides with toilet training, and then returns to a baseline value of between 1% and 2%.

The signs and symptoms of UTI in an older child are those seen in adults: voiding dysfunction, dysuria, hematuria, incontinence, suprapubic or flank tenderness, lethargy, and fever. In the neonate, however, the symptoms are much more subtle. Weight loss is most often the prominent symptom, followed by irritability, fever, cyanosis, and central nervous system (CNS) disorders. Thus, nonspecific complaints or problems should raise the suspicion of a UTI in a newborn but should not lead to hasty conclusions. Fewer than 20% of infants with nonspecific complaints and only 18% of children with specific voiding complaints actually have a UTI.

Documentation of UTI requires that a specimen be properly obtained and cultured. Urinalysis may suggest the presence of an infection, but the final determination should rest on bacterial growth on a culture. Of the several ways to collect an aliquot of urine from a child, the easiest, if a child is toilet-trained, is the midstream clean-catch specimen. If a child is not toilet-trained, that option is unavailable. Three methods remain, each with its advantages and disadvantages. The simplest but least reliable is the U-bag. A negative culture from a U-bag is meaningful, but, if the culture grows, the bacteria may be a contaminant from the rectum, skin, or prepuce. Therefore, whenever this method produces a positive culture, the culture should be repeated using a more accurate method. Two other procedures are available; both are somewhat more involved, but each should provide an uncontaminated aliquot of bladder urine. The first is a percutaneous bladder tap. In the neonate and infant, the bladder's intra-abdominal position makes the procedure easier than in older patients. Still, the bladder should be full and preferably palpable. The second method is urethral catheterization. In the small girl, visualizing the urethra may be difficult, but, with practice, the procedure can be mastered easily. A small feeding tube (5F or 8F) is most appropriate for catheterization. There should be little risk of urethral trauma or introduction of bacteria into the bladder if routine care and antisepsis are used.

Any treatment program should be based on an accurate culture and sensitivity. Consequently, the culture must be obtained before antibiotics are started, because a single dose of medication can give a false-negative result.

UTIs are often divided into categories based on the presumed location of the inflammation. Cystitis is a UTI confined to the bladder, whereas pyelonephritis involves the kidney. Accurate delineation between the two is difficult; clinical signs and symptoms offer the most meaningful clues. High fever, nausea, vomiting, flank pain, and lethargy are usually associated with acute pyelonephritis, whereas dysuria, frequency, urgency, enuresis, suprapubic pain, and a low-grade fever are more common with cystitis, although crossover is common. 2,3 dimercapto-succinic acid renal scanning offers an objective alternative to the subjectivity of clinical acumen, but final determination of the scan's sensitivity is still pending.

It is recommended that all children with a documented UTI undergo adequate studies to evaluate the anatomy of the urinary tract. Generally, studies should be done to evaluate both the lower tract (urethra and bladder) by way of voiding cystourethrogram and the upper tracts by way of renal ultrasound, intravenous pyelogram, or nuclear medicine renal scan. This recommendation is based on the clinical observation that children most likely to sustain renal parenchymal damage from infection are those who have an anatomical defect of the urinary tract. For the older girl with symptoms of simple cystitis, it can be argued that performing only an upper tract study is sufficient because it will reveal any significant pathology. The yield for these evaluations is age- and sex-dependent and ranges up to 50% in young girls with pyelonephritis (primarily from discovery of vesicoureteral reflux). If an anatomical anomaly such as obstruction or reflux is discovered, it must be addressed.

Most UTIs can be treated adequately on an outpatient basis with a 7- to 10-day course of antibiotics. If shorter courses are used, there is a higher recurrence rate. Initial treatment should be begun only after a urine specimen for culture and sensitivity has been obtained. A broad-spectrum generic agent such as amoxicillin (in three divided doses) or trimethoprim-sulfamethoxazole is then begun empirically; therapy is adjusted, if necessary, after the culture and sensitivity results are available. A repeat culture to confirm eradication of the infection should be obtained about 1 week after the completion of treatment. Occasionally a child with severe symptoms accompanying pyelonephritis will require hospitalization for parenteral antibiotics and control of nausea. For the child with frequently recurring infections (at least four per year), a long-term, low-dose daily prophylactic antibiotic is appropriate, usually nitrofurantoin or trimethoprim-sulfamethoxazole at one-quarter to one-half the therapeutic dose. Usually the medications are given for 9 to 12 months. Subsequent follow-up should include regular urinalyses and cultures when indicated.

■ UPPER TRACT INFECTION

Spread of bacteria into the upper tract is a much more serious problem. First, children with pyelonephritis tend to be very ill and appear toxic. They often require hospitalization for initial control of the fever, nausea, and vomiting. Second, the ultimate outcome may be a focal scar in the renal parenchyma, with subsequent tissue atrophy and loss of segmental renal function.

The potential for bacteria to ascend into the upper urinary tract is a combination of decreased patient resistance and bacterial virulence. Although some bacteria can infect the kidney because of their intrinsic virulence, especially those that are P-fimbriated, all bacteria are more likely to cause pyelonephritis rather than cystitis when anatomical abnormalities are present. When children with UTI present with significant fever, 60% are found to have structural abnormalities, most often vesicoureteral reflux. In addition, children with structural abnormalities are more likely to have pyelonephritis when they have a recurrence than are children who present with symptoms of pyelonephritis but whose initial workup was normal. However, the natural history and ultimate outcome of any episode of pyelonephritis do not seem to differ between children with normal anatomy and those with vesicoureteral reflux.

Not all children who develop pyelonephritis develop renal scars. Among children with vesicoureteral reflux, about 40% have renal scarring. However, most of these scars are noted on their initial evaluation; if additional infections occur, subsequent scarring is often minimal or does not seem to result despite symptoms compatible with renal infection. These observations have led to a theory that the risk of renal scarring depends on the anatomy of the renal papilla. Some papilla ("compound papilla") are more likely to develop severe inflammatory atrophy, and some kidneys have a greater proportion of compound papilla than others. However, the likelihood of developing a renal scar has been shown to correlate with the number of episodes of pyelonephritis.

■ CONCLUSION

The recognition of UTI in children requires sufficient workup to place children in categories of "at risk" or "minimal risk." The former are those with structural anomalies, because these children are most likely to develop severe recurrences and renal atrophy. The latter may have multiple recurrences, but with little or no risk of upper tract infection or damage. Their treatment is symptomatic and is driven by social as well as medical factors.

(Abridged from David R. Roth and Edmond T. Gonzales Jr., Urinary Tract Infections, in Oski, DeAngelis, Feigin, McMillan, Warshaw: *Principles and Practice of Pediatrics, Second Edition*, J.B. Lippincott, 1994.)

Oski's Essential Pediatrics,
edited by Kevin B. Johnson and Frank A. Oski.
Lippincott–Raven Publishers,
Philadelphia © 1997

140

Chronic Renal Failure

The incidence of chronic renal disease in children is unknown, but data suggest that 1.5 to 3 children per 1 million population per year develop end stage renal disease (ESRD). This incidence may increase as more infants with chronic renal failure (CRF) are recognized and treated.

■ SIGNS OF PROGRESSIVE LOSS OF RENAL FUNCTION

The most common finding that should alert the pediatrician to the possibility of chronic renal disease is growth impairment. Short stature, particularly if associated with other symptoms such as polyuria, frequent bouts of dehydration, salt craving, bone deformities, abnormal tooth development, or anemia, should suggest that the affected patient may have chronic renal disease. A previous history of urinary tract infections or glomerulonephritis adds further support to this suspected diagnosis.

■ ETIOLOGY

The etiologies of CRF in children are listed in Table 140–1. Most authors agree that different forms of obstructive uropathy are collectively the most common cause of renal failure in children.

■ ABNORMALITIES ASSOCIATED WITH LOSS OF RENAL FUNCTION

With progressive loss of renal function, many metabolic changes occur (Table 140–2). The inability of patients with CRF to tolerate excess protein or nitrogen intake is well recognized. The measure of blood urea nitrogen (BUN) is a function of dietary protein intake and renal clearance. Therefore, if protein intake remains constant as renal function declines, the BUN will increase.

Sodium intolerance in patients with CRF is well recognized. However, some children with CRF secondary to obstructive uropathy or cystic diseases may not be able to conserve sodium. Children with loss of renal function must maintain sodium intake within a narrow range. A normal adult may tolerate a dietary sodium intake of 2 to 1000 mEq/day. A patient with CRF and only 10% residual renal function may become sodium-depleted if dietary intake is less than 40 mEq/day. Conversely, the same patient may become hypertensive if sodium intake exceeds 80 mEq/day.

Potassium balance can become positive in patients with CRF. Hyperkalemia usually is not seen until residual renal function is well below 10% of normal. Hyperkalemia may be seen earlier in the course of CRF if the patient is sodium-depleted. Hyperkalemia may occur with greater than 10% residual function in the rare patient who has defective renin release secondary to renal damage. Hypokalemia can occur in some patients with CRF because of renal potassium wasting, but usually results from anorexia, emesis, and inadequate potassium intake.

Anemia, a well-known consequence of CRF, is the result of defective erythropoietin production by the damaged kidney. Patients with renal failure also have reduced gastrointestinal (GI) absorption of iron. Therefore, when evaluating these patients, iron deficiency as a cause for anemia must be considered. Exogenous erythropoietin is available; through its use and avoidance of iron deficiency, the anemia of CRF can be reversed.

TABLE 140-1. Etiology of CRF in Children*

Obstructive uropathy, including reflux nephropathy or renal dysplasia secondary to obstruction

Renal hypoplasia/dysplasia

Glomerulopathy/glomerulonephritis (all forms)

Hereditary disease, including hereditary nephritis or renal cystic diseases

*In order of frequency.

TABLE 140-2. Metabolic Abnormalities Associated With CRF

Elevated BUN—protein intolerance

Decreased phosphate excretion

Decreased sodium excretion

Reduced ability to conserve sodium

Decreased hydrogen ion excretion

Decreased potassium excretion

Reduced production of 1,25-dihydroxycholecalciferol

Reduced production of erythropoietin

Neuropathy is a recognized part of the uremic syndrome. In children, especially infants, this consequence of CRF is of special importance. CRF early in life may delay brain development and lead to permanent neurologic impairment. Careful neurologic and frequent developmental evaluation of these children is required. Decisions concerning the timing of dialysis or transplantation may depend on the results of these examinations.

■ TREATMENT

Once CRF is recognized and the physiology of lost renal function is understood, treatment is required. The nondialytic treatment of a child with renal insufficiency is in a state of flux. Numerous changes in recommended therapy have been made over the past few years and will continue to be made as more information becomes available about the metabolic abnormalities and the requirements for growth in these children (Table 140–3).

Patients with CRF may develop hyperlipidemia if fats are used as a caloric supplement instead of glucose. Whether this causes increased morbidity in infants and children is unknown.

Treatment of the anemia associated with chronic renal disease is difficult, and a cure may be impossible. As stated before, many children with CRF become iron-deficient secondary to persistent microscopic blood loss in stools and to low dietary iron intake. If iron deficiency is present, it should be corrected; however, the anemia usually persists despite iron therapy. One of the many functions of the kidney is to produce erythropoietin, and this is lost in patients with severe renal damage. Without this hormone, erythrocyte production is reduced and a hypoplastic anemia results. Recombinant human erythropoietin is available for the treatment of children with CRF. This agent corrects the anemia in patients with CRF and thus eliminates the need for costly and potentially dangerous blood transfusions.

Hypertension is a common sign of progressive loss of renal function and most often results from excessive blood volume. The most effective treatment is to reduce sodium intake or to increase sodium excretion. Patients with renal failure become intolerant of both excessively high and low sodium intakes. If sodium restriction is too rigid, the patient may become hypovolemic, and this can exacerbate other signs of CRF. Sodium intake must be adjusted carefully to avoid both of these extremes. Occasionally, patients with CRF develop hypertension that is not volume-related but is due rather to an excessive production of renin. These children can be treated successfully with an angiotensin-converting enzyme inhibitor that will block the conversion of angiotensin I to angiotensin II, lower peripheral resistance,

TABLE 140-3. Nondialytic Therapy of CRI/CRF

DIET

Provide at least 100% RDA caloric intake

Protein intake controversial; range 0.5–1.5 g/kg/d

RENAL OSTEODYSTROPHY

1,25-dihydroxycholecalciferol (dose variable)

Calcium carbonate (as a calcium supplement and PO_4 binder)

ANEMIA

May require iron

Erythropoietin

HYPERTENSION

Control sodium intake

If hyperreninemic, consider ACE inhibitor

ACIDOSIS

May improve with reduced protein intake

Sodium citrate or $NaHCO_3$, 2–4 mEq/kg/d

and normalize blood pressure. When the patient with CRF develops hypertension, especially because of excessive blood volume, it may mean the child will soon require dialysis.

■ GROWTH FAILURE

Growth failure is a common and often untreatable consequence of CRF in children. Growth failure is particularly severe in children who develop renal insufficiency in the first year of life. Infants with CRF grow poorly between birth and age 2. Even if normal growth velocity can be achieved from age 2 onward, so much growth potential has been lost that dwarfism is the result. Growth retardation could be avoided if catch-up growth were achieved after successful renal replacement therapy. However, accelerated growth only rarely occurs after a successful renal transplantation. To affect growth in this population, early recognition of CRF is essential.

To correct growth failure, one must attempt to correct all the metabolic abnormalities mentioned. Adequate dietary intake is important, especially in infants with renal failure. Several infants with CRF were identified early in life and aggressive nutritional therapy was initiated. Dietary intake was given by tube feedings (either nasogastric or transpyloric) in an amount to provide at least 100% of the recommended daily allowance (RDA) for calories and 1 to 2 g/kg/day of protein. Although data are sparse, near-normal growth has been achieved in some patients. Providing adequate nutrition to older dialysis patients has also affected growth favorably.

Many children with CRF cannot conserve sodium. If sodium is restricted in these patients, poor growth may result; conversely, greater sodium intake by these patients will improve growth. Acidosis is often a complication of CRF, and correction and control of the acidosis are essential to normal growth in this population. Early and aggressive therapy of renal osteodystrophy with vitamin D metabolites and calcium carbonate is required for optimal growth in these children. The anemia seen secondary to CRF may slow growth in these patients. Growth potential can be improved by careful attention to maintaining acid–base, electrolyte,

and water balance in these patients. Treating renal osteodystrophy and providing adequate nutrition are essential in maintaining normal growth velocity. It has been suggested that children with CRF may have improved growth when given supraphysiologic doses of recombinant human growth hormone, and early published results of the use of this therapy are encouraging.

(Abridged from Edward C. Kohaut, Chronic Renal Failure, in Oski, DeAngelis, Feigin, McMillan, Warshaw: *Principles and Practice of Pediatrics, Second Edition*, J.B. Lippincott, 1994.)

Oski's Essential Pediatrics,
edited by Kevin B. Johnson and Frank A. Oski.
Lippincott–Raven Publishers,
Philadelphia © 1997

141

Glomerulonephritis and Nephrotic Syndrome

GLOMERULONEPHRITIS

Glomerulonephritis (GN) is the result of an immune process that injures the glomeruli of the kidney. This heterogenous group of diseases appears to be mediated primarily by immune mechanisms that invoke inflammatory reactions that cause alteration of glomerular structure and function throughout both kidneys. Impairment of tubular function may be present but is not predominant and results from either glomerular injury or direct immunologic injury similar to that affecting the glomeruli.

■ CLINICAL PRESENTATIONS

GN may present clinically in a variety of ways. Classification by clinical presentation (Table 141–1) is helpful in narrowing the differential diagnosis and directing the diagnostic evaluation.

The *acute nephritic syndrome* is the sudden onset of hematuria, either gross or microscopic, proteinuria, decreased glomerular filtration rate (GFR), occasionally oliguria and retention of salt and water, which may be associated with edema, circulatory volume overload, and hypertension. The hallmark of this syndrome is hematuria and red blood cell casts in the urine, with only minimal to moderate proteinuria.

Some patients with *chronic GN* have few overt symptoms. Asymptomatic hematuria or proteinuria discovered on routine urinalysis may be the presenting signs. Malaise, fatigue, anemia, and failure to grow normally may be the only signs of slowly progressive chronic GN with chronic renal failure.

If the clinical course is one of nephritis with rapid decline in renal function to uremia and often permanent loss of renal function, the presentation is termed *rapidly progressive GN*. Renal biopsies from these patients frequently show glomerular crescent formation alone or in addition to identifying characteristics of a specific histopathologic type of GN.

Patients with the *nephrotic syndrome* have massive proteinuria (in excess of 40 mg/m^2/hour in children), hypoproteinemia, hyperlipidemia, and edema. Hematuria, either

TABLE 141-1. Clinical Presentation of Glomerulonephritis

Acute nephritis syndrome
Chronic glomerulonephritis
    Asymptomatic hematuria or proteinuria
    Chronic renal failure
Rapidly progressive glomerulonephritis
Nephrotic syndrome

gross or microscopic, may be present but is not the prominent feature.

This chapter will discuss the many kinds of GN of children and adolescents under the major headings of these clinical presentations. Because most of the disease entities that present with the acute nephritic syndrome may also have an insidious onset characteristic of chronic GN, acute and chronic GN are grouped together.

ACUTE AND CHRONIC GLOMERULONEPHRITIS OF CHILDHOOD

■ ACUTE POSTSTREPTOCOCCAL GN

Acute poststreptococcal GN (APSGN) is the most common form of immune-mediated nephritis in children. It is, by far, the most common form of postinfectious nephritis, although infection with a variety of other bacterial, viral, parasitic, rickettsial, and fungal agents may be followed by an acute nephritic syndrome similar to that following infections with nephritogenic strains of group A beta-hemolytic streptococci. In contrast to "rheumatogenic" strains of group A streptococci, which cause acute rheumatic fever associated with pharyngeal infection, nephritogenic strains of group A streptococci may cause either pharyngeal or skin infections.

Susceptibility to APSGN may be genetically determined as well as dependent on favorable host factors. The disease occurs most often in elementary-school children (mean age 7 years), affects twice as many males as females, and is rare before age 3 years. An episode of group A streptococcal throat or skin infection precedes all cases of APSGN. In most instances, the interval between the infection and the onset of clinical GN is about 8 to 14 days, although both longer and shorter intervals have been reported.

Clinical Features

The clinical expression of APSGN is variable and extends from a completely asymptomatic form to the most severe manifestations of acute renal failure, including edema, oliguria, congestive heart failure (CHF), hypertension, and encephalopathy. The most common presenting symptoms are hematuria, proteinuria, and edema, often accompanied by rather nonspecific findings of lethargy, anorexia, vomiting, fever, abdominal pain, or headache.

Gross hematuria is present in only 30% to 50% of children with APSGN. The urine is usually described as smoky, tea-colored, cola-colored, or occasionally dirty greenish-colored. At least two thirds of hospitalized patients have edema, which is

initially mild and may be noted only periorbitally, but can become marked, especially if normal fluid intake occurs over several days at the height of the disease. Evidence of circulatory congestion such as orthopnea, dyspnea, cough, auscultatory rales, and gallop rhythms are apparent on physical examination in many children with edema. The chest x-ray usually shows cardiomegaly and pulmonary edema of varying degrees. Severe CHF is rare. Hypertension is common in inpatients (50% to 90%), but hypertensive encephalopathy, characterized by headache, somnolence, convulsions, coma, confusion, aphasia, transient blindness, agitation, or combativeness, occurs in only a few (5%).

Laboratory Features

Laboratory investigation should begin with a careful analysis of the urine. The specimen may be yellow, slightly discolored, or grossly bloody, and usually has a high specific gravity and a low pH. Microscopic hematuria with predominantly dysmorphic erythrocytes in the centrifuged urinary sediment is present in virtually all cases, and leukocyturia is almost as common. Red blood cell casts are found very often (60% to 85%) in centrifuged specimens where the resuspended sediment is freshly examined and is of acid pH. Leukocyte casts as well as hyaline and granular casts are often seen. The presence of leukocytes and leukocyte casts should not be considered evidence of superimposed urinary tract infection, but rather of glomerular inflammation. Proteinuria occurs in most cases and correlates qualitatively with the amount of blood in the urine, reaching nephrotic proportions in less than 5% of patients.

A laboratory evaluation for streptococcal infection is mandatory. Serum ASO, AHT, and anti-DNase B titers are most helpful for confirming previous recent infection. Throat and skin lesion cultures may also be positive at the time of nephritis and should be treated with appropriate antibiotics. Asymptomatic family members may also have positive cultures. Family screening for subclinical streptococcal disease and nephritis has been recommended.

One of the most important diagnostic laboratory findings in APSGN is a depressed serum concentration of C3. Activation of the alternative pathway of complement occurs in most cases, resulting in reduced serum C3 levels in at least 90% of patients examined in the early phase of their nephritis. Serum C4 is occasionally also depressed. Serum C3 returns to normal concentrations 10 days to 8 weeks after the onset of the nephritis. If the serum C3 is not measured within the first few days of presentation of the nephritis, the concentration may already have returned to normal, and its depression will have been missed. Prior treatment of the streptococcal infection with penicillin may attenuate the period of depression of serum C3 so that serum C3 appears normal at the time of presentation of the nephritis. The degree of serum C3 depression bears no relationship to the severity of the disease.

GFR is usually depressed during the acute stage of moderate to severe nephritis. Serum urea nitrogen may be elevated disproportionately to serum creatinine. Even when GFR is normal or only slightly decreased, severe salt and water retention may occur. Urine volume is usually reduced, but severe oliguria is uncommon. Urine concentrating ability is well preserved. The fractional excretion of sodium is usually less than 1%, even in the presence of reduced GFR. The acutely inflamed kidney of APSGN retains sodium even in the face of acute renal failure, unlike the high fractional excretion of sodium that occurs in acute tubular necrosis. If a child with APSGN is allowed free access to fluids, dilutional hyponatremia may develop. When acidosis and hyperkalemia occur, they are the result of aldosterone suppression caused by extracellular volume expansion, as well as of reduced GFR, if severe.

Pathogenesis

Based on morphologic, serologic, and clinical parameters, it is widely accepted that APSGN is immune complex-mediated, although the precise mechanism is unknown. It is also speculated that streptococci may produce glomerular injury and set the stage for inflammatory changes, or that streptococci induce autologous IgG/anti-IgG complexes through neuraminidase desialation of host IgG and neoantigen formation.

Differential Diagnosis

Many renal disorders may at their onset mimic APSGN, but only a few do so commonly and with great synonymity. Other disorders frequently confused with APSGN include benign hematuria, IgA nephropathy, hereditary nephritis, idiopathic hypercalciuria, and resolving episodes of previously undiagnosed postinfectious GN.

Treatment

All therapy for ASPGN is supportive and directed toward treating the clinical manifestations of acute nephritis. Hypertension, although usually only mild to moderate in severity, may be severe and require emergency treatment. Loop diuretics and fluid restriction are important adjunct therapies and usually suffice alone for mild hypertension, as well as relieving edema and circulatory congestion. Restricting fluid intake to an amount equal to insensible water loss may obviate the need for diuretic therapy. On the other hand, the use of diuretics may allow the patient to have a more palatable diet and avoid the psychological tension associated with severe fluid restriction. Patients with oligoanuria may respond poorly to diuretics and thus require strict fluid restriction for control of edema and hypervolemia. In these patients, hyperkalemia should be anticipated and treated with dietary potassium restriction, binding resins, or dialysis as needed.

All patients should receive a course of penicillin or other antistreptococcal antibiotic if there is evidence of ongoing throat or skin infection. This in no way influences the course or prognosis of the nephritis.

Prognosis

Overall, the prognosis of APSGN is excellent, with full recovery expected in more than 98% of affected children. The resolution must be documented at follow-up office visits over time. Most children spend no more than 5 days in the hospital, but the disease resolves slowly over many months. Few children develop chronic renal failure. Hypertension usually resolves within 3 weeks, as does gross hematuria. The latter may be exacerbated by exercise or intercurrent infections, but its reappearance is of no prognostic significance. Microscopic hematuria persists for many months and has been documented for as long as 3 years in a few patients. Proteinuria resolves within a few months; its persistence should raise concern regarding the possibility of an incorrect

diagnosis or chronicity. The serum C3 concentration must be measured again 6 to 8 weeks after the acute episode. Failure of C3 to increase into the normal range during this period of time strongly suggests the diagnosis of membranoproliferative GN, and a renal biopsy should be done for confirmation.

■ IgA NEPHROPATHY

IgA nephropathy is characterized histologically by the presence of mesangial IgA deposits and clinically by chronic hematuria and normal renal function early in the course. Once considered a benign disease, IgA nephropathy is now known to progress to chronic renal failure in adulthood in as many as 40% of patients.

Clinical Features

Almost three fourths of the children who present with IgA nephropathy are males. The mean age of presentation for both sexes combined is 9 years. Hematuria is the most common initial sign, occurring microscopically in 100% and macroscopically in 85% of the children with biopsy-proven IgA nephropathy. Gross hematuria may be a constant feature or it may occur episodically, usually in association with a febrile illness unrelated to the urinary tract. Proteinuria unrelated to gross hematuria occurs in about 40% to 50% of the affected children, reaching the nephrotic range in some. Isolated proteinuria is not a sign of IgA nephropathy in children. Patients with moderate to severe proteinuria are at greater risk of developing renal insufficiency. Hypertension, found in about 10%, is not a prominent feature, even when patients are followed for many years; its occurrence usually coincides with the development of chronic renal failure. About 20% of the patients have a mild decrease in GFR during episodic gross hematuria. Complaints of fever, malaise, and loin or abdominal pain are common at that time as well. Renal function usually returns to normal after the acute episode.

Laboratory Features

Laboratory studies, other than a renal biopsy examination, will not confirm the diagnosis of IgA nephropathy. Serum IgA levels are elevated in no more than half of the patients and appear to bear no relationship to the disease severity or activity. Serum IgG, IgM, and C3 concentrations are seldom abnormal.

Differential Diagnosis

The presence of microscopic hematuria with or without mild proteinuria between episodes of gross hematuria also occurs in hereditary nephritis (Alport's syndrome), in benign hematuria, and in idiopathic hypercalciuria, occasionally in membranoproliferative GN (MPGN), and rarely in membranous GN.

IgA nephropathy is easily confused with acute poststreptococcal GN, especially if the initial presentation is an episode of gross hematuria and mild systemic complaints. In IgA nephropathy, unlike acute poststreptococcal GN, there is no latent period between the infection and the onset of hematuria, and the serum C3 concentration is normal. Gross hematuria persists only a few days in patients with IgA nephropathy, usually resolving when the associated fever remits.

Therapy

The potential for progression of IgA nephropathy to chronic renal failure and end-stage renal disease has led to uncontrolled trials of prednisone and even cytotoxic drug therapy in patients with severe symptoms, advanced renal biopsy lesions, heavy proteinuria, or already apparent renal failure. Prednisone therapy appears to improve urinary findings in some patients, a few of whom also appear to have had improvement or stabilization of histopathologic lesions in subsequent renal biopsies. Data are too limited to determine if the progression of renal failure can be retarded by therapy. Until controlled therapeutic trials are done, no specific drug therapy can be recommended. Medical management of hypertension and chronic renal failure, when it occurs, are the treatment measures of choice.

Prognosis

Most children with IgA nephropathy have either a very slowly progressive or completely benign course until adulthood. Predicting which 5% to 10% will develop end-stage renal disease in childhood or adolescence is difficult. Heavy proteinuria, hypertension, and a renal biopsy showing glomerular proliferative lesions with crescents, sclerosis, or glomerular basement membrane (GBM) alterations suggest a poor prognosis.

■ HENOCH-SCHÖNLEIN PURPURA NEPHRITIS

Henoch-Schönlein purpura (HSP) nephritis is a systemic vasculitis that typically affects children and presents as a triad of purpuric rash, crampy abdominal pain, and arthritis. Signs and symptoms of nephritis may not appear until days or several weeks into the course of the disease. Because of the unproven assumption that these children are allergic to drugs, food, microorganisms, or some other unidentified antigens, the term *anaphylactoid purpura* has been applied to this disease. Although children with HSP do not appear to be more allergic than others, the term has persisted.

HSP is probably mediated by IgA, which can be identified by immunofluorescence staining of renal and skin biopsies from affected patients. The renal lesion is identical to that seen in IgA nephropathy, raising the question of whether IgA nephropathy and HSP may be a spectrum of the same disease.

Clinical Features

Most affected children are white boys between the ages of 3 and 10 years. Two thirds of patients report the onset of an upper respiratory tract infection 1 to 3 weeks before the onset of purpura. The incidence of HSP is seasonal, with its peak in winter.

The disease usually begins with an acute erythematous macular rash, most often on the ankles and spreading to the dorsum of the legs, the buttocks, and the ulnar surfaces of the arms. The trunk is spared. Within a day, the lesions become purpuric and may coalesce. The skin lesions disappear in about 2 weeks, although in some children the rash comes and goes over a period of days to weeks. Many patients experience edema of the scalp, face, and dorsum of the hands and feet with the rash. Joint pain, with or without edema, occurs in 60% to 75% of cases. Colicky abdominal pain with melena or bloody diarrhea occurs in one half of the affected children and mimics other gastrointestinal diseases. Severe vasculitis of the bowel may result in gastrointestinal hemorrhage, perforation, or intussusception.

The renal manifestations of HSP are clinically important in a few patients, but, if the urine is examined over the duration of the disease, abnormalities will be found in almost every case. The spectrum of renal disease in HSP is broad, ranging from asymptomatic hematuria and proteinuria to full-blown acute nephritic syndrome with the nephrotic syndrome. Hypertension is uncommon.

Laboratory Features

No laboratory test is diagnostic of HSP. Leukocytosis occurs early in the course. Hemoglobin, hematocrit, and the peripheral blood smear are normal, as are the platelet count, bleeding time, and coagulation studies. The erythrocyte sedimentation rate may be elevated. Microscopic hematuria and proteinuria are often present in the urinalysis. Gross hematuria may be seen in 20% to 30% of cases. Azotemia occurs in up to 20% but is usually transient. Uremia requiring acute dialysis for a short time is rare.

Serum IgA concentration is elevated in 50% of the children with HSP. The elevation often occurs during the acute phase only, with levels returning to normal as symptoms resolve. Serum C3 concentration is normal, but breakdown products of complement are increased in the serum, indicating complement activation, presumably by circulating immune complexes or cryoglobulins, which have been identified in many patients.

Pathology

If the clinical signs and symptoms of HSP are atypical, the diagnosis can be confirmed by microscopic examination of skin and renal biopsy specimens. Skin lesions typically show a leukocytoclastic vasculitis, characterized by transmural and perivascular infiltration with polymorphonuclear leukocytes, histiocytes, and sometimes eosinophils. The renal lesion is identical to that seen in IgA nephropathy (see above) and ranges from no identifiable abnormalities by light microscopy to mesangial proliferation, focal and segmental proliferative lesions, and diffuse proliferative lesions with or without crescents. Brightly staining deposits of IgA are always found in the mesangium by immunofluorescence. Electron microscopic examination shows dense deposits in the same location.

Differential Diagnosis

The purpuric nature and distribution of the skin lesions of HSP can be quite characteristic. If the rash is atypical in distribution, other causes of purpura such as leukemia, septicemia, hemolytic-uremic syndrome, systemic lupus erythematosus, and idiopathic thrombocytopenic purpura must be considered. The abdominal symptoms mimic many infectious and inflammatory bowel diseases. HSP may actually cause an acute surgical emergency secondary to bowel perforation or intussusception. Pancreatitis is uncommon. Vasculitis of the testis may resemble torsion of the testis, orchitis, or incarcerated hernia. Joint symptoms are difficult to distinguish from those seen in rheumatoid arthritis, lupus, and acute rheumatic fever. The renal manifestations of HSP may appear identical to those seen in acute poststreptococcal GN, bacterial endocarditis, systematic lupus erythematosus, polyarteritis, and membranoproliferative GN.

Clinical Course and Therapy

The clinical course varies from very mild to severe. Most patients have several bouts of rash and abdominal pain over the first month of disease. Recurrences over a longer period of time may be associated with a poorer prognosis. The main determinant of the overall prognosis is the persistence and severity of the renal disease. Children with minor urinary abnormalities have an excellent prognosis for complete recovery, whereas those who present with a severe acute nephritic syndrome or the nephrotic syndrome may develop chronic renal failure and even end-stage renal disease. Patients who have renal disease should have long-term follow-up until the urinalysis is normal for several years. Those showing persistent urinary abnormalities or evidence of progressive renal failure should be seen by a pediatric nephrologist.

Therapy is limited to supportive measures. Careful monitoring to detect serious abdominal complications is of paramount importance in patients with abdominal pain. When abdominal pain is severe and incapacitating even after administration of analgesics, corticosteroids may provide relief. The use of analgesics and steroids is not without risk, because they may mask symptoms of gastrointestinal perforation. There is no evidence that corticosteroids have any beneficial effect on the clinical course of the renal disease.

NEPHROTIC SYNDROME

The nephrotic syndrome (NS) is a clinical condition resulting from the loss of large amounts of protein from the blood into the urine. The amount of proteinuria is usually sufficient to cause hypoproteinemia and consequent edema. Hyperlipidemia and lipiduria are also part of the fully expressed NS. The NS may be a feature of any form of childhood GN or may be secondary to other systemic diseases, nephrotoxins, or allergic reactions (Table 141–2).

■ OVERVIEW

Primary NS has been reported to occur with an annual incidence as high as 7 cases per 100,000 children under age 16 years, but an incidence of 2 per 100,000, the figure determined in a 16-year population survey in Erie County, New York, seems more likely to represent the usual incidence rate.

In early childhood, about 80% of the children with primary NS have minimal change nephrotic syndrome (MCNS). Of these, 60% are between ages 2 and 6 years. MCNS is uncommon in infants under age 1 year and accounts for only 30% of adolescent and 15% to 20% of adult cases. Because older children are more likely to have underlying histopathologic types of GN other than MCNS, a diagnostic renal biopsy is usually performed early in their disease course. The histopathologic type, more than age at onset or any other feature of the NS, determines the clinical outcome.

Clinical Consequences of Proteinuria

Many proteins appear in the urine of nephrotic patients, but albumin is found in greatest abundance. Albuminuria is the primary cause of hypoalbuminemia, which is the main

---

TABLE 141-2. Causes of the Nephrotic Syndrome

PRIMARY NEPHROTIC SYNDROME

Minimal change disease

Diffuse mesangial proliferative glomerulonephritis

Focal segmental glomerulosclerosis

Membranoproliferative glomerulonephritis

Membranous glomerulonephritis

SECONDARY NEPHROTIC SYNDROME

Other Renal Diseases
Hemolytic-uremic syndrome, anti-GBM disease, IgA nephropathy, idiopathic RPGN, diffuse mesangial sclerosis

Infectious
Bacterial (poststreptococcal, infective endocarditis, shunt nephritis, leprosy, syphilis), viral (hepatitis B, cytomegalovirus, Epstein-Barr, varicella, HIV), protozoal (malaria, toxoplasmosis), parasitic (schistosomiasis, filariasis)

Neoplasia
Lymphoma leukemia, Wilms' tumor, pheochromocytoma, others

Medications
Mercurials, gold, penicillamine, trimethadione, mephenytoin

Systemic Diseases
Systemic lupus erythematosus, Henoch-Schönlein purpura, polyarteritis nodosa, Takayasu syndrome, dermatitis herpetiformis, sarcoidosis, Sjögren syndrome, amyloidosis, diabetes mellitus

Allergic Reactions
Insect stings, poison oak and ivy, serum sickness

Familial Disorders
Alport syndrome, Fabry disease, nail-patella syndrome, sickle-cell disease, Finnish nephrosis

Circulatory Disorders
Constrictive pericarditis, congestive heart failure, renal vein thrombosis

Miscellaneous
Chronic renal allograft rejection, preeclampsia, malignant hypertension

---

determinant of reduced plasma colloid oncotic pressure in primary NS. Reduction of oncotic pressure causes a shift of fluid from the intravascular compartment to the interstitial space, with consequent edema. In response to a loss of vascular volume, the kidney increases its reabsorption of sodium and water and worsens the edema.

Historically, nephrotic patients were thought to reabsorb sodium avidly by way of the renin–angiotensin–aldosterone axis in response to decreased intravascular volume associated with low plasma oncotic pressure. Recently, investigators have shown that some nephrotic patients actually have increased or normal plasma volume and normal or suppressed serum renin and aldosterone levels, suggesting that salt and water retention may be a primary renal disturbance, as in acute GN. Each explanation may be valid for some patients with NS, depending on their underlying renal disease or the stage of their disease at the time of study.

Laboratory Features

Proteinuria is the hallmark of NS. The urinalysis shows qualitatively large amounts of protein (2 to 4+ by dipstick), a high specific gravity, and hyaline and granular casts. To be classified as nephrotic-range proteinuria, the protein excretion rate should exceed 40 mg/m^2/hr in a 24-hour urine collection. In children, especially the very young, reliable 24-hour urine collections are difficult to obtain. Alternative measurements, such as a random urine protein:creatinine ratio of above 1.0, may be substituted. A low serum albumin concentration correlated with a series of strongly positive (2+ or more) dipstick tests for albumin in random urinalyses may also suffice.

The massive proteinuria of NS usually causes hypoalbuminemia. Hypoalbuminemia becomes clinically significant when the serum albumin is 2.5 g/dL or less and edema occurs. In addition, the concentration of other plasma proteins, such as coagulation inhibitors and vitamin D-binding globulin (Table 141–3), is decreased because of increased urinary losses, decreased synthesis, or increased catabolism.

Serum cholesterol, triglycerides, and total lipids are elevated in most cases of primary NS of childhood. Total cholesterol levels are usually very elevated, exceeding 400 mg/dL in two thirds of the children with MCNS. The degree of hypercholesterolemia is inversely related to the serum albumin concentration.

Lipiduria, a common urinary abnormality, is best appreciated by polarized light microscopy. Oval fat bodies, which are lipid-laden renal tubular cells sloughed into the urine, may be easily identified in the urinary sediment, even without a polarized microscope.

Hematuria occurs in some children with primary NS, and it may be helpful in narrowing the differential diagnosis. Transient microscopic hematuria occurs in only 25% of the children with MCNS, and gross hematuria is almost never encountered. In children with other forms of primary NS, either gross or microscopic hematuria is present more than half the time.

Renal function measured by creatinine or inulin clearance is normal or increased in most patients with NS, although one third of the children with MCNS show transient depression of GFR at the onset of their disease, probably due to hypovolemia and poor renal perfusion. If GFR remains low after NS has been treated and the affected child has improved clinically, the child should be evaluated for an underlying diagnosis other than MCNS. Renal tubular wasting of glucose, bicarbonate, amino acids, or phosphate, typical of partial or complete Fanconi's syndrome, is extremely uncommon and suggests the diagnosis of focal segmental glomerulosclerosis (FSGS).

Extrarenal Complications and General Management

Each protein abnormality of NS causes specific clinical consequences. Hypoalbuminemia causes edema, which usually begins insidiously with unexpected weight gain and early morning periorbital swelling that shifts during the day to the lower legs and feet. Therapy for severe edema includes intravenous or oral furosemide, alone or in combination with intravenous albumin infusions or oral metolazone. These therapies should be used judiciously, because they may produce profound electrolyte disturbances and cause hypovolemic shock or venous thromboses in patients already predisposed to these complications.

Decreased serum concentrations of immunoproteins are thought to be the basis of the predisposition of nephrotic patients to infection with encapsulated bacteria. The exact mechanism for serum IgG depression, an almost universal finding in patients with primary NS, is unknown. Primary peritonitis is a particular problem: 6% of nephrotic children suffer at least one episode of bacterial peritonitis. Aggressive antibiotic therapy, specific for the common bacterial pathogens listed above, should be given at the first suspicion of systemic or peritoneal infection. Pneumococcal and *Haemophilus influenzae* B vaccines may be effective long-term deterrents to infection, but can be given only to patients who are in remission and on no immunosuppressive medications at the time of vaccination to achieve an effective antibody response. The use of prophylactic antibiotics during relapses is controversial but advocated by some clinicians. Nephrotic patients ordinarily tolerate viral infections well, unless they are receiving high-dose immunosuppressants.

Numerous defects in hemostasis occur in NS. Alterations in almost every coagulation factor and clotting inhibitor, as well as increased platelet adhesiveness and defects in the fibrinolytic system, have been reported. Systemic anticoagulation is indicated for all patients who develop thromboembolic disease and for those at high risk because of immobilization. Avoidance of bed rest, volume depletion, diuretics, and deep venous or arterial punctures are important aspects of the management of patients at risk for thrombosis.

■ MINIMAL CHANGE DISEASE

MCNS is characterized by the onset of NS without systemic disease, hypocomplementemia, or other serious signs of renal disease. Although nephritic features (hematuria, azotemia, and hypertension) occur in 10% to 30% of children with MCNS, these signs seldom occur together and are almost never severe or persistent. Patients with MCNS are notably young—two thirds of them present between ages 2 and 6 years. For this reason, preadolescents with NS and no nephritic signs, hypocomplementemia, or signs of systemic disease do not need a kidney biopsy before the initiation of therapy. Steroid therapy effectively induces a remission in most patients. Prompt and sustained remissions correlate well with minimal changes of glomerular morphology. Clinical and laboratory features and pathophysiology are those of NS described above.

Therapy and Outcome

The diagnosis of NS is usually first suspected in the outpatient setting. Hospitalization for a new nephrotic patient is strongly recommended for dietary and, if needed, diuretic management of edema, for initiation of steroid therapy, and for parent and patient education about the disease. At least 24 hours before starting steroid therapy, a tuberculin skin test should be done; if the result is negative, treatment may be safely started.

Corticosteroids are the mainstay of therapy for patients with minimal change nephrotic syndrome. The typically

TABLE 141-3. Common Plasma Protein Concentration Derangements in Patients With the Nephrotic Syndrome

INCREASED LEVELS	DECREASED LEVELS
Alpha-2 globulins	Albumin
Beta globulins	Alpha-1 globulins
Coagulation factors	IgG
Antifibrinolysins	Coagulation inhibitors
Most lipoproteins	Transferrin
	Transcortin
	Thyroxine-binding globulin
	Vitamin D-binding globulin

responsive patient loses the proteinuria within the first 3 weeks of therapy. Relapses occur in 80% of affected children, often during the period of slow prednisone tapering. During this time, the urine should be checked routinely at home for protein, using a dipstick daily or at least three times a week to screen for early signs of relapse, before the onset of edema. Patients who have fewer than two relapses in a 6-month period may be treated as described above for each relapse. Those who have more than two relapses in a 6-month period are called frequent relapsers and may do well on longer courses of alternate-day prednisone. Patients who cannot tolerate cessation of steroid therapy without a relapse are called steroid-dependent.

Frequent relapsers and steroid-dependent patients may require a diagnostic renal biopsy. If the biopsy shows MCNS and additional therapy to control the NS is desirable, a 2-month course of chlorambucil or cyclophosphamide may produce a sustained remission. Patients with frequently relapsing NS have more prolonged remissions than steroid-dependent patients after cytotoxic therapy. During therapy, patients should have a weekly complete blood count to monitor for signs of bone marrow depression that might require altering or stopping the drug dosage. Before beginning therapy with cytotoxic drugs, patients and parents should also be warned of other potential drug side effects, such as sterility in males after long-term cyclophosphamide therapy. Cyclosporine has also been effective in inducing a remission in steroid-dependent patients, but the relapse rate after discontinuation of this drug has been substantial.

The long-term prognosis for MCNS is excellent. Most patients (80%) enter a sustained remission during adolescence. The overall death rate in a large group of patients with MCNS followed by the International Study of Kidney Disease in Children (ISKDC) for 5 to 15 years was 2.6%.

(Abridged from Phillip L. Berry and Eileen D. Brewer, Glomerulonephritis and Nephrotic Syndrome, in Oski, DeAngelis, Feigin, McMillan, Warshaw: *Principles and Practice of Pediatrics, Second Edition*, J.B. Lippincott, 1994.)

Oski's Essential Pediatrics,
edited by Kevin B. Johnson and Frank A. Oski.
Lippincott–Raven Publishers,
Philadelphia © 1997

142

Progressive Hereditary Nephritis

■ ALPORT'S SYNDROME

Among progressive hereditary nephritis syndromes, Alport's syndrome is the most common, with an estimated gene frequency of 1 in 5000 in the United States. This diagnosis accounts for as much as 3% of all childhood chronic renal failure and for 0.6% of all patients in Europe who are starting renal replacement therapy. Patients with Alport's syndrome come from all geographic and racial backgrounds. The vast majority present with microscopic or macroscopic hematuria, but patients may rarely present with deafness, hypertension, proteinuria, edema, or renal failure.

Individuals with a gene for Alport's syndrome are considered to be affected only if they exhibit hematuria. Hematuria is present in most affected family members by the time they reach 6 years of age. Microscopic hematuria may be found at birth, it may be intermittent in females and younger males, and it may not be discovered until adulthood in some females. Episodes of macroscopic hematuria are frequent; they usually appear a few days after the onset of an upper respiratory infection and rarely last longer than 1 to 2 weeks. Proteinuria may appear during the first decade of life; it is often intermittent in young males and in females of all ages. The onset of proteinuria is considered a poor prognostic sign because it is often present and progressive in patients who eventually develop renal failure, and because it can result in nephrotic syndrome in young adults (usually males).

Virtually all males with Alport's syndrome develop chronic renal failure. In affected males with adult types of Alport's syndrome, early chronic renal failure progresses steadily to end stage renal disease (ESRD) over the course of a few years. Affected females are less likely to develop chronic renal failure.

Kindreds with type IV Alport's syndrome have normal hearing, but kindreds with all other types of Alport's syndrome exhibit bilateral cochlear deafness. Affected individuals have hearing loss at frequencies between 2 and 8 kHz, which is easily demonstrated by audiometric screening. The use of this screening tool shows that up to 85% of males and 18% of females with Alport's syndrome have significant hearing loss by 15 years of age. Hearing loss is often progressive and is more severe in males. In some kindreds, progression of hearing loss portends progression of renal failure. Although some affected individuals with ESRD have socially normal hearing, most patients with milder hearing loss have less severe renal involvement.

Ocular defects are found in individuals with Alport's syndrome. Lenticonus anterior, a protrusion of the anterior lens into the chamber, may occur in these patients and can lead to significant visual impairment; it is sometimes present with cataracts. Other patients have bilateral, multiple whitish spots surrounding the fovea. Some authors associate these perimacular spots with more severe renal involvement.

■ PATHOLOGY

The glomerular basement membrane (GBM) of patients with Alport's syndrome has a distinct appearance by electron microscopy. In some areas, the GBM is thin, measuring 50 to 150 nm wide compared with the normal 200 to 350 nm. In other areas, the membrane is thick, measuring 300 to 550 nm wide. These thick areas have a characteristic split appearance formed by a crisscrossing network of 100-nm-wide bands of lamina densa. Some capillary loops have only thin segments, some only thick segments, and others have both. The frequency of thin segments seems to decrease with age, whereas thick segments increase. Split, thick segments may be found as early as 1 year of age but are sometimes absent from the first biopsy specimen. Segments of thick and split GBM are more frequent in males but occur in both sexes. Some investigators argue that an increase in thick segments on biopsy correlates clinically with increased proteinuria. The observation that strongly suggests the diagnosis of Alport's syndrome is the finding of thin, normal, and thickened segments of GBM in the same biopsy specimen.

Basement membranes in nonrenal tissues are also abnormal in affected individuals.

Gene linkage studies have mapped the three X-linked Alport's syndrome types (types II, III, and IV) to a single area on the X chromosome, within region Xq21.2–22.1 near the centromere. Thus, these three phenotypes appear to result from different mutations of a single genetic locus. However, genes for the two main structural proteins of basement membrane, the alpha-1 and alpha-2 chains of type IV collagen, do not seem to be involved, because both are located on chromosome 13.

■ DIAGNOSIS AND DIFFERENTIAL DIAGNOSIS

Children found to have hematuria in multiple urine samples over an interval of a few weeks should be evaluated for the possibility of a progressive hereditary nephritis. Personal and extended family histories of hematuria, proteinuria, hypertension, ophthalmologic abnormalities, deafness, renal failure, and bleeding tendencies must be thoroughly documented. Physical examination and laboratory evaluation should seek evidence for renal failure, hearing loss, lenticonus anterior, perimacular spots, and thrombocytopenia. In addition, all family members should be tested on multiple occasions for hematuria. If the workup suggests the presence of familial hematuria, the differential diagnosis would include epidemic acute poststreptococcal glomerulonephritis (APSGN), familial idiopathic hypercalciuria, Alport's syndrome, other progressive hereditary nephritis syndromes, IgA nephropathy, and familial benign hematuria. APSGN should be evaluated by careful history, appropriate serologic testing, and serum complement levels; hypercalciuria is evaluated by the measurement of 24-hour urinary calcium excretion. The possibility of Alport's syndrome may be evaluated by screening affected family members with audiometry and, if necessary, by ophthalmologic consultation. Renal biopsy is usually reserved for patients with proteinuria or renal insufficiency, but it can be justified for prognostic purposes because biopsy evaluation can be diagnostic for IgA nephropathy and strongly suggestive of Alport's syndrome. New kindreds with Alport's syndrome are still diagnosed using the criteria outlined at the beginning of this chapter. Other progressive hereditary nephritis syndromes have a family history of renal failure in affected individuals but do not meet the criteria for Alport's syndrome. In contrast, familial benign hematuria is a diagnosis of exclusion, and family members must be followed for the development of proteinuria, renal failure, and deafness. Patients with persistent hematuria but without evidence of familial involvement must also be followed closely because Alport's syndrome is associated with a new mutation rate of 17% and because 7% of female obligate carriers do not have hematuria. Tests designed to detect mutations in the Alport's syndrome *COL4A5* gene are on the horizon and will probably be used in the near future as part of the workup for persistent hematuria.

Prenatal diagnosis is not yet routinely available for any of the progressive hereditary nephritis syndromes, although it can potentially be performed now for a few Alport's syndrome kindreds with known *COL4A5* gene mutations.

■ TREATMENT

No specific therapy is available for patients with hereditary nephritis. Hearing aids temporarily benefit patients with Alport's syndrome and hearing loss. Chronic renal failure is treated with dialysis or renal transplantation. Some patients with Alport's syndrome develop anti-GBM antibodies after receiving a renal transplantation, presumably because the donor kidney contains the *COL4A5* antigen that is absent in the host. However, severe anti-GBM nephritis is rare, and graft survival in patients with Alport's syndrome is not different from that of patients without Alport's syndrome.

(Abridged from David R. Powell, Progressive Hereditary Nephritis, in Oski, DeAngelis, Feigin, McMillan, Warshaw: *Principles and Practice of Pediatrics, Second Edition,* J.B. Lippincott, 1994.)

Oski's Essential Pediatrics,
edited by Kevin B. Johnson and Frank A. Oski.
Lippincott–Raven Publishers,
Philadelphia © 1997

143

Nail Patella Syndrome

■ CLINICAL FEATURES AND BIOPSY FINDINGS

Nail patella syndrome (NPS) is inherited as an autosomal dominant disorder, probably with full penetrance but variable expressivity. The locus for NPS is on chromosome 9, linked to the loci for both adenylate kinase 1 and the ABO blood group. The cardinal features of NPS are dysplastic nails and hypoplastic patellae; some patients have iliac horns, knee and elbow abnormalities, cataracts, and renal disease.

Nephropathic and nonnephropathic forms of NPS apparently exist, because renal disease aggregates in some NPS kindreds while sparing others. In kindreds with a history of nephropathy, 48% of the family members develop renal disease and 14% go on to renal failure; interestingly, the presence of nephropathy or renal failure in parents with NPS does not appear to increase the risk of the same complication in their children. Most patients present with proteinuria, which may lead to nephrotic syndrome, and occasionally NPS is associated with congenital nephrosis. Chronic renal failure has been reported in children under age 10 years but usually develops in teenagers and young adults, sometimes after years of asymptomatic proteinuria.

Kidney biopsy specimens from NPS patients have characteristic findings by electron microscopy. The glomerular basement membrane is irregularly thickened with electron lucent areas in the lamina rara externa and interna, and fibrillar or periodic collagenlike material is present in these membranes and in mesangial matrix. This collagenlike material was not found in a biopsy specimen from a relative free of NPS. Recent work suggests that some of these patients have an abnormal antigenicity of the glomerular basement membrane similar to that found in patients with Alport's syndrome. These findings suggest that the basic abnormality of NPS involves disordered connective tissue metabolism, but how this leads to renal failure is unclear.

The degree of electron microscopic abnormality does not seem to correlate with a loss of kidney function in NPS, because changes were present in biopsy specimens of some NPS patients who had no clinical evidence of renal dysfunction. Patients with NPS and a normal glomerular filtration rate, including those with nephrosis, do not demonstrate significant findings by light microscopy. However, patients with renal failure often demonstrate the nonspecific changes of proliferative and chronic glomerulonephritis.

Patients with NPS, especially those from kindreds with a history of renal disease, must be monitored periodically for the development of nephrosis and renal failure. No specific therapy exists for renal involvement in NPS; treatment of nephrosis and renal insufficiency are symptomatic.

(Abridged from David R. Powell, Nail Patella Syndrome (Hereditary Onycho-Osteodysplasia), in Oski, DeAngelis, Feigin, McMillan, Warshaw: *Principles and Practice of Pediatrics, Second Edition,* J.B. Lippincott, 1994.)

Oski's Essential Pediatrics,
edited by Kevin B. Johnson and Frank A. Oski.
Lippincott–Raven Publishers,
Philadelphia © 1997

144

Renal Tubular Acidosis

Renal tubular acidosis (RTA) is a biochemical syndrome characterized by a persistent hyperchloremic (nonanion gap) metabolic acidosis and is caused by abnormalities in the renal regulation of bicarbonate concentration. The glomerular filtration rate is usually normal: it may be mildly to moderately depressed but is never severely abnormal. Clinical manifestations suggesting the possibility of RTA include unexplained acidosis, failure to thrive and grow, profound weakness, polyuria, nephrolithiasis, nephrocalcinosis, and rickets.

■ CLASSIFICATION AND PATHOGENESIS

A classification of RTA is shown in Table 144–1.

Proximal RTA is a defect in the proximal tubular reabsorption of filtered bicarbonate. Ordinarily about 85% (somewhat less in infants) of filtered bicarbonate is reabsorbed in the proximal tubule and 15% (somewhat more in infants) in the distal nephron. In proximal RTA, the tubular maximum for bicarbonate reabsorption is abnormally low, so that at normal plasma levels of bicarbonate more than 15% of filtered bicarbonate is delivered to the distal nephron for reabsorption, resulting in the urinary excretion and lowering of the bicarbonate concentration in the body fluids. Proximal RTA represents a defect in the sodium/hydrogen ion exchange mechanism in this segment of the nephron.

The mechanisms of transport impairment in proximal RTA have not been defined. Possibilities include a defective sodium/potassium ATPase activity in the basolateral membrane, which normally provides the gradient for maximal efficiency of the luminal sodium/potassium antiporter; a defect in the sodium/hydrogen antiporter itself; or deficiency or inhibition of carbonic anhydrase activity.

Patients with proximal RTA spill bicarbonate into the urine at lower-than-normal plasma bicarbonate concentrations (ie, the renal threshold for bicarbonate is reduced). Because the amount of bicarbonate filtered per day varies from hundreds to thousands of milliequivalents, depending on the patient's size, there is the potential for very large losses of this most important buffer from the body stores. In proximal RTA, the distal mechanisms of acidification are intact.

Distal RTA (see Table 144–1) is seen in two major forms. Type 1 is usually associated with hypokalemia or normokalemia (secretory defect or gradient defect) or rarely with hyperkalemia (voltage-dependent defect). Type 4 RTA is always associated with hyperkalemia. Distal RTA type 1 results from a reduced rate of hydrogen ion secretion by the distal nephron, which may be due to a primary disorder of the hydrogen ion secretory pump (classic distal RTA), increased back-leak of secreted hydrogen ion from lumen to cell (gradient defect), or a decrease in the lumen-negative electrical potential difference that normally promotes hydrogen ion secretion (voltage-dependent RTA). Patients with distal type 1 cannot lower their urine pH below 5.5 regardless of the degree of the acidosis. Patients have also reduced total acid excretion, principally because of a low rate of ammonium secretion. Hypokalemic distal RTA most likely involves reduced function or inhibition of H,K-ATPase. Type 4 RTA is usually observed in children with either a deficiency in circulating aldosterone or unresponsiveness of the renal tubular transport sites to aldosterone.

Distal RTA type 1 may be seen in an incomplete or partial form. This is probably true of the other types, but clinical descriptions of partial defects have been limited to distal type 1. Transient instances of RTA have been described for all three major types of RTA. RTA may be inherited (eg, type 1 autosomal dominant trait) or acquired. Disorders associated with RTA types 2 and 1 are shown in Tables 144–2 and 144–3. Proximal RTA can occur as an isolated abnormality either sporadically or as an inherited disorder. However, it is much more common for proximal RTA to be seen as part of Fanconi's syndrome with associated glycosuria, aminoaciduria, hyperphosphaturia, and so forth.

■ CLINICAL CHARACTERISTICS

Proximal RTA Type 2

Most patients with proximal RTA type 2 manifest this tubular abnormality as part of Fanconi's syndrome, a syndrome of multiple proximal tubular dysfunctions (see Chapter 145). The clinical manifestations in these instances may be related to the condition causing Fanconi's syndrome or to some of the other tubular abnormalities that are a part of the syndrome. Patients with proximal RTA type 2 as an isolated disorder usually present either with unexplained acidosis or with failure to thrive and grow properly. The acidosis, as with all types of RTA, is a hyperchloremic metabolic acidosis. Usually at presentation the patient is in a reasonably steady-state condition; the extent of lowering of the plasma bicarbonate is determined by the severity of the proximal tubular defect in bicarbonate reabsorption. This steady state has been reached because the filtered load of bicarbonate has decreased to a point at which the amount that escapes reabsorption by the impaired proximal tubule is small enough to be completely reabsorbed by the distal nephron. Therefore, on presentation, there is usually no bicarbonate in the urine, and because the distal acidification mechanisms are intact in proximal RTA, the urine is acid ($pH < 5.5$). If the patient with proximal RTA type 2 is then treated with sufficient base, the plasma bicarbonate will increase and the amount of bicarbonate filtered will increase. This will overwhelm the impaired proximal tubules with bicarbonate, resulting in a large increase in delivery of bicarbonate to the distal nephron. The urine will, therefore, contain increasing amounts of bicarbonate as the plasma level increases and the urine becomes alkaline, even though the plasma bicarbonate may still be below normal.

In summary, patients with proximal RTA type 2 have severe bicarbonate wasting when plasma bicarbonate levels are normal, but during the untreated or acidotic state, their bicarbonaturia ceases, urinary pH becomes acid, and urinary net acid excretion approximates net acid production. Patients with proximal RTA type 2 often have hypokalemia, but serum potassium levels may be normal. Patients with this form of RTA seldom manifest the complications of nephrocalcinosis, nephrolithiasis, or rickets, which are common manifestations in patients with untreated distal RTA type 1. They may, however, manifest with muscle weakness and polyuria, both caused by hypokalemia.

TABLE 144-1. Pathophysiologic Classification of RTA

Type	Pathophysiology
Proximal RTA (type 2)	Impaired proximal tubular HCO_3^- reabsorption
Distal RTA (type 1)	Impaired distal tubular H^+ secretion
Secretory defect ("classic distal RTA")	H^+ pump failure
Gradient defect	Increased back-leak of secreted H^+
Voltage-dependent defect	Reduced luminal electronegativity
Hyperkalemic distal RTA (type 4)	Impaired ammoniagenesis
Hypoaldosteronism	
Primary	
Secondary	
Pseudohypoaldosteronism	
Total	
Partial	Increased NaCl reabsorption in ascending
Chloride shunt	loop of Henle

Distal RTA Type 1

Patients with this type of RTA may present with unexplained acidosis or with failure to thrive and grow, hypokalemia, or one or more of the complications of RTA such as nephrolithiasis, nephrocalcinosis, rickets, or polyuria. Hypercalciuria is also common, and urinary citrate excretion is low. These abnormalities, along with the persistently alkaline urine, are instrumental in the development of nephrocalcinosis and nephrolithiasis in these patients. It is unknown whether the low urinary citrate excretion is primary or is secondary to the prolonged metabolic acidosis. In the inherited variety of distal RTA type 1, metabolic acidosis may occur in the first few months of life. Most preadolescent children with distal RTA type 1 waste bicarbonate and have a significantly higher fractional excretion of bicarbonate than do adults with this type of RTA. Most patients with distal RTA type 1 have either hypokalemia or normokalemia.

Distal RTA Type 4 (Hyperkalemic)

Hyperkalemic distal RTA (type 4) is thought to be the most common type of RTA in both children and adults. It represents an abnormality of distal tubular function in regard to the renal handling of hydrogen and potassium ions. It manifests with a persistent hyperchloremic (nonanion gap) metabolic acidosis and hyperkalemia. The hyperkalemia is probably the most distinctive clinical characteristic of this type of RTA when compared with types 1 and 2, because both of these types usually have either normal, or frequently low, serum potassium concentrations. Patients with type 4 RTA usually can make an acid urine ($pH < 5.5$), but total acid excretion is low due to very low rates of ammonia excretion, the urine anion gap is positive, and the renal excretion of potassium is inappropriate to the serum concentration of potassium. The defects in urinary potassium and hydrogen ion excretion appear to be secondary to hypoaldosteronism or to end-organ resistance to aldosterone (pseudohypoaldosteronism). Hypoaldosteronism can be primary or secondary (Table 144–4).

Primary hypoaldosteronism is seen in patients with acute adrenal insufficiency, Addison's disease, and salt-losing congenital adrenal hyperplasia. Patients may show all the signs of adrenal insufficiency, including salt wasting, tendency to low blood volume and low blood pressures, metabolic acidosis, hyponatremia, and hyperkalemia. Peripheral renin activity (PRA) is usually increased, but there is a virtual absence of circulating aldosterone. Renal function in these patients, including renal tubular function, is within normal limits.

Secondary hypoaldosteronism results from decreased production or release of the active form of renin due to destruction of the cells of the juxtaglomerular apparatus, as seen in patients with intrinsic renal disease such as lupus nephropathy, diabetic nephropathy, obstructive uropathy, and interstitial nephritis. Reduction in overall renal function can be demonstrated, but the hyperkalemia and metabolic acidosis are out of proportion in severity to the degree of renal insufficiency. These patients do not demonstrate salt wasting or tendency to low blood volume, and their blood pressure may be either normal or elevated.

Another form of type 4 RTA occurs in both children and adults and is associated with salt retention. Its pathogenesis has been attributed to an abnormally increased reabsorption of sodium chloride in the thick ascending limb of Henle (chloride shunt), which causes salt retention, tendency to increase blood volume, and hypertension. This entity has also been called Gordon syndrome, and seems to be in many ways a mirror image of Bartter's syndrome. Short stature is common, and most patients appear to have inherited the syndrome by way of an autosomal dominant mode of transmission. The PRA and plasma aldosterone levels are both reduced.

■ DIAGNOSIS

Patients with all forms of RTA have a hyperchloremic metabolic acidosis. This type of acidosis must be differentiated from an anion-gap type of acidosis by measuring the plasma undetermined anion gap* (Figure 144–1). Once a hyperchloremic (nonanion gap) metabolic acidosis has been demonstrated, it is important to rule out other causes of this type of acidosis before making a diagnosis of RTA. The chief

---

*Undetermined anion gap= NA^+ - (Cl^- + HCO_3^-) (Normals: Neonates, 18 or less; older infants and children, 16 or less; adolescents and adults, 14 or less)

TABLE 144-2. Disorders Associated With RTA Type 2

ISOLATED DEFECT
Sporadic
Hereditary
Use of carbonic anhydrase inhibitors

FANCONI SYNDROME
Primary, Secondary

Inherited
Cystinosis
Tyrosinemia
Lowe syndrome
Hereditary fructose intolerance
Wilson disease
Glycogen storage disease
Metachromatic leukodystrophy
Osteopetrosis with carbonic anhydrase deficiency
Cytochrome-c-oxidase deficiency

Defect in Calcium Metabolism
Hyperparathyroidism
   Primary
   Secondary

Dysproteinemic States
Multiple myeloma
Light chain diseases
Monoclonal gammopathy
Amyloidosis

Interstitial Renal Disease
Sjögren disease
Medullary cystic disease
Renal transplant rejection
Chronic renal vein thrombosis
Balkan nephropathy

Drugs and Toxins
Outdated tetracycline
Maleic acid
Cadmium
Lead
Mercury

Miscellaneous
Malignancy
Chronic nephrotic syndrome
Congenital heart disease

TABLE 144-3. Disorders Associated With Distal RTA Type I

PRIMARY
Sporadic
Hereditary

SECONDARY (ACQUIRED)
Genetic Diseases
Ehlers-Danlos
Wilson disease
Hereditary elliptocytosis
Fabry disease
Sickle-cell nephropathy
Osteopetrosis with carbonic anhydrase deficiency
Medullary cystic disease
Hereditary hypercalciuria
Marfan syndrome
Sensorineural deafness

Disorders Causing Nephrocalcinosis
Idiopathic hypercalciuria
Medullary sponge kidney
Primary hyperparathyroidism
Hyperthyroidism
Vitamin D intoxication

Autoimmune Diseases
Sjögren syndrome
Systemic lupus erythematosus
Chronic active hepatitis
Fibrosing alveolitis
Primary biliary cirrhosis
Hyperglobulinemic purpura
Thyroiditis
Cryoglobulinemia

Tubulointerstitial Diseases
Obstructive uropathy
Balkan nephropathy
Chronic pyelonephritis
Leprosy
Transplant rejection

Drugs and Toxins
Amphotericin B
Lithium
Toluene

Miscellaneous
Hepatic cirrhosis
Malnutrition

differential diagnosis is usually diarrhea with bicarbonate loss in the stools, because this is, by far, the most common cause of hyperchloremic metabolic acidosis. In patients with consistently alkaline urine, it is wise to consider the possibility of a urinary tract infection (UTI) with a urea-splitting organism. If there is any suspicion of a UTI, a urine culture should be done. The plasma pH, partial pressure of carbon dioxide (PCO_2), and total carbon dioxide must be measured several times to document the persistence of the acidosis. All urine passed should be tested for pH; at least some of these should be done with a pH meter, which is more accurate than dipsticks.

Again, the urine anion gap is a good way to estimate urinary ammonium excretion—the most important component of total acid excretion—but direct measurement of NH_4 is better. The urine anion gap is obviously not as reliable if the urine contains large amounts of unmeasured anions such as ketoacids, penicillin, and salicylates, which will lead to underestimation of urinary ammonium excretion. Glomerular function should be evaluated with a serum creatinine, and several serum potassium concentrations should be done.

TABLE 144-4. Clinical Spectrum of Distal Type IV Hyperkalemic RTA

| Mechanism Designation | PRA | Aldo | Plasma | | Salt Wasting |
			BV	BP	
Hypoaldosteronism					
Primary mineralocorticoid deficiency, no intrinsic renal disease	Increase	Decrease	Nor/decr.	Nor/decr.	Yes
Primary hyporeninemic, secondary hypoaldosteronism due to intrinsic renal disease	Decrease	Decrease	Nor/incr.	Nor/incr.	No
Pseudohypoaldosteronism, end-organ resistant to aldosterone					
Total resistance	Increase	Increase	Decrease	Nor/decr.	Yes
Partial resistance associated with renal immaturity	Nor/incr.	Nor/incr.	Normal	Normal	No
Chloride shunt or Gordon syndrome	Decrease	Decrease	Increase	Increase	No

PRA, *plasma renin activity;* Aldo, *aldosterone;* BV, *blood volume;* BP, *blood pressure;* Nor/incr., *normal or increased;* Nor/decr., *normal or decreased.*

Modified from McSherry E. Renal tubular acidosis in childhood. Kidney Internat. *1981:20:799.*

■ THERAPY

General

Administration of alkali is common to the therapy of almost all types of RTA. The most frequently used alkalis are sodium bicarbonate and sodium citrate, the latter usually given as Shohl's solution. Each gram of $NaHCO_3$ provides 12 mEq of bicarbonate, and Shohl's solution contains 1 mEq of citrate per milliliter of solution. In patients with hypokalemic types of RTA, a percentage of alkali can be given as the potassium salt. Plasma bicarbonate, either direct or indirect (from pH and PCO_2), and serum potassium deter-minations should be performed every 2 to 4 days during alkali dosage adjustment. After correction of the acidosis, bicarbonate and potassium levels should be measured every 2 weeks for 1 to 2 months and then monthly for several more months. Ultimately, these determinations are done three to six times a year, depending on the difficulty encountered in controlling the metabolic acidosis. Normal stature can usually be attained if the metabolic acidosis is well controlled over a prolonged period.

(Abridged from L. Leighton Hill and Myra Chiang, Renal Tubular Acidosis, in Oski, DeAngelis, Feigin, McMillan, Warshaw: *Principles and Practice of Pediatrics, Second Edition,* J.B. Lippincott, 1994.

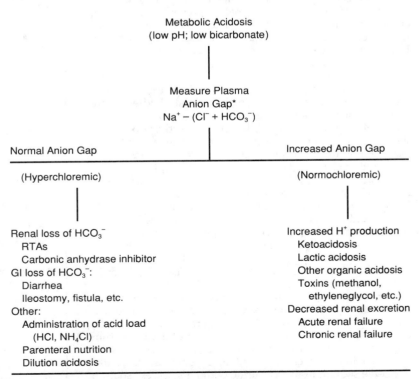

Figure 144-1. The differentiation of metabolic acidosis into hyperchloremic and normochloremic types.

*Normals: Neonates—18 or less, older infants and children—16 or less, adolescents—14 or less.

Oski's Essential Pediatrics,
edited by Kevin B. Johnson and Frank A. Oski.
Lippincott–Raven Publishers,
Philadelphia © 1997

145

Fanconi's Syndrome

Fanconi's syndrome (FS) is the result of generalized transport dysfunction of the proximal renal tubule. It is characterized classically by excessive urinary losses of amino acids, glucose, bicarbonate, and phosphate, and also calcium, magnesium, uric acid, and other organic acids, low-molecular-weight (tubular) proteins, sodium, potassium, and water. The urinary losses can result in metabolic acidosis, dehydration, hypokalemia, hypophosphatemia, rickets, and growth retardation in children. Many inherited and acquired disorders can lead to FS in adults and children (Table 145–1). When FS occurs in childhood, however, the cause is usually hereditary and related to an inborn error of metabolism.

■ CLINICAL AND LABORATORY FINDINGS

The general clinical manifestations of FS depend on the patient's age and the type and chronicity of the underlying disease. Infants and children most often present with failure to thrive. Many features of FS, including chronic acidosis, volume contraction, hypokalemia, hypophosphatemia, and abnormal vitamin D metabolism, contribute to impaired linear growth.

Episodic vomiting, anorexia, polydipsia and polyuria, chronic constipation, and unexplained fevers are nonspecific symptoms of chronic FS. Constipation probably results from chronic volume depletion associated with the polyuria, hypokalemia, and chronic metabolic acidosis of untreated FS. Unexplained fevers, which occur especially frequently in infants and young children with cystinosis, may reflect episodic dehydration.

The laboratory findings of FS mostly reflect abnormal proximal renal tubular function. In normal children, more than 98% of the filtered amino acids are reabsorbed in the proximal renal tubule. In FS, hyperaminoaciduria occurs in the presence of normal plasma amino acid levels and is an exaggeration of the normal excretory pattern of each amino acid, with the percentage of tubular reabsorption of each amino acid decreased below normal. Because urinary losses are trivial compared to intake, hyperaminoaciduria is not clinically significant, but it is an important clinical marker for FS. Plasma and urinary amino acids should be sampled simultaneously as part of the clinical evaluation of patients with FS.

Urinalysis often reveals glucosuria, abnormally high urine *p*H (>5.5), specific gravity 1.010 to 1.015, even in the presence of dehydration; and mild albuminuria (1 to 2+ or 30 to 100 mg/dL) with normal serum protein and albumin.

Serum chemistries are often abnormal in fully expressed FS. Besides hyperchloremic metabolic acidosis with a normal anion gap, patients may have hyponatremia, hypokalemia, hypophosphatemia, and, in some cases, hypouricemia. Serum calcium and magnesium are usually normal, despite increased losses of calcium and magnesium in the urine. Excessive sodium loss in the urine without sufficient sodium intake can eventually result in hyponatremia, although increased delivery of sodium to the distal renal tubule and

high levels of renin and aldosterone caused by volume depletion will increase distal tubular sodium reabsorption to avoid hyponatremia.

■ TREATMENT

Table 145–1 lists many of the causes of FS (most of these disorders are discussed elsewhere in this text). Identification of the underlying cause for FS is crucial to direct therapy. In some cases, specific therapy or withdrawal of an offending substance may normalize the tubular dysfunction. When no specific therapy exists, symptomatic treatment of the electrolyte disturbances and bone disease of FS is the only alternative.

TABLE 145-1. Causes of Fanconi's Syndrome

HEREDITARY

Primary
Idiopathic

Secondary
Cystinosis

Lowe syndrome

Tyrosinemia type 1

Galactosemia

Hereditary fructose intolerance

Glycogen storage disease

Wilson disease

Other (cytochrome-c-oxidase deficiency, metachromatic leukodystrophy, Alport syndrome)

ACQUIRED

Intoxications
Drugs

    Gentamicin and other aminoglycosides

    Outdated tetracycline

    Cephalothin

    Valproic acid

    Streptozolocin

    6-Mercaptopurine

    Azathioprine

    Cisplatin

Toxins

    Heavy-metals (lead, mercury, cadmium, uranium, platinum)

    Glue (toluene) sniffing

    Paraquat

    Maleic acid (experimental in animals)

Disease states
Nephrotic syndrome

Sjögren syndrome

Multiple myeloma

Light chain nephropathy

Hypergammaglobulinemia

Amyloidosis

Interstitial nephritis with antitubular basement membrane antibody

Renal vein thrombosis

Malignancy (lymphoma, carcinoma)

Renal transplantation

Proximal renal tubular acidosis may be severe, requiring large amounts of alkali therapy divided into four to six daily doses. Potassium supplementation is almost always necessary when alkali therapy is given. Administration of the potassium salt of citrate, bicarbonate, or acetate fulfills the dual purpose of treating acidosis and preventing hypokalemia. Mixtures of sodium and potassium citrate or potassium citrate alone are available commercially for oral use. Sodium wasting and dehydration are treated with combinations of sodium bicarbonate, citrate, and chloride, depending on the degree of acidosis. Prevention of dehydration from obligatory polyuria is best handled by allowing the patient free access to fluids. If the patient is vomiting and cannot readily ingest adequate fluid, dehydration may occur rapidly and will require early intervention with intravenous replacement therapy.

Hypophosphatemia and impaired renal vitamin D metabolism are the factors leading to rickets and other bone complications. The simultaneous administration of phosphate and alkali supplements may lead to tetany from acute hypocalcemia, so phosphate supplements should be added with caution in patients receiving alkali therapy. In some patients, supplementation with 1,25-dihydroxyvitamin D or dihydrotachysterol, neither of which requires further renal metabolism for biologic activity, is necessary to heal and sustain healing of rickets and osteomalacia. Hypercalciuria and transient hypercalcemia are toxic side effects of excessive vitamin D metabolite therapy.

(Abridged from Eileen D. Brewer and David R. Powell, Pan Proximal Tubular Dysfunction (Fanconi Syndrome), in Oski, DeAngelis, Feigin, McMillan, Warshaw: *Principles and Practice of Pediatrics, Second Edition*, J.B. Lippincott, 1994.)

Oski's Essential Pediatrics, edited by Kevin B. Johnson and Frank A. Oski. Lippincott–Raven Publishers, Philadelphia © 1997

146

Nephrogenic Diabetes Insipidus

Nephrogenic diabetes insipidus (NDI) is a hereditary or acquired disorder characterized by renal tubular resistance to antidiuretic hormone (ADH). The inability to concentrate the urine because of this tubular disease leads to marked polyuria with compensatory polydipsia. The pattern of inheritance in the great majority of cases is consistent with a sex-linked dominant transmission with complete expression only in the afflicted male and variable penetrance in the female. Even in males there may be variation in the degree of severity of the defect; most are diagnosed in early infancy because of a severe defect, but some have a mild enough disease to escape detection until the second or third decade of life.

The defect in hereditary NDI, at least in males with the severe defect, usually is more severe than that seen in the acquired types. There are two general causes of the acquired types. The first is the loss of the concentration gradient in the medullary interstitial tissues as a result of the tissue destruction occurring with obstructive uropathy, vesicoureteral

reflux, sickle-cell nephropathy, cystic disease, pyelonephritis, interstitial nephritis, and nephrocalcinosis. The second cause is the decreased responsiveness to ADH by the distal tubules and collecting ducts, although the concentration gradient in the medullary interstitial tissues remains intact. Conditions that cause this alteration include hypokalemic states, hypercalcemia, amyloidosis, sarcoidosis, and various drugs that interfere with the action of ADH, such as lithium, demeclocycline, cisplatin, vinblastine, methoxyflurane, amphotericin B, colchicine, and propoxyphene. This second group of conditions more closely resembles hereditary NDI than does the first group. NDI can also be seen as part of Fanconi's syndrome, most likely because of the chronic hypokalemia that often occurs.

■ CLINICAL FEATURES

The most common clinical manifestations of NDI are shown in Table 146–1. Polyuria is constant even during periods of dehydration. Elevated body temperature, a consequence of the dehydration, often leads to multiple investigations attempting to identify possible bacterial, viral, or parasitic infections. The large fluid ingestion may interfere with attaining adequate calorie intake; this, along with the deleterious effects of the chronic hypernatremia, leads to failure to thrive. The constant need for intake of liquids interferes with normal sleep patterns. Chronic severe constipation is another result of the constant tendency to negative water balance that characterizes NDI. When a child with NDI is well hydrated, a dramatic reversal in the condition is seen: the signs and symptoms of dehydration disappear, the fever abates, and the vomiting, irritability, and other manifestations disappear until dehydration recurs.

■ LABORATORY FINDINGS

Hypernatremia and hyperchloremia are commonly seen when the patient has been in negative water balance. The urinalysis is usually normal, except for being inappropriately dilute (ie, specific gravity <1.006 and urine osmolality <200 mOsm/kg) despite evidence of dehydration. Small amounts of protein and a few red blood cells may be found in the urine, and the blood urea nitrogen (BUN) may be elevated during dehydration. With rehydration, the sodium, chloride, BUN, and creatinine levels return to normal and, although the urine remains dilute, the protein and red blood cells disappear. When the patient is in water balance, the glomerular filtration rate and all other renal function tests, aside from the inability to conserve water, are normal.

TABLE 146-1. Clinical Manifestations

Polyuria and polydipsia
Growth and developmental failure
Recurrent bouts of dehydration
Unexplained fever
Thirst
Vomiting
Constipation
Onset during infancy
Positive family history
Irritability

In the infant with NDI, the serum sodium is often elevated early in the morning because of insufficient fluid intake during the night, but may return to normal during the day concomitant with adequate fluid intake. Ultrasound examination may reveal marked dilatation of the urinary tract in NDI because of extremely high water turnover. This is usually minimal at the time of diagnosis in very young infants, but it may be found to be massive later if control of water balance is not good. Marked dilatation of the urinary tract may also be seen in patients not identified as having NDI until later in childhood.

■ DIAGNOSIS

The diagnosis of NDI is suspected because of polyuria, polydipsia, bouts of dehydration, hypernatremia, dilute urines, and a positive family history. The differential diagnosis includes other causes of polyuria such as central diabetes insipidus, diabetes mellitus, psychogenic water drinking, and chronic renal insufficiency. The chief differential is often between central (ADH-deficient) diabetes insipidus and nephrogenic (vasopressin-resistant) diabetes insipidus. An attempt to assess and document the magnitude of the polyuria and polydipsia by measuring intakes and outputs is essential. The most important test is a well-controlled water deprivation or concentration test in the hospital during the day and under close medical supervision. A urine:plasma osmolality ratio of 2.0 or more is sufficient to rule out both nephrogenic diabetes insipidus and central (ADH-deficient) diabetes insipidus.

The next step in the diagnostic process is to test the renal tubular response to antidiuretic substances. The testing substance of choice is desmopressin acetate (DDAVP), a synthetic analogue of 8-arginine vasopressin. DDAVP should be given intranasally. Urine should be measured for volume and for concentration (specific gravity and osmolality) at 1- to 2-hour intervals after administration. If there is no response in terms of decrease in volume of urine and increase in the osmolality of the urine, then a second dose should be given and additional urine samples collected for volume and concentration. Serum sodium and osmolality should be obtained before and 4 hours after the administration of DDAVP. A urine:plasma ratio for osmolality of 1.5 or greater would indicate an adequate tubular response to antidiuretic substances. If the patient fails to concentrate the urine with the water deprivation test and also after DDAVP or aqueous vasopressin USP (Pitressin) stimulation, then a diagnosis of NDI is indicated.

■ THERAPY OF HEREDITARY NDI

The daily water turnover of infants and children with NDI can be enormous, equalling half or more of the patient's total body water each day. The intake of volumes of this magnitude may be very difficult to achieve purely from a mechanical point of view. Fluid intake as high as 300 to 400 mL/kg/day may be required just to maintain water balance. This high free water intake should be spaced fairly evenly over the 24-hour period, even at night to prevent early-morning dehydration and hypernatremia. A diet that will result in a low renal solute load is of major importance in reducing the obligatory renal water requirement. Such a diet is reasonably low in protein and sodium chloride. In the infant, breast milk is preferable, but, if it is unavailable, a low-protein, low-electrolyte commercial formula will suffice. Roughly 6% of the total calories should come from protein, and the daily sodium intake should not exceed 1 mEq/kg of body weight. In older children, the daily protein intake should be about 2 g/kg, and the total daily sodium content should be in the range of 1 to 2 g.

The importance of a low renal solute load in determining the volume of obligatory urine water is shown in Table 146–2. Two disease states, chronic renal insufficiency and NDI, are compared with the normal patient. The same diet is assumed for each of these three children (ie, a diet yielding about 600 mOsm of solute for renal excretion per day). The normal child should be able to concentrate to 1200 mOsm/L of urine water, the patient with chronic renal failure can usually concentrate to about 300 mOsm/L, and the patient with NDI can concentrate in the vicinity of 100 mOsm/L. The obligatory urine volume is determined by dividing the total solute load for excretion by the maximum ability to concentrate. As can be seen in this theoretical example, the person with no disease would have an obligatory renal water requirement of 0.5 L; the patient with chronic renal insufficiency would have a mild polyuria, with an obligatory water excretion of 2 L/day; and the patient with NDI would have severe polyuria, with an obligatory renal water excretion of 6 L/day. If the diet of the patient with NDI were reduced in protein and sodium chloride content so that the renal solute load was decreased to 300 mOsm/day, then the obligatory renal water excretion would be only 3 L/day instead of 6 L/day, a dramatic decrease.

The thiazide diuretics can be used to diminish the polyuria further. The thiazide diuretics increase sodium excretion, thereby producing a borderline low blood volume. As a result, increased proximal tubular reabsorption of salt and water occurs, and there is less delivery of water to the concentrating sites in the kidney. With a slower flow rate

TABLE 146-2. Water Turnover Related to Inability to Concentrate Urine

Disease	Solute Load (SL)*	Maximum Ability to Concentrate (c)	V = SL/C†	Obligatory Renal Water in Liters (V)	Degree of Polyuria
None	600	200 mOsm/kg	V = 600/1200	0.5	None
Chronic renal failure	600	300 mOsm/kg	V = 600/300	2.0	Mild
NDI	600	100 mOsm/kg	V = 600/100	6.0	Severe
NDI	300	100 mOsm/kg	V = 300/100	3.0	Moderate

*Average diet might yield 600 mOsm of solute/m² to be excreted by kidney (principally urea, electrolytes, and other nitrogenous products).

†V = SL/C where V = obligatory urine volume in liters; SL = 24-hour renal solute load, and C = concentration of urine in mOsm/kg of water.

through the collecting ducts, some water diffuses from the collecting duct lumen to the medullary interstitial tissues despite the lack of effect of ADH. The thiazide may decrease urine volume by as much as 20% to 40%. Therefore, these drugs are valuable in the very young infant who has a great physical problem in taking in the volume of free water required to stay in water balance. The decrease in urine volume also prevents or lessens the degree of dilatation of the urinary tract, which is almost inevitable at the high water turnover rates these patients experience when untreated. Because the effect of the thiazide is almost completely nullified by a high sodium intake, sodium restriction to the level previously recommended is vital.

The other agents that appear to be helpful in the management of NDI are prostaglandin synthetase inhibitors (eg, indomethacin). The effects of prostaglandins on renal function are complex and appear to vary with the particular prostaglandin involved and the particular situation under which it is tested. In general, however, it appears that prostaglandin synthetase inhibitors usually inhibit water excretion.

Obviously, the treatment of the acquired types of NDI varies depending on the therapy necessary to treat the underlying disease causing the secondary tubular defect. However, many of the principles outlined for the therapy of hereditary NDI also apply to patients with the acquired variety. In particular, these patients benefit from the provision of extra free water and a diet that will yield a low renal solute load.

(Abridged from L. Leighton Hill, Nephrogenic Diabetes Insipidus, in Oski, DeAngelis, Feigin, McMillan, Warshaw: *Principles and Practice of Pediatrics, Second Edition,* J.B. Lippincott, 1994.)

Oski's Essential Pediatrics,
edited by Kevin B. Johnson and Frank A. Oski.
Lippincott–Raven Publishers,
Philadelphia © 1997

147

Renal Hypertension

RENOVASCULAR HYPERTENSION

Renovascular hypertension (RVH) results from the impairment of blood flow to part or all of one or both kidneys and accounts for between 4.5% and 11.5% of sustained secondary hypertension during childhood. Main renal arteries or smaller intrarenal arteries may be affected. The incidence of RVH is substantially lower in black than in white patients.

Table 147–1 outlines the major causes of renovascular hypertension.

■ CLINICAL FINDINGS

Table 147–2 contains clinical clues that suggest a renovascular origin for hypertension. RVH should be considered in any case of severe or refractory hypertension in a child, especially in the first decade of life. The presence of retinopathy, signs of secondary hyperaldosteronism (hypokalemia,

mild metabolic alkalosis), and an abdominal bruit should lead to a consideration of RVH. Hypertension associated with a unilateral small kidney and an excellent response to angiotensin-converting enzyme (ACE) inhibitors also merits consideration of RVH.

The preliminary workup should include a urinalysis, serum creatinine, serum calcium, and electrolytes. An electrocardiogram (ECG) and chest radiograph can be obtained to look for evidence of left ventricular hypertrophy. Many nephrologists recommend an echocardiogram for evaluating cardiac status because it is more sensitive in demonstrating left ventricular hypertrophy. Either ultrasonography (preferred) or an intravenous urogram should be part of the preliminary workup to search for abnormalities such as obstructive uropathy, mass lesions, renal scarring, cystic disease, and abnormal renal size. Renal scans are helpful in screening for renal scarring.

■ DIAGNOSTIC STUDIES

Screening Tests

Renal Imaging Studies

Ultrasonography provides accurate information on renal location, size, volume, and contour and should be done as part of the preliminary workup to rule out some of the renal parenchymal diseases mentioned previously. However, it gives no information as to renal function. In newborns, it may be useful in visualizing aortic thrombosis associated with umbilical artery catheters.

Doppler imaging of renal arterial flow at the time of ultrasonography is being evaluated. Preliminary figures in adults are encouraging, but there are limitations in the ability to get an adequate study. There are insufficient data in children to evaluate its potential usefulness.

Intravenous urograms are preferred over sonograms by some, but "rapid sequence urograms" are no longer performed routinely because of a high rate of false-positive results.

ACE inhibitors have been used with serum renin levels, radionuclide imaging, and renal vein renin determinations to improve the predictive values of these tests. Renal function in a kidney that has renal artery stenosis depends on an elevated efferent arteriole tone that is maintained by high renin levels. This tone is depressed when an ACE inhibitor is given. With radionuclide imaging, there is a decreased uptake and clearance of the isotope from the kidney after

TABLE 147-1. Intrinsic Renal Artery Disease

Fibromuscular lesions:
    Intimal
    Medial
    Perimedial
Arteritic lesions
Thrombotic and embolic lesions
Aneurysms
Arteriovenous malformations (fistulas)
Neurofibromatosis (intimal lesion, nodular lesion)
Abdominal coarctation with renal artery involvement
Arteriosclerotic lesions

TABLE 147-2. Clinical Clues That Suggest Renovascular Hypertension

Abrupt onset of severe hypertension

Epigastric, subcostal, or flank bruit

Progression to malignant-phase hypertension

Retinopathy

Hypokalemia

Plasma bicarbonate high-normal to elevated

Hypertension refractory to intensive antihypertensive regimen

Hypertension with unilateral small kidney

Excellent response to angiotensin-converting enzyme inhibitors

Transient impairment in renal function in response to angiotensin-converting enzyme inhibitor

captopril (an ACE inhibitor) is given. This test has been useful in improving sensitivity and specificity in adults, but the experience in children has been limited. The captopril challenge test measures the rise in peripheral renin after the administration of oral captopril. Positive predictive values in adults have ranged from 32% to 92%, with one study in children having a positive predictive value of 43%. Captopril has also been given before obtaining renal vein renins. The ultimate usefulness of the captopril challenge test and captopril renography in children is yet to be determined, but it appears that a negative captopril challenge test or captopril renography will provide strong evidence against renal vascular hypertension.

Confirmatory Tests

Renal arteriography with renal vein renins remains the gold standard in the diagnosis of renovascular hypertension. These studies are usually done concomitantly and provide both anatomical and functional information. The purpose of these studies is to visualize a functionally significant lesion. The presence of collateral vessels with a stenotic lesion implies a significant lesion. Recognizing a branch lesion may be helpful in renal vein sampling.

Differential renal vein renins are obtained from effluent venous blood from each renal vein and from the inferior vena cava. In unilateral RVH, the affected (ischemic) kidney should have a renal vein renin activity at least 1.5 times greater than that from the renal vein of the contralateral kidney. In addition, a renal/systemic index should be calculated, looking at the renal vein renin levels in comparison to the inferior vena cava (IVC). Obviously, sampling errors can occur that will negate the value of the study. Because higher renal vein renin activities increase the reliability of the study, the differential renal vein studies usually are done after some maneuver designed to stimulate renin production, such as sodium depletion, the administration of loop diuretics, or the administration of ACE inhibitors. The presence of a significant difference in renal vein activity predicts benefit of surgery in 90% of the patients; however, a significant number of patients with negative studies also will benefit from surgery.

■ CLINICAL MANAGEMENT

Pharmacologic management of the blood pressure in RVH has improved greatly with the introduction of the beta blockers in the 1970s and the ACE inhibitors in the 1980s.

ACE inhibitors block the conversion of angiotensin I to angiotensin II, thereby lowering angiotensin II concentration and reducing the degree of vasoconstriction and the secretion of aldosterone. An ACE inhibitor is usually the drug of choice in RVH. ACE inhibitors must be used with extreme caution if there is bilateral renal artery stenosis or evidence of stenosis in a solitary kidney: patients have presented with renal failure subsequent to initiating ACE inhibitor therapy in these circumstances. Because ACE inhibitor therapy is frequently initiated before bilateral renal artery stenosis is diagnosed, a cautious approach is prudent. The patient should be monitored for evidence of azotemia or hyperkalemia after beginning therapy with captopril, enalapril, or lisinopril (ACE inhibitors). There is some concern about the long-term effects of ACE inhibitor therapy for renovascular disease because these drugs decrease systemic blood pressure at the expense of decreased perfusion to the stenotic kidney.

Long-term medical therapy is indicated in the patient whose vascular lesion is not amenable to surgical correction. Medical therapy also may be useful in other situations, such as in very young children to allow the renal vasculature to grow sufficiently to permit revascularization procedures. Under these circumstances, renal function must be followed closely because it may deteriorate from progressive arterial disease, even though blood pressure control is successful. If renal function does deteriorate, then reconsideration must be given to surgery or to percutaneous transluminal renal angioplasty.

(Abridged from L. Leighton Hill and Seth Paul Kravitz, Renal Hypertension, in Oski, DeAngelis, Feigin, McMillan, Warshaw: *Principles and Practice of Pediatrics, Second Edition*, J.B. Lippincott, 1994.)

Oski's Essential Pediatrics, edited by Kevin B. Johnson and Frank A. Oski. Lippincott–Raven Publishers, Philadelphia © 1997

148

Urolithiasis

There is a marked variation worldwide in the incidence of stones in children. In some countries, such as Turkey and Thailand, urolithiasis is endemic; bladder stones predominate and dietary factors are postulated to play a causative role. In contrast, stones are uncommon in children in the United States, where less than 1% of all renal stones occur in children under age 10 and less than 3% in children under age 19, and where most stones have a metabolic origin. In the United States, boys with stones outnumber girls by 2:1, stones are very uncommon in black children, and bladder stones are much less common than upper tract stones. Although the two conditions may coexist, a distinction should be made between urolithiasis (stones in the urinary tract) and nephrocalcinosis (an increase in the calcium content of the renal tissue).

■ FORMATION OF STONES

Urinary calculi consist of a very small glycoprotein matrix with surrounding organic or inorganic crystals. Urinary crystalloids capable of being crystallized include calcium, phosphorus, oxalates, cystine, uric acid, xanthine, and ammonium. Supersaturation of the urine with various ionic species eventually leads to precipitation, with subsequent crystal growth. Urine volume, through its effect on dilution and concentration, obviously plays a critical role in determining the degree of saturation. Urine pH is an important factor in determining solubility. Theoretically, any factor that increases the number of nuclei in tubular fluid or urine, such as epithelial injury, could lower the metastable limit, the supersaturation at which crystals first form. There are also inhibitor substances that inhibit crystallization.

■ CLINICAL FEATURES

The presentation in children, especially young children and infants, may be very nonspecific. Gross or microscopic hematuria may be the only manifestation, or hematuria may be accompanied by nonspecific abdominal pain or by fever, pyuria, and abdominal pain. Signs and symptoms might be those of a urinary tract infection (UTI). Typical renal colic is unusual in the small child but can be present in the older child. In some instances, the stone or gravel already has been passed spontaneously. Frequently the patient has a family history of stones. Urinary stones can cause obstruction of the urinary flow, dilatation of the urinary tract, and, ultimately, renal parenchymal damage. Stones can predispose to UTIs; conversely, UTIs can be important in the formation of stones.

■ DIAGNOSIS

A high index of suspicion frequently is required to make the diagnosis of urolithiasis. Demonstration of the stone can be done by imaging techniques such as a plain radiograph of the abdomen, intravenous urograms, an ultrasound study of the urinary tract, or tomograms. All stones containing calcium are radiopaque. Cystine stones are slightly radiopaque because of the sulfur present in cystine. Struvite stones also are radiopaque. The stones that are most frequently radiolucent are those resulting from disorders of purine metabolism (Table 148–1).

The diagnosis of urolithiasis also can be made by the proven passage of a stone, gravel, or sludge. Whenever urolithiasis is considered, any passed material must be saved and the urine must be strained, whether at home or in the hospital, in an attempt to obtain a stone.

The laboratory workup is suggested in Table 148–2. The metabolic evaluation of stone formers should begin 4 to 6 weeks after stone diagnosis and passage, because passage may cause transient changes in urinary chemistry. The serum calcium determines the possible presence of hypercalcemia. Serum phosphorus may be low in hyperparathyroidism, in one type of hypercalciuria, and in renal tubular acidosis (RTA), and may be elevated in the tumor lysis syndrome. Serum creatinine estimates glomerular function. The electrolytes, pH, PCO_2, and urine pH are used to investigate the possibility of RTA. All children with stones should have a spot chemical urine test for cystine to rule out cystinuria and a quantitative amino acid analysis if the spot test is positive. A timed urine sample (at 6, 8, 12, or preferably 24 hours) is collected for quantitative measurement of calcium and uric acid. Quantitative urinary calcium excretion or a spot urine for calcium:creatinine ratio will provide information as to the possible presence of hypercalciuria. Hyperuricosuria can occur without hyperuricemia.

TABLE 148-1. Urolithiasis Classification Based on Stone Composition

I. Calcium stones (calcium oxalate and calcium phosphate)
  A. Hypercalciuria
    1. Hypercalcemic hypercalciuria
       Hyperparathyroidism
       Thyrotoxicosis
       Vitamin D intoxication
       Idiopathic infantile hypercalcemia
       Sarcoidosis
       Neoplastic deposits in bones
       Immobilization
    2. Normocalcemic hypercalciuria
       Idiopathic or familial hypercalciuria
         Absorptive
         Renal
         1,25-dihydroxycholecalciferol-induced
       Distal RTA (type 1)
       Acetazolamide use
       Loop diuretic use
       Immobilization
       Vitamin D excess
       Cushing's syndrome
  B. Hyperoxaluria (calcium oxalate)
    1. Primary hyperoxaluria types 1 & 2
    2. Secondary hyperoxaluria
       Inflammatory bowel disease
       Pyndoxine deficiency
       Massive doses of vitamin C
  C. Hyperglycinuria (calcium oxalate stones)
  D. Idiopathic urolithiasis
II. Magnesium ammonium phosphate (struvite) plus basic calcium phosphate (apatite)
  A. Urinary tract infection with urea-splitting organisms (mostly *Proteus* species)
  B. Foreign body plus urinary stasis plus infection
III. Uric acid stones*
  A. Hyperuricosuria
    1. Gout
    2. Lesch-Nyhan syndrome
    3. High purine diet
    4. Type I glycogen storage disease
    5. Leukemia-lymphoma
    6. Leukemia-lymphoma cytotoxic prescription
IV. Xanthine stones*
  A. Primary xanthinuria
  B. Allopurinol therapy
V. Dihydroxyadenine stones*
VI. Cystine stones
  A. Cystinuria

Disorders of purine metabolism.

TABLE 148-2. Laboratory Workup for Urolithiasis

BLOOD DETERMINATIONS

Calcium, repeat 2 or 3 times

Phosphorus

Alkaline phosphatase

Creatinine

Electrolytes

pH and P_{CO_2}

Uric acid

URINE STUDIES

Urinalysis, repeat 2 or 3 times

Urine culture

Spot urine for cystine (cyanide-nitroprusside test)

Urine pHs, repeat 4–6 times

Spot urine for calcium/creatinine ratio

24-hour urine for calcium, creatinine, oxalate, and uric acid. Add xanthine if patient has hypouricemia and quantitative amino acids if spot test for cystine is positive.

OTHER STUDIES

Ammonium chloride loading test may be necessary to assess renal ability to acidify.

■ TREATMENT

One of the most important measures in preventing the formation or further growth of any stone regardless of etiology is to increase urine volume, which reduces the urinary concentrations of calcium, phosphorus, oxalates, cystine, uric acid, and other possible constituents of stones. This dilution of the urine can be accomplished by raising the fluid intake to 1.5 to 2 times normal (2400 mL/m^2/day or more). The high fluid intake should be distributed as much as possible throughout the 24 hours, including at bedtime and during the night if the patient awakens. Early morning urines should be kept at a specific gravity of less than 1.014. UTI, if present, must be treated and a search for anatomical abnormalities completed. Any urologic abnormalities predisposing to infections or stones should be corrected.

Stone Removal

Many stones will pass through and out of the urinary tract spontaneously. Others may dissolve slowly (eg, uric acid stones) or at least not grow as a result of medical treatment. Some stones must be removed: struvite stones, stones causing prolonged obstruction with obstructive nephropathy, and stones causing significant chronic pain or resistant UTI. The traditional surgical management of patients with calculus disease in the past consisted of endoscopic manipulation with stone baskets or loops for stones in the lower part of the ureter (below the pelvic brim) or open surgical procedures for calculi higher in the urinary tract. These traditional methods of stone removal are being replaced by a variety of new modalities, including extracorporeal shock-wave lithotripsy, percutaneous nephrostolithotomy, and the use of percutaneously placed endoscopes to fragment calculi with

ultrasound waves or lasers. These techniques, used first in adults, are finding widespread application in children and represent a dramatic advance in medical therapy.

Specific Therapeutic Measures

The treatment for pediatric hypercalciuria and stones due to hypercalcemia is elimination of the cause of the hypercalcemia; that is, parathyroidectomy (for patients with hyperparathyroidism), treatment of thyrotoxicosis or Cushing's disease, withdrawal of vitamin D therapy, at least partially mobilizing immobilized patients, and so on. Distal RTA, a form of normocalcemic hypercalciuria, can be treated with appropriate amounts of sodium bicarbonate or sodium citrate plus potassium citrate, striving to keep the serum bicarbonate concentration in the range of 22 to 28 mEq/L (see Chapter 144).

The therapy of urolithiasis due to familial or idiopathic hypercalciuria is controversial. It is probably no longer necessary to try to distinguish the various types of hypercalciuria in regards to therapy; rather, all patients with stones from idiopathic or familial hypercalciuria should be treated similarly, with increased fluid intake and reduced calcium intake and sodium intake. Thiazide diuretics, which enhance renal tubular reabsorption of calcium, are effective in reducing calcium excretion and preventing recurrent stone formation. Because high sodium chloride intakes tend to negate this effect of thiazides, restriction of sodium intake to a maximum of 2 g/day is indicated. The addition of potassium citrate to this regimen is advised. Whether to use thiazide drugs for long-term therapy depends on the number of recurrences of stones and the complications encountered. Dietary calcium restriction can be tried but must be used cautiously in a growing child. The use of phosphate compounds (cellulose phosphate, orthophosphate) in children is poorly tolerated and has generally been abandoned.

Of the therapies for familial hypercalciuria, the thiazide diuretics have been the most successful, but long-term use of a thiazide would be considered only in those patients with recurrent stones. The therapy of familial hypercalciuria is not completely clear at this time. Thiazides reduce stone formation in patients with recurrent idiopathic urolithiasis, even though urinary calcium before treatment was normal.

Allopurinol therapy is very effective in patients with uric acid and dihydroxyadenine stones. A high urine output is also valuable in treating these two types of stones. Alkalinization of the urine to a pH of 6.5 with sodium bicarbonate or sodium citrate is important in treating and preventing uric acid calculi. Hemodialysis may be necessary to control the extreme hyperuricemia seen in patients with the tumor lysis syndrome.

Dilution of the urine decreases the saturation of cystine, and alkalinization will increase the solubility of cystine. The alkali therapy must be divided over the entire day and night so as to ensure a pH above 7 (ideally above 7.4). Of these two treatments, increasing the fluid intake is much more important. D-penicillamine is another effective therapy, but it is seldom used because it is expensive and has many side effects.

(Abridged from L. Leighton Hill, Urolithiasis, in Oski, DeAngelis, Feigin, McMillan, Warshaw: *Principles and Practice of Pediatrics, Second Edition*, J.B. Lippincott, 1994.)

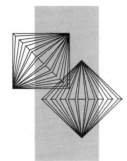

SECTION 11

Gastrointestinal Diseases

Oski's Essential Pediatrics,
edited by Kevin B. Johnson and Frank A. Oski.
Lippincott–Raven Publishers,
Philadelphia © 1997

149

Developmental Disorders of Gastrointestinal Function

■ EMBRYOLOGY

Structural developmental anomalies are important causes of neonatal gastrointestinal disease. Several fundamental processes must occur during fetal development for normal intestinal structure to be present at birth (Table 149–1). Failure of these developmental events to occur may result in major defects in gut structure and function.

■ GASTROINTESTINAL OBSTRUCTION IN THE NEONATE

The symptoms and signs suggesting obstruction are several. The immediate inability of the neonate to swallow secretions and saliva or his or her failure to tolerate the attempt at first feeding is the first manifestation of high esophageal mechanical obstruction. Alternatively, infants with intestinal obstruction may be seen acutely in a morbid state with either vomiting or abdominal distention, as obstruction may become apparent only several hours after the initiation of feedings. Bilious vomiting or obstipation in the neonate always demands immediate, careful, and comprehensive evaluation and care. As important, the infant who apparently tolerates early feedings but then fails to pass meconium in the first 48 hours of life must be investigated for distal bowel obstruction.

TABLE 149-2. Common Causes of Gastrointestinal Obstruction in the Neonate

Type	Time of Presentation
Tracheoesophageal fistula (may be part of VACTERL association)	Birth—respiratory difficulty, aspiration
Gastric web	May present later in infancy or early childhood
Pyloric stenosis	First 4 weeks of life, males (first born)
Intestinal malrotation—extrinsic obstruction or volvulus	70% present in neonates, 3/4 of these in first month of life
Jejunal/ileal atresia	Most common causes of obstruction in first 2 weeks of life
Meconium ileus	First 48 hours of life present with clinical features consistent with intestinal obstruction and failure to pass meconium
Hirschsprung's disease (colonic aganglionosis)	Usually presents in first 48–72 hours, but may have recurrent obstruction during neonatal period
Imperforate anus	Present at birth

The pathophysiology of obstruction in the newborn may be functional or mechanical. Functional obstruction may be mediated by aberrant bowel innervation, inflammation, or a lumen impacted with abnormal meconium. Mechanical obstruction may be at any level of the gastrointestinal tract, from the esophagus to the anus. The latter may be intrinsic, as with an atretic or obliterated gut lumen, or extrinsic, as in the case of a constricting band. Obstruction, moreover, may be complicated; mechanical and functional obstruction may coexist.

TABLE 149-1. Principles of Normal Gut Development and Major Developmental Anomalies

Principle	Developmental Mechanism	Developmental Anomaly
Growth	Gut elongation, rotation, and mesenteric fixation	Malrotation
Lumen formation	Recanalization from solid cell phase	Duodenal atresia, stenosis
Separation	Proximal: pulmonary tract	Tracheoesophageal fistula
	Distal: genitourinary tract (formation of rectum and anus)	Exstrophy, imperforate anus
Motility	Innervation for propulsion of fecal stream	Hirschsprung's disease
Regression	Closure of fetal remnant accessory intestine, the vitelline system	Meckel's diverticulum

Complete evaluation and intervention can be performed on an acute basis for all disorders producing gastrointestinal obstruction in the neonate. The benefits of a good history and a complete physical examination cannot be understated. Historically, polyhydramnios, a positive family history of other neonates with obstruction, and birth weight are helpful indicators. During the examination, it is essential that an attempt be made to pass a catheter into the stomach, that the presence of bowel sounds be sought, that the neonate's abdomen be palpated for the presence of a mass, and that the anus be examined carefully for patency. Documentation of extraintestinal anomalies may offer additional information to the clinician in the process of diagnosing the cause of gastrointestinal obstruction. Table 149–2 lists many of the common causes of gastrointestinal obstruction presenting during the neonatal period.

(Abridged from William M. Belknap and Colston F. McEvoy, Developmental Disorders of Gastrointestinal Function, in Oski, DeAngelis, Feigin, McMillan, Warshaw: *Principles and Practice of Pediatrics, Second Edition,* J.B. Lippincott, 1994.)

Oski's Essential Pediatrics,
edited by Kevin B. Johnson and Frank A. Oski.
Lippincott–Raven Publishers,
Philadelphia © 1997

150

Neonatal Cholestasis

Neonatal cholestasis, defined as prolonged conjugated hyperbilirubinemia, is the end result of impaired bile flow and excretion. The cumulative incidence of neonatal cholestasis is about 1 in 2500 live births. Liver dysfunction in the neonate, regardless of the cause, commonly is associated with bile secretory failure and cholestatic jaundice. The potential mechanisms by which bile secretion may be impaired are many. Hepatocellular injury, such as that noted in neonatal hepatitis, may cause functional impairment of bile secretion. Mechanical obstruction to bile flow also may occur, as noted in extrahepatic biliary atresia. Although many disorders can present as neonatal cholestasis, neonatal hepatitis and biliary atresia are the most common syndromes, accounting for 70% to 80% of all cases of prolonged conjugated hyperbilirubinemia in infants (Figure 150–1). Table 150–1 lists the differential diagnosis of conjugated hyperbilirubinemia in neonates.

Identification of the infant with cholestasis begins with measurement of total and conjugated bilirubin fractions. The cholestatic infant will have an elevated conjugated fraction, generally at a level above 2 mg/dL and accounting for more than 15% to 20% of the total bilirubin. The possibility of liver or biliary tract disease must be considered in any neonate who is jaundiced beyond 2 weeks of age. Indeed, jaundice after 11 days in term infants and after 14 days in premature infants is unusual, occurring in only 0.5% of infants in one study. Subsequent efforts must be directed toward rapid diagnosis of and therapy for potentially treatable disorders, such as sepsis, galactosemia, and hypothyroidism or panhypopituitarism, in which delay of diagnosis may have catastrophic consequences; differentiation of biliary atresia from neonatal hepatitis, because the former will require surgical intervention; and effective management of the consequences of chronic cholestasis. Early in the workup of any cholestatic infant, vitamin K should be given in an effort to prevent life-threatening hemorrhage. Further description of specific diagnostic modalities is included with the discussion of each entity.

■ BILIARY ATRESIA

Extrahepatic biliary atresia, which occurs in about 1 in 8000 live births, consists of atresia or hypoplasia of any portion of the extrahepatic biliary system. The obstruction may occur as a discrete distal lesion, allowing surgical drainage of patent portions of bile duct proximal to the atresia. In the most common form, however, the atretic area extends to above the level of the porta hepatis and often affects intrahepatic bile ducts, making surgical drainage difficult.

The clinical presentation of this disorder is similar to that of neonatal hepatitis. Typically, infants are born at term and are of normal birth weight. Jaundice develops at 3 to 6 weeks of age in otherwise well-appearing, thriving infants, and the stool eventually becomes acholic. About 15% of infants may have associated defects, including polysplenia, cardiovascular anomalies, and malrotation of the intestine. There is no apparent genetic predisposition, and familial recurrence is rare. Hepatic pathology will vary with the age of the infant; early biopsy samples may feature the presence of multinucleated giant cells, which decrease in number with age. Classic features of biliary atresia include bile ductular proliferation, bile plugs, and portal or perilobular fibrosis and edema.

Biliary atresia appears to be an evolving lesion with progressive obliteration of bile ducts; this is supported by the fact that several infants with previously documented patent extrahepatic biliary ducts have been found, on reexploration, to have biliary atresia. Thus, it is possible to speculate that neonatal hepatitis and extrahepatic biliary atresia represent different manifestations of hepatocyte or biliary tract injury by a single agent. However, the etiology of the disorder is unknown.

The diagnosis of biliary atresia involves the exclusion of other known causes of neonatal cholestasis. Differentiation of biliary atresia from neonatal hepatitis remains difficult. Clinical features aiding in discrimination include birth weight (biliary atresia is more common in term infants, whereas infants with neonatal hepatitis often are born prematurely or are small for gestational age); the presence of associated anomalies or an enlarged, firm liver (suggestive of biliary atresia); and the consistent absence of stool pigment (associated with biliary atresia). Duodenal fluid may be collected and assayed for the presence of bilirubin pigment or bile acids, the presence of which virtually excludes the diagnosis of biliary atresia. An abdominal ultrasound examination permits evaluation for the presence of a gallbladder, which often is absent in biliary atresia. Further studies should be directed at ruling out endocrine, metabolic, and other miscellaneous causes of cholestasis, as listed in Table 150–1.

Hepatobiliary imaging, using imidodiacetic acid derivatives, may be employed. The radionuclide is given intravenously. In patients with biliary atresia, uptake into the liver is rapid, but no excretion into the intestine occurs. Conversely, in patients with neonatal hepatitis, uptake is slow, but excretion does occur. This study typically is performed after phenobarbital has been given orally for 3 to 5 days to enhance biliary excretion of the isotope.

TABLE 150-1. Differential Diagnosis of Conjugated Hyperbilirubinemia (Neonatal Cholestasis)

BILE DUCT OBSTRUCTION

Cholangiopathies

    Extrahepatic biliary atresia

    Nonsyndromic paucity of intrahepatic bile ducts

    Choledochal cyst

    Neonatal sclerosing cholangitis

    Spontaneous perforation of common bile duct

    Bile duct stenosis

    Caroli's disease

Other

    Inspissated bile/mucous plug

    Cholelithiasis

    Tumors/masses (intrinsic and extrinsic)

NEONATAL HEPATITIS

Idiopathic

Viral

    Cytomegalovirus

    Rubella

    Reovirus type 3

    Herpesviruses

        Simplex

        Zoster

        Human herpesvirus type 6

    Adenovirus

    Enteroviruses

    Parvovirus B19

    Hepatitis B

    Hepatitis C

    ? Non A, non B, non C

    Human immunodeficiency virus

Bacterial and parasitic

    Bacterial sepsis

    Syphilis

    Listeriosis

    Tuberculosis

    Toxoplasmosis

IDIOPATHIC CHOLESTATIC SYNDROMES

Arteriohepatic dysplasia (Alagille syndrome)

Byler's syndrome

Hereditary cholestasis with lymphedema (Aaqenaes)

Benign recurrent cholestasis

Familial cholestasis of North American Indians

METABOLIC DISEASES

Disorders of amino acid metabolism

    Tyrosinemia

Disorders of lipid metabolism

    Niemann-Pick disease

    Gaucher disease

    Wolman's disease

Disorders of the urea cycle

    Arginase deficiency

Disorders of carbohydrate metabolism

    Galactosemia

    Fructosemia

    Type IV glycogenosis

Disorders of bile acid synthesis

Peroxisomal disorders

    Zellweger's syndrome

Disorders of oxidative phosphorylation

Other

    Alpha-1-antitrypsin deficiency

    Cystic fibrosis

    Hypopituitarism (Septo-optic dysplasia)

Hypothyroidism

Neonatal hemochromatosis

Toxic

Drugs

Parenteral nutrition

MISCELLANEOUS ASSOCIATIONS

Shock/hypoperfusion

Histiocytosis X

Intestinal obstruction

Erythrophagocytic lymphohistiocytosis

Neonatal lupus erythematosus

Indian childhood cirrhosis

Extracorporeal membrane oxygenation

Autosomal trisomies

Graft vs. host disease

Veno-occlusive disease

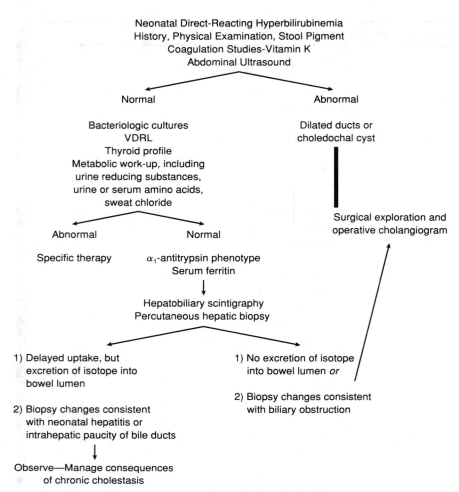

Figure 150-1. Flow chart for the work up of neonatal cholestasis.

Percutaneous hepatic biopsy is of great value in the differentiation of neonatal hepatitis and extrahepatic biliary atresia. This procedure may be performed safely using the Menghini technique. Pathologic findings favoring the diagnosis of extrahepatic biliary atresia include bile duct proliferation, bile plugs, and portal and perilobular fibrosis.

If the diagnosis of extrahepatic biliary atresia cannot be ruled out definitively after the evaluation described above has been performed, operative exploration and cholangiography should be undertaken. This procedure enables recognition of biliary atresia as well as exclusion of other forms of extrahepatic bile duct disease (stenosis or perforation of the common bile duct). The surgeon should avoid transection of a biliary tree that is patent but small because of biliary hypoplasia or the diminished bile flow that is associated with intrahepatic cholestasis. Resection is *not* indicated in these cases. Correctable forms of atresia (distal obstruction), as mentioned previously, also may be found.

In about 80% of cases, however, a "noncorrectable" atresia will be found. In these patients, further exploration is indicated and an attempt to establish biliary drainage should be made, using the hepatoportoenterostomy procedure of Kasai. This procedure consists of transection of the porta hepatis, with subsequent apposition of a Roux-en-Y loop of intestine. The rationale is to drain any small, persisting bile duct remnants. Prognosis after this procedure is affected by the age of the patient at the time of operation, with success rates of 90% in infants less than 2 months of age decreasing to less than 20% in patients greater than 90 days of age. Also

important is the size of the lumina of the residual ducts that are encountered at surgery; those with diameters of less than 150 μm are associated with a poor prognosis. This operation rarely is definitive in patients with noncorrectable atresia, and most patients will have progressive hepatic disease as well as repeated episodes of bacterial cholangitis. Therapy of the patient after the hepatoportoenterostomy (Kasai) operation consists of prompt and vigorous treatment of the episodes of cholangitis and consistent attention to nutritional support. Patients in whom bile flow was attained initially after the Kasai operation, but who subsequently stop draining, probably should undergo reoperation in an effort to establish bile flow again. Multiple attempts at reexploration and revision of a nonfunctional conduit should be avoided, however. Regardless of the eventual outcome, one beneficial effect of the Kasai procedure often is to provide adequate time for the patient to grow before hepatic transplantation becomes necessary. Biliary atresia without intervention is universally fatal, with the mean age of death being less than 1 year. Liver transplantation is essential in the treatment of children whose operation is not successful in restoring bile flow, in those who are referred late (probably at 120 days of age or later), and in those in whom liver failure eventually develops despite some degree of bile drainage.

(Abridged from Donald A. Novak, Frederick J. Suchy, and William F. Balistreri, Neonatal Cholestasis, in Oski, DeAngelis, Feigin, McMillan, Warshaw: *Principles and Practice of Pediatrics, Second Edition,* J.B. Lippincott, 1994.)

Oski's Essential Pediatrics,
edited by Kevin B. Johnson and Frank A. Oski.
Lippincott–Raven Publishers,
Philadelphia © 1997

151

Gastroesophageal Reflux

Gastroesophageal reflux is defined as the retrograde movement of gastric contents from the stomach into the esophagus. Such episodes frequently occur physiologically, and the event is brief, asymptomatic, and self-limited. It is well established that infants, particularly premature infants, have a greater frequency and duration of reflux episodes in both the sleeping and the awake states. The pathologic consequence of gastroesophageal reflux in the full-term and premature newborn usually is minimal.

The physiologic barriers for preventing reflux of gastric contents into the esophagus include the following. The first is a functional lower esophageal sphincter at the level of the gastroesophageal junction. It is most likely that the lower esophageal sphincter is the principal barrier against gastroesophageal reflux. The basal tone or pressure achieved at this specific anatomic site probably maintains gastric contents within the stomach. The second factor preventing gastroesophageal reflux is the ability to clear fluid actively from the distal esophagus by maintaining active motility. When normal distal esophageal motility is present, fluid entering the distal esophagus results in prompt clearance or return to the stomach. This prevents a peptic injury to the esophagus by the acidic contents of the stomach. This clearance is aided cooperatively by gravity, the ready flow of saliva from the mouth, and intact neuromuscular function of the distal esophagus. Thus, the ability of the distal esophagus to evoke local propulsive waves to clear its distal third is an essential reflux barrier. A third function important in maintaining normal upper gastrointestinal function is intrinsic gastric motility. Gastric emptying, the ability of the stomach to discharge efficiently and completely a milk feeding into the duodenum after it is emulsified and acidified, is a fundamental aspect of upper intestinal function and digestion. Failure of prompt and efficient emptying will overwhelm the reservoir capacity of the stomach and potentiate gastroesophageal reflux.

When examined closely, virtually all newborn infants are observed to have gastroesophageal reflux. This usually is manifested clinically at the time of feeding as the effortless regurgitation of a portion of the feeding. Dysfunction in or incoordination of the mechanisms of upper gastrointestinal motility cited above probably plays a role; this phenomenon is the result of a physiologic delay in the maturation of this function. Occasionally, unforced regurgitation of an entire feeding may occur, and should not occasion alarm. Rarely, either the overall frequency of reflux or the marked duration of single episodes may cause problems in a neonate, particularly a premature infant. Such reflux is problematic most often in infants with other diseases, such as chronic pulmonary disease or symptomatic congenital heart disease. In a minority of infants, reflux may occur excessively frequently or be of such duration as to create primary problems in the absence of a concomitant illness. Reflux may occasion reluctance to feed in the caretaker, and caloric deprivation may result, with failure of the infant to grow and thrive. In addition, the physical action of reflux of feedings may prevent the retention of sufficient intake to support normal growth. Reflux, by virtue of its frequency or duration, may

result in peptic esophagitis. Infants with esophagitis will have frequent regurgitation, general irritability or colic, or reflux of small amounts of blood-tinged formula. The presence of esophagitis is a very important indicator for pathologic gastroesophageal reflux.

Much discussion has occurred about the role of gastroesophageal reflux in precipitating major respiratory events in neonates. Frequently, reflux events will result in coughing or choking. These commonly are associated with the feeding or occur in the immediate postprandial period. It is apparent that, on rare occasion, reflux may be a cause of obstructive apnea. The rarest and most serious complication of gastroesophageal reflux is tracheal aspiration.

Evaluation for the presence of esophageal reflux begins with excluding partial upper intestinal obstruction. Reflux never should be confused with such disorders as pyloric stenosis, gastric antral web, duodenal stenosis, annular pancreas, or malrotation. Vomiting secondary to increased intracranial pressure, metabolic disease manifesting acidosis or hyperammonemia, and drug toxicity, as well as the presence of infections such as pneumonia, otitis media, or urinary tract infection must be considered carefully and excluded. In general, the normal health of the infant, the absence of bloody or bilious vomiting, and a history of normal weight gain indicate that gastroesophageal reflux is physiologic and benign. If regurgitation of entire feedings has occurred and is of sufficient frequency, upper gastrointestinal obstruction or other causes of frank vomiting must be considered.

Barium contrast studies of the pharynx, esophagus, and upper gastrointestinal tract should be performed to confirm that anatomy and motility are normal. This study may demonstrate the occurrence of gastroesophageal reflux in roughly 50% of cases; unfortunately, reflux on barium swallow may be artifactual. This point is particularly relevant in small infants when the study is performed under stressful circumstances with an indwelling nasogastric tube. A very sensitive modality with which to define the actual frequency and duration of gastroesophageal reflux is the use of an indwelling *p*H monitor. Such a study may be performed in very small infants for as long as 12 to 24 hours. In addition, concomitant monitoring for cardiopulmonary dysfunction or recording of the cessation of active respiration occasionally is used in problem cases when reflux is thought to cause respiratory dysfunction in hospitalized infants.

Choking during feedings should not be attributed to gastroesophageal reflux; swallowing dysfunction may be present. Nasal–pharyngeal incoordination and other causes of swallowing dysfunction should be differentiated from gastroesophageal reflux in the infant who presents with feeding difficulties. The investigation for aspiration may include performing technetium–sulfur colloid scintiscanning of gastric emptying. In this case, the actual gastric emptying can be quantified, in addition to visualization and documentation of gastroesophageal reflux and actual aspiration.

Therapy for gastroesophageal reflux is individualized. In the uncomplicated patient with postprandial regurgitation of small amounts of the feeding, simple observation and reassurance are indicated. An upright, prone posture, taking advantage of gravity, is the next level of therapy. Formally placing the infant in a 30-degree posture after the time of feeding, or maintaining very difficult cases nearly continuously in this position, will minimize reflux. Frequent, small feedings are advantageous, in contrast with larger and less frequent feedings. Thickened feedings also have been advocated in some cases, but the utility of this practice recently has been brought into question. Documentation of esophagitis calls for prompt, aggressive therapy, including antacid administration after feedings; severe or unresponsive cases are treated pharmacologically with an H_2-receptor–blocking agent. Agents to enhance gastroduodenal motility and increase distal gastroesophageal sphincter pressure have been advocated. These drugs include bethanechol and metoclopramide; the latter agent has been associated with the undesirable side effects of restlessness and oculogyric crisis, particularly in newborn or premature infants. The routine use of these drugs in neonates cannot be advocated.

Because gastroesophageal reflux results from immaturity of the mechanisms necessary to maintain normal upper gastrointestinal motility, it will resolve rapidly in most infants. Indeed, most infants achieve normal function by 6 to 7 weeks of age; a minimum of 60% to 70% of infants with obvious gastroesophageal reflux achieve complete functional maturity without specific therapy. Because prolonged gastroesophageal reflux may occur during sleep as absent voluntary swallowing and salivation, resulting in prolonged episodes, placing the infant in a prone, upright position during sleep may be advantageous. In the remaining infants, continued reflux will improve or resolve by the time they are 6 months old; in 90% of them, it will resolve completely by the time they are 18 months old.

Intractable gastroesophageal reflux may occur in the neurologically impaired infant. In such cases, surgical fundoplication and gastrostomy tube placement may be indicated. Surgical therapy for gastroesophageal reflux also may be necessary in cases in which documented aspiration pneumonia has occurred on two occasions. Although surgical therapy may be of some benefit, it rarely is indicated. Surgical fundoplication is associated with postoperative complications in up to 10% to 20% of patients. In addition, a repeat surgical procedure may become necessary.

Patients who have undergone repair of a tracheoesophageal fistula commonly have distal esophageal dysmotility and gastroesophageal reflux. Reflux may be very problematic in such cases.

(Abridged from William M. Belknap and Colston F. McEvoy, Sucking and Swallowing Disorders and Gastroesophageal Reflux, in Oski, DeAngelis, Feigin, McMillan, Warshaw: *Principles and Practice of Pediatrics, Second Edition*, J.B. Lippincott, 1994.)

Oski's Essential Pediatrics,
edited by Kevin B. Johnson and Frank A. Oski.
Lippincott–Raven Publishers,
Philadelphia © 1997

152

Distended Abdomen

Abdominal distention in the newborn may result from several causes, including organomegaly, intestinal obstruction, pneumoperitoneum, hemoperitoneum, ascites, and an abdominal mass. Intestinal obstruction is discussed in Chapter 149. This chapter focuses on abdominal masses, which are a common cause of distended abdomens in newborns.

■ ABDOMINAL MASS IN THE NEWBORN

The lesions causing abdominal masses that present in the neonatal period usually are benign; only 10% to 15% rep-

TABLE 152-1. Causes of Abdominal Mass in the Newborn*

RENAL
Unilateral cystic dysplastic kidney
Hydronephrosis
Renal vein thrombosis
Nephromegaly
Renal polycystic disease
Wilms' tumor
Mesoblastic nephroma
Neurogenic bladder

ADRENAL
Adrenal hemorrhage
Abscess
Neuroblastoma (calcification 50%)
Teratoma (calcification 75%)

RETROPERITONEAL
Lymphangioma
Neuroblastoma
Sacrococcygeal teratoma
Ganglioneuroma
Leiomyosarcoma
Pancreatic cyst

GASTROINTESTINAL
Intestinal duplication
Segmental intestinal dilatation
Mesenteric cyst (± intestinal malrotation)
Lymphangioma
Intraperitoneal meconium cyst

HEPATIC
Hepatomegaly
Infantile hemangioendothelioma (calcification)
Hepatoblastoma (calcification 40%)
Mesenchymal hamartoma
Subcapsular hematoma
Epidermoid cyst
Benign teratoma
Focal nodular hyperplasia (rare)
Angiosarcoma, undifferentiated sarcoma
Metastatic disease (neuroblastoma)

BILIARY
Hydropic gallbladder
Choledochal cyst
Spontaneous perforation of the common bile duct

GENITAL TRACT
Hydrometrocolpos
Ovarian cyst
Ovarian teratoma
Urachal cyst
Inguinal masses: hernia, hydrocele, calcified meconium

See text for relative frequency.

resent malignant tumors (Table 152–1). Two thirds of abdominal masses in the neonate are retroperitoneal in location; the kidneys predominate as the most common origin of an abdominal mass presenting in the newborn period. Renal mass lesions, therefore, are the single most common diagnostic category of abdominal mass in the newborn, as well as the most common of the masses that arise specifically from the retroperitoneal space. The remainder of the regional abdominal masses detected in this age group originate in gastrointestinal, mesenteric, hepatobiliary, or genital tracts; many of the specific aspects of these disorders in the newborn are discussed elsewhere in this text.

(Abridged from William M. Belknap, Distended Abdomen, in Oski, DeAngelis, Feigin, McMillan, Warshaw: *Principles and Practice of Pediatrics, Second Edition*, J.B. Lippincott, 1994.)

Oski's Essential Pediatrics, edited by Kevin B. Johnson and Frank A. Oski. Lippincott–Raven Publishers, Philadelphia © 1997

153

Necrotizing Enterocolitis

Necrotizing enterocolitis is the most common gastrointestinal emergency in the infant. This disorder encompasses several distinct disease entities, which may be characterized according to their clinical presentation and course. The most common form of the disease is idiopathic neonatal necrotizing enterocolitis. Although its etiology is unknown, specific precipitating factors may be implicated in many instances. The clinical manifestations of idiopathic neonatal necrotizing enterocolitis may mimic the symptoms and signs of various neonatal gastrointestinal disorders, and may be indistinguishable from those of sepsis neonatorum. Necrotizing enterocolitis has become the single most common surgical emergency among neonatal intensive care units. Early recognition and aggressive treatment of this disorder during the last 10 years have led to a markedly improved clinical outcome.

■ ETIOLOGY AND PATHOGENESIS

The precise etiology of neonatal necrotizing enterocolitis is unknown, but it probably is caused by multiple factors in a susceptible host. The features most commonly implicated in the pathogenesis of the disease are ischemic insult to the gut, the presence of bacterial or viral organisms in the intestinal tract, the availability of intraluminal substrate (usually formula or human milk) to promote bacterial proliferation or induce mucosal injury, and altered host defense. The first three factors (ischemia, infectious agents, and milk feedings) are thought to be the predisposing variables that initiate the pathogenesis of necrotizing enterocolitis. Other factors, such as inflammatory mediators (cytokines), oxygen radicals, and bacterial fermentation products and toxins, are thought to propagate the disease process. Despite recent advances, the pathogenesis of necrotizing enterocolitis remains an enigma.

■ EPIDEMIOLOGY

The overall incidence of necrotizing enterocolitis is 2.4:1000 live births (range, 0.0:1000 to 7.2:1000) or 2.1% (range, 1.0% to 4.1%) of all admissions to neonatal intensive care units (Table 153–1). The incidence of necrotizing enterocolitis averages 3% to 4% in infants whose birth weight is less than 2000 g, and decreases significantly to 1% in infants whose birth weight is greater than 2000 g. Males and females are affected equally. Black and white infants are affected more commonly than are those of Hispanic origin, but the racial patterns reflect the populations served by individual neonatal centers. Seasonal variation does not affect the incidence of necrotizing enterocolitis. Periodic clusters of cases or epidemics have been reported, however.

■ CLINICAL FEATURES

Nearly three fourths of all infants with necrotizing enterocolitis are born prematurely, with a gestational age of less than 37 weeks and a birth weight of less than 2000 g (Table 153–2). Full-term infants in whom necrotizing enterocolitis develops generally have congenital heart disease, congestive heart failure, or protracted diarrhea of unknown etiology that is complicated by malnutrition. The onset of symptoms occurs within the first 5 days of life in 44% of infants, although symptoms may occur as early as the first day and as late as the fourth week after birth (Table 153–3). Generally, the postnatal age at diagnosis is related inversely to the gestational age.

Significant maternal or perinatal risk factors may be present at the time of diagnosis; many of these factors, however, occur equally in premature infants in whom necrotizing enterocolitis does not develop. Most infants who are seen in the first week of life are recovering from their initial acute illness at the time of onset of this disorder, and many are considered to be "growing" premature infants.

Feedings with either human milk or commercial formulas have been instituted in 98% of infants in whom necrotizing enterocolitis develops. The feedings are tolerated poorly, however, and generate gastric retention, the earliest presenting symptom of the disease (Table 153–4). Other gastrointestinal symptoms and signs, including regurgitation, vomiting, abdominal distention, diminished bowel sounds, reducing substances in the stools, and hematochezia (with either guaiac-positive stools or frank blood), follow rapidly. Diarrhea is an infrequent finding. Systemic manifestations of necrotizing enterocolitis, including temperature instability,

TABLE 153-1. Epidemiology of Neonatal Necrotizing Enterocolitis

INCIDENCE	
Cases/1000 live births	2.4
Percentage of NICU admissions	2.1
Percentage of live births	
Birth weight < 1000 g	3.4
Birth weight 1000–2000 g	3.9
Birth weight > 2000 g	1.0
Sex (Male: Female) Ratio	1:1
Racial (White: Black: Hispanic: Other) Ratio	14:18:1:1

TABLE 153-2. Proposed Risk Factors Associated With Necrotizing Enterocolitis

GROUP I: PRETERM INFANTS < 2000 G

Prenatal
Maternal age > 35 y

Maternal infection treated with antibiotics

Premature rupture of membranes > 24 h before delivery

Perinatal
Maternal anesthesia at delivery

Normal Apgar score at 1 min, low at 5 min

Postnatal
Patent ductus arteriosus

Administration of intravenous glucose or total parenteral nutrition before onset of disease

Gavage feeding

Absence of prophylactic oral antibiotics before the onset of disease

Transport to community hospital from regional neonatal intensive care unit

Cocaine exposure

GROUP II: OLDER INFANTS > 2000 G

Perinatal
Polycythemia

Respiratory distress

Hypoglycemia

Postoperative repair of abdominal wall defects and cut lesions

TABLE 153-4. Presenting Symptoms and Signs of Necrotizing Enterocolitis

Finding	Incidence (%)
GASTROINTESTINAL	
Abdominal distention	89
Hematochezia	
Guaiac-positive stools	80
Grossly bloody stools	43
Fecal reducing substances (3+, 4+)	71
Gastric residual	73
Vomiting	37
Diarrhea	25
SYSTEMIC	
Lethargy	84
Temperature instability	81
Apnea	66
Respiratory failure	40
Hypotension	37

lethargy, apnea, respiratory failure, and hypotension, also may be apparent at the onset of the disease.

Subclinical necrotizing enterocolitis is suspected, but not confirmed, in about 25% of cases, and the symptoms resolve gradually. In 25% to 40% of cases, there is fulminant progression of the disease, with evidence of perforation and peritonitis that is characterized by abdominal tenderness on palpation, a feeling of fullness or a mass (particularly in the right lower quadrant), and erythema, ecchymosis, or necrosis of the abdominal wall. Lethargy, severe acidosis, sepsis, disseminated intravascular coagulation (DIC), and shock may supervene rapidly.

Premorbid risk factors associated with death from necrotizing enterocolitis have been proposed. Poor prognostic factors include premature rupture of membranes, low Apgar scores at 5 minutes, a prolonged oxygen requirement at birth, abdominal distention, portal vein gas on radi-

TABLE 153-3. Clinical Features of Necrotizing Enterocolitis: Age at Diagnosis

Gestational Age (wk)	Age at Diagnosis* (d)	Postnatal Age at Diagnosis (d)	Frequency (%)
26–30	20 ± 4	0–1	5
31–33	14 ± 2	1–3	18
34–37	5 ± 1	3–5	21
		6–12	23
		>12	23

*Mean ± SEM.

ographic studies, *Klebsiella* septicemia, blood transfusion, and surgical intervention.

■ LABORATORY AND RADIOGRAPHIC STUDIES

Laboratory studies of infants with necrotizing enterocolitis may demonstrate a decreased platelet count, increased prothrombin and partial thromboplastin times, and serum factor V concentrations of less than 40%, all of which are consistent with the diagnosis of DIC. Platelet counts of less than 50,000/mm^3 have been found in 38% of infants with necrotizing enterocolitis and may lead to significant bleeding complications, such as intracranial hemorrhage. A serial decrease in platelets to levels less than 100,000/mm^3 is thought to correlate closely with gangrenous bowel and impending perforation. A complete blood count and differential are of little assistance in the diagnosis of necrotizing enterocolitis, but an absolute neutrophil count of less than 1500/mm^3 is associated with a poor prognosis.

The presence of 3+ or 4+ reducing substances, α_1-antitrypsin, or blood in the stool may be an early, but nonspecific, presenting sign of necrotizing enterocolitis. Similarly, levels of C-reactive protein, α_1-acid glycoprotein (orosomucoid), lysosomal acid hydrolase, and urinary D-lactate, a metabolite of carbohydrate fermentation produced by enteric microflora, are increased in infants with this disease and may serve as useful markers to discriminate between necrotizing enterocolitis and other intestinal insults. Elevated breath hydrogen levels may be useful to detect the onset of necrotizing enterocolitis 24 hours before symptoms appear in a premature infant who is at risk for the development of this disorder.

Blood cultures may show bacterial growth in one third of all specimens obtained. Cerebrospinal fluid (CSF) cultures may be warranted if sepsis or meningitis is suspected. Stool cultures generally show the presence of normal enteric flora. Additional cultures for *Clostridium difficile* and assays for its toxins may be indicated, however, when the history and physical findings support the clinical impression. When abdominal paracentesis is performed in infants with sus-

TABLE 153-5. Presenting Radiographic Features of Necrotizing Enterocolitis

Finding	Incidence (%)
Pneumatosis intestinalis	91
Dilatation of bowel loops	83
Persistent "fixed loop"	33
Peritoneal fluid (ascites)	29
Portal venous gas	23
Pneumoperitoneum	17

pected peritonitis, Gram's stain and culture of the peritoneal fluid demonstrate enteric organisms in one third of the cases. Usually, these organisms are the same as those recovered from blood culture.

Radiographic features characteristic of necrotizing enterocolitis may be seen in 87% of patients before a definitive diagnosis is made (Table 153–5). An abdominal film in the supine, decubitus, or upright position may show the presence of pneumatosis intestinalis, edema of the bowel wall, dilatation of loops of bowel, ascites, portal vein gas, or free air in the peritoneum. Serial films may reveal the presence of fixed loops of bowel, which is an ominous feature suggesting the presence of intestinal perforation.

The diagnosis of necrotizing enterocolitis is confirmed when the following triad of clinical features is present: abdominal distention, hematochezia, and pneumatosis intestinalis. Pneumatosis intestinalis may not be identified, however, in nearly 15% of surgically or autopsy-confirmed cases. Similarly, portal vein gas, once thought to be a poor prognostic feature of necrotizing enterocolitis, may be a transient finding on radiographic examination. Newer radionuclide scanning techniques that use technetium 99m diphosphonate may facilitate earlier detection of this disorder.

■ DIFFERENTIAL DIAGNOSIS

The differential diagnosis of necrotizing enterocolitis includes anal fissures, pneumatosis coli, infectious enterocolitis, neonatal appendicitis, intestinal obstruction, spontaneous perforation, and Hirschsprung's disease (Table 153–6).

TABLE 153-6. Differential Diagnosis of Necrotizing Enterocolitis

ANAL FISSURES

PNEUMATOSIS COLI

INFECTIOUS ENTEROCOLITIS

Salmonella, Shigella, Campylobacter

Pseudomembranous colitis (Clostridium)

NEONATAL APPENDICITIS

SPONTANEOUS PERFORATION

INTESTINAL OBSTRUCTION

Congenital (intussusception, meconium ileus, ileal atresia, volvulus)

Acquired (milk curds)

HIRSCHSPRUNG'S DISEASE

■ TREATMENT

The treatment of infants with necrotizing enterocolitis is based on a method of clinical staging at the time of diagnosis (Table 153–7). Infants classified as having stage I or II disease require appropriate diagnostic studies and vigorous medical therapy, whereas those categorized as having stage III disease require surgical intervention.

The medical treatment of necrotizing enterocolitis primarily is supportive. When the diagnosis is suspected, oral feedings should be withheld and nasogastric suction and intravenous fluid should be instituted. Initial laboratory studies should include a complete blood count and differential, a platelet count, prothrombin and partial thromboplastin time determinations, serum electrolyte measurements, and blood urea nitrogen, creatinine, and acid–base studies. Routine cultures of the blood, urine, stool, and CSF should be obtained. Additional stool specimens should be sent for viral and fungal studies when appropriate. The stools should be checked routinely for pH, glucose, occult blood, and α_1-antitrypsin. Total parenteral nutrition should be provided to maintain the nutritional status of the infant. Parenteral antibiotics that cover a broad spectrum of aerobic and anaerobic organisms should be administered for 10 to 14 days. Although the choice of antibiotic therapy will depend on the resistance patterns of individual institutions, the antibiotics recommended include ampicillin, aminoglycosides (eg, gentamicin and amikacin), clindamycin, and the newer cephalosporins (eg, cefotaxime). Although the administration of topical antibiotics such as gentamicin and colistin diminishes the bacterial flora of the gut, this therapy is not recommended in the treatment of necrotizing enterocolitis because of the development of resistant bacterial strains of significant virulence and the equivocal outcome of morbidity and mortality.

Serial abdominal films of the infant in the supine and decubitus positions are recommended every 6 to 8 hours as needed, and serve as the best guide in following the course of the disease. If there is no further progression of illness and the pneumatosis resolves, nasogastric suction may be discontinued. Oral feedings may be resumed gradually within 7 to 14 days after the acute illness.

Surgical intervention is necessary when the disease progresses clinically or when the complications of necrotizing enterocolitis become apparent (Table 153–8). The indications for surgery include rapid clinical deterioration manifested by thermal instability, bradycardia, persistent metabolic acidosis, progressive hyponatremia, and thrombocytopenia; intestinal perforation manifested by pneumoperitoneum on abdominal flat plate; a palpable abdominal mass; intestinal obstruction; or peritonitis manifested as abdominal tenderness and rigidity, erythematous discoloration of the abdominal wall, or the radiographic appearance of a fixed and unchanging collection of intraluminal gas, usually in the right lower quadrant. Abdominal paracentesis and lavage have been recommended to identify infants with intestinal gangrene and impending perforation. The presence of brown, fecal-stained peritoneal fluid that contains bacteria on Gram's stain suggests intestinal gangrene and may be an indication for early operative intervention.

Preventive measures have been advocated to reduce the frequency or minimize the severity of necrotizing enterocolitis. These recommendations include delaying oral feedings for 1 week in low-birth-weight infants with a history of perinatal asphyxia; avoiding hypertonic formulas, medications, and diagnostic agents in sick newborn infants; performing a phlebotomy and exchange transfusion with plasma when polycythemia becomes critical (hematocrit greater than

TABLE 153-7. Staging Criteria for the Treatment of Necrotizing Enterocolitis

Stage	Systemic	Intestinal	Radiologic	Treatment
I. Suspect	Lethargy, temperature instability, apnea, bradycardia	Gastric residual, emesis, abdominal distention, hematochezia	Ileus, intestinal dilatation	Parenteral nutrition, nasogastric suction, antibiotics
II. Definite—same features as stage I plus:				
A. Mildly ill	—	Absent bowel sounds	Pneumatosis intestinalis	—
B. Moderately ill	Metabolic acidosis, thrombocytopenia	Abdominal tenderness	Portal vein gas	$NaHCO_3$
III. Advanced—same features as stage II plus:				
A. Shock	Respiratory arrest, hypotension, disseminated intravascular coagulation, combined respiratory metabolic acidosis	Peritonitis	Ascites	Intravenous fluids, isotropic agents, paracentesis
B. Bowel perforation	—	—	Pneumoperitoneum	Surgery

70%); placement of arterial umbilical catheters in the aorta distal to the renal arteries; and avoidance of placement of venous umbilical catheters in the portal vein. More recent studies suggest that the administration of oral immunoglobulin (IgA-IgG) preparations may prevent the development of necrotizing enterocolitis in premature infants at risk for this disorder. Further studies that document the benefit of prophylactic immunoglobulin therapy are warranted.

■ COMPLICATIONS

The complications of necrotizing enterocolitis may occur early or late in the course of the disease, and vary in the frequency of their appearance. The acute complications include sepsis (60%), peritonitis (20% to 30%), meningitis, abscess formation, thrombocytopenia, DIC, and intestinal or extraintestinal bleeding. Antibiotic therapy provides coverage for the treatment of the infectious complications of necrotizing enterocolitis. Fresh-frozen plasma, platelet concentrates, or an exchange transfusion may be necessary for the hematologic complications. Shock, hypotension, respiratory arrest, hypoglycemia, and metabolic acidosis require aggressive resuscitative efforts in the early stages of advanced disease.

The late complications of necrotizing enterocolitis include stenosis, stricture formation, intestinal atresia, pericolic abscess, enterocele, enterocolic fistula, and short-gut syndrome. Intestinal stenoses and strictures are the most common complications of necrotizing enterocolitis, occurring in 11% to 36% of infants treated medically, and less frequently in those treated surgically. The interval during which a stricture may develop ranges from 1 to 20 months; the average abnormality is detectable by 2 months after the acute episode. About 80% of strictures occur in the colon, predominantly on the left side, but strictures also may be seen in the terminal ileum and jejunum. Multiple strictures may be seen in individual patients. Birth weight, gestational age, disease severity, or the presence of pneumatosis intestinalis does not correlate with the likelihood of stenosis or stricture developing after an episode of necrotizing enterocolitis. Barium enema studies should be considered about 4 weeks after the acute episode of necrotizing enterocolitis, to avoid significant delays in the diagnosis of strictures. About 60% of infants have asymptomatic stenoses, of which half may progress to overt symptoms. However, about 20% resolve spontaneously.

Significant malabsorption may occur postoperatively in about 8% of patients with necrotizing enterocolitis because the amount of small bowel remaining after surgery is insufficient. Prolonged parenteral or enteral nutrition may be required for survival. Vitamin B_{12} malabsorption without megaloblastic anemia has been described in children after ileocecal valve and terminal ileal resection has been performed for neonatal necrotizing enterocolitis. Prolonged vitamin B_{12} therapy may be necessary in these circumstances.

■ PROGNOSIS

The prognosis for necrotizing enterocolitis has improved considerably in the last 10 years as a result of advances in the care of the critically ill infant, earlier diagnosis and treatment, and the institution of a standard aggressive approach in the

TABLE 153-8. Indications for Surgery in Necrotizing Enterocolitis

Clinical deterioration
Peritonitis
Perforation
Abdominal mass
Obstruction

TABLE 153-9. Survival Rates of Infants With Necrotizing Enterocolitis

Birth Weight (g)	Survival Rate (%)
<1000	43
1000–1500	67
1500–2000	82
2000–2500	44
>2500	80

treatment of this disorder. The overall survival rate is 70% to 80%. When classified on the basis of medical or surgical management, the survival rates are 71% and 65%, respectively. The prognosis is affected adversely by the degree of prematurity (Table 153–9) and the persistence of respiratory problems requiring ventilatory support. Late-onset necrotizing enterocolitis has a better prognosis than does the early onset form.

About 50% of the survivors of necrotizing enterocolitis become normal, healthy children. Fifteen percent have neurologic impairment. Neurologic morbidity probably is not related to the occurrence of necrotizing enterocolitis, however, but rather is part of the spectrum of complications associated with prematurity and asphyxia. Late gastrointestinal morbidity is seen in about 10% of infants with necrotizing enterocolitis. Long-term follow-up (1 to 10 years) of these infants demonstrates that, in the absence of major intestinal resection (less than 25%), complete recovery of gastrointestinal function is expected. A small number of children with extensive resection may have the persistence of loose stools or increased frequency of bowel movements, however, as a result of lactose intolerance or the short-gut syndrome.

(Abridged from Kathleen J. Motil, Necrotizing Enterocolitis, in Oski, DeAngelis, Feigin, McMillan, Warshaw: *Principles and Practice of Pediatrics, Second Edition*, J.B. Lippincott, 1994.)

Oski's Essential Pediatrics,
edited by Kevin B. Johnson and Frank A. Oski.
Lippincott–Raven Publishers,
Philadelphia © 1997

154

Functional Constipation

Constipation is a common complaint in children and is one of the problems most frequently referred to the pediatric gastroenterologist. Because stool habits are a major concern of many parents, the physician or health care worker should become familiar with both normal and abnormal patterns of defecation to advise parents properly.

Constipation refers to both the frequency of defecation and the consistency of the stool. Both of these parameters change with age and diet, enhancing concern among parents who compulsively monitor their children's stool habits. The normal infant tends to pass a stool after each feeding, but this varies considerably. Breast-fed infants and those fed elemental diets have less frequent stools than infants fed conventional formulas. Children older than 6 months of age tend to pass a stool at least once a day. Less frequent stools should be of concern if they are hard, dry, unusually large, or difficult to pass.

Many general causes exist for constipation. It is often a familial complaint, and the parents of constipated children often report being constipated when they were children. This implies a genetic component to constipation and may be the result of an increased efficiency of water extraction from fecal material due to either a congenitally long or hypomotile large bowel. Diet plays a role in the volume and hard-

ness of fecal material throughout life. Some dietary residue such as plant fiber tends to make stools soft, whereas other residue, such as the calcium salts in cow's milk, tends to make stools firm. Elemental and chemically defined diets decrease dietary residue and thus decrease stool frequency.

Hospitalized children may become constipated due to a decreased stimulus for defecation resulting from inactivity. Diseases associated with fever may result in acute constipation. Some chronic diseases, such as hypothyroidism, are associated with constipation. The differential diagnosis of constipation is discussed below.

■ PATHOPHYSIOLOGY

For defecation to proceed, a normal rectum and puborectalis muscle, normal internal and external anal sphincters, and normal innervation of these structures through both the autonomic and somatic nervous systems must be present. The rectum functions not as a storage area for fecal material but rather as a sensing organ that initiates the process of defecation. When stool moves into the rectum from the sigmoid colon, pressure is put on the wall and the rectal valves. This pressure initiates an impulse within the intrinsic nervous system of the rectum, resulting in relaxation of the internal anal sphincter, which is experienced as the urgency felt just before defecation. If it is inconvenient to defecate, contraction of the external sphincter is initiated first by reflex and then intentionally. The external sphincter is assisted by contraction of the puborectalis muscle, which helps constrict the anal canal. If the external sphincter is held contracted long enough, the reflex to the internal sphincter wanes and the urge to defecate disappears. When it is convenient to defecate, the external sphincter is consciously relaxed and stool is propelled by colonic peristalsis through the open anal canal. As stool enters the anal canal, a secondary reflex is initiated via the somatic nervous system that results in contraction of the abdominal musculature and assists in emptying the lower colon.

Children who develop functional constipation associate discomfort with defecation. The most common reason for discomfort is an anal fissure resulting from either hard stool or the use of suppositories, enemas, or a rectal thermometer. Occasionally, the sense of discomfort results from a bad toilet-training experience. Whatever the cause, the result is the same. Whenever the child feels the sensation associated with relaxation of the internal anal sphincter, he or she aggressively contracts the external sphincter to prevent expulsion of stool and the pain it is expected to bring. Stool collects in the rectum, and, over a period of months, the rectum gradually dilates. As it enlarges, it becomes less capable of propulsive peristaltic activity, resulting in more stool retention. As the rectal volume increases, its sensory capacity diminishes, making retention easier. Eventually, the constipation becomes self-perpetuating.

■ CLINICAL FINDINGS

The most common symptom associated with constipation is chronic recurrent abdominal pain, which occurs in about 60% of the patients. The pains are intermittent and localized to the periumbilical region and resemble functional abdominal pain.

Stools of very large caliber are another associated symptom. Parents often must break up stools mechanically to flush the toilet. The size of the stool is a function of the size of the colon.

Poor appetite and poor growth are occasionally seen in association with constipation. This may be a consequence of early satiety due to the sensation of fullness of the colon. Parents frequently describe their constipated children as lethargic.

■ DIAGNOSIS

The diagnosis of functional constipation is made from the history and physical examination. Stool is often palpable in the abdomen, particularly in the left lower quadrant. Rectal examination reveals a short anal canal associated with a large dilated rectum, full of stool. The external sphincter is intact, and the child can squeeze the examiner's finger. The anus should be properly positioned about midway between the scrotum and tip of the coccyx in males and about one third the distance from the vaginal fourchette in females. It should also be centered within the perianal skin pigmentation.

If a barium enema is done, no bowel preparation should be used so that the large rectum dilated with stool can be appreciated. Dilatation of the rectum to the anal verge is diagnostic of functional constipation and rules out Hirschsprung's disease.

Rectal manometry can be helpful in distinguishing functional constipation from Hirschsprung's disease and sacral nerve abnormalities. Functional constipation is associated with normal relaxation of the internal anal sphincter and no contraction of the external anal sphincter in response to considerable distention of the rectal ampulla. Normal contraction of the external anal sphincter should be elicited by stimulation of the perianal skin to rule out the possibility of abnormalities of sensory input.

■ DIFFERENTIAL DIAGNOSIS

Functional constipation must be differentiated from Hirschsprung's disease, anterior displacement of the anus, and sacral nerve abnormalities (usually associated with spina bifida occulta). Other causes of constipation are listed in Table 154–1.

■ TREATMENT

Simple constipation in the neonate is best treated with a nonabsorbable carbohydrate such as that present in dark corn syrup or Maltsupex. In the treatment of older children and adolescents with simple constipation, stool softeners such as Colace or bulk agents are suggested.

In children with longstanding functional constipation associated with a megarectum, a laxative program is required. Treatment is initiated by emptying the rectal vault with an enema. A large-volume enema preparation such as soapsuds is usually more effective than a small-volume enema such as phospho-soda (Fleet enema). If stool in the rectal vault is firm, a preliminary mineral-oil enema will act as a softener and lubricant.

Once the rectum has been cleared of stool, a program of daily laxatives should be initiated to prevent reaccumulation of fecal material and to allow the rectum to return to normal size. Laxatives should be taken only once a day, preferably in the morning so that the day's activity can enhance the effect. The preferred laxative is concentrated, flavored milk of magnesia. The dose is titrated up or down, depending on the daily response. If a bowel movement did not occur in the previous 24 hours, the dose is increased; if diarrhea occurred in the previous 24 hours, the dose is decreased. Adjustments are

made daily until a dose is found that stimulates one or two normal bowel movements per day. It may take 3 to 4 weeks to establish the proper dose of laxative. Other laxatives shown to be effective include senna, given along with mineral oil and lactulose. Whatever laxative is used, the parents should be given the necessary instructions on how to manage the dose themselves.

TABLE 154-1. Causes of Constipation

FUNCTIONAL CONSTIPATION AND ENCOPRESIS

DIETARY CAUSES
Protracted vomiting
Excessive intake of cow's milk
Lack of bulk in diet

DRUGS THAT AFFECT MOTILITY

STRUCTURAL DEFECTS OF THE ANUS OR RECTUM
Anterior displacement of the anus
Anal or rectal stenosis
Presacral teratoma
Rectal prolapse

SMOOTH MUSCLE DISEASE
Scleroderma
Dermatomyositis
Systemic lupus erythematosus
Primary chronic intestinal pseudo-obstruction

ABNORMAL MYENTERIC GANGLION CELLS
Hirschsprung's disease
Chagas' disease
von Recklinghausen disease
Multiple endocrine neoplasia type 2B

ABSENCE OF ABDOMINAL MUSCULATURE
SPINAL CORD DEFECTS
Spina bifida occulta
Myelomeningocele
Meningocele
Diastematomyelia
Paraplegia
Cauda equina tumor
"Tethered cord" syndrome

METABOLIC AND ENDOCRINE DISORDERS
Hypothyroidism
Hypoparathyroidism
Renal tubular acidosis
Diabetes insipidus
Vitamin D intoxication
Idiopathic hypercalcemia
Hypokalemia

NEUROLOGIC AND PSYCHIATRIC CONDITIONS
Myotonic dystrophy
Amyotonia congenita
Mental retardation
Psychosis

Patients should be reexamined at 1- to 2-month intervals, and a rectal examination should be done to determine rectal vault size. Laxatives can be tapered when the rectal vault returns to normal size, which may take 6 months to 1 year. At that time, parents and children should be instructed about proper diet and the use of bulk agents to avoid hard stools. During laxative therapy, attempts should be made to establish a bowel habit. Once the parent determines when the laxative begins to stimulate, the child should be asked to sit on the toilet at that approximate time each day. This behavior should continue after the laxative has been discontinued.

(Abridged from William J. Klish, Functional Constipation, in Oski, DeAngelis, Feigin, McMillan, Warshaw: *Principles and Practice of Pediatrics, Second Edition,* J.B. Lippincott, 1994.)

Oski's Essential Pediatrics,
edited by Kevin B. Johnson and Frank A. Oski.
Lippincott–Raven Publishers,
Philadelphia © 1997

155

Chronic Nonspecific Diarrhea of Childhood

Chronic nonspecific diarrhea of childhood (also called protracted diarrhea or irritable bowel syndrome) is a common and often frustrating problem seen in children between 6 and 36 months of age. It is characterized by a pattern of two or more loose, voluminous stools per day lasting for more than 4 weeks, unassociated with other symptoms such as pain or growth failure. Children with this syndrome usually are not bothered by the diarrhea. Their parents, however, have difficulty dealing with this symptom because most of the affected children are still in diapers and the stool volume is so great that it spills from the diapers, making a mess.

■ ETIOLOGY

Although chronic nonspecific diarrhea of childhood is the most common form of chronic diarrhea without failure to thrive in young children, the etiology remains unknown. Because malabsorption of nutrients is not a factor in this disease, the cause of the diarrhea is either enhanced secretion of fluid in the distal bowel or interference with absorption of water and electrolytes from the colon. Chronic nonspecific diarrhea is frequently initiated by an acute infection that is usually treated with a broad-spectrum antibiotic such as ampicillin, so alteration of bacterial flora in the colon may play a role in the etiology of the diarrhea.

Some investigators have thought that the diarrhea might be induced by the increased intake of fluids observed in these children. However, the increased thirst is more likely to be the effect rather than the cause of the diarrhea. Some children drink large amounts of fruit juice, such as apple juice. This undoubtedly plays some role in the perpetuation of the diarrhea, because apple juice contains enough nonabsorbable carbohydrate such as sorbitol to induce colonic fermentation, resulting in the stimulus for diarrhea, as seen in other forms of carbohydrate intolerance.

A low dietary fat intake has been hypothesized to play a role in the persistence of the diarrhea, but this observation has not held up under scrutiny. However, because many of these children eventually are placed on strict elimination diets, dietary restriction of fiber and other residue may help perpetuate the loose stools.

One group of investigators has suggested that disordered small intestine motility plays a role in the etiology of chronic nonspecific diarrhea of childhood. They showed that the migrating motor complex of the duodenum was not suppressed as it normally should be with the introduction of glucose into the bowel. This implies that children with this disorder have relative hypermotility of the intestine during meals.

■ DIFFERENTIAL DIAGNOSIS

The diagnosis of chronic nonspecific diarrhea of childhood should be suspected if the following criteria are met: child's age between 6 and 36 months; two or more loose, voluminous stools per day, frequently containing undigested food particles; diarrhea lasting for more than 4 weeks; absence of abdominal pain; absence of failure to thrive; and absence of a definable cause for the chronic diarrhea.

Disaccharide intolerance, infection, protein hypersensitivity, and occasionally inflammatory bowel disease can mimic chronic nonspecific diarrhea in presenting symptoms. Carbohydrate intolerance can be diagnosed by placing the patient on a totally unrestricted diet with milk and testing several stools for the presence of sugar or acid. Unabsorbed disaccharide (lactose or sucrose) will appear in the stool either unchanged or partially fermented to the monosaccharides, including glucose. Their presence can be determined through the use of Clinitest tablets or glucose test tape. Completely fermented sugars result in the production of organic acids such as acetic and butyric acids. Their presence can be found by testing the stool pH with nitrazine paper. A pH of less than 5.5 is considered suggestive of carbohydrate intolerance.

Stools should be cultured for bacteria. Most pathogenic bacteria cannot produce diarrhea for longer than several weeks. However, *Campylobacter jejuni* has been implicated in several cases of chronic diarrhea and must be ruled out. The presenting symptoms of *Giardia lamblia* infection can be identical to those of chronic nonspecific diarrhea, and this infection must also be ruled out.

A complete blood count with differential, reticulocyte count, and a stool guaiac test might give a clue to the presence of either protein hypersensitivity or inflammatory bowel disease. Eosinophilia is occasionally present in protein hypersensitivity. If this diagnosis is suspected, a carefully constructed elimination diet should be initiated, making certain that the child receives adequate intake to thrive.

■ TREATMENT

Before initiating treatment, it is important to stress that, although the diarrhea is hard for the parents to deal with, it does not threaten the child's well-being. Treatment fails in 10% to 20% of children regardless of the form of therapy. The syndrome improves with age, and most children have outgrown it by age 3 years.

Therapy should be initiated by placing the child on a normal diet for his or her age. If the diet has been restricted, many children will normalize their stool pattern due to an increase in dietary residue. If large amounts of fruit juices are being given, attempts should be made to substitute other liquids.

Psyllium bulk agents are very effective at minimizing the diarrhea. It can be mixed with other foods for palatability. If a good response is obtained, the psyllium can usually be discontinued without return of the diarrhea. Cholestyramine has been used successfully to treat this syndrome. Because there is some potential for side effects from cholestyramine, this should not be tried until after psyllium therapy fails. Occasional children will respond to a 7- to 10-day course of metronidazole.

(Abridged from William J. Klish, Chronic Nonspecific Diarrhea of Childhood, in Oski, DeAngelis, Feigin, McMillan, Warshaw: *Principles and Practice of Pediatrics, Second Edition*, J.B. Lippincott, 1994.)

Oski's Essential Pediatrics, edited by Kevin B. Johnson and Frank A. Oski. Lippincott–Raven Publishers, Philadelphia © 1997

156

Gastrointestinal Bleeding

Gastrointestinal (GI) bleeding in children is common, and occasionally it is life-threatening. This chapter outlines an approach to managing a child who may have bled.

■ ESTABLISHING BLOOD LOSS

It must first be determined if blood loss has occurred. Many substances ingested by children may be mistaken for blood. Red food coloring, fruit-flavored drinks, fruit juices, and beets may color the vomitus or stool reddish. Stools can acquire a black color from ingested iron, bismuth subsalicylate, grape juice, spinach, and blueberries. The vomitus is tested by Gastroccult (*p*H-buffered) and the stool by guaiac, Hemoccult, or Hematest for the presence of blood. If a child presents in the office with anemia for which there is no clear explanation, several stools should be tested for occult blood.

■ TYPE OF BLEEDING

A description of the color, location, and amount of blood is usually helpful. Did the child cough up blood (hemoptysis) or vomit up blood (hematemesis) following epistaxis? Gastric acid will turn the blood a brown color. Bright-red blood (hematochezia) or blood streaking in the stool is most often due to polyps, proctitis, or constipation with anal fissures or hemorrhoids. Bright-red blood on the outside of the stool accompanied by pain on passage of the stool is usually from an anal fissure. Bright-red blood mixed with mucus in a loose stool is typical of chronic ulcerative colitis. The classic currant jelly stool occurs from ileocolic intussusception and may occur with midgut volvulus. Melena (black or dark-maroon stool) suggests a lesion proximal to the right colon, such as a Meckel's diverticulum. A bleeding duodenal ulcer may present with red bloody stools instead of melena because of rapid transit through the GI tract.

If the patient enters the emergency department with melena or hematochezia with evidence of anemia or hypotension, gastric contents must be aspirated to look for evidence of upper GI bleeding.

■ ETIOLOGIES

Certain causes of GI bleeding are more common in specific age groups, but there is considerable overlap (Table 156–1). At all ages, stress (burns, central nervous system trauma) and aspirin ingestion may lead to gastric stress erosions and ulcerations. Thrombocytopenia and coagulopathies must be considered. Intestinal bleeding is not uncommon in children with cancer who develop thrombocytopenia secondary to chemotherapy. Chemotherapy may be followed by esophagitis, gastritis, and enterocolitis.

In addition to these age-independent etiologies, children of different ages may have an etiology that is typical of patients in a specific age range.

Neonatal

In the first few days of life, hematemesis or the passage of bloody stools in a healthy newborn is most likely due to swallowed maternal blood, which can be differentiated from fetal hemoglobin by the Apt alkali denaturation test. If the red blood denatures with alkali to a brown color, the hemoglobin is of adult origin.

Hemorrhagic disease of the newborn with prolongation of the prothrombin time must be considered when vitamin K has not been given. Breast-fed infants are particularly susceptible to this complication.

An anal fissure is a common cause of bleeding, usually initiated by the passage of a firm stool that makes a small tear along the anal canal.

Irritation from nasogastric tube feedings is a common cause of small amounts of blood in the gastric aspirate or stool.

The First 6 Months

Nonspecific colitis has recently been shown to be a common cause of hematochezia in infants younger than 6 months old. Gastroesophageal reflux in the infant is very common and may cause reflux esophagitis with blood loss.

Milk- or soy-protein–induced enteropathy is a common cause of blood-streaked stools early in infancy. This may also occur in breast-fed infants, and the mother may be tried on a milk- or soy-free diet.

6 Months to 5 Years

Epistaxis must always be considered as a cause of blood in vomitus. The blood loss from gastroesophageal reflux associated esophagitis may be associated with "coffee grounds" (dark brown) emesis but is generally occult; it may cause chronic anemia.

Intussusception occurs most often during the first 2 years of life and usually presents with brief, frequent spasms of severe abdominal pain. The process may progress to vomiting, lethargy, currant jelly stools, and complete intestinal obstruction. A sausage-shaped mass may be felt in the abdomen. Diagnosis is confirmed by barium enema or ultrasound, and reduction with air, water, or barium under mild pressure is successful in most cases. In patients over age 2, a mass acting as a lead point is often present.

TABLE 156-1. Etiologies of GI Bleeding

NEONATE
Swallowed maternal blood
Hemorrhagic disease of the newborn
Anal fissure
Hemorrhagic gastritis
Stress ulcers
Infection enterocolitis
Protein-sensitive enterocolitis
Hirschsprung's enterocolitis
Duplication cysts
Midgut volvulus
Vascular malformations

FIRST 6 MONTHS OF LIFE
Nonspecific colitis
Anal fissure
Esophagitis
Infective enterocolitis
Protein-sensitive enterocolitis
Intussusception
Lymphonodular hyperplasia
Duplication cysts
Hirschsprung's enterocolitis
Vascular malformations

6 MONTHS TO 5 YEARS
Epistaxis
Esophagitis
Esophageal varices
Gastritis
Infective enterocolitis
C difficile colitis
Lymphonodular hyperplasia
Intussusception
Meckel's diverticulum
Vascular malformations
Henoch-Schönlein purpura
Hemolytic-uremic syndrome
Neutropenic typhlitis
Polyps
Anal fissure

5 TO 18 YEARS
Same as 6 mo–5 yr, plus
Mallor-Weiss tear
Gastritis
Peptic ulcer
Chronic ulcerative colitis
Crohn's disease
Hemorrhoids

Meckel's diverticulum, a remnant of the oomphalome-senteric duct located about 30 cm from the ileocecal valve, is often asymptomatic; however, when it contains gastric mucosa, acid secretion can cause ulceration of the adjacent ileum with subsequent painless bleeding presenting as black or maroon stools and anemia. The diagnosis is made by 99mTc pertechnetate radionuclide scan. Some radiologists use intravenous histamine-2 receptor blockers (H$_2$ blocker) to enhance visualization. Pertechnetate is taken up by epithelial cells of the gastric mucosa. Surgery is indicated for bleeding. A Meckel's diverticulum may act as a lead point for intussusception.

Henoch-Schönlein purpura is a systemic vasculitis in which abdominal cramps and intestinal bleeding may precede the purpuric skin manifestations. Hemolytic-uremic syndrome may follow a variety of infections such as *Escherichia coli* 0157:H7, causing a severe colitis with frequent bloody stools before the onset of uremia and anemia. Neutropenic typhlitis is a necrotizing enterocolitis involving the cecum and right colon in immunosuppressed patients.

Juvenile colonic polyps (inflammatory hamartomas) are the most common cause of intermittent painless hematochezia in children 2 to 5 years old. Most polyps are solitary and located within 30 cm of the anus. The diagnosis is made by digital rectal examination, barium enema, sigmoidoscopy, or colonoscopy. Snare cauterization polypectomy through the colonoscope is appropriate.

5 to 18 Years of Age

Although the following diagnoses may be made before a patient is 5 years old, these diagnoses are more common afterward.

Epistaxis is more common in older children. An episode of forceful vomiting may cause a small linear (Mallory-Weiss) tear at the gastroesophageal junction, with minimal or moderate blood loss. Ingestion of caustic medications may irritate the esophageal mucosa.

The inflammatory bowel diseases—Crohn's disease and chronic ulcerative colitis—are of unknown etiology and are characterized by a remitting–relapsing symptom pattern. In mild stages of Crohn's disease, chronic ulcerative colitis, or ulcerative proctitis, there may be only occult blood or small amounts of visible blood in the stool. Crohn's disease that involves only the small intestine may be accompanied only by occult blood in the stool. The nearer the lesions are to the anus, the more likely it is that hematochezia will occur. Tenesmus is more common in ulcerative colitis, whereas Crohn's disease may present with painless bright-red bleeding. Severe blood loss is more common in ulcerative colitis, but occurs in both. Both usually have other signs and symptoms, including diarrhea, weight loss, fever, abdominal pain, anorexia, malaise, joint pain, and decreased growth. Diagnosis is suspected by history, physical examination, the presence of microcytic anemia, thrombocytosis, elevated erythrocyte sedimentation rate, or hypoalbuminemia, and is confirmed by intestinal radiographs, colonoscopy, and biopsy. Sulfasalazine (or the newer acetylsalicylate derivatives) and corticosteroids are the mainstays of treatment.

Peutz-Jeghers syndrome consists of diffuse GI hamartomas, most marked in the small bowel, associated with melanotic areas on the buccal mucosa and lips. Other chronic polyposes include juvenile polyposis coli, familial adenomatous polyposis, and Gardner's syndrome (familial adenomatous polyposis associated with bony lesions, subcutaneous tumors, and cysts). The latter two conditions have clear malignant potential, and colectomy in late childhood is advised.

Vascular lesions take a variety of forms. Telangiectasias may be associated with Turner's syndrome. Small angiodysplasias, hemangiomas, or arteriovenous malformations may occur, and arteriography may be helpful in diagnosis. Hemorrhoids are relatively uncommon in children, so portal hypertension should be considered. A rare cause of monthly bleeding in an adolescent female is ectopic endometrium in the GI tract.

■ DIAGNOSIS

A careful history and physical examination will be helpful in most cases (Figure 156–1). The child's condition will determine the rapidity of the approach to diagnosis. If the child is pale and weak with tachycardia and hypotension, immediate stabilization of the cardiovascular status is paramount, and history, physical examination, diagnosis, and therapy must be done rapidly.

Important elements of the history include the child's age, amount and character of the bleeding in vomitus or stool, associated abdominal or rectal pain, diarrhea, drug ingestion, fever, systemic symptoms such as joint pain or aphthous ulcerations, growth pattern, recent illnesses, foreign travel, and family history of GI or bleeding disorders.

Important components of the physical examination are general appearance; vital signs; examination of skin for telangiectasias, purpura, or melanotic spots on lips; evidence of epistaxis, abdominal organomegaly, tenderness, or masses; and anorectal examination to verify the presence of blood in the stool and to identify fissures, fistulas, and distal polyps.

If there is upper GI bleeding on gastric aspiration, upper endoscopy is attempted when the gastric aspirate following lavage is almost clear. Small-diameter endoscopes allow examination of infants. If upper GI bleeding has stopped or has been minimal, an upper GI radiologic examination or upper endoscopy may be done. Upper GI bleeding usually is accompanied by melena; however, if the bleeding has been abrupt, the stool guaiac may still be negative. Also, bleeding from a duodenal ulcer may result in red blood in the stools if the transit through the intestinal tract is rapid.

Upper GI bleeding is more likely to be massive than is lower GI bleeding. Massive lower GI bleeding may come from a Meckel's diverticulum, arteriovenous malformation, or intestinal duplication, but occasionally occurs with the inflammatory bowel diseases. Currant jelly stool with abdominal pain and tenderness suggests infarction of the bowel secondary to intussusception. Similar findings may be present secondary to intestinal volvulus or an incarcerated internal hernia, which are also surgical emergencies.

Melena may signify upper or lower GI bleeding. Meckel's diverticulum commonly presents as painless melena in a healthy 18- to 24-month-old child who has a significant decrease in hematocrit. If bleeding is ongoing, visualization through the colonoscope may be hindered by the blood. In these situations, a 99mTc sulfur colloid-labeled red cell scan or angiography may be helpful in identifying a site of bleeding. If these do not identify a lesion, colonoscopy can be attempted following a large-volume cleansing electrolyte lavage. Computed tomography or magnetic resonance imaging scanning is helpful only when the bleeding is from an identifiable mass.

If hematochezia is accompanied by diarrhea, a sigmoidoscopy is helpful in determining friability or visualizing the pseudomembranes associated with *Clostridium difficile* infection. Biopsies may reveal amebae or distinguish between chronic and acute inflammatory changes. Stool cultures for *Shigella, Salmonella, Campylobacter jejuni, Yersinia, E coli* 0157:H7, and *C difficile* toxin should be considered.

Colonoscopy is most helpful in the diagnosis of inflammatory bowel disease, arteriovenous malformations visible through the mucosal surface, lymphonodular hyperplasia, and polyps. Barium enemas are valuable for detecting polyps, inflammatory bowel disease, lymphonodular hyperplasia, Hirschsprung's disease, and colonic duplication, and for the diagnosis and treatment of intussusception.

■ THERAPY

Therapy of a massive GI hemorrhage is aimed at resuscitating the patient, localizing the site of bleeding, and deciding on a treatment plan to stop the hemorrhage. If orthostatic or frank hypotension is present, an intravenous catheter is inserted to obtain blood for laboratory studies and for the infusion of normal saline or colloid until properly typed and crossmatched blood is available. Blood is sent for complete blood count, type and crossmatch, erythrocyte sedimentation rate, platelet count, clotting functions, liver function

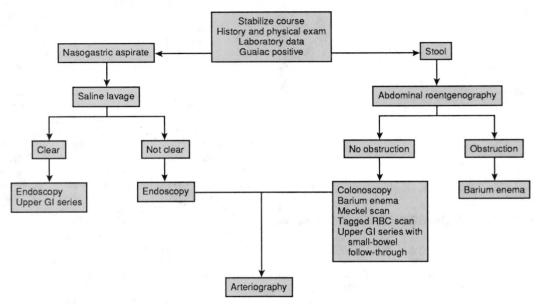

Figure 156-1. Approach to acute GI bleeding.

tests, blood urea nitrogen, and serum electrolytes. A large-bore nasogastric tube is placed into the stomach, and gastric contents are aspirated. An aspirate of red blood or "coffee grounds" material from the stomach indicates bleeding above the ligament of Treitz, although absence of blood does not rule out bleeding just distal to the pylorus. If fresh blood is present, saline lavage is done until bleeding ceases. Abdominal roentgenograms taken in the upright, supine, and cross-table lateral positions are taken to look for signs of obstruction and air outside the GI tract.

Further therapy for severe upper GI bleeding consists of blood replacement and neutralization of gastric acid. An intravenous infusion of an H_2-receptor antagonist such as cimetidine may be used to decrease gastric acidity.

After endoscopy and intravenous administration of an H_2 blocker, antacids and sucralfate may be given through the nasogastric tube to keep the gastric pH above 5 and to coat the irritated mucosal surfaces. If bleeding esophageal varices are seen, or if the bleeding site cannot be identified and bleeding continues, intravenous vasopressin is given.

If bleeding cannot be controlled, sclerotherapy or rubber-banding for varices, endoscopic heater probe (or laser) coagulation of bleeding sites, selective angiography with embolization, or surgery is the next step.

Therapy for mild bleeding depends on the lesions found.

In an intensive care unit, GI bleeding occurs in 5% to 10% of the children. Significant bleeding requiring transfusion occurs most often in children with coagulopathy.

(Abridged from Marilyn R. Brown, Gastrointestinal Bleeding, in Oski, DeAngelis, Feigin, McMillan, Warshaw: *Principles and Practice of Pediatrics, Second Edition,* J.B. Lippincott, 1994.)

Oski's Essential Pediatrics,
edited by Kevin B. Johnson and Frank A. Oski.
Lippincott–Raven Publishers,
Philadelphia © 1997

157

Peptic Ulcer Disease

Peptic ulcer disease (PUD) is an ulcerative condition of the stomach or duodenum that may be acute or chronic. It is classified as primary peptic (idiopathic) ulcer disease when it occurs in otherwise healthy individuals and as secondary (stress) ulcer disease when there are underlying disorders associated with injury, illness, or drug therapy. Most primary peptic ulcers are chronic and more often duodenal in origin; most stress ulcers are acute and more often gastric in location (Table 157–1).

■ EPIDEMIOLOGY

The incidence of PUD in children is unknown (Table 157–2). The prevalence is estimated to be 1.7% in large general pediatric practices and 3.4 per 10,000 pediatric hospital admissions. The male:female ratio is 1.5:1. Primary PUD occurs at any age, but its frequency is higher in older children and adolescents. Primary and stress ulcers occur in a ratio of 7:1 in children more than 6 years old. Secondary stress ulcers are more common in infants less than 6 months

TABLE 157-1. Patterns of PUD and Their Frequency in Children

Clinical Feature	Frequency (%)	
	Primary Peptic Ulcer	Secondary Stress Ulcer
Duration of symptoms		
Acute	17	96
Chronic	83	4
Location of ulcer		
Gastric	16	30
Duodenal	33	21

old and are equal in frequency to primary peptic ulcers in children aged 6 months to 6 years.

■ PREDISPOSING FACTORS

Several entities have been implicated as predisposing factors for PUD in children (Table 157–3).

Drugs and systemic illnesses have been associated with the production of secondary ulcers. Corticosteroid therapy often is complicated by the appearance or reactivation of stress ulcers, presumably due to the inhibition of phospholipase A and prostaglandin synthesis. Similarly, aspirin and nonsteroidal anti-inflammatory agents inhibit prostaglandin synthesis, thereby increasing the risk of ulcer formation. Stress ulcers in children can occur in conjunction with systemic illnesses such as sepsis, hypotension, respiratory distress, extensive burns (Curling's ulcer), and brain injury (Cushing's ulcer). These ulcers may result from a low-flow state (ie, a shunting of blood from the superficial epithelium during stress, leading to a relative hypoxemia and depletion of nutrients necessary for the energetics of cellular metabolism).

A spiral, urease-producing bacterium, *Helicobacter pylori,* has been associated with primary antral gastritis and peptic ulcerations in children. The gastritis is characterized by infiltrates of polymorphonuclear leukocytes in the acute stage, followed by infiltrates of lymphocytes and plasma cells in the chronic stage. *H pylori* is not present in secondary gastritis associated with disorders such as Crohn's disease or eosinophilic gastroenteritis. The organism may be found in ulcers located in the esophagus or duodenum, but only in the presence of gastric metaplasia. *H pylori* is a major predispos-

TABLE 157-2. Epidemiology of Peptic Ulcer Disease in Children

Feature	Occurrence
Incidence	?
Prevalence (%)	1.7
Sex (male:female) ratio	1.5:1
Age distribution (%)	
Birth to 6 mo	14
6 mo to 2 y	8
2 to 5 y	17
5 to 10 y	30
10 to 15 y	31

TABLE 157-3. Factors Predisposing to Peptic Ulcer Disease in Children

PRIMARY PEPTIC ULCER

Genetic factors

Psychological factors

Alcohol

Caffeine

Cigarette smoking

Helicobacter pylori

SECONDARY STRESS ULCER

Drugs (corticosteroids, aspirin, nonsteroidal agents)

Complications of systemic illness (sepsis, hypotension, respiratory distress)

Injury (burns, brain injuries)

TABLE 157-4. Presenting Features of Peptic Ulcer Disease in Children

Clinical Features	Frequency (%)
SYMPTOM	
Abdominal pain	71
Epigastric	57
Periumbilical	32
"Typical"	9
Nausea	25
Vomiting	18
Hematemesis	18
Melena	13
Anorexia	17
Headache	11
Failure to thrive	3
SIGN	
Abdominal tenderness	58
GI bleeding	53
Acute abdomen	22
Perforation	18
Obstruction	7
Anemia	11

ing factor to PUD, but infection alone is insufficient to cause ulcer formation. Little is known about the source and spread of *H pylori,* but transmission from infected family contacts has been suggested. The eradication of *H pylori* results in a rapid resolution of the acute inflammatory component of the gastritis, but the chronic inflammatory component may persist for as long as 1 year. The eradication of the organism also is associated with a pronounced reduction in the relapse rate of duodenal ulcers. Ulcer relapse is associated with either reinfection or recrudescence of *H pylori* infection.

■ CLINICAL FEATURES

The clinical picture of PUD in children is variable and depends on the classification of the ulcer and the patient's age. Abdominal pain, generally localized to the epigastric or periumbilical area, is the most common presenting symptom (Table 157–4). Typical ulcer pain that worsens with fasting, is relieved with meals, and wakens the patient at night is uncommon in children. Nausea, vomiting, and anorexia occur in 25% or less of the children with ulcer disease, and hematemesis and melena occur in less than 20%. Frontal headaches are present in about 10% of children. Failure to thrive is rarely associated with PUD.

Abdominal tenderness and overt gastrointestinal (GI) bleeding are found on physical examination in at least half the children with PUD. An acute abdomen with features of abdominal distention, decreased bowel sounds, and peritoneal irritation, consistent with the diagnosis of intestinal perforation or obstruction, occurs in nearly one fourth of children at presentation.

In general, infants and children less than 6 years old are more likely to have an acute secondary ulcer in conjunction with illness, surgery, or trauma; older children and adolescents tend to display features of primary PUD. The features of primary PUD generally are chronic symptoms of abdominal pain and vomiting, whereas secondary ulcers are more frequently associated with acute GI bleeding and vomiting.

■ LABORATORY AND RADIOLOGIC STUDIES

Laboratory studies in PUD generally are normal unless overt or occult bleeding is a prominent feature. About 10% of children with PUD have an iron-deficiency anemia. Hemoglobin, hematocrit, serum iron, and ferritin levels may be low, whereas the reticulocyte count and total iron-binding capacity may be elevated with chronic blood loss. Red blood cell smears may show hypochromic, microcytic morphology, and stool smears may be positive for occult blood.

An upper GI series is the most readily available test for the diagnosis of PUD in children. Roentgenographic signs of PUD in the duodenum are characterized by a filling defect or a deformity of the duodenal bulb. In some instances, duodenal irritability may be the only finding because the barium moves too rapidly out of the bulb or a fibrin clot covers the ulcer. Ulcer craters also may be found in the pyloric region, leading to outlet obstruction. The diagnosis of PUD should not be made unless a persistent crater is demonstrated. Deformity of the duodenal bulb with scar formation suggests the presence of a previous ulcer and does not imply the presence of currently active disease.

Primary gastric ulcers usually are located on the lesser curvature of the stomach. The crater is sharply delimited and surrounded by edematous, radiating gastric folds that may obstruct the pyloric channel. In contrast, stress ulcer craters are shallow and often multiple, and may be present in both the stomach and duodenum.

Overall, upper GI series detect PUD in 70% of the children who are studied. The frequency of detection for duodenal ulcer, however, is 89%, compared with 50% for gastric ulcers. Air contrast imaging may enhance the features of primary and secondary PUD and lead to more accurate diagnosis.

Endoscopy

Fiberoptic endoscopy has become the diagnostic procedure of choice for the detection of PUD in children. Gastroesophagoduodenoscopy is indicated to determine the source of upper GI bleeding and to make the initial diagnosis of PUD, or when roentgenographic findings are absent in symptomatic patients. Endoscopy confirms the diagnosis of PUD in 97% of the patients examined for this purpose. Detection of *H pylori* requires cultures, measurement of urease activity (CLO test, Delta West, Australia), or Warthin-Starry silver stains of the antral biopsy tissue specimens.

■ DIFFERENTIAL DIAGNOSIS

The diagnosis of PUD in children may be difficult to make because the symptoms often mimic those of other diseases. Indeed, errors in diagnosis may be as high as 12%; the most common incorrect diagnoses are appendicitis and Meckel's diverticulum. The principal conditions to consider in the differential diagnosis are gastroduodenitis, Zollinger-Ellison syndrome, chronic recurrent (functional) abdominal pain, gastroesophageal reflux, esophagitis, pancreatitis, cholelithiasis, appendicitis, Meckel's diverticulum, intussusception, inflammatory bowel disease, and infectious diarrhea (Table 157–5). The symptoms of abdominal pain, vomiting, and rectal bleeding may be common to all of these entities and lead to a significant diagnostic dilemma. Therefore, the diagnosis of PUD depends primarily on the physician's awareness and should be considered early in the differential diagnosis of abdominal pain.

■ TREATMENT

The goal of medical therapy in PUD is to promote ulcer healing, relieve pain, and prevent complications. The control of gastric acid production by drugs, diet, and the avoidance of factors that stimulate acid secretion is essential (Table 157–6).

The mainstay of medical management includes antacids (Maalox II, Mylanta II) and H$_2$-receptor antagonists (cimetidine, ranitidine, famotidine). Antacids promote the healing of ulcers and provide relief of symptoms by neutralizing gastric acid. In the presence of stress ulcers, acute bleeding can be controlled by a nasogastric drip of antacids. The side effects of antacid therapy—diarrhea and constipation—can be ameliorated by adjusting the proportion of magnesium and aluminum in the dosing regimen. Calcium antacids and sodium bicarbonate are considered unsuitable for chronic use because of the potential for increased acid secretion after buffering capacity ceases or systemic alkaline and sodium loading, respectively.

H$_2$-receptor antagonists are potent inhibitors of basal and food-stimulated acid production. Their use is associated with a healing rate of 90% in children with PUD. H$_2$-receptor antagonist therapy may be a useful nighttime adjunct to antacid therapy if night pain occurs. In the presence of complications of PUD, cimetidine or ranitidine may be given intravenously to minimize acid production. H$_2$-receptor therapy also is effective in the prophylaxis of GI bleeding after critical illness, brain injury, or surgery. Side effects asso-

TABLE 157-5. Differential Diagnosis of Peptic Ulcer Disease

Gastroduodenitis	Cholelithiasis
Zollinger-Ellison syndrome	Appendicitis
Chronic recurrent abdominal pain	Meckel's diverticulum
Gastroesophageal reflux	Intussusception
Esophagitis	Infectious diarrhea
Pancreatitis	Inflammatory bowel disease

TABLE 157-6. Treatment of Peptic Ulcer Disease in Children

MEDICAL

Hospitalization

Nasogastric suction and lavage

Blood transfusion

Medications (antacids, H$_2$-receptor antagonists, anticholinergics)

Diet (avoid snacks)

Abstinence (cigarette smoking, alcohol, aspirin)

SURGICAL

Truncal or selective vagotomy

Pyloroplasty

Antrectomy

ciated with these drugs are uncommon; rebound hypersecretion of hydrochloric acid may occur after discontinuation of the medication. Compliance with H$_2$-receptor antagonist therapy has been better than compliance with antacids alone. Maintenance therapy with H$_2$-receptor antagonists does not protect entirely against a recurrence of primary PUD. Therapy with these drugs beyond 1 year is not recommended, although serious long-term side effects have not been documented.

Other medications such as sucralfate and anticholinergic drugs may be added to the therapeutic regimen. Sucralfate binds to the erosive surface of the ulcer and protects the mucosa from further damage. Anticholinergics such as propantheline bromide decrease acid secretion, but the effective dose often produces side effects such as blurred vision and dry mouth. Cytoprotective drugs have not been studied sufficiently in children to warrant their use.

Dietary intervention also may promote ulcer healing. Milk feedings have been found to raise the gastric *p*H and to prevent GI bleeding in hospitalized children. The factors responsible for the reduction of gastric acidity are unknown, although several peptides and hormones found in bovine and human milk have been implicated. Frequent snacks should be avoided to minimize food-stimulated acid secretion. Alcoholic beverages, cigarette smoking, aspirin, and other drugs that damage the gastric mucosal barrier are contraindicated.

The surgical management of PUD is reserved for patients with complications of ulcers, including intractable pain, perforation, hemorrhage, and obstruction. Truncal or selective vagotomy with pyloroplasty, or, in some instances, antrectomy, is the most common procedure performed in children with PUD.

■ COMPLICATIONS

Hospitalization for PUD usually is unnecessary unless the complications of intractable pain, obstruction, active bleeding, or perforation are present. If signs of gastric outlet obstruction are found, food should be withheld and nasogastric suction applied for several days. Surgical intervention should be considered if the obstruction does not resolve within 72 hours of nasogastric drainage. If GI bleeding is present, a large-bore nasogastric tube should be inserted and the stomach should be lavaged repeatedly with ice-cold normal saline. Vital signs, central venous pressure, and hematocrit values should be monitored carefully to determine whether blood transfusions are necessary. During severe hemorrhage, selective abdominal angiography may be necessary to identify the site of bleeding. Intravenous vasopressin, 0.3 to 0.4 units/1.73 m²/min for 48 hours, may control active bleeding. Surgical intervention should be considered when one third to one half of the total blood volume has been replaced.

■ PROGNOSIS

The prognosis of primary PUD in children and adolescents is less than optimal. Disease recurs within 1 year in 35% to 50% of all patients, and at least two thirds have repeated relapses over the years. About 60% of children with recurrences require surgery, although the availability of H₂-receptor antagonists may reduce this rate. However, the benefits of safe and effective surgical intervention may outweigh the long-term inconvenience, cost, and disability associated with chronic relapsing PUD.

The prognosis of secondary stress ulcers is affected by the precipitating illness or injury. The outcome in the neonate with gastric hemorrhage and perforation is poor. Healing generally occurs in infants and children who develop an acute ulcer, although emergency surgery may be necessary for hemorrhage or perforation. Recurrences of stress ulcers are unlikely with resolution of the underlying illness.

(Abridged from Kathleen J. Motil, Peptic Ulcer Disease, in Oski, DeAngelis, Feigin, McMillan, Warshaw: *Principles and Practice of Pediatrics, Second Edition*, J.B. Lippincott, 1994.)

Oski's Essential Pediatrics,
edited by Kevin B. Johnson and Frank A. Oski.
Lippincott–Raven Publishers,
Philadelphia © 1997

158

Intussusception

Intussusception is the most common cause of intestinal obstruction in infants aged 3 months to 1 year. It is rare in the first month of life. There is great regional variation in the incidence of intussusception, from less than 0.5 to 4 per 1000 live births.

■ PATHOPHYSIOLOGY

Intussusception is the result of invagination or telescoping of a portion of the bowel into the more distal bowel (Figure 158–1). The portion of the bowel that invaginates into the more distal bowel, the *intussusceptum,* is pulled along with its mesentery by peristaltic waves. As the proximal bowel is pulled into the lumen of the *intussuscipiens,* or distal bowel, the mesentery is compressed and angled, resulting initially in lymphatic obstruction and subsequently in venous obstruction. The intussuscepted mass quickly obstructs the intestinal lumen, with resulting distention and peristaltic rushes proximal to the obstructing mass. With each peristaltic rush, the patient experiences colicky pain. Early in the course of illness, the affected infant will reflexively evacuate the distal colon and pass several partially formed stools. As reflex ileus and pylorospasm develop, the infant begins to

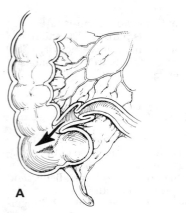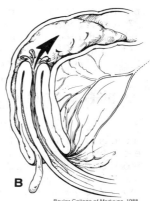

Baylor College of Medicine 1988

Figure 158-1. The development of an ileocolic intussusception. (**A**) The invagination typically begins several centimeters proximal to the ileocecal valve. As the ileum is drawn into the more distal bowel, the lumen is obstucted and the mesenteric vessels become compressed. (**B**) Edema and venous engorgement devlop, with accumulation of blood and mucus ("currant jelly") in the lumen of the colon. If not reduced, infarction of the intussusceptum occurs.

vomit. Initially the vomitus is clear, but, as signs of intestinal obstruction develop, the vomitus becomes bile-stained and eventually fecaloid. The peristaltic rushes and colicky pain first occur at intervals of several minutes and last only a few seconds. During the intervals between peristaltic rushes, the infant appears to be in no discomfort, and the abdomen is soft and scaphoid.

At this time, a mass is almost always palpable. Because 95% of the cases of intussusception are ileocolic, with the invaginating bowel beginning just proximal to the ileocecal valve, the sausage-shaped mass can be found in the distribution of the colon, commonly in the area of the hepatic flexure but occasionally more distally. In 3% of the cases, the intussuscepting intestine prolapses through the rectum.

As the edema from lymphatic obstruction and venous engorgement increases, the hydrostatic pressure within the intussusception increases until it equals the arterial pressure, at which time arterial inflow ceases. During this process, the intestinal mucosa becomes ischemic, with a transition of the endothelial cells to goblet cells and an outpouring of mucus into the intestinal lumen. Venous engorgement results in leakage of blood into the intestinal lumen, and the blood and mucus form "currant jelly" stools. Currant jelly stools are a fairly late sign of intussusception, usually requiring several hours to develop. They have been reported in 85% of the patients in some series and are more common in younger patients.

If complete intestinal obstruction ensues, the child may develop abdominal distention, fluid loss from vomiting and sequestration of intraluminal fluid, and continuous abdominal pain. If there is a further delay in diagnosis and treatment, infarction of the intussusceptum will occur. In most cases, this is associated with generalized peritonitis; if untreated, death of the patient occurs within 2 to 5 days.

■ CLINICAL PRESENTATION

Nearly all affected infants present with vomiting and colicky pain. However, because these two symptoms are nonspecific and common, they are less likely to prompt a visit to the physician. Infants typically are seen later in the course of illness, at which time they are more likely to have currant jelly stools and high fever. Intussusception in infants less than 3 months old is less likely to be reduced by barium enema.

■ DIAGNOSIS

The diagnosis of intussusception frequently is made from a clinical history of intermittent, colicky pain lasting only a few seconds and extending over the course of several hours, after which the patient becomes lethargic, vomits, and shows signs and symptoms of intestinal obstruction. On physical examination, a palpable sausage-shaped mass in the distribution of the colon, typically in the area of the transverse colon, confirms the diagnosis. If currant jelly stools are noted in association with a sausage-shaped mass and intermittent colicky pain, the diagnosis is no longer in doubt. At times, the intussusception mass will be located medial to the lateral edge of the rectus abdominis muscle and below the edge of the liver, making palpation difficult. This is particularly true when some degree of intestinal obstruction and abdominal distention has developed. In addition, only 65% of infants with intussusception will have currant jelly stools. For these reasons, any infant or young child with signs and symptoms of distal small bowel or colonic obstruction, intermittent colicky pain, currant jelly or guaiac-positive stools, or a sausage-shaped mass in the distribution of the colon should undergo a diagnostic barium enema examination. The diagnosis will be confirmed in 100% of the patients in whom the intussusceptum extends through the ileocecal valve into the colon.

■ DIFFERENTIAL DIAGNOSIS

Intussusception should be included in the differential diagnosis of any condition characterized by abdominal pain, blood in the stool, or an intra-abdominal mass. Intussusception is often confused with gastroenteritis. Although intermittent colicky abdominal pain is typical of both, the pain associated with intussusception is more constantly episodic. Early in the illness, the infant with intussusception appears well between paroxysms of pain.

Intussusception, particularly cecal-colic intussusception, occasionally results in partial intestinal obstruction and presents with liquid, blood-streaked, loose stools similar to those seen with infectious enterocolitis. Guaiac-positive and blood-streaked stools are common in infants with gastroenteritis. The bloody-mucoid or currant jelly stools are the result of venous-congested, vascularly compromised intestine; they may also be seen in other processes such as volvulus and incarcerated internal hernia.

■ TREATMENT

The modern treatment protocol and guidelines for the use of barium enema are described in Table 158–1. The primary concern is rapid resuscitation of the volume-depleted child. This requires placement of a large intravenous plastic catheter for intravenous administration of fluids and, if necessary, of blood products. Gastric aspiration through a nasogastric tube prevents further vomiting and enteric accumulation of fluid. Antibiotics are reserved for patients with peritoneal signs or evidence of compromised bowel. As soon as the diagnosis is made, the operating room should be prepared for emergency surgery, as it would be in the case of an incarcerated hernia. If the patient's hemoglobin is low, blood should be typed and crossmatched, because bowel resection may be necessary.

Only after resuscitation has been initiated should the patient be taken to the radiology suite for a diagnostic and therapeutic contrast enema examination with fluoroscopy. Contrast materials used include air, water-soluble contrast, and barium. If the risk of perforation is increased, air or water-soluble contrast is a better choice than barium.

TABLE 158-1. Principles of Barium Enema Reduction of Intussusception

1. Notify OR to prepare for emergency operation if barium reduction is not successful.

2. Initiate resuscitation with intravenous fluids and nasogastric suction.

3. Insert ungreased Foley catheter in rectum, distend balloon, and pull down against levators. Tape catheter in place and hold buttocks tightly together. Wrap legs.

4. Let barium run from a height of 3'6" above the table while intermittently fluoroscoping the patient.

5. Abandon procedure if barium column is stationary and its outline is unchanged for 10 minutes.

6. Reduction is marked by: free flow of barium well into ileum; expulsion of feces and flatus with the barium; disappearance of the mass on physical examination; and clinical improvement of the child.

7. Failure to reduce the intussusception requires prompt operative intervention.

(Modified from Ravitch MM. Intussusception. In: Welch KJ, Randolph JG, Ravitch MM, et al, eds. Pediatric surgery. Chicago: Year Book Medical Publishers, 1987:868).

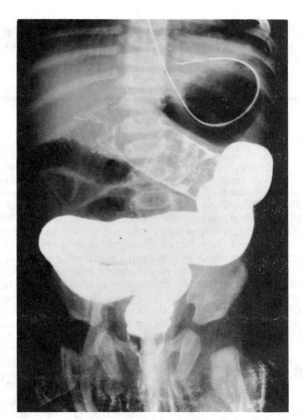

Figure 158-2. Barium enema study showing the coiled-spring pattern of barium around the intussusceptum in the transverse colon.

Once the diagnosis is confirmed by contrast enema, a decision must be made whether to attempt hydrostatic reduction (Figure 158–2). The only absolute contraindications to hydrostatic reduction are free intraperitoneal air or peritoneal signs and systemic signs of compromised intestine. Relative contraindications include intestinal obstruction as evidenced by multiple air–fluid levels with dilated segments of small bowel. Several cases have been reported in which patients with high-grade bowel obstruction developed perforation and barium spillage during attempted hydrostatic reduction. If a filling defect suggesting a lead point is seen after reduction, laparotomy should be done.

At present, 30% to 70% of the patients with intussusception are successfully treated by hydrostatic reduction of the intussusception. The recurrence rate after both hydrostatic reduction and surgical reduction is close to 5%; recurrences usually occur shortly after the successful reduction.

Patients with free air or peritoneal signs and patients in whom hydrostatic reduction is unsuccessful should be taken directly to the operating room for operative reduction. Because the intussusceptum causes vascular compromise, these are true surgical emergencies. Successful operative reduction is possible in most patients; however, nearly 25% of infants requiring surgery require resection because reduction is impossible or the intestine is nonviable. The compromised bowel may be excised and a primary ileocolostomy performed.

(Abridged from William J. Pokorny, Intussusception, in Oski, DeAngelis, Feigin, McMillan, Warshaw: *Principles and Practice of Pediatrics, Second Edition,* J.B. Lippincott, 1994.)

Oski's Essential Pediatrics,
edited by Kevin B. Johnson and Frank A. Oski.
Lippincott–Raven Publishers,
Philadelphia © 1997

159

Anorectal Malformations

Embryonic development of the anus and rectum with separation from the urogenital tract primarily occurs between the 4-mm (4th week) and 16-mm (6th week) stage of embryonic development but continues to the 56-mm stage. Major anorectal malformations occur in 1 per 5000 live births, with minor anomalies reported in as many as 1 per 1500 live births. Imperforate anus has been reported in siblings and in members of one family over three generations.

Lesions close to the anus are more common than high and intermediate lesions in girls; high lesions are more common in boys. Nearly 80% of the boys with a high lesion have a fistula to the urinary tract, and nearly all girls with a high lesion have a fistula to the vagina, bladder, or cloaca (Figures 159–1 and 159–2).

■ DIAGNOSIS

The level of the anorectal anomaly cannot be predicted from the appearance of the perineum. However, several findings on physical examination suggest the level of an imperforate anus. A flat bottom with no crease or anal dimple and

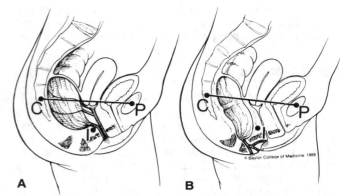

Figure 159-1. Anorectal anomalies in the female. (**A**) High lesions usually have a fistula to the vagina, whereas intermediate lesions may have a fistula to the vagina or outside the hymen at the vestibule. (**B**) Low lesions may also have a fistula to the vestibule or to the fourchette or perineum.

no evidence of an external sphincter predicts a high imperforate anus (Figure 159–3). On the other hand, a well-developed anal dimple is not always associated with a low anomaly. Nevertheless, a well-developed raphe, anal dimple, and bucket-handle raphe suggest a low lesion. Ninety percent of the boys with a low lesion have a fistula to the perineum. Whitish inspissated mucus (perineal pearls) or meconium-stained material may be expressed from the fistula in the subcuticular tract along the raphe of the perineum, scrotum, or even ventral surface of the penis (Figure 159–4). Often the perineal fistula is not obvious at birth but becomes evident with the passage of a small fleck of meconium during the first 24 hours of life (Figure 159–5). The passage of flatus or meconium in the urine is diagnostic of a high or intermediate anomaly with a fistula to the urethra or bladder.

In most girls, the lesion is low (Figure 159–6) Nearly all of these girls have a fistula to the perineum, as an anterior or ectopic anus (Figure 159–7) to the fourchette or to the vestibule, which is between the posterior fourchette and the hymenal ring (Figure 159–8). Openings into the vestibule may be associated with low lesions or high lesions with long fistulas. The complete absence of an external fistula indicates a high or intermediate lesion. Most girls with high lesions have a fistula to the vagina; fistulas to the urinary tract are rare. In patients with a single opening, a cloacal anomaly must be considered.

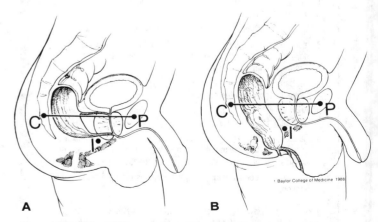

Figure 159-2. Anorectal anomalies in the male. (**A**) 80% of high and intermediate lesions have fistulas to the bulbar or membranous urethra. (**B**) 90% of males with low lesions have a fistula to the perineum or median raphe.

Initial diagnostic studies are designed to identify the level of descent of the rectum and to detect associated anomalies, including fistulas. Ultrasound is useful to evaluate the anatomical integrity of the urinary tract. If there is no evidence of a genitourinary anomaly at birth, intravenous pyelography and voiding cystourethrography should be done before discharge or when the child is 6 weeks old and better able to concentrate the dye.

The urine should be examined for meconium or squamous epithelial cells. A chest radiograph may be obtained with a nasogastric tube in place to rule out esophageal, cardiac, and vertebral anomalies. If cardiomegaly is present, cardiac evaluation should be done. An abdominal-pelvic radiograph may reveal anomalies of the gastrointestinal tract as well as of the lumbosacral spine.

If the patient exhibits no evidence of a fistula to the perineum, a Wangensteen-Rice radiograph (invertogram) should be obtained after 12 hours of life; this allows sufficient time for air to reach the rectum.

■ ASSOCIATED MALFORMATIONS

Associated anomalies are reported in 40% to 50% of the patients with imperforate anus. Associated anomalies must be sought in infants with all forms of anorectal malformations. In addition to imperforate anus, esophageal atresia, vertebral anomalies, and radial and renal anomalies make up the VATER association. The association has been expanded to VACTERL, where "C" represents cardiac lesions and "L" represents limb deformities. When one of these anomalies is seen, the others should be sought.

Nearly 40% of the infants with imperforate anus have genitourinary anomalies, ranging from minor genital anomalies such as hypospadias to renal agenesis. Unilateral renal agenesis is the most common defect, occurring in 8% to 25% of the patients with imperforate anus.

Gastrointestinal anomalies, most notably esophageal atresia, occur in 10% to 15% of the children with imperforate anus.

Cardiovascular anomalies are reported in 7% to 12% of the patients with imperforate anus. Ventricular septal defect and tetralogy of Fallot are two of the more common anomalies.

Skeletal anomalies are found in 6% to 20% of the patients with anorectal malformations. Vertebral anomalies,

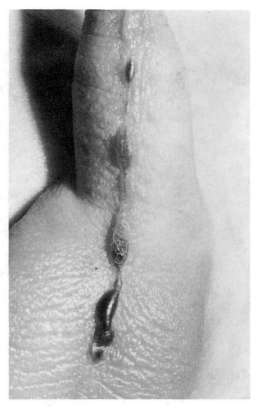

Figure 159-4. Male with a low lesion and fistula to the median raphe. Note meconium along the median raphe. A perineal anoplasty was done shortly after birth.

usually sacral, are the most common defect. As many as 50% of the patients with high lesions have sacral vertebral anomalies. All patients with anorectal malformations should be evaluated by ultrasonography, computed tomography, or magnetic resonance imaging to identify lesions of the lumbosacral spine and cord.

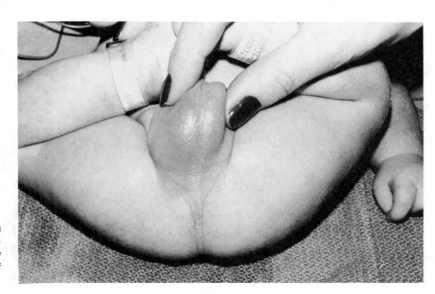

Figure 159-3. Perineum of a male with a high lesion and a rectourethral fistula. After 24 hours, there is no evidence of a fistula to the perineum or raphe. A colostomy was done on the second day of life, and reconstruction of the anus and rectum was performed at 1 year.

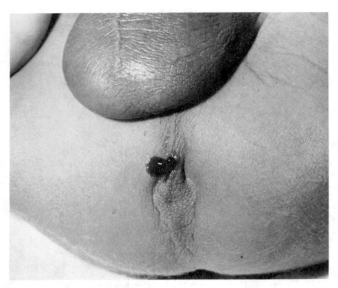

Figure 159-5. Male with anoperineal fistula. Meconium did not appear until 18 hours after birth. A perineal anoplasty was done on the second day of life.

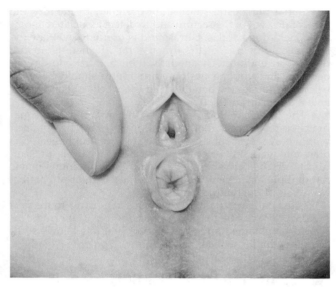

Figure 159-7. Ectopic perineal anus located posterior to the fourchette but anterior to the external sphincter. The patient did well with dilations until 6 months of age, when the anus was moved to the normal location.

■ TREATMENT

The treatment of imperforate anus depends on the level of descent of the rectum and on the presence or absence of a fistula to the urinary tract, vagina, or perineum. Children with ectopic or anterior anus are usually asymptomatic during infancy but become constipated when their diet changes and their stools become more formed and solid. At that time, the anus should be surgically moved posteriorly to its normal location.

Infants with low lesions and perineal fistulas may require only dilation of the tract to allow fecal evacuation. Openings into the vestibule in girls may be either high with a long fistula or low. Low openings may be treated by dilatation and, at age 6 months, by translocation of the anus to its normal position. High lesions with a long fistula require a diverting colostomy.

Children with high and intermediate lesions should undergo diverting colostomies as soon as the diagnosis is confirmed. This is particularly important in patients with fistulas

to the urinary tract. Failure to completely divert the feces from the fistula will result in recurrent urinary tract infections.

■ PROGNOSIS

Nearly all patients with low malformations have normal rectal function. The outcome of patients with high and intermediate malformations varies: a good outcome has been reported in 33% to 80% of the patients. Toilet training may be difficult until the child is older, often 5 or 6 years of

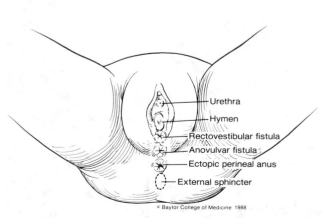

Figure 159-6. Appearance of fistulas on the female perineum.

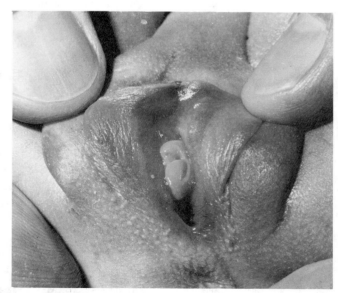

Figure 159-8. Rectovestibular fistula located between the hymen and fourchette in the fossa navicularis. A colostomy was done on the second day of life, and anorectal reconstruction was performed at 1 year.

age. The rectal function and fecal continence continue to improve into early adolescence. If the patient and his or her family can be supported through the early postoperative years, rectal function nearly always improves to an acceptable level.

In the early postoperative period, constipation may be due to stenosis and, rarely, to Hirschsprung's disease, but it is more often due to a lack of rectal sensation for fecal material, which leads to fecal impaction. Attention must be given to regular evacuations to prevent impactions. Once impaction develops, the rectum and distal colon become overdistended and lose their muscular tone and peristaltic function. This must be prevented. In some instances, daily laxatives or enemas are required.

(Abridged from William J. Pokorny, Anorectal Malformations, in Oski, DeAngelis, Feigin, McMillan, Warshaw: *Principles and Practice of Pediatrics, Second Edition,* J.B. Lippincott, 1994.)

Oski's Essential Pediatrics,
edited by Kevin B. Johnson and Frank A. Oski.
Lippincott–Raven Publishers,
Philadelphia © 1997

160

Crohn's Disease

Crohn's disease is a transmural inflammatory process that may affect any segment of the gastrointestinal (GI) tract from mouth to anus in a discontinuous fashion. The small bowel is involved in 91% of the cases, particularly the distal ileum (71%), usually (52%) in combination with colitis (ie, ileocolitis). Isolated colonic disease without clinical or radiologic evidence of small bowel involvement occurs in 9% of patients. The small bowel involvement is responsible for many of the specific nutritional complications of Crohn's disease, whereas the colonic involvement poses the greatest challenge for differentiation from other infectious and inflammatory bowel diseases.

■ PATHOLOGY

Table 160–1 outlines the distinctions between Crohn's disease and ulcerative colitis. Unlike the findings in ulcerative colitis, the inflammation in Crohn's disease usually does not involve a continuous segment of bowel and often appears as discrete focal ulcerations (ie, aphthae) with relatively intact intervening mucosa. As the disease progresses, in the 61% of cases involving the colon, right-sided inflammation predominates, with relative sparing of the rectum. Anal involvement, in the form of skin tags, anal fissures, abscesses, and fistulas, is more common in Crohn's disease than in ulcerative colitis and occurs in approximately 25% of the patients.

■ ETIOLOGY

As in ulcerative colitis, the cause of Crohn's disease is unknown. The familial clustering of Crohn's disease supports a genetic predisposition.

■ EPIDEMIOLOGY

The incidence of Crohn's disease has risen to an estimated 3.5 new cases per 100,000 population per year, making Crohn's disease more common than ulcerative colitis in pediatric practice. The epidemiology is similar to that of ulcerative colitis, with an increased prevalence among Caucasians (especially in the Jewish population), approximately equal male and female representation, and a bimodal age at onset, with peaks in the second and third and again in the sixth decades of life. Although there is an increased prevalence of Crohn's disease among first-degree relatives, there is no specific heritable pattern.

■ CLINICAL PRESENTATION

The presentation of Crohn's disease in children depends on the location and extent of inflammation. In many cases, the onset is insidious with nonspecific features of GI involvement or extraintestinal manifestations leading to delayed or incorrect diagnosis. There is an average delay of 13 months from the onset of symptoms to diagnosis. Diarrhea, abdominal pain (most frequently postprandial periumbilical cramping), fever, and weight loss are the most common presenting features. Rectal bleeding, seen in 30% Crohn's disease cases, is much less common than in ulcerative colitis and usually signifies colonic involvement.

The three general patterns of clinical presentation based on anatomical involvement show considerable overlap. Patients with the first pattern present with nonspecific extraintestinal manifestations and growth retardation (Table 160–2). Overt clinical signs of GI involvement may not appear for years, although this inflammation may be extensive enough to cause early satiety, nausea, poor feeding, and malabsorption syndromes. Over time, net energy and protein deficits are reflected in decreased weight velocity followed by decreased height velocity and delayed skeletal and sexual maturation. Certain extraintestinal features that may be clues indicating the presence of Crohn's disease include perianal disease, oral aphthae, erythema nodosum, arthritis, uveitis, and digital clubbing. Abdominal radiographs may show an unusual gas pattern with some small bowel dilatation. Recognizing this insidious mode of presentation leads to timely use of specific tests to confirm the diagnosis.

Another pattern of presentation is produced by small bowel involvement, which probably is responsible for much of the postprandial cramping, early satiety, nausea, and poor feeding that patients report. Rarely, the esophagus or stomach may be affected.

Colonic involvement may present as diarrhea, often associated with cramps and urgency to defecate after any distention of the inflamed colon by the fecal stream. Other signs of colitis may be indistinguishable from those seen in ulcerative colitis and consist of an inflammatory exudate of neutrophils into the lumen and occult or overt rectal bleeding. Perianal disease and relative sparing of the rectum are more frequent in Crohn's colitis than in ulcerative colitis and may be the only differentiating features. A rare complication, toxic dilatation with risk of perforation and sepsis, known as toxic megacolon, has been reported in Crohn's colitis; treatment is the same as outlined for toxic megacolon complicating severe ulcerative colitis (see Chapter 161).

With Crohn's disease, these three patterns of anatomical involvement overlap to produce a clinical presentation unique for each patient, and a clinical diagnosis alone usually is not possible or sufficient.

TABLE 160-1. Comparative Features of Ulcerative Colitis and Crohn's Disease

	Ulcerative Colitis	Crohn's Disease
Site of disease		
Upper GI	0%	20%
Ileum alone	0%	19
Ileum and colon	Backwash ileitis	52%
Colon alone	90% (distal colon predominant)	9% (proximal colon predominant)
Rectum	~ 100%	Rare (< 5%); perianal disease in 25%
Cross pathology/radiology	Hemorrhagic mucosa, diffuse continuous inflammation, pseudopolyps, loss of haustra, no perirenal disease	Segmental involvement, skip regions, focal aphthae, thickened bowel wall, serosal fat, narrow separate bowel loops, anal tags, fistulas
Histology	Mucosal and submucosal inflammation, cryptitis, crypt abscess and distortion, depletion of goblet cells	Transmural inflammation, noncaseating granulomas, prominent lymphoid tissue, preserved goblet cells, fibrosis

Extraintestinal Signs

The systemic nature of Crohn's disease is apparent in the range of potential involvement of extraintestinal organs. Arthritis and arthralgias may occur in as many as 11% of cases and usually present as a seronegative monoarticular arthritis of a knee or ankle or as a migratory polyarthritis. Arthritis is more common in patients with colonic involvement (eg, colitis, ileocolitis) and seems to parallel disease activity, although occasionally it precedes overt GI signs. Sacroiliitis and ankylosing spondylitis are rare and occur predominantly in patients with histocompatibility gene HLA-B27.

Approximately 5% of the patients develop cutaneous lesions of erythema nodosum, erythema multiforme, or pyoderma gangrenosum. Management requires control of the underlying bowel disease, often with the addition of metronidazole, topical cromolyn sulfate, and occasional skin grafting.

Signs of liver disease occur in fewer than 8% of patients with Crohn's disease. Liver involvement correlates with bowel disease activity but rarely progresses to cirrhosis or chronic active hepatitis.

Undernutrition and Growth Failure

Weight loss occurs in as many as 87% of the children presenting with Crohn's disease and may be as much as 12.5

TABLE 160-2. Crohn's Disease: Patterns of Involvement

EXTRAINTESTINAL SIGNS AND GROWTH RETARDATION
Anorexia, malaise, fatigue
Perianal disease, stomatitis
Erythema nodosum, pyoderma gangrenosum
Anemia, hepatitis renolithiasis, arthritis clubbing

SMALL BOWEL INVOLVEMENT
Diarrhea
Abdominal mass, postprandial cramps, nausea
Malabsorption
Mineral and vitamin deficiencies (Fe, Zn, Mg, folate, vitamin B_{12})

COLONIC FEATURES
Diarrhea, urgency
Rectal bleeding fecal leukocytes
Perianal fistula, abscess

kg. Often accompanying the weight loss are impaired linear growth, retarded bone development and mineralization, and delayed sexual maturation. These changes initially may be subtle and often precede overt bowel disease by months or years (Figure 160–1). Most of these effects seem to be caused by undernutrition because they can be reversed by nutritional supplementation.

Most endocrine tests are normal in patients with growth retardation and short stature associated with Crohn's disease. Although bone age may be delayed and serum insulin-like growth factor-1 levels depressed, both respond to nutritional therapy, and pituitary, thyroid, adrenal, and growth hormone studies are normal. Similarly, arrested sexual maturation, with delayed puberty and menarche, responds to nutritional therapy and control of the disease.

Over time, the patient with longstanding disease may adapt to a state of chronic undernutrition and become a "nutritional dwarf," characterized by height stunted below expected percentiles, appropriate weight for height, and normal to subnormal linear growth velocity. The consequences of untreated chronic undernutrition in a child with Crohn's disease are poor disease control, increased complications, delayed puberty, and permanent short stature.

■ COMPLICATIONS

The major intestinal complications of Crohn's disease are caused by the transmural nature of the inflammation, extending from mucosa to serosa. Contiguous loops of bowel or other organs may be enveloped in inflammation. Adhesions, strictures, and abscesses may develop, with a risk of obstruction or bacterial overgrowth. Fistulas may form to any abdominal or pelvic structure and should be suspected to underlie any chronic draining ulcer or sinus. Enterocutaneous, enteroenteric, perirectal, labial, enterovaginal, and enterovesical fistulas may pose a nutritional hazard, because they are conduits for major losses of protein and other nutrients. Perianal disease occurs in 25% of the patients with Crohn's disease, most often in the context of colonic inflammation and fistula formation. Skin tags, anal fissures, and perianal or perirectal abscesses may precede other signs of intestinal Crohn's disease or develop during an exacerbation of colitis.

The risk of malignancy of all types appears to be increased in patients with Crohn's disease, estimated as 20 times greater than normal for patients with Crohn's disease diagnosed before the age of 21 years.

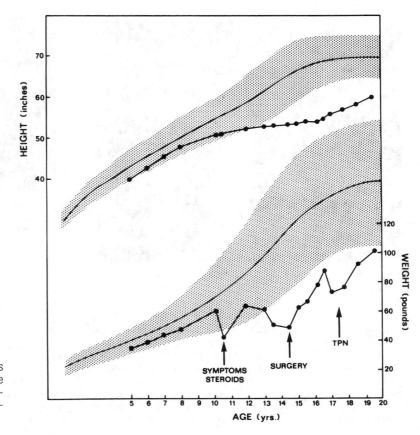

Figure 160-1. Growth curve of an adolescent with Crohn's disease. The reduction in linear growth preceded the acute weight loss and onset of symptoms. Although growth accelerated after steroid treatment, limited resection, and parenteral nutrition, premorbid percentiles were not achieved.

■ DIAGNOSIS

The diagnosis of Crohn's disease is based on clinical presentation, radiologic findings, and mucosal appearance and histology and on exclusion of alternative causes. A complete history should be obtained, with attention to family history, exposure to infectious agents or antibiotic treatment, extraintestinal manifestations, and retardation in growth rate or in sexual development. Physical examination should include assessment of hydration, nutritional status, signs of peritoneal inflammation, and signs of systemic chronic disease. Features suggesting Crohn's disease are stomatitis, perianal skin tags or inflammation, and clubbing. Fever, orthostasis, tachycardia, and abdominal tenderness, distention, or mass should be considered indications for admission to the hospital.

Laboratory Evaluation

A complete blood cell count can detect leukocytosis or identify anemia. The erythrocyte sedimentation rate is elevated in 90% of the patients and may be useful as a marker of inflammatory activity. Serum total protein and albumin levels may be low as a consequence of severe undernutrition and enteric protein losses. Serum magnesium, iron, and plasma zinc levels may be low due to poor intake coupled with cumulative losses from sloughed intestinal epithelial cells or bleeding. Ileal dysfunction may be revealed by a low vitamin B_{12} and low fat-soluble vitamin levels. Urinalysis may reveal pyuria. Fresh stool should be obtained for examination of blood, leukocytes, and parasites and cultured for infectious pathogens. Microbiologic studies should include culture for *Yersinia enterocolitica* and assay for *Clostridium difficile* toxin. Serologic titers may help exclude *Entamoeba histolytica*. Detection of pathogens may not exclude the existence of underlying Crohn's disease, but the infections must be treated first.

Radiology

Although the extent of radiographic involvement has not correlated with clinical disease activity, radiologic studies are often essential to diagnosis and management.

Upright and supine radiographs of the abdomen and a chest x-ray will demonstrate the extent of bowel dilatation and help exclude ileus, intestinal obstruction, or pneumoperitoneum, signifying perforation. If clinical colitis is present and colonoscopy is unavailable, a barium enema study with air contrast to reveal mucosal detail may demonstrate characteristic aphthous lesions and show cecal or segmental involvement or right-sided predominance (Figures 160–2 and 160–3). If Crohn's disease is suspected but difficult to demonstrate or if complications are suspected, computed tomography often can demonstrate the bowel wall thickening, fat wrapping, or abscesses (Figure 160–4). Radionuclide scans lack the resolution and specificity required for diagnosis.

Endoscopy

Colonoscopy with biopsy of the colon and terminal ileum is the most sensitive and specific test for evaluating Crohn's ileocolitis. As reflected in its pathology, the lesions of Crohn's disease may appear as discrete ulcerations or

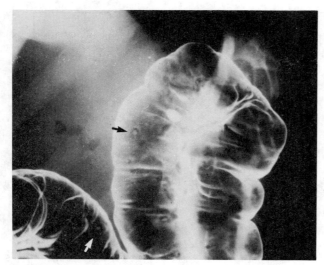

Figure 160-2. Air contrast barium enema in a patient with Crohn's diease demonstrating aphthae (*arrows*) in the splenic flexure.

aphthae of the mucosa, often with a central exudate and corona of erythema. Intervening areas may be normal in appearance and histologic characteristics. In more than 60% of the patients with colonic involvement, disease is more active in the proximal colon and cecum. Because the histology of regions that appear grossly normal may show signs of nonspecific chronic inflammation, biopsies must be obtained from multiple sites, regardless of gross endoscopic appear-

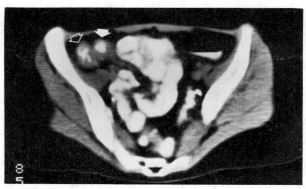

Figure 160-4. Computed tomogram of the lower abdomen of a 12-year-old girl with Crohn's ileocolitis. Notice the thickened bowel wall of terminal ileum (*soild arrow*) and cecum (*open arrow*), and thickened mesentery. No abscesses or fistulas were demonstrated.

ance. Endoscopy to explore the esophagus, stomach, and duodenum is indicated when involvement is suspected on clinical or radiologic grounds.

■ DIFFERENTIAL DIAGNOSIS

Crohn's disease appears in many forms, which makes diagnosis and differentiation from other entities challenging. Signs of inflammation (*eg*, fever, abdominal cramps, tenderness), extraintestinal lesions, or an elevated sedimentation rate can often differentiate inflammatory causes of growth failure from endocrine or psychogenic syndromes such as growth hormone deficiency, hypopituitarism, and anorexia nervosa. Signs of colitis on stool examination, barium study, or colonoscopy with biopsy or the presence of oral aphthae or perianal disease can localize the inflammation to the GI tract. The presence of extracolonic disease or granulomas on biopsy favors Crohn's disease over ulcerative colitis, although, in the absence of such features, Crohn's disease cannot be excluded. In some cases, Crohn's colitis clinically and histologically may be indistinguishable from ulcerative colitis until extracolonic or histologic features appear. There is even a report of the co-occurrence of the two disease patterns. Occasionally, evidence of Crohn's disease does not appear until inflammation develops in the ileostomy or ileoanal pouch of a patient who has had a colectomy for what was presumed to be ulcerative colitis.

GI disorders are common in pediatric patients, with as many as 10% of children between the ages of 7 and 11 years seeking medical attention for the complaint of recurrent abdominal pain, usually periumbilical in location. Unless there are signs of inflammation or growth disturbance, extensive evaluation for inflammatory bowel disease is contraindicated. Nevertheless, the periumbilical nature of the pain is nonspecific and not pathognomonic for functional abdominal pain because it is characteristic of most children presenting with inflammatory bowel disease. In uncomplicated recurrent abdominal pain, discomfort due to stool retention, lactose intolerance, peptic disease, urinary tract infection, pelvic inflammatory disease, or psychosocial causes should be considered and eliminated.

Rectal bleeding is more common in ulcerative colitis than in Crohn's disease and has many causes in addition to colitis, such as Meckel's diverticulum, hemolytic-uremic syndrome, Henoch-Schönlein purpura, intestinal polyps, or hemorrhoids. Anal fissures secondary to constipation usually pre-

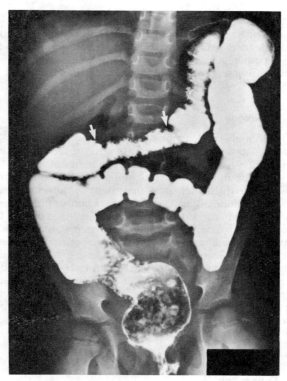

Figure 160-3. Barium enema study in an 8-year-old girl with Crohn's disease reveals segmental colitis involving discrete regions of the transverse colon (*between arrows*). Notice the irregular mucosal margins consistent with active ulceration and edema. The rectum, shown with residual stool, was spared.

sent without signs of colitis or chronic perianal inflammation and skin tags.

Pathogens such as *C difficile, Y enterocolitica,* enteropathogenic *Escherichia coli, Aeromonas hydrophila, Giardia lamblia,* and *Entamoeba histolytica* must be excluded, along with the customary *Salmonella, Shigella,* and *Campylobacter* cultured in the setting of enterocolitis. These agents are often overlooked in the initial evaluation and may produce a chronic inflammatory picture resembling Crohn's ileocolitis. Tuberculosis, *Yersinia,* and lymphoma may involve the small bowel, predominantly the terminal ileum, which is rich in lymphoid tissue, and may resemble Crohn's disease clinically and radiographically.

Unlike most other rheumatologic diseases of childhood, the arthritis of inflammatory bowel disease is usually asymmetric, involving large joints of the lower extremities without deformity.

■ THERAPY

Because no pharmacologic regimen has been shown to alter the long-term outcome of Crohn's disease, the goals of treatment are to minimize the morbidity of disease exacerbations without introducing iatrogenic morbidity.

Pharmacologic Therapy

Corticosteroids can effect short-term remissions of active small bowel disease in 70% of the patients. Unfortunately, symptoms may recur with reduction of the dosage such that 70% of these patients suffer relapse within 1 year. Continuous low-dose treatment does not seem to prevent relapse, but higher-dose, alternate-day steroids may allow control of symptoms with a minimum of side effects and a lower risk of growth retardation. Indications for steroid therapy are limited to symptoms refractory to other agents, extensive small bowel disease, severe or persistent systemic and extraintestinal complications, and postoperative recurrences.

In as many as 75% of the patients who cannot be managed without high-dose or prolonged corticosteroids or who are at risk for complications of steroid therapy, immunosuppressive agents (*eg,* azathioprine, 6-mercaptopurine) are useful in maintaining remission and allowing reduction in steroid dosage. The role of cyclosporine in acute exacerbations of Crohn's disease has not been determined decisively, but early experience suggests that short-term benefits may be achieved.

Nutritional Therapy

Because of the limitations and morbidity of medical treatment and the nutritional impact of Crohn's disease, increased emphasis has been placed on nutritional rehabilitation and therapy as a way of altering the course of Crohn's disease. Optimal prospective management in patients with inflammatory bowel disease should include regular assessment of growth and nutritional status. Maintenance of optimal nutritional status with aggressive support of energy and protein intake may prolong remission or allow reduced corticosteroid treatment. The goals of nutritional therapy in Crohn's disease must include recovery of metabolic homeostasis by correcting specific nutrient deficits and replacing ongoing losses; provi-

sion of sufficient energy and protein for positive nitrogen balance (*ie,* protein synthesis) and healing; and promotion of catch-up growth toward premorbid percentiles.

The optimal nutritional therapy serves as an adjunct to medical therapy in controlling symptoms and inducing remission. Short-term remissions have been achieved by aggressive elemental enteral or parenteral nutritional support alone. Elemental diets have been advocated as primary initial therapy to induce remission until immunosuppressive agents become effective. They have been variably ineffective in closing fistulas, but most eventually require surgery. After nutritional rehabilitation and disease remission have been achieved, efforts should continue to ensure catch-up growth rates of at least 0.5 cm each month and 1 kg each month toward premorbid percentiles.

Surgery

Unlike ulcerative colitis, in which disease is limited to the colon and can be cured by total colectomy, there is no definitive surgical cure for Crohn's disease. For these reasons and because of the high incidence of complications requiring repeat operation, surgery is reserved for the acute and chronic complications of Crohn's disease refractory to medical or nutritional therapy. Indications include intestinal obstruction, fistula, abscess, uncontrolled hemorrhage, toxic megacolon, perforation, and growth failure in the setting of localized disease. Local resection is more successful in isolated small bowel disease than in the presence of colitis. Intractable colitis is managed by total proctocolectomy or segmental colectomy with anastomosis. The endorectal pull-through operation used for intractable ulcerative colitis never should be used for Crohn's disease because of the risk of perirectal or pelvic abscess or perianal disease. Perianal abscesses often need draining with probing or contrast agent injection to exclude underlying fistulas; proctectomy is rarely required to control perianal disease; and anal tags should not be excised.

■ PROSPECTIVE MANAGEMENT AND PROGNOSIS

Crohn's disease is a chronic incurable disease requiring careful surveillance, patient education, and expert management by a team consisting of a pediatrician, gastroenterologist, nutritionist, psychiatrist or psychologist, social worker, and nurse. An alliance with a pediatric surgeon familiar with inflammatory bowel disease is essential for management of potential complications. The success of long-term management is determined in part by the degree to which the patient and family understand and participate in the treatment.

The management of Crohn's disease in children is complex and requires adaptation of the patient to the lifelong unpredictable nature of this disease, the morbidity of chronic medication and hospital visits, and the demands of adolescent development. A willingness to become active in the management of his or her condition and to work with the team involved in each case is probably the patient's best prognostic feature.

(Abridged from W. Daniel Jackson and Richard J. Grand, Crohn's Disease, in Oski, DeAngelis, Feigin, McMillan, Warshaw: *Principles and Practice of Pediatrics, Second Edition,* J.B. Lippincott, 1994.)

Oski's Essential Pediatrics,
edited by Kevin B. Johnson and Frank A. Oski.
Lippincott–Raven Publishers,
Philadelphia © 1997

161

Ulcerative Colitis

Ulcerative colitis (UC) is a chronic relapsing inflammatory disease of the colon and rectum of unknown etiology.

■ PATHOLOGY

A comparison of the patterns of pathologic involvement in UC and Crohn's disease can be found in Chapter 160 (see Table 160–1). The distal colon is most severely affected, and the rectum is involved in most patients with UC. Inflammation is limited primarily to the mucosa and consists of continuous involvement along the length of the bowel with varying degrees of ulceration, hemorrhage, edema, and regenerating epithelium. Although considered to be limited to the colon, inflammation may extend uninterrupted to the cecum and up to 25 cm into the terminal ileum as "backwash" ileitis without stenosis or distortion.

■ ETIOLOGY

The cause of UC is unknown. No infective agent has been found, although the lesions resemble changes seen with infectious colitis. There is evidence of autoimmunity in terms of serum antibodies, immune-complex complement activation, and lymphocytes directed against colonic epithelium, but these phenomena are not consistently observed and do not correlate with disease activity. Although there are no specific heritable patterns, 15% to 40% of the patients may have other family members with inflammatory bowel disease, with an incidence about 10 times greater when there is a positive family history. However, concordance between monozygotic twins is low, and human leukocyte antigen (HLA) patterns have not been specific.

■ EPIDEMIOLOGY

The incidence of UC in children has gradually increased. The incidence in the general population ranges from 3.9 to 7.3 cases per 100,000, with a prevalence ranging from 41.1 to 79.9 cases per 100,000 population. The disease is more prevalent in Caucasians, with increased representation among those of Jewish backgrounds. UC occurs more commonly in Northern Europe and North America, with an urban predominance. Affected females outnumber affected males by about 50%. The distribution of age at onset is bimodal, with the major peak in the second and third decades and a second peak in the fifth and sixth decades. Between 15% and 40% of all the patients with UC present before age 20 years, with a peak onset in adolescence. The disease is rare in children less than 2 years old, although cases in infants have been reported. Most cases of infantile colitis are due to cow's milk or soy protein allergy and are transient.

■ CLINICAL PRESENTATION

There are at least four patterns of presentation of UC, differing in the extent of mucosal inflammation and systemic disturbance (Table 161–1). The most common presentation is the insidious onset of diarrhea and hematochezia (overt rectal bleeding), usually without systemic signs of fever, weight loss, or hypoalbuminemia. In these patients, the disease is often confined to the distal colon and rectum; the physical examination is normal, without abdominal tenderness; and the course remains mild, with intermittent exacerbations.

About 30% of the patients have moderate signs of systemic disturbance and present with bloody diarrhea, cramps, urgency, anorexia and weight loss, malaise, mild anemia, and low-grade or intermittent fever. Physical examination may reveal abdominal tenderness, and stool will show varying amounts of blood and leukocytes.

■ COMPLICATIONS

The most serious complication of UC, toxic megacolon, occurs in less than 5% of the patients and is a medical and surgical emergency. In this entity, dilatation of the diseased colon is accompanied by fever, tachycardia, hypokalemia, hypoalbuminemia, and dehydration. A leukocytosis with a predominance of immature neutrophils may be present. Some of these signs, particularly fever and tenderness, may be masked by high-dose steroid treatment. The patient with toxic megacolon is at risk for colonic perforation, gram-negative sepsis, and massive hemorrhage.

With longstanding disease, a colonic stricture may occur. In adults, this may be due to carcinoma; in children, benign postinflammatory fibrotic stricture is more likely. Intra-abdominal and hepatic abscesses occur less often than with Crohn's disease, except after perforation or colectomy.

■ DIAGNOSIS

The diagnosis of UC is based on clinical presentation, radiologic findings, mucosal appearance, and histology, as well as on the exclusion of other known etiologies of colitis. A complete history should be obtained, with attention to family history, exposure to infectious agents or antibiotic treatment, retardation in growth or sexual development, and extrain-

---

TABLE 161-1. UC Patterns of Presentation

EXTRAINTESTINAL (<5%)

Growth failure, arthropathy, erythema nodosum, occult fecal blood, elevated sedimentation rate, nonspecific abdominal pain, altered bowel pattern, cholangitis

MILD DISEASE (50%–60%)

Diarrhea, mild rectal bleeding, abdominal pain

No systemic disturbance

MODERATE DISEASE (30%)

Bloody diarrhea, cramps, urgency, abdominal tenderness

Systemic disturbance: anorexia, weight loss, mild fever, mild anemia

SEVERE DISEASE (10%)

More than six bloody stools per day, abdominal tenderness, ±distention, tachycardia, fever, weight loss, significant anemia, leukocytosis, hypoalbuminemia

testinal manifestations. The physical examination should include assessment of hydration, nutritional status, and systemic and extraintestinal signs of chronic disease. The presence of fever, orthostasis, tachycardia, abdominal tenderness, distention, or masses indicates moderate to severe disease and the need for hospitalization.

Laboratory Evaluation

A complete blood cell count will disclose leukocytosis or anemia. The erythrocyte sedimentation rate is elevated in about 70% of the patients and is a marker of inflammatory activity. Elevated serum transaminases and alkaline phosphatase may signify sclerosing cholangitis. Stool should be examined for blood, leukocytes, and ova and parasites. Culture of fresh stool should rule out common enteric pathogens. An assay for *Clostridium difficile* toxin should be obtained on all patients regardless of prior antibiotic treatment. Finding a pathogen does not exclude underlying inflammatory bowel disease in which the incidence of secondary infections is increased.

Radiology

Chest and abdominal radiographs, both upright and supine, will show the extent of colonic dilatation and help exclude obstruction due to stricture and pneumoperitoneum from perforation. These films form a baseline for later comparisons. A barium enema examination can be used to assess the character and extent of colonic disease but should never be performed in patients with acute, active colitis. In cases of mild to moderate colitis without dilatation, an air contrast barium enema study will reveal the mucosal detail necessary to detect ulcerations. Even without air contrast, a barium enema may reveal the chronic changes of foreshortening, loss of haustrations, pseudopolyps, and strictures as well as spasm (Figure 161–1). In moderately to severely ill patients with dilated bowel, extensive bleeding, persistent fever, or an abdominal mass, abdominal ultrasound or computed tomography (CT) scanning may demonstrate abscesses. Radionuclide studies are rarely helpful unless barium studies cannot be safely done.

Endoscopy

Flexible sigmoidoscopic or colonoscopic inspection of the colon and ileum, in conjunction with mucosal biopsies, is the most sensitive and specific means of evaluating intestinal inflammation. In many cases, it may make barium contrast studies unnecessary. Active disease is characterized by diffuse continuous involvement of the mucosa with edema, erythema, and friability. Erosions may be seen in the acute stages, followed by mucosal regeneration forming pseudopolyps in the atrophic mucosa of chronic disease. In UC, proctitis is usually present, and, although the entire colon may be involved, the distal colon usually is affected more severely. Biopsies should be obtained from multiple colonic levels, including the rectum.

■ DIFFERENTIAL DIAGNOSIS

Gastrointestinal (GI) complaints are prevalent in children: up to 10% of children, particularly those aged 7 to 11 years, may seek medical attention for the complaint of recurrent abdominal pain, usually periumbilical in location. In

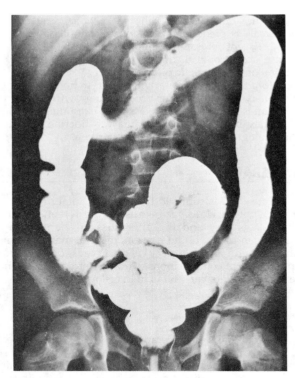

Figure 161-1. Single-contrast barium enema study in a 10-year-old boy with ulcerative colitis. There is continuous involvement of the entire colon with reflux of barium into the terminal ileum through a normal ileocecal valve. The small caliber, shortening and loss of haustra of the transverse and distal colon indicate long-standing disease. The irregular mucosal margins of the cecum and transverse colon suggest active ulceration. The poor coating and dilatation of the terminal ileum may represent backwash ileitis. There are no strictures or signs of obstruction.

most of these cases, extensive evaluation for inflammatory bowel disease is contraindicated unless there are associated features of fever, diarrhea, growth disturbance, or other extraintestinal manifestations. On the other hand, the periumbilical location of the pain is nonspecific and should not be considered pathognomonic for functional abdominal pain, because it is also characteristic of most cases of inflammatory bowel disease. In cases of uncomplicated recurrent abdominal pain, constipation, lactose intolerance, urinary tract infection, peptic disease, or psychosocial causes should be considered.

Rectal bleeding may be due to Meckel's diverticulum, hemolytic-uremic syndrome, polyposis, hemorrhoids, or anal fissures. The bleeding from Meckel's diverticulum is usually painless, copious, and without fecal leukocytes. Hemolytic-uremic syndrome can often be excluded by inspecting the blood smear and measuring the blood urea nitrogen. Polyps may be detected by sigmoidoscopy or barium enema. Fissures may be secondary to constipation or may be the perianal manifestations of Crohn's disease, particularly if inflammation is prominent.

Colitis, characterized by fecal leukocytes accompanying the bleeding and sigmoidoscopic evidence of inflammation, may be caused by infection or allergy. Infection with *Salmonella, Shigella, Campylobacter, Yersinia, Aeromonas*, certain strains of *Escherichia coli,* and *Entamoeba histolytica* may resemble UC and should be excluded. *C difficile* pseudomembranous colitis may be present even in the absence of a history of antibiotic treatment and seems to be more prevalent in patients with inflammatory bowel disease. Food proteins, usually cow's milk or soy protein in infancy, may produce an allergic colitis distinguished from UC only by histology, which in allergic disease reveals a predominant eosinophilic infiltration of the mucosa. Except for rare eosinophilic gastroenteritis, such a response occurs only in infancy and responds promptly to exclusion of the allergenic protein.

Before the onset of overt GI manifestations of UC, the patient may be followed for prodromal growth retardation or extraintestinal disease. For example, extraintestinal signs of UC may be mistaken for primary endocrine disorders, rheumatologic diseases, or anorexia nervosa.

■ THERAPY

Because UC is confined to the colon, total proctocolectomy is curative. However, because of the potential complications of surgery and the difficulties in adapting to an ileostomy and life without a colon, medical management is attempted initially. Surgery is reserved for failure to respond, severe complications, chronic steroid dependence, or excessive risk of carcinoma in longstanding disease.

Medical Therapy

The goals of medical therapy of UC in children are to control inflammation and symptoms and to prevent relapses. The choice of therapy depends on the severity of the inflammation.

Mild cases of colitis unaccompanied by systemic signs can be managed on an outpatient basis with rest, low-residue diet, and the gradual introduction of sulfasalazine or a non-sulfa 5-aminosalicylate alternative (Table 161–2). Response to treatment is expected within 2 weeks, with reduction in stool frequency, bleeding, and cramps. Subsequently, activity and diet may be liberalized as tolerated.

Moderate disease, when colitis is accompanied by systemic signs, requires hospitalization for proper evaluation, observation for complications, and management. In addition to bed rest and a low-residue diet, corticosteroids are given.

TABLE 161-2. Pharmacologic Therapy for UC

MODERATE TO SEVERE COLITIS

Methylprednisolone or prednisone: 1–2 mg/kg/day divided bid for 2 weeks; taper to 1–2 mg/kg/day qd over 4–6 weeks, depending on clinical response. When clinical remission is achieved, taper to qod and discontinue over another 4 weeks

Sulfasalazine: 40–50 mg/kg/day divided bid to qid initiated gradually during steroid taper in daily 250-mg increments until full dose is achieved (maximum, 3–4 g/day).

(Non-sulfa 5-amino salicylates (dose varies according to product used)

Folate supplementation: 1 mg/kg

MILD OR LOCALIZED DISTAL COLITIS

Sulfasalazine: 40–50 mg/kg/day divided bid to qid

Non-sulfa 5-amino salicylates (dose varies according to product used)

Folate: 1 mg/day

Hydrocortisone enemas

REFRACTORY DISEASE

Azathioprine: 2 mg/kg/day

6-Mercaptopurine: 1 mg/kg/day

PREVENTIVE MAINTENANCE

Sulfasalazine: 40–50 mg/kg/day divided bid to qid

Non-sulfa 5-amino salicylates (dose varies according to product used)

Folate: 1 mg/day

Sulfasalazine or a non-sulfa 5-aminosalicylate alternative may be used as an adjunct, although additional benefits have not been proved in disease of moderate or greater activity. Failure to respond to this regimen warrants a trial of bowel rest with nutritional support by elemental formula or parenteral nutrition. The immunosuppressant azathioprine or its active metabolite 6-mercaptopurine is useful in refractory disease dependent on chronic steroid therapy.

After blood has been drawn for culture and stool obtained for bacterial culture, parasite examination, and *C difficile* toxin assay, broad-spectrum antibiotic coverage should be instituted. Intravenous adrenocorticotropin or high-dose steroid treatment is essential. Serial abdominal radiographs should be obtained for surveillance of complications, which may be masked by steroid treatment. CT, radionuclide-labeled leukocyte scans, or ultrasound examination to search for abscesses is indicated in patients who fail to respond to treatment.

Nutritional Therapy

The goals of nutritional therapy are to restore metabolic homeostasis by correcting nutrient deficits and replacing ongoing losses, to provide sufficient energy and protein for positive nitrogen balance or net protein synthesis, and to promote catch-up growth toward premorbid percentiles. The provision of adequate nutrients is essential for optimal healing. In UC, where malabsorption is unlikely and increased metabolic requirements are small or unproved, the undernutrition is caused by a reduced voluntary intake of calories and protein. Guidelines for supplementation are to provide at least 140% of the recommended daily allowance (RDA) for height and age for both energy and protein. Continuous nocturnal nasogastric infusions of enteral formula through a soft Silastic catheter may be necessary for patients who cannot voluntarily increase their intake. For severe disease, when bowel rest is desired as an adjunct to medical treatment, parenteral nutrition through a central venous catheter or elemental diet is necessary to achieve nutritional goals.

Surgery

Surgery is indicated when medical and nutritional therapies fail to control the disease or prevent significant morbidity due to either disease or treatment. Although in most cases medical management is successful in controlling UC and prolonged remissions are possible, a cure can be obtained only by surgical excision.

Indications for colectomy in acute UC include uncontrolled hemorrhage, severe colitis that fails to respond within 2 weeks to intensive treatment (including corticosteroids, antibiotics, bowel rest, and nutritional support), and complications of toxic megacolon, stricture, or perforation. The morbidity and mortality of elective colectomy in a patient whose disease activity is controlled and whose nutritional status has been optimized are much less than in the acutely ill patient, whose risk of mortality can be up to 23% and who faces a greater prospect of postoperative complications.

■ PROSPECTIVE MANAGEMENT AND PROGNOSIS

UC is a chronic disease requiring careful surveillance, patient education, and expert management by a team consisting of a pediatrician, gastroenterologist, nutritionist, psychiatrist or psychologist, social worker, and nurse. An alliance with a pediatric surgeon familiar with inflammatory bowel disease is essential for the management of potential complications. The success of management depends on the degree to which the patient and family understand and participate in the treatment. Nutrition and growth, sexual maturation, psychosocial adjustment to disease, and compliance with therapy should all be monitored as carefully as one monitors the clinical signs and symptoms of disease activity outlined above.

The frequency of follow-up depends on the course and on activity, but intervals should be no greater than 6 months. Most children have the potential for a full active life with good general health. Ten percent of the patients will experience only the presenting episode of colitis but must be followed carefully because of the risk of cancer in later life. Some 20% of the patients will have intermittent symptoms, 50% will have chronic disease, and the remaining 20% will have chronic, active, incapacitating disease.

The risk of colonic carcinoma in pediatric-onset UC increases by an estimated 10% to 20% per decade after the first 10 years of disease, depending on the extent of involvement. Because the risk is cumulative, patients with persistent symptoms and pancolitis of early onset in youth are at greatest risk. The risk of carcinoma appears to be less in patients with left-sided colitis or proctitis. Most tumors arise in the distal colon and rectum and may be preceded by histologic signs of dysplasia. Histologic evidence of dysplasia warrants consideration of proctocolectomy.

The advent of steroids and potent immunosuppressants has dramatically altered the prognosis for medical management of UC, with fewer patients requiring surgery to control the disease. Most patients can resume full activities, including school attendance and athletics. UC has no specific effect on fertility and poses no risk to the fetus.

Despite the successes of medical management, there is no medical cure. The medications used to control the disease have potential morbidity, and the risk of colonic carcinoma is significant and cumulative, warranting careful surveillance.

(Abridged from W. Daniel Jackson and Richard J. Grand, Ulcerative Colitis, in Oski, DeAngelis, Feigin, McMillan, Warshaw: *Principles and Practice of Pediatrics, Second Edition*, J.B. Lippincott, 1994.)

Oski's Essential Pediatrics,
edited by Kevin B. Johnson and Frank A. Oski.
Lippincott–Raven Publishers,
Philadelphia © 1997

162

Chronic Recurrent Abdominal Pain

Chronic, recurrent abdominal pain is undoubtedly the most frustrating problem a pediatrician must manage. It is also common. Unless the diagnosis is dealt with in a positive manner and the parents develop confidence in that diagnosis, they will constantly seek medical advice and frequently shop around for answers.

It is imperative that the physician approach the diagnosis of chronic recurrent abdominal pain with confidence. The pediatrician must never doubt that the child is in actual pain and must build a trusting relationship with the parents.

■ DIFFERENTIAL DIAGNOSIS

The common entities that cause chronic recurrent abdominal pain of childhood, listed in their approximate order of frequency, are functional abdominal pain, lactose intolerance, simple constipation, musculoskeletal pain, parasitic infection, reflux esophagitis, peptic ulcer disease, and inflammatory bowel disease. Most of these diagnoses can be screened without a multitude of laboratory and x-ray examinations.

Lactose intolerance is probably the second most common cause of abdominal pain in childhood. If a child is genetically programmed to become lactase deficient, the activity of this enzyme gradually begins to decrease around 4 to 6 years of age. Early in the development of lactose intolerance, pain may be the sole symptom.

Dietary restriction may be the easiest way to establish lactose intolerance as a cause of abdominal pain. The child should be given a lactose-free diet for about 2 weeks. If the abdominal pain disappears, the diagnosis can be suspected. However, it should be confirmed by giving the child lactose again and observing for reexacerbation of symptoms. This cycle should be completed twice to ensure that lactose intolerance is present.

Musculoskeletal pain arising from the abdominal muscles is a diagnosis that can be overlooked easily. School-age children are frequently engaged in competitive sports and subjected to intensive exercise training programs. These can result in strained muscles and chronic myositis of specific muscle bundles. The pain is usually described as sharp or knifelike and may be triggered by various activities or body positions. It is usually located at or near the insertion of the rectus or oblique muscles into the costal margin or iliac crest. If the abdominal muscles are tightened during the physical examination and the pain still is reproduced by palpation, the origin is undoubtedly musculoskeletal.

Many other diseases can cause abdominal pain in children, but most of the other diagnoses are associated with other symptoms. If the child complains only of abdominal pain and results of all of the tests suggested earlier are negative, the physician should feel comfortable in making the diagnosis of functional abdominal pain.

■ TREATMENT

If the diagnosis of functional abdominal pain is made, it is helpful to discuss this diagnosis with the parents in the same manner as organic disease. The physician must convey the message that the pain is real but is not caused by a process that will become progressively worse and threaten the life of the child. The analogy of a headache in an adult is useful. The pain of a headache is real, but it is treated only as pain, and, under normal circumstances, it is not allowed to interfere with daily responsibilities. A child's responsibility is to go to school, and pain should not prevent this from happening. If the pain is severe, it should be treated with medications, such as acetaminophen. Antimotility agents are usually ineffective. Using a hot pad or hot water bottle as a counterirritant is sometimes helpful. Above all, the physician should instill confidence in parents that the pain is not threatening to their child's well-being and will disappear as the child matures.

(Abridged from William J. Glish, Chronic Recurrent Abdominal Pain, in Oski, DeAngelis, Feigin, McMillan, Warshaw: *Principles and Practice of Pediatrics, Second Edition*, J.B. Lippincott, 1994.)

Oski's Essential Pediatrics,
edited by Kevin B. Johnson and Frank A. Oski.
Lippincott–Raven Publishers,
Philadelphia © 1997

163

Henoch-Schönlein Syndrome

Henoch-Schönlein syndrome, also known as anaphylactoid, allergic, or rheumatoid purpura, Henoch-Schönlein purpura, and the Schönlein-Henoch syndrome, is primarily a disorder of childhood.

■ CLINICAL MANIFESTATIONS

Most cases of Henoch-Schönlein syndrome occur in children younger than 7 years of age, although adult cases have been reported. The entity is uncommon in infants younger than 1 year of age. Males are affected more frequently than females in most reported series. Although all races are susceptible, Caucasians predominate in most series.

The syndrome usually presents in a previously healthy child. The onset may be acute, with many features appearing at once, or gradual, with symptoms appearing over days to several weeks. The frequency of signs and symptoms is listed in Table 163–1. Low-grade fever and malaise are common early in the illness. Half of the patients present with a skin rash, which is central to the diagnosis. Occasionally, the rash appears several weeks after other signs are noticed. The time of appearance of other features varies, although, in most cases, involvement of the joints, gastrointestinal (GI) tract, and skin occur within several days of onset.

Skin lesions, which occur in all patients, may be urticarial at the onset, occasionally developing hemorrhagic centers similar to erythema multiforme. More often, a reddish, nonpruritic, maculopapular rash subsequently appears, frequently coalescing to form larger purpuric areas. Scattered petechial lesions may be seen. The rash is typically located on the lower extremities and buttocks, but may involve the trunk, face, and upper extremities. The lesions arise in crops and follow the usual evolution of ecchymoses, turning brown, then yellow, and fading over several days. Ulceration and scarring are rarely seen.

Subcutaneous edema of the dorsum of the hands, feet, scalp, ears, and periorbital region occurs in as many as half of the patients. This nonpitting, localized swelling may be tender and distorting. It is more common in children younger than 3 years of age.

GI involvement occurs in as many as 85% of patients (see Table 163–1). Colicky abdominal pain occurs in as many as 70% of patients and in 14% of patients may precede other symptoms by several weeks. The diagnostic difficulties may prompt a laparotomy. Other common symptoms are melena or guaiac-positive stools (56%), ileus (40%), vomiting (25%), and hematemesis (10%). Life-threatening complications such as massive GI hemorrhage and intussusception may occur in 5% and 3% of cases, respectively. Hemorrhage from the stomach has been reported frequently and may require surgical intervention. In Henoch-Schönlein syndrome, intussusception is more common in older children and is frequently ileoileal; the lead point may be formed by submucosal hemorrhages. Surgical reduction is usually recommended. The more usual presentation seen in children younger than 3 years of age is

ileocolic intussusception. Other, less common modes of GI involvement include pancreatitis, intestinal perforation, vasculitis of the gallbladder, and protein-losing enteropathy. Hepatomegaly of uncertain cause has been described in as many as 10% of patients.

Joint pains with periarticular swelling occur in two thirds of patients with Henoch-Schönlein syndrome. In approximately 25%, joint symptoms may precede the rash. Large joints are most frequently affected; less commonly, fingers and wrists may be involved. The joint space is normal, and warmth and effusions are rare. Joint involvement is the most transient feature of Henoch-Schönlein syndrome and resolves without residual damage. The incidence of renal disease varies from 40% to 60% in different studies. The spectrum of findings ranges from microscopic hematuria in 50% of those with renal involvement to gross hematuria (40%), nephrotic syndrome (30%), mild proteinuria (25%), and acute nephritis with hypertension (15%); in 5% of patients, the renal disease progresses to chronic renal failure.

Renal involvement appears before other symptoms in only 3% of patients. In some cases, renal disease occurs as the other manifestations are resolving; this pattern is thought by some to herald a more complicated renal course. More severe renal disease seems to occur in older children and is often associated with the increased severity of other symptoms.

The clinical course is favorable if microscopic hematuria alone is noticed. If diffuse involvement with crescent formation in more than 50% of glomeruli occurs, the clinical manifestations are more severe, and the frequency of progression to chronic renal failure is higher.

Acute scrotal involvement is seen in 10% to 15% of males. Scrotal involvement occasionally is severe enough to suggest testicular torsion, but surgical exploration usually reveals local hemorrhage or hematoma of the scrotum and its contents. Technetium 99m pertechnetate imaging has been used to differentiate the two entities. Hyperemia is seen in Henoch-Schönlein syndrome, but the tracer activity is absent in testicular torsion.

The incidence of neurologic symptoms varies with the definition used. It has been estimated at 2% to 8% in most series, but, if behavioral changes and headaches are included, as many as 43% of patients may be affected. Other manifestations of central nervous system (CNS) involvement include seizures in half of patients with neurologic symptoms, focal neurologic deficits in a third, and peripheral nerve involvement in only a few.

Seizures may be associated with cerebral ischemia secondary to the vasculitis, or with subarachnoid, subdural, cortical or intraparenchymal hemorrhages. Hypertension associated with renal disease is an additional complication. Most symptoms are transient, although permanent deficits can result from hemorrhage or rarely from infarction.

Rare complications attributed to Henoch-Schönlein syndrome have included pulmonary hemorrhages, cardiac involvement, intramuscular hemorrhage, and ureteral vasculitis with stenosis.

■ LABORATORY DATA

No pathognomonic laboratory tests are available for Henoch-Schönlein syndrome. There is usually a leukocytosis of 10,000 to 20,000/mm^3 with a left shift. Normochromic anemia is frequent, possibly reflecting intestinal blood loss. The erythrocyte sedimentation rate is mildly elevated in as many as 75% of patients. Platelet counts are usually normal, although thrombocytosis has been reported; coagulation studies are normal.

The total hemolytic complement levels are low in a third of patients, associated with normal C3 and C4 but with low properdin levels. Serum immunoglobulins are raised early in the course and return to normal after several months. Assays for antinuclear antibodies and IgG rheumatoid factors are negative. Factor XIII (ie, fibrin-stabilizing factor) is lower in Henoch-Schönlein syndrome than other types of vasculitis. Concentrations lower than 50% of normal reportedly herald complications, and levels normalize with resolution of the disease. Abdominal symptoms are particularly associated with low Factor XIII levels.

Renal disease may be implicated on urinary microscopy by the demonstration of blood, casts, and protein in the urine. Serum creatinine and blood urea nitrogen levels may be elevated, and electrolyte alterations and hypoalbuminemia may be found. In more severe cases of nephritis or nephrotic syndrome, a renal biopsy may be indicated.

Radiologic studies with contrast agents show abnormalities most often in the small intestine, predominantly the duodenum and jejunum. Hypomotility, thickened folds, pseudotumors, and "thumbprinting" characteristic of submucosal hemorrhages may be seen. The terminal ileum may show changes resembling those of Crohn's ileitis. Residual damage may later manifest as small intestinal strictures. Colonic involvement is unusual. Intussusception is sometimes demonstrated. Ultrasound has been advocated for the diagnosis intussusception; the bowel forms a characteristic "Swiss roll" pattern.

Endoscopy may reveal erosive gastritis and duodenitis, and punctate, erythematous lesions may coalesce, giving rise to purpuric lesions. Colonic aphthoid ulcers and rectal ulcers have been observed. Sigmoid biopsies have shown only nonspecific acute and chronic inflammatory changes that are most prominent around the vessels.

■ DIFFERENTIAL DIAGNOSIS

For the complete syndrome, the diagnosis is rarely in question. Because single manifestations can appear before the characteristic rash, other causes of acute abdominal pain must be considered, and the child must be evaluated for nephritis or arthritis.

Similar rashes may be seen with septicemia, coagulopathies, systemic lupus erythematosus, hemolytic uremic syndrome, and after streptococcal glomerulonephritis. Blood cultures, low C3 levels, and positive assays for antinuclear antibodies, abnormal platelet counts, and clotting studies can differentiate these entities from Henoch-Schönlein syndrome.

Nephritis with mesangial IgA deposits may be seen in Iga nephropathy (ie, Berger's disease), systemic lupus erythematosus, and cirrhosis. More severe renal involvement usually occurs after other manifestations have appeared, readily differentiating Henoch-Schönlein syndrome from other causes of glomerulonephritis. However, some authorities think that Henoch-Schönlein syndrome is the systemic form of IgA nephropathy. This view is supported by the observations that both diseases may occur in the same patient, within the same family or in identical twins of which one developed IgA nephropathy and the other Henoch-Schönlein syndrome. Immunologic and genetic differences and different clinical courses of the two diseases suggest that they are distinct disorders with common renal pathology.

Rheumatoid arthritis and rheumatic fever may cause joint pains with skin rashes but are easily differentiated from Henoch-Schönlein syndrome. Polyarteritis nodosa involving skin, kidneys, joints, and GI tract may be difficult to differentiate from Henoch-Schönlein syndrome. Muscles are often involved, and cardiac involvement should be sought.

TABLE 163-1. Frequency of Signs and Symptoms in Henoch-Schönlein Syndrome

Manifestation	% of Patients
Rash	100
Abdominal pain	70
Joint pain	60–90
Guaiac-positive stools	56
Subcutaneous edema	50
Fever	50
Ileus	40
Hematuria	30–40
Vomiting	25
Proteinuria	10–20
Scrotal involvement	10–15 of males
Hematemesis	10
Hepatomegaly	10
CNS involvement	2–8
GI hemorrhage	5
Intussusception	3

■ TREATMENT

Treatment is supportive. In acute cases, adequate hydration should be provided, and the patient should be monitored for possible complications. Frequent assessment of vital signs and hematocrit, stool examination for blood, and abdominal examinations are important. Any sudden increase in abdominal symptoms may be secondary to intussusception or perforation of the bowel or to pancreatitis. Because the location of intussusception in Henoch-Schönlein syndrome is more commonly in the small bowel, surgical intervention is usually required. Intracranial complications may be manifested by sudden changes in behavior or level of consciousness. The nephropathy is treated with attention to fluid balance, electrolyte status, salt intake, and the possibility of hypertension.

Optimal nutrition should be maintained, especially during more prolonged courses. Salicylates may alleviate joint discomfort, but they should be used with caution if abdominal symptoms appear prominent, especially if the possibility of GI bleeding exists.

Considerable controversy has surrounded the use of corticosteroids, particularly for abdominal pain. Anecdotal evidence suggests a role for a short course of prednisone for 5 to 7 days to hasten resolution of pain. Steroid administration has been advocated by some to reduce the likelihood of intussusception. The response in individual cases has been striking, and no ill effects of use of prednisone in this manner have been reported. No controlled, prospective trials have been performed to address this problem, and retrospective studies leave the optimal management in doubt. Many patients improve without specific intervention, and corticosteroids are not recommended for skin rash, edema, joint pains, or renal disease. Major manifestations of localized vasculitis in the lungs, testes, and CNS should be treated with corticosteroids.

Severe renal involvement has been treated with aza-thioprine or cyclophosphamide in combination with pred-nisone to reduce long-term renal disease. However, the use-fulness of this therapy has not been established by a controlled study. The clinical manifestations of Henoch-Schönlein syndrome, especially abdominal symptoms, were significantly improved between 1 and 3 days after adminis-tration of Factor XIII concentrate. Relapse of abdominal symptoms was associated with a subsequent fall in plasma Factor XIII levels.

■ CLINICAL COURSE AND PROGNOSIS

In the absence of renal disease and major CNS involve-ment, the prognosis is excellent. The illness lasts for 4 to 6 weeks in most cases, although approximately half of the patients have one or more recurrences, usually within 6 weeks but sometimes as late as 7 years after the onset of ill-ness. Children younger than 3 years of age tend to have a shorter, milder course and fewer recurrences.

In rare cases, long-term morbidity is accounted for by residual CNS damage. Chronic renal disease develops in 10% to 25% of those who have nephritis initially (5% of all patients). Long-term follow-up is usually necessary in patients with renal involvement, because progression of renal disease may not occur for many years. Microscopic hematuria alone is asso-ciated with good long-term prognosis. The outcome of more severe renal involvement is less predictable. Although nephrotic syndrome with crescent formation in more than 50% of glomeruli is more often associated with a poor outcome, as many as 40% of these patients may have normal long-term renal function.

(Abridged from Steven R. Martin, David A. Bross, and W. Allan Walker, Henoch-Schönlein Syndrome, in Oski, DeAngelis, Feigin, McMillan, Warshaw: *Principles and Practice of Pediatrics, Second Edition,* J.B. Lippincott, 1994.)

Oski's Essential Pediatrics,
edited by Kevin B. Johnson and Frank A. Oski.
Lippincott–Raven Publishers,
Philadelphia © 1997

164

Protein Intolerance

An *adverse reaction* to food is a general term implying any abnormal response to food or food additives. *Food intolerance* means any physiologic abnormality attributed to food ingestion, including immunologic and nonimmuno-logic (*eg,* toxic, metabolic, or pharmacologic) mechanisms. *Food allergy, food hypersensitivity,* or *protein intolerance* implies an immunologic reaction to a protein component of the diet that can be reproduced in food challenges. *Food anaphylaxis* is a subset of food allergies in which an IgE-mediated (type I) hypersensitivity reaction occurs. This chapter focuses on the latter two categories, with emphasis on the allergic enteropathies likely to come to the attention of pediatricians; allergic processes causing systemic reac-tions are described elsewhere in this book.

■ COMMON FOOD ANTIGENS

Whether because of the widespread use of cow's milk–based formulas or because of the antigenic potential of their proteins, allergic reactions to cow's milk proteins are clearly the most clinically important in infancy. Patients with cow's milk allergy react to multiple milk proteins, of which more than 20 have been identified. Food processing tech-niques, such as pasteurization and homogenization, can alter protein structure and the antigenicity of these proteins. Soy proteins can induce allergic disease, with clinical symp-toms and intestinal biopsies resembling those of cow's milk allergy. The enteropathy associated with gluten sensitivity (*ie,* celiac disease) is a special type of food intolerance and is discussed in Chapter 166.

An important aspect of food allergy is the impact of age and illness. Immaturity seems to favor priming the systemic immune response in the face of antigen uptake instead of the development of tolerance, which is a more mature response. In states of intestinal inflammation, ulceration, immunodefi-ciency, or malnutrition, intact proteins more readily cross the intestinal mucosa barrier. The immature or damaged barri-ers allow increased antigen uptake, with the risk of sensiti-zation and subsequent allergic response.

■ COW'S MILK PROTEIN INTOLERANCE

Allergy to cow's milk proteins was first described early in this century. The prevalence of this disorder is believed to be 0.5% to 7.5% among European and North American infants. Risk factors include a family history of atopy and early dietary exposure to cow's milk. The age of onset is directly correlated with the time of introduction of artificial formulas. Even exclusively breast-fed infants can develop symptoms of protein intolerance, which may respond to elimination of the offending agent from the mother's diet.

Gastrointestinal Manifestations

Symptoms referable to the gastrointestinal (GI) tract are among the most common in cow's milk allergy, occurring in 50% to 80% of patients. Several clinical entities have been described. These are probably related to a variety of immune responses other than type I, IgE-mediated disease (*eg,* Arthus reactions, T-cell cytotoxic reactions).

Colitis

The presentation of milk-induced colitis can range from asymptomatic GI blood loss with anemia to explosive bloody diarrhea and hypovolemic shock. Depending on the clinical setting, the differential diagnosis is broad and can include infectious gastroenteritis (*eg, Salmonella, Shigella, Yersinia, Campylobacter, Clostridium difficile*), necrotizing ente-rocolitis, sepsis, inflammatory bowel disease, intussuscep-tion, volvulus, and bowel infarction. Structural causes of GI bleeding such as polyps, Meckel's diverticulum, and arteri-ovenous malformations may need to be considered. Historic features suggesting allergic colitis include recent ingestion of cow's milk and a family history of allergic disease.

Evaluation of these infants should include a thorough search for infectious agents, a complete blood count with a differential count, and coagulation studies. Peripheral eosinophilia is often seen, and a Wright's stain of the stool can reveal eosinophils. The diagnosis can be confirmed by flexible sigmoidoscopy.

Eosinophilic Enteritis

Controversy exists about the role of protein intolerance in the pathogenesis of eosinophilic enteritis, a clinicopathologic entity distinct from allergic enterocolitis and the enteropathy described earlier. These patients often respond to treatment similar to that given to children with milk-induced colitis or enteropathy. This syndrome is discussed fully in Chapter 165.

Other Gastrointestinal Symptoms

Symptoms and syndromes ranging from irritable bowel syndrome, abdominal migraine, gastroesophageal reflux, and chronic aphthous ulcerations have been ascribed to protein intolerance, but usually without convincing proof of an immunologic basis. Colic is often treated by dietary manipulation, although its relation to true protein intolerance is rarely documented. Food intolerance or allergy may be the cause of colic in 10% to 12% of otherwise healthy infants, and a change of formulas may improve symptoms. The resolution of colic coincident with a change in formula is a necessary but not sufficient condition to prove an allergic cause for these symptoms. Because frequent formula changes during infancy can convince the parents that their children are particularly susceptible to allergies and other illnesses, any treatment of colic by a formula change should be done with the reassurance that food allergy in infants is usually a short-lived phenomenon and that many factors may contribute to colic.

Nongastrointestinal Manifestations

Shock due to anaphylactic reactions to food represents a true hypersensitivity reaction, although it is the least common form of all food allergies. Unlike the enteropathies described earlier, whose clinical expressions uniformly lessen with advancing age, a small percentage of patients with IgE-mediated reactions retain their allergy for life. Because anaphylaxis can occur with ingestion of minute amounts of antigen, any diagnostic challenge of a patient with purported allergens must occur with venous access ensured and epinephrine, antihistamines, and steroids available. Other immediate reactions include urticarial rashes, lip swelling, and laryngeal edema. A study of a series of 13 fatal or near-fatal anaphylactic reactions to food found that two thirds of the fatal but none of the nonfatal reactions occurred at school, emphasizing the need for heightened public awareness of and preparedness for these emergencies.

■ EVALUATION OF SUSPECTED FOOD ALLERGY

The utility of radioallergosorbent testing (RAST) to detect food allergy is limited by the technique's measurement of IgE antibodies, which are the immunologic mediators in only a select group of patients. In patients with acute-onset dermatologic or respiratory manifestations of cow's milk allergy, the sensitivity and specificity of RAST are approximately 80%. In patients with GI symptoms, RAST testing is usually much less helpful.

Skin tests in the assessment of food allergy have similar degrees of sensitivity and specificity as RAST, but they are usually less expensive than RAST. However, skin testing can be technically difficult when performed on infants and is more reliable in children older than 3 years of age. A negative skin test in older children is helpful in ruling out disease, although a positive test does not confirm the diagnosis.

The use of food challenges has greatly aided the scientific study of protein intolerance, and double-blind, placebo-controlled challenges have become the gold standard for diagnosis.

■ TREATMENT OF PROTEIN INTOLERANCE

The therapeutic mainstay in protein intolerance is strict dietary avoidance of the offending antigen. In the case of cow's milk intolerance, soy-based or casein hydrolysate formulas may be used, although as many as 25% of the infants who exhibit intolerance to cow's milk protein are intolerant of soy. Casein hydrolysate formulas, in which the in vitro breakdown of casein leads to small peptides with molecular weights less than 1200, are recommended by the American Academy of Pediatrics Committee on Nutrition for the treatment of protein intolerance. Unfortunately, these formulas are expensive and unpalatable, two factors that detract from their effectiveness.

■ PREVENTION

Because many of the symptoms of cow's milk protein intolerance occur most frequently in the first year of life, exclusive breast-feeding during this time, with delayed introduction of solid foods until 4 to 6 months of age, helps to prevent the onset of this food allergy. This advice should be given to parents of infants with a strong family history of atopy, and it is in keeping with the American Academy of Pediatrics recommendations for infant nutrition. Whether exclusive breast-feeding early in infancy protects against the development of other allergic diseases or merely delays their onset remains controversial.

(Abridged from Christopher Duggan and W. Allan Walker, Protein Intolerance, in Oski, DeAngelis, Feigin, McMillan, Warshaw: *Principles and Practice of Pediatrics, Second Edition*, J.B. Lippincott, 1994.)

Oski's Essential Pediatrics, edited by Kevin B. Johnson and Frank A. Oski. Lippincott–Raven Publishers, Philadelphia © 1997

165

Eosinophilic Gastroenteritis

Eosinophilic gastroenteritis is a rare clinicopathologic entity that occurs during infancy, childhood, and adolescence. The clinical manifestations include vomiting, abdominal pain, malabsorption, gastrointestinal (GI) obstruction, and ascites. The cause is unknown, but the disease has been associated with allergic symptoms. In the appropriate clinical setting, the diagnosis of eosinophilic gastroenteritis requires a histologic demonstration of markedly increased numbers of eosinophils in the GI tract.

■ DIAGNOSIS

Physical findings are usually nonspecific. Hepatosplenomegaly and lymphadenopathy have been reported, and longstanding disease may produce malnutrition.

Peripheral eosinophilia is an inconsistent finding, occurring in 13% to 85% of patients. Eosinophilia usually does not occur in circumscribed disease. IgE levels appear to be elevated in patients with more severe disease but not consistently. Charcot-Leyden crystals, derived from eosinophils, can sometimes be found in the stool. In diffuse disease, malabsorption may occur, and the bone marrow may be infiltrated with eosinophils.

GI biopsies, usually obtained at endoscopy, are the cornerstone of diagnosis. Involved tissue may appear erythematous, granular, nodular, or ulcerated but often looks normal. Because the lesions may appear normal and involvement is often patchy, it is essential to obtain multiple biopsy specimens, which include the antrum, for histologic evaluation. Occasionally, the diagnosis is made at exploratory laparotomy; serosal disease may present with an acute abdomen or if muscular disease causes complete obstruction.

■ DIFFERENTIAL DIAGNOSIS

The nonspecific symptoms seen in cases of eosinophilic gastroenteritis make the diagnosis difficult unless a high index of suspicion is maintained. Peripheral eosinophilia may be helpful, but other conditions such as collagen vascular diseases, especially polyarteritis nodosa, and enteroinvasive parasitic infestation should be excluded.

■ TREATMENT

No specific treatment or consistently effective diet is available. An elimination diet should be attempted if the clinical symptoms are mild and the allergen can be identified. If a clear association between the disease and the ingestion of specific foods has been demonstrated, symptoms can improve markedly after the offending agents are discontinued. The use of elimination diets in patients without a clear precipitant has not been particularly useful, although there are reports of long-lasting responses. If elimination diets are used for prolonged periods, care should be taken to ensure a complete and well-balanced diet.

■ PROGNOSIS

The prognosis varies according to the type and extent of eosinophilic infiltration. For circumscribed and muscle layer disease, the prognosis is excellent, particularly if surgical intervention alleviates the symptoms.

For diffuse mucosal disease, the prognosis varies. Some patients have long-term remissions, but others have chronic disease requiring prolonged steroid therapy. Complications include small bowel bacterial overgrowth, hemorrhage, and perforation. No malignant transformation has been reported.

(Abridged from Glenn T. Furuta and W. Allan Walker, Eosinophilic Gastroenteritis, in Oski, DeAngelis, Feigin, McMillan, Warshaw: *Principles and Practice of Pediatrics, Second Edition*, J.B. Lippincott, 1994.)

Oski's Essential Pediatrics, edited by Kevin B. Johnson and Frank A. Oski. Lippincott–Raven Publishers, Philadelphia © 1997

166

Malabsorption States

Impaired intestinal absorption of nutrients may result from several clinical conditions, including short bowel syndrome, small bowel bacterial overgrowth, celiac disease, and various immunodeficiency states. Malabsorption of carbohydrate can result in failure to thrive, diarrhea, and weight loss, but, unlike malabsorption of essential amino acids, fatty acids, vitamins, or minerals, it does not lead to specific nutrient deficiencies.

■ SHORT BOWEL SYNDROME

Short bowel syndrome can be caused by prenatal events, such as congenital short bowel, volvulus, small bowel atresia, or gastroschisis. Acquired causes of the syndrome include volvulus, necrotizing enterocolitis, meconium ileus, and Crohn's disease. Because most cases occur in the perinatal period, the remaining length of bowel must be sufficient to allow the nutrient absorption required for growth. Despite the compensatory intestinal growth, dominated by villous hyperplasia, that usually occurs, various degrees of nutrient malabsorption may persist.

The adaptation phase that follows massive resection of the intestine can last as long as 3 years. Total oral or enteral nutrition ultimately may be feasible if at least 20 to 30 cm of small bowel remains and the ileocecal valve is intact. During the adaptation period and sometimes during periods of accelerated growth, intravenous nutrition may be mandatory. When a patient is being weaned from intravenous nutrition, prolonged enteral feedings administered as a constant infusion through a nasogastric tube or a gastrostomy may be necessary. The degree of carbohydrate, protein, and fat malabsorption that results from a short bowel is related to the extent of the resection, the segment of bowel resected, and the existence of the ileocecal valve.

After proximal small bowel resection, iron, zinc, and folate deficiency may occur in addition to decreased absorption of calcium, magnesium, and phosphorus. Resection of the colon may result in water and sodium losses. The small bowel may compensate for the absence of the colon through an increased capacity to reabsorb water and electrolytes. Calcium and magnesium soaps may form in the lumen of the bowel in cases of fat malabsorption and lead to hypocalcemia and hypomagnesemia. Pancreatic secretions may be decreased after a proximal resection because of the loss of stimulation by cholecystokinin.

The treatment of short bowel syndrome includes the use of lactose-free, elemental diets with low osmolality. If small bowel bacterial overgrowth occurs, it must be treated.

■ SMALL BOWEL BACTERIAL OVERGROWTH

In healthy persons, the stomach, duodenum, and upper small bowel are sterile or the number of organisms never surpasses 10^5 colony-forming units per milliliter (CFU/mL). Mechanisms such as gastric acidity, secretions of the intestine and pancreas, immunoglobulins, and especially intestinal peristalsis aid in maintaining a low bacterial count. The distal ileum contains as many as 10^9 CFU/mL, including gram-negative bacilli and anaerobes. The ileocecal valve is important in preventing an anaerobic, colonic-type flora in the distal small bowel. Impairment of any of these mechanisms may result in small bowel bacterial overgrowth. The clinical entities in which bacterial overgrowth may occur are listed in Table 166–1.

Small bowel bacterial overgrowth frequently leads to malabsorption of carbohydrate because of intraluminal use by bacteria. Presenting symptoms are abdominal distention as a result of gas formation, vomiting, and diarrhea. Diarrhea can result from bacterial degradation of brush border disacchari-dases and from a decrease in small bowel villous height and a consequent decrease in the transport of monosaccharides.

The diagnosis of small bowel bacterial overgrowth is made by intestinal intubation, aspiration, culture, and colony count of intestinal fluid. High fasting breath hydrogen levels may herald bacterial overgrowth. Treatment includes the correction of the underlying abnormality by resection of intestinal strictures or adhesions or the use of sulfonamides or oral antibiotics, such as kanamycin, neomycin, or gentamicin. In older children, metronidazole or tetracyclines may be used. An ion exchange resin such as cholestyramine may help bind bacterial products such as bile acids.

■ CELIAC DISEASE

Celiac disease is characterized by villous atrophy of the proximal small bowel, and it responds to the withdrawal of gluten from the diet. The fraction of gluten called gliadin has been identified as the agent responsible for the disease. The relation between celiac disease and intolerance to dietary wheat and rye was recognized by Dicke in 1950. The highest rate of celiac disease occurs in Ireland, where 1 in 300 persons is affected. The prevalence in some areas of the United States is estimated to be 1 in 2000. For unknown reasons, the prevalence of this disease is slowly decreasing.

TABLE 166-1. Factors Predisposing to Small Bowel Bacterial Overgrowth

CONGENITAL BOWEL ABNORMALITIES	CHANGES IN PERISTALSIS
Gastroschisis	Chronic diarrhea
Small bowel atresia	Pseudo-obstruction
Meconium ileus	Scleroderma
Malrotation	Diabetes
Duodenal webs	**NUTRITIONAL FACTORS**
ABDOMINAL SURGERY	Celiac disease
Postoperative adhesions	Malnutrition (severe)
Intestinal bypass surgery	Hypokalemia
Roux-en-Y procedures	**HYPOCHLORHYDRIA**
Short bowel	
Gastrectomy	**OTHER**
Vagotomy	Nasojejunal tubes
ACQUIRED BOWEL ABNORMALITIES	Antacids, H²-receptor blockers
Crohn's disease	
Tumors	Cystic fibrosis
Fistulas	

The age at which cereal is introduced into the diet and the amount and type of cereal ingested may affect the presentation of the disease. Precocious presentation may occur between 10 to 18 months of age with frothy, liquid, foul-smelling stools. The child acquires the celiac aspect, characterized by wasting and severe abdominal distention, at approximately 1 year of age. The other form of presentation occurs at 2 to 3 years of age with poor feeding, lack of weight gain for several months or actual weight loss, irritability, and diarrhea consisting of foul-smelling, bulky stools. Mono-symptomatic forms may present with constipation or severe, recurrent abdominal pain.

Laboratory analyses are nonspecific, and serum abnormalities, such as low hemoglobin, iron, albumin, cholesterol, calcium, phosphate, vitamin A, or carotene levels, are related to the malabsorption but are nonspecific for the disease. Fat globules may be identified in a stool smear, and fat malabsorption can be quantified by means of a 72-hour stool collection (ie, normal absorption >95% of ingested fat). After ingestion of D-xylose, the serum level 1 hour later remains low. However, this test is not sensitive and is not specific for celiac disease. Intestinal permeability tests using small-molecular-weight sugars can detect alteration of the small bowel mucosa. Although elevated serum levels of antigliadin antibodies and antireticulin antibodies may indicate the disease, the diagnosis requires a peroral small bowel biopsy. Endomysial antibodies seem to be the most sensitive and specific of the noninvasive tests for the diagnosis of celiac disease.

A small bowel biopsy can demonstrate moderate to severe villous atrophy and a chronic inflammatory infiltrate of the lamina propia. If the biopsy results support the clinical and laboratory findings, the patient is placed on a gluten-free diet for 6 to 12 months. Small bowel biopsy repeated at the end of this period should demonstrate normalization of the villous architecture. To confirm the diagnosis, the patient is reexposed to gluten for 2 years or until symptoms recur, at which time a third biopsy is recommended. This biopsy should demonstrate recurrence of villous atrophy and chronic inflammatory infiltrate. The strict diagnostic criteria have been revised.

■ IMMUNODEFICIENCY STATES INCLUDING GASTROINTESTINAL MANIFESTATIONS OF AIDS

The gastrointestinal (GI) manifestations observed in patients with acquired immunodeficiency syndrome (AIDS) include esophagitis and diarrhea with or without parasitic, viral, or bacterial infections. Nutrient malabsorption is not always a factor in the illness, although children may have nutrient malabsorption even if they do not have overt symptoms.

Organisms commonly associated with the diarrhea in AIDS patients are *Candida albicans*, *Cryptosporidium*, cyto-megalovirus, atypical mycobacteria, and *Salmonella typhimurium*. Even in the absence of systemic or enteric infections or malignancy, many adult and pediatric AIDS patients suffer from chronic diarrhea, anorexia, and weight loss. *Mycobacterium avium-intracellulare* has been found in the small bowel of patients with AIDS and has been associated with diarrhea.

AIDS may be expressed as a failure to thrive, with or without diarrhea. Diarrhea and malabsorption are more prevalent in patients with documented GI infections. Increased fecal fat, diminished appetite, and weight loss are frequently observed in these patients. A small bowel biopsy can identify infiltration of the lamina propria with chronic inflammatory cells and occasional subtle villous atrophy. Nonspecific inflammatory cell infiltrate can also be seen in the colon. These histologic and functional abnormalities have been referred to as AIDS enteropathy.

Feedings can be administered through a nasogastric tube if children are too debilitated to take food orally. This technique may also facilitate gastric emptying and formula tolerance.

■ IgA DEFICIENCY

Selective IgA deficiency is the most common of the primary immunodeficiency states, affecting approximately 1 in 700 of the population. Because other immunoglobulins, such as IgM, may compensate for the deficiency, only 13% of the patients have significant GI symptoms. The GI manifestations of IgA deficiency are chronic diarrhea, steatorrhea, lactose malabsorption, milk-protein intolerance, and those secondary to infestation by *Giardia lamblia*. Small bowel villous atrophy has been observed in patients with IgA deficiency and giardiasis. Diarrhea and malabsorption usually improve after treatment for *G lamblia*.

(Abridged from Carlos H. Lifschitz, Malabsorption States, in Oski, DeAngelis, Feigin, McMillan, Warshaw: *Principles and Practice of Pediatrics, Second Edition*, J.B. Lippincott, 1994.)

Oski's Essential Pediatrics,
edited by Kevin B. Johnson and Frank A. Oski.
Lippincott–Raven Publishers,
Philadelphia © 1997

167

Appendicitis

Appendicitis is the most common illness in childhood for which emergency surgical consultation is sought. In older children, the signs and symptoms are frequently typical and the diagnosis is quickly made. However, the classic syndrome may not be evident and the correct diagnosis may be obscure in the preschool-age population, in whom a delay in diagnosis results in an incidence of rupture at the time of surgery approaching 65%, and in adolescent girls, 40% of whom may have a normal appendix at laparotomy despite a preoperative diagnosis of appendicitis or acute right lower quadrant pain. The presentation of appendicitis varies with age, and the incidence of other illnesses whose presentation may be confused with this diagnosis varies with age. The annual incidence of appendicitis is 4 per 1000 children, and it is diagnosed two to three times per week on the pediatric surgical services of large city or county hospitals and children's hospitals. Appendicitis is most common in adolescents and young adults but is also reported during infancy.

The progression of appendicitis to necrosis and perforation occurs in only 10% of the patients by 24 hours but in almost 50% by 48 hours. To avoid a high incidence of perforation, it is important that the diagnosis be made and the patient operated on in the first 24 hours.

■ DIAGNOSIS

Course and Symptoms

The diagnosis of appendicitis depends on an understanding of the pathogenesis and progression of the disease. In the first few hours after onset, the child may have only umbilical pain and tenderness poorly localized to the right lower quadrant. Pylorospasm may not have developed, and bowel sounds may be normal. Because there is no ileus, abdominal radiographs may be normal, as may the leukocyte count and temperature. By 12 hours, reflex ileus and pylorospasm typically have developed with loss of appetite, vomiting, and decreased bowel sounds. The inflammatory process typically reaches the peritoneum, and the pain and tenderness become localized to the right lower quadrant. The leukocyte count and temperature are mildly increased. Early in the syndrome, abdominal radiographs typically show scoliosis with curvature of the spine concave to the right due to muscle spasm and a dilated cecum containing an air–fluid level. By 24 hours, the full syndrome has developed in most patients, and 10% have progressed to perforation. By 48 hours after onset, 50% have perforated appendixes. These children appear ill, and they do not like to move or even cry because of the peritoneal irritation. They are most comfortable lying on their sides with hips and knees flexed. When asked to walk, they do so slowly with a shuffling gait and in a bent-over position. By this time, the leukocyte count is above 15,000/mm^3, and the temperature is elevated. After perforation occurs, abdominal radiographs show a paucity of bowel gas in the right lower quadrant and the development of generalized ileus with multiple small bowel air–fluid levels.

The location of the appendix in the abdomen explains the variation of symptoms seen with appendicitis. If the appendix is anterior and in contact with the anterior abdominal wall, very early localization to the right lower quadrant occurs. A distended, firm appendix often can be palpated if the child is seen early before abdominal guarding due to pain and intestinal distention due to ileus develop. If the appendix is retrocecal or located in the posterior portion of the abdomen, localization of the pain and tenderness on examination occur late, if at all. If the appendix is posterior in the pelvis, the pain may localize only to the lower abdomen, and tenderness to palpation is poorly localized. However, point tenderness can be elicited, and a palpable appendix or mass may be found on rectal examination. The psoas sign, elicited by extension of the hip to stretch the psoas muscle, is positive if the appendix is posterior and in contact with the psoas muscle.

The most confusing symptom attributed to appendicitis is diarrhea. Many instances of delay in obtaining surgical consultation have occurred because the child had "diarrhea" and was considered to have gastroenteritis. Almost 15% of children with appendicitis have diarrhea, but it is a specific form of diarrhea and should not be confused with that seen with gastroenteritis. During the early stages of appendicitis, before the development of ileus, patients may reflexively evacuate the distal colon. Parents may give a child with "stomach pain" laxatives, which can also cause frequent soft or liquid stools. The diarrhea of appendicitis is most common in patients with a low-lying appendix in proximity to the sigmoid colon and rectum. The inflammatory process extends to the muscular wall of the sigmoid colon, and any distention of the sigmoid colon by fluid or gas may cause tenesmus; the child goes to the toilet and passes gas and small amounts of stool. This relieves the symptoms until the sigmoid colon again becomes distended with gas or fluid a few minutes later. In contrast, the child with gastroenteritis typically has voluminous liquid stools. If the child or parent is asked only about the frequency of stools and not about the volume and character, the two conditions may be confused. The child with frequent stools due to sigmoid colon irritation and a pelvic appendix typically has tenderness on rectal examination; the child with gastroenteritis does not.

Processes in the urinary tract, including infection and ureteral stones, can mimic appendicitis, and appendicitis can manifest with signs and symptoms of urinary tract infection and pain. This may occur when the inflamed retrocecal appendix lies over the right ureter, causing partial obstruction and inflammation of the ureter. Dilatation of the right collecting system, right flank and back pain, and leukocytes in the urine are observed. The inflamed appendix may also lie against the bladder and cause inflammation of the bladder wall. As the bladder contracts, the patient experiences pain that may be referred to the groin or penis; the child stops voiding after evacuating only a small volume of urine. The bladder refills, the child again has a sense of urgency, and the cycle repeats. This results in urgency and frequency with only small amounts of urine voided. Inflammation of the bladder wall is associated with pyuria, but the leukocytes are not as numerous as in cystitis. Exquisite anterior tenderness may be elicited on rectal examination, and the condition can be confused with acute prostatitis. However, acute prostatitis is rare in childhood.

Approximately 65% of preschool-age children have perforated appendixes at surgery. Perforation may result from a delay in diagnosis because the young child does not exhibit the symptom complex typical of appendicitis in older children and adults. Pain localizes poorly in young children, and periumbilical generalized pain and tenderness, rather than right lower quadrant pain, may be reported. Vomiting is a nonspecific symptom in a young child and frequently is associated with gastroenteritis. Because appendicitis is not common in the young child, but vomiting and abdominal pain associated with gastroenteritis are common, appendicitis often is not considered. This may delay diagnosis. In our own experience with preschool-age children, if the correct diagnosis was considered at initial medical consultation, the perforation rate was 35%. In children diagnosed and treated for some other disease during the first medical consultation, the perforation rate was 83%. This indicates the importance of maintaining a high index of suspicion when treating children with abdominal pain. Any child in whom appendicitis is a possibility should be admitted for observation. Young children with perforation of the appendix more commonly present with generalized peritonitis, and older children and adults commonly have a localized inflammatory process and develop a para-appendiceal abscess.

Although constipation may occur at any age and cause abdominal pain, it is most often confused with appendicitis in children 4 to 10 years of age. A report of a bowel movement on the day of admission does not exclude this diagnosis, because children of this age frequently are unwilling to describe their bowel function. This diagnosis usually can be confirmed on rectal examination, but some children have a normal rectal examination with evidence of fecal accumulation on an abdominal radiograph. The pain associated with constipation usually is colicky but may be dull and steady. The pain tends to vary in intensity to a much greater extent than the pain of appendicitis, which is usually persistent and progressively worsening. On physical examination, the child with constipation may exhibit mild voluntary guarding and tenderness, but often the tenderness is poorly localized to the periumbilical area. Depending on the amount of voluntary guarding, a fecal mass may be palpable. An enema given in the emergency cen-

ter can relieve symptoms. However, the distention and peristalsis of the colon and cecum associated with an enema in a child with appendicitis increases abdominal pain.

Appendicitis in adolescent girls is sometimes difficult to diagnose because other causes of abdominal pain, including ovarian cyst, menstrual and ovulatory pain, and pelvic inflammatory disease, may mimic appendicitis. Although not proved, it is generally accepted that perforation of the appendix in a young adolescent girl may be associated with scarring of the fimbriae and fallopian tubes, increasing the likelihood of infertility.

The differential diagnosis of appendicitis includes viral syndromes, gastroenteritis, mesenteric adenitis, right lower lobe pneumonia, and Meckel's diverticulitis. Differentiation of these diagnoses is readily apparent by the absence of associated symptoms in patients with appendicitis, although patients with symptoms localized to the abdomen can be confusing.

Laboratory Findings

The diagnosis of appendicitis depends primarily on the history and physical findings. The leukocyte count, hematocrit, and hemoglobin should be determined and a urinalysis performed before a child with suspected appendicitis is taken to the operating room. The leukocyte count can be normal in early appendicitis, but usually it is increased. If neutropenia is detected, a viral syndrome must be ruled out. Neutropenia that develops late in the course of appendicitis and is associated with generalized peritonitis is a poor prognostic sign. Urinalysis is helpful in excluding urinary tract infection. Serum electrolytes, blood urea nitrogen, and serum creatinine levels should be determined in any patient with persistent vomiting or peritonitis to help assess the general state of hydration and electrolyte balance. Any patient in whom the diagnosis is uncertain should undergo further diagnostic evaluation, including abdominal and chest radiography and abdominal ultrasound examination. In the child with classic signs and symptoms of appendicitis, these studies need not be done.

Abdominal ultrasound examination commonly reveals an enlarged, inflamed appendix, periappendiceal abscess, or phlegmon, but a normal appendix cannot be identified. Many centers rely on ultrasound to diagnose difficult cases. Barium enema examinations may be helpful in a patient with persistent abdominal pain but without a typical history or physical findings of appendicitis and for whom the diagnosis remains in doubt. The appendix may fill in 80% of the normal patients who are examined by barium enema. The radiographic findings in appendicitis include cecal spasm, partial filling of the appendix with a paracecal mass, and a cut-off of the contrast within the appendix. Although the proximal appendix may fill even in the setting of a distal obstruction and appendicitis, an astute radiologist usually can identify the exact location of the appendix, and tenderness to palpation can be elicited at that location.

■ TREATMENT

The treatment of appendicitis is appendectomy. Patients with appendicitis and no evidence of metabolic derangement should be taken directly to the operating room. Patients with significant fluid losses due to vomiting or sequestration of intraluminal or intraperitoneal fluid should be given intravenous fluids containing 5% dextrose in 0.5 N saline or lactated Ringer's solution. A patient with evidence of a perforated appendix should be given appropriate antibiotics preoperatively to ensure adequate tissue antibiotic concentrations during surgery. Gentamicin, ampicillin, and clindamycin commonly are used, but other combinations of antibiotics that provide adequate coverage for anaerobic and aerobic microorganisms can be used. Peritoneal fluid should be routinely cultured for aerobic and anaerobic microorganisms in patients with gangrenous or perforated appendixes.

We operate on all patients with appendicitis as promptly as possible. Some surgeons recommend nonoperative treatment of a child with a localized para-appendiceal abscess, if the course is one of progressive resolution of the para-appendiceal abscess and improvement of symptoms with antibiotic therapy; the patients undergo surgery 8 to 12 weeks later as an interval appendectomy. In most centers, primary surgical drainage of the abscess with initial appendectomy is preferred. Most patients with simple acute appendicitis can be cared for with intravenous fluids and without a nasogastric tube for approximately 12 to 24 hours, at which time oral intake can be resumed. Most patients can be discharged within 3 days of surgery. Patients with a perforated appendix typically have ileus that lasts 3 to 5 days, requiring continuous nasogastric drainage. They commonly receive a 4- to 7-day course of intravenous antibiotic therapy that resolves the symptoms. Although postoperative intra-abdominal infections and wound infections are rare in patients with acute appendicitis, almost 5% of the patients with ruptured appendixes develop postoperative intra-abdominal sepsis and form an abscess, and 3% to 7% develop wound infections if the wounds are closed primarily. Many surgeons close only the fascia in the case of a perforated appendix, which virtually eliminates the problem of wound infection, but care of the open wound is more difficult for the patient's family. Most patients with ruptured appendixes are discharged from the hospital 5 to 10 days after surgery.

(Abridged from William J. Pokorny, Appendicitis, in Oski, DeAngelis, Feigin, McMillan, Warshaw: *Principles and Practice of Pediatrics, Second Edition,* J.B. Lippincott, 1994.)

Oski's Essential Pediatrics,
edited by Kevin B. Johnson and Frank A. Oski.
Lippincott–Raven Publishers,
Philadelphia © 1997

168

Ascites

Ascites is the accumulation of fluid in the peritoneal cavity. Ascites is a manifestation of an underlying disorder, such as cirrhosis, congestive heart failure (CHF), nephrotic syndrome, protein-losing enteropathy, or malnutrition associated with hypoalbuminemia. Ascites has been a recognized entity since the time of Hippocrates, who stated, "When the liver is full of fluid and this overflows into the peritoneal cavity so that the belly becomes full of water, death follows." Although the predicted outcome is less bleak today, much controversy remains about the pathogenesis and treatment of ascites.

■ PATHOGENESIS

The presumed initiating factor in the development of ascites in cases of CHF is increased hydrostatic pressure. In patients with the nephrotic syndrome, protein-losing enteropathy, or malnutrition, the associated hypoalbumine-

mia results in a decreased oncotic pressure. These alterations in Starling forces cause fluid to move from the intravascular space to the extravascular space. When the rate of extravascular fluid production exceeds the ability of the lymphatic system to reabsorb this fluid and transport it back to the vascular system, the fluid accumulates in the peritoneal cavity resulting in ascites.

The exact role of hypoalbuminemia in the development and maintenance of ascites is controversial, because many patients with hypoalbuminemia or analbuminemia do not have ascites. Approximately 50% of patients with serum albumin concentrations less than 2.5 g/dL develop ascites. The pathogenesis of ascites in cirrhosis is less well defined and remains an area of active research.

■ DIFFERENTIAL DIAGNOSIS

The differential diagnosis of ascites is subdivided into eight major categories: portal hypertension, hypoalbuminemia, infectious, chylous, urinary, gastrointestinal, miscellaneous, and pseudoascites (Table 168–1). Portal hypertension, the most common cause of ascites in North America, can have a prehepatic, hepatic, or posthepatic origin. The major cause of prehepatic portal hypertension is portal vein thrombosis or occlusion, which can result in the development of esophageal varices but rarely causes ascites. Hepatic-origin portal hypertension is often secondary to hepatic fibrosis or cirrhosis. These disorders can result from congenital hepatic fibrosis, neonatal hepatitis, biliary atresia, α_1-antitrypsin deficiency, cystic fibrosis, chronic active hepatitis, or one of several storage diseases. Although primary and metastatic hepatic tumors may cause portal hypertension and ascites, the incidence is rare. Hepatic cysts, which may result in ascites, commonly occur with polycystic kidney disease. Posthepatic causes of portal hypertension include the Budd-Chiari syndrome (*ie,* hepatic vein thrombosis), constrictive pericarditis, or CHF. The latter two possibilities emphasize the importance of a thorough cardiac examination when evaluating a patient with ascites.

Physical Examination

The clinical hallmark of ascites is abdominal distention (Figure 168–1). Other potential physical findings of ascites include bulging flanks, protrusion of the umbilicus, and scrotal swelling. Patients with portal hypertension may have a prominent abdominal venous pattern (Figure 168–2).

When there is massive ascites (see Figure 168–1), the patient's condition is obvious. In less dramatic presentations, three physical signs can help detect ascites: flank dullness, shifting dullness, and fluid wave. Flank dullness is verified with the patient in the supine position. In patients with ascites, the gas-filled loops of bowel float to the center of the abdomen on top of the ascitic fluid. When the physician percusses the abdomen, it is tympanitic at the umbilicus and dull below the level of fluid into the flanks. Shifting dullness can be assessed by percussing the abdomen while the patient is in the supine position and then in the right and left lateral decubitus positions. Ascites is suggested if the point of dullness shifts with the changes in position. A fluid wave is elicited by having the patient place the lateral aspect of his or her hands longitudinally on the abdomen. The examiner taps the lateral abdominal wall lightly while feeling the opposite wall for a fluid wave. Flank dullness and shifting dullness have the greatest sensitivity, and the fluid wave has the greatest specificity.

TABLE 168-1. Categories in the Differential Diagnosis of Ascites

Portal hypertension
    Prehepatic
        Portal vein thrombosis or occlusion
    Hepatic
        Fibrosis
        Cirrhosis
        Tumors
        Cysts
    Posthepathic
        Budd-Chiari syndrome
        Constrictive pericarditis
        Congestive heart failure
Hypoalbuminemia
    Nephrotic syndrome
    Protein-losing enteropathy
    Malnutrition
    Hydrops fetalis
Infectious causes
    Bacterial peritonitis
    Fungal peritonitis
    Tuberculous peritonitis
    Cytomegalovirus
    Toxoplasmosis
    Syphilis
Chylous
    Traumatic
    Lymphatic obstruction
    Lymphatic abnormalities
Urinary causes
    Posterior urethral valves
    Bladder perforation
    Ureteral stenosis
    Urethral stenosis
    Neurogenic bladder
Gastrointestinal causes
    Pancreatic causes
    Intestinal atresia
    Meconium peritonitis
    Bile peritonitis
Miscellaneous causes
    Gynecologic disorders
    Ventriculoperitoneal shunts
    Eosinophilic peritonitis
    Hypothyroidism
Pseudoascites
    Omental cysts
    Mesenteric cysts
    Enteric duplication

orrhoids, peripheral edema, scleral icterus, spider telangiectasia, and splenomegaly. Other aspects of a physical examination that require particular attention in patients with ascites are the cardiac and chest examination. There are several potential cardiac causes of ascites. Patients with massive ascites may be tachypneic due to compromised intrathoracic volume. Some patients may develop sympathetic pleural effusions.

A physical assessment of nutritional status should be performed. Patients with ascites may be compromised nutritionally because of the underlying disorder that caused the ascites. Patients with massive ascites may experience early satiety, resulting in inadequate intake, or they may have malabsorption secondary to an edematous intestinal tract; both of these conditions can adversely affect their nutritional status. Patients with cirrhosis also may develop deficiencies of fat-soluble vitamins or essential fatty acids, nutritional signs for which the physician must be alert.

Radiologic Evaluation

Because physical examination is not sensitive enough for detecting submassive ascites, other means are required. Plain radiographs of the abdomen may be helpful. The classic radiographic findings of ascites include separation of and floating bowel loops; abdominal haziness; indistinct psoas muscle shadows; and increased pelvic density in the upright position. These nonspecific signs are not sufficiently sensitive to detect ascites. More reliable signs include an increased distance (>2 mm) between the properitoneal fat stripe and the right colon (ie, McCort or flank stripe sign), a radiolucent shadow between the lateral wall of the liver and the abdominal wall (ie, Hellmen sign), radiodensity superior and lateral to the bladder (ie, dog's ear sign), and obliteration of the lower lateral hepatic angle. Of these four signs, the flank stripe sign and obliteration of the lower hepatic angle are the most sensitive and reliable indicators of ascites in 55% and 85% of patients, respectively.

Ultrasound, unlike plain radiography, is sensitive and specific for ascites. Ultrasound can demonstrate as little as 150 mL of fluid in vivo. Ultrasound can differentiate free from loculated fluid or detect causes of pseudoascites such as an omental cyst. Abdominal ultrasound scans should be obtained during the initial evaluation of every patient with ascites before paracentesis. This helps to differentiate true ascites from pseudoascites, for which paracentesis may be detrimental. Ultrasound is the diagnostic procedure of choice because of its sensitivity, specificity, and noninvasive nature.

Computed tomography is extremely sensitive in the detection of ascites, but it should be performed only in special circumstances, because of the expense and exposure to radiation.

Analysis of Ascitic Fluid

Ascitic fluid for diagnostic evaluation is obtained by abdominal paracentesis. Paracentesis is indicated in patients who present with new onset of ascites after performing an abdominal ultrasound, in those with suspected peritonitis, in patients with cirrhosis and ascites who deteriorate suddenly, and possibly in the assessment of patients with blunt abdominal trauma. Paracentesis also can be used therapeutically in certain situations.

Paracentesis is a safe procedure with a complication rate of 1% to 3%. Potential complications include persistent leak-

The physical examination alone is not sufficiently accurate or sensitive enough to detect ascites. In one study of patients with equivocal ascites, the physical examination alone had an accuracy rate of only 56%.

Patients in whom ascites is secondary to cirrhosis may have physical signs of chronic liver disease, such as large hem-

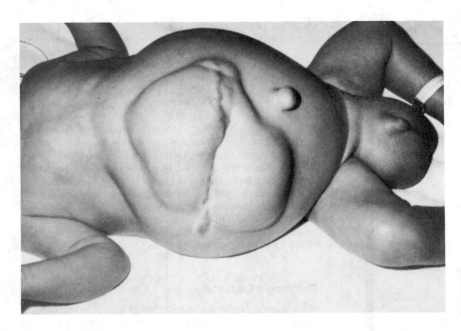

Figure 168-1. A 6-month-old infant with severe neonatal hepatitis. Note the marked abdominal distention, bulging of the flanks, wound and umbilical herniation, and scrotal swelling.

age, bladder or intestinal perforation, scrotal swelling, pneumoperitoneum and bleeding. Paracentesis is not contraindicated for patients with coagulopathies. It has been estimated that the risk of bleeding, which would require a transfusion, from paracentesis is less than the risk of acquiring hepatitis from a transfusion of fresh-frozen plasma, which does not need to be given to a patient with a coagulopathy before paracentesis.

Various tests can be performed to classify the ascitic fluid further and determine its cause. Traditionally, peritoneal fluid had been separated into transudative and exudative categories. Most often, ascitic fluid is a transudate and is associated with an increased hydrostatic pressure in the portal system or with decreased serum oncotic pressure. Typically, transudative ascitic fluid is clear or straw colored, with total protein concentrations less than 2.5 to 3.0 g/dL or less than one half the plasma total protein concentration. The concentrations of electrolytes, urea, creatinine, glucose,

triglycerides, cholesterol, and hydrogen ions are almost identical to plasma levels. Trace elements tend to be present in lower concentrations than in plasma. There may be an increased level of fibrin split products in ascitic fluid relative to plasma. The leukocyte count is less than 250 to 500 cells/mm³; less than one third of the cells are neutrophils. Gram's stain and cultures reveal no organisms.

Exudative ascitic fluid is secondary to inflammation of the peritoneum or abdominal viscera (*ie*, peritonitis, pancreatitis) or caused by leakage of lymph or chyle into the peritoneal cavity. Exudative peritoneal fluid is usually turbid or cloudy. Characteristically, the protein content is elevated, with the total protein concentration typically above 3 g/dL. The protein content may be less in patients with hypoproteinemia. The ratio of ascitic protein to plasma protein can be determined in these patients and tends to be greater than 0.5 with exudative ascites. Lactate dehydrogenase (LDH) is elevated relative to plasma; the ratio of ascitic fluid LDH to

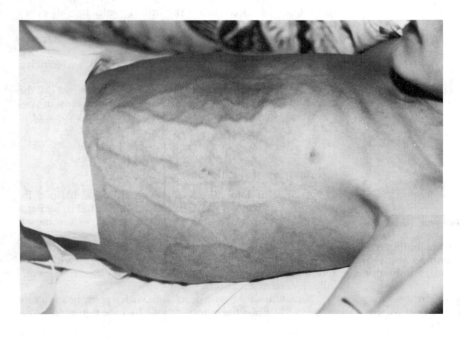

Figure 168-2. An 11-year-old child with portal vein obstruction. Note the prominent abdominal vasculature.

plasma LDH is greater than 0.6. An elevated leukocyte count is common in patients with peritonitis; the count is greater than 500 leukocytes/mm³, and more than 50% of the cells are neutrophils (ie, absolute neutrophil count of >250/mm³). Initial studies found that the pH of ascitic fluid from a patient with peritonitis tended to be low, less than 7.31, and the lactate level elevated. It was proposed that a pH gradient of greater than 0.1 between arterial blood and ascitic fluid indicated peritonitis. However, ascitic fluid pH and lactate levels and their gradients between blood and ascitic fluid are not sensitive predictors of peritonitis, although they are specific. A low ascitic fluid pH is associated with a high mortality rate. The single best predictor of peritonitis is a neutrophil count greater than 250 cells/mm³. The leukocyte count in ascites can increase during diuretic treatment, but the neutrophil count does not. Peripheral leukocytosis does not affect the leukocyte or neutrophil count of ascites.

Classification of ascites into transudative and exudative categories based on total protein and LDH levels is suboptimal. Many patients with cirrhosis and ascites have elevated protein concentrations in their ascitic fluid. The protein concentration can be increased in the ascitic fluid by diuretic therapy. It has been proposed that the serum–ascites albumin gradient is superior in differentiating transudative and exudative ascites. If the serum–ascites albumin concentration is greater than 1.1 g/dL, transudative ascites is likely. Exudative ascites typically has a serum–ascites albumin concentration gradient less than 1.1 g/dL. It is important to simultaneously measure the serum and ascites albumin concentration. The physician should always obtain a Gram's stain and culture of the ascitic fluid when a paracentesis is performed. The sensitivity of ascitic fluid cultures are greatly increased if 10 mL of fluid is placed into aerobic and anaerobic blood culture bottles at the bedside. If tuberculosis is a consideration, the sensitivity is increased if a greater amount of fluid is obtained, centrifuged, and then appropriately cultured.

Malignant ascites, rare in children, is characterized by elevated protein and LDH levels. The serum–ascites albumin concentration gradient is less than 1.1 g/dL in 93% of these patients. The glucose level may be low, and the fluid may be bloody. Ascitic fluid secondary to the nephrotic syndrome has the characteristics of ascitic fluid associated with cirrhosis. It is straw colored with a total protein concentration less than 2.5 g/dL and an albumin gradient of greater than 1.1 g/dL.

■ TREATMENT

Several medical and surgical therapeutic modalities can be used to treat ascites. The initial therapy must be directed at the underlying disorder, after which the ascites may be treated. The mere presence of ascites does not mandate therapy. Therapy should be instituted if secondary complications develop, such as patient discomfort, reduced mobility, or impaired respiratory, cardiovascular, or gastrointestinal function. The treatment of patients should focus on reducing symptoms with a minimum of complications induced by the treatment.

Medical treatment consists primarily of nutritional and diuretic therapies. Bed rest is recommended frequently for adults with ascites, because of the theoretical possibility that an upright position activates the renin–angiotensin–aldosterone and sympathetic nervous systems, which increases tubular reabsorption of sodium. Prolonged bed rest for pediatric patients is not a practical therapeutic modality, and the goal of normalizing the lives of pediatric patients to promote sound psychological development is poorly served by enforced bed rest.

Salt restriction is the mainstay of nutritional therapy in the treatment of ascites and should be instituted immediately. Sodium retention, whether primary or secondary, is responsible for maintaining ascites. Moderate to marked salt restriction alone can result in significant diuresis in 10% to 20% of patients.

Therapy must be directed at the normalization and maintenance of nutritional status. Patients with massive ascites may have early satiety because of gastric compression, or they may have gastroesophageal reflux, which can limit intake, ultimately producing malnutrition. Patients with ascites and hypoalbuminemia may have an edematous intestinal tract, which causes malabsorption and a deterioration in their nutritional status. Patients with ascites caused by liver disease may malabsorb fat and fat-soluble vitamins and require specific therapy.

Although water intake may have to be restricted in some patients with cirrhosis, water intake need not be a concern for most of those who can excrete the amount of fluid normally consumed. Excessive fluid intake should be discouraged. Fluid restriction of 50% to 70% of maintenance should be instituted if the serum sodium decreases much below 130 mEq/L. Diuretics are frequently used in the management of patients with ascites. Rational use of these agents requires a thorough understanding of the pathophysiology of ascites and knowledge of the diuretics. Spironolactone, the first diuretic to be employed, inhibits sodium reabsorption in the distal and collecting tubules by inhibiting the effect of aldosterone. It is a weak natriuretic agent that increases sodium excretion by only 2%; it does not cause hypokalemia. Potential side effects include hyperkalemia, gynecomastia, and metabolic acidosis. The latter complication develops as a result of spironolactone inhibition of renal hydrogen ion secretion.

If sodium restriction and spironolactone do not result in adequate diuresis, furosemide should be added. Furosemide is a potent natriuretic agent that increases sodium excretion by 20% to 25% by inhibiting sodium reabsorption in the ascending limb of the loop of Henle. Furosemide should be used only in conjunction with spironolactone, because without the latter agent, the sodium not absorbed in the loop of Henle would be absorbed in the distal and collecting tubules because of the hyperaldosteronemia of these patients. The major complication associated with furosemide is a marked kaluresis, which can cause hypokalemia and metabolic alkalosis. Hypokalemia may result in arrhythmias and growth failure. Hypokalemia may precipitate hepatic encephalopathy, because hypokalemia causes increased renal production of ammonium. Other potential complications of furosemide use include hyponatremia, hypochloremia, and azotemia.

Diuresis should be induced gradually. After diuretic therapy is begun, fluid comes initially from the intravascular space and then is replaced by edema or ascitic fluid. Edema fluid is mobilized more readily than ascitic fluid, which can be mobilized at a maximal rate of 900 mL/day in adults. Patients with ascites and edema can be diuresed aggressively as long as edema is present. Patients without edema probably should not be diuresed more than 300 to 500 mL/day. Aggressive diuresis should be avoided in patients with decreased renal function because of the possible development of hypovolemia, further reduction in renal function, and development of the hepatorenal syndrome. All patients who receive diuretic therapy should be monitored closely for electrolyte, urea, and creatinine levels.

Albumin can be infused intravenously in conjunction with furosemide to achieve a more rapid diuresis in patients who are acutely symptomatic. Because albumin enters the peritoneal fluid, the effect is transient. This therapy is expensive, may result in increased portal pressure, and may cause variceal bleeding. Autogenous ascitic infusion has been done with variable success and has limited applicability.

Nonsteroidal anti-inflammatory agents should be used with caution in patients with cirrhosis and ascites. These agents inhibit renal prostaglandin synthesis, which causes a marked reduction in renal blood flow, glomerular filtration rate, and free water clearance. These agents also reduce the natriuretic activity of furosemide.

Two peritoneovenous shunts are used: the LeVeen and Denver shunts. The LeVeen shunt, which has been the shunt of choice, consists of a perforated tube connected to another tube with a one-way, pressure-sensitive valve. The perforated portion is placed in the abdominal cavity; the other end is tunneled subcutaneously over the chest and inserted into the superior vena cava. When abdominal pressure exceeds superior vena cava pressure, ascitic fluid is drawn into the circulatory system. The Denver shunt is similar except that it has a bulb that can be pumped to transfer ascitic fluid to the circulatory system. Although experience with these shunts in children has been limited, the results have been successful.

Both types of shunts are associated with a high rate of complications. Patients with peritoneovenous shunts may develop infections, most commonly *Staphylococcus*, which cannot be eradicated from the shunt, requiring the shunt to be removed. The incidence of bacterial infections can be decreased by giving prophylactic antibiotics before procedures. Intravascular coagulation occurs in approximately 25% of persons with shunts, probably because of the large amount of fibrin split products and other clotting factors in the ascitic fluid transported to the vascular system. This high incidence of intravascular coagulation can be decreased by removing all of the ascites at the time of shunt surgery. The postoperative use of aspirin decreases the incidence of this significant complication. The shunts also frequently become occluded: 40% at 3 months and 80% at 2 years. Other potential complications include pulmonary embolism, CHF, bleeding varices, and small bowel obstruction. The high incidence of complications and occlusion limit the usefulness of the shunts.

■ COMPLICATIONS

Complications associated with ascites can be secondary to the presence of ascites or to the therapeutic modalities used to treat the ascites. Massive ascites can impair respiratory function by pushing up the diaphragm, decreasing intrathoracic volume, or by the presence of pleural effusions. Ascites can increase intra-abdominal pressure, resulting in gastroesophageal reflux or early satiety. Massive ascites can cause patient discomfort and reduce mobility. The multiple complications of diuretic therapy, paracentesis, and peritoneovenous shunt were discussed in the previous section.

Spontaneous bacterial peritonitis (SBP) is a complication that occurs when the ascitic fluid becomes infected (*ie*, peritonitis) in the absence of a local source of infection such as a perforation. The incidence of SBP is approximately 15%, but it occurs most commonly in patients with cirrhosis and ascites and occurs much less frequently when the ascites is caused by the nephrotic syndrome or CHF. The reticuloendothelial system phagocytic activity is decreased in cirrhosis, accounting for the increased incidence of SBP. The ascitic fluid of these persons has lower total protein and complement levels, which predispose them to developing SBP. Aerobic gram-negative organisms are most commonly recovered and are responsible for approximately 72% of cases. *Escherichia coli* is the most common aerobic gram-negative organism, followed by *Klebsiella*. Aerobic gram-positive organisms are detected in 29% of patients, with *Streptococcus* and enterococcal species accounting for most of these infections. Anaerobes are responsible for fewer than 8% of SBP cases. If multiple organisms are recovered from the ascitic fluid, a secondary cause for the infection should be sought.

Patients with SBP most commonly present with fever, abdominal pain, and no other source of infection. They may also present with hypotension, diarrhea, portosystemic encephalopathy, or unexplained deterioration despite previously stable cirrhosis. Ten percent of patients with SBP are totally asymptomatic at the time of presentation. The key to making the correct diagnosis is to be alert to the possibility and perform paracentesis if the patient has any symptoms compatible with SBP.

Therapy should be instituted for any patient if the neutrophil count of the ascitic fluid is greater than 500 cells/mm^3 or if the clinical condition is compatible with SBP and the neutrophil count is greater than 250 cells/mm^3. Treatment should not wait until cultures are positive, because patients with SBP deteriorate rapidly if appropriate treatment is not instituted promptly. Ampicillin and an aminoglycoside provide good coverage, but it may not be advisable to give a patient with cirrhosis and diminished renal function a nephrotoxic drug. Cefotaxime is considered the drug of choice for presumed SBP. Therapy should be continued for 10 to 14 days. Blood and urine cultures should be obtained before starting therapy, because 50% and 40%, respectively, are positive.

SBP is associated with a mortality rate of 25% to 50%. There is a high recurrence rate of SBP in those who survive the initial episode, with the probability of recurrence of 70% within 1 year. Because of the high mortality rate and frequent recurrence of SBP, patients with cirrhosis who recover from the initial episode of SBP should be considered for liver transplantation after the infection has resolved.

(Abridged from William J. Cochran, Ascites, in Oski, DeAngelis, Feigin, McMillan, Warshaw: *Principles and Practice of Pediatrics, Second Edition,* J.B. Lippincott, 1994.)

Oski's Essential Pediatrics,
edited by Kevin B. Johnson and Frank A. Oski.
Lippincott–Raven Publishers,
Philadelphia © 1997

169

Pancreatitis

ACUTE PANCREATITIS

Acute pancreatitis is the second-most common pancreatic disorder in children after cystic fibrosis. Blunt abdominal trauma and viral infections, especially mumps, account for most cases. Other causes are much less common (Table 169–1). Child abuse is a major cause of traumatic pancreatitis in young children. More recently defined causes of pancreatitis include refeeding after starvation, Kawasaki disease, and Reye's syndrome. Improved techniques have increased the recognition of congenital abnormalities associated with pancreatitis.

TABLE 169-1. Causes of Acute Pancreatitis in Children

Drugs and toxins	Cholelithiasis and
Alcohol	choledocholithiasis
Azathioprine	Duplication cyst
L-Asparaginase	Complication of endoscopic
Corticosteroids	retrograde
Estrogen	cholangiopancreatography
Furosemide	Pancreas divisum
6-Mercaptopurine	Pancreatic ductal
Methyldopa	abnormalities
Pentamidine	Pancreatic pseudocyst
Scorpion bites	Postoperative
Sulfasalazine	Tumor
Tetracycline	Systemic disease
Thiazides	Bone marrow transplantation
Valproic acid	Cystic fibrosis
Hereditary pancreatitis	Diabetes
Idiopathic causes	Head trauma
Infectious causes	Hemolytic uremic syndrome
Coxsackievirus B	Hyperlipoproteinemia types
Epstein-Barr virus	I and IV
Hepatitis A virus	Hyperparathyroidism
Influenza A virus	Kawasaki disease
Measles	Malnutrition
Mumps	Periarteritis nodosa
Mycoplasma	Peptic ulcer
Rubella	Refeeding after malnutrition
Reye's syndrome	Systemic lupus erythematosus
Obstructive	Traumatic causes
Ampullary disease	Blunt injury
Ascariasis	Child abuse
Biliary tract malformations	Scoliosis surgery
	Surgical trauma

The sequence of events leading to pancreatitis has not been adequately defined. Many investigators think that activation of proteolytic pancreatic proenzymes after colocalization with lysosomal hydrolases within the acinar cell leads to autodigestion and further activation and release of active proteases. Lecithin is activated by phospholipase A_2 into the toxic lysolecithin. Prophospholipase is unstable and can be activated by minute quantities of trypsin. The healthy pancreas is protected by three factors: pancreatic proteases are synthesized as inactive proenzymes; digestive enzymes are segregated into secretory granules; and the presence of protease inhibitors.

The histopathologic findings of acute pancreatitis are related to the release of activated proteolytic and lipolytic enzymes. Interstitial edema appears early. As the episode of pancreatitis progresses, localized and confluent necrosis, blood vessel disruption leading to hemorrhage, and an inflammatory response in the peritoneum may develop.

The definition of acute pancreatitis and its differentiation from chronic pancreatitis have been subjects of much dispute. The most widely accepted definition holds that acute pancreatitis is an isolated episode with complete morphologic and histologic resolution. Acute pancreatitis may recur, but unless structural damage occurs, it rarely becomes chronic.

■ CLINICAL MANIFESTATIONS

The child with acute pancreatitis has continuous midepigastric and periumbilical abdominal pain, often radiating to the back, with vomiting and, frequently, fever. He appears acutely ill and is restless and uncomfortable. He may lie on his side. The pain increases in severity for 24 to 48 hours. During this interval, vomiting may increase, and the patient may require hospitalization for fluid and electrolyte therapy. The acute case is usually self-limited, and the prognosis is excellent.

In more severe cases, jaundice, ascites, and pleural effusions may occur. Acute hemorrhagic pancreatitis, the most severe form of acute pancreatitis, is rare in children. In this life-threatening condition, the child is severely ill with intractable nausea, vomiting, and abdominal pain. The pancreas may become necrotic and transformed into an infected, inflammatory, hemorrhagic mass or phlegmon. The mortality rate from shock, renal failure, infection, massive gastrointestinal bleeding, and other complications approaches 50%. Several classification systems have been devised to predict the outcome of pancreatitis, but none is relevant for pediatric patients.

■ LABORATORY FINDINGS

Because no test is accepted as a reference standard for the diagnosis of pancreatitis, many tests have been recommended. The most widely used tests are determinations of serum amylase and lipase activities. The serum amylase level is typically elevated for 4 to 5 days, and the lipase is elevated longer. False-positive and false-negative results occur. Many nonpancreatic conditions have been associated with hyperamylasemia. False-positive results may occur in testing patients with diabetic ketoacidosis, renal failure, burns, and an elevation of salivary amylase, as occurs in mumps. Fractionation of serum amylase into the salivary and pancreatic components can be readily done in most clinical laboratories. We prefer to determine the serum lipase, which may be more specific than amylase for acute pancreatitis. Its use in the past was limited by technical difficulties that have been overcome.

The levels of another serum enzyme, immunoreactive cationic trypsin (IRT), increase in acute pancreatitis and decrease in pancreatic insufficiency. Experience with this technique in children is still limited. Newer tests, such as those for serum pancreatic elastase 1 and phospholipase A_2, are being studied.

Commonly found laboratory abnormalities include leukocytosis, hyperglycemia, glucosuria, hypocalcemia, and hyperbilirubinemia. Radiologic findings are usually nonspecific. A sentinel loop of small bowel or a segmental ileus may be seen. Ultrasonography and computed tomography (CT) are cornerstones in the diagnosis and management of pancreatitis. These studies may demonstrate diffuse pancreatic enlargement, indeterminate pancreatic masses, pancreatic and extrapancreatic fluid collections, and peripancreatic abscesses, but at least 20% of patients with acute pancreatitis have normal CT examinations.

■ TREATMENT

Treatment of mild and moderate episodes of acute pancreatitis is supportive and expectant. The aims of therapy are to relieve pain and restore homeostasis. Meperidine is given as necessary for pain control. Fluid and electrolyte balance is maintained. Nasogastric suction is useful to control vomiting but does not speed resolution of the underlying pancreatitis. Antibiotics are used only for the treatment of a specific infection. Improvement usually occurs in 2 to 4 days. The patient with acute pancreatitis may be refed after clinical symptoms have resolved and the serum amylase and lipase have returned to near normal. Surgery is rarely required. The treatment of severe acute pancreatitis usually is prolonged and may require total parenteral nutrition and surgical drainage.

CHRONIC PANCREATITIS

The cause of chronic or recurrent pancreatitis in children is usually hereditary, traumatic, or anomalies of the pancreatic or biliary ductal systems. Many kindreds have been described in which the disease is transmitted as an autosomal dominant trait with incomplete penetrance. Symptoms frequently begin in the first decade but are usually mild at onset. Although spontaneous recovery from each attack occurs in 4 to 7 days, episodes become progressively more severe. Hereditary pancreatitis is diagnosed if the disease affects successive generations of a family. Evaluation during symptom-free intervals may be unrewarding until calcifications, pseudocysts, or pancreatic insufficiency develop. Other conditions associated with chronic relapsing pancreatitis are hyperlipoproteinemia (ie, types I and V), hyperparathyroidism, ascariasis, and cystic fibrosis. Most cases of recurrent pancreatitis in childhood are associated with anatomical abnormalities.

Every child who has experienced more than one episode of pancreatitis must be thoroughly evaluated. Serum lipid, calcium, and phosphorus levels are determined. In the appropriate clinical setting, stools are evaluated for *Ascaris*. A sweat test is performed. Plain abdominal films are evaluated for the presence of pancreatic calcifications. Ultrasound or CT scans are performed to detect a pseudocyst. The biliary tract is evaluated for the presence of stones.

Experience with endoscopic retrograde cholangiopancreatography (ERCP) in children is growing. ERCP, which defines the anatomy of the gland, should be considered in the evaluation of children with idiopathic, nonresolving, or recurrent pancreatitis and before surgery in patients with pseudocysts. In these cases, ERCP may detect unsuspected anatomical defects that are amenable to surgical therapy. This technique is useful and safe even in very young children if performed by experienced investigators. Pancreatograms from a normal child and from a child with chronic pancreatitis are shown in Figure 169–1.

■ DISORDERS OF THE DUCTS AND SPHINCTER

Although a variety of anatomical defects leading to pancreatitis have been described in case reports, only two, choledochal cysts and pancreas divisum, are commonly seen in practice.

Choledochal Cysts

A choledochal cyst is a congenital dilatation of the extrahepatic biliary tract and usually causes symptoms of biliary tract obstruction, such as nausea, vomiting, and fever, with the classic triad of pain, jaundice, and an abdominal mass. These features are thought to be caused by an anomalous long common channel of the pancreatic and common bile ducts. The presentation sometimes may be that of pancreatitis. The diagnosis is usually easily made by ultrasound or CT scans.

A choledochocele, an intraduodenal choledochal cyst, frequently can only be diagnosed by ERCP. The symptoms of choledochocele may be those of pancreatitis or biliary tract obstruction. The treatment of all forms of choledochal cyst is surgical resection.

Pancreas Divisum

In normal embryologic development, the dorsal and ventral pancreatic anlage fuse by the end of the sixth week of gestation. Incomplete fusion may lead to pancreas divisum, a condition in which the dorsal and ventral portions of the pancreas drain into the duodenum independently, and a variety of other anomalies. A large body of literature has developed about whether these anomalies predispose the

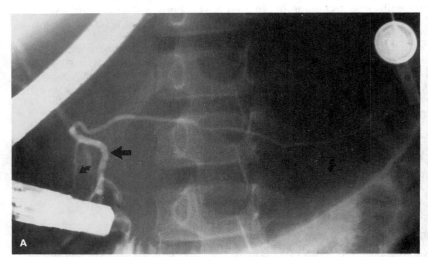
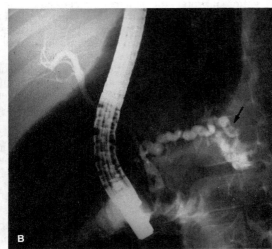

Figure 169-1. (A) Normal pancreatogram. Notice the excellent visualization of the side branches *(small arrows)* and the main pancreatic duct *(large arrow)*. (Courtesy of Anthony Bohorfoush, MD, Medical College of Wisconsin, Milwaukee, WI.) **(B)** Chronic pancreatitis. Notice the dilatation and tortuosity of the main pancreatic duct. Filling defects represent intraductal stones *(arrow)*.

patient to pancreatitis. Various anomalies of the ductal system exist in 30% to 40% of normal persons, and pancreas divisum is seen in 5% to 15%. Although the controversy is not settled, the consensus opinion is that pancreas divisum predisposes to pancreatitis only when it is associated with an anomaly, such as stenosis of the accessory sphincter. Several surgical and therapeutic endoscopic procedures have been recommended with only mixed success.

(Abridged from Steven L. Werlin, Pancreatitis, in Oski, DeAngelis, Feigin, McMillan, Warshaw: *Principles and Practice of Pediatrics, Second Edition*, J.B. Lippincott, 1994.)

Oski's Essential Pediatrics,
edited by Kevin B. Johnson and Frank A. Oski.
Lippincott–Raven Publishers,
Philadelphia © 1997

170

Disorders of the Liver and Biliary System

VIRAL HEPATITIS

Viral hepatitis in children is a major health concern throughout the world. Multiple hepatotropic viruses causing disease in humans have been identified. These include hepatitis A, hepatitis B, the delta agent (*ie*, hepatitis D), and the more recently described hepatitis C and E. Other viruses capable of causing hepatitis include Epstein-Barr virus (EBV), cytomegalovirus (CMV), varicella virus, herpes simplex virus, rubella, and coxsackievirus B; typically these organisms cause hepatitis as part of a multisystem presentation, and they are discussed in other chapters.

■ HEPATITIS A

Hepatitis A virus (HAV), a member of the picornavirus family, is an RNA virus. Hepatitis A accounts for as many as 25% of cases of hepatitis in the developing world. Transmission is usually through the fecal–oral route, although parenteral transmission has been recorded. Consumption of contaminated food or water is usually implicated. There is no known carrier state, and transmission is by person-to-person spread during the preicteric stage of disease. Fecal viral shedding is maximal during the late incubation period (28 days), immediately before or after symptom onset. As a result of this method of spread, infants may be ideal vectors of HAV infection, with spread to other family members or to other children at day care centers. Institutionalized children are also at high risk for disease acquisition.

Clinical symptoms of HAV infection may be absent or, especially in children younger than 2 years of age, may consist of nausea, vomiting, and diarrhea. The patient is often anicteric. In adults, symptoms of acute hepatitis predominate. Approximately two thirds of those with symptoms become jaundiced. Prodromal symptoms of fever, headache, and anorexia may occur. In most patients, HAV infection

has a mild course and clinical improvement occurs rapidly. Aminotransferase levels, which peak within 1 week of disease onset, usually normalize within several weeks but may remain elevated for several months (Figure 170–1). Diagnosis may be made through the demonstration of anti-HAV IgM in serum; anti-HAV IgG develops later and persists for life. The disorder invariably resolves. There is no evidence of chronic hepatitis due to HAV. A small percentage of patients may develop fulminant hepatitis due to HAV, accounting for a fatality rate for those infected with HAV of less than 1%.

Treatment of HAV infection is symptomatic. Infected infants should not return to their day care center until 2 weeks after onset of symptoms to minimize the exposure of others to fecal shedding. If HAV is documented in a day care center attendee, parent, or employee, intravenous immune globulin should be given to all employees and children.

■ HEPATITIS B

The hepatitis B virus (HBV) is a DNA virus of the hepadnavirus family. HBV-related viral particles can be found in serum and tissue of infected persons. Transmission of HBV usually occurs by the parenteral route, through exchange of blood or body secretions. The virus has been demonstrated in blood, semen, saliva, and breast milk. Transmission may occur through intimate contact of any type and through vertical (*ie*, mother to infant) transmission. Persons at high risk include those with frequent exposure to blood or blood products. Children at greatest risk in the United States include those born to mothers who had acute hepatitis B in the third trimester or are chronic HBsAg carriers. Institutionalized children, hemophiliacs, hemodialysis patients, and intravenous drug abusers are at risk for disease. The prevalence of the HBsAg carrier state in the United States is approximately 0.1%.

The incubation period of HBV is estimated at 60 to 180 days, and the subsequent infection is often subclinical, but symptoms occur in 25% to 30% of patients (Figure 170–2). Early symptoms may be systemic and include fever, symmetric arthropathy, and skin eruptions, and urticarial or, in some children, a papular acrodermatitis known as Gianotti-Crosti syndrome. The disease is often anicteric. Malaise, right upper quadrant pain, and a variety of nonspecific gastrointestinal (GI) complaints may occur. Diagnosis of acute hepatitis B is made in the proper clinical setting through the demonstration of HBsAg and anti-HBc IgM in serum. HBsAg positivity in the absence of anti-HBc IgM suggests chronic infection.

The outcome of HBV infection varies. Adults and older children infected with HBV typically have a benign course with complete resolution. Approximately 1% of patients may suffer from fulminant hepatitis. A chronic carrier state may ensue after HBV infection in fewer than 1% to 10% of older patients. At least 20% of preschool-age children with acute HBV infection become chronic carriers. Virtually all infants born to HBsAg-positive mothers contract HBV unless intervention is initiated; of these, approximately 90% become chronic carriers. Transmission in the neonatal period may occur at delivery when the infant is in contact with large amounts of maternal blood. Infants may become infected postnatally from the mother or from infected siblings. In each case, development of the chronic carrier state is common. Infection acquired during the neonatal period is typically asymptomatic. Less commonly, a mild icteric hepatitis may occur. In rare cases, fulminant hepatic failure may occur, particularly after infection with a precore defective variant of HBV.

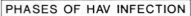

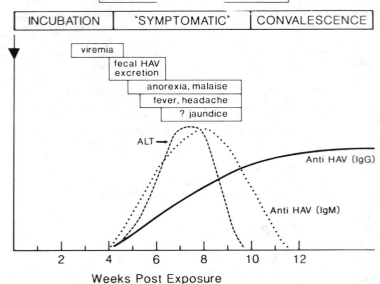

Figure 170-1. Typical course of hepatitis A infection. The period of viremia, which occurs during the incubation phase, is brief. The duration of fecal excretion overlaps this prodromal phase and is present early in the symptomatic phase. Jaundice may occur up to 6 weeks after exposure but is not present in all cases. The aminotransferase ALT (SGPT) elevation also precedes the development of clinical symptoms; values usually remain abnormal after serum bilirubin returns to normal. Anti-HAV is detectable early in the acute "symptomatic" phase of the illness; the initial response is anti-HAV IgM, which peaks shortly after the onset of symptoms and progressively declines. This is succeeded by a gradual rise in anti-HAV of the IgG class, which peaks after the symptomatic phase and remains detectable indefinitely (*arrow* = exposure). (From Balistreri WF. Viral hepatitis. *Pediatr Clin North Am.* 1988;35:640.)

Children who are chronic HBsAg carriers are often asymptomatic and seldom have a history of previous hepatitis. Problems inherent in the chronic carrier state include risk of disease transmission to others and increased risk for the development of cirrhosis and of hepatocellular carcinoma. Chronic infection may be associated with asymptomatic infection, chronic persistent hepatitis, or chronic active hepatitis. The diagnosis of chronic HBV infection rests on the demonstration of elevated transaminases and HBsAg positivity, often accompanied by HBV DNA or HBeAg seropositivity.

Studies of adults and children suggest a role for interferon-A in the treatment of chronic hepatitis B virus infection. The duration of interferon therapy is usually 6 months; side effects include fever (predominantly in the first month of therapy), malaise, autoimmune phenomena, and bone marrow suppression. Patients with decompensated HBsAg-positive liver disease may develop hepatic failure during treatment.

Because of the limitations of treatment, attention must continue to focus on disease prevention. Infants of infected mothers should be given hepatitis B immune globulin and hepatitis B vaccine. Universal vaccination of children against hepatitis B virus has been recommended by the American Academy of Pediatrics. Despite current uncertainty concerning optimal immunization schedules and the duration of protection, this step should dramatically decrease new cases of hepatitis B virus infection and its complications, including hepatocellular carcinoma, in the years to come.

■ HEPATITIS DELTA INFECTION

The hepatitis delta virus (HDV) is a defective RNA virus that requires the hepatitis B virus to cause infection. HDV infection does not occur without acute or chronic hepatitis B infection. The modes of transmission of the delta agent appear to be similar to those discussed for hepatitis B. Endemic areas include the Amazon Basin (*ie*, Labrea hepatitis), the Mediterranean basin, areas of European Russia, and developing tropical areas. In the United States, risk factors for HDV infection are those associated with HBV infection, especially percutaneous transmissions.

The presence of delta virus coinfection usually does not modify the underlying severity of the HBV infection. In most cases, the disease is self-limited, but coinfection may be associated with a higher rate of fulminant hepatitis. HBV and HDV coinfection is responsible for as much as 30% of fulminant hepatitis worldwide; in this specific form of infection, there are frequently two peaks of serum aminotransferase activity, usually a few weeks apart. Presumably, the first peak corresponds to HDV and HBV infection and the second to HBV replication, which is no longer inhibited by HDV replication.

The diagnosis of HDV infection rests on a high level of clinical suspicion; all patients with fulminant hepatic failure and patients known to be carriers of HBsAg who suffer acute exacerbation of disease activity must be studied serologically. The presence of delta antigen or of IgM antibodies to HDV (anti-HDV) is evidence of infection. There has been no specific treatment for this disease, but data suggest a role for interferon therapy. Preventive measures are aimed at the prevention of HBV infection.

■ NON-A, NON-B HEPATITIS

Non-A, non-B (NANB) hepatitis refers to hepatitis for which no other cause (*ie*, viral hepatitis type A, B, or D; CMV; EBV; drug reactions) can be documented. It is likely that several NANB viral agents exist. Two have been delineated: hepatitis C and E.

Epidemic Non-A, Non-B Hepatitis: Hepatitis E

The E form of hepatitis appears to be enterically transmitted, probably through fecally contaminated water supplies. Epidemics may involve large numbers of cases. Outbreaks have occurred in Asia, Africa, and Russia. The incubation period appears to be 35 to 45 days, with a peak age of incidence between 15 and 40 years. The disease may be mild to severe in intensity, with an approximately 20% incidence of fatality in pregnant women. The responsible agent appears to be a 32- to 34-nm viruslike particle that is also transmissible to animals.

The viral genome of these particles, designated hepatitis E, has been partially cloned and suggests that hepatitis E may be a member of the calicivirus family. No commercial sero-

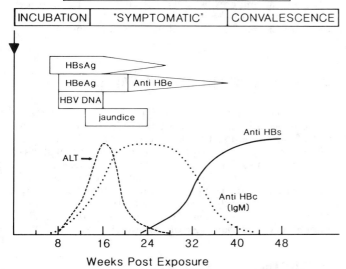

Figure 170-2. Typical course of hepatitis B infection. After exposure to HBV (*arrow*), the earliest detectable serum marker is a rise in HBsAg, which may appear at any time (weeks 1–10) postexposure; HBV DNA and HBeAg follow closely. HBsAg is detectable 2 to 8 weeks before the onset of the symptomatic phase, which is heralded by an increase in aminotransferase (ALT) levels, serum bilirubin concentrations, and constitutional signs. Clearance of HBsAg by immune aggregation with anti-HBc occurs by 6 to 8 months postinfection; those who fail to clear are termed HBsAg carriers. Anti-HBc, which appears just before the symptomatic phase, is the first detectable host-induced immunologic marker of hepatitis B infection. Anti-HBc of the IgM class may be the only marker of HBV infection in serum after clearance of HBsAg, and before a rise in anti-HBs. Anti-HBc is not a neutralizing antibody and therefore, in contrast to anti-HBs, is not protective. (From Balistreri WF. *Pediatr Clin North Am.* 1988;35:647.)

logic assays for this agent are available. There is no evidence to suggest that hepatitis E causes chronic infection. No treatment is available.

Parenteral Non-A, Non-B Hepatitis: Hepatitis C

Hepatitis C virus (HCV) is the major cause of post-transfusion and community-acquired non-A, non-B hepatitis. The virus consists of a single-stranded RNA genome and shares some similarities in nonstructural proteins with the flavivirus family. Cloning of the agent and ongoing refinement of HCV-specific serologic assays have led to rapid advances in our understanding of the clinical course of acute and chronic infection and in the seroepidemiology of the virus. The overall prevalence in the United States of antibody against HCV is about 0.6%. Transmission has occurred primarily by blood or blood products. Serologic screening of blood donors has led to a dramatic decrease in cases associated with blood transfusion, but transmission by intravenous drug use and sexual contact remains important. Vertical transmission from mother to infant may occur, particularly in the setting of maternal human immunodeficiency virus (HIV) infection, but probably much less often than with hepatitis B. Household spread is not frequent.

The clinical manifestations of acute HCV infection are usually mild and may be missed unless tests of liver dysfunction are serially evaluated after a possible exposure. The virus does not appear to be an important cause of fulminant hepatitis, but

chronic infection develops in more than 50% of the patients. The illness in these patients is often characterized by a fluctuating pattern of aminotransferase elevations and few symptoms, but as many as 25% of these patients ultimately develop cirrhosis. There is also a strong association between HCV infection and the development of hepatocellular carcinoma.

The serodiagnosis of HCV infection relies on a second-generation enzyme immunoassay (*ie*, ELISA-2) and recombinant immunoblot assay (*ie*, RIBA-2), which detect antibody against several viral antigens. Serial measurement of anti-HCV antibodies may be required to exclude infection. Moreover, 90% to 95% of the patients with chronic non-A, non-B hepatitis have anti-HCV antibodies using the second-generation assays.

Treatment of chronic hepatitis C infection with interferon-A for 6 months improves liver tests and histopathologic abnormalities in about 50% of adults. Half of these patients can be expected to relapse after discontinuation of therapy, but they usually respond to retreatment. There is little information on the treatment of chronic HCV infection in children.

The efficacy of prophylaxis against hepatitis C with standard immune globulin is unproven. However, a single injection of immune globulin may be reasonable after percutaneous exposure to anti-HCV–positive blood.

CHRONIC HEPATITIS

Chronic hepatitis may occur as a result of persistent hepatic viral infection, as seen in conjunction with hepatitis B, D, and C. Drugs that have been cited as the cause of chronic hepatitis include oxyphenisatin, nitrofurantoin, methyldopa, isoniazid (INH), dantrolene, and acetaminophen. Chronic lupoid or autoimmune chronic hepatitis, first described by Waldenström, may be responsible for chronic hepatitis with rapid progression to cirrhosis. Metabolic disorders such as Wilson's disease and α_1-antitrypsin deficiency may present with clinical and histologic features similar to those found in chronic hepatitis. Biliary tract disease, particularly primary sclerosing cholangitis, must be considered in the differential diagnosis.

Chronic hepatitis is a prolonged necroinflammatory process involving the liver. The clinical manifestations have an insidious onset. The diagnosis rests on the finding of abnormally elevated serum aminotransferase levels, typically for a period of at least 6 months. Other investigators suggest the appropriateness of applying the label "chronic" to hepatic disease after a shorter observation period, perhaps 4 months, particularly if signs of chronic hepatic disease are present. Between 30% and 50% of pediatric patients present with acute illness. The onset of ascites, encephalopathy, hypoalbuminemia, hypergammaglobulinemia, and hypoprothrombinemia may be sudden.

Regardless of the mode of onset, a liver biopsy is required to establish the diagnosis of chronic hepatitis and the severity of the underlying histopathologic process, which are essential to establish for appropriate treatment. The biopsy may reveal changes consistent with chronic persistent hepatitis, chronic lobular hepatitis, or chronic active hepatitis, each of which implies a different prognosis. Characteristic pathologic findings of specific disease entities may be found. In infection secondary to HBV, hepatocytes have a "ground glass" appearance with orcein-positive inclusions. Biopsies from hepatitis C patients may exhibit fatty infiltration, acidophilic bodies, bile duct damage, and lymphoid aggregates. Hepatitis due to drug toxicity histologically resembles viral disease, and the biopsy specimen in autoimmune hepatitis frequently contains an infiltrate of plasma cells.

■ CHRONIC PERSISTENT HEPATITIS

Chronic persistent hepatitis is most often observed after episodes of HBV or NANB viral infection. Patients are asymptomatic or may have vague complaints such as fatigue and anorexia. Hepatomegaly and right upper quadrant tenderness may be minimal. The patient may have a history of drug abuse. Serum aminotransferase values remain mildly increased after an acute episode of hepatitis. Other tests of liver function, including alkaline phosphatase, bilirubin, albumin, and serum globulin, usually are normal. If serum aminotransferase values remain elevated for more than 6 months, a liver biopsy should be performed. Findings suggestive of chronic persistent hepatitis include infiltration of the portal tracts with lymphocytes and a lack of significant fibrosis. The "limiting plate" of hepatocytes about the portal area remains intact.

■ CHRONIC ACTIVE HEPATITIS

Chronic active hepatitis is characterized by hepatic inflammation, necrosis, and fibrosis, which may progress to cirrhosis and eventually liver failure. Prolonged HBV infection accounts for 15% to 20% of cases of chronic active hepatitis. In addition, 30% to 50% of cases of hepatitis C infection may result in chronic active hepatitis.

Up to 20% of chronic active hepatitis cases are ascribed to autoimmune chronic hepatitis, a disorder most frequently diagnosed in young women aged 15 to 25 years. The disease may be associated with other disorders of presumably immunologic origin, including thyroiditis, arthritis, rash, and Coombs-positive hemolytic anemia. Presenting features commonly resemble those of acute viral hepatitis and may include weakness, nausea, vomiting, behavioral changes, malaise, and jaundice. Conversely, and less commonly, patients may be asymptomatic, and the disease may be discovered when liver function abnormalities are uncovered in the course of routine evaluations. Laboratory features include elevated serum aminotransferases, often in the range of 500 to 1000 IU. Coagulation defects and hypergammaglobulinemia usually exist. Serologic abnormalities include positive LE cell tests in approximately 15% of cases, and antinuclear and anti-smooth muscle antibodies in 70%. In addition, some cases of chronic active hepatitis in children and adults are associated with the presence of anti-liver-kidney microsome (anti-ER) antibodies. These patients may form a distinct subset of patients with autoimmune chronic hepatitis, characterized by early age at onset and rapidly progressive hepatic disease. HLA types B8 and DRW3 appear to be associated with the development of autoimmune chronic active hepatitis. Findings on physical examination often include jaundice, mild hepatomegaly, and splenomegaly. Signs of chronic liver disease, including spider telangiectasias and palmar erythema, may be present. In advanced cases, findings may reflect underlying hepatic cirrhosis and may include edema, ascites, variceal hemorrhage, and hepatic encephalopathy.

Pathologic findings in chronic active hepatitis, regardless of cause, include the characteristic finding of piecemeal necrosis. In this histopathologic process, portal inflammation breeches the portal-parenchymal interface (limiting plate), and necrosis of bordering hepatocytes is present. In more severe disease, bands of necrosis may spread from portal area to portal area, central area to portal area, or central area to central area (bridging necrosis). Fibrosis extends into the lobule, eventually causing cirrhosis. The presence of bridging or of multilobular necrosis usually denotes severe, progressive disease. Cirrhosis may be present at the time of diagnosis.

FULMINANT HEPATIC FAILURE

Fulminant hepatic failure (FHF) results from acute, massive hepatocellular necrosis or from sudden, severe impairment of hepatocellular function. Patients typically have no evidence of prior hepatic dysfunction. Hepatic encephalopathy is a prerequisite for the diagnosis of FHF. In cases of viral hepatitis, encephalopathy must occur within 8 weeks of onset. Hepatic failure complicating chronic liver disease may present with similar clinical and laboratory features. In FHF, all hepatic functions are usually impaired, including hepatic synthetic, excretory, and detoxifying functions.

■ ETIOLOGY

Approximately 50% of FHF cases are caused by acute viral hepatitis. Hepatitis A, B, C, D, and E may all cause FHF, as may Epstein-Barr virus, herpes simplex virus, and enteroviral infections. Other non-A, non-B agents may be involved as well. Hepatotoxic drugs may be responsible for 25% of cases of FHF. Acetaminophen toxicity is a common cause. Less commonly associated agents include intravenous tetracycline, halothane, sodium valproate, ethanol, carbon tetrachloride, methyldopa, and isoniazid. Poisoning due to ingestion of the mushroom *Amanita phalloides* may be responsible. Hepatic ischemia due to endotoxic shock, vascular occlusion, or congenital heart disease may result in massive necrosis. In childhood, metabolic disorders including galactosemia, tyrosinemia, hereditary fructose intolerance, and Wilson's disease may cause FHF.

■ CLINICAL FEATURES

The patient may have had a recent episode of viral hepatitis or recent drug and toxin ingestion. Patients or their parents may report the onset of lethargy, nausea, vomiting, fever, lack of appetite, and abdominal pain. Jaundice may have developed. Hepatic encephalopathy may initially manifest with minor behavioral or motor disturbances. Infants may become irritable, eat poorly, and exhibit disturbed sleep patterns; older children may be confused and exhibit slurred speech. Asterixis, elicited through dorsiflexion of the hand at the wrist, may be demonstrable. Hepatic encephalopathy may progress to deep coma. Fetor hepaticus is often present. Ascites may develop, and there may be frequent episodes of bleeding. Hyperventilation may be an early sign, with hypoventilation becoming a problem in more advanced stages of disease. Cardiac arrhythmias (eg, tachycardia, bradycardia) and hypotension often occur. Hepatomegaly may occur, and a rapidly decreasing hepatic size is an ominous sign.

■ LABORATORY FEATURES

Laboratory features include elevation of conjugated and unconjugated serum bilirubin. Serum aminotransferases may be dramatically elevated initially, although a subsequent decrease may occur as the patient's condition worsens. Indices of hepatic synthetic function are commonly altered. Serum albumin concentrations may be normal at presentation but may decrease with time. The prothrombin time is markedly elevated and usually does not improve with vitamin K administration; values over 50 seconds have been associated with poor outcome. The serum concentrations of clotting factors synthesized in the liver (ie, Factors I, II, V, VII, IX, and X) are usually low, and Factor VIII levels are normal or increased. Levels of Factor VII, which has a short plasma half-life, below 8% of normal have been associated with a very poor outcome. Platelet concentrations may be diminished secondary to bone marrow suppression, disseminated intravascular coagulation, or hypersplenism. Platelet function may also be abnormal.

Serum ammonia may be elevated, but the onset of encephalopathy may precede this rise, which presumably is caused by an inadequacy of urea cycle function. Serum sodium values are frequently diminished in the setting of renal resorption of sodium and elevated total-body sodium values. Hypokalemia may result from increased renal excretion of potassium. Hypoglycemia may occur, particularly in children, presumably because of depletion of hepatic glycogen, inadequacy of gluconeogenesis, and hormonal dysfunction. Azotemia may occur; serum creatinine values rise, and blood urea nitrogen values may remain stable or fall because of deficient urea synthesis. Hypophosphatemia, hypocalcemia, and hypomagnesemia may occur. Hyperventilation may cause systemic alkalosis, but cell necrosis may result in systemic acidosis. Hepatic biopsy, which is seldom possible in patients with FHF because of marked coagulopathy, reveals massive hepatocellular necrosis, which may be patchy or zonal. Bridging necrosis and sparse inflammation may also be seen. In cases of tetracycline toxicity or of acute fatty liver of pregnancy, microvesicular fatty infiltration of hepatocytes occurs. Hepatic failure in these cases is presumably secondary to hepatocyte organelle dysfunction.

■ PROGNOSIS

If recovery from FHF occurs, it is usually complete, with no residual hepatic dysfunction. Patients with FHF due to HBV and especially those (45%) HBV with HDV coinfection may have chronic active hepatitis after recovery.

The survival rate is best for patients with FHF due to HAV (60% to 70%) and acetaminophen intoxication (50%). Lowest survival rates are found for those with FHF secondary to non-A, non-B hepatitis and idiosyncratic reactions to halothane (10% to 20%). Multiple prognostic indicators have been proposed. The following factors are associated with a poor prognosis:

Acetaminophen toxicity associated with a pH less than 7.3 (95% mortality), prothrombin time of more than 100 seconds, and a creatinine level of more than 300 μmol/L with grade 3 encephalopathy (77% mortality)

Viral hepatitis and drug reactions associated with an age of less than 11 or more than 40 years, jaundice more than 7 days before onset of encephalopathy, bilirubin levels higher than 300 μmol/L, and a prothrombin times greater than 50 seconds

Other proposed variables have included Factor V levels less than 20% or Factor VII levels of less than 8% of controls. Grade 4 coma, renal failure, and major episodes of GI bleeding have been identified as poor prognostic signs in the pediatric population. The decision to transplant is a difficult one

and must be based on relative outcomes of FHF and of transplantation. Twenty-eight percent of transplantation candidates die awaiting organs. For those who receive organs, the survival rate is approximately 60%. Transplantation is usually curative. Although patients transplanted secondary to fulminant hepatitis B infection may remain serologically positive, they rarely have clinical disease, unlike those transplanted for chronic HBV. One group suggested the need for transplantation be determined by grade 4 encephalopathy and the need for continued fresh frozen plasma (FFP) infusions to keep the prothrombin time within 10 seconds of control values.

Hepatocellular failure is the cause of death of 20% of the patients with FHF, and 80% of the deaths are caused by complications, including cerebral edema, GI hemorrhage, and sepsis.

PORTAL HYPERTENSION

■ ETIOLOGY AND CLINICAL PRESENTATION

Portal hypertension occurs in children because of obstruction to blood flow at one of several sites. An extrahepatic or presinusoidal block most often occurs in children as a result of obstruction to blood flow in the portal vein or one of its branches. In approximately 40% of children with this lesion, a history of portal vein injury may be elicited. Causes of injury include umbilical vein catheterization, neonatal omphalitis, or surgical trauma. Older children may have a history of abdominal trauma or pancreatitis. Clinical signs at presentation may include abdominal pain, diarrhea, and abdominal distention. Splenomegaly is usually found, although the liver size is normal. Ascites and GI hemorrhage, usually from esophageal varices, may occur. Multiple congenital anomalies, including biliary, cardiovascular, and urinary tract abnormalities, have been associated with this syndrome. Laboratory findings are consistent with hypersplenism: thrombocytopenia, neutropenia, or anemia. Abnormalities of coagulation factors may be detected.

■ DIAGNOSIS

Diagnosis is by ultrasound, angiography of the portal venous system, and magnetic resonance imaging, all of which are useful in demonstrating the anatomy of the portal venous system. Because intrinsic liver disease must be excluded, hepatic biopsy may be required.

■ PROGNOSIS

Hemorrhage from esophageal varices is frequently observed in cases of extrahepatic portal hypertension; in one series, the incidence was 79% of children. Presumably because of relatively intact hepatocellular function, most of these bleeding episodes are well tolerated and may be treated conservatively and with endoscopic sclerotherapy. Portosystemic shunt procedures have also been used, but shunt surgery in young children carries a high rate of failure because of shunt thrombosis. In addition, the long-term risk of encephalopathy exists. In affected children, bleeding episodes usually decrease in frequency with age, often ceasing entirely in the third decade of life, presumably because of the development of effective collateral circulation.

HEPATORENAL SYNDROME

The hepatorenal syndrome denotes the occurrence of unexplained progressive renal disease in patients with hepatic disease. The hepatorenal syndrome occurs in patients with ascites and portal hypertension after a precipitating event, most often one producing a decrease in circulating plasma volume. Laboratory features include a low urine sodium in conjunction with azotemia. The differential diagnosis of oliguria in the cirrhotic patient also includes prerenal causes and acute tubular necrosis; if acute tubular necrosis is present, support with dialysis is necessary until renal function returns.

There is no specific therapy for hepatorenal syndrome, but sodium and fluid intake should be limited. Dialysis may be useful for patients with acute hepatic dysfunction in whom adequate hepatic function is expected to return. The prognosis of the patient with hepatorenal syndrome and chronic liver disease is poor, and transplantation should be considered.

HEPATIC TRANSPLANTATION

With the availability of the immunosuppressive agent cyclosporine, liver transplantation has become a viable option for many patients with acute fulminant hepatic failure and chronic hepatic disease. Potential candidates for liver transplantation include those with the following conditions:

Diseases after a progressive, irreversible, downhill course, such as biliary atresia after a failed Kasai procedure

Decompensated hepatic disease, especially if accompanied by life-threatening complications, such as ascites with spontaneous bacterial peritonitis and variceal hemorrhage

Intractable pruritus or severe metabolic bone disease with resultant social invalidism

Diseases for which no alternative therapy is available, such as the type I Crigler-Najjar syndrome.

Contraindications to liver transplantation include unresectable extrahepatic primary malignancy, malignancy metastatic to the liver, or terminal disease uncorrectable by liver transplantation. Disorders in children for which liver transplantation may be required include biliary atresia, tyrosinemia, α_1-antitrypsin deficiency, neonatal hepatitis (rarely), fulminant hepatic failure, and Wilson's disease with fulminant hepatic failure.

Survival rates after liver transplantation range from 60% to 90%. Slightly lower rates of survival are reported for infants younger than 1 year of age and weighing 5 to 10 kg. Size is a major limiting factor in transplantation because of technical difficulties and because of the lack of donors weighing less than 10 kg. Newer technologies, including split liver transplantations and the use of living related donors, are partially ameliorating the problem.

Potential complications of liver transplantation include hepatic artery thrombosis, graft necrosis, biliary anastomotic leakage, GI bleeding, and GI perforation. Viral and bacterial sepsis may occur. Despite immunosuppression with cyclosporine, episodes of rejection may occur. Treatment of these episodes includes bolus administration of corticosteroids and, if needed, additional immunosuppressive agents, including monoclonal antilymphocyte antibody preparations.

Despite these limitations, liver transplantation is a life-saving and potentially curative procedure for many patients with hepatic disease. Follow-up of children who have undergone liver transplantation entails careful monitoring of cyclosporine levels and hypertension, which often occurs after liver transplantation. Episodes of rejection must be quickly differentiated from episodes of viral hepatitis, ordinarily by percutaneous hepatic biopsy. Additional psychosocial issues arise as the patient and his or her family returns to their social environment. The use of newer immunosuppressive agents, including FK506, may further enhance the success of hepatic transplantation and allow multiple organ (ie, gut and liver) transplantation.

CHOLEDOCHAL CYSTS

■ CLINICAL FEATURES

Choledochal cysts occur in as many as 2% of infants with obstructive jaundice. This potentially correctable lesion must be sought in all cholestatic infants.

Choledochal cysts may manifest at any age. There is a 3:1 female predominance. The infantile form usually presents in the first few months of age with jaundice and acholic stools; hepatomegaly may develop. A palpable abdominal mass may be found in as many as 60% of these patients. Approximately 50% of infants experience vomiting and failure to thrive. Infants with choledochal cysts have various degrees of hepatic impairment at diagnosis. Those with cirrhosis and portal hypertension usually have a poor prognosis despite cyst resection.

Children older than 2 years of age may present with the classic signs of abdominal pain (often secondary to pancreatitis), jaundice, and an abdominal mass, but all three findings are present in fewer than 25% of affected patients. Episodes of recurrent cholangitis may also occur. Hepatic injury due to obstruction caused by the cyst is usually less severe in patients who are first seen at an older age; their prognosis is better. Abnormalities of the pancreatic duct are common in patients with late-onset choledochal cysts, as are coexisting hepatic and biliary anomalies, including double common duct, double gallbladder, and accessory hepatic ducts. Biliary and pancreatic calculi may be detected.

■ DIAGNOSIS

The diagnosis of choledochal cysts is usually made with ultrasonography, which has demonstrated choledochal cysts in utero. Other potentially useful techniques include radionuclide scintigraphy, computed tomography scans, endoscopic retrograde cholangiopancreatography, and percutaneous transhepatic cholangiography.

■ THERAPY

Therapy usually involves surgical excision of the cyst. A Roux-en-Y loop of jejunum is used to drain the proximal duct system. Cholangitis may occur postoperatively, and the development of malignancy in retained cystic tissue is a risk.

(Abridged from Donald A. Novak, Frederick J. Suchy, and William F. Balistreri, Disorders of the Liver and Biliary System Relevant to Clinical Practice, in Oski, DeAngelis, Feigin, McMillan, Warshaw: *Principles and Practice of Pediatrics, Second Edition*, J.B. Lippincott, 1994.)

Oski's Essential Pediatrics,
edited by Kevin B. Johnson and Frank A. Oski.
Lippincott–Raven Publishers,
Philadelphia © 1997

171

Neonatal Hyperbilirubinemia

Jaundice is one of the most common conditions found in the newborn infant, and measurement of the serum bilirubin concentration probably is the laboratory test performed most often in the newborn nursery. Although the cause of most neonatal jaundice is developmental and the clinical course nearly always is benign, physicians caring for newborn infants must be alert for the minority of cases in which the cause of hyperbilirubinemia is pathologic or the clinical course is atypical, with exaggerated and possibly harmful levels of hyperbilirubinemia. Observation and follow-up of the newborn infant must be diligent to identify such cases early enough in the clinical course to ensure prompt and adequate treatment.

■ DEFINITION

The term *hyperbilirubinemia* implies an excessive level of serum bilirubin, potentially associated with a pathologic cause or outcome. In fact, during the first few days of postnatal life, most newborns have maximum serum bilirubin levels exceeding the upper limits of normal for adults, even when no disease is present. The reason for this "physiologic" hyperbilirubinemia is a developmental delay in the conjugation and excretion of bilirubin as the infant achieves a postnatal transition from dependence on maternal clearance of fetal bilirubin by reexcretion across the placenta and maternal conjugation of the unconjugated pigment, to a more mature and self-contained enzymatic and excretory pathway for bilirubin conjugation and elimination.

In the first 3 to 4 postnatal days, normal infants have a physiologic increase in serum bilirubin from cord bilirubin levels of 1.5 mg/dL or less at birth to a mean value of 6.5 ± 2.5 mg/dL (mean ± SD) on the third or fourth postnatal day. There is a difference in mean serum bilirubin levels even within the first 3 or 4 days between breast-fed infants (7.3 ± 3.9 mg/dL) and formula-fed infants (5.7 ± 3.3 mg/dL). This difference persists for the next several days, with clinically significant hyperbilirubinemia developing more frequently in breast-fed infants during the first week.

Although most newborns have hyperbilirubinemia by normal adult standards, physiologic jaundice is an event that is linked to normal development, is benign and self-limited, resolves by the end of the first week, and requires no treatment. Virtually all newborns manifest a phase of physiologic jaundice; during this time, the serum bilirubin level rises to between 6 and 8 mg/dL. This elevation, which results almost exclusively from an increase in the amount of unconjugated bilirubin (UCB), occurs in the absence of hemolytic disease and is more marked in premature infants. Classically, neonatal unconjugated hyperbilirubinemia has been attributed primarily to defective bilirubin conjugation and, indeed, low levels of glucuronyl transferase activity are detected in the human fetal and neonatal liver. However, a variety of other factors may contribute to the genesis of physiologic jaundice.

In addition, bilirubin appears to undergo a significant enterohepatic circulation in the newborn. Conjugated bilirubin in the intestinal tract of the adult is reduced by anaerobic intestinal flora to poorly absorbable urobilinogen. These flora are not present in the fetal and neonatal intestine. Instead, β-glucuronidase activity, present in the neonatal intestine, hydrolyzes bilirubin diglucuronide into UCB, which subsequently is reabsorbed into the portal circulation, contributing to the "bilirubin overload" and further taxing already stressed metabolic and excretory pathways. Thus, delayed passage of meconium can cause an elevation in the serum bilirubin level.

Some newborns show an unusually early onset, exaggerated and sustained levels, or an uncommonly long duration of hyperbilirubinemia, and these infants may require medical attention. About 3% of term newborns may have exaggerated or sustained hyperbilirubinemia as part of the normal postnatal development of their ability to conjugate and excrete bilirubin, whereas another 3% to 5% of these infants may have clinically significant hyperbilirubinemia associated with some other identifiable cause. Even with exaggerated hyperbilirubinemia, about half of the cases encountered appear to be developmental, self-limited, and presumably benign. Hyperbilirubinemia, therefore, is a frequent observation in the nursery, and the term used by itself indicates only that the level of jaundice observed is greater than that expected for a healthy infant. Further observation and diagnostic studies may be necessary to arrive at a specific cause for the hyperbilirubinemia, or to alert the pediatrician that it is of pathologic origin and potentially is hazardous.

Because visible cutaneous and scleral jaundice in the newborn usually is noted only when the serum bilirubin level exceeds 7 to 8 mg/dL, most self-limited developmental jaundice with a maximum serum bilirubin level at or below the mean value for newborns remains undetected. There is no indication for routine serum bilirubin determination in newborns who are not clinically jaundiced. However, visible jaundice develops in about 15% of newborns with serum bilirubin levels in the range of 10 to 12 mg/dL or greater. The differential diagnosis of jaundice in these infants may be assisted by noting the rapidity of onset, the presence of major or minor blood group incompatibility between the mother and her newborn, the presence of associated findings such as hematomas or evidence of infection, the method of feeding being used, and the duration and clinical course of jaundice beyond the third day. If the presence of visible jaundice in the range of 13 to 15 mg/dL is accepted as a working definition of exaggerated hyperbilirubinemia, about 3% of the newborn population will have jaundice in this range as a result of a detectable cause potentially requiring treatment and follow-up, whereas about 3% will represent the statistical upper limits of normal. Strictly speaking, the term *hyperbilirubinemia* in the newborn should be reserved for cases that exceed the expected limits of normal or are associated with an unusual rapidity of onset, unexpected persistence beyond the first few days, or a recognized pathologic cause.

■ CAUSES OF HYPERBILIRUBINEMIA

Table 171–1 lists many common causes of neonatal jaundice. Many of these conditions are discussed elsewhere in this book. About 2% of breast-fed infants have a prolonged (2- to 8-week) course of moderate unconjugated hyperbilirubinemia, usually in the range of 10 to 15 mg/dL, while they are feeding adequately on breast milk and have normal weight gain and no other abnormal clinical findings. Arias and colleagues showed that, in a group of infants with breast-milk jaundice, high levels of 3α-, 20β-pregnanediol in

TABLE 171-1. Differential Diagnosis of Neonatal Jaundice

Cause	Associated Findings
UNCONJUGATED ("INDIRECT") HYPERBILIRUBINEMIA	
Hemolytic Disease (Isoimmune)	
ABO incompatibility	Positive Coomb's antiglobulin test (anti-A or anti-B); microspherocytes
Rh incompatibility	Maternal anti-Rh titer; positive Coomb's test; nucleated RBCs
Other minor blood group incompatibility	Positive Coomb's test; RBC morphology variable
*Structural or Metabolic Abnormalities of RBCs**	
Hereditary spherocytosis	Family history; splenomegaly; microspherocytes
Glucose-6-phosphate dehydrogenase (G6PD) deficiency	Family history; recent exposure to an oxidant in food or drug; with or without splenomegaly
Hereditary Defects in Bilirubin Conjugation	
Crigler-Najjar syndrome	Complete lack of glucuronyl transferase; severe, lifelong unconjugated hyperbilirubinemia
Gilbert's disease (Arias syndrome)	Family history; partial defect of glucuronyl transferase; sometimes responds to phenobarbital
Bacterial Sepsis	History and findings compatible with neonatal infection; often an increase in direct bilirubin as well
"Breast-Milk" Jaundice	Mild to moderate, but persistent, hyperbilirubinemia; usually improves when breast milk is discontinued
Physiologic Jaundice	Usually mild to moderate; no predisposing factors; self-limited (duration <1 wk)
CONJUGATED ("DIRECT") HYPERBILIRUBINEMIA	
Congenital Biliary Atresia	Dilated intrahepatic ducts; no bile excretion
Extrahepatic Obstruction	Extrahepatic mass or cyst; dilated main or common bile ducts
Neonatal Hepatitis	
Bacterial	Findings compatible with neonatal sepsis
Viral	Inflammatory changes; other systemic signs of a specific viral infection
Nonspecific	Inflammatory changes without a specific viral etiology
"Inspissated Bile Syndrome"	Persistent direct hyperbilirubinemia associated with isoimmune hemolytic disease
Post-Asphyxia	Compatible history, plus increased hepatocellular enzyme concentrations
α_1-Antitrypsin Deficiency	Deceased, α_1-antitrypsin levels; reduction or "chronic" lung disease
Neonatal Hemosiderosis	Hemosiderin-filled macrophages in biopsy

*Only the two most common disorders listed, as examples. RBCs, *red blood cells.*

their mothers' milk were associated with decreased hepatic conjugation of bilirubin and persistent hyperbilirubinemia, and they proposed that the ingestion of pregnanediol in breast milk was the specific cause of this condition. In more recent investigations of breast-milk jaundice, however, not all infants exposed to high milk levels of pregnanediol have had hyperbilirubinemia, and not all cases of breast milk jaundice have been associated with high pregnanediol levels. Other possible contributing factors to breast-milk jaundice, proposed by some investigators but not confirmed by multiple independent studies, include high concentrations of lipase, β-glucuronidase, or polyunsaturated fatty acids in breast milk. Multiple hormonal or enzymatic factors may be involved in suppressing the conjugation of bilirubin or cleaving bilirubin conjugates in the small bowel in certain mother–baby pairs, thereby promoting the reabsorption and enterohepatic recirculation of UCB. Although the pathogenesis of breast-milk jaundice is controversial, most patients are asymptomatic and have only mild hyperbilirubinemia, and the majority respond to temporary cessation of breast-feeding for 36 to 48 hours with a prompt decrease in the serum bilirubin level.

The early onset of hyperbilirubinemia in breast-fed infants may be abetted by hospital feeding practices, which frequently call for an 8- to 12-hour period of postnatal observation without feeding, followed by a schedule of feeding every 4 hours. This type of scheduling may not allow sufficient nursing time during the first few days, resulting in the delayed onset of adequate lactation, suboptimal volume intake, and a delay in the normal bilirubin excretion that takes place as meconium is expelled, followed by normal neonatal stools that are rich in bile pigments.

■ BILIRUBIN TOXICITY

High circulating concentrations of bilirubin are toxic to the central nervous system (CNS), with the basal ganglia being the most vulnerable areas and cortical damage occurring relatively infrequently. The reason for the susceptibility of the basal ganglia to bilirubin toxicity is not known, and the metabolic abnormalities underlying bilirubin toxicity in the CNS are not understood. Clinical manifestations of bilirubin toxicity most frequently involve the basal ganglia and cranial nerve nuclei. The most characteristic findings are opisthotonos, extensor rigidity, tremors, ataxic gait, oculomotor paralysis, and hearing loss. Fatal cases in the newborn period often are characterized by loss of the suck response and lethargy, followed by hyperirritability, then seizures and death. The acute phases of bilirubin toxicity in severely affected infants often have been accompanied also by gastric and pulmonary hemorrhages. In fatal cases, the meninges and cortical surfaces may be stained lightly with bilirubin, but dense regional staining with bilirubin is found in the basal ganglia, globus pallidus, hippocampus, and, sometimes, cerebellum. In later deaths, scarring and gliosis may be found in these or adjacent areas that presumably were sites of bilirubin deposition. Neurologic damage in survivors corresponds to injury in the areas found to be stained in many autopsies. Intelligence and higher cortical functions are relatively spared, whereas ataxia, choreoathetosis, tremors, oculomotor palsy, and central hearing loss persist.

In general, the serum UCB concentrations associated with overt bilirubin encephalopathy (or kernicterus, the pathologic term for nuclear staining with bilirubin) are substantially higher than the indirect bilirubin levels normally seen among infants with hyperbilirubinemia in ordinary clinical practice. Bilirubin levels generally associated with clinical signs of kernicterus in term infants tend to be in the range of 25 to 30 mg/dL, or even higher. In epidemiologic surveys of bilirubin encephalopathy associated with Rh hemolytic disease, basal ganglion staining or clinical signs of bilirubin encephalopathy were encountered occasionally when the serum indirect bilirubin level reached or slightly exceeded 20 mg/dL. In most proven cases, however, the serum bilirubin level was considerably higher, often approaching 30 mg/dL. On the other hand, there are well-documented cases of patients with serum indirect bilirubin levels in the range of 30 to 35 mg/dL who did not experience serious long-term sequelae. Therefore, no precise bilirubin level has been established clearly at which either safety or permanent harm can be guaranteed.

Premature infants, especially those with a birth weight of less than 1500 g, and some infants with sepsis or metabolic complications of asphyxia or respiratory distress may be vulnerable to bilirubin toxicity at lower indirect bilirubin concentrations. During the 1960s and 1970s, numerous cases of basal ganglion staining at maximum serum bilirubin levels of 10 to 15 mg/dL, along with other, more perplexing, cases of generalized cortical and subcortical bilirubin staining, were reported in preterm infants or in larger infants with a complicated postnatal course often marked by sepsis or asphyxia. A few such patients had overt neurologic findings of bilirubin encephalopathy, but, in many cases, "low bilirubin kernicterus" was an incidental finding at autopsy, unsuspected from the clinical course. The clinical significance of low bilirubin kernicterus and its implication for follow-up of jaundiced preterm infants are uncertain, but the incidence of bilirubin staining in the CNS discovered at autopsy seems to have decreased in the 1980s. Moderate hyperbilirubinemia in the range of 15 to 20 mg/dL poses little or no acute or long-term developmental risk for otherwise normal infants. Term infants with hyperbilirubinemia in this range show, at most, only subtle and short-term behavioral changes, with no detectable long-term developmental or neurologic sequelae on follow-up. In the range of 20 to 25 mg/dL, some term infants become less active and responsive, and also show reversible increases in conduction time and occasional decreases in wave amplitude on determinations of auditory brain stem evoked potentials. The long-term significance of abnormalities in brain stem evoked potentials is not clear, but the study tracings return to normal as bilirubin concentrations fall back into the normal range or respond to treatment.

In summary, uncontrolled levels of severe hyperbilirubinemia produce a characteristic pattern of damage in the basal ganglia, manifested by basal ganglion staining at autopsy or by a subcortical neurologic deficit in survivors. In the range of 20 to 25 mg/dL of indirect bilirubin, some term infants show subtle but reversible sensory and behavioral changes of uncertain prognostic significance. Low bilirubin kernicterus in preterm infants remains a diagnostic and developmental puzzle, with a definitive solution becoming less likely as the incidence of low bilirubin kernicterus declines in this high-risk group.

The mechanism of bilirubin toxicity is not clear, but it probably is mediated by the entry of UCB into susceptible areas of the CNS. There are two possible mechanisms for bilirubin entry into the brain: diffusion of UCB, a somewhat lipophilic compound, across an intact blood–brain barrier, or damage to the blood–brain barrier with significant entry of plasma contents into the brain. Nearly all the bilirubin in the circulation is bound tightly to serum albumin, but at the very high bilirubin levels that usually are found in term infants with kernicterus, the total bilirubin concentration in the plasma may exceed the albumin concentration available to bind it, with increased diffusion of "free" bilirubin across the blood–brain barrier into the brain extravascular space. Because of the fact that, in most cell models of bilirubin toxicity, free bilirubin (ie, that which is not bound to plasma albumin) produces the abnormal metabolic or neurologic effect, whereas bilirubin bound to an equimolar concentration of albumin in the same system usually fails to produce the same effect, it is a plausible, but still unproven, hypothesis that the free fraction of UCB is the species responsible for the observed toxicity in patients with severe hyperbilirubinemia. In very immature or high-risk infants, however, especially those with kernicterus or cortical bilirubin staining as an incidental finding at autopsy, it also is plausible that injury to the blood–brain barrier allows quantitative entry of albumin-bound bilirubin, with incidental staining of susceptible structures, but without clinical evidence of bilirubin toxicity. The controversy regarding the relative contributions of "free" bilirubin and of underlying injury to the brain or blood–brain barrier in the finding of kernicterus at autopsy, or in the observation of neurologic abnormalities in the clinical setting, remains unresolved at this time.

■ DIAGNOSIS

Determination of the serum bilirubin concentration is indicated only for visible jaundice in healthy term infants, unless prenatal or delivery room screening procedures reveal the presence of a hemolytic anemia with a positive Coombs' test. Daily inspection of the baby, undressed and in adequate light, allows early recognition of cutaneous or scleral jaundice in most cases. For nonwhite infants, part of the examination can include brief compression with the examiner's thumb of the skin over a firm surface such as the forehead, sternum, or upper thigh; briefly blanching the skin may help to reveal an underlying yellow color. Skin reflectance by means of a commercially available transcutaneous bilirubinometer is another aid to the evaluation of clinically evident jaundice in the nursery. The reflectance of jaundiced skin correlates well enough with serum bilirubin levels to be used as a screening test for hyperbilirubinemia with proper standardization of the technique and the instrument. Again, the correlation of skin reflectance with serum bilirubin levels is better in white than in nonwhite infants with jaundice.

Both clinical observation and skin reflectance document that cutaneous jaundice progresses from the face downward in term infants. Scleral and facial jaundice become visible at bilirubin levels of 6 to 8 mg/dL, jaundice of the shoulders and trunk becomes apparent at 8 to 10 mg/dL, jaundice of the lower body is noticeable at 10 to 12 mg/dL, and generally distributed jaundice can be seen at 12 to 15 mg/dL. Although this is only the roughest of guidelines, it serves to emphasize that daily observation of newborns for signs of jaundice often permits the timely recognition of developing hyperbilirubinemia, with the advantages that early detection may provide for timely diagnosis, intervention, and follow-up. Sometimes, the nurse is the first observer to note jaundice in the clinical record, and nurses' notes or messages should be followed up by reexamination of the infant and performance of appropriate laboratory studies when indicated. Visible jaundice on the first day is always abnormal and requires prompt evaluation and follow-up. Faint jaundice, first appearing only on the third or fourth hospital day or on the day of discharge, usually is consistent with the average bilirubin levels expected in term infants who are otherwise well, and it may require no intervention.

In addition to a laboratory request for the measurement of total and direct (or conjugated) bilirubin, the clinical detection of hyperbilirubinemia should prompt a thorough examination of the infant's abdomen with palpation of the liver and spleen, and a review of the maternal and neonatal hospital records for evidence of blood group incompatibility, a positive antibody titer or Coombs' test, or a family history of neonatal or childhood jaundice in siblings or other relatives. All women who are receiving prenatal care or are admitted to a hospital for delivery should have their major (A,B,O) and minor (Rh) blood groups determined. If the mothers are Rh negative, they also should have a titer for anti-Rh antibodies determined during the course of prenatal care. At birth, a cord blood specimen for each infant should be sent to the hospital serology laboratory or blood bank. If the mother's blood type is group O, or if she is Rh negative (with any major group), the infant's major and minor blood groups should be determined and an antibody screen performed if the maternal and neonatal major or Rh blood groups are incompatible.

Although 25% of pregnancies potentially are ABO incompatible, only a minority (10% to 15%) have hemolytic anemia as documented by a positive Coombs' test. In the absence of a positive antibody test, it is not possible to confirm the diagnosis of hemolytic anemia in the newborn. If prenatal or postnatal screening tests reveal the presence of a Coombs-positive hemolytic anemia, or if splenomegaly is present, then, in addition to serum bilirubin measurement, determination of hemoglobin, hematocrit, red cell indices, reticulocyte count, and red cell morphology should be undertaken. For the more common instance of benign, self-limited developmental hyperbilirubinemia, a complete blood count is not necessary unless there is strong reason to suspect hemolysis or infection as the source of hyperbilirubinemia. For known cases of Rh sensitization, hemoglobin, hematocrit, and bilirubin determinations should be performed on the cord blood as well as on subsequent postnatal specimens. For most cases of suspected ABO hemolytic disease, cord blood determinations are not needed because ABO incompatibility seldom causes significant jaundice or anemia at birth.

■ MANAGEMENT

The clinical course in most cases of neonatal jaundice defines the problem as benign and self-limited. Unless the infant has clear evidence of a hemolytic anemia or some other significant perinatal or postnatal abnormality, most cases of "physiologic hyperbilirubinemia" can be managed with observation, serial bilirubin determinations, and reassurance. Despite an extensive differential diagnosis for neonatal jaundice, the vast majority of cases are attributable to a small number of causes that usually are detectable by serial bilirubin determinations, examination of the patient, and review of maternal and neonatal blood type and antibody studies. The benign and self-limited course of most cases of nonhemolytic hyperbilirubinemia makes it unnecessary to pursue further diagnostic studies in the first few days.

ABO Incompatibility

ABO hemolytic disease is more common than Rh hemolytic disease, but it is more benign. In nearly all cases, the mother's blood type is group O (the major blood type in 40% of the North American population) and the infant's blood type is group A or B. Prenatal detection of ABO incompatibility is not feasible and generally is not necessary. Instead of sensitization during pregnancy, preformed maternal anti-A or anti-B antibodies of the IgG class are transferred passively to the infant late in pregnancy or at parturition. Rapid early hemolysis of fetal cells occurs, with splenic recognition and removal of antigen–antibody complexes. Because fetal red cells have only about 7500 to 8000 A or B antigen sites per cell (versus 15,000 to 20,000 in the adult), the fetal cells do not agglutinate, and they may not be destroyed completely. Splenic removal of the antibody may damage the cell membrane, which then repairs and reenters the circulation as a microspherocyte. Likewise, the decreased number of antigen–antibody sites on fetal cells may give a weakly positive or even a negative direct Coombs' reaction. The antibody may be identified correctly by incubation of the neonatal serum with incompatible adult red cells and performance of an *indirect* Coombs' test. Because not all ABO-incompatible pregnancies result in neonatal hemolysis, a positive Coombs' test (direct or indirect) is necessary to confirm the diagnosis.

ABO incompatibility seldom presents with severe jaundice or severe anemia at birth, but the rate of increase in bilirubin on the first postnatal day may lead to preparations for an exchange transfusion in some cases. If the initial rate of increase exceeds 1 mg/dL/h, if the infant is significantly anemic (hemoglobin 10 g/dL or less), or if the serum bilirubin level reaches the range of 15 to 20 mg/dL within the first 24 hours, a double volume exchange transfusion is indicated after the indirect bilirubin level has exceeded 15 mg/dL and before it exceeds 20 mg/dL. After the first postnatal day, the rate of red cell degradation and the subsequent rate of increase in the serum bilirubin level begin to diminish as the antigen–antibody complexes are cleared and the rate of hemolysis slows. This often will be reflected in a rapid early increase in the serum bilirubin level to the range of 10 to 15 mg/dL or slightly higher, followed by a plateau level at 15 to 20 mg/dL on the second hospital day. In this case, blood may be crossmatched and preparations made for an exchange transfusion, but the transfusion need not be done unless the hemolytic anemia becomes more severe or the serum bilirubin concentration exceeds 20 mg/dL.

As a general policy, exchange transfusion should be considered for any newborn with an indirect serum bilirubin level in the range of 20 to 25 mg/dL from any cause. Sustained hyperbilirubinemia within this range is potentially hazardous, as evidenced by changes in brain stem conduction time, changes in feeding behavior and responsiveness as noted anecdotally by many observers, and occasional cases of overt kernicterus at these bilirubin levels. It also is significant that, after prolonged exposure to UCB at 25 mg/dL, the amount of extravascular bilirubin may represent 30% to 50% of the body's total bilirubin stores. After an initial double volume exchange transfusion at 25 mg/dL has been performed, the immediate decline in the serum bilirubin level to 12 to 13 mg/dL is followed rapidly by a rebound to the range of 16 to 17 mg/dL. If the source of hyperbilirubinemia remains untreated or if the failure of bilirubin excretion persists at these levels, within a few hours, the serum bilirubin level may rise again to its preexchange level, making a second exchange transfusion necessary. If the infant is treated with earlier exchange transfusions to maintain the postexchange bilirubin concentration between 10 and 20 mg/dL, however, the risk of a second exchange transfusion becoming necessary is diminished somewhat, and the duration of exposure to extreme levels of hyperbilirubinemia is shortened.

■ PHOTOTHERAPY

Just as bilirubin probably is the most common laboratory determination performed in the newborn nursery, phototherapy probably is the most common treatment performed. The systematic use of fluorescent light to lower serum bilirubin levels followed the observations of Cremer, Perryman, and Richards in 1958 that jaundice was less frequent in a well-lighted nursery in a new wing of their hospital than in a dimly lighted one in an older wing. The mechanism of phototherapy, once thought to be the degradation of bilirubin and excretion of its degradation products as smaller molecules, now is found to proceed through the light-induced formation of configurational and structural isomers of UCB. These isomeric forms of bilirubin are more water-soluble than the parent compound, bilirubin IX-α; therefore, they are transported through the liver more rapidly than is the predominant form of UCB. The dose applied to the skin, ideally 5 to 10 $\mu W/cm^2/nm$ in the spectral range of 400 to 500 nm, rapidly converts UCB to its isomers in a dose-dependent fashion at the level of the skin. Doses lower than 3 to 4 $\mu W/cm^2/nm$ produce inefficient photoconversion, whereas the effectiveness of doses above 10 to 12 $\mu W/cm^2/nm$ is limited by a plateau effect in the photoconversion response and by practical limits on achieving higher light doses in the nursery setting. The photoconversion to isomers is rapid, followed by slower distribution of the isomers from the skin into the circulation and subsequent excretion of the isomers by the liver.

■ OTHER THERAPEUTIC CONSIDERATIONS

Feeding promotes peristalsis and colonization of the bowel. Peristalsis increases the rate of bilirubin excretion as the stools change from meconium to transitional to the bilirubin-rich yellowish brown stools that are apparent at several days of life, whereas bowel colonization with normal flora promotes the enzymatic conversion of bilirubin to other bile products that cannot be reabsorbed or reconverted to UCB. Unfed or underfed newborns tend to have more persistent jaundice than do those who are fed adequately, so the underfed nursing infant may show improvement rather than worsening of jaundice with increased frequency of nursing and a rise in milk intake within the first few days. It is possible to reduce the enterohepatic circulation of bilirubin by feeding agar or charcoal to the newborn, but these approaches have not gained widespread popularity. On the other hand, phenobarbital in low doses stimulates the conjugating enzymes and the hepatic excretory system for bilirubin; thus, infants with a family history of significant neonatal hyperbilirubinemia or those with contraindications to exchange transfusion (*eg*, for religious reasons) may benefit from the maternal or early neonatal administration of phenobarbital in low doses—usually lower than would be required to achieve therapeutic levels for seizure control. This is an approach to hyperbilirubinemia that can be used selectively, but has not found widespread acceptance in North America.

Future therapy for unconjugated hyperbilirubinemia, both that seen in the neonate and that occurring in the older patient with Crigler-Najjar syndrome, may focus on the inhibition of bilirubin formation from its hemoglobin precursor. The synthetic heme analogue tin-protoporphyrin has been shown to inhibit competitively heme oxygenase, the rate-limiting enzyme in the degradation of hemoglobin to bilirubin. Experiments using animal models and some preliminary clinical studies have shown that administration of this agent results in decreased biliary excretion of bilirubin, with concomitant increases in the excretion of heme pigment into bile. In addition, when it is given to neonatal animals or human newborns shortly after delivery, hyperbilirubinemia is prevented. Thus, with further development and documentation of its safety and efficacy, this approach may offer a specific therapy for unconjugated hyperbilirubinemia.

Management of Breast-Milk Jaundice

Most breast-fed infants have normal postnatal serum bilirubin levels that do not require any specific diagnostic or treatment measures. Early hyperbilirubinemia in breast-fed newborns may be associated with suboptimal feeding schedules and milk intake, resulting in excessive weight loss, infrequent stools, and inadequate excretion of bilirubin. No fixed interval between birth and the first breast-feeding should be necessary if the mother and baby are in good condition immediately after delivery. During the first several days postpartum, nursing on demand or at intervals more frequent than every 4 hours may help to stimulate lactation, avert excessive weight loss, and aid the transition from meconium to normal stools. Routine supplementation of breast-feeding with bottled water may be counterproductive, diminishing the thirst response between nursing periods while providing inadequate substrate for hepatic function and inadequate bulk for peristalsis. Water supplementation should be reserved for those few infants in whom milk intake and hydration are clearly inadequate and weight loss is obviously excessive.

Preterm infants of 35 to 37 weeks' gestation and weighing 2500 to 3000 g may appear healthy at birth, but may not nurse as well as term infants and still may have immature liver function. This group includes some infants delivered by elective cesarean section before term, with the smooth initiation of nursing complicated further by the mother's postoperative condition. Hepatic immaturity and inadequate intake may increase the likelihood of hyperbilirubinemia in such infants. Formula or water supplementation may be needed for adequate hydration and nutrition until lactation is well established, and phototherapy for hyperbilirubinemia in the range of 15 to 20 mg/dL may be used during the first several days, until hepatic function matures and adequate excretion of bilirubin begins.

The discontinuation of breast-feeding in a well baby with persistent hyperbilirubinemia is largely a matter of clinical judgment. Many cases of breast-milk jaundice are mild enough to require no intervention except for bilirubin determinations once or twice in the first several weeks after discharge, to follow the resolution of the problem. More severe cases, which often appear toward the end of the first week and then fail to resolve or progress to still higher levels of hyperbilirubinemia, may benefit from the therapeutic test of discontinuing breast-feeding for 36 to 48 hours. Discontinuation of nursing in the first few days, however, may not lower the bilirubin level or establish the probability of a breast milk inhibitor; the hormonal or enzymatic factors associated with persistent jaundice may not become operative until nursing is well established.

Hyperbilirubinemia caused by breast milk factors usually responds to the temporary cessation of nursing with a prompt decline of 2 to 4 mg/dL in the serum bilirubin level, after which nursing usually can be resumed with little or no further increase in bilirubin. In most cases, it appears that even temporary removal of the inhibiting factor allows an improvement in hepatic function and in the intestinal excretion of bilirubin. Only in rare cases is hyperbilirubinemia severe and persistent enough to require the complete discontinuation of breast-feeding. Phototherapy is indicated for

TABLE 171-2. Anticipatory Management of Neonatal Jaundice

1. Know maternal blood type
2. Know baby's blood type if mother is Rh-negative or Group O
3. Identify jaundice (especially if early onset)
4. Identify risk factors present by
   Serum bilirubin
                   and/or
   Coomb's test, Hgb, Hcrit, RBC indices and morphology
5. Observe, repeat, and discharge if jaundice is nonprogressive and no risk factor is present; or,
6. Start therapy as described below, if indicated by
   a. Approaching threshold
                   or
   b. Risk factors present
7. Start phototherapy when unconjugated bilirubin is below expected exchange transfusion level
8. Exchange Transfusion
   a. Early, if conditions are met
   b. Later, if phototherapy fails to control serum BR

Oski's Essential Pediatrics,
edited by Kevin B. Johnson and Frank A. Oski.
Lippincott–Raven Publishers,
Philadelphia © 1997

172

Cholecystitis

Cholecystitis is an inflammatory disease of the gallbladder that may be acute or chronic. In some instances, acute cholecystitis may be superimposed on the preexisting chronic form of the disease. Acute and chronic cholecystitis may be classified further as calculous or acalculous, based on the presence or absence of gallstones, which, if present, occur in 80% to 85% of children who have this disorder. Chronic cholecystitis with cholelithiasis is the most common pattern, occurring in almost two thirds of children with this diagnosis. The frequencies of the patterns of cholecystitis are shown in Table 172–1.

■ EPIDEMIOLOGY

The incidence of cholecystitis in children ranges from less than 1% to 4%. Although this disorder is less common in children than in adults, its frequency in childhood appears to be increasing. Girls are affected more commonly than boys after adolescence. Both sexes are affected equally before this age (Table 172–2). Several entities have been implicated as predisposing factors for cholecystitis in children and are listed in Table 172–3.

■ CLINICAL FEATURES

The clinical presentation of cholecystitis varies from total absence of symptoms to florid illness. The symptoms of cholecystitis in children are similar to those in adults and are summarized in Table 172–4.

■ LABORATORY AND RADIOGRAPHIC STUDIES

Although leukocytosis and elevated serum bilirubin and alkaline phosphatase levels may be found in many patients, laboratory studies, including liver function tests, are of limited diagnostic value. A complete blood cell count

only a small minority of breast-fed infants with hyperbilirubinemia that persists above 15 mg/dL and is unresponsive to the temporary discontinuation of breast-feeding.

Some authorities suggest that term breast-fed infants without other risk factors require no treatment until the serum indirect bilirubin exceeds 20 mg/dL, and that exchange transfusion is not indicated in these low-risk infants until the serum bilirubin level reaches or exceeds 25 mg/dL. Medical supervision and even daily follow-up of infants with "borderline," but still increasing, bilirubin levels is important. Undetected, unsupervised hyperbilirubinemia in breast-fed infants thought to be at no risk occasionally may progress to levels of 25 to 30 mg/dL or greater. Besides the uncertain risk of later neurologic damage from prolonged extremely high bilirubin levels, some unsupervised infants with extreme hyperbilirubinemia later are found to have risk factors that were not recognized at birth, and some of these are at risk for the development of clinically evident bilirubin encephalopathy.

■ CONCLUSION

In summary, most cases of neonatal hyperbilirubinemia are developmental, benign, and self-limited. Significant hyperbilirubinemia may occur in a few normal infants, in a somewhat larger number of breast-fed infants, and in many infants with hemolytic anemia of prenatal or neonatal origin. The typical case of physiologic jaundice may be managed with serial bilirubin determinations, close observation, and reassurance. For more severe or more complicated cases, after initial neonatal stabilization and specific diagnosis, exchange transfusion is the treatment of choice for indirect hyperbilirubinemia with levels in excess of 20 mg/dL or levels that are rising rapidly in association with hemolysis. Phototherapy can be used to stabilize indirect hyperbilirubinemia resulting from any cause, and potentially may offer the brain additional protection by isomerization of UCB. Long-term follow-up of persistent hyperbilirubinemia is necessary for a minority of infants who have jaundice associated with breast-feeding. Table 171–2 outlines a suggested approach to the anticipatory management of neonatal jaundice.

(Abridged from William J. Cashore, Neonatal Hyperbilirubinemia, in Oski, DeAngelis, Feigin, McMillan, Warshaw: *Principles and Practice of Pediatrics, Second Edition,* J.B. Lippincott, 1994.)

TABLE 172-1. Patterns of Cholecystitis and Their Frequency

Type	Frequency (%)
ACUTE CHOLECYSTITIS	
Calculous	19
Acalculous	5
CHRONIC CHOLECYSTITIS	
Calculous	64
Acalculous	12

TABLE 172-2. Epidemiology of Cholecystitis in Childhood

Sex distribution	
Female: male ratio	2:1
Race distribution	
White: black: Hispanic ratio	2:1:1
Age distribution (% of cases)	
Birth–5 y	22
6–10 y	19
11–15 y	30
16–20 y	29

TABLE 172-4. Clinical Features of Cholecystitis in Childhood

Finding	Frequency (% of Cases)
SYMPTOM	
Abdominal pain	67
Right upper quadrant	79
Epigastrium	19
Radiation to back, shoulder	38
Vomiting	41
Dietary fat intolerance	33
SIGN	
Abdominal tenderness	68
Jaundice	35
Fever	27
Mass	17

and hemoglobin electrophoresis may be indicated to determine the presence of an underlying hemolytic disorder.

Abdominal ultrasonography is the most effective, non-invasive method of delineating gallbladder dilation, thickened walls, and the presence of stones in the gallbladder or common bile and hepatic ducts. Significant abnormalities can be demonstrated in at least 90% of the children tested.

Hepatobiliary imaging with a ^{99m}Tc-labeled iminodiacetic acid derivative may be useful to demonstrate a nonfunctioning gallbladder in acute cholecystitis. Although performed infrequently, endoscopic retrograde cholangiopancreatography (ERCP) may suggest cystic or common bile duct obstruction in the absence of visualization of the gallbladder.

■ DIFFERENTIAL DIAGNOSIS

The principal conditions to consider in the differential diagnosis of cholecystitis are appendicitis, pancreatitis, gastroesophageal reflux, esophagitis, peptic ulcer disease, hepatitis, hepatic abscess or tumor, intussusception, pyelonephritis or nephrolithiasis, and pneumonitis (Table 172–5). Acute appendicitis is the disease most often confused

with acute cholecystitis. Generally, abdominal tenderness, fever, and leukocytosis progress more relentlessly in appendicitis than in cholecystitis. Laparotomy can resolve the diagnostic dilemma.

■ TREATMENT

The treatment of acute cholecystitis includes hospitalization, hydration with intravenous fluids, correction of electrolyte abnormalities, discontinuation of oral feedings, and insertion of a nasogastric tube for suction (Table 172–6). Medications (eg, meperidine, morphine) should be considered for pain relief. Antibiotics have no therapeutic value in early acute cholecystitis, because the illness has an uncomplicated course, but, if the clinical condition worsens (eg, fever, chills, increased pain, abdominal mass), antibiotic therapy is recommended.

Although the management of uncomplicated acute cholecystitis is controversial, cholecystectomy is the treatment of choice. Cholecystectomy can be performed safely and without delay even in children who are seriously ill. If the child's condition is precarious, cholecystostomy may be the preferred temporary procedure. One exception to this treatment plan is the child with sickle-cell anemia whose course is complicated by acute cholecystitis or an abdominal pain crisis. Urgent cholecystectomy under these circumstances has been associated with a high rate of surgical complications.

TABLE 172-3. Factors Associated With Cholecystitis in Childhood

Factors	Frequency (% of Cases)
Hemolytic disease	37
Ileal abnormalities	37
Pregnancy	31
Obesity	27
Total parenteral nutrition	19
Infection	12
Family history of biliary disease	12
Previous abdominal surgery	9
Cystic fibrosis	7
Biliary tract anomalies	6
Cirrhosis	4
Trauma	1
Other (congenital anomalies, drugs, ventilatory support)	<1

TABLE 172-5. Differential Diagnosis of Cholecystitis in Childhood

Appendicitis	Hepatic abscess, tumor
Pancreatitis	Intussusception
Gastroesophageal reflux	Pyelonephritis
Esophagitis	Nephrolithiasis
Peptic ulcer disease	Pneumonitis
Hepatitis	

TABLE 172-6. Treatment of Cholecystitis in Childhood

Medical	Surgical
Hospitalization	Cholecystectomy
Intravenous hydration	Exploration of the common duct
Correction of electrolyte abnormalities	
Nasogastric suction	
Analgesics	
Antibiotics	

■ COMPLICATIONS

The major complication of acute cholecystitis is perforation, which may manifest as a localized pericholecystic abscess, an extension into the peritoneal cavity with generalized peritonitis, or the formation of a cholecystenteric fistula, primarily with the duodenum or the hepatic flexure of the colon. Surgical intervention is indicated for these complications. Less frequently, ascending cholangitis, liver abscess, or sepsis may complicate the clinical course of acute cholecystitis.

The complications of chronic cholecystitis in the absence of cholelithiasis are minimal. Patients with gallstones are at risk for recurrent bouts of acute cholecystitis, pancreatitis, perforation, bile peritonitis, biliary obstruction, biliary cirrhosis, and cancer of the gallbladder.

■ PROGNOSIS

The prognosis after surgery for children with cholecystitis but without underlying hemolytic disease is excellent. The overall mortality rate for acute and chronic cholecystitis is less than 2% for children. Ten-year follow-up of children with gallbladder disease detected no further illness after cholecystectomy in 97% of patients. In children with hemolytic disorders, 82% had resolution of their episodes of abdominal pain and jaundice for as long as 6 years after cholecystectomy.

(Abridged from Kathleen J. Motil, Cholecystitis, in Oski, DeAngelis, Feigin, McMillan, Warshaw: *Principles and Practice of Pediatrics, Second Edition,* J.B. Lippincott, 1994.)

Oski's Essential Pediatrics,
edited by Kevin B. Johnson and Frank A. Oski.
Lippincott–Raven Publishers,
Philadelphia © 1997

173

Short Bowel Syndrome

Short bowel syndrome is perhaps the most common indication for the chronic use of parenteral nutrition in pediatrics. In the neonatal period, massive small-bowel resection often is necessary because of either congenital anomalies of the gastrointestinal tract or advanced ischemic injury from necrotizing enterocolitis. A smaller number of patients require resection later in life as a result of vascular injury of the small intestine, usually secondary to midgut volvulus, or

they have short bowel syndrome as a result of surgical management of advanced inflammatory bowel disease. Long-term survival without parenteral nutrition depends on the ability of the small intestine to increase its absorptive capacity so the patient's nutritional needs can be provided through the enteral route.

Many patients with a surprisingly short segment of small intestine eventually develop the ability to live without parenteral nutrition as a result of a compensatory increase in mucosal surface area caused by the adaptive response to massive resection. This compensatory growth is dominated by villus hyperplasia, although some dilatation and lengthening of the remaining small intestine do occur.

As might be expected, increases in villus length and in the number of enterocytes available for absorption per centimeter of bowel are accompanied by a gradual increase in the absorption of nearly all nutrients.

Stimulation of the adaptation process becomes the primary goal of therapy in the treatment of patients with short bowel syndrome. The importance of intraluminal nutrition in stimulating this process has been well documented in previous studies. The intraluminal nutrients not only are necessary to produce adaptation, but also are essential to maintain the structural and functional integrity of the small intestine.

The clinical management of short bowel syndrome can be considered best in three phases. Phase I consists of nutritional repletion with total parenteral nutrition (TPN). Phase II includes the gradual introduction of enteral nutrition, usually by continuous infusion. During phase III, continuous enteral nutrition is reduced incrementally as the patient is weaned over gradually to bolus or solid feeding.

Chronic bacterial overgrowth is a frequent complication of short bowel syndrome, further exacerbating malabsorption. Bacterial overgrowth is likely to occur when the ileocecal valve is absent, when a tight anastomosis or partial obstruction is present, or when a dilated segment of bowel with poor motility exists. Bacterial overgrowth exacerbates malabsorption because of injury of the intestinal mucosa and deconjugation of bile acids, facilitating their reabsorption and reducing bile acid availability for solubilization of long-chain fats. Such patients may respond to intermittent broad-spectrum antimicrobial therapy. I have found the combination of metronidazole with trimethoprim-sulfamethoxazole to be particularly helpful; clindamycin, because of its efficacy against anaerobic organisms, or oral gentamicin also may be useful. In some instances, continuous administration of cyclic antibiotics is required to control bacterial overgrowth. If possible, resecting a tight anastomosis or performing an intestinal tapering procedure is useful in alleviating bacterial overgrowth, and often results in marked improvement in absorption.

Metabolic acidoses have developed in some patients as a result of the production of excessive D-lactate by intestinal bacteria. Although both D-lactate and L-lactate are produced by intestinal bacteria, only the L form can be metabolized in humans. D-lactic acidosis is correctable by elimination of bacterial overgrowth and should be considered in patients with short bowel syndrome who have repeated attacks of dyspnea and drowsiness.

Gastric acid hypersecretion is common in infants with short bowel syndrome. Cimetidine has been shown to decrease stool mass as well as fecal excretion of sodium and potassium in adults with short bowel syndrome.

A number of surgical procedures have been devised to improve absorption in patients with short bowel syndrome. Most involve slowing intestinal transit. The most direct approach is construction of a valve or sphincter that functions in a manner similar to the ileocecal valve, causing constriction of the lumen and creating a partial mechanical obstruction. The intent also is to prevent retrograde reflux of bacterial contents into the small intestine. Clinical experience has been somewhat limited, and results usually are unsatisfactory. Antiperistaltic segments of small intestine also have been used.

Intestinal tapering or lengthening surgery occasionally may be helpful. A markedly dilated intestine often develops in patients with short bowel syndrome secondary to both partial chronic obstruction and adaptation. Tapering dilated segments reduces stasis and bacterial content, improves intestinal function, and preserves intestinal length. Intestinal tapering procedures have proven to be a valuable adjunct in patients with dilated segments of bowel who respond poorly to antibiotic therapy for bacterial overgrowth.

The ultimate cure for short bowel syndrome probably rests with intestinal transplantation. Improvements in immunosuppression with cyclosporine and FK506 suggest that intestinal transplantation ultimately may be possible. Substantial experience has been gained in performing intestine transplantations in experimental animals. In excess of 30 intestinal transplantations have been performed in children at a number of centers throughout North America and Europe. Most have been performed for short bowel syndrome with severe TPN-induced liver disease and have included concurrent liver transplantation. Early reports are encouraging, but adequate early diagnosis of small-intestinal rejection remains a problem, and early reports of the development of intestinal lymphomas are worrisome. Although denervation of the small intestine and lymphatic disruption occur, these do not appear to be major negative factors.

The prognosis for short bowel syndrome has been altered markedly through the use of parenteral nutrition. Advances in parenteral therapy, including changes in catheter techniques, solutions, understanding of the importance of intraluminal nutrition, and, finally, use of parenteral nutrition in the home, have altered markedly the way in which patients with short bowel syndrome are treated. In 1972, the classic paper by Wilmore defined the prognosis for short bowel syndrome in infants. Of 20 infants with a jejunoileal segment length of 38 to 75 cm, 95% survived. Infants with 15 to 38 cm of jejunum and ileum survived 50% of the time, provided the ileocecal valve was intact. Those without an ileocecal valve died, as did infants with less that 15 cm of small intestine, including all those with intact ileocecal valves. This paper pointed out the importance of the ileocecal valve in determining the prognosis for short bowel syndrome. Because this organ delays transit through the small intestine and reduces bacterial overgrowth at this site, it is the key to survival in many patients with short bowel syndrome.

Other data suggest that advances in parenteral nutrition have significantly changed the prognosis regarding short bowel syndrome in the 1980s. It was concluded that ultimate survival, including normal growth, without parenteral nutrition is possible with as little as 11 cm of jejunum and ileum and an intact ileocecal valve, and with as little as 25 cm of jejunum and ileum without an ileocecal valve. Patients with short bowel syndrome now die of the complications of parenteral nutrition, such as severe TPN cholestasis or fulminant septicemia, rather than of malnutrition. Intestinal transplantation likely will alter the prognosis further.

(Abridged from Jon A. Vanderhoof, Short Bowel Syndrome, in Oski, DeAngelis, Feigin, McMillan, Warshaw: *Principles and Practice of Pediatrics, Second Edition*, J.B. Lippincott, 1994.)

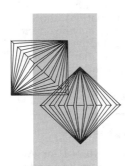

SECTION 12
Endocrinology and Metabolism

Oski's Essential Pediatrics, edited by Kevin B. Johnson and Frank A. Oski. Lippincott–Raven Publishers, Philadelphia © 1997

174

The Parathyroid Glands

Advances in understanding calcium homeostasis have revealed a rigidly controlled system involving the liver, bone, intestines, kidneys, and parathyroid glands. This system is remarkable for its inherent stability, but diseases of the parathyroid gland or the other organs in this system may cause significant clinical and metabolic disorders in children.

■ PHYSIOLOGY

Parathyroid hormone (PTH) indirectly activates the osteoclasts in the bone and increases resorption of mineralized bone, which mobilizes calcium and phosphorus. PTH activates the proximal and distal tubular cells in the kidney to promote calcium resorption and to inhibit phosphorus resorption. PTH stimulates the production of 1,25-dihydroxyvitamin D_3 in the kidney.

An understanding of calcium homeostasis must include an explanation of the actions of vitamin D. Vitamin D has two entry points into the body: from the skin and from dietary supplementation. The skin contains a previtamin D compound, 7-dehydrocholesterol. Ultraviolet energy from the sun or other sources converts this substance to a previtamin D compound, which is converted by heat-sensitive reactions to vitamin D. Vitamin D is transferred by a serum-binding protein to the liver. Dietary sources may include irradiated ergosterol, vitamin D_2, or vitamin D_3. Vitamins D_2 and D_3 differ slightly in their structure, but they have similar functions.

Vitamins D_2 and D_3 are hydroxylated in the liver at the 25 position by a 25-hydroxylase enzyme. Diseases of the liver and pharmacologic agents, including phenytoin and phenobarbital, have been reported to interfere with this important hydroxylation step. Interference in this step may result in vitamin D deficiency. The 25-hydroxyvitamin D is transported to the kidney, where another hydroxylation step occurs at the 1 position. 1,25-dihydroxyvitamin D_3 is the most active metabolite and is responsible for most actions of vitamin D. The 1 hydroxylation is stimulated through the actions of PTH, estrogen, growth hormone, prolactin, and insulin.

HYPOPARATHYROIDISM

Hypoparathyroidism in children is a rare entity, excluding transient hypoparathyroidism in neonates. This disease is recognized clinically by its accompanying hypocalcemia. The clinical manifestations of hypocalcemia are secondary to neuromuscular instability. The most common presentation is a seizure, which may be preceded by numbness and tingling sensations in the extremities. Chvostek's sign (ie, stimulation of the upper lip by tapping the facial nerve in front of the ear), Trousseau's sign (ie, carpopedal spasm produced by inflation of the blood pressure cuff greater than the systolic blood pressure for 2 minutes), laryngospasm, bronchospasm, and prolonged QT intervals on the electrocardiogram (ECG) can occur.

■ DIGEORGE'S ANOMALY

DiGeorge's anomaly (formerly DiGeorge's syndrome) was first described in infants with congenital absence of the thymus, absence of the parathyroid glands, and deficient cell-mediated immunity. Later descriptions included cardiovascular malformations (eg, truncus arteriosus and aortic arch syndromes). Typical dysmorphic features of the face have been reported. These include low-set ears, short philtrum, micrognathia, and a small fishlike mouth. Pathologic findings include absent, aplastic, and hypoplastic parathyroid glands.

■ ACUTE ILLNESSES

Acute illnesses in children, such as gram-negative sepsis, have been associated with hypocalcemia secondary to a relative hypoparathyroidism. The cause of the relative hypoparathyroidism in critically ill children is unknown, but it may be related to macrophage-generated interleukins, which may act as calcium ionophores. The critically ill child admitted to an intensive care unit is a prime candidate. Recognition may be delayed in some severe illnesses because of the concern for the primary problem. However, correction of the hypocalcemia is a requisite for patient improvement, because many cardiovascular agents require appropriate concentrations of calcium. Ionized calcium levels rather than total serum calcium levels reflect the child's true status, because disturbances in total calcium determination from hypoalbuminemia, fluctuations in the bicarbonate ion, and radiographic contrast media may complicate total serum calcium measurements.

■ LABORATORY FINDINGS

The characteristic laboratory findings of hypoparathyroidism include hypocalcemia and hyperphosphatemia. The PTH level is low in most of the situations described earlier. Radiographs of bones do not usually show any diagnostic features. The differential diagnosis includes hypocalcemia for other reasons, such as phosphate-induced hypocalcemia, renal failure, and hypocalcemic rickets. The clinical history, laboratory assessment, and radiographs can facilitate the evaluation. Children with pseudohypoparathyroidism present with hypocalcemia and hyperphosphatemia, but their PTH levels are elevated.

■ TREATMENT

The immediate treatment of hypoparathyroidism can be generalized if modifications are made for each specific cause. All untreated patients with hypoparathyroidism have hypocalcemia, which requires immediate medical intervention. The hypocalcemia is treated with intravenous calcium. Oral treatment with calcium supplementation may be initiated when the patient becomes stable. The amount of calcium supplementation administered should be regulated closely by serum calcium determinations.

HYPERPARATHYROIDISM

Hyperparathyroidism is an uncommon disorder among pediatric patients, but it is important because an aggressive approach must be undertaken to prevent chronic renal diseases from nephrocalcinosis. The clinical manifestations of hypercalcemia from any cause are similar. The neuromuscular and gastrointestinal organs are affected initially. Muscle weakness, paralysis, hyporeflexia, constipation, anorexia, and vomiting may be observed. The kidney may be affected adversely with resulting polyuria and polydipsia. Nephrocalcinosis may occur later. The cardiovascular symptoms may reveal bradycardia and a reduced QT interval.

■ ETIOLOGY

Multiple Endocrine Neoplasia Type I

Multiple endocrine neoplasia type I (MEN I) or Wermer's syndrome is an autosomal dominant form of an inherited disease in which hyperparathyroidism, pancreatic tumors, and pituitary adenomas occur. Almost all affected patients have hyperparathyroidism secondary to enlargement and hyperplasia of all parathyroid tissue. The cause is unknown, but studies using restriction fragment link polymorphisms have located a potential MEN I gene on chromosome 11. Some cases have been reported among neonates and children. The diagnosis is confirmed by hypercalcemia, elevated levels of PTH, and the familial incidence. Treatment consists of subtotal parathyroidectomy ($3\frac{1}{2}$ glands) with autotransplantation of a small amount of parathyroid tissue to the muscles of one of the extremities.

■ LABORATORY FINDINGS

Hyperparathyroidism from any cause can be recognized by elevated levels of PTH concomitant with hypercalcemia and hypophosphatemia. The newer assays for the intact (1-84) PTH molecule have facilitated the measurements that previously were difficult to obtain.

■ TREATMENT

Treatment of hypercalcemia secondary to hyperparathyroidism must include treatment of the underlying disorder. The immediate treatment requires hydration, which can be done orally in cooperative children or by intravenous methods in uncooperative ones. Sunlight, any form of vitamin D, and dairy products should be avoided during hypercalcemia. These treatments usually suffice in children, but additional treatment can be undertaken with calcitonin, phosphorus, mithramycin, peritoneal dialysis, and bisphosphonates. The latter forms of treatment have been used in adults, and the experience in treating children is nonexistent or limited.

(Abridged from John L. Kirkland, The Parathyroid Glands, in Oski, DeAngelis, Feigin, McMillan, Warshaw: *Principles and Practice of Pediatrics, Second Edition*, J.B. Lippincott, 1994.)

Oski's Essential Pediatrics,
edited by Kevin B. Johnson and Frank A. Oski.
Lippincott–Raven Publishers,
Philadelphia © 1997

175

Puberty and Gonadal Disorders

■ PRECOCIOUS SEXUAL DEVELOPMENT

Causes of precocious or inappropriate sexual development are listed in Table 175–1. In evaluating a child for sexual precocity, a careful medical and family history is imperative. Does the child have any history of a central nervous system (CNS) disorder? What is the child's growth pattern? Is there evidence of linear growth acceleration? Previous growth measurements are valuable. When did the various pubertal changes begin? How fast have these changes progressed? Is the child outgrowing clothes and shoes rapidly? Has the child's appetite increased? When did the parents and siblings have pubertal changes? Is there a history of early sexual development in any relatives? Questions regarding exposure to any exogenous source of sex steroids must be asked. Creams and pills can contain sex steroids, especially estrogens, and oral contraceptives are readily found in many homes. Are any athletes in the home taking anabolic steroids?

The physical examination should include a careful examination of the fundi. The child's skin should be inspected for signs of oiliness, acne, and café au lait spots. The thyroid should be palpated. The presence of axillary hair and odor, the amount of breast tissue, and whether the nipples and areolae are enlarging and thinning should be evaluated. The abdomen should be carefully palpated for masses. The amount, location, and character of pubic hair should be noted.

In girls, the clitoris, labia, and vaginal orifice should be examined carefully. Is there evidence of maturation of the labia minora? Does the vaginal mucosa look red and shiny (prepubertal) or pink and dull (estrogenized)? Is the clitoris of normal size? Are vaginal secretions evident on the genitalia or on the child's underwear?

In boys, the stretched length and width of the penis should be measured. Careful palpation and measurement of the testes are key. Are the testes prepubertal in length (<2.5 cm), or are they enlarging? Is there a difference in size and consistency of the two testes, suggesting a unilateral mass? Transillumination of the testes may be helpful, especially if there are size discrepancies. Is the scrotum thinning, or does it look thick and nonvascular (*ie*, prepubertal)? Are the results of the neurologic examination normal?

True or Central Precocious Puberty

True or central precocious puberty is caused by early maturation of hypothalamic GnRH secretion. This form of precocious puberty is much more common in girls than in boys.

A search for an underlying CNS abnormality should be made by imaging of the CNS with computed tomography (CT) or magnetic resonance imaging (MRI). CNS tumors, especially hypothalamic hamartomas, are known causes of central precocious puberty. Neurofibromas, gliomas, and other tumors have been found with some frequency. Other CNS lesions, such as hydrocephalus, post-trauma, and postinfectious encephalitis or meningitis, are associated with precocious puberty.

In many cases, no definable CNS abnormality can be found, and the problem falls into the idiopathic category, which occurs more frequently in girls than in boys. In idiopathic precocious puberty, although the onset is at an early age, the pattern and timing of progression of pubertal events are normal.

Children with central precocious puberty have accelerated linear growth, advanced bone ages, and pubertal levels of luteinizing hormone (LH), follicle-stimulating hormone (FSH), and the sex steroids, estradiol and testosterone.

In boys, the finding of bilateral pubertal-sized testes almost always indicates central precocious puberty. This is an extremely important point in the physical examination, because it determines the diagnostic workup.

Treatment with GnRH analogues produces a prepubertal hormonal state, and growth acceleration, bone age advancement, and the progression of secondary sex characteristics cease.

In some patients with severe prolonged untreated primary hypothyroidism, precocious sexual development may be seen and is associated with pubertal levels of LH and FSH. These patients exhibit poor linear growth and usually delayed bone age. If the thyroid-stimulating hormone (TSH) overproduction is suppressed by exogenous thyroxine, the LH and FSH concentrations decrease to prepubertal levels, and the pubertal changes regress.

Precocious Puberty Independent of Pituitary Gonadotropins

Girls

Girls with precocious puberty independent of pituitary gonadotropins have a non–gonadotropin-stimulated or independent source of estrogens producing their pubertal changes. An exogenous source of estrogens must be sought. The use of skin creams and medications must be pursued and the labels read to see whether they contain estrogen. Birth control pills are widely used, and, although they may not be in the child's home, grandparents, friends, and babysitters may keep them in unprotected locations. In some

TABLE 175-1. Precocious or Inappropriate Sexual Development

TRUE OR CENTRAL PRECOCIOUS PUBERTY (CENTRAL GONADOTROPIN SECRETION)

Idiopathic

Central nervous system (CNS) tumors: hamartomas, other

Other CNS disorders: trauma, postinfectious, hydrocephalus

Severe primary hypothyroidism

PRECOCIOUS PUBERTY INDEPENDENT OF PITUITARY GONADOTROPINS

Girls

    Exogenous estrogen exposure

    Estrogen-secreting tumors (adrenals or ovaries)

    Ovarian cysts

    McCune-Albright syndrome

Boys

    Exogenous androgen exposure

    Adrenal androgen secretion

        Congenital adrenal hyperplasia

        Adrenal tumors

    Testicular androgen secretion

        Tumors

        Familial Leydig cell hyperplasia

    Gonadotropin-secreting tumors

    McCune-Albright syndrome

HETEROSEXUAL DEVELOPMENT

Virilization in girls

    Congenital adrenal hyperplasia

    Adrenal tumors

    Ovarian tumors

Feminization in boys

    Adrenal tumor

    Testicular tumor

    Increased peripheral conversion of androgens to estrogens

VARIATIONS OF NORMAL PUBERTY

Premature thelarche

---

cases, ingestion of animal protein, especially poultry, has been reported to produce estrogenization in a child if the animal received estrogens.

Estrogen-producing tumors of the ovary and adrenal gland must be considered. Adrenal estrogen-producing tumors are rare and are associated with high estradiol levels and increased levels of other adrenal sex hormones. They should be visible with abdominal CT or MRI scans. Estrogen-producing ovarian tumors are more common and may be palpable during careful bimanual examination. As with adrenal tumors, estradiol levels are usually high. Ultrasound and CT scans usually demonstrate the ovarian mass. Ovarian cysts, associated with high levels of estradiol, are another cause of gonadotropin-independent precocious puberty and are demonstrable with imaging. Sometimes ovarian cysts are recurrent.

Treatment entails removal of the estrogen source if exogenous exposure is the cause. If an adrenal or ovarian tumor is found, surgical excision and, if the tumor is malignant, additional treatment are indicated. Ovarian cysts are difficult to treat because they may recur, and surgical excision may make no difference in the patient's long-term clinical course.

McCune-Albright syndrome is an unusual syndrome of irregular café au lait spots, polyostotic fibrous dysplasia, and precocious puberty. It is seen in both sexes. The cause is likely to be an abnormality in a subunit of the G-protein of the receptor.

Boys

Boys with gonadotropin-independent precocious puberty have a source of androgens independent of central gonadotropin secretion. Exogenous androgen exposure must be considered. With the widespread abuse of androgens (ie, anabolic steroids) by athletes, young children are at risk for exposure.

An adrenal source of androgens, including an adrenal tumor or an adrenal biosynthetic defect (eg, 21-hydroxylase deficiency, 11-hydroxylase deficiency) causes precocious puberty in boys. Those with an adrenal or exogenous androgen source show clinical virilization, including linear growth acceleration and bone age advancement, but have prepubertal testes on examination.

Testicular tumors may produce elevated androgens and cause precocious puberty. On examination, the testes show a size discrepancy; the testis with the tumor is larger and often has an irregular consistency.

Treatment of gonadotropin-independent precocious puberty in boys entails removal of the androgen source in exogenous exposure. Excision of adrenal or testicular tumors is indicated, with additional treatment if the lesions are malignant. Adrenal enzyme deficiencies require appropriate glucocorticoid replacement.

■ VARIATIONS OF NORMAL PUBERTY

Three variations of normal pubertal development occur frequently and must be differentiated from progressive and pathologic processes. These are premature thelarche (in girls), premature adrenarche (in girls and boys), and pubertal gynecomastia (in boys).

Premature Thelarche

Premature thelarche is a common entity in which there is clinical evidence of mild estrogenization in girls, typically between 1 and 4 years of age. Breast enlargement occurs, often without nipple and areolar development. No sexual hair develops, and there is no linear growth acceleration. This is an isolated phenomenon, and lack of progression is the hallmark. Laboratory tests show incomplete estrogenization of the vaginal mucosa, a normal bone age, and prepubertal gonadotropin patterns. Estradiol levels are usually prepubertal but may be slightly increased.

Postulated causes include ovarian cysts and transient pituitary gonadotropin secretion. No treatment is necessary. Close follow-up is important, because the early stages of precocious puberty may be clinically indistinguishable from premature thelarche.

Premature Adrenarche

Premature adrenarche is caused by early activation of adrenal androgens, producing pubic and axillary hair development and axillary odor. In girls, the pubic hair often begins on the labia. There are no other signs of pubertal changes and no signs of abnormal virilization. If signs of gonadarche are observed, an evaluation for precocious puberty is indicated. If virilization occurs, a workup for virilizing lesions is necessary. Some children with this diagnosis may have mild neurologic problems. Height and bone age are often slightly greater than the mean but fall within two standard deviations. Plasma adrenal androgens and urinary androgen metabolites (17-ketosteroids) are increased to the early pubertal range.

Typically, premature adrenarche occurs in 6- to 8-year-old children, but it may be seen in much younger children. The sexual hair gradually increases. Evidence suggests that a substantial percentage of children with this diagnosis may have mild 21-hydroxylase deficiency, and an adrenocorticotropic hormone (ACTH) stimulation test may be useful for diagnosing some patients.

Pubertal Gynecomastia

Pubertal gynecomastia is common in teenage boys, typically beginning in Tanner stage 2 or 3 and lasting for about 2 years. In some boys, the ratio of estradiol to testosterone may be elevated. Severely affected boys may require surgical reduction.

Tamoxifen and testolactone may be effective for treating gynecomastia in moderate cases.

Pathologic causes of gynecomastia must be considered. Hypogonadism (eg, Klinefelter's syndrome [47XXY]); partial androgen insensitivity; partial blocks in testosterone biosynthesis; hyperthyroidism; adrenal, testicular, or LH and human chorionic gonadotropin (hCG)-producing tumors; liver tumors or disease; and chronic debilitating illness causing malnutrition have all been associated with gynecomastia. A variety of drugs can cause gynecomastia: androgens, estrogens, hCG, psychoactive drugs (eg, phenothiazines), street drugs and alcohol, testosterone antagonists (eg, ketoconazole, cimetidine, spironolactone), and antituberculosis and cytotoxic agents.

Obese teenage boys may present with large breasts that are only adipose tissue and of no pathologic consequence. However, determining whether glandular breast tissue exists in an extremely obese boy may be difficult.

■ DELAYED PUBERTY

The causes of delayed puberty are listed in Table 175-2. An evaluation for pubertal delay is indicated if no signs of puberty are observed in a girl by 13 years of age or in a boy by 14 years of age. Evaluation is also indicated if there is an arrest in pubertal maturation.

The differential diagnosis of delayed or absent puberty rests on the initial gonadotropin levels. If LH and FSH levels are high, a primary gonadal abnormality exists. If LH and FSH levels are normal or low, a search for central hormonal abnormalities or chronic disease must be undertaken.

Elevated Gonadotropin Levels

Patients with elevated LH and FSH levels have evidence of bilateral gonadal failure and lack of appropriate sex steroid levels to feed back centrally. After LH and FSH levels are found to be elevated, a karyotype should be determined.

TABLE 175-2. Causes of Delayed Puberty

ELEVATED GONADOTROPIN LEVELS

Gonadal failure: autoimmune, chemotherapy or radiation, traumatic, infectious, postsurgical, torsion, "vanishing testes," pure gonadal dysgenesis, myotonic dystrophy

Complete androgen insensitivity syndrome

Complete 17α-hydroxylase deficiency

Chromosomal abnormalities

    Turner's syndrome

    Klinefelter's syndrome

NORMAL OR LOW GONADOTROPIN LEVELS

Constitutional delay of growth and adolescence

Hypopituitarism

    Isolated LH/FSH deficiency associated with hyposmia or anosmia (Kallmann's syndrome)

    Multiple hormone deficiencies

Chronic disease

Syndromes

    Prader-Willi

    Laurence-Moon-Biedl

Common causes of delayed puberty are chemotherapy, radiation therapy, and autoimmune glandular failure.

Girls with the XY karyotype who have complete androgen insensitivity develop breasts at the appropriate age, but no sexual hair develops, and no menses occur. Girls with the XY karyotype and complete 17-hydroxylase deficiency (ie, no sex steroids can be formed) have no secondary sex characteristics. If these syndromes are partial, enough androgen is present to cause genital ambiguity in the neonate or virilization during puberty.

Turner's syndrome is a common cause of delayed breast development and elevated gonadotropin levels. It is invariably associated with short stature and often with other anomalies, including webbed neck, increased nevi, high-arched palate, shield chest, coarctation of the aorta, renal anomalies, an increased arm-carrying angle, and edema of the hands and feet. Most girls with this syndrome have a 45X karyotype, but many have a mosaic pattern (45X/46XX) or an X-chromosomal structural abnormality (eg, ring or isochrome). Buccal smears are not adequate for this diagnosis. Sexual hair develops in girls with Turner's syndrome because adrenal androgens are not affected.

Boys with *Klinefelter's syndrome* (47XXY) usually come to attention because of gynecomastia and small testes (ie, inadequate masculinization). They are usually clinically normal at birth, and throughout childhood, they are tall with slim builds and long limbs. They may also have mosaic chromosome patterns (eg, 46XY/47XXY) or multiple X chromosomes.

Treatment of patients with gonadal failure involves replacing sex steroids. Depending on the age of the patient and whether height is an issue, this can be done gradually over several years or more abruptly.

(Abridged from Leslie P. Plotnick, Puberty and Gonadal Disorders, in Oski, DeAngelis, Feigin, McMillan, Warshaw: *Principles and Practice of Pediatrics, Second Edition,* J.B. Lippincott, 1994.)

Oski's Essential Pediatrics,
edited by Kevin B. Johnson and Frank A. Oski.
Lippincott–Raven Publishers,
Philadelphia © 1997

176

Growth, Growth Hormone, and Pituitary Disorders

■ GROWTH

Problems related to normal or abnormal growth are common in pediatric practice. Short stature can be defined as height more than two standard deviations (2 SD) below the mean and tall stature as height more than 2 SD above the mean. Three percent of children are at or more than 2 SD below the mean, and 3% are at or more than 2 SD above the mean.

In addition to actual height and weight at any one time, the rate of growth over time is essential in deciding which children may have pathologic growth and which do not.

Bone age is important in evaluating a child for a growth problem. Children with normal bone ages are unlikely to have a systemic chronic disease or a hormonal abnormality as the cause of the growth problem. Significantly delayed or advanced bone ages (*ie,* >2 SD from the mean) may indicate pathology and require evaluation.

■ SHORT STATURE OR POOR LINEAR GROWTH

A child with a height below the 3rd percentile or whose growth curve has been crossing percentiles downward should be carefully examined for a pathologic cause of poor growth (Table 176–1).

Probably the largest category of causes of poor growth is *major organ system disease.* Most patients in this category have a disorder that is not subtle, and the history and physical examination disclose the problem without extensive laboratory testing. However, some disorders may not be evident from history and physical examination and require laboratory studies for diagnosis. Examples include renal tubular acidosis, inflammatory bowel disease, and celiac disease.

Chromosomal disorders are often associated with poor growth. These usually are evident from characteristic dysmorphic features and developmental delay.

Familial or genetic short stature is a common cause of short stature in children. Usually the parents' heights are in the lower normal percentiles for adults. This is not a disorder, because these children are entirely normal. Their heights are usually at or slightly below the 3rd percentile but not at or more than 3 SD below the mean. They have normal growth velocities, and their height curve parallels the 3rd percentile. Their bone ages are normal, and their pubertal growth spurt is normal in timing and magnitude.

One or both of the parents may be short for a pathologic reason, which the child may have inherited, such as familial growth hormone (GH) deficiency or mild chondrodysplasias. If a parent's height is more than 2 SD below the mean (*ie,* less than 3rd percentile) or if the parent is disproportionately short for the family, both parent and child may have pathologic short stature.

TABLE 176-1. Causes of Short Stature or Poor Linear Growth

Major organ system disease
  Central nervous system
  Cardiac
  Pulmonary
  Hematologic
  Renal
  Gastrointestinal or nutritional
Chromosomal disorders: Turner's syndrome
Inborn errors of metabolism
Intrauterine growth retardation
Familial or genetic short stature
Constitutional delay of growth and adolescence
Endocrine disorders
  Cortisol excess (exogenous or endogenous)
  Hypothyroidism
  Pseudohypoparathyroidism
  Poorly controlled diabetes
  Growth hormone deficiency (*eg*, idiopathic, organic, familial, psychosocial)
Shifting linear percentiles
Skeletal disorders
Deprivation or psychosocial dwarfism
Medications

Constitutional slow growth with delayed adolescence, called *constitutional delay,* is another common diagnostic category. This variant of normal growth is seen much more frequently in boys than in girls. Typically, affected children lag 2 to 4 years behind average in height, bone age, and pubertal development. There is often a positive family history in parents, older siblings, or other family members.

If growth rate is normal, the height is at or slightly below the 3rd percentile, there is a positive family history, and the bone age is delayed by 2 to 4 years, no additional evaluation is needed. However, if there is any concern about a subnormal growth velocity, further evaluation is indicated. Patients with early inflammatory bowel disease or with milder degrees of GH deficiency may initially resemble children with constitutional delay. Because growth velocity gradually drops with age and is at its lowest just before the pubertal growth spurt begins (Figure 176–1), teenagers with constitutional delay may spend a prolonged time at this low rate. Growth velocity should be assessed in relation to bone age and chronologic age.

Endocrine abnormalities are another diagnostic category of short stature. Cortisol excess (*ie,* cortisol in greater amounts than physiologic needs) produces short stature, whether the excess cortisol is exogenous, due to oral, topical, or inhalant glucocorticoids, or endogenous, as in Cushing's disease. Children with cortisol excess have a subnormal linear growth rate, delayed bone age, and typical cushingoid clinical features: round, plethoric "moon" face, centripetal obesity, increased dorsal fat pad ("buffalo hump"), and proximal muscle weakness. When the source of excess glucocorticoids is removed, the growth rate increases, but the ultimate height can be compromised by years of glucocorticoid excess.

Hypothyroidism is a distinct endocrine cause of short stature, characterized by a subnormal linear growth rate, increased weight gain, and a delayed bone age. When the

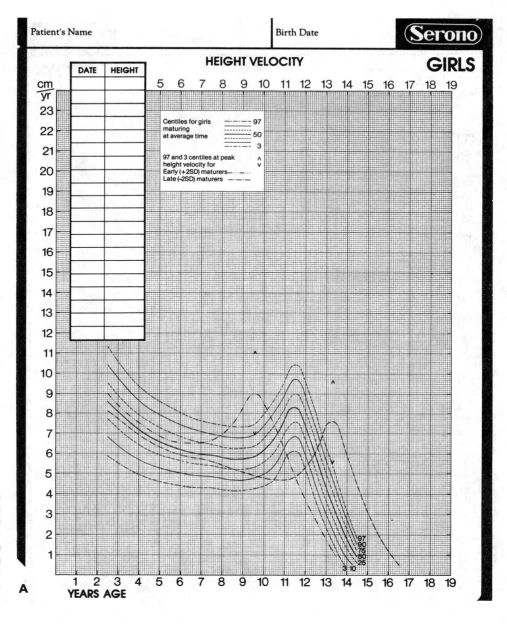

Figure 176-1. Growth velocity curves for girls **(A)** and boys **(B)**, including early and late pubertal patterns. (North American growth and development longitudinal standards. Height: distance and velocity for girls and boys. From Tanner JM. *J Pediatr.* 1985;107. Distributed by Serono Laboratories, Randolph, MA.)

diagnosis is made and appropriate treatment given, children undergo catch-up growth. The threshold for performing thyroid function tests should be low for a child with a question of poor growth rate, because the diagnostic tests and treatment are of minimal risk, inexpensive, and effective. Treatment often has dramatic effects on clinical signs and symptoms and growth. Patients with pseudohypoparathyroidism have a characteristic phenotype that includes short stature.

Poorly controlled insulin-dependent diabetes mellitus may be associated with short stature and poor linear growth rate. The growth retardation in poorly controlled diabetes can be severe. Improving metabolic control usually normalizes the growth rate.

GH deficiency is a diagnostic category that has undergone considerable flux in recent years. GH deficiency may be idiopathic, organic, or familial; it is occasionally psychosocial and reversible. It may occur alone or with other pituitary hormone deficiencies. Children with classic GH deficiency have short stature, poor linear growth rate, and delayed

bone age, and they are usually chubby. They may have fasting hypoglycemia, and boys may have small penises. They fail to release normal amounts of GH in response to certain standard pharmacologic stimuli.

Various degrees of GH deficiency occur; there is a continuum from normal GH secretion to classic GH deficiency, and where a physician draws the line between normal and abnormal is arbitrary. Some patients respond normally to pharmacologic tests but have low physiologic 24-hour GH secretion, and some have borderline responses to pharmacologic tests; both groups of patients have partial GH deficiency or neurosecretory defects. Other patients secrete normal amounts of immunologically active GH that is biologically subactive. Patients in these categories may have been previously classified as having constitutional delay. The level of somatomedin-C in some of these patients may be borderline or low.

The diagnosis of classic GH deficiency remains clear-cut, but the standards of diagnosis of the lesser degrees of GH compromise or of biologically subactive GH are in flux. Because some or many of these patients may benefit from

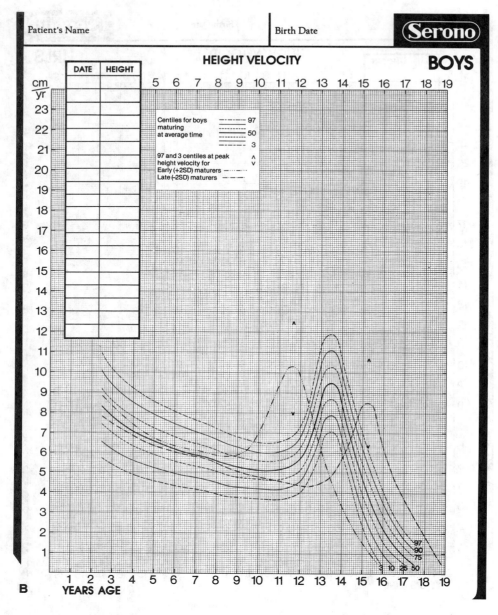

Figure 176-1. (Continued.)

treatment with exogenous GH, this is an important question for pediatric endocrinologists.

Specific causes of GH deficiency, isolated or associated with other pituitary hormone deficiencies, are congenital abnormalities (including septo-optic dysplasia), trauma, central nervous system (CNS) infections, vascular abnormalities, irradiation for malignancies, tumors (eg, craniopharyngiomas), and infiltrative processes such as histiocytosis.

Craniopharyngiomas are the most common tumors associated with pituitary and hypothalamic deficiencies. They are tumors of the Rathke pouch and are usually suprasellar but may be entirely intrasellar. Patients with craniopharyngiomas usually present with headache, visual abnormalities and neurologic symptoms. They may also have symptoms of diabetes insipidus and growth failure.

On physical examination, they may have visual defects (eg, field cuts, optic atrophy, papilledema) and signs of pituitary hormone deficiencies. CNS imaging shows calcifications in most patients and identifies the tumors. Treatment is surgical excision, often followed by radiation therapy, and appropriate hormonal replacement therapy.

Some children who are born smaller or larger than their genetic growth potential gradually *shift percentiles*, up or down, for height and weight. A typical example is a child who at birth is in the 90th percentile for length and weight but whose parents are in the 10th percentile for height. During the first 1 to 2 years of life, this child gradually decelerates to approximately the 10th percentile. Sometimes it is difficult to differentiate this pattern from pathologic growth. The key points are a gradual deceleration of height and weight proportionally, deceleration not below the genetically anticipated percentile, and once the percentile is reached, velocities normalizing and height and weight remaining at that percentile. If the deceleration is abrupt and falls to less than the 5th percentile or to a percentile below the parents' percentile, further evaluation is needed.

Skeletal dysplasias, including rickets, are obvious causes of poor growth. The skeletal abnormalities are usually evident on physical examination, as are abnormal arm spans and upper and lower segment ratios. Radiologic studies can help identify the specific abnormalities.

Psychological factors have been associated with poor growth. The growth abnormality can be caused by severe deprivation of caloric intake. Children in disturbed families may have psychosocial dwarfism, with disturbed eating and sleeping behaviors and transient pituitary hormone deficiencies, especially of GH and adrenocorticotropic hormone (ACTH). When the child is removed from the adverse home environment, catch-up growth occurs, and the hormonal levels normalize.

Various *medications* may produce poor growth. Glucocorticoids were discussed earlier in this chapter. Stimulants such as amphetamines and methylphenidate, especially in high doses, have been associated with impairment of weight and height.

■ TALL STATURE AND EXCESSIVE LINEAR GROWTH

Most children with tall stature (*ie*, heights more than 2 SD above the mean) have familial or genetic tall stature; their parents or other family members are tall. This, like familial short stature, is not pathologic. These children grow above the 95th percentile, but their growth curves are parallel to it. Their linear growth velocities are normal, and their bone ages are normal. Their pubertal growth spurt is normal in timing and magnitude, although they tend to grow in the upper normal velocity percentiles.

Certain syndromes are associated with tall stature and should be sought on examination. Marfan's syndrome, cerebral gigantism, homocystinuria, Klinefelter's syndrome (XXY), and XYY karyotypes are associated with tall stature.

Nutritional obesity is often associated with tall stature. Obese children typically show linear growth in the upper normal percentiles and may also have bone ages at the upper limits of normal (*ie*, approximately 1 to 2 SD above the mean). This is in contrast to the weight gain associated with endocrine abnormalities such as hypothyroidism, Cushing's disease, and GH deficiency, in which linear growth rate is subnormal and bone age is delayed.

Endocrine abnormalities can cause tall stature. Children with hyperthyroidism may have an excessive linear growth rate during the hyperthyroid period, but this finding is usually not a presenting complaint.

GH excess (*ie*, pituitary gigantism) causes excessive linear growth rates. GH excess is rare in childhood and adolescence and is usually caused by a pituitary GH-producing tumor or sometimes by excess GH-releasing factor production from a hypothalamic or peripheral tumor, such as a pancreatic tumor.

Many children with tall stature and excessive linear growth rates probably have precocious sex hormone secretion due to central precocious puberty or a variety of gonadal or adrenal abnormalities (see Chapter 175). Children with precocious sex hormone secretion have excessive linear growth rates initially. However, the hormones also cause rapid bone age advancement and early epiphyseal fusion, which compromise adult stature.

High doses of sex steroids can be used to treat tall stature if the predicted adult height is excessive.

■ WORKUP FOR SHORT STATURE OR POOR LINEAR GROWTH VELOCITY

The evaluation of a child with poor growth begins with a careful history. Height and growth patterns and the timing of puberty in parents, siblings, and other relatives should be

asked about. Gestational age and length and weight at birth are important. Anything in the history to suggest major organ system pathology should be heeded, remembering that renal and gastrointestinal (GI) disorders can be subtle. The child's psychological adjustment to his stature should be investigated, as should the overall family functioning. Nutritional issues should be discussed.

The child's growth curve should be carefully evaluated. If no previous growth data are available, questions about changes in shoe and clothing sizes and about how the child's growth compares with that of siblings and peers can be helpful. For example, "He used to be a head taller than his sister, who's 3 years younger, but now they're the same height," is revealing information. Every effort should be made to obtain previous growth data.

The entire physical examination is important. Any features of chronic disease should be elicited. Accurate height and weight measurements are mandatory. Careful fundoscopic examination looking for evidence of optic nerve abnormalities, and confrontation visual fields, should be done. Because dentition reflects bone age, the age appropriateness of primary and secondary teeth should be assessed. Are there any dysmorphic features of the face or body habitus or extremities? The thyroid should be carefully palpated. Are there signs of sexual maturation? In boys, is the penis abnormally small? Are there any clinical features of cortisol excess or of Turner's syndrome? Is the child's appearance proportionate or disproportionate for arm span and for upper and lower segment ratios?

If there are clues to a specific diagnosis, a complete laboratory workup is unnecessary. For example, if the child appears normal on examination and the history and growth curve strongly suggest familial short stature, no workup is necessary. Perhaps only a bone age evaluation to assess predicted height should be done. If the child is clearly cushingoid, the specific cause of this should be pursued.

In the many children in whom no clear cause is evident after history and physical examination, we recommend the following starting laboratory workup: complete blood count with erythrocyte sedimentation rate, chemistry panel including electrolytes, urinalysis with specific gravity and *p*H (urine culture if any signs of infection are present), bone age, thyroid hormone levels (*ie*, T_4, T_3RU, TSH), screening GH test (*eg*, exercise), IGF-I, and banded karyotyping for girls.

Any specific abnormalities found should be investigated further, but, if nothing abnormal is seen other than perhaps a significant bone age delay, the next step depends on the clinical impression and on the child's growth curve and current growth rate. Growth is an ongoing dynamic process, and evaluation over time is useful. If a child's growth rate is persistently subnormal such that he or she gradually or abruptly falls away from a normal curve, a repeat investigation or a more detailed look (*eg*, 24-hour GH monitoring, repeat definitive GH testing, pursuit of subtle GI pathology) may be indicated.

Despite the sophisticated diagnostic testing available, some children have clearly negative workup results, do not fit the diagnosis of constitutional delay, and are left with a diagnosis of idiopathic short stature. Children in this category need careful follow-up, because a specific cause may become evident with time.

■ DISORDERS OF ANTIDIURETIC HORMONE

Antidiuretic hormone (ADH, vasopressin) is released from the posterior pituitary by neurons originating in the hypothalamic supraoptic and periventricular nuclei. ADH release is mediated through osmoreceptors and baroreceptors, and secretion increases in response to hypovolemia and hyperosmolality. ADH acts by means of the kidney to reabsorb water, which decreases urine volume and increases urine osmolality.

Diabetes Insipidus

Diabetes insipidus is a disorder of subnormal ADH secretion or reduced kidney responsiveness to ADH. Renal responsiveness can be established by monitoring the response to exogenous vasopressin. ADH deficiency may be genetic but more often is caused by lesions in the hypothalamic area, commonly tumors and infiltrative disorders, such as histiocytosis. Trauma, inflammatory processes, and vascular abnormalities are also causes of ADH deficiency.

ADH deficiency manifests with symptoms of polyuria and polydipsia with large volumes of dilute urine. Symptoms are often dramatic and may be abrupt in onset. The search for an organic cause requires head computed tomography or magnetic resonance imaging scans, a search for histiocytosis, and an evaluation for dysfunctions of other areas of the hypothalamic–pituitary axis.

The best diagnostic test is water deprivation. This test should be done under careful observation in a well-hydrated child. Body weight, urine and serum sodium and osmolality, urine volumes, and ADH levels should be measured at baseline, frequently during the test, and at the end of the test. The ADH level is not essential for the diagnosis. If serum osmolality and serum sodium values rise above normal in the context of poor urine concentration, the diagnosis of diabetes insipidus is made. A weight loss of a maximum of 5% is allowed. At the end of the water deprivation test, exogenous ADH (ie, injection of aqueous vasopressin) is given to assess renal responsiveness.

Children with psychogenic or neurogenic polydipsia as the primary problem must be differentiated from those with diabetes insipidus. These children usually have low serum sodium and osmolality.

Diabetes insipidus due to ADH deficiency is treated with exogenous ADH. The best mode of treatment is with intranasal DDAVP, a long-acting analogue of arginine vasopressin. To eliminate nighttime awakening to urinate and drink, treatment is begun with low doses initially that are gradually increased. DDAVP can also be given parenterally. In most patients, DDAVP can be given every 12 hours. A long-acting preparation given by injection (ie, pitressin tannate in oil, duration 2 to 4 days) was successful before DDAVP became available and can still be used in the rare patient unable to take DDAVP. Because infant diets have a low solute load, their urine should remain dilute, and long-acting ADH preparations are contraindicated. A shorter-acting spray (ie, lysine vasopressin, duration 4 to 6 hours) can be given before bedtime to produce short-lasting antidiuresis during the night.

An intact thirst mechanism allows patients on ADH preparations to easily regulate their fluid balance on their own as long as they have free access to water. In the unusual patient with abnormal thirst, regulation becomes difficult, and strict prescriptions of fluid intake must be given.

Syndrome of Inappropriate Antidiuretic Hormone Secretion

Excess endogenous or exogenous ADH without fluid restriction leads to water intoxication: water retention and weight gain, hyponatremia, and production of a small amount of concentrated urine. The typical symptoms are lethargy, weakness, nausea, vomiting, headaches, and seizures.

In children, the most likely causes of the syndrome of inappropriate antidiuretic hormone secretion are intracranial disease (eg, meningitis), neurosurgery, head trauma, and pulmonary disease. Malignancies producing excess ADH are uncommon in children.

The treatment is fluid restriction. In severe cases, use of hypertonic saline with diuretic therapy (eg, furosemide) may be indicated. Slow and steady correction is required.

(Abridged from Leslie P. Plotnick, Growth, Growth Hormone, and Pituitary Disorders, in Oski, DeAngelis, Feigin, McMillan, Warshaw: *Principles and Practice of Pediatrics, Second Edition,* J.B. Lippincott, 1994.)

Oski's Essential Pediatrics,
edited by Kevin B. Johnson and Frank A. Oski.
Lippincott–Raven Publishers,
Philadelphia © 1997

177

Insulin-Dependent Diabetes Mellitus

Insulin-dependent diabetes mellitus (IDDM) is a common, serious disease of childhood and adolescence. The diagnosis is usually straightforward, but long-term management is a major challenge for the child, the family, and the health care team. Developments in the past decade have made the attainment of metabolic control a technical possibility, but diabetes management is stressful to the family, and psychological and behavioral issues often interfere with the goal of metabolic control. Few other diseases require the extensive self-care management needed to care for IDDM.

■ DEFINITION AND DIAGNOSTIC CRITERIA

Since the statement from the National Diabetes Data Group in 1979, diabetes has been classified as two main types. Type I or IDDM is the type most commonly found in children and adolescents. This type has also been called juvenile-onset, ketosis-prone, or brittle diabetes. Patients with IDDM are insulinopenic and need exogenous insulin to prevent ketosis and to preserve life.

Type II or non–insulin-dependent diabetes mellitus (NIDDM) is most commonly found in adults and in obese persons. This type has also been called adult-onset, maturity-onset, ketosis-resistant, or stable diabetes. Affected patients are not insulin dependent or ketosis prone, but they may use exogenous insulin, and they can develop ketosis in certain situations. Some patients with type II diabetes have insulin resistance and hyperinsulinemia.

For diabetes to be diagnosed, a child must have the classic symptoms with a random plasma glucose level above 200 mg/dL (11.1 mmol/L), or, if the child is asymptomatic, an oral glucose tolerance test must show elevated fasting values (·140 mg/dL in venous plasma or ·120 mg/dL in venous whole blood) and elevated postglucose values on more than one occasion. After a dose of 1.75 g of glucose per 1 kg of ideal body weight (maximum, 75 g), the 2-hour glucose value and an intervening value must be elevated (≥200 mg/dL in venous plasma; ≥180 mg/dL in venous whole blood).

The diagnosis of IDDM in a child is rarely subtle. Most present with the classic symptoms of polyuria, polydipsia, polyphagia, weight loss, and lethargy. Glucose tolerance testing is rarely necessary for diagnosis.

■ EPIDEMIOLOGY

The prevalence of IDDM in the United States in children and adolescents varies somewhat according to different sources, with most studies reporting a rate of 1.2 to 1.9 cases per 1000 members of the population of this age group.

■ CLINICAL PRESENTATION

Most children with IDDM present with the classic symptoms of polyuria, polydipsia, polyphagia, and weight loss; many also complain of lethargy. If the diagnosis is not made and treatment is not begun, further metabolic decompensation occurs, with worsening diabetic ketoacidosis (DKA).

In young children and infants, the diagnosis is more likely to be missed in its early stages because of difficulty in recognizing early symptoms, and children of these ages are more likely to present with severe ketoacidosis. If pediatricians inquire specifically about the classic symptoms in patients with nonspecific signs of illness and weight loss, this diagnosis is more likely to be made quickly. Early diagnosis avoids further metabolic decompensation and the risks of DKA.

Most children with new-onset IDDM have symptoms of less than 1 month's duration, but some have had mild to moderate symptoms for several months. Questions about bed wetting, nocturia, number of diapers used, or leaving class to use the bathroom may help uncover polyuria.

IDDM must be considered in any child with clinical dehydration who continues to urinate regularly. Too often, frequent urination leads the parent or physician to incorrectly conclude that the child is not dehydrated. Routine dipstick testing for urine glucose and ketones in patients with nonspecific symptoms such as lethargy, weight loss, nausea, and vomiting and in those with specific IDDM symptoms could greatly enhance the early diagnosis of this disease before severe metabolic decompensation has occurred.

New-onset IDDM may be managed in an inpatient or outpatient setting, depending on the severity of the patient's metabolic abnormalities and the health care resources available.

■ CLINICAL COURSE

After the initial presentation, most newly diagnosed children with IDDM undergo a honeymoon period or remission phase. During this period, the remaining functional β cells regain the ability to produce insulin, possibly as a result of elimination of hyperglycemia. Measurement of C-peptide levels has demonstrated that improved insulin secretion occurs during this phase. Because endogenous insulin secretion increases, requirements for exogenous insulin decrease, usually dropping to less than 0.5 U/kg/day. Hypoglycemia becomes a potential problem. This phase usually begins within 1 to 3 months after diagnosis and lasts for several months, sometimes as long as 12 to 24 months. It is a period

of relative well-being, with metabolic normalcy as indicated by normal glycosylated hemoglobin (HbA$_{1C}$) levels. Education about the honeymoon period must be included in the education of the newly diagnosed patient, because denial of disease and subsequent failure to monitor are likely to occur unless patients and families learn about this phase and expect its occurrence and its end.

As this phase ends, the remaining β cells lose their capacity to secrete insulin, and requirements for exogenous insulin rise. This usually occurs gradually but, as in cases of acute infection, it may be abrupt. Careful monitoring and frequent dose adjustments are extremely important during the end of the remission phase, and close contact between the patient and physician is necessary.

■ GOALS OF TREATMENT

Normal Development

Normal growth in height and weight and normal timing of adolescent pubertal development are important goals of long-term management. Chronically undertreated children with poorly controlled IDDM often fail to grow normally and have delayed skeletal maturation (ie, bone age) and delayed sexual maturation. The growth retardation can be severe. Growth is an important factor to follow, and height, weight, and pubertal development should be monitored carefully. The causes for deviations from normal velocities should be sought.

Children receiving excessive insulin doses may gain weight too rapidly. Excessive insulin doses, which can cause rebound hyperglycemia and ketosis, can produce the same degree of growth retardation as chronically inadequate doses. Mauriac syndrome (ie, IDDM, growth retardation, and hepatomegaly) is caused by poor diabetic control, and, although patients with this syndrome are usually receiving inadequate insulin doses, excessive doses have also been associated with this clinical picture.

Management of Insulin-Dependent Diabetes Mellitus

Education of the patient and family with the goal of independent management of IDDM at home is important. Some families achieve independence quickly. Others require intensive and repeated education on a one-to-one basis or in group programs. Independent decision making by patients and families who are well educated about diabetes and its management enhances independence, feelings of control, and self-esteem, and it is important for long-term psychological success. Most day-to-day decisions regarding hyperglycemia, hypoglycemia, illness, ketonuria, unusual activities, or eating schedules can be handled appropriately by knowledgeable families. Frequent blood glucose monitoring, which is discussed later in this chapter, is the cornerstone of management.

Children and adolescents with IDDM should be encouraged to participate in any activities that are appropriate to their age and interest. An adolescent with sports practice three times a week after school can learn how to increase calories or decrease insulin doses and to keep her blood glucose levels in an acceptable range during the activity. Certain precautions must be taken. For example, a source of calories must be readily available during a physical activity. When adolescents drive, a readily available glucose source must be in easy reach, not locked in the glove compartment. Medic-Alert bracelets or necklaces should be worn.

The diet should be designed around the child's and family's food preferences and habits using sound nutritional principles. It is important that families participate in the planning of the diet and that the amount of food be adequate for satiety to maximize adherence.

Avoiding Metabolic Abnormalities

Avoidance of metabolic abnormalities is another important goal. Blood glucose monitoring several times a day along with urinary ketone checks are mainstays of management. Significant hyperglycemia and hypoglycemia should be avoided. In young children, especially preschoolers, blood glucose levels vary widely. To avoid serious hypoglycemia in this age group, compromises may have to be made in tolerating hyperglycemia.

HbA_{1C} levels should be monitored regularly usually every 3 to 4 months with a goal of achieving a level in or near the normal range. Normal values vary depending on the laboratory method used. Blood lipids should be monitored and dietary modifications made if hyperlipidemia occurs.

Ketonuria should be treated early. In most patients who monitor regularly, DKA can be avoided by responding to hyperglycemia, ketosis, and periods of illness by adjusting insulin doses.

The demands of the diabetes management regimen are high and require care and understanding on the part of the families and the health care team to maximize the child's chances for successful emotional development.

■ MANAGEMENT

Insulin

Regular insulin is rapid acting and is the insulin used to rapidly treat hyperglycemia, ketosis, and DKA. Semilente is another short-acting insulin. NPH or Lente are intermediate in peak and duration of action. Ultralente is a long-acting insulin with duration of more than 24 to 36 hours. However, human Ultralente may have a much shorter duration of action (Table 177–1).

Most children and adolescents require two injections per day of short- and intermediate-acting insulin to achieve satisfactory metabolic control; the injections are administered shortly before breakfast and dinner. Absorption may vary from different injection sites and is more rapid in exercised sites and at higher temperatures. Injection into hypertrophied sites may slow absorption.

Frequent blood glucose monitoring is necessary so patients can respond to the levels by adjusting their insulin doses.

Dietary Management

Diet is a cornerstone of diabetes management. Children and adolescents with IDDM require a nutritionally balanced diet with adequate calories and nutrients for normal growth. The recommended diet usually contains 50% to 55% carbohydrate calories, 20% protein, and approximately 30% fat. Most carbohydrate calories are complex carbohydrates, and the fat portion should emphasize low levels of cholesterol and saturated fats. Timing of meals and snacks should minimize blood glucose variability. In addition to the usual three meals, midafternoon snacks are necessary, particularly because they are timed to coincide with the typical peak of

TABLE 177-1. Timing of Action of Available Insulins

Insulin	Onset (hours)	Peak (hours)	Usual Duration (hours)
Regular			
Human	0.5–1.0	2–3	3–6
Pork	0.5–2.0	3–4	4–6
NPH/Lente			
Human	2–4	4–10	10–16
Pork	4–6	8–14	16–20
Ultralente			
Human	6–10	Minimal (?)	18–20
Animal	8–14	Minimal	24–36
Mixed (70% NPH, 30% regular)			
Human	0.5	2–12	24

the morning NPH insulin dose and with most after-school sports activities. Bedtime snacks are important for most children receiving evening NPH doses. Midmorning snacks are useful in preschool-age children, but most school-age children find them disruptive to their school routine. This snack usually is not recommended after a child begins elementary school.

Exercise

Physical fitness and regular exercise are important for all patients with IDDM. Insulin requirements may be lower, metabolic control improved, and self-esteem and body image better in the physically fit child. During periods of exercise, extra calories or lower insulin doses may be needed to prevent hypoglycemia. Blood glucose monitoring to assess the effects of exercise on blood glucose and the response to these therapeutic maneuvers should be done to arrive at an effective regimen for the individual patient. Regular exercise is to be encouraged at any age, because it then can become part of the child's health care regimen.

Monitoring

One of the major advances of the last decade has been the technique of self-monitoring of blood glucose. Numerous reagent strips, glucose meters, and finger puncture devices are available. Current glucose meters are small, portable, and accurate. Improvements and advances include memory storage at 300 readings with the date and time of the reading. A noninvasive blood glucose meter is expected to become available in the future.

The measurement of HbA_{1C} levels is another major advance in diabetes management. This is an objective level that measures an average blood glucose reading over approximately the previous 2 months. Various methods are available, and normal ranges vary. The upper limit of normal in our hospital laboratory is 7.9%. Levels below 9% are considered very good control, and levels below 10% are reasonable.

Urinary ketones also should be monitored. Even patients who do accurate and regular blood glucose monitoring need to check urinary ketones, particularly when the blood glucose levels are above 250 mg/dL, when they have a fever, when they feel nauseous or are vomiting, or when they are just not feeling well. This is important in achieving the goal of aborting DKA episodes by treating early ketosis.

Education

Education is fundamental to diabetes management and control. Patients and families need to understand all aspects of diabetes, including acute and long-term complications. They must understand details of insulin action, including duration and timing, injection techniques, dietary information, blood glucose monitoring, and urinary ketone checks. They must gain skills in integrating the demanding clinical regimen into their schedules so they can achieve emotional stability and ongoing psychological growth.

Education must be appropriate to the child's age and the family's educational background, and it must be ongoing. Shifting responsibility from parent to child for diabetes self-care skills (eg, insulin injections) should be done gradually and when the child shows interest and readiness to do so. Premature shifting of responsibility may be a cause of deterioration in metabolic control.

The life of the entire family is affected by having a child with IDDM. Sharing responsibilities and attending support groups and camps for IDDM children can help with psychological adjustment.

Teaching about and managing diabetes are best handled by a diabetes management team, including a physician, nurse educator, dietitian, and psychologist or psychiatric social worker.

■ COMPLICATIONS

Acute Effects

Hypoglycemia

Hypoglycemia (ie, blood glucose less than 50 to 60 mg/dL) occurs in patients on insulin whether they are or are not in tight metabolic control, but it occurs more frequently when blood glucose levels are kept close to normal. Hypoglycemic symptoms may be mild (ie, adrenergic symptoms of tremors, sweating, hunger, palpitations); moderate (ie, adrenergic plus neuroglycopenic symptoms of headache, irritability or other mood change, sleepiness, confusion, inattentiveness, impaired judgment, weakness), or severe (ie, unresponsiveness, coma, convulsions). Mild and moderate reactions can be treated by ingesting simple sugars (ie, 10 to 15 g of glucose). Moderate reactions may require assistance by another person and additional carbohydrate. Severe reactions require treatment with intravenous glucose or parenteral glucagon. All patients' families and day care providers, teachers, coaches, and others should learn the signs and symptoms of hypoglycemia, have a readily available source of glucose to treat it (eg, a tube of cake frosting), and ideally have and know how to use glucagon injections to treat severe reactions. Evidence suggests that a longer duration of disease and tight metabolic control are associated with a diminished counter-regulatory hormone response to hypoglycemia, and some patients have hypoglycemic unawareness. These factors increase the risk of severe hypoglycemia. Young children often cannot notify their parents of hypoglycemic symptoms, and goals for metabolic control may need to be loosened. There is also concern that hypoglycemia may have deleterious effects on learning. Fear of hypoglycemia, particularly after a severe reaction, may cause long-lasting acceptance by patients and

families of unacceptably high blood glucose levels (>200 mg/dL).

Hyperglycemia and Ketosis

Patients with IDDM and their families must learn how to adjust insulin doses to treat the inevitable hyperglycemia that occurs with IDDM or when to call their health care provider for assistance with this. Ketosis may occur occasionally or more frequently, and patients must know how to respond.

Diabetic Ketoacidosis

DKA is a common and potentially life-threatening, acute complication of IDDM. It is the most common cause of death in patients with IDDM younger than their midtwenties. Mortality rates may be as high as 6% to 10%. DKA can be defined as a blood glucose level usually greater than 250 mg/dL, pH less than 7.2 or 7.3, and plasma bicarbonate level of 15 or less. Severe DKA is defined as a pH of 7.1 or less and a bicarbonate level of 10 or less; milder forms may be seen. Careful monitoring of blood glucose and urinary ketones and appropriate treatment responses to early metabolic abnormalities can prevent a significant number of DKA episodes in established IDDM patients. In new-onset IDDM, attention to early signs and symptoms of diabetes by the primary health care providers and families may help lower the number of newly diagnosed patients presenting with severe DKA.

The basic cause of DKA is absolute or relative insulin deficiency. There are also elevated levels of counter-regulatory or stress hormones (eg, glucagon, cortisol, growth hormone, catecholamines) that antagonize insulin. These hormonal abnormalities produce hyperglycemia (by increased glucose production and decreased use), which leads to an osmotic diuresis and dehydration, lipolysis and hyperlipidemia, acidosis due to the production of ketones (ie, acetoacetate, β-hydroxybutyate) from fatty acids, and electrolyte abnormalities due to intracellular–extracellular shifts and urinary losses. Table 177–2 lists the common errors in DKA diagnosis and management.

■ PRESENTATION AND DEFINITION

The usual manifestations of DKA include a history of classic signs and symptoms of polyuria, polydipsia, and weight loss. After patients are sufficiently ketotic and acidotic, they have the fruity breath odor of ketosis. Many also exhibit nausea, vomiting, and lethargy. State of consciousness may vary from awake and alert (with mild DKA) to drowsiness or coma. Hyperventilation and dehydration also occur. Abdominal pain and an elevation in leukocytes may be due solely to DKA and may be confused with an acute abdomen. These clinical findings usually resolve with therapy of DKA, but, if not, an underlying cause (eg, appendicitis) must be sought. DKA must be considered in children who are vomiting and appear dehydrated but who continue to urinate excessively.

In a known diabetic patient, DKA may be precipitated by an acute infection but is usually caused by omission of insulin. This may be deliberate or be based on a misconception that insulin doses should be eliminated or significantly decreased because of anorexia or vomiting. Careful monitoring of blood glucose levels and urinary ketones and appropriate therapeutic response can help avoid many DKA episodes.

Recurrent DKA in most cases is thought to be caused by deliberate insulin omission, sometimes by a child without the parents' knowledge and sometimes by the child and par-

TABLE 177-2. Common Errors in Diabetic Ketoacidosis Diagnosis and Management

Using good urine output to mean the patient is not significantly dehydrated (usually occurs with new-onset IDDM)

Delay in starting insulin: waiting for all laboratory values to be done or waiting for infusion pump

Letting the blood glucose drop too low by not adding enough glucose to the intravenous fluids

Too aggressive fluid intake (too rapid or too much)

Feeding patient too early, causing nausea and vomiting before gastric peristalsis normalizes

Decreasing the intravenous insulin rate or discontinuing intravenous insulin when the blood glucose has decreased but the patient is still acidotic

Not anticipating cerebral edema

Not heeding and treating symptoms of cerebral edema (eg, worsened sensorium, severe headache)

Not carefully reviewing clinical and laboratory data and adjusting the treatment plan as needed (ie, rigidly adhering to a predetermined treatment regimen)

Stopping the intravenous insulin before starting subcutaneous insulin

Not giving subcutaneous insulin before a meal or snack

ents in collusion. Putting a responsible adult in charge of the insulin injections and using a simplified regimen (eg, one or two shots per day) may be successful in lowering the number of or eliminating the DKA episodes.

The degree of hyperglycemia does not correlate with the degree of acidosis, and patients may be severely acidotic but only minimally hyperglycemic. The diagnosis of DKA can be rapidly established at the bedside with a meter glucose reading and a urinary or serum ketone determination using strips or tablets.

■ TREATMENT

The basic components of DKA treatment are fluid and electrolyte replacement (with careful attention to potassium) and insulin. This must be done with frequent monitoring of clinical and laboratory factors, using a flow sheet (Table 177–3) and paying careful attention to details and trends.

Fluid Replacement

Dehydration affects virtually all patients with DKA. Water and electrolyte losses occur because of polyuria caused by the osmotic diuresis produced by glycosuria, hyperventilation, vomiting, and diarrhea. The best measure of dehydration is the patient's current weight compared with a recent, healthy weight. Dry mucous membranes, poor skin turgor, and orthostatic hypotension are clinical indications of dehydration. Most patients with DKA are 5% to 10% dehydrated. Patients in shock may have greater degrees of dehydration.

Adequate intravenous fluid replacement is extremely important and should begin as soon as the diagnosis of DKA is established. Normal saline (NS) or Ringer's lactate, an isotonic solution, is recommended initially because they help to restore the intravascular volume and, therefore, maintain blood pressure and kidney perfusion, which enhances glucose loss through the kidney, resulting in a lower blood glucose level.

Insulin

For more than a decade, continuous low-dose insulin infusion has been the method of choice. Short-acting (regular) insulin is the only type used. The advantages of a continuous intravenous insulin infusion are the elimination of the problem of poor absorption from subcutaneous and intramuscular sites in a dehydrated patient and rapid clearance, allowing easy dose adjustment, which makes management more controllable.

The usual recommended dose is 0.1 U/kg/hour. Sometimes a bolus of the same dose is given before starting the insulin infusion. Running the infusate (30 to 50 mL) through the tubing to saturate binding sites on the tubing is recommended.

A decrease in glucose should occur at a rate of about 75 to 100 mg/dL/hour. In the first hour or two of treatment, there is a decrease in glucose level from the initial rehydration fluids as intravascular volume expands.

The blood glucose level corrects to normal levels more quickly than the acidosis, and it is necessary to continue intravenous insulin until the acidosis is cleared. Continuing the intravenous insulin infusion until urinary ketones are cleared may enable easier management after the infusion is discontinued and subcutaneous insulin is started. If the blood glucose level decreases to 250 mg/dL and acidosis is still detected, glucose should be added to intravenous fluids, starting with 5% dextrose and increasing as needed to 7.5% or 10% dextrose to keep the blood glucose approximately 250 mg/dL. If the blood glucose level is less than 300 at the onset of treatment, it is useful to add 5% dextrose at the onset of therapy. In some patients, despite the use of 10% dextrose, the blood glucose may fall too low (perhaps <100 mg/dL), and it becomes necessary to decrease (not discontinue) the intravenous insulin infusion rate.

Potassium

Patients with DKA have total-body potassium depletion, but the measured serum potassium may be high, nor-

TABLE 177-3. Diabetic Ketoacidosis Flow Sheet

Feature	Monitoring Schedule
Clinical data	
Weight	Onset of treatment and every
Vital signs	1–2 h initially
State of consciousness	
Laboratory data	
Electrolytes (Na, K, Cl, HCO$_3$), venous pH	Every 1–2 h for the first 4–8 h and then every 2–4 h until DKA is cleared
Glucose	Hourly
Blood urea nitrogen, creatinine, calcium, phosphate levels	Every 4–8 h depending on initial levels and type of fluids used
Urinary ketone level	Every void
Fluids	Type and rate; record hourly input
Urine output	Record every void
Potassium, phosphate, bicarbonate	Record amounts added to fluid
Insulin	Dose, rate, and route

mal, or low. There is an exchange of intracellular potassium ions for extracellular hydrogen ions. Treatment with insulin causes potassium to move intracellularly, causing a decrease in serum potassium. Both hypokalemia and hyperkalemia are potential causes of death, and the serum potassium, therefore, must be monitored every 1 to 2 hours, and potassium should not be added to the intravenous fluids until the serum potassium level is known and the patient is voiding. An electrocardiogram can help assess whether hypokalemia or hyperkalemia is present while awaiting the potassium level.

Phosphate

Phosphate depletion occurs in DKA because of poor food intake, the catabolic state, and urinary losses. Insulin treatment causes phosphate to move intracellularly, lowering serum phosphate levels. In clinical studies, routine phosphate administration has not been demonstrated to have any advantage in DKA treatment. There are potential theoretical benefits for phosphate use; phosphate depletion can impair central nervous system (CNS) and myocardial function and cause insulin resistance and shift the hemoglobin–oxygen dissociation curve to impair oxygen delivery to the tissues.

Bicarbonate

Treatment of DKA with bicarbonate to help correct acidosis has been controversial. The treatment of DKA with insulin generates bicarbonate as ketones are metabolized, and there is no need to use bicarbonate in mild or moderate DKA. These patients gradually correct their acidosis as insulin and fluid treatment proceed. Potential risks of bicarbonate include overtreatment producing a metabolic alkalosis, greater risks of hypokalemia and paradoxic cerebrospinal fluid acidosis. Clinical trials of bicarbonate in severe DKA have not shown improvement in DKA outcome whether or not bicarbonate was used.

Bicarbonate use should be reserved for patients who are severely acidotic if the acidosis may threaten respiratory or cardiac function (eg, pH ≤ 7.0 to 7.1 and bicarbonate ≤ 5) and to administer enough bicarbonate only for a small partial correction (eg, to raise the pH to 7.2, maximum). The pH should be rechecked approximately 30 minutes after the infusion. Do not give bicarbonate to hypokalemic patients until treatment with potassium is ongoing.

Converting to Subcutaneous Insulin

Patients should be continued on intravenous fluids and an intravenous insulin infusion until they are clinically stable with normal sensorium and normal vital signs, until the acidosis is cleared (ie, normal venous pH and bicarbonate), and until they can take fluids and food orally without vomiting. Any identified precipitating factor (eg, infection) should have been treated.

Regular insulin is used for the first day or so after a DKA episode. Subcutaneous insulin takes time to take effect, and the intravenous insulin infusion must be continued for 30 to 60 minutes after the first subcutaneous dose of insulin is given. This prevents insulin levels from becoming too low, which would allow recurrence of lipolysis and ketogenesis. A dose between 0.10 to 0.25 U/kg is given before a meal.

The switch from intravenous to subcutaneous insulin is best done during the daytime. The subcutaneous insulin doses should all be followed within approximately 0.5 hour by a meal or snack, and doses of regular insulin are needed about every 4 to 6 hours. During this period of dose adjustment, frequent blood glucose measurements and urinary ketone checks are important. Dose adjustment depends on the patient's blood glucose response to previous subcutaneous doses. When the patient's usual insulin requirement is known and the precipitating factor of the DKA is cleared, the patient may be able to resume his or her usual dose of insulin as soon as normal caloric intake is reestablished. For example, a well-controlled child who had an episode of moderate DKA due to a skipped insulin dose with a viral gastroenteritis could probably resume the usual insulin schedule fairly soon after her DKA has cleared and she can eat normally; DKA is cleared at approximately 1 AM, the intravenous fluids and intravenous insulin are continued through the night, vomiting has ceased and the child can eat and drink without nausea. The usual morning dose may be satisfactory before breakfast. Some patients may need lower insulin doses after a DKA episode due to decreased caloric intake, but some may need more. Frequent monitoring of blood glucose and urinary ketones is imperative. Newly diagnosed patients need to have their current insulin requirements established.

There are two common errors that occur during this transition period. First, the intravenous insulin infusion is discontinued without giving subcutaneous insulin, and the patient becomes hyperglycemic, ketotic, and even acidotic within several hours. This is done because the blood glucose is normal or low and the acidosis is cleared. If this condition occurs during the night, it may be 4 to 8 hours before it is appreciated that the patient's metabolic control has deteriorated. The second common error is to withhold regular insulin before a meal because the blood glucose is normal or low. When this is done, the blood glucose increases to high levels after eating, and the general response is then to give regular insulin to lower the blood glucose level, which may fluctuate over a wide range during the remainder of the day. The best approach is to give regular insulin before eating to prevent a postprandial glucose rise.

Prevention

Many episodes of DKA can be prevented by vigilance and careful monitoring of blood glucose and urinary ketones. Urinary ketones should be checked whenever blood glucose is elevated to approximately 250 mg/dL or higher and if the patient is feeling ill. This cannot be overemphasized. When ketone tests become positive (moderate to large), extra regular insulin can be given until the ketones are clear. Failure to monitor, failure to recognize or pay attention to symptoms of illness, and failure to contact the health care team early may lead to episodes of DKA that could have been prevented. Proper sick-day management can prevent DKA.

■ COMPLICATIONS

Cerebral edema is an unpredictable, often fatal, and uniformly feared complication of treating DKA. It usually occurs when biochemical abnormalities are improving. Cerebral edema probably accounts for half or more of DKA-associated deaths. Subclinical brain swelling occurs often during DKA treatment. Factors implicated but not pinpointed as possible causes of cerebral edema are too rapid a drop in blood glucose, dropping the blood glucose to an excessively low level, excessive fluid administration, tonicity of intravenous fluids, failure of the serum sodium to rise during treatment, and the use of bicarbonate.

Chronic Effects

Autoimmune Disease

Associated autoimmune disease, particularly thyroid dysfunction, occurs with greater frequency with IDDM. Thyroid function should be monitored periodically (every few years at a minimum) in IDDM patients.

Joint Dysfunction

Limited joint mobility, perhaps due to glycosylation of tissue proteins, is a marker for long-term poor control and is associated with other complications (*eg*, retinopathy, nephropathy and neuropathy). The hands and other joints should be examined.

Growth Disturbances

Linear growth is negatively affected by poor diabetic control. Decreased growth velocity, crossing percentiles downward for height and weight, eventual short stature, and delayed skeletal and sexual maturation are associated with chronic undertreatment with insulin. An extreme form of this, the Mauriac syndrome or diabetic dwarfism, occurs rarely and is usually associated with hepatomegaly. Careful height and weight measurements should be obtained every 3 to 4 months and plotted on growth curves so deviations from normal velocities can be detected early. Alternatively, treatment with excessive insulin doses often leads to excessive weight gain, causing the weight curve to cross percentiles upward. The maintenance of normal growth curves for height and weight is an important goal of diabetes management.

Retinopathy

Most patients with IDDM develop background retinopathy after 15 to 20 years of the disease. The percentage of patients developing proliferative retinopathy is less, with studies reporting incidences of 20% to 50%. About 5% to 10% of IDDM patients become blind. Early treatment with laser photocoagulation can significantly reduce the rate of progression to blindness. All patients with IDDM should be evaluated yearly by an ophthalmologist, with regular-interval eye examinations by the child's pediatrician and diabetes physician. These yearly examinations should begin within 5 years of the onset of the disease. Intensive blood glucose control delayed onset and slowed progression of retinopathy.

Nephropathy

About 30% to 40% of patients with IDDM eventually develop end-stage renal disease and need dialysis or transplantation. End-stage renal disease is an important cause of morbidity and mortality. Diabetic nephropathy is characterized by proteinuria, which may be severe, producing a nephrotic syndrome, hypertension, initial hyperfiltration (*ie*, increased glomerular filtrate rate [GFR]), and progressive renal insufficiency (*ie*, increasing serum creatinine and urea nitrogen, decreasing GFR). Glomerular damage, especially mesangial expansion and basement membrane thickening, is the most characteristic histologic finding. Researchers have shown the importance of tight metabolic control to prevent nephropathy or slow its progression.

A genetic predisposition may be an important underlying factor. All patients with IDDM should be monitored by urinalysis, with a check for protein, serum creatinine, and blood urea nitrogen at least annually for the first few years of the disease. Twenty-four-hour urine samples for quantitative protein and, if possible, tests for microalbuminuria should be done at least yearly, preferably starting in the first year after the diagnosis. Blood pressure should be monitored accurately several times a year. After hypertension, overt proteinuria, or elevation in serum creatinine or urea nitrogen is found, monitoring of renal function several times each year and consultation with a nephrologist is warranted. Microalbuminuria (<200 to 250 mg/day) may be a marker for the early stages of nephropathy. Low-protein diets have been successful in slowing or preventing progression of renal insufficiency in IDDM, but there are concerns about their use in growing children.

Hypertension is an extremely important factor that is known to accelerate the progression of nephropathy. It should be aggressively treated. Angiotensin-converting enzyme (ACE) inhibitors are recommended. It is not known whether using ACE inhibitors to lower blood pressures already in the normal range are useful in preventing or retarding nephropathy. It is also important for patients to avoid other risk factors, such as smoking.

Neuropathy

Symptomatic diabetic neuropathy, peripheral or autonomic, is uncommon in children and adolescents with IDDM, although changes in nerve conduction may be measured after 4 to 5 years of the disease. Overall, neuropathy is a common IDDM complication, and its frequency increases with the duration of disease and degree of hyperglycemia. Improvements in glycemic control may help neuropathic symptoms. Clinical trials of aldose reductase inhibitors have reported serious side effects.

Macrovascular Complications

Patients with IDDM tend to have coronary artery, cerebrovascular, and peripheral vascular disease more often, at an earlier age, and more extensively than the nondiabetic population. Hypertension, elevated blood lipid levels, and cigarette smoking are other risk factors for developing macrovascular complications. Risk factor assessment, including lipid panels, blood pressure measurements, and determining if the patient smokes, should be done, and treatment should be instituted as indicated. A strong admonition against smoking and referral to an appropriate program for patients who are already smokers are indicated.

(Abridged from Leslie P. Plotnick, Insulin Dependent Diabetes Mellitus, in Oski, DeAngelis, Feigin, McMillan, Warshaw: *Principles and Practice of Pediatrics, Second Edition*, J.B. Lippincott, 1994.)

Oski's Essential Pediatrics,
edited by Kevin B. Johnson and Frank A. Oski.
Lippincott–Raven Publishers,
Philadelphia © 1997

178

The Thyroid Gland

Abnormalities of the thyroid gland may result from altered function (*eg,* hypothyroidism, hyperthyroidism), altered structure (*eg,* enlargement, nodule), or nonthyroidal causes (*eg,* drugs, other illnesses).

HYPOTHYROIDISM

Hypothyroidism is defined as a state in which the thyroid gland fails to secrete sufficient quantities of thyroid hormone. Primary hypothyroidism results from a problem inherent to the gland itself, and secondary or central hypothyroidism results from the failure of pituitary stimulation of the thyroid gland. Primary and central hypothyroidism can be congenital or acquired.

■ CONGENITAL HYPOTHYROIDISM

Congenital hypothyroidism is a disease with an overall prevalence of 1 of 4000 live births, including 1 of 2000 persons of Far Eastern or Hispanic descent, 1 of 5500 persons of European descent, and 1 of 32,000 persons of African descent. Ninety-five percent of all cases are sporadic, and 5% are genetic, most often reflecting a dyshormonogenesis. There is a 2:1 female-to-male predominance, and associations with specific human lymphocyte antigen (HLA) types have been reported in certain populations. Newborn screening for congenital hypothyroidism is carried out in all 50 states in the Unites States, but the methods of screening vary. Healthy, premature infants have lower T_4 concentrations than term infants of the same chronologic age. This must be kept in mind when evaluating the results of the newborn screen. If the newborn screen blood sample is obtained within the first day of life, and the thyroid-stimulating hormone (TSH) level may be falsely elevated because of the peripartum TSH surge.

Diagnosis

Congenital hypothyroidism rarely is diagnosed from clinical abnormalities. These children have normal birth weight and length and a slightly larger than average head circumference at birth, and one third of them have longer than average gestation. Most cases are detected as a result of newborn screening tests, which must be confirmed by thyroid function tests using a venous blood sample. The dried filter paper test does not suffice as the confirmatory test.

Certain clinical features of hypothyroidism, listed in Table 178–1, may suggest the diagnosis before the results of the newborn screening tests are available. Features that suggest the possibility of hypopituitarism (*eg,* midline defects, hypoglycemia, micropenis) should lead to an evaluation for central hypothyroidism. Goiters are rarely present in

patients with congenital hypothyroidism, even in cases of dyshormonogenesis. They may be seen in cases of placental transmission of a goitrogen, and they may be large enough to produce upper airway obstruction.

The hormonal patterns found in congenital hypothyroxinemia are summarized in Table 178–2. In true hypothyroidism, other tests may be helpful in determining the cause of the disease, including thyroid scanning; urinary iodine if iodine toxicity or deficiency is suspected; bone age, which may be delayed in longstanding hypothyroidism; thyroglobulin level, which may help differentiate ectopic from dysplastic glands; and α-fetoprotein levels, which may be elevated in longstanding disease.

Treatment

The treatment of congenital hypothyroidism consists of replacement of thyroid hormone with oral levothyroxine. In primary hypothyroidism, several months of treatment may be necessary before the TSH level normalizes. Rarely, the pituitary set point for TSH release may be elevated in these patients, causing the TSH level to remain high despite normal free T_4 and T_3 levels.

With prompt and adequate treatment, children with congenital hypothyroidism have the potential for normal somatic and intellectual growth and development. If hypothyroidism is left untreated, severe mental retardation and neurologic dysfunction ensue, which are more severe in children with primary than with central hypothyroidism. Patients in whom treatment is begun before 6 weeks of age have an average IQ of 100. If treatment is begun at 6 weeks to 3 months, the average IQ decreases to 95; if begun at 3 to 6 months, the average IQ is 75. After 6 months, the average IQ is 55 or less.

■ ACQUIRED HYPOTHYROIDISM

Acquired hypothyroidism appears after the newborn period in a child who did not have congenital hypothyroidism. The estimated prevalence is 1 per 500 to 1000 school-age children, with a female-to-male preponderance of 4:1. Certain types of acquired hypothyroidism are familial.

The most common cause is chronic lymphocytic thyroiditis (CLT), also known as Hashimoto's thyroiditis. A defect in cell-mediated immunity results in lymphocytic infiltration and enlargement of the thyroid gland. Titers of antithyroglobulin and antimicrosomal antibodies are elevated in more than 80% of patients. Patients with CLT present with nontender enlargement of the gland, which may be

TABLE 178-1. Signs and Symptoms of Congenital Hypothyroidism

Large fontanelles	Prolonged jaundice
Umbilical hernia	Constipation
Macroglossia	Lethargy
Mottled, dry skin	Difficulty feeding
Hypotonia	Cool skin
Abdominal distention	Sleeps through night (newborn period)
Hoarse cry	Hypothermia
Respiratory distress	Goiter (rare)

TABLE 178-2. Hormonal Patterns in Congenital Hypothyroxinemia

Cause	First Newborn Screen		Follow-up Confirmation			
	T_4	TSH	T_4	T_3RU	TSH	Free T_4
Primary hypothyroidism	Low	High	Low	Low/Nl	High	Low
Central hypothyroidism	Low	Nl*	Low	Low/Nl	Nl*	Low
Transient hypothyroidism	Low	High	Nl	Nl	Nl	Nl
Thyroid-binding globulin deficiency†	Low	Nl	Low	High	Nl	Nl

Nl, *normal;* T_4, *thyroxine;* TSH, *thyroid-stimulating hormone;* T_3RU, *triiodothyronine resin uptake.*

The normal level of TSH seen in central hypothyroidism is inappropriately low for the decreased levels of T_4 and free T_4.

†*The diagnosis of thyroid-binding globulin (TBG) deficiency is most accurately made by demonstration of a low TBG level.*

asymmetric. The patients are often euthyroid, but some may present with transient hyperthyroidism or have signs and symptoms of hypothyroidism.

Diagnosis

The diagnosis of hypothyroidism is usually straightforward. The clinical features are listed in Table 178–3. The earliest sign of hypothyroidism in a child is often a slowing of the linear growth rate, because skeletal growth is sensitive to thyroid hormone levels.

Except in the rare cases of peripheral resistance to thyroid hormone, circulating levels of T_4 and T_3 are low in hypothyroidism. Tests that assess concentrations of thyroid hormone-

binding proteins (*eg,* T_3RU, TBG level) or free T_4 levels must be performed before therapy is initiated. TSH levels help differentiate primary from secondary hypothyroidism.

Treatment

The treatment of acquired hypothyroidism is thyroid hormone replacement with a single daily dose of oral levothyroxine. In cases of hypothyroidism due to goitrogen exposure, it may be possible to treat the hypothyroidism by removing exposure to the goitrogen.

It is important to monitor the growth rate and T_4 levels in all patients and TSH levels in patients with primary hypothyroidism. Many children who commence treatment after longstanding hypothyroidism may experience school and behavioral problems, which may be related to a decrease in attention span and an increase in energy level as they become euthyroid.

HYPERTHYROIDISM

Hyperthyroidism occurs when the thyroid gland secretes excessive amounts of thyroid hormone. The clinical manifestation is called thyrotoxicosis. Like hypothyroidism, hyperthyroidism may be congenital or acquired. Hyperthyroidism in childhood is rare and accounts for fewer than 5% of all cases of hyperthyroidism.

■ CONGENITAL HYPERTHYROIDISM

Congenital hyperthyroidism, more often called neonatal thyrotoxicosis, is seen almost exclusively in infants of mothers with Graves' disease. Neonatal thyrotoxicosis may be transient, lasting up to several weeks, or prolonged, lasting over 6 months. It is a serious illness requiring prompt and aggressive management. This disease occurs in as many as 1 of 70 infants of mothers with Graves' disease. It has an equal sex distribution, unlike the later-onset form of thyrotoxicosis, which has a female preponderance. If maternal thyroid-stimulating immunoglobulin (TSI) titers are more than five times the normal values, regardless of whether she has had ablative thyroid therapy, the risk of neonatal thyrotoxicosis

TABLE 178-3. Signs and Symptoms of Acquired Hypothyroidism

Short stature, decreased growth velocity

Obesity, myxedema

Goiter (primary hypothyroidism)

Delayed skeletal and dental age

Cold intolerance

Constipation

Dry, cool skin

Thinning of hair

Lethargy

Delayed reflex return

Bradycardia

Delayed puberty

Abnormal menses

Precocious puberty (rare)

Muscular pseudohypertrophy (rare)

Galactorrhea (rare)*

Hypothalamic thyroid-releasing hormone (TRH) stimulates prolactin release from the posterior pituitary. In primary hypothyroidism, increased TRH may produce hyperprolactinemia and galactorrhea.

is greatly increased. Neonatal thyrotoxicosis accounts for about 1% of all cases of pediatric thyrotoxicosis.

Diagnosis

The diagnosis is made on the basis of clinical findings combined with elevated levels of T_4, free T_4, and T_3. The diagnosis may sometimes be available prenatally through cordocentesis for fetal thyroid hormone levels. Fetal tachycardia and intrauterine growth retardation may suggest the diagnosis. Affected patients often have low birth weight and microcephaly. They also exhibit marked irritability and hyperactivity, tachycardia, tachypnea, prominent eyes, thyroid enlargement, and a failure to gain weight despite marked hyperphagia. The glandular enlargement may be so marked that it causes respiratory distress requiring endotracheal intubation. Other features include vomiting, severe diarrhea, hepatosplenomegaly, jaundice, thrombocytopenia, and cardiac failure. The mortality rate in untreated cases is 15% to 25%, and death is most often caused by cardiac failure. The severity of the disease does not correlate with the size of the goiter, but it may be related to maternal TSI levels.

Treatment

The treatment of neonatal thyrotoxicosis is directed toward immediate management of the symptoms and reduction in the amount of thyroid hormone produced. This treatment must be initiated in the newborn or intensive care nursery with adequate cardiopulmonary monitoring and venous access.

Therapy consists of a combination of Lugol's solution (5% iodine and 10% potassium iodide), propylthiouracil, and propranolol. Treatment with dexamethasone is helpful in some cases. If no improvement occurs within 24 hours, the doses of Lugol's solution and propylthiouracil should be increased by at least 50%. If evidence of cardiac failure arises, the infant should be digitalized promptly. Adequate caloric intake is vital in these hypermetabolic infants. Serum levels of thyroid hormone must be carefully monitored to ensure adequate therapy and to avoid hypothyroidism. In milder cases, Lugol's solution and propranolol may not be needed.

Long-term complications of neonatal thyrotoxicosis can occur even in patients who receive prompt and adequate treatment. These include premature craniosynostosis and neurodevelopmental defects, particularly intellectual impairment; both may be caused by intrauterine thyrotoxicosis. The intellectual impairment usually correlates with premature craniosynostosis, but a direct effect of thyrotoxicosis on the developing brain cannot be ruled out.

■ ACQUIRED HYPERTHYROIDISM

Acquired hyperthyroidism is most often due to Graves' disease (ie, autoimmune thyrotoxicosis). The female-to-male ratio ranges from 3:1 to 5:1. There is a familial tendency and an association with HLA types B8 and DR3. Emotional stress as a precipitating factor of thyrotoxicosis has been described frequently.

Diagnosis

The diagnosis of Graves' disease is based on the combination of clinical findings (Table 178–4) and the characteristic elevations of thyroid hormone levels. The thyroid gland is almost invariably enlarged, and tachycardia, nervousness, and widened pulse pressure are seen in more than 80% of patients. Most patients experience weight loss, although weight gain may occur because of a significantly increased appetite. Proptosis or exophthalmos is a common finding, but the Graves' ophthalmopathy in children usually is less severe than in adults.

The thyroid hormone profile characteristically shows elevated total T_4, free T_4, and T_3 levels, accompanied by very low or undetectable levels of TSH. In some cases, the T_3 level is elevated with a normal level of T_4 (ie, T_3 toxicosis). The source of T_3 in patients with T_3 toxicosis is direct secretion by the gland. In these patients, the contribution of T_3 secreted by the gland may equal or exceed that of peripheral T_4 deiodination to the total circulating T_3.

In patients with hyperthyroidism without exophthalmos, it may be difficult to differentiate among early CLT, subacute thyroiditis, and Graves' disease. If TSI levels are not elevated, a radioactive iodine uptake scan aids in the diagnosis. Characteristically, patients with Graves' disease have elevated uptake that is not suppressed with administration of T_3. Patients with CLT or subacute thyroiditis generally have normal or decreased uptake of ^{123}I.

Treatment

The three forms of treatment for Graves' disease are medical, surgical, and radioactive iodine ablation. The mainstay of medical management is antithyroid medication, with methimazole (Tapazole) or propylthiouracil. Both are equally effective in decreasing the production of T_4 and T_3 by the thyroid gland, but propylthiouracil also blocks the peripheral deiodination of T_4 to T_3. Propylthiouracil is not known to significantly decrease thyroid gland secretion of T_3 and may, therefore, not provide significant advantage over methimazole in patients with T_3 toxicosis.

Approximately 5% to 10% of patients treated with antithyroid medication experience side effects from the medication. Most of these side effects are minor and include erythematous skin rashes, urticaria, and arthralgias. Granulocytopenia is the most frequently seen serious side effect and is generally heralded by a fever or sore throat. Vasculitis, at times severe, is another serious side effect. If side effects occur, discontinuation of the drug generally reverses the problem. The patient may then be treated with a different antithyroid preparation; however, the same reaction may occur.

TABLE 178-4. Signs and Symptoms of Hyperthyroidism

Goiter
Anxiousness, nervousness
Tachycardia
Widened pulse pressure
Increased appetite
Weight loss or gain
Tremor
Proptosis
Heat intolerance
Increased growth velocity
Diarrhea
Sleep disturbances

Surgical subtotal thyroidectomy is effective and has low morbidity when performed by an experienced surgeon. The patient must be euthyroid for surgery, and preoperative treatment with iodides such as Lugol's solution is often recommended to decrease vascularity of the gland. The risks include hypothyroidism (up to 50%), transient hypocalcemia (10% to 20%), and, rarely, hypoparathyroidism, recurrent laryngeal nerve damage, or recurrence of thyrotoxicosis. [131]I ablation has been widely used to treat thyrotoxicosis in adults. Its use in children has been limited because of a theoretical risk of the later development of thyroid or other malignancies. However, available data suggest that ^{131}I treatment in childhood or adolescence does not affect the risk of developing thyroidal or nonthyroidal cancers or leukemia and does not increase the risk of birth defects in the patient's offspring. Remission from thyrotoxicosis should occur within several weeks, and it is often followed by permanent hypothyroidism after several months or years.

Prognosis

The prognosis for children with Graves' disease is generally good. Evidence suggests that with antithyroid medication alone, remission of Graves' disease, defined as being euthyroid for 1 year after stopping medication, occurs at a rate of approximately 25% every 2 years. In some cases, relapse of hyperthyroidism or spontaneous hypothyroidism may occur after remission.

A rare but life-threatening complication of Graves' disease is thyroid storm, also called thyrotoxic crisis. This is a clinical diagnosis based on the manifestations of exaggerated and uncontrolled hyperthyroidism. Patients generally present with marked hyperthermia and tachycardia and may develop cardiac failure, vomiting, diarrhea, and central nervous system (CNS) abnormalities, including confusion, apathy, and coma. Thyroid storm can be precipitated by many events but most often is associated with infection, surgery, or trauma. The therapy includes aggressive antithyroid treatment including propylthiouracil or Tapazole, Lugol's solution, or lithium carbonate; prevention of thyroid hormone action with β-blockade; antipyretics; support of life-threatening conditions using intravenous hydration, oxygen, and digitalis; and treatment of any underlying infection.

TABLE 178-5. Causes of Thyromegaly

Diffuse	Nodular
Hashimoto's thyroiditis	Hashimoto's thyroiditis
Thyrotoxicosis	Thyroid cyst
Graves' disease	Thyroid adenoma
Thyroiditis	Hyperfunctional (hot)
TSH-secreting adenoma	Hypofunctional (cold)
Pituitary resistance	Thyroid carcinoma
Goitrogen exposure	Papillary
Dyshormonogenesis	Follicular
Iodine deficiency (endemic)	Mixed papillary or follicular
Idiopathic (simple) goiter	Anaplastic
Acute, subacute thyroiditis	Medullary
	Nonthyroidal masses

TSH, *thyroid-stimulating hormone.*

■ DIFFUSE THYROMEGALY

Diffuse thyromegaly is most often caused by autoimmune thyroid diseases, including Hashimoto's thyroiditis (*ie*, CLT) and Graves' disease. Autoimmune thyroid disease accounts for more than 90% of the patients with diffuse thyromegaly. There is a female preponderance among children with diffuse thyromegaly. The cause, diagnosis, and treatment of these two diseases were discussed previously.

In some cases of diffuse thyromegaly, particularly in adolescent girls, no cause can be determined and the diagnosis of *idiopathic (simple) goiter* is made. Other causes of enlargement of the thyroid gland (Table 178–5) are ingestion of a goitrogen including antithyroid medication, other drugs, and certain foods, familial dyshormonogenesis, and rare pituitary abnormalities, such as pituitary resistance to thyroid hormone or a TSH-secreting pituitary adenoma.

(Abridged from Patricia A. Donohoue, The Thyroid Gland, in Oski, DeAngelis, Feigin, McMillan, Warshaw: *Principles and Practice of Pediatrics, Second Edition*, J.B. Lippincott, 1994.)

Oski's Essential Pediatrics,
edited by Kevin B. Johnson and Frank A. Oski.
Lippincott–Raven Publishers,
Philadelphia © 1997

179

The Adrenal Cortex

ADRENOCORTICAL ABNORMALITIES

■ CONGENITAL ADRENAL HYPERPLASIA

Congenital adrenal hyperplasia (CAH) is a family of diseases caused by an inherited deficiency of any of the enzymes necessary for the biosynthesis of cortisol (Figure 179–1). These enzymes, with the exception of 3β-hydroxysteroid dehydrogenase, are members of the cytochrome P-450 family. The cytochromes P-450 are microsomal or mitochondrial terminal oxidases involved in electron transport and require NAD and flavoproteins as cofactors. Deficiency of any one of these enzymes results in decreased production of cortisol and increased secretion of adrenocorticotropic hormone (ACTH). With stimulation by ACTH, the adrenal cortex becomes hyperplastic, and steroid precursors preceding the enzymatic block accumulate. These accumulated precursors are shunted, if possible, to a steroidogenic pathway that is unaffected by the enzymatic block. Each particular form of CAH is manifested by the clinical features produced by deficient end products (*eg*, glucocorticoid, mineralocorticoid, androgen) and by accumulated or shunted precursors (*eg*, mineralocorticoid or androgen excess). CAH is inherited as an autosomal recessive disorder and has an equal sex distribution. A summary of these diseases and their clinical features is given in Table 179–1. The severity of the clinical features varies among families.

The most common form of CAH is caused by 21-hydroxylase (21-OH) deficiency, accounting for more than 90% of the cases. The most severe form, the salt-losing form, is caused by complete absence of 21-OH activity and results

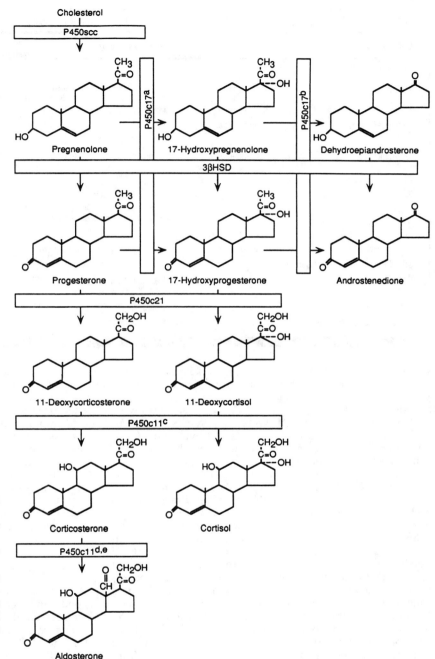

Figure 179-1. Adrenal steroid biosynthetic pathways. Enzyme names: P450scc, 20-hydroxylase, 22-hydroxylase, 20,22-desmolase; P450c17, [a]17α-hydroxylase, [b]17,20-desmolase (lyase); 3β-HSD, 3β-hydroxysteroid dehydrogenase, $\triangle^5\triangle^4$-isomerase; P45c21, 21-hydroxylase; P45c11, [c]11β-hydroxylase, [d]18-hydroxylase (CMOI), [e]18-dehydrogenase (oxidase) (CMOII); CMOI, corticosterone methyl oxidase I; CMOII, corticosterone methyl oxidase II. The 20-hydroxylase, 22-hydroxylase, and 20,22-desmolase are activities of the same P450scc enzyme. Both 17α-hydroxylase and 17,20-desmolase activities are properties of the same P450c17 enzyme. However, 11β-hydroxylase and CMO activities are properties of two different isozymes of P450c11, encoded by different genes. In addition, several isoforms of 3β-HSD exist.

in cortisol and mineralocorticoid deficiencies. Affected girls have ambiguous genitalia at birth due to hypersecretion of adrenal androgens, which are converted to testosterone. Affected and untreated girls and boys usually present with symptoms of acute adrenal insufficiency, known as a salt-losing crisis, at 1 to 3 weeks of age.

The simple virilizing form is caused by a partial 21-OH deficiency. Patients with this disease produce adequate amounts of cortisol and aldosterone under the stimulation of excess ACTH and elevated plasma renin activity (PRA) levels, but at the expense of excess androgen production. Girls may present with ambiguous genitalia or postnatal virilization, and boys may present with suspected isosexual precocious puberty, although the testes remain prepubertal in size. The combined frequencies of the salt-losing and simple virilizing forms approximates 1 in 10,000 to 13,000 births among Caucasians. The incidence among Asian and black populations is somewhat lower.

A mild degree of 21-OH deficiency, the attenuated form, manifests as hirsutism or menstrual irregularities in adolescent or adult females. In an asymptomatic form, there are biochemical abnormalities consistent with 21-OH deficiency, but no clinical features are evident.

Diagnosis

The diagnosis of CAH due to 21-OH deficiency is made when elevated levels of hormones preceding the enzymatic block (see Figure 179–1) are demonstrated in a child with the typical clinical findings. A female infant with virilization of the external genitalia or a male infant with a salt-losing cri-

TABLE 179-1. Clinical Features of the Different Forms of Congenital Adrenal Hyperplasia at Diagnosis

Deficient Enzyme	Clinical Form	Elevated Levels	Abnormal Sexual Development
21-Hydroxylase			
Complete deficiency	Salt-losing	Urinary 17-ketosteroids, plasma 17-hydroxyprogesterone, plasma androstenedione, plasma renin activity (PRA), ACTH	Females: ambiguous genitalia
Partial deficiency	Simple virilizing	Same as above	Females: ambiguous genitalia
			Males and females: postnatal virilization
Mild deficiency	Attenuated	Same, but milder elevations	Female adolescents: hirsutism, menstrual irregularities
11-Hydroxylase	Hypertensive	Urinary 17-hydroxycorticosteroids, urinary 17-ketosteroids, plasma 11-deoxycorticosterone (DOC), plasma 11-deoxycortisol, plasma androstenedione	Females: ambiguous genitalia
			Males and females: postnatal virilization
17-Hydroxylase	Hypertensive	Plasma DOC, plasma corticosterone	Males: absent or incomplete virilization
3β-Hydroxysteroid dehydrogenase			
Complete deficiency	Salt-losing	Plasma dehydroepiandrosterone (DHA), 17-hydroxypregnenolone, PRA, ACTH	Males and females: ambiguous genitalia
Partial deficiency	Mild	Plasma DHA, 17-hydroxypregnenolone	Female adolescents: hirsutism
Cholesterol side-chain cleavage	Salt-losing "lipoid"	No steroids produced	Males: absent virilization

sis (dehydration with hyponatremia, hyperkalemia, and acidosis) has elevated plasma 17-hydroxyprogesterone, progesterone, and androstenedione levels, increased urinary 17-ketosteroids, elevated PRA and ACTH levels, and low or undetectable serum cortisol. Older children who present with inappropriate virilization (*ie*, simple virilizing form) have normal cortisol and electrolyte levels, but with the same elevated hormone levels as described for the younger group. These children also have growth acceleration and advanced skeletal age due to the effects of sex steroids.

In the salt-losing form, treatment is first directed at correcting the life-threatening metabolic abnormalities of adrenal crisis by correction of dehydration with intravenous saline and dextrose, correction of hyperkalemia with insulin and glucose if necessary, and, after a blood sample is obtained for steroid hormone measurements, glucocorticoid replacement with the rapidly acting intravenous glucocorticoid, hydrocortisone, at a "stress" dosage, which is three times the calculated dose for daily physiologic replacement. Because parenteral mineralocorticoid preparations are no longer available, prolonged treatment with high-dose glucocorticoids is necessary until oral mineralocorticoids can be tolerated. This allows enough mineralocorticoid effect from the glucocorticoid preparation to achieve a lowering of the serum potassium concentration and adequate urinary sodium retention. In many cases, supplemental sodium chloride must be added for infants to maintain normal serum electrolyte levels.

Treatment

Treatment with glucocorticoids promptly decreases the ACTH level and the excess androgen production. Children with the salt-losing form of CAH have a lifelong requirement for glucocorticoid replacement but may tolerate discontinuation of daily mineralocorticoid therapy when they reach adulthood. Careful titration of glucocorticoid therapy is necessary, because the balance between undertreatment (*ie*, androgen excess) and overtreatment (*ie*, cushingoid fea-

tures) may be within a narrow dosage range and varies significantly from patient to patient.

For the simple virilizing form of 21-OH deficiency, mineralocorticoid therapy is not needed. However, mineralocorticoid supplementation has been successfully employed to decrease the required glucocorticoid dose for adequate suppression of adrenal androgen levels. Glucocorticoid therapy must be titrated for optimal results, as in the salt-losing form.

In treating both forms of this disease, as for all children receiving glucocorticoid therapy, the dosage must be increased during times of stress and the parents must be trained to administer intramuscular hydrocortisone during times when the child cannot take the medication orally.

Prognosis

The prognosis for children with 21-OH deficiency is good with careful follow-up and titration of hormonal replacement therapy. Some degree of morbidity is associated with surgical correction of the external genitalia in girls, and this may be significant if multiple surgical procedures are needed. Fertility is normal in males with the salt-losing form, but females with this form may have decreased fertility, for unknown reasons. In the simple virilizing form, fertility is unaffected in adequately treated males and females.

Prenatal Diagnosis

The prenatal diagnosis of 21-OH deficiency is available for families at risk. The diagnosis is based on the presence of elevated amniotic fluid levels of 17-hydroxyprogesterone combined with human leukocyte antigen (HLA) typing of fetal cells. The genes for 21-OH lie within the HLA complex on chromosome 6 and are inherited with the HLA complex. If the HLA haplotypes of a previously affected sibling are known and no HLA recombination has occurred, the 21-OH status of the fetus can be determined by the HLA type. In some centers, chorionic villus biopsy specimens can be analyzed for HLA and by hybridization with deoxyribonucleic acid (DNA) probes for the HLA and 21-OH genes, allowing prenatal diagnosis much earlier in pregnancy.

■ PRIMARY ADRENAL INSUFFICIENCY

Primary adrenal insufficiency or failure is most often due to Addison's disease. The most common cause of Addison's disease is autoimmune destruction of the adrenal cortex, as is seen in the autoimmune polyglandular syndromes. Approximately 45% of patients with autoimmune Addison's disease (ie, caused by antiadrenal antibodies) develop one or more other autoimmune endocrinopathies, most often thyroid disease. Other, rarer causes of primary adrenal failure are congenital adrenal hypoplasia, bilateral adrenal hemorrhage (as in the Waterhouse-Friderichsen syndrome), trauma, thrombosis, infection (eg, tuberculosis), destruction due to tumor metastases, or degeneration, as is seen in adrenoleukodystrophy.

In primary adrenal failure, there is decreased or absent production of all three groups of adrenal steroid hormones. In most cases, the signs and symptoms of adrenal insufficiency develop slowly, particularly the hyperpigmentation associated with increased ACTH. These features are listed in Table 179–2.

The diagnosis is based on demonstration of elevated ACTH levels combined with decreased or absent cortisol and mineralocorticoid production. The fasting 8 AM cortisol level is low and fails to rise with ACTH stimulation. The fasting glucose value may be low, and hyponatremia with hyperkalemia may be present. PRA is usually elevated. Adrenal androgen levels may be below normal in adolescent patients. Antiadrenal antibody levels and antibodies to other endocrine glands should be measured.

Treatment includes physiologic replacement with glucocorticoid and mineralocorticoid. Glucocorticoid dosage must be increased during times of stress.

■ SECONDARY ADRENOCORTICAL INSUFFICIENCY

Secondary adrenocortical insufficiency is most often due to ACTH deficiency. Rarely, resistance to ACTH may occur.

ACTH deficiency may be due to idiopathic hypopituitarism (congenital), congenital malformations of the pituitary or hypothalamus, destruction of the pituitary or hypothalamus (infection, hemorrhage, tumor, irradiation, infiltrative disease), or iatrogenic causes (glucocorticoid treatment of the mother prenatally or pharmacologic glucocorticoid treatment postnatally).

In the absence of primary adrenal disease, ACTH deficiency does not result in mineralocorticoid deficiency. Therefore, hyponatremia, hyperkalemia, and dehydration are not seen as manifestations of ACTH deficiency. In fact, cortisol deficiency may result in decreased renal clearance of free water, resulting in fluid retention. This is often apparent in patients with diabetes insipidus, who may appear to have improvement of their disease if ACTH deficiency develops.

The diagnosis of ACTH deficiency is based on absence of the 8 AM peak in serum cortisol and on lack of response to tests of ACTH secretion (insulin-induced hypoglycemia, glucagon stimulation, metyrapone). In cases of partial ACTH deficiency, the patient may produce enough ACTH for normal daily physiologic needs (normal 8 AM cortisol, normal 24-hour urinary 17-hydroxycorticosteroids) but be unable to respond to stress and fail the tests of stimulated ACTH secretion. In any child with ACTH deficiency, the secretion of other anterior and posterior pituitary hormones must be carefully assessed.

ACTH deficiency is treated with glucocorticoid at physiologic replacement doses. The dosage must be carefully titrated to prevent overtreatment, which seems to occur at lower doses in children with ACTH deficiency than in those with primary adrenal failure. Mineralocorticoid treatment is unnecessary.

■ ADRENOCORTICAL HYPERFUNCTION

Adrenocortical hyperfunction is most often manifested by the effects of glucocorticoid excess, called Cushing's syndrome.

Etiology

The most common cause of Cushing's syndrome is iatrogenic administration of pharmacologic doses of a glucocorticoid as an anti-inflammatory or immunosuppressive agent. Other causes of Cushing's syndrome are rare in child-

---

TABLE 179-2. Signs and Symptoms of Adrenal Insufficiency

GLUCOCORTICOID DEFICIENCY

Fasting hypoglycemia

Increased insulin sensitivity

Decreased gastric acidity

Gastrointestinal symptoms (eg, nausea, vomiting)

Fatigue

MINERALOCORTICOID DEFICIENCY

Muscle weakness

Weight loss

Fatigue

Nausea, vomiting, anorexia

Salt craving

Hypotension

Hyperkalemia, hyponatremia, acidosis

ANDROGEN DEFICIENCY (IE, OLDER CHILDREN, ADULTS)

Decreased pubic and axillary hair

Decreased libido

Increased ACTH and β-Lipotropin

Hyperpigmentation

TABLE 179-3. Causes of Cushing Syndrome

ACTH INDEPENDENT

Iatrogenic (eg, glucocorticoid therapy)

Andrenocortical tumors (eg, adenoma, carcinoma, micronodular disease)

ACTH DEPENDENT

Hypothalamic CRF-producing tumor

Pituitary ACTH-producing tumor

Ectopic CRF-producing tumor (eg, pancreas, lung)

Ectopic ACTH-producing tumor (eg, lung, bronchus, gut)

Iatrogenic (eg, ACTH therapy)

Increased serotonin levels (eg, idiopathic)

TABLE 179-4. Clinical Features of Hypercortisolism

Obesity with violaceous striae
  Generalized in infants
  Truncal in older children with moon facies or buffalo hump
Decreased height velocity
  Short stature
  Delayed bone age
Plethora, increased hematocrit
Easy bruisability
Hypertension
Osteoporosis
Glucose intolerance
Poor wound healing
Increased frequency of infections
Renal stones, hypercalciuria
Weakness, muscle wasting (unusual in infants)
Depression

hood (Table 179–3). These include ACTH-dependent hypercortisolism (Cushing's disease) and primary adrenal hypercortisolism. Among children with hypercortisolism who are not receiving exogenous glucocorticoids, those who are less than 7 years old are more likely to have a primary adrenal cause. Those over 7 years old are more likely to have ACTH-dependent hypercortisolism. The clinical features of hypercortisolism are listed in Table 179–4.

Diagnosis

The diagnosis of Cushing's syndrome is based on demonstration of hypercortisolism and determination of its source in patients not receiving glucocorticoid treatment.

Measurement of serum cortisol levels at 8 AM and in the evening may fail to show the normal diurnal variation. However, the diurnal pattern may not mature in normal children until after 3 years of age. Serum ACTH levels are of some value. Low levels do not rule out the possibility of an ACTH-producing tumor, but high levels usually rule out a primary adrenal cause. The 24-hour urinary 17-hydroxycorticosteroid levels and free cortisol levels are usually elevated, as are 17-ketosteroids in some cases.

In children with equivocal clinical features and baseline static test results, an overnight dexamethasone suppression test may be the most advantageous dynamic screening test. After a single dose of dexamethasone, the 8 AM serum cortisol should be less than 5 µg/dL in a normal child. If the child fails the overnight test, a low-dose and then a high-dose dexamethasone suppression test (Table 179–5) should be performed. Failure to respond to the low-dose test in conjunction with appropriate suppression on the high-dose test suggests an ACTH-producing pituitary adenoma. Failure to respond to the high-dose dexamethasone test suggests an ectopic ACTH-producing tumor or an adrenal tumor.

If a pituitary, adrenal, or ectopic ACTH-producing tumor is suspected, radiologic imaging studies must be performed to visualize the tumor. Many ACTH-producing pituitary tumors are microadenomas, visible only at the time of transsphenoidal pituitary exploration.

Treatment

The treatment of Cushing's syndrome is removal of the cause of hypercortisolism. In iatrogenic disease, this is not always possible, because of the nature of the disorder, which requires glucocorticoid treatment.

In ACTH-dependent disease, the source of ACTH production usually must be removed surgically. In pituitary Cushing's disease, medications such as cyproheptadine and

TABLE 179-5. Normal Plasma and Urinary Steroid Hormone Levels With Static and Dynamic Tests

Test	Values
RESTING LEVELS	
Plasma cortisol*	8 AM: 11 ± 2.5 µg/dL; 8 PM: 3.5 ± 1.5 µg/dL
Urinary 17-hydroxycorticosteroids (17-OHCS)	2.9 ± 1.2 mg/m^2/24 h
Urinary free cortisol	25–65 µg/m^2/24 h
ADRENAL CAPACITY	
IV test: 25 USP U Acthar over 6 h	Plasma cortisol: 40 ± 5 µg/dL at 6 h
IV test: 0.25 mg Cortrosyn stat	Plasma cortisol: 32 ± 4 µg/dL at 2 h
IM test: 20 U/m^2 Acthar gel every 8 h for 3 days	Urinary 17-OHCS: 85 ± 15 mg/m^2/24 h after 3 days
ACTH CAPACITY†	
Oral metyrapone: 300 mg/m^2 every 4 h for 24 h	Urinary 17-OHCS increase >9 mg/m^2/24 h
Oral metyrapone: 300 mg/m^2 at midnight	8 AM: 11-deoxycortisol, 7–22 µg/dL
IV metyrapone: 500 mg/m^2 (max, 1 g) over 4 h	Plasma 11-deoxycortisol: 5–15 µg/dL at 5 h, with plasma cortisol level decreasing to near zero
Regular insulin 0.1 U/kg IV or glucagon 0.1 mg/kg IM	Rise in serum cortisol >20 µg/dL, or a twofold increase from baseline
PITUITARY SUPPRESSION TEST	
Low-dose dexamethasone: 1.25 mg/m^2/24 h (in 3 divided doses) for 3 d	Urinary 17-OHCS <1 mg/m^2/24 h or decrease in plasma or urinary androgens in hyperandrogenic states
High-dose dexamethasone: same, with 3.75 mg/m^2/24 h	Same

*Stress or anxiety may cause elevation of cortisol levels far above the stated normal range.

†Metyrapone will no longer be available for diagnostic testing in the near future. Insulin-induced hypoglycemia or glucogen stimulation will be the tests of choice for ACTH capacity. The specifics of these tests are detailed in Vandershueren-Lodenweyck M, et al. J. Pediatr. 1974;85:182.

bromocriptine have been more effective in lowering ACTH levels in adults than in children. Bilateral adrenalectomy was once the only treatment for ACTH-dependent disease, but most patients then developed Nelson's disease (ie, pituitary enlargement, hyperplasia of ACTH-producing cells).

In primary adrenal disease, adrenalectomy, unilateral in the case of a tumor and bilateral in micronodular disease, is the treatment of choice.

The most commonly encountered side effect of these treatments is adrenal insufficiency, due to ACTH deficiency or to adrenalectomy. In the case of unilateral adrenalectomy, the contralateral adrenal gland will need time to recover from prolonged lack of ACTH stimulation. Patients who undergo pituitary exploration have a small risk of developing panhypopituitarism.

Prognosis

The prognosis for patients with Cushing's syndrome is based on the underlying cause. Patients with adrenal or pituitary adenomas have a good prognosis after adequate surgical resection. Those who have adrenal or ectopic ACTH-producing carcinomas have a poorer prognosis.

Hypersecretion of adrenal androgens may be caused by CAH or by an adrenal tumor. In addition, feminizing adrenocortical tumors have been described. Adrenal tumors, including adenomas and carcinomas, are rare in childhood; they are treated by surgical resection and, in some cases, adjunctive therapies.

Hypersecretion of mineralocorticoids may be caused by the hypertensive form of CAH (see Table 179–1) or by primary hyperaldosteronism. In 11-OH or 17-OH deficiency, glucocorticoid replacement therapy results in lowering of mineralocorticoid levels. Hyperaldosteronism is rare in childhood and is treated with the aldosterone inhibitor, spironolactone.

Rare causes of apparent mineralocorticoid excess include an inherited defect in the conversion of cortisol to cortisone and licorice ingestion.

(Abridged from Patricia A. Donohoue, The Adrenal Cortex, in Oski, DeAngelis, Feigin, McMillan, Warshaw: *Principles and Practice of Pediatrics, Second Edition*, J.B. Lippincott, 1994.)

Oski's Essential Pediatrics,
edited by Kevin B. Johnson and Frank A. Oski.
Lippincott–Raven Publishers,
Philadelphia © 1997

180

The Adrenal Medulla

ABNORMALITIES OF THE ADRENAL MEDULLA

Abnormalities of the adrenal medulla are caused by benign or malignant tumors that secrete catecholamines.

■ PHEOCHROMOCYTOMA

Pheochromocytoma is rare in childhood but must be considered in a child with hypertension or other symptoms of catecholamine excess. This tumor may arise from any chromaffin tissue, but it is most often found in the adrenal medulla. Bilateral adrenal or extra-adrenal tumors are a more common feature in pediatric pheochromocytomas than adult pheochromocytomas, and they are often associated with the familial multiple endocrine neoplasia (MEN) syndromes. The neoplasias associated with the various MEN syndromes are listed in Table 180–1. Features consistent with these associated tumors (eg, medullary carcinoma of the thyroid) should be sought in any patient with pheochromocytoma. The MEN syndromes are inherited in an autosomal dominant manner and have variable expression. Pheochromocytomas are also associated with neuroectodermal dysplasias (eg, neurofibromatosis).

Pheochromocytoma is benign in more than 90% of pediatric patients. There is a male preponderance among children with this tumor, but the sex ratio is reversed in adults. The peak incidence occurs between 9 and 12 years in the pediatric group.

The signs and symptoms of pheochromocytoma are those of catecholamine excess (Table 180–2). These features are highly variable and are likely to be paroxysmal, but the hypertension may be sustained. Hypertensive crisis may occur during anesthesia.

Diagnosis

The diagnosis of pheochromocytoma is based on demonstration of increased catecholamines and their metabolites in a 24-hour urine sample and in blood. These substances urinary free epinephrine and norepinephrine, metanephrine, and VMA. Urinary VMA levels may be falsely elevated with certain drugs such as aspirin, penicillin, and sulfa preparations. If these test results are inconclusive, a clonidine suppression test may be useful. Clonidine causes a decrease in blood catecholamine levels only if they are not elevated due to secretion from an autonomous source. If suspected from the biochemical tests, the tumor can usually be localized by ultrasound, computed tomography, magnetic resonance imaging, or intravenous pyelography. Venography to demonstrate elevated levels of catecholamines should only be performed after adequate A-blockade with Regitine to prevent a hypertensive crisis. Scintigraphic imaging with ^{131}I-metaiodobenzylguanidine (MIBG scan) has been used to demonstrate the presence of a pheochromocytoma. MIBG is similar in structure to norepinephrine and is concentrated in tissues that are synthesizing catecholamines by means of norepinephrine in storage granules.

TABLE 180-1. The Multiple Endocrine Neoplasia Syndromes

Neoplasia	MEN Type I*	MEN Type IIa†	MEN Type IIb
Pheochromocytoma		+‡	+
Medullary thyroid carcinoma		+	+
Multiple neural tumors			+
Parathyroid or hyperplasia	+	+	
Pancreatic islet tumors	+		
Anterior pituitary tumors	+		

Also known as Wermer's syndrome.
†Also known as Simple's syndrome.
‡The + indicates that the tumor is associated with the syndrome.

TABLE 180-2. Signs and Symptoms of Pheochromocytoma

Hypertension

Sweating and flushing

Palpitations and tachycardia

Emotional lability

Headache

Nausea and vomiting

Constipation

Polyuria and polydipsia

Treatment

The treatment of pheochromocytoma is surgical excision. This requires extensive preoperative treatment with α- and β-blockade and with α-methyltyrosine if needed. If bilateral adrenalectomy is necessary, treatment for primary adrenal insufficiency must be promptly instituted. Postoperative recording of blood pressure and catecholamine levels is needed to monitor for tumor recurrence. Malignant tumors are diagnosed on the basis of functional tumor in nonchromaffin tissue areas. Benign tumors may cause blood vessel or capsular invasion but do not spread beyond chromaffin tissue areas. Malignant tumors grow slowly and are resistant to irradiation and chemotherapy; symptoms are treated medically, with various degrees of success.

(Abridged from Patricia A. Donohoue, The Adrenal Medulla, in Oski, DeAngelis, Feigin, McMillan, Warshaw: *Principles and Practice of Pediatrics, Second Edition*, J.B. Lippincott, 1994.)

Oski's Essential Pediatrics,
edited by Kevin B. Johnson and Frank A. Oski.
Lippincott–Raven Publishers,
Philadelphia © 1997

181

Signs and Symptoms of Inborn Errors of Metabolism

The typical newborn infant has a limited repertoire of reactions to use in response to adversity. Many of the signs and symptoms associated with inborn errors also may be typical of other more common disorders. It is essential, however, for the clinician to keep in mind that inborn errors do occur in infants and may cause problems. If appropriate laboratory tests are not pursued, the diagnosis may be missed and a treatable disorder could go unrecognized. Furthermore, failure to identify patients with inborn errors obviates the possibility of genetic counseling and prenatal diagnosis.

■ EVALUATION

Vomiting, jaundice, diarrhea, seizures, lethargy, apnea, coma, abnormal hair, abnormal eyes, dysmorphic features, unusual odor, hypoglycemia, and metabolic acidosis may be seen in patients with inborn errors of metabolism (Table 181–1). Vomiting may reflect dietary protein or carbohydrate intolerance and is often seen in association with the adrenal failure of congenital adrenal hyperplasia. Vomiting may be projectile and mimic pyloric stenosis or may be attributed to gastroesophageal reflux. It is usually responsive to withdrawal of the offending nutrient. Jaundice is seen in a number of inborn error conditions and may be associated with intrinsic hepatocellular disease or may be due to increased production or decreased removal of bilirubin. Diarrhea is a relatively rare sign but may be a clue in those conditions indicated in Table 181–1. Seizures or altered mental status, which often produces notable and worrisome symptoms, is seen in many inborn errors. Trauma, asphyxia, intracranial hemorrhage, infection, and central nervous system malformations may be more common, but if these etiologies are not positively established, then metabolic disorders must be considered carefully. Abnormal hair or eyes or dysmorphic features are typical of some heritable defects of metabolism. Unusual odors are detected in some infants with inborn errors characterized by excretion of volatile organic acids. Such olfactory clues are enhanced by slightly acidifying a sample of urine or by smelling the patient's hair or the nape of his or her neck where sweat-derived organic acids may localize. Diagnosis of an inborn error should never be excluded based on absence of pathognomonic odor. A variety of physiologic and environmental factors may influence the ability to detect these odors. Finally, any unexplained biochemical alteration such as acidosis or hypoglycemia may be an indication for a more vigorous search for an underlying primary hereditary defect.

Initial laboratory evaluation of patients with suspected inborn errors of metabolism often include general measurements and spot tests indicated in Table 181–2. Hypoglycemia is a prominent feature of glycogen storage diseases types I and III as well as of defects of the gluconeogenic pathway. Secondary hypoglycemia is seen in maple syrup urine disease, organic acidemias, and disorders of fatty acid oxidation due to many mechanisms. Bilirubin levels, liver function studies, serum copper determinations, sweat chloride levels, and α_1-antitrypsin quantitation or phenotyping may be clinically indicated. Blood pH should be assessed for evidence of metabolic acidosis. Many patients partially compensate for increased acid production with hyperpnea and lower PCO_2. Thus, plasma bicarbonate concentrations and calculated base deficit often need to be evaluated as well. Measuring electrolyte levels is also useful. Reduced serum sodium and elevated potassium values may reflect relative mineralocorticoid deficiency or resistance to mineralocorticoid activity. The most common of these disorders is 21 hydroxylase deficiency, a diagnosis of which usually can be established by finding elevated 17 hydroxyprogesterone levels. Such patients often present in adrenal crisis at 1 or 2 weeks of age. Girls with this disorder may have undergone some virilization of external genitalia, but affected boys are notoriously difficult to diagnose by physical examination alone unless there is already a high index of suspicion.

■ METABOLIC ACIDOSIS

Metabolic acidosis is a frequent finding in sick newborn infants. Patients with hypoxemia, shock, poor perfusion, sepsis, and renal dysfunction, among others, may exhibit this laboratory finding. The magnitude of the anion gap is a useful measurement when determining etiology. Hyperchloremic acidosis without much expansion of the anion gap

TABLE 181-1. Signs and Symptoms of Inborn Errors in Newborns

VOMITING	**SEIZURES, LETHARGY, APNEA, COMA**
Disorders of steroid biosynthesis	Nonketotic hyperglycinemia
Urea cycle disorders	β-Alaninemia
Organic acidemias	Organic acidemias
Galactosemia	Other aminoacidopathies
Hereditary fructose intolerance	Disorders producing hypoglycemia
Wolman's disease	Menke's syndrome
Various amino acid disturbances	Urea cycle disorders
JAUNDICE	Fatty acyl-CoA dehydrogenase deficiency
Galactosemia	Neonatal adrenoleukodystrophy
Hereditary fructose intolerance	**ABNORMAL HAIR**
Tyrosinemia	Menke's syndrome
α_1-Antitrypsin deficiency	Argininosuccinic aciduria
Hypothyroidism	Phenylketonuria
Wolman's disease	Lysinuric protein intolerance
Red blood cell membrane defects	**ABNORMAL ODOR**
Immune hemolytic anemias	Maple syrup urine disease
Glycolytic defects	Isovaleric acidemia
Crigler-Najjar syndrome	Methionine malabsorption
DIARRHEA	Phenylketonuria
Congenital disaccharidase deficiencies	β-Methylcrotonyl-CoA carboxylase deficiency
Glucose-galactose malabsorption	Tyrosinemia
Familial chloridorrhea	**COARSE OR DYSMORPHIC FEATURES**
Wolman's disease	GM_1 gangliosidosis
Tyrosinemia	β-Glucuronidase deficiency
Cystic fibrosis	Fucosidosis
HYPOGLYCEMIA	Neuraminidase deficiency
Branched-chain amino acid disorders	I cell disease
Organic acidemias	Glutaric acidemia II
Fatty acyl-CoA dehydrogenase deficiencies	Zellweger syndrome
Galactosemia	Neonatal adrenoleukodystrophy
Hereditary fructose intolerance	**ABNORMAL EYE FINDINGS**
Gluconeogenic defects	Galactosemia
Glycogen storage disease types I, III, VI	Sulfite oxidase deficiency
METABOLIC ACIDOSIS	GM_1 gangliosidosis
Organic acidemias	β-Glucuronidase deficiency
Type I glycogen storage disease	I cell disease
Primary lactic acidoses	Neuraminidase deficiency
Pyruvate carboxylase deficiency	Zellweger syndrome
Gluconeogenic enzyme defects	
Pyruvate dehydrogenase deficiency	
Galactosemia	
Hereditary fructose intolerance	
Pyroglutamic aciduria	

is often of renal origin. Identification of specific acids contributing to the gap is the most useful adjunct. Lactate levels are readily measured in most clinical laboratories. Results expressed as mEq/L can be used to estimate the extent to which lactate contributes to anions that are unaccounted for. Elevated lactate levels are seen secondary to hypoxemia or as a result of primary disturbances in lactate or pyruvate metabolism. Measurement of lactate-pyruvate ratios and plasma alanine levels may help in discriminating between these possibilities. A growing number of mitochondrial electron transport defects has been defined in recent years, but there is still a large number of infants with primary genetic lactic acidosis in whom specific etiologies are difficult to establish. If lactate does not account for most or all of the excessive anion gap, an organic acidemia should be pursued by measuring organic acid in urine by gas chromatography or volatile organic acids in plasma. A modest elevation of blood lactate level should be expected as a secondary event

TABLE 181-2. Laboratory Evaluation of Patients With Suspected Inborn Errors of Metabolism

GENERAL METHODS
Blood glucose
Lactate
pH
Electrolytes
Ammonia
Bilirubin
Liver function
Serum copper
Sweat chloride
α_1-Antitrypsin
17 Hydroxyprogesterone
Ketone bodies
Free fatty acids

SPOT TESTS
Ferric chloride
Dinitrophenylhydrazine
Clinitest
Mucopolysaccharides
Cyanide nitroprusside
Methylmalonic acid

CARBOHYDRATES
Reducing substances in urine
Oligosaccharide chromatography
Glycogen content of red blood cells, liver, or muscle
Mucopolysaccharide fractionation

AMINO ACID CHROMATOGRAPHY
Plasma
Urine

ORGANIC ACID ANALYSIS
Volatiles
Nonvolatiles

FATTY ACID CHAIN LENGTHS

SPECIFIC ENZYME ASSAYS

DNA-BASED DIAGNOSTIC TESTS

in many of the organic acidemias, but it usually does not account for the entire deficit of measured anions. When organic acidemia is suspected, urine and plasma samples should be frozen for subsequent analysis. These specimens should be obtained when the patient is acutely ill and likely to be excreting large amounts of abnormal metabolites.

■ HYPERAMMONEMIA

Hyperammonemia is often a clinical sign of an underlying metabolic disturbance. Figure 181–1 shows elevated blood ammonia in a newborn is most often due to a primary genetic disorder of one of the urea cycle enzymes, transient hyperammonemia of the newborn, or some other inborn error that produces metabolites that interfere with waste nitrogen disposal.

The latter conditions often can be suspected through detection of metabolic acidosis, which is usually not observed in primary urea cycle disturbances unless the patient develops shock or critical circulatory embarrassment. Plasma amino acids then provide useful data for subdividing the primary hyperammonemias. Elevated citrulline, argininosuccinic acid, or arginine levels are usually seen in citrullinemia, argininosuccinic acidemia, or hyperargininemia, respectively. Very low plasma citrulline values are found with blocks proximal to this metabolite in the urea cycle. Transient hyperammonemia of the newborn is probably a developmental defect in which elevated ammonia levels with normal levels of citrulline due to a maturational delay in expression of urea cycle enzymes are found.

■ DISORDERS OF FATTY ACID OXIDATION

Abnormalities of fatty acid oxidation are disorders recognized with increasing frequency. Patients with these disorders often present with alterations in mental status, hypoglycemia, fatty infiltration of the viscera, and a clinical picture reminiscent of Reye's syndrome. Disorders of fatty acid oxidation have been found in a significant proportion of victims of sudden infant death syndrome. Cellular oxidation of fatty acids requires their transport into mitochondria after the formation of acyl-carnitine esters, the production of acyl-CoA intermediates, and the subsequent activity of chain-length-specific acyl-CoA dehydrogenases. Finally, intact electron transport mediated by an electron transport flavoprotein (ETF) and ETF dehydrogenase is required. Defects in each of these steps have been recognized. In general, all result in an elevation of circulating free fatty acids, a relative inability to procedure β-hydroxybutyrate and acetoacetate (ketone bodies), even in response to fasting, and in a diversion of fatty acids from the normal pathway of β oxidation to ω oxidation, resulting in generation of measurable levels of dicarboxylic acids. Defects in ETF or ETF dehydrogenase may also produce accumulations of other organic acids such as glutaric acid or ethylmalonic adipic acid because their oxidation requires ETF-dependent acyl-CoA dehydrogenase as well.

■ OTHER CONSIDERATIONS IN INBORN ERRORS

A number of spot tests (see Table 181–2) are used to detect inborn errors. They are useful but nonspecific and require more experience for accurate interpretation than is generally believed. Both false-positive and false-negative results are fairly frequent; thus, spot tests are relatively crude screening tests. The ferric chloride reaction may be positive in a number of disorders. The dinitrophenylhydrazine test yields a visible precipitate with urine containing significant amounts of α ketoacids such as in patients with maple syrup urine disease. Clinitest tablets can be used to detect glucose, galactose, or other reducing substances in urine. The cyanide nitroprusside test is positive in the presence of sulphur-containing amino acids such as homocystine or cystine. Caution must be used in the newborn period, because of the relatively reduced tubular reabsorptive capacity for cystine and the dibasic amino acids. Most inborn errors require sophisticated equipment and expertise for their definitive diagnosis. Gas chromatography, mass spectrometry, and specific enzyme assays may be needed. Increasingly, defects may be detected at a nucleic acid level, but the need for enzymatic activity assessment probably will persist in most of these conditions because of molecular heterogeneity.

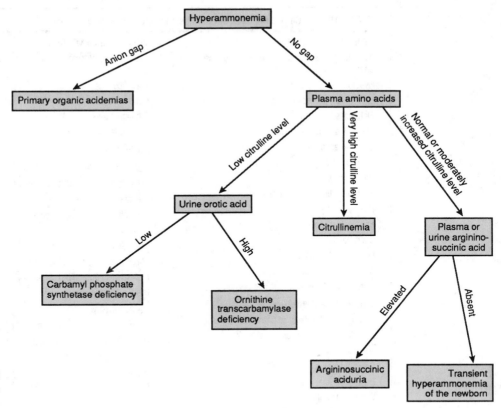

Figure 181-1. Hyperammonemia in the newborn. (Adapted from Batshaw, et al. *Pediatrics.* 1981; 68:291.)

Patients with inborn errors of metabolism may be detected by newborn screening. Most states mandate testing for phenylketonuria and hypothyroidism. Some states have more comprehensive programs that detect an array of conditions, potentially in a presymptomatic state. Implementation of these tests, however, differs according to regional priorities due to economic and other issues. For most inborn errors, screening tests of suitable sensitivity, specificity, and cost are not available, so clinical acumen is essential.

Treatment of hereditary metabolic disorders must be tailored to the clinical situation. Avoiding noxious nutrients, restricting dietary protein intake, and administering pharmacologic amounts of vitamins or cofactors may be beneficial. For a number of conditions, hepatic transplantation may be the only treatment consonant with a reasonable chance of success and an acceptable quality of life. Often, highly complex dietary manipulations are required. These depend on sophisticated nutritional and laboratory analytical services available at a limited number of centers. Acutely, in cases of suspected organic acidemias or urea cycle disorders, dietary protein should be restricted and sufficient calories provided to attempt to suppress endogenous tissue catabolism. If this treatment is continued, a protein-free intake cannot be maintained. Sufficient essential amino acids and nitrogen must be supplied to support growth and anabolism. This level of protein intake often must be determined empirically, but decisions are aided by careful measurement of relevant metabolites. Occasionally, dialysis may help in the emergent therapy of life-threatening inborn errors. In those conditions associated with hyperammonemia, alternative means of waste nitrogen excretion through administration of compounds such as sodium benzoate or sodium phenylacetate may be of considerable benefit. Many inborn errors of metabolism associated with cellular storage of bipolymers are not responsive

to dietary therapy and await development of treatment such as gene replacement.

■ CHROMOSOMAL DISORDERS

About 1 in 200 liveborn infants have detectable chromosomal disorders. Collectively, they account for a sizable fraction of malformations, morbidity, and mortality in the newborn period. Nearly all recognizable chromosomal defects are associated with aneuploidy for all or some segment of a chromosome. *Aneuploidy* means that some number of genes in a portion of the genome is present in other than the expected diploid complement. Duplications of chromosomal material produce trisomies (or, occasionally, tetrasomies, for example), and deletions or deficiencies produce monosomic conditions. In either event, the imbalance of gene expression

TABLE 181-3. Indications for Chromosome Studies

Features suggestive of a known chromosomal syndrome

Ambiguous genitalia

Stillborn infants or fetuses with no obvious cause of death or with multiple malformations

Infants with two or more major congenital abnormalities or multiple dysmorphic features

Neurologic defects with major or minor malformations

Parents, siblings, and other appropriate family members of infants found to have translocations, duplications, or deletions

Parents who have had multiple (three or more) spontaneous pregnancy losses of unknown etiology

TABLE 181-4. Clinical Features in Chromosome Disorders in Newborn Period

DOWN'S SYNDROME

Trisomy 21; Trisomy for Part of 21; Mosaicism for Trisomy 21

Hypotonia

Excess skin on back of neck

Flat facies

Upslanting palpebral fissures

Simian crease

Hip dysplasia

Heart disease

Gastrointestinal abnormalities

Brachycephaly

Brushfield's spots

Short hands

Ulnar loop dermatoglypia

Distal axial triradius

Increased gap between first and second toes

TRISOMY 18 SYNDROME

Trisomy for All or Most of Chromosome 18

Intrauterine growth retardation

Microcephaly

Polyhydramnios

Decreased fetal activity

Short palpebral fissures

Small mouth and mandible

Overlapping third and fifth fingers

Low-arch dermal ridge pattern

Hypoplasia of nails

Short sternum

Cryptorchidism

Cardiac defects

Renal abnormalities

TRISOMY 13 SYNDROME

Trisomy for All or a Large Part of Chromosome 13

Holopresencephaly

Encephalocele

Microcephaly

Microphthalmia with coloboma

Cleft lip or palate

Capillary hemangiomas

Scalp defects

Polydactyly

Thin ribs

Cardiac defects

Cryptorchidism

Hypertonia or hypotonia

TRISOMY 8 SYNDROME

Usually Mosaicism for Trisomy 8 or Partial Trisomy 8 Due to Translocation

Thick lips

Deep-set eyes

Prominent ears

Camptodactyly

TRIPLOIDY

69XXY or 69XXX Karyotype

Placental with hydatidiform changes

Prenatal growth retardation

Microphthalmia with coloboma

Syndactyly

Heart defects

Stillborn or early neonatal death

Hypospadias and cryptorchidism

Brain malformations

4p⁻SYNDROME

Partial Deletion of the Short Arm of Chromosome 4

Marked intrauterine growth deficiency

Microcephaly

Hypotonia

Seizures

Hypertelorism

Posterior scalp defects

Cleft lip

Hypospadias and cryptorchidism

Simian crease

Abnormal dermatoglyphics

Posterior mouth

CRI DU CHAT SYNDROME

Partial Deletion of the Short Arm of Chromosome 5

Low birth weight

Typical cry

Hypotonia

Microcephaly

Hypertelorism

Low-set ears

Abnormal facies

Congenital heart defects

Abnormal dermatoglyphics

(Continued)

---

created by these structural aberrations is presumed to produce clinical consequences. In few, if any, chromosomal disorders is it known which genes are implicated or even what number of genes is involved.

High-resolution banding procedures for karyotype analysis and molecular methods applied to clinical samples detect ever smaller degrees of abnormalities. Very small cytologically detectable deletions have been found in Prader-Willi syndrome, Miller-Dieker syndrome, DiGeorge's syndrome, Langer-Giedion syndrome, aniridia-Wilms' tumor association, and retinoblastoma. The number of genes minimally needed to be deleted to produce these

TABLE 181-4. Clinical Features in Chromosome Disorders in Newborn Period *(Continued)*

13q⁻ SYNDROME

Deletion of Part of the Long Arm of Chromosome 13

Intrauterine growth retardation

Microcephaly

Brain malformations

Prominent nasal bridge

Hypertelorism

Small or absent thumbs

Cardiac defects

Hypospadias and cryptorchidism

Retinoblastoma

Short neck

18p⁻ SYNDROME

Deletion of Part of the Short Arm of Chromosome 18

Mild growth deficiency

Mild microcephaly

Ptosis

Hypertelorism

Micrognathia

Large ears

Small hands and feet

18q⁻ SYNDROME

Partial Deletion of the Long Arm of Chromosome 18

Mild growth retardation

Hypotonia

Nystagmus

Microcephaly

Midface hypoplasia

Deep-set eyes

Abnormal dermatoglyphics

Cryptorchidism

Cardiac defects

Skin dimples at joints

Narrow or atretic ear canals

Long hands with tapering fingers

21q⁻ SYNDROME

Partial Deletion of the Long Arm of Chromosome 21

Low birth weight

Hypertonia

Redundant eyelids

Large external ears

Micrognathia

Dysplastic nails

Delayed bony development

TURNER'S SYNDROME

XO Karyotype, but Many Patients Are Mosaic for Some Other Cell Line Including XO/XY; May Be Associated With Structural Abnormalities of X Chromosome

Small stature

Ovarian dysgenesis

Lymphedema of hands and feet

Wide-spread nipples

Narrow maxilla

Low posterior hairline

Webbed neck

Short fourth metacarpal

Hyperconvex fingernails

Pigmented nevi

Renal anomalies

Cardiac defects

Cubitus valgus

XXXXY SYNDROME

Karyotype as Stated

Hypotonia

Low birth weight

Abnormal facies

Radioulnar synostosis

Abnormal dermatoglyphics

Small penis and testes

phenotypes is not known. Some monogenic disorders, however, clearly are associated with smaller intragenic deletions or loss of DNA that involves only a single gene (*eg,* some types of thalassemia). Thus, single-gene disorders and "chromosomal conditions" are likely to be considered simultaneously.

Down's Syndrome

The chromosome disorder most often observed in the newborn period is Down's syndrome, which accounts for about one third of detected abnormalities. The constellation of facial, limb, and internal abnormalities found in this disorder is well known and virtually pathogenomic. Low birth weight, brachycephaly, small ears, upslanting palpebral fissures, redundant skin at the nape of the neck, Brushfield's spots, short and broad hands, clinodactyly of the fifth finger, simian creases, wide space between the first and second toes, and profound hypotonia are seen in most infants. As many

as half of the children with Down's syndrome have congenital heart defects. Ventricular septal defects and endocardial cushion defects account for two thirds of the abnormalities. About 5% of patients have gastrointestinal anomalies, including duodenal atresia and Hirschsprung's disease. Various immunologic abnormalities are detectable later in life with a high incidence of leukemias. In the newborn period, leukemoid reactions are frequently noted and may be associated with fetal hydrops. Mental retardation is an invariant concomitant of Down's syndrome.

As with most other chromosome disorders, a presumptive diagnosis often may be made based on physical findings. Because of the lifelong and severe implication of these disorders, however, documentation with suitable cytogenetic studies should be carried out as soon as is feasible. This documentation confirms the diagnosis, assists in medical decision making, and rules out the possibility of a translocation, partial trisomy 21, or other unusual karyotypic constitution that might alter the recurrence risk. If rapid information is essential for making a therapeutic decision, bone marrow-derived chromosomes or cord blood lymphocyte chromosomes can be harvested after short-term culture, and slides can be prepared within hours. The morphologic findings and resolution of chromosomes studied with rapid harvesting may not permit detection of subtle abnormalities, but altered numbers of chromosomes should be readily recognizable.

The risk of Down's syndrome and other aneuploidies increases with increasing maternal age, for reasons that are unclear. About half of all children with Down's syndrome are born to mothers older than 35 years of age, although this group of women has only 5% to 7% of all liveborn infants. Trisomy 21 is present in 90% to 95% of patients with Down's syndrome. The remainder have chromosomal translocations that may be de novo events in the infants examined or may represent the outcome of pregnancies of balanced translocation carrier parents. The latter group of parents may be at a significantly increased risk of having additional offspring with unbalanced karyotypes. Potential indications for undertaking cytogenetic analyses are listed in Table 181–3.

Other Chromosomal Abnormalities

Trisomy 18 is often characterized by microcephaly, small palpebral fissures, overriding of the second and fifth fingers, and omphalocele (Table 181–4). Trisomy 13 should be suspected when a sloping forehead, holoprosencephaly, polydactyly, cleft lip and palate, and cystic kidneys are seen. Trisomy for all or parts of other chromosomes may be observed but much less frequently (see Table 181–4).

In addition to the disorders described here that are characterized by extra autosomal chromosomal material, partial deletions of autosomes are seen. Although many of these disorders have reasonably consistent phenotypes, there is, perhaps, more variability in clinical features because the precise extent of the deletion may differ from one individual to another. The features of some of the more commonly seen deletion syndromes are listed in Table 181–4.

Abnormality of structure or number of the sex chromosomes are particularly common. Based on karyotypes of early abortuses, Turner's syndrome due to an XO karyotype may be present in as many as 4% of all human conceptions. Despite the relatively mild phenotype of the syndrome postnatally, perhaps only 1 in 100 of these XO embryos survives. Those female fetuses who do make it to term often have lymphedema of the hands and feet with or without cystic hygromas. Also of consequence in the newborn period may be cardiac (coarctation of the aorta or aortic stenosis) or renal (eg, horseshoe kidneys) abnormalities. Later, typical features of short stature, gonadal dysgenesis, cubitus valgus, low posterior hairline, typical facies, widely spaced nipples, multiple pigmented nevi, hyperconvex fingernails, and short fourth metacarpals may become more apparent. Klinefelter's syndrome due to an XXY karyotype occurs in about 1 of 1000 newborn boys. Clinical detection in infancy of this syndrome or the equally frequent XYY syndrome is unusual. The greater the degree of aneuploidy, the more marked the dysmorphic features may be, rendering them more easily detectable in the newborn period. Thus, the XXXXY syndrome with its characteristic midface hypoplasia, genital abnormalities, and radioulnar synostosis may often be detected in infancy.

(Abridged from Larry J. Shapiro, Signs and Symptoms of Inborn Errors of Metabolism, in Oski, DeAngelis, Feigin, McMillan, Warshaw: *Principles and Practice of Pediatrics, Second Edition*, J.B. Lippincott, 1994.)

Oski's Essential Pediatrics,
edited by Kevin B. Johnson and Frank A. Oski.
Lippincott–Raven Publishers,
Philadelphia © 1997

182

Disorders of Amino Acid Metabolism

■ PHENYLKETONURIA

Phenylketonuria, the most important paradigm of the inborn errors of metabolism, was discovered in the early 1930s by Folling.

Patients with disorders of phenylalanine metabolism usually appear to be normal at birth. Some of them may have vomiting episodes, occasionally to the point of having a diagnosis and surgical correction of pyloric stenosis. Psychomotor development will be impaired such that, despite normal performance at birth, at the age of 1 year, the intelligence quotient will be about 50 and, at the age of 3 years, it will average about 20. Beginning at several months of age, the patient may manifest the mousey, pungent odor responsible for the disorder first being elucidated. Although the infant's pigmentation at the time of birth will be normal for infants in the family, melanization will not progress as would be expected ("dilute" pigmentation). The majority of affected persons will show poor head growth, and abnormal electroencephalograms and seizures are common. An indolent, eczema-like rash may develop, particularly in the perineal region. Until newborn screening programs were developed, the diagnosis usually was made during the workup of a mentally retarded young child. Dilute pigmentation, rash, and seizures in addition to the retardation helped to indicate phenylketonuria. The urinary findings of increased phenylpyruvic acid and other metabolites of phenylalanine, coupled with a significant increase in the plasma phenylalanine concentration but a low or, at most, normal tyrosine concentration, are diagnostic. Unfortunately, enzyme studies have not been carried out very frequently because the activity is present only in the liver and intestinal tract. The few studies that have been done have shown essentially no enzyme activity in the fully developed classic cases with relatively high phenylalanine concentrations.

Treatment consists of administering a diet that is selectively low in its phenylalanine content. Because phenylalanine is an essential amino acid, controlling the dietary intake will permit the patient to have only that amount of phenylalanine that is necessary for normal protein synthesis. This is achieved by giving one of several commercial formulas that are phenylalanine-poor or phenylalanine-free and supplementing it with a standard formula and low-protein foods. It is imperative that the phenylalanine concentration be monitored at appropriate intervals so that it is maintained within the limits of 2 and 8 mg/dL for optimum results. Although dietary control will not result in the restoration of damaged neurologic function, it will prevent further neurologic deterioration and correct the dilute pigmentation, odor, and skin eruption. The patient should be maintained on the diet for his or her lifetime. This frequently is difficult to achieve, however, after late childhood or adolescence. It is particularly important for females to remain on dietary control.

Newborn screening programs have been successful. After demonstration that the phenylalanine concentration even in phenylketonuric infants is essentially normal at birth, it was hypothesized that, if cases were detected and appropriate treatment instituted in the first days of life, mental retardation and other manifestations would be prevented. This was demonstrated first on siblings of known cases. Further extension of this hypothesis was enabled by the development by Guthrie of an inexpensive test that could be applied to all newborns. At preferably 3 to 5 days of age, the age at which the initial data were obtained, a few drops of blood are allowed to flow onto a special filter paper. When the blood is dry, the paper can be transported to a laboratory and its phenylalanine concentration determined. When the phenylalanine concentration is above a specified level (in most laboratories, 4 mg/dL), further studies are done and, if the diagnosis is made, a low-phenylalanine diet is instituted immediately, ideally before 2 weeks of age.

All forms of phenylketonuria are inherited on an autosomal recessive basis. Classic phenylketonuria has its highest incidence of 1:4500 in Celtic peoples, an incidence of about 1:12,000 in mixed populations such as that of the United States, and low to virtually no incidence in Asians, Finns, black Africans, and Ashkenazi Jews. Hyperphenylalaninemia and biopterin disorders are distributed more evenly.

Diagnosis of the carrier state may be achieved by the administration of deuterium-labeled phenylalanine and subsequent measurement of labeled tyrosine in the blood. It is an expensive procedure, however, because of the requirement for a deuterated reagent and the high-resolution mass spectrometry necessary to assay the specimens. More recently, recombinant DNA techniques in informative families have been used for carrier detection and prenatal diagnosis.

■ DISORDERS OF AMMONIA METABOLISM

Excess dietary or waste nitrogen, remaining after that needed for protein synthesis and tissue maintenance is used, normally is not stored in the body, but is converted into urea by a series of reactions known as the urea cycle (Figure 182–1). Disorders of the urea cycle are associated with the accumulation of ammonia and its precursors, such as glutamine, glutamic acid, aspartic acid, and glycine. Elevated plasma ammonia levels that exceed three times the upper limits of normal are toxic and are associated with cytotoxic changes in the brain and liver. With rising ammonia levels, patients show poor feeding, anorexia, behavioral changes, irritability, vomiting, lethargy, ataxia, and seizures. As the hyperammonemia progresses, the child becomes comatose and ventilatory support may be needed. Circulatory collapse and cerebral edema may occur. The classic cases are neonates who have been asymptomatic for 24 to 48 hours and then

have a rapidly progressing course with neurologic deterioration. Milder forms of the disorders may be detected later in the neonatal period, produce intermittent symptoms over a period of years, or be detected in older children or adults as a result of neurologic problems or psychomotor retardation. As a group, they are estimated to occur in about 1:30,000 live births. All the disorders of ammonia metabolism are inherited as autosomal recessive traits, except for ornithine-trans-carbamylase (OTC) deficiency, which is associated with an X-linked pattern of inheritance, and transient hyperammonemia of the newborn, which is not genetic in nature.

Diagnosis of a specific urea cycle disorder usually can be made on the basis of the pattern of plasma and urine amino acid abnormalities and the presence or absence of orotic aciduria. Confirmation of specific enzymatic deficiencies requires only erythrocytes or cultured skin fibroblasts for some of the disorders, but necessitates liver biopsy for others. Secondary hyperammonemia, caused by organic acidurias, usually can be excluded by the absence of acidosis, but urinary organic acid determination is suggested to rule out the rare case that might be detected initially with only hyperammonemia.

Treatment of acute hyperammonemia, either as the initial presenting episode or as a subsequent intercurrent episode, is a medical emergency. With the initial episode, blood and urine samples should be collected for diagnostic testing, but treatment should be started immediately, before a specific diagnosis is established. Therapy should include the removal of all exogenous protein sources and the administration of intravenous glucose to prevent protein catabolism. Drugs that employ alternate pathways for waste nitrogen excretion, such as sodium benzoate and sodium phenylacetate, may be used intravenously to control mild to moderate hyperammonemia (less than 350 μM). Reduction of markedly elevated plasma ammonia and ammonia precursors is carried out most effectively by hemodialysis. Alternatively, peritoneal dialysis may be employed. If there is a temporary delay in dialysis, exchange transfusion, which is the least effective, may be done. Because the duration of time in coma is related inversely to outcome, prompt referral to a tertiary medical center is indicated if dialysis is not readily available.

Even with prompt and aggressive medical therapy, only 30% to 50% of neonates who have hyperammonemic coma survive the neonatal period. Most of those who do survive have significant neurologic deficits and psychomotor retardation. Seizure disorders, cortical atrophy, and spastic quadriparesis are common. Later acute episodes, usually precipitated by intercurrent infections or excessive protein intake, also may lead to further neurologic sequelae or death.

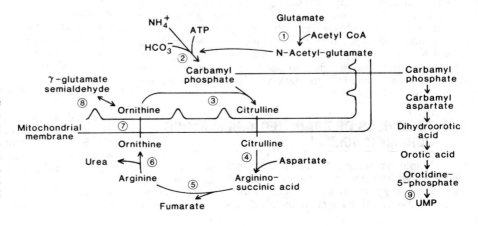

Figure 182-1. Urea cycle. *1*, N-acetyl-glutamate synthetase (NAGS); *2*, carbamyl phosphate synthetase I (CPS I); *3*, ornithine transcarbamylase (OTC); *4*, argininosuccinate synthetase (AS); *5*, argininosuccinate lyase (AL); *6*, arginase; *7*, mitochondrial ornithine transport defect (HHH); *8*, ornithine aminotransferase; *9*, decarboxylase, site of allopurinol block in pyrimidine pathway. *ATP*, adenosine triphosphate; *CoA*, coenzyme A; *UMP*, uridine monophosphate.

■ ORNITHINE-TRANSCARBAMYLASE DEFICIENCY

OTC deficiency probably is the most common of the urea cycle disorders and is inherited as an X-linked trait. Affected males usually have massive hyperammonemia in the neonatal period. Plasma citrulline levels are reduced markedly; plasma glutamine, glycine, and alanine levels are elevated, along with other nonspecific elevations associated with massive hyperammonemia, such as lysine and proline levels. Urinary orotic acid is elevated markedly. Plasma ammonia levels often exceed 1,000 μM. Even with aggressive management, many patients do not survive the neonatal period. The enzymatic deficiency may be confirmed with liver biopsy. Males with 10% to 25% of normal enzymatic activity and a milder clinical course have been reported. Therapy for those males who survive the neonatal period is similar to that for CPS I deficiency and includes a restricted dietary protein intake (0.4 to 0.7 g/kg/d), supplemental essential amino acids and L-citrulline, use of nonprotein caloric and other nutrient supplements, and either combined sodium benzoate and sodium phenylacetate or high-dose phenylbutyrate.

Females who are heterozygous for OTC deficiency have a wide clinical spectrum, ranging from being affected as severely as are hemizygous affected males to being asymptomatic. The degree of relative lyonization (random X chromosome inactivation) in hepatocytes of normal and abnormal OTC genes in the individual female determines the clinical severity of her disease. At least three severely affected females have not survived the neonatal period. More often, affected females have 10% to 20% of normal OTC activity and have the disorder diagnosed initially during childhood with symptoms of intermittent hyperammonemia, such as cyclic vomiting, lethargy, and coma, or with protein intolerance or avoidance. Neurologic problems such as strokes, cerebral atrophy, dementia, or other encephalopathic processes may be seen. Therapy for heterozygous females depends on the degree of severity of their disease.

It is important that female relatives of affected patients be evaluated to determine if they are carriers for OTC deficiency. Approximately two thirds of mothers of affected males will be carriers for the disorder. Carrier detection may allow early identification of females at risk for hyperammonemic episodes and also may be helpful in reproductive planning. Measurement of urinary orotic acid or orotidine while taking allopurinol, which inhibits the pyrimidine pathway beyond orotic acid, will detect most OTC carriers. Urinary orotic acid measurement during protein loading should be avoided because it is less accurate and carries a risk of producing symptomatic hyperammonemia in partially affected females. DNA probes have been established and are available for both carrier detection and prenatal diagnosis. Using this technique, a few predicted affected males have been treated from birth with varying outcomes. Even with aggressive therapy, some have died with hyperammonemia in the neonatal period. At least four male patients, three of whom were treated from birth, and one severely affected female patient have undergone successful liver transplantation resulting in correction of their urea cycle disorder.

■ DISORDERS OF BRANCHED-CHAIN AMINO ACID METABOLISM

Maple syrup urine disease varies greatly in its degree of severity, which is inversely proportional to the residual activity of the enzyme involved (Figure 182–2). In the severest cases, patients will have acute metabolic disease in the early

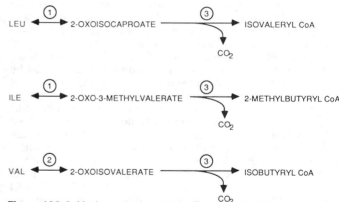

Figure 182-2. Maple syrup urine disease. The amino acids accumulate as well as the oxo acids because of the ready reversibility of the transaminases. Note that here are two transaminases; rare disorders have been associated with each. *1*, leucine-isoleucine transaminase; *2*, valine transaminase; *3*, branched-chain oxo acid dehydrogenase complex, the enzyme deficient in this disorder.

neonatal period, will progress to seizures, and, if untreated, will die within a matter of days to weeks. Severe acidosis, hypoglycemia, and hyperammonemia occur, and these infants may require dialysis. The characteristic odor of maple syrup, although not present uniformly, has led to the diagnosis in a number of these infants. Milder cases may not be detected until later in infancy or even in childhood when there is an intercurrent illness or some other source of metabolic stress that results in decompensation and the findings of dullness, lethargy, and acidosis of varying degrees. Plasma and urine studies will show an increase in both the branched-chain amino acids leucine, isoleucine, and valine, and their corresponding oxo acids (keto acids). The disorder is caused by reduced activity of branched-chain oxo acid dehydrogenase, which may be demonstrated in cultured skin fibroblasts. Management in patients with milder forms of the disease who have appreciable residual enzyme activity may be accomplished with the administration of thiamine in pharmacologic doses and prescription of a low-protein diet. Severely affected patients will require a milk substitute that is free of the branched-chain amino acids, with supplementation of small but appropriate amounts of the individual branched-chain amino acids to achieve a normal or near-normal concentration of all amino acids. At initial diagnosis and in times of catabolism, they may require dialysis or special hyperalimentation mixtures to achieve control of their disorder. The isoleucine concentration is the first to change when its intake is varied, but it is felt that the leucine concentration is related most to symptomatology. If all three of the "noxious" amino acids as well as all the other amino acids are not monitored, there tends to be an amino acid imbalance, which may result in severe nutritional difficulties, which of themselves may be a severe and potentially fatal problem.

Prenatal diagnosis has been accomplished using cultured amniotic fluid cells, but carrier detection is not reliable. The disorder has an incidence of about 1:200,000 and is inherited on an autosomal recessive basis. It is believed that the various degrees of severity in different families are caused by different alleles at the same locus. Newborn screening may be carried out using filter paper specimens to measure the blood leucine concentration.

(Abridged from Rebecca S. Wappner and Ira K. Brandt, Disorders of Amino Acid Metabolism, in Oski, DeAngelis, Feigin, McMillan, Warshaw: *Principles and Practice of Pediatrics, Second Edition*, J.B. Lippincott, 1994.)

Oski's Essential Pediatrics,
edited by Kevin B. Johnson and Frank A. Oski.
Lippincott–Raven Publishers,
Philadelphia © 1997

183

Disorders of Fatty Acid Oxidation

During fasting, mitochondrial beta-oxidation of fatty acids is an important source of energy production. After fatty acids are mobilized from adipose tissue, they are transported bound to albumin to the liver and other tissues, where they are taken across the plasma membrane by fatty acid binding proteins. The fatty acids then are "activated" to their coenzyme A (CoA) esters by cytosolic acyl-CoA synthase, transported across the mitochondrial membrane by a carnitine-mediated system, and oxidized to ketone bodies in the mitochondrial matrix. Thus, the disorders involving mitochondrial beta-oxidation of fatty acids are characterized by faulty formation of ketone bodies, impaired energy production, and the accumulation of partially oxidized fatty acid metabolites during periods of stress and fasting. The disorders have widely varying clinical manifestations. All are thought to be inherited as autosomal recessive traits.

Long-chain (C10 to C18) fatty acids are activated by cytosolic acyl-CoA synthase at the outer aspect of the mitochondrial membrane to form long-chain acyl-CoA esters, which then are transesterified with carnitine by carnitine palmityl transferase (CPT) I to form long-chain acyl-carnitine esters at the inner aspect of the outer mitochondrial membrane. The long-chain acylcarnitines then cross the inner mitochondrial membrane by a process that is mediated by carnitine translocase. At the matrix side of the inner mitochondrial membrane, the long-chain acyl-carnitines are reesterified to long-chain acyl-CoA esters by CPT II. Medium-chain (C6 to C12) and short-chain (C4 and C6) fatty acids do not appear to need carnitine-mediated transport to enter the mitochondrial matrix, where they are activated to form their acyl-CoA esters. The acyl-CoA esters then enter into the betaoxidation pathway, as shown in Figure 183–1. With each cycle through the pathway, the fatty acid-CoA ester is reduced in length by two carbons, and an acetyl-CoA group is generated that can be metabolized further to ketone bodies in the liver and kidneys or can enter the tricarboxylic acid cycle. The beta-oxidation pathway includes a series of chain length–specific acyl-CoA dehydrogenases, enoyl-CoA hydratase, 3-hydroxyacyl-CoA dehydrogenase, and 3-ketoacyl-CoA thiolase. The acyl-CoA dehydrogenases are flavoproteins that transfer the electrons that are generated to electron transfer flavoprotein and subsequently to the mitochondrial respiratory chain. Long-chain acyl-CoA dehydrogenase (LCAD) catalyzes the reaction for fatty acid chain lengths of 12 to 18 carbons, medium-chain acyl-CoA dehydrogenase (MCAD) catalyzes the reaction for fatty acid chain lengths of 4 to 14 carbons, and short-chain acyl-CoA dehydrogenase (SCAD) catalyzes the reaction for fatty acid chain lengths of 4 or 6 carbons. Fatty acid acyl-CoA esters with odd chain lengths are oxidized similarly until the three-carbon propionyl-CoA is formed. Unsaturated fatty acids require two additional enzymes, 3-*cis*, 2-*trans*-enoyl-CoA isomerase and 2,4-dienoyl-CoA reductase, for complete beta-oxidation of these compounds.

The acetyl-CoA and acyl-CoA esters formed as a result of beta-oxidation exit the mitochondrial matrix by carnitine-mediated transport similar to that for the entrance of long-chain acyl-CoA esters. Acetylcarnitine is formed by carnitine acetyltransferase and is transported by a translocase from the mitochondrial matrix to the cytosol.

Carnitine (L-*carnitine)* is involved in the transport of long-chain fatty acid acyl-CoA esters into the mitochondria and the transport of products of beta-oxidation from the mitochondrial matrix. It also functions as a "trap" for by-products of faulty mitochondrial beta-oxidation or other abnormal organic acids by forming carnitine esters with these compounds. Plasma carnitine measurements usually report total, free, and esterified values. In some patients with organic acidemias or disorders of beta-oxidation, the total plasma carnitine level may be normal, but the esterified fraction will be abnormally high, resulting in a relative deficiency of free carnitine, which is needed for appropriate fatty acid utilization. In other patients, the total and free carnitine levels will be low and the esterified carnitine level will be elevated inappropriately.

Dietary sources of carnitine include meats and dairy products. Endogenous carnitine can be synthesized from lysine. Deficiency states usually are associated with organic acidemias or faulty beta-oxidation. Secondary deficiencies also may be seen with renal tubular disorders, vitamin C and pyridoxine deficiencies, strict vegetarian diets, total parenteral nutrition, hemodialysis, and valproate anticonvulsant therapy.

Systemic carnitine deficiency, regardless of the etiology, results in faulty fatty acid oxidation and has been associated with inability to tolerate fasting, hypoketotic hypoglycemia, liver dysfunction, hypotonia, myopathies, and cardiomyopathies. Because our knowledge of carnitine deficiency preceded our understanding of fatty acid oxidation, many of the patients reported to have systemic carnitine deficiency in the past subsequently have been found to have defects in fatty acid oxidation.

MCAD deficiency is the most common of the disorders and is estimated to occur in 1:10,000 births. Most patients are seen between 5 and 24 months of age with repeated episodes of vomiting, lethargy, and hypotonia after a decreased carbohydrate intake associated with an intercurrent illness or fasting. Mild hepatomegaly and seizures may occur. Hypoglycemia and mildly elevated ammonia and liver enzyme levels usually are noted. A mild metabolic acidosis may be present. Urine ketones may be absent or present in trace amounts, which has led to the term *hypoketotic hypoglycemia* for this group of disorders. However, some patients are able to make ketone bodies with stress. The amount of ketones produced, though, as determined by plasma β-hydroxybutyrate levels, is inappropriately low for the degree of hypoglycemia and the marked elevation of plasma-free fatty acids mobilized in response to fasting. The pathophysiologic reason for the hypoglycemia is not understood completely, but is thought to result from failure of the normal gluconeogenic response to fasting, which normally occurs as a response to increased acetyl-CoA and ketone body production.

There is wide variability in clinical presentation. Some patients have had the disorder diagnosed in the newborn period, whereas others are asymptomatic and are detected only by family screening. Some patients have a rapidly deteriorating course with an episode that progresses to coma and death from cardiorespiratory collapse or cerebral edema. The accumulation of acyl-CoA compounds, especially those with chain lengths of three carbons or more, is associated with encephalopathies and may result in cerebral edema. The mortality rate is highest between 15 and 26 months of age, when it is reported to be 59%. About 25% of patients die with their first episode, which frequently is unrecognized as being caused by a disorder of fatty acid oxidation until the disorder is diagnosed in a second child in the family. Many of the

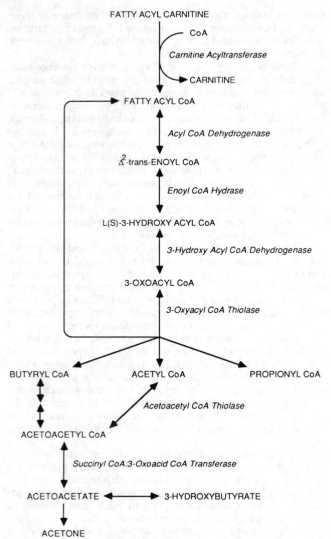

FATTY ACYL CARNITINE

CoA

Carnitine Acyltransferase

CARNITINE

FATTY ACYL CoA

Acyl CoA Dehydrogenase

Δ^2-trans-ENOYL CoA

Enoyl CoA Hydrase

L(S)-3-HYDROXY ACYL CoA

3-Hydroxy Acyl CoA Dehydrogenase

3-OXOACYL CoA

3-Oxyacyl CoA Thiolase

BUTYRYL CoA   ACETYL CoA   PROPIONYL CoA

Acetoacetyl CoA Thiolase

ACETOACETYL CoA

Succinyl CoA:3-Oxoacid CoA Transferase

ACETOACETATE ◀──▶ 3-HYDROXYBUTYRATE

ACETONE

Figure 183-1. Hepatic mitochondrial metabolism of fatty acids. *CPT II*, carnitine palmitoyl transferase II; *ETF*, electron transport flavoprotein; HMG, 3-hydroxymethylglutaryl; *CoA*, coenzyme A; *FAD*, flavin adenine dinucleotide, *FADH₂*, reduced form of FAD.

deaths have been thought to be the result of Reye's syndrome or sudden infant death syndrome. Autopsy findings include fatty infiltration of the liver, which may be macrovesicular or microvesicular in pattern. Mitochondrial changes in the liver on electron microscopy differ from those seen in Reye's syndrome and may show a condensed appearance of the Mit with increased matrix density and intracristal widening, or enlarged and abnormally shaped Mit with an increase in the number of cristae and crystalloids in the matrix.

With episodes, affected individuals accumulate metabolites of medium chain length (C6 to C12), especially octanoic acid and 4-decenoic acid. With the accumulation of fatty acyl-CoA intermediates of medium chain length with the Mit, alternative pathways of microsomal (omega and omega-1) oxidation and peroxisomal beta-oxidation become involved and lead to excessive production of (omega-1)-hydroxy acids and medium-chain dicarboxylic acids such as adipic, suberic, and sebacic acids. These metabolites may be detected in the blood or urine of patients during episodes by organic acid analysis employing gas chromatography-mass spectrometry. Acyl-CoA compounds may be conjugated with glycine as well as carnitine. Abnormal metabolite patterns may be detected by either urinary acyl-glycine profiles (stable isotope dilution gas chromatography-mass spectrometry) or plasma or urine acyl-carnitine profiles (fast atom bombardment with tandem mass spectrometry). These latter two tests are more sophisticated and sensitive than are routine organic acid measurements, and are available in only a limited number of laboratories. They are indicated in the evaluation of all patients suspected of having a defect in fatty acid oxidation, however, because asymptomatic patients may have normal routine organic acid analysis (gas chromatography-mass spectroscopy) between episodes, but frequently will have abnormal profiles by acyl-glycine or acyl-carnitine techniques. Patients usually have abnormal plasma and urinary carnitine levels, with lowered total and elevated esterified fractions. An oral carnitine load, followed by measurement of urinary acyl-carnitines, may assist in the diagnosis of patients who are carnitine depleted. Patients should not be subjected to a provocative fast because of the possibility of inducing a fatal acute episode. The recent availability of acyl-carnitine profiles from blood filter paper dots will allow retrospective diagnosis in children who have died and will make newborn screening for this group of disorders feasible in the future. Deficient activity of MCAD may be shown in cultured skin fibroblasts or leukocytes. The complementary DNA has been cloned, and DNA diagnosis may be done using blood filter paper dots in most patients. Prenatal diagnosis and carrier detection are available.

The basis for treatment is the avoidance of fasting and lipolysis. Frequent meals or feedings, with a high carbohydrate and relatively lowered fat intake is recommended. MCT (medium-chain triglyceride) oil in any form should be avoided. Treatment should be started as soon as the diagnosis is considered, even if test results are not available yet. L-carnitine supplementation is indicated in symptomatic patients. Only the prescription form of L-carnitine should be used and not the D,L form that is available in health food stores. Episodes should be treated promptly with intravenous glucose and hydration, to which most patients respond. Once the disorder is recognized and treated, many patients do well. However, residual neurologic dysfunction from severe episodes will persist.

(Abridged from Rebecca S. Wappner and Ira K. Brandt, Disorders of Mitochondria, in Oski, DeAngelis, Feigin, McMillan, Warshaw: *Principles and Practice of Pediatrics, Second Edition*, J.B. Lippincott, 1994.)

Oski's Essential Pediatrics,
edited by Kevin B. Johnson and Frank A. Oski.
Lippincott–Raven Publishers,
Philadelphia © 1997

184

Defects in Carbohydrate Metabolism

DISORDERS OF GLYCOGEN SYNTHESIS AND DEGRADATION

■ GLYCOGEN STORAGE DISORDERS

The disorders associated with abnormal synthesis and degradation of glycogen vary widely in their clinical spectrum. Table 184–1 lists the disorders according to their currently accepted type and specific enzymatic defect. The disorders may have primarily hepatic or muscle involvement.

Hepatic Glycogen Storage Disorders

The frequency of hepatic glycogen storage disorders is estimated to be 1:60,000 births. The pathogenesis of the various disorders often may by predicted by the site of their associated enzymatic defects. All cause some degree of hepatomegaly and usually hypoglycemia. Functional testing may help to distinguish between the disorders. The presence of fasting hypoglycemia, the response to glucagon in the fasting and fed state, the response of blood glucose to the administration of other carbohydrates such as galactose, and the type of glucose response noted with a glucose tolerance test may be used to help differentiate between the disorders. All fasting and tolerance testing should be done with caution and close observation of the patient. For the severe disorders, the presence of lactic acidosis and hypoglycemia may be considered a relative contraindication to proceeding with fasting, glucagon stimulation, and other tests in the classic fashion. Liver and muscle biopsies may be done to assess the total content of glycogen and the type of glycogen structure present, and to document deficient activity of specific enzymes. Open liver biopsies and muscle biopsies, rather than punch biopsies, are preferred because of the sample size needed for these analyses. Muscle biopsy should be done at the same time as open liver biopsy, regardless of the suspected clinical type of glycogen storage. It is most important that an experienced laboratory be contacted before obtaining the samples to ensure appropriate handling. Because many of the disorders may be documented in leukocytes, erythrocytes, or cultured skin fibroblasts, these less invasive procedures should be done first, if possible.

All the disorders are inherited as autosomal recessive traits except for type IXb, which is inherited as an X-linked trait. Carrier detection and prenatal diagnosis vary depending on the tissue distribution of the enzyme involved in the specific disorder.

Type Ia Glycogen Storage Disease (von Gierke's Disease)

Type Ia glycogen storage disease (GSD), also known as hepatorenal GSD, is associated with deficient activity of glu-

cose-6-phosphatase in liver, kidney, and intestine. Patients have marked hepatomegaly, lactic acidosis, and hypoglycemia, and the disorder often is diagnosed in the neonatal period. Milder forms may be discovered later with hepatomegaly and short stature. Other clinical features include a doll-like appearance, decreased motor mass, renal enlargement, failure of maturation in puberty, vomiting, and diarrhea. Many infants are obese as a result of demanding frequent feedings, including nocturnal feedings beyond the time this behavior usually disappears (Figure 184–1).

Fasting hypoglycemia may be profound and often is without clinical symptoms in the untreated patient. This tolerance of hypoglycemia is thought to be the result of the ability of these patients to use alternative substrates for glucose in the brain. Glucose-6-phosphatase is essential for the normal release of hepatic free-glucose, whether it is the product of glycogenolysis or gluconeogenesis. Dietary carbohydrates other than glucose also cannot be converted to glucose because the conversion involves glucose-6-phosphatase as the final step. The fasting hypoglycemia results in activation of phosphorylase and hepatic glycogenolysis, which leads to the formation of glucose-6-phosphate. The glucose-6-phosphate then is metabolized to lactate by glycolysis. Gluconeogenesis also is stimulated, and there occurs a recycling between lactate and glycogen, which results in a net increase in lactate. Stimulation of the glycolytic and gluconeogenic pathways also results in elevated triglyceride, cholesterol, very–low-density lipoprotein, free fatty acid, and uric acid levels. Xanthomas, lipemia retinalis, gout, and uric acid nephropathy may occur. Within the liver parenchyma, adenomatous nodules may appear, which can develop into hepatic carcinoma. Abnormal bleeding tendencies occur; these are thought to be caused by decreased platelet adhesiveness from the hypoglycemia.

Because patients with GSD I frequently become hypoglycemic after 2 to 3 hours of fasting, any tolerance or stimulation test should be done cautiously and with intravenous glucose at hand. Glucose tolerance testing gives a diabetic-type early response. Insulin levels are low. There is no glycemic response to galactose (1 to 2 g/kg of 20% solution, orally or intravenously). Glucagon stimulation occasionally will produce a response, which is defined as a rise in blood glucose of 50% more than baseline. Lactic acid levels will rise with fasting and with glucagon or galactose administration. Glycogen content is elevated in liver, kidney, and intestine. Glycogen structure is normal. On liver biopsy, the hepatocytes are noted to have glycogen in the nuclei and lipid droplets of varying size in the cytoplasm. There are no signs of cirrhosis. The diagnosis may be confirmed by measurement of glucose-6-phosphatase in liver or intestinal biopsy samples. Prenatal diagnosis and carrier detection are not readily available.

Treatment is directed at supplying continuous exogenous glucose. Infants are given a formula with glucose or glucose polymers as the only carbohydrate source. Older children are given similar enteral supplements and are restricted in their intake of natural sources of galactose and fructose. Frequent daily feedings, every 2 to 3 hours, are supplemented with nocturnal nasogastric or gastrostomy drip feeding. Uncooked cornstarch slurries may be used with older children. There is remarkable clinical and laboratory improvement with dietary therapy. Tolerance of hypoglycemia may be present no longer, however, and clinical symptoms of hypoglycemia may occur. The patients continue to be at risk for significant acidosis and hypoglycemia with intercurrent illnesses or if enteral feedings are interrupted.

TABLE 184-1. Classification of Glycogen Storage Disorders

Type	Enzyme Affected	Major Tissue Involved	Clinical Features
0	Glycogen synthetase	Liver	Hypoglycemia, ketosis, no hepatomegaly
Ia	Glucose-6-phosphatase	Liver, kidney, intestine	Hypoglycemia, lacticacidosis, hepatomegaly
Ib	Transport defect of glucose-6-phosphate	As in Ia, plus neutrophils	As in Ia, plus Crohn's disease
Ic	Transport defect of inorganic phosphate	As in Ia	As in Ia, juvenile diabetes
II	Lysosomal α-glucosidase	Muscle, generalized	Lysosomal storage disease
III	Debrancher	Liver, muscle	Milder Ia, cirrhosis, ketosis, ± muscle
IV	Brancher	Liver, muscle	Hepatomegaly, cirrhosis, ± muscle
V	Muscle phosphorylase	Muscle	Weakness, cramps, myoglobinuria
VI	Hepatic phosphorylase	Liver	Hepatomegaly
VII	Muscle phosphofructokinase	Muscle	Weakness, cramps, myoglobinuria
VIII	Loss of activation of phosphorylase	Liver, brain	Hepatomegaly, progressive CNS dysfunction
IX	Phosphorylase kinase	Liver, ± muscle	Hepatomegaly, ketosis
X	cAMP-dependent kinase	Liver, muscle	Hepatomegaly, ± mild muscle
XI	Unknown	Liver, kidney	Hepatomegaly, renal tubular dysfunction

■ DISORDERS OF GALACTOSE METABOLISM

Galactose-1-Phosphate Uridyl Transferase Deficiency (Classic Galactosemia)

Galactose-1-phosphate uridyl transferase deficiency is the most common group of the disorders of galactose metabolism and is inherited as an autosomal recessive trait. In its classic form, it occurs in about 1:62,000 births. Affected infants appear normal at birth. Shortly after the ingestion of dietary galactose, symptoms appear, which usually are evident by 1 week of age. Failure to thrive, vomiting, diarrhea, and lethargy are noted. There may be prolonged physiologic jaundice or the appearance of hepatotoxic jaundice after 1 week of age with increased direct bilirubin. Exchange transfusion and phototherapy may be indicated. Hepatomegaly and abnormal liver function tests are common. Extrahepatic biliary atresia may have been considered. Nuclear cataracts appear within days or weeks and may become irreversible. Often, the cataracts are evident only on slit-lamp examination. Renal tubular dysfunction with generalized aminoaciduria, proteinuria, and galactosuria develops. Marasmus and increasing central nervous system (CNS) involvement develop. The symptoms are rapidly progressive, and most untreated infants do not survive past 6 weeks of age. Deaths are due most commonly to liver failure and septicemia, especially with *Escherichia coli*. The cataracts are thought to be the result of lenticular accumulation of galactitol, as with the kinase deficiency. Galactose-1-phosphate levels are elevated markedly in the tissues and are thought to be responsible for the hepatic, renal, and CNS manifestations of the disorder.

The presence of non-glucose reducing substances in the urine may be demonstrated, as in galactokinase deficiency. Care should be taken because false-negative results may be obtained in those infants with poor intake, vomiting, or marasmus, or in those receiving a galactose-free diet. Galactose tolerance testing is dangerous and should be avoided. The disorder may be confirmed by demonstrating deficient activity of galactose-1-phosphate uridyl transferase in erythrocytes. If the child has received a transfusion or an exchange transfusion, a falsely elevated level of erythrocyte enzymatic activity may be obtained. The disorder also may be detected by newborn screening programs that test for elevated blood galactose (Paigen test) or galactose-1-phosphate

(Paigen test) or screen for the transferase by spot enzyme assay (Beutler test). All screening tests should be confirmed with quantitative enzymatic testing and electrophoresis, which can be done with erythrocytes or cultured skin fibroblasts. Because of the seriousness of the disorder, however, it is recommended that patients who are presumed to be affected based on newborn screening or on clinical grounds be changed promptly to a galactose-free diet while awaiting the results of confirmatory testing. Carrier testing and prenatal diagnosis are available.

Treatment includes strict dietary restriction of all galactose and lactose sources, as for galactokinase deficiency. There is gradual and dramatic improvement when the child is placed on the diet. Markedly elevated galactose-1-phosphate intracellular levels decrease slowly, but may remain elevated for 10 to 15 days. Some persistent mild elevation of erythrocyte galactose-1-phosphate may be seen in well-controlled patients, which is thought to occur as a result of in vivo formation from uridine diphosphate galactose (UDP-galactose). The hepatic and renal manifestations improve slowly and may be reversed entirely. There is significant improvement in the cataracts, but residua may remain, which usually do not interfere with vision. About 50% of patients who are treated early may have later psychomotor difficulties and specific learning disabilities, especially in expressive language, mathematics, and spatial relationships. Behavioral problems with attention deficits and other psychological problems may occur. Females may have hypergonadotropic hypogonadism with ovarian atrophy, which can occur prenatally or at any later time. Males have normal gonadal function. Because there is no improvement in galactose tolerance with age, the dietary restriction must continue indefinitely. Intermittent erythrocyte galactose-1-phosphate determinations may help to guide clinical management. Failure to comply with dietary restriction also will lead to poor physical growth.

Milder forms of classic galactosemia may present with a less severe clinical picture without failure to thrive and may not be detected until the patient is more than 4 months of age. Some children may present even later in childhood with a history of intermittent milk aversion or partial treatment. The findings of cataracts, hepatic involvement, and psychomotor difficulties should raise the possibility of this diagnosis.

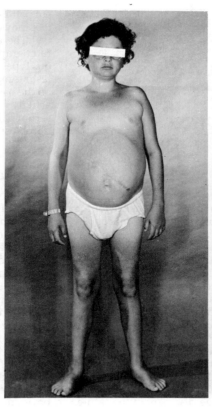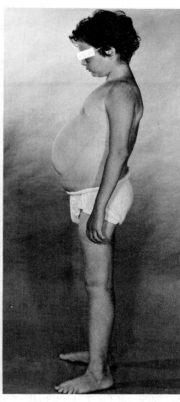

Figure 184-1. Glycogen storage disease IA, age 13 years.

■ DISORDERS OF FRUCTOSE METABOLISM

Fructose-1-Phosphate Aldolase B Deficiency (Hereditary Fructose Intolerance)

The autosomal recessive disorder fructose-1-phosphate aldolase B deficiency is associated with reduced activity of aldolase B in the liver, renal cortex, and small intestine. There is considerable heterogeneity in residual activity among affected patients, who usually have less than 15% of normal hepatic aldolase B activity. The true incidence of the disorder is unknown; it is estimated to occur in 1:20,000 individuals in Switzerland and also is seen in North America and Europe.

The symptoms of this disorder, which occur only after the ingestion of dietary fructose, are related to acute hypoglycemia and chronic hepatic and renal dysfunction. In young infants, the symptoms usually do not start until weaning or the introduction of fruits, vegetables, and juices. Symptoms may occur before this time if the infant is taking a formula with fructose or sucrose as the carbohydrate source. The symptoms of an acute ingestion, which are more severe in young infants than in older children and adults, are associated with hypoglycemia and include sweating, trembling, emesis, lethargy, coma, seizures, and even shock and death. With acute fructose ingestion, there is depletion of intracellular Pi and adenosine triphosphate (ATP), and secondary inhibition of gluconeogenesis and glycolysis. More chronic symptoms include poor feeding, failure to thrive, vomiting, diarrhea, irritability, tremors, hepatomegaly, hepatic dysfunction leading to cirrhosis and hepatic failure, and proximal renal tubular dysfunction of the Fanconi type. The accumulation of fructose-1-phosphate in the liver, kidney, and small intestine is thought to be responsible for these manifestations. The pattern of these chronic symptoms with intermittent acute episodes, associated with the ingestion of fructose-containing foods, point to the disorder clinically. Older children and adults will have a nutritional his-

tory of avoidance of fructose and may be referred for bizarre eating patterns.

Laboratory findings associated with acute episodes will include hypoglycemia, hypophosphatemia, hypermagnesemia, hyperuricemia, hyperkalemia, lactic acidosis, and fructosemia and fructosuria. The presence of a non-glucose reducing substance in the urine should be confirmed as fructose by sugar chromatography. Fructosuria will not be present in those patients with intake of foods or fluids with other carbohydrate sources and may not be seen in patients with poor intake or those without recent exposure to fructose. Laboratory findings from chronic exposure are those associated with hepatic dysfunction and proximal renal tubular dysfunction. Liver biopsy samples reveal diffuse steatosis, scattered hepatic necrosis, periportal and intralobular fibrosis, and cirrhosis in later stages. Renal biopsy reveals granulation and vacuolization of epithelial cells with dilated proximal tubules. Small-intestinal biopsy samples may exhibit submucosal or serosal hemorrhages.

Treatment with avoidance of all dietary sources of fructose, including foods and medications, should be instituted once the disorder is suspected. There is prompt cessation of symptoms with intravenous glucose in acute episodes. Once a fructose-restricted diet is started, clinical improvement usually is evident within days. Small children may have persistent hepatomegaly, and some in the later stages of liver failure may die. After several weeks of treatment, an intravenous fructose tolerance test may be done with caution. An oral fructose tolerance test may lead to a severe acute episode and should be avoided. The disorder also can be documented by enzymatic assay of aldolase B in biopsy samples from the liver or small intestine. Because aldolase B is not expressed in cultured skin fibroblasts or amniocytes, carrier and prenatal testing are not available.

(Abridged from Rebecca S. Wappner and Ira K. Brandt, Defects in Carbohydrate Metabolism, in Oski, DeAngelis, Feigin, McMillan, Warshaw: *Principles and Practice of Pediatrics, Second Edition,* J.B. Lippincott, 1994.)

Oski's Essential Pediatrics,
edited by Kevin B. Johnson and Frank A. Oski.
Lippincott–Raven Publishers,
Philadelphia © 1997

185

Lysosomal Storage Disorders

Lysosomes are cytoplasmic, single membrane–bound organelles that contain hydrolytic enzymes responsible for the degradation of a variety of compounds, including mucopolysaccharides (MPS), sphingolipids, and glycoproteins.

The pattern of clinical findings seen with the various disorders is related to the type of compound stored and its natural distribution in the body. The disorders usually are classified according to the type of compound stored. All the disorders are inherited as either autosomal recessive or X-linked traits. Carrier testing and prenatal diagnosis are available for most of the disorders, but only in a limited number of experienced laboratories. Exact enzymatic diagnosis is essential for accurate carrier and prenatal studies.

Current therapy consists of symptomatic and supportive therapy for the patient and family. Enzyme replacement therapy is available only for type I Gaucher's disease, but it may be available for other lysosomal storage disorders in the future. Bone marrow transplantation with tissue-typed identical siblings may be considered, especially for those disorders that do not have central nervous system (CNS) involvement and for the mucopolysaccharidoses. Animal models are available that can be used for the investigation of new therapies. For many of the disorders, the associated genes have been mapped and cloned. Heterogeneity has been noted in the molecular basis for many of the disorders and, at times, has been correlated with varying clinical presentations.

■ MUCOPOLYSACCHARIDOSES

The mucopolysaccharidoses are associated with lysosomal accumulation of partially degraded acid MPS. MPS, also termed *glycosaminoglycans,* are large molecules composed of repeating sulfated hexuronate or hexosamine disaccharide units attached to a protein core. Radiographs may show a distinct pattern that is termed *dysostosis multiplex.* The skull is enlarged and elongated (dolichocephaly), and the calvarium is thickened. The sella may be J-, wooden-shoe-, or boot-shaped (Figure 185–1). The vertebral bodies in the lower thoracic and upper lumbar areas have a "beaking" of the anterior inferior surface caused by hypoplasia of their anterosuperior areas (Figure 185–2). A dorsal kyphosis, or gibbus deformity, develops. The ribs are thickened, except where they join the spine, and they have an oar-shaped appearance (Figure 185–3). The metacarpals have a proximal narrowing with distal widening, giving them a "baby-bottle" appearance. The distal humerus and ulna may show an abnormal angulation called a *Madelung's deformity* (Figure 185–4). The pelvis may have flaring of the iliac bones, shallow acetabular areas, and progressive coxa valga. The long bones become shortened, thickened, and may have signs of expansion of the medullary cavity. Hypoplasia of the odontoid process may occur. Radiographs in Morquio syndrome, which is associated with keratan sulfate and chondroitin-6-sulfate storage, show a differ-

ent pattern, with platyspondyly, which resembles the spondyloepiphyseal dysplasias (Figure 185–5).

The age of onset, severity, and pattern of clinical and radiographic findings help to distinguish between the various types of mucopolysaccharidoses. Although urinary MPS testing may be helpful in some cases, the diagnosis is made on the basis of enzymatic testing. Demonstration of deficient activity of a specific lysosomal hydrolase may be done with serum or leukocytes for most of the disorders. Cultured skin fibroblasts may be required for others.

Hurler's Syndrome (MPS I-H)

Hurler's syndrome is associated with deficient activity of α-L-iduronidase and excessive storage of heparan and dermatan sulfates. It is inherited as an autosomal recessive trait and occurs in about 1:100,000 births. Hurler's syndrome is considered to be the most severe of the mucopolysaccharidoses and is the prototype for the group.

Children with this disorder appear normal at birth. Between 6 and 12 months of age, they have the onset of gradual coarsening and prominence of the facial features, with flattening of the midfacial areas and widening of the nasal bridge. Clouding of the corneas is present. Gingival hyperplasia and thickening of the alveolar ridge develop. Dental eruption is delayed. Deafness may occur and often is helped transiently by amplification. Respiratory involvement results from thickening of the soft tissues in the nasal and pharyngeal areas. Initially, the child may have persistent rhinorrhea or noisy breathing. Gradual upper airway obstruction may result in sleep apnea and cor pulmonale. Cardiac involvement usually develops between 2 and 5 years of age, and may result in thickened valve leaflets, pseudo-atheromatosis of the coronary arteries, cardiomyopathy, and congestive heart failure. Hepatosplenomegaly develops during the first year. There usually are no associated physiologic problems except for occasional hypersplenism with thrombocytopenia or pancytopenia. Umbilical and inguinal hernias often require surgical correction (Figures 185–6 and 185–7).

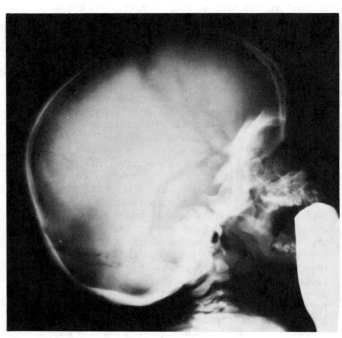

Figure 185-1. Lateral skull radiogram in Hurler's syndrome.

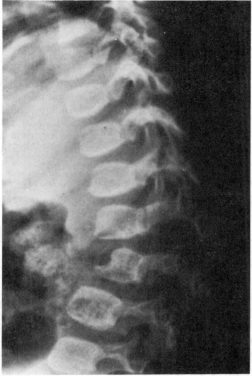

Figure 185-2. Lateral spine radiogram in Hurler's syndrome.

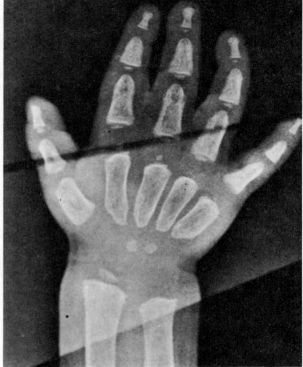

Figure 185-4. AP hand and wrist radiogram in Hurler's syndrome.

Bone growth is delayed, and there usually is minimal linear growth after 2 to 3 years of age. The gibbus deformity, a dorsolumbar kyphosis, develops during the first year and may progress. The head becomes enlarged and dolichocephalic, with prominence of the frontal areas and suture lines. Radiographs show a progression of the dysostosis multiplex as described previously.

Overproduction of collagen and elastin may accompany the MPS storage and result in joint stiffness, carpal tunnel syndrome, thickening of the meninges with hydrocephalus, and decreased compliance of the thoracic cage.

Psychomotor development appears normal for the first year, remains on a plateau for 1 to 2 years, then regresses

gradually. Physical limitations are noted as a result of the joint stiffness and bone involvement. Contractures in the lower extremities lead to a "jockey stance," and the hands become stiff and clawlike in appearance with limited manual dexterity. Physical therapy may be prescribed, with the restriction that flexion and extension of the neck should not be done because of possible hypoplasia of the odontoid process. Adaptive equipment may be of benefit. Most children eventually become wheelchair-bound and do not live past their early teenage years. Death may occur earlier from cardiopulmonary involvement.

Hurler's syndrome may be confirmed by demonstrating deficient activity of α-L-iduronidase in leukocytes or cultured skin fibroblasts. Carrier detection is available, but there is considerable overlap between carriers and noncarriers. Prenatal diagnosis is available with both chorionic villi sampling and cultured amniotic fluid cells.

Hunter's Syndrome (MPS II)

Hunter's syndrome is associated with deficient activity of iduronosulfate sulfatase and storage of heparan and dermatan sulfate. It is inherited as an X-linked trait. There are both severe (type A) and mild (type B) forms. The clinical features of the severe form are very similar to those of Hurler's syndrome except that the onset is between 1 and 2 years of age, the course of the disease is somewhat slower, and there is no corneal clouding (Figure 185–8). Deafness is common. Skin lesions, consisting of ivory raised papules, often are noted on the upper back and on the lateral upper arms and thighs. Patients commonly survive until the second or third decades. The milder type of this disorder is usually associated with normal intelligence and survival into the sixth or seventh decade of life. Deficient activity of iduronosulfate sulfatase

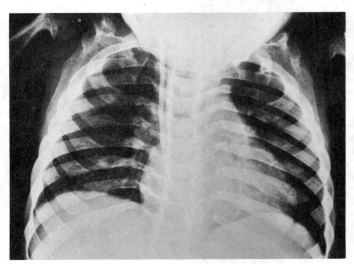

Figure 185-3. AP chest radiogram in Hurler's syndrome.

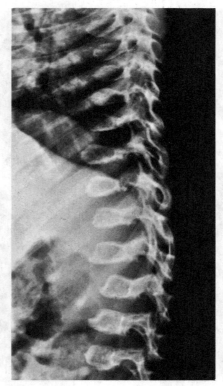

Figure 185-5. Lateral spine radiogram in Morquio syndrome.

may be noted in serum, leukocytes, and cultured skin fibroblasts. Carrier detection is difficult because of lyonization in the female; there is considerable overlap between carriers and noncarriers. Prenatal diagnosis is available using chorionic villi sampling and cultured amniotic fluid cells.

■ THE SPHINGOLIPIDOSES

The sphingolipidoses are associated with lysosomal accumulation of glycosphingolipids, gangliosides, and sphingomyelin. Faulty degradation of the molecules results from deficient activity of lysosomal acid hydrolases as a result of gene mutations at the enzyme loci or a missing sphingolipid activator protein needed for enzyme–lipid stabilization and interaction.

Tay-Sachs Disease, GM₂ Gangliosidosis, Type I

Tay-Sachs disease is associated with the storage of GM_2 ganglioside in the nervous system. Affected children usually are normal at birth. Between 6 and 12 months of age, hypotonia and psychomotor retardation are noted. Children may display an exaggerated startle response to stimuli that is termed *hyperacusis*. After 1 year of age, there is a steady progression of CNS degeneration with spasticity and blindness. Seizures and macrocephaly occur. Cherry-red spots in the macular area may be seen as early as 3 months of age and represent a normal red macular area surrounded by a white area of storage. Later in the disorder, the spots appear darker, with brown coloration, as macular degeneration advances. Most children require nasogastric or gastrostomy feedings and have problems with oral secretions after 18 to 24 months of age. Intercurrent respiratory problems are frequent. Most die between 3 and 4 years of age. The diagnosis can be confirmed by measurement of hexosaminidase A in serum, plasma, leukocytes, or cultured skin fibroblasts. There is severe deficiency of hexosaminidase A, which may be expressed in specific activity units or as a percentage of the total enzyme. Because hexosaminidase B is not affected

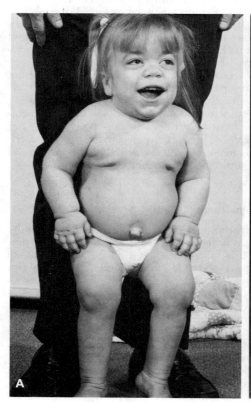
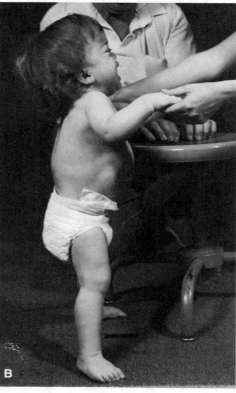

Figure 185-6. Children with Hurler's syndrome. **(A)** Age 37 months; **(B)** age 27 months. Note the dolichomacrocephaly and dorsal kyphosis.

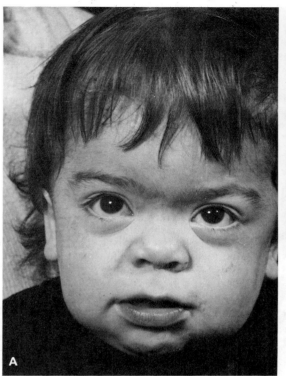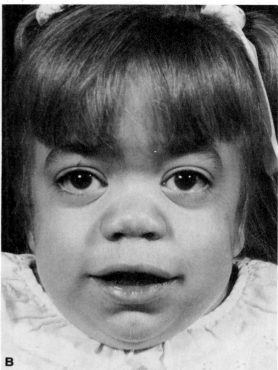

Figure 185-7. Face in Hurler's syndrome. (**A**) Age 27 months; (**B**) age 37 months.

and may be increased, the total amount of β-hexosaminidase is normal.

The disorder is most common in individuals of Eastern European Jewish ancestry, among whom the carrier rate is 1:27. Since the 1970s, community education and carrier testing have allowed more than one half million individuals to be tested. At-risk couples, in which both individuals are carriers for Tay-Sachs disease, have been identified before the birth of an affected child. It is recommended that all couples of Eastern European Jewish ancestry have carrier testing performed before conception. Because the carrier rate among individuals of other backgrounds is about 1:200, the possibility of Tay-Sachs disease cannot be excluded in non-Jewish families. Prenatal diagnosis is available using chorionic villi sampling or amniocentesis.

Gaucher's Disease (Glucocerebrosidosis)

Gaucher's disease is an autosomal recessive disorder associated with deficient activity of β-glucocerebrosidase (β-glucosidase) and storage of sphingolipid with terminal glucosyl residues in β linkage, glucocerebroside (glucosylceramide), in the reticuloendothelial system.

Type 1, the adult, chronic, non-neuronopathic form, may have the onset of symptoms at any age. This is the most common of the sphingolipid storage disorders and is found most often among individuals of Eastern European Jewish ancestry. The initial symptoms usually are splenomegaly with pancytopenia from hypersplenism. Hepatomegaly is common, with mildly elevated liver function test results, but usually no significant dysfunction. Infiltration of the bone marrow also interferes with bone growth and mineralization, and may lead to a leukoerythroblastic anemia. Radiographs show an expanded cortex of the distal femur termed an *Erlenmeyer-flask*

deformity; bone erosion with cystlike changes of varying sizes may occur. Patients also may have avascular crises, pseudo-osteomyelitis, and avascular necrosis of the femoral heads. Pulmonary storage may lead to abnormal pulmonary function test results and cor pulmonale. Older patients may have a yellow or brown discoloration of the exposed skin or pingueculae on the conjunctiva. Although CNS disease is not common, oculomotor apraxia may occur. The disorder is very slowly progressive, and many patients who are seen initially in childhood live well into adult life.

Bone marrow and other tissues from the reticuloendothelial system have large, lipid-laden, fusiform histiocytes with dense eccentric nuclei and are said to resemble "wrinkled tissue paper" or "crumpled silk" (Gaucher's cells). Serum acid phosphatase levels may be elevated.

Although it is extremely expensive, enzyme replacement therapy should be considered for any symptomatic patient with type 1 disease. Bone marrow transplantation also has resulted in clinical improvement, but it is associated with considerable risks when compared to enzyme replacement therapy.

Before enzyme replacement therapy was available, many patients required splenectomy for persistent thrombocytopenia and bleeding diatheses. Postsplenectomy management should include prophylactic antibiotics and immunization, as for other asplenic individuals. Orthopedic problems are often difficult to treat and should be referred to specialists who are experienced with these patients. Two other types of Gaucher's disease deserve mention.

Type 2, the acute neuronopathic or infantile form of Gaucher's disease, has its onset between birth and 18 months of age. Hepatosplenomegaly is accompanied by rapidly progressing CNS deterioration. Trismus, strabismus, and retroflexion of the head are pathognomonic. Spasticity, hyperreflexia, and seizures occur. Feeding and respiratory prob-

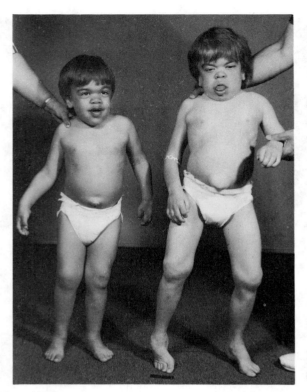

Figure 185-8. Brothers, ages 5 and 15 years, with Hunter's syndrome.

lems are common. Death usually occurs by 2 years of age. Treatment is symptomatic and supportive.

Type 3, the subacute neuronopathic or juvenile form of Gaucher's disease, has features of both types 1 and 2. Behavioral changes, oculomotor apraxia, extrapyramidal and cerebellar signs, seizures, and developmental regression are common. Many patients live into early adulthood.

The diagnosis of all three types of Gaucher's disease is established by the demonstration of deficient activity of β-glucosidase in leukocytes or cultured skin fibroblasts in experienced laboratories. Carrier detection and prenatal diagnosis are available. Molecular genetic studies may help to differentiate between type 1 and type 3 disease in young patients.

(Abridged from Rebecca S. Wappner and Ira K. Brandt, Lysosomal Storage Disorders, in Oski, DeAngelis, Feigin, McMillan, Warshaw: *Principles and Practice of Pediatrics, Second Edition,* J.B. Lippincott, 1994.)

Oski's Essential Pediatrics,
edited by Kevin B. Johnson and Frank A. Oski.
Lippincott–Raven Publishers,
Philadelphia © 1997

186

Disorders of Metal Metabolism

Inorganic metallic cations require carrier-mediated transport mechanisms to cross cell membranes during intestinal absorption and for uptake into tissues. They also require transport proteins to carry them to their sites of tissue utiliza-

tion or storage. The metals have associated intracellular ligands, such as metallothioneins, that function as a means for storage of the metals, prevent the tissue injury that may result from toxicity of the ions in the free state, and appear to be involved with regulation of the intracellular metabolism of the metals. Inherited defects may occur in any of these mechanisms associated with the absorption, transport, cellular uptake, storage, function, and excretion of cationic metals.

■ DISORDERS OF IRON METABOLISM

The body of the normal, healthy adult contains 3 to 5 g of iron. About two thirds of this is found in hemoglobin and myoglobin, and 25% to 30% is stored as ferritin and hemosiderin. The remainder exists in transferrin, heme, and flavin enzymes, and in other iron-containing compounds. Dietary iron is absorbed in the duodenum and upper jejunum. Iron is stored in the body in the liver, spleen, skeletal muscle, and bone marrow in the form of ferritin and hemosiderin.

Familial (Idiopathic) Hemochromatosis

Familial (idiopathic) hemochromatosis is a fairly common disorder associated with excessive intestinal uptake and transfer of iron, and progressive storage of hemosiderin in parenchymal cells throughout the body. The exact biochemical defect and pathogenesis are unknown. The intestinal absorption and transfer of iron across the intestinal mucosal cells is disproportionately high for the degree of iron storage in the body. There is a low iron concentration in the intestinal mucosal cells and reticuloendothelial cells, suggesting that a defect in the regulation of iron uptake and transfer may be involved. Because the gene for hemochromatosis is located on chromosome 6 near the human leukocyte antigen region, and because the genes for transferrin and ferritin are located on other chromosomes, it is unlikely that genetic mutations at the transferrin or ferritin locus are directly responsible for this disorder. The major site of hemosiderin deposition is in the parenchymal cells of the liver, pancreas, heart, gonads, skin, and joints. There is minimal storage in the reticuloendothelial system, which is the major site for hemosiderin deposition in other nongenetic forms of hemosiderosis. The mechanism by which tissue damage occurs is unknown but may be related to increased lysosomal fragility or free radical production in response to elevated levels of hemosiderin.

The disorder is inherited as an autosomal recessive trait and has an incidence of about 1:250 persons. There is great variability in clinical manifestations among affected individuals. Most often, the patient is a male more than 40 years of age. Because of the slow progression of iron storage, the disorder usually is not seen in childhood and is infrequent in women before menopause as a result of the protective effect of body iron loss through menses and with pregnancy.

The clinical manifestations are related to the slowly progressive storage of hemosiderin in parenchymal cells. The classic triad of hepatic cirrhosis, bronze hyperpigmentation of the skin, and diabetes mellitus is characteristic for the later stages of the disorder. In addition, patients may have abdominal pain, hypogonadism, other endocrine abnormalities, myocardial disease, osteoporosis, and arthropathies. Untreated, the majority die within 10 years of their diagnosis from hepatoma, other malignancies, or hepatic or cardiac failure. The reason for the increased risk of malignancies, especially hepatoma and cholangioma, is unknown.

Treatment by repeated phlebotomy is effective in reducing iron stores. It is done weekly initially, for up to 2 years, and must be continued throughout life at periodic intervals. Phlebotomy is more effective than chelators in removing parenchymal hemosiderin storage. With treatment, there is improvement in all clinical signs except advanced cirrhosis with portal hypertension, hypogonadism, arthropathy, and diabetes. The cardiomyopathy usually regresses, and hyperpigmentation disappears.

The diagnosis is established by finding elevated serum iron concentrations, an elevated percentage saturation of transferrin (more than 62%), and elevated serum ferritin levels. Urinary excretion of iron after deferoxamine will be elevated. Liver biopsy samples will reveal hemosiderin deposition and an elevated iron concentration. Heterozygotes may have abnormal serum and urine testing and elevated liver iron stores, but usually not to the extent seen in affected homozygotes. The majority of heterozygotes are unaffected clinically; long-term studies are being conducted to determine if they should take any special precautions with dietary sources of iron, however.

Because relatives, especially siblings, of affected individuals also may be affected, but preclinical in manifestation, it is important to screen them so treatment may be started before the development of the irreversible features of the disorder. Human leukocyte antigen (HLA) typing may be helpful, in addition to the usual blood and urine testing described previously.

Secondary hemosiderosis may result from other causes of cirrhosis, increased dietary iron intake, hemolytic anemias, multiple transfusions, and porphyria cutanea tarda. In these forms, the hemosiderin storage usually is in the reticuloendothelial system and less is seen in the parenchymal cells.

■ DISORDERS OF COPPER METABOLISM

Copper is an essential trace mineral that is a component of many biologically important enzymes, such as cytochrome oxidase, superoxide dismutase, tyrosinase, dopamine hydroxylase, lysyl oxidase, and ceruloplasmin. Nutritional copper deficiency is associated with clinical features related to decreased function of the referenced enzymes. Dietary copper is absorbed in the small intestine and is transported to the liver bound to albumin and, to a lesser extent, to free amino acids. There are at least three hepatic pools of copper. One copper pool, bound to a high–molecular-weight ceruloplasminlike protein, is destined for homeostatic excretion in bile. A second copper pool exists as the ferroxidase ceruloplasmin. About 90% to 95% of serum copper also is in the form of ceruloplasmin. In the third hepatic pool, copper appears to be stored in association with metallothionein, a low–molecular-weight protein that is involved principally with zinc metabolism and is important in binding excess metal ions in cells throughout the body. This store of copper is bound to heavy lysosomes. Free copper ions are very reactive and toxic, and there probably exist yet-undescribed transport molecules that deliver copper to tissues where it is needed for incorporation into the copper enzymes.

Wilson's Disease

Wilson's disease (hepatolenticular degeneration) is an autosomal recessive disorder associated with progressive intracellular accumulation of copper in the liver and subsequently throughout the body. The basic defect is yet to be characterized, but it appears to occur in the liver and is associated with defective incorporation of copper into apoceruloplasmin and with defective biliary secretion of copper.

Similarity of the hepatic copper deposition to that seen in normal neonates has suggested that the defect may be caused by an altered controller gene, which fails to switch the metabolism of copper from that of the fetus to that of the postnatal period. Indeed, studies in patients with Wilson's disease have shown a reduction in transcription of the ceruloplasmin gene and also deficiency of a high–molecular-weight ceruloplasminlike protein, which is responsible for the biliary excretion and decreased intestinal reabsorption of copper in normal individuals.

The major clinical manifestations of Wilson's disease involve the liver and central nervous system. Hepatic dysfunction may occur at any age but often is the presenting manifestation in children. The onset may occur as early as 4 years of age but usually is between 8 and 16 years of age. A slow hepatic accumulation of copper begins at birth. Symptoms often are insidious, but they also may occur as acute hepatic and renal failure with hemolysis caused by toxicity from acute hepatic free copper release. These episodes often are difficult to treat, even with plasmapheresis and peritoneal dialysis, and many patients have frank hepatic failure and die. The disorder may be indistinguishable clinically from chronic active hepatitis. Wilson's disease should be considered in any patient who has recurrent episodes of jaundice and hemolysis, and in any child who has cirrhosis after 8 years of age.

Copper storage also is prominent in the brain and results in the gradual onset of dysarthria, dystonia, choreoathetosis, tremors, ataxia, peripheral neuropathy, and seizures. Late in the disorder, intellectual deterioration develops, and pseudobulbar palsies may lead to death. Patients also may have behavioral and psychiatric problems. The neurologic manifestations of Wilson's disease are rare before 14 years of age and are seen most frequently between 20 and 40 years of age. Patients may have degeneration of basal ganglia, cortical atrophy, and ventricular dilatation on computed tomographic (CT) scanning. All patients, regardless of whether they experience neurologic symptoms, have elevated hepatic copper stores. The hepatic copper may result in storage in other tissues throughout the body, and anemia, neutropenia, thrombocytopenia, osteoarthropathy, renal calculi, renal tubular acidosis, pancreatic disease, cardiomyopathy, and hypoparathyroidism may develop. Storage of copper in the cornea may result in the pathognomonic Kayser-Fleischer rings, which are brownish green, granular copper deposits in Descemet's membrane extending a few millimeters centrally from the corneal limbus. Many may be seen directly, but others require slit-lamp examination. "Sunflower" cataracts also may develop. Patients with neurologic involvement often have Kayser-Fleischer rings; patients with hepatic involvement frequently do not.

The disorder usually is associated with reduced total serum copper levels, reduced ceruloplasmin concentrations, elevated nonceruloplasmin copper levels, and elevated urinary copper excretion, which may be augmented by the administration of D-penicillamine. Ninety-five percent of adult patients and 80% to 85% of affected children may be detected by these tests. Elevation of liver copper levels may be detected with liver biopsy and may be needed to establish the diagnosis. Care should be taken in handling samples because copper contamination may occur if proper containers and technique are not used. Elevated liver copper levels also may occur with other disorders that are associated with hepatic dysfunction and decreased biliary function. Reduced in vitro incorporation of radiolabeled copper into ceruloplasmin is perhaps the most sensitive and accurate testing method available. Partial reduction of incorporation of radiolabeled copper may be noted in heterozygotes and in patients with other liver disorders. About 10% to 20% of heterozygotes will have lowered ceruloplasmin levels; a few also will have reduced total serum copper concentrations and elevated copper excretion with D-penicillamine, electroencephalographic abnormalities, and neurologic manifestations. All siblings of patients should be evaluated thoroughly because they may be affected, but asymptomatic.

Treatment includes the use of D-penicillamine to promote urinary copper excretion and decreased body copper stores. Dosages are determined by monitoring 24-hour urinary copper excretion levels. Pyridoxine supplementation should be given with D-penicillamine due to the known interference with pyridoxal phosphate-dependent enzymes during chelation therapy. Zinc deficiency may result, and zinc also should be given to induce the formation of metallothionein, a metal-binding protein, which may help sequester copper in the gut and prevent copper reabsorption. Trientine hydrochloride also may be used for chelation if significant side effects or toxicity from D-penicillamine occur. Clinical improvement in the neurologic symptoms may be seen in several weeks, but they may take up to 2 years to resolve completely. Hepatic dysfunction also may improve, but more slowly, and cirrhosis and portal hypertension persist. Even with aggressive management, late-stage hepatic dysfunction may continue to progress, and liver transplantation should be considered. Prenatal diagnosis is not possible.

■ DISORDERS OF ZINC METABOLISM

Acrodermatitis Enteropathica

Acrodermatitis enteropathica is a rare, autosomal recessive disorder associated with severe systemic zinc deficiency caused by impaired intestinal absorption. The basic metabolic defect is unknown, but it may be related to a zinc binding factor or ligand such as metallothionein, which facilitates zinc uptake or transport in intestinal mucosa. Numerous zinc-dependent enzymes function in many important biologic pathways, including those involved with nucleic acid and protein synthesis, regulation of cell division, antioxidant activity, stabilization of macromolecules and polymers, and association of hormones with receptors on cell surfaces or in the nuclei. Zinc also appears to be necessary for wound healing and intact chemotaxis in response to infections.

Most affected infants have acrodermatitis, failure to thrive, irritability, anorexia, and diarrhea before 1 year of age. Because breast milk has more bioavailable zinc than do infant formulas, children who are breast-fed are detected later than are those who are fed formula. The clinical manifestations in breast-fed infants often appear after weaning. The earliest sign usually is maceration and fissures at the angles of the mouth. This is associated with a vesicobullous and eczematoid dermatitis, which extends from the mouth to symmetric, well-demarcated lesions on the face and behind the ears. The rash also appears on the distal extremities, which has given the disorder its name. The diaper area, areas subject to irritation, knees, elbows, and trunk may be affected. Initially, the dermatitis is intensely erythematous and erosive, but later it becomes dry, hyperkeratotic, and psoriasislike in appearance. The hair is sparse, fine, and brittle, and it often has a reddish color. Alopecia is seen frequently. Ocular manifestations include photophobia, conjunctivitis, blepharitis, and a corneal dystrophy, which may be seen with slit-lamp examination. Other features include paronychia, nail dystrophy, personality changes, superficial and systemic moniliasis, repeated bacterial infections, tremor, ataxia, and reversible cerebral atrophy. The failure to thrive is progressive and may lead to marasmus and death if it is not treated. Milder cases with later onset have been reported. Depression, apathy, and paranoia may be seen in older children and adults. Untreated adult females may have a history of miscarriages and children born with anencephaly and congenital skeletal dysplasias.

The diagnosis is established by finding low serum zinc levels. Occasionally, normal zinc levels are noted in clinically affected infants; with therapy, there is improvement in growth, which increases the requirement for zinc and may cause the serum zinc level to decrease, confirming the diagnosis. Alkaline phosphatase, a zinc-requiring enzyme, usually is present in low levels. Plasma ammonia concentrations may be elevated, and a hypobetalipoproteinemia with an altered lipid profile will be noted.

Treatment with oral zinc preparations (sulfate, acetate, or gluconate) will result in clinical improvement in a matter of days. The dosage must be individualized in accordance with the patient's clinical response and blood levels. Treatment is needed for life. Increased requirements occur at times of increased growth, such as puberty, and with infections. Pregnancies in treated women have resulted in normal infants. There are no means for carrier detection or prenatal diagnosis.

Zinc deficiency also may be seen with malnutrition, synthetic diets, chronic hyperalimentation without zinc supplementation, chronic enteritis, cirrhosis, extensive burns, and chelation therapy for other metals.

Familial Hyperzincemia

Familial hyperzincemia has been reported in a family with an autosomal dominant pattern of inheritance. Plasma zinc concentrations were elevated up to five times normal. Because the zinc was complexed with albumin, no clinical symptoms were noted.

(Abridged from Rebecca S. Wappner and Ira K. Brandt, Disorders of Metal Metabolism, in Oski, DeAngelis, Feigin, McMillan, Warshaw: *Principles and Practice of Pediatrics, Second Edition,* J.B. Lippincott, 1994.)

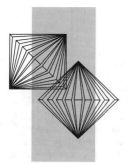

SECTION 13

Immunology and Allergy

Oski's Essential Pediatrics,
edited by Kevin B. Johnson and Frank A. Oski.
Lippincott–Raven Publishers,
Philadelphia © 1997

187

The Primary Immunodeficiency Diseases

The immune system is composed of a variety of cells (B lymphocytes, T lymphocytes, monocytes, and neutrophils) and their secretory products (antibodies, complement, and cytokines), which all recognize foreign antigens and react to them. The first primary immunodeficiency disease, X-linked agammaglobulinemia, was recognized in 1952 by Ogden C. Bruton. Since then, disorders involving nearly all components of the immune system have been identified. This chapter reviews the normal physiology of the immune system, discusses the clinical presentation of immunodeficient patients, and outlines the laboratory tests that are most useful in their diagnosis.

■ THE CLINICAL PRESENTATION OF PRIMARY IMMUNODEFICIENCY DISEASES

The primary immunodeficiency diseases were originally viewed as rare disorders, presenting early in life with severe clinical symptoms. It has become increasingly clear, however, that these diseases are not as uncommon as originally suspected, that their clinical expression can sometimes be mild, and that they may present at any age. Furthermore, although the initial description of patients with primary immunodeficiency diseases focused on their increased susceptibility to infection, these patients may present with a variety of other clinical manifestations. These include autoimmune or chronic inflammatory disorders and syndrome complexes in which immunodeficiency may occur but is often not the presenting feature.

Increased Susceptibility to Infection

Children with primary immunodeficiency diseases most commonly present with an increased susceptibility to infection. Respiratory tract infections and diarrhea are characteristic, but sepsis, meningitis, and osteomyelitis can occur as well. Individual infections may not be more severe than in a normal host, but the striking clinical feature of immunodeficiency is the chronic or recurring nature of infections. However, not all patients with immunodeficiency are diagnosed after a long series of recurrent infections. In some instances, the initial infection is so severe (*eg,* pneumonia with empyema) or is caused by such an unusual organism (*eg, Pneumocystis carinii*) that the diagnosis of immunodeficiency is made.

Autoimmune and Inflammatory Disorders

Just as immunodeficiency can lead to defects in the protective functions of the immune system and an increased susceptibility to infection, immunodeficiency can also lead to abnormal immunoregulatory mechanisms with the result being autoimmune or chronic inflammatory diseases. Thus, patients with primary immunodeficiency diseases sometimes present with autoimmune hemolytic anemia or immune thrombocytopenia, autoimmune endocrinopathy, juvenile rheumatoid arthritis, a lupuslike illness, or inflammatory bowel disease. This type of presentation is most often seen in patients with common variable immunodeficiency, selective IgA deficiency, chronic mucocutaneous candidiasis, and deficiencies of the classical complement pathway.

Immunodeficiency Syndromes

Immunodeficiency can also be seen as one part of a constellation of signs and symptoms in a syndrome complex (Table 187–1).

■ LABORATORY EVALUATION OF THE CHILD WITH SUSPECTED IMMUNODEFICIENCY

One of the most important aspects of the diagnostic workup for immunodeficiency is deciding which patients should be screened, not how to proceed with the evaluation. As discussed previously, indications for screening include the history of severe or chronic/recurrent infections, infection caused by an opportunistic organism, autoimmune disorders, or recognition of specific syndromes that have been associated with immunodeficiency. In addition, a diagnostic evaluation should be considered for any child in whom problems with infection exceed the norm for the clinician's own experience with children of the same age. Selection of screening tests for immunodeficiency should be based on the spectrum of problems in a given patient and the relative frequencies of primary immunodeficiencies in the population. Finally, whenever immunodeficiency disease is suspected, consideration must also be given to secondary causes for immunodeficiency (*eg,* human immunodeficiency virus [HIV] infection or complications of drug therapy [corticosteroids, trimethoprim/sulfamethoxazole, phenytoin]).

Examination of the Peripheral Blood Smear

The complete blood count with examination of the blood smear is an inexpensive, readily available test that provides important diagnostic information relating to a number of immunodeficiency diseases.

Neutropenia may occur secondary to immunosuppressive drugs, infection, malnutrition, autoimmunity, or as a primary problem (congenital or cyclic neutropenia). A persistent neutrophilia with a predominance of immature forms is characteristic of leukocyte adhesion molecule deficiency, and abnormal cytoplasmic granules may be seen in the peripheral blood smear of patients with Chédiak-Higashi syndrome.

The blood is predominantly a "T cell organ" (ie, the majority [50% to 70%] of peripheral blood lymphocytes are T cells whereas only 5% to 15% are B cells). Therefore, lymphopenia sometimes may be a presenting feature of T cell or combined immunodeficiency disorders such as severe combined immunodeficiency disease or DiGeorge's syndrome.

Thrombocytopenia may occur as a secondary manifestation of immunodeficiency but is often a presenting manifestation of the Wiskott-Aldrich syndrome. A unique finding in the latter group of patients is an abnormally small platelet volume, a measurement that is made easily by automated blood counters.

Examination of red blood cell morphology yields important clues about splenic function. Howell-Jolly bodies may be visible in peripheral blood in cases of splenic dysfunction or asplenia. The converse is not always true, and absence of Howell-Jolly bodies does not guarantee that splenic function is normal.

Evaluation of Humoral Immunity

Measurement of serum immunoglobulin levels is an important screening test to detect immunodeficiency for three reasons:

1. More than 80% of patients with primary disorders of immunity will have abnormalities of serum immunoglobulins.

2. These measurements yield indirect information about several disparate aspects of the immune system because immunoglobulin synthesis requires the coordinated function of B lymphocytes, T lymphocytes, and macrophages.

3. The measurement of serum immunoglobulin levels is readily available, highly reliable, and relatively inexpensive.

The initial screening test for humoral immune function is the quantitative measurement of serum immunoglobulins. Neither serum protein electrophoresis nor immunoelectrophoresis is sufficiently sensitive or quantitative to be useful for this purpose. Quantitative measurements of serum IgG, IgA, and IgM identify patients with panhypogammaglobulinemia as well as those with deficiencies of an individual class of immunoglobulins, such as selective IgA deficiency. Interpretation of results must be made in view of the marked variations in normal immunoglobulin levels with age. Therefore, age-related normal values must always be used for comparison.

There are four subclasses of IgG, and selective deficiencies of these have been described. IgG_1 and IgG_3 are the principal subclasses used for responses to protein antigens; IgG_2 is the principal subclass used for responses to polysaccharide antigens. In some instances, the total serum IgG may be normal or near normal, but the patient may still have an IgG subclass deficiency. Thus, in a child in whom there is a strong suspicion of humoral immunodeficiency but total serum IgG is normal, quantitative measurements of individual IgG subclasses should be performed.

In addition to measurement of immunoglobulin levels, assessment of antibody function should always be included as part of the evaluation of humoral immunity. Antibody titers generated in response to childhood immunization with diphtheria and tetanus toxoids are usually the most convenient to measure. In children older than ages 18 to 24 months, it is also important to assess the antibody response to polysaccharide antigens, because these responses may be deficient in some patients who can respond normally to protein antigens (eg, Wiskott-Aldrich syndrome or IgG_2 subclass deficiency). Antibody can be measured in response to immunization with pneumococcal (Pneumovax) or meningococcal capsular polysaccharide vaccines. Alternatively, because the ABO blood group antigens are polysaccharides, antipolysaccharide antibody can be assessed by quantitating isoagglutinin titers. Their value in the young child is limited, however, because even normal children of this age may not have significant isoagglutinins.

If immunoglobulin levels and antibody titers are decreased, the evaluation should proceed with enumeration of B lymphocytes in the peripheral blood. Further specialized tests may be necessary to specifically delineate the functional B cell defect. These may include in vitro studies of mitogen or antigen-driven B cell proliferation and immunoglobulin secretion.

Evaluation of Cell-Mediated Immunity

Testing for defects of cell-mediated immunity is difficult because of the lack of good screening tests. Because T lymphocytes make up 50% to 80% of peripheral blood mononuclear cells, lymphopenia is suggestive of T lymphocyte deficiency. However, lymphopenia is not always present in patients with T lymphocyte functional defects. Similarly, the lack of a thymus silhouette on chest x-ray is a helpful sign in some T lymphocyte disorders, but the thymus of normal children may involute after stress and may give the appearance of thymic hypoplasia.

Delayed type hypersensitivity skin testing with a panel of antigens is an excellent screening method for older children. A standardized panel of antigens prepared for delayed-type hypersensitivity testing should be used. The presence of one or more positive delayed-type skin tests is generally indicative of intact cell-mediated immunity. There are significant limitations to this testing:

Prior exposure to antigen is a prerequisite.

A positive skin test to some antigens does not ensure that the patient has normal cell-mediated immunity to all antigens (eg, patients with chronic mucocutaneous candidiasis have a lacunar defect in which cell-mediated immunity is generally intact except for their response to Candida).

Normal patients may have transient depression of delayed-type hypersensitivity with acute viral infections.

Normal children younger than age 12 months frequently are unresponsive to all of the antigens in the panel.

The test is, therefore, least helpful when it is most needed, namely in young infants in whom a congenital

TABLE 187-1. Examples of Congenital Syndromes in Which Immunodeficiency Occurs as Part of a Symptom Complex

Syndrome	Clinical Presentation	Immunologic Abnormality
Acrodermatitis enteropathica	Dermatitis	Variable B- and T-lymphocyte deficiency
	Alopecia	
	Diarrhea	
Ataxia-telangiectasia	Ataxia	Variable B- and T-lymphocyte deficiency
	Telangiectasia	
Autoimmune polyglandular syndrome	Hypofunction of one or more endocrine organs	Variable B- and T-lymphocyte deficiency
Cartilage hair hypoplasia	Short-limbed dwarfism	Neutropenia
	Sparse hair	T-lymphocyte deficiency
Centromeric instability syndrome	Dysmorphic facies	Variable B- and T-lymphocyte deficiency
	Ataxia	
	Developmental delay	
Chédiak-Higashi syndrome	Oculocutaneous albinism	Abnormal neutrophil function
DiGeorge's anomaly	Hypoparathyroidism	T-lymphocytic deficiency
	Congenital heart disease	
	Elfin facies	
Hyperimmunoglobulin E syndrome	Coarse facies	Neutrophil chemotactic defect
	Eczematoid rash	
	Elevated IgE	
Ivemark syndrome	Bilateral right-sidedness	Congenital asplenia
	Bilateral three-lobed lungs	
	Bilateral morphologic right atria	
Wiskott-Aldrich syndrome	Thrombocytopenia	Variable B- and T-lymphocyte deficiency
	Eczema	

abnormality of T lymphocytes (*eg*, severe combined immunodeficiency) is suspected. In conclusion, delayed-type hypersensitivity testing has poor positive or negative predictive value when applied to children for evaluation of immunodeficiency.

Indirect information about T cell function may be obtained by enumerating peripheral blood T lymphocytes, using fluorescein-conjugated monoclonal antibodies to cell surface determinants. Total T ($CD2^+$ or $CD3^+$), T helper ($CD4^+$) and T killer/suppressor ($CD8^+$) cells can be quantitated with the appropriate monoclonal antibodies. Patients with severe combined immunodeficiency and DiGeorge's anomaly generally have decreased numbers of both $CD4^+$ and $CD8^+$ T lymphocytes. Patients infected with the human immunodeficiency virus have decreased T lymphocytes because there are decreased numbers of $CD4^+$ lymphocytes, whereas patients infected with the Epstein-Barr virus characteristically have elevated numbers of $CD8^+$ cells.

Other specialized tests of cell-mediated immunity include the measurement of lymphocyte proliferate in vitro after stimulation with mitogens, antigens, or allogeneic cells. Production of lymphokines and cytotoxic effector function can be measured as well.

Evaluation of Phagocytic Cells

Evaluation of phagocytic cells usually entails assessment of both their number and their function. Disorders that are characterized by a deficiency in phagocytic cell number, such as congenital agranulocytosis or cyclic neutropenia, usually can be detected by using a white blood cell count and differential.

Assessment of phagocytic cell function depends on a variety of assays. In vitro measurement of directed cell motility (chemotaxis), ingestion (phagocytosis), and intracellular killing (bactericidal activity) can be performed. In addition, there are assays that indirectly assess bactericidal activity by measuring the metabolic changes in the cell that accompany or are responsible for intracellular killing. The most readily available tests assess the oxidative metabolic responses of phagocytes by measuring the reduction of nitroblue tetrazolium to formazan (NBT test; see Chapter 190), the production of reduced forms of molecular oxygen (peroxide, superoxide, hydroxyl radicals), and chemiluminescence. Each of these functions is reduced markedly in disorders of intracellular killing such as chronic granulomatous disease.

Evaluation of the Complement System

Most of the genetically determined deficiencies of the classical activating pathway of C3 (C1, C4, and C2), of C3 itself, and of the terminal components (C5, C6, C7, C8, and C9) can be detected using antibody-sensitized sheep erythrocytes in a total serum hemolytic complement (CH_{50}) assay. Because this assay depends on the functional integrity of C1 through C9, a severe deficiency of any of these components leads to a marked reduction or absence of total hemolytic complement activity. Deficiencies of factor H, factor I, and properdin of the alternative pathway can be detected by a hemolytic assay that assesses lysis of rabbit erythrocytes. The serum of patients with deficiencies of C3 or C5–9 is abnormal when tested in the rabbit erythrocyte assay (as well as in the CH_{50} assay), because the lysis of rabbit erythrocytes depends on these components as well as components of the alternative activating pathway.

The identification of the specific component that is deficient usually rests on both functional and immunochemical tests, and highly specific assays have been developed for each of the individual components. In most cases, both functional and immunochemical assessment of the specific component will demonstrate the deficiency. There are some exceptions. For example, one form of C1 inhibitor deficiency and one form of C1q deficiency are characterized by dysfunctional proteins that can be detected by using immunochemical assays but are markedly reduced in functional activity.

(Abridged from Howard M. Lederman and Jerry A. Winkelstein, The Primary Immunodeficiency Diseases, in Oski, DeAngelis, Feigin, McMillan, Warshaw: *Principles and Practice of Pediatrics, Second Edition*, J.B. Lippincott, 1994.)

Oski's Essential Pediatrics,
edited by Kevin B. Johnson and Frank A. Oski.
Lippincott–Raven Publishers,
Philadelphia © 1997

188

Disorders of Humoral Immunity

Antibodies play a critical role in the host's defense against infection. Many of the protective functions of antibody, such as neutralization of viruses and toxins and inhibition of microbial adherence, can be performed without the participation of other components of the immune system. In addition, there are antibody-mediated functions such as the activation of complement and the ability to opsonize foreign particles for phagocytosis that depend on the recruitment of nonspecific host defense mechanisms. Together these effector mechanisms form a defense network that is particularly effective against a variety of extracellular pathogens. Most notably, these include encapsulated bacteria such as *Haemophilus influenzae* and *Streptococcus pneumoniae*. Antibody also participates in host defense against many viruses. Humoral immunity generally is not as important in the host's defense against intracellular bacteria (*eg*, mycobacteria), fungi, or protozoa. The biologic significance of antibody in host defense against microorganisms is largely defined by recognition of the specific infections that occur in patients with inborn errors of humoral immunity.

■ X-LINKED AGAMMAGLOBULINEMIA

X-linked agammaglobulinemia (X-LA) is the prototypic disorder of humoral immunity. Males with this disease have severe panhypogammaglobulinemia with little or no humoral immune function, but intact cell-mediated immunity. These patients have B lymphocyte precursors (pre-B cells) but do not have mature B lymphocytes or plasma cells. T lymphocytes and all other components of the immune system are normal.

It appears that X-LA results from a developmental arrest of B lymphocyte maturation, although the precise pathophysiologic basis of this disorder is unknown. The defective gene has been mapped to the X chromosome, and X-LA,

therefore, is not the result of abnormal structural genes on the somatic chromosomes that encode the immunoglobulins. The X-chromosome effect on B-lymphocyte differentiation is observed in the female carriers of X-LA, all of whom are immunologically normal. Generally, inactivation of one X chromosome occurs at random in female cells. However, among carriers for X-LA, all mature B lymphocytes have inactivated the abnormal X chromosome. Evidently, lack of expression of the normal gene (or possibly expression of the X-LA gene) blocks B-cell differentiation. Analysis of X-chromosome activation patterns of peripheral blood can be used to determine carrier status.

The differential diagnosis of panhypogammaglobulinemia in infancy includes transient hypogammaglobulinemia of infancy, immunoglobulin deficiency with increased IgM, combined immunodeficiency disorders and rare cases of human immunodeficiency virus (HIV) infection. Quantitation of B and T lymphocytes in peripheral blood helps distinguish among these possibilities. Boys with X-LA have normal numbers of T lymphocytes but have no detectable B lymphocytes. In contrast, infants with transient hypogammaglobulinemia or common variable immunodeficiency generally have normal numbers of B and T lymphocytes; children with severe combined immunodeficiency have decreased numbers of T lymphocytes with normal, decreased, or increased numbers of B cells; and children with HIV infection have decreased numbers of CD4+ T lymphocytes.

Boys with X-LA are usually protected by transplacentally acquired maternal IgG for the first 3 to 4 months of life. Thereafter, chronic and recurrent infections are the predominant clinical manifestation of X-LA. Otitis media, pneumonia, diarrhea, and sinusitis occur most often, usually in combination with each other. Clues to the diagnosis of immunodeficiency include the chronic or recurrent nature of infections, and the occurrence of those infections at more than one anatomic site. *S pneumoniae*, *H influenzae*, and *Staphylococcus aureus* are the most frequently identified bacterial pathogens, but nontypeable *H influenzae*, *Salmonella*, *Pseudomonas*, and *Mycoplasma* infections occur with increased frequency, as do viral infections. Infections are not limited to mucosal surfaces. Bacterial meningitis, sepsis, and osteomyelitis occur in as many as 10% to 15% of untreated patients. Other sentinel symptoms that should prompt consideration of X-LA include the presentation of oligoarticular arthritis or dermatomyositis in a young male.

Patients with X-LA have an increased susceptibility to infections throughout life. Gamma globulin replacement therapy is highly effective in reducing the incidence of systemic bacterial infections such as meningitis and sepsis. It is sometimes less effective in preventing infections along mucosal surfaces. Chronic infections develop in a large proportion of X-LA patients, particularly those who had severe recurrent or chronic infections before the recognition of immune deficiency and initiation of gamma globulin prophylaxis. The respiratory tract and contiguous mucosal surfaces including the paranasal sinuses are the most common sites of chronic disease. Gamma globulin therapy should allow normal or near-normal growth velocity. Persistently impaired linear growth should prompt evaluation of growth hormone levels because X-LA has occurred in association with growth hormone deficiency in a few kindreds.

Enterovirus infections are a particularly difficult problem in X-LA patients. This group of viruses (coxsackie, echo, and polio viruses) tend to cause chronic diarrhea, hepatitis, pneumonitis, and meningoencephalitis in patients with X-LA. In some instances, the infection takes the form of a dermatomyositislike syndrome consisting of rash, edema of subcutaneous tissue, and muscle weakness. Enterovirus infections often are fatal in X-LA patients, although therapy with huge doses of gamma globulin containing virus-specific antibodies has been helpful.

Therapeutic management of patients with X-LA includes the use of gamma globulin prophylaxis and an aggressive approach to the diagnosis and therapy of febrile or inflammatory illnesses. Early recognition of the disease and adequate gamma globulin replacement leads to a good prognosis in most patients. Although there are no controlled studies, gamma globulin prophylaxis appears to be most effective in patients who have not yet incurred structural damage to target organs of the respiratory or gastrointestinal (GI) tract. Most reported deaths of X-LA patients are attributed to recurrent lower respiratory tract infections with resulting chronic pulmonary disease or to chronic enterovirus infections. Early diagnosis is critical to initiate gamma globulin therapy before the onset of any of these problems and to provide families with appropriate genetic counseling.

■ COMMON VARIABLE IMMUNODEFICIENCY

The phrase common variable immunodeficiency (CVID) describes a heterogeneous group of disorders characterized by hypogammaglobulinemia. In distinction from X-LA, B lymphocytes frequently are found in the peripheral blood of CVID patients, and the hypogammaglobulinemia may be less profound. Additional immunologic abnormalities such as T cell dysfunction and autoimmune diseases are expressed variably. Many patients with CVID appear to have defects intrinsic to the B lymphocyte, but other patients have excessive T lymphocyte suppressor function, inadequate T lymphocyte helper function, or anti-B lymphocyte antibodies. Most patients do not manifest symptoms until after the first decade of life, but some patients present in early childhood or infancy. It has long been assumed that CVID patients have acquired hypogammaglobulinemia, although there are only a few reports in which the acquisition is documented. There is no recognizable pattern of inheritance in most patients, but other disorders of humoral immunity (eg, IgA deficiency and transient hypogammaglobulinemia of infancy) occur at higher frequency among family members of CVID patients than among the general population.

As in X-LA, the most frequent manifestations of CVID are chronic or recurrent infections of the upper and lower respiratory tracts. Recurrent pneumonia, chronic bronchitis, and sinusitis occur in the majority of patients, and some eventually develop chronic pulmonary dysfunction. Most of the identified respiratory tract pathogens are encapsulated bacteria. There is an almost equal incidence of obstructive and restrictive lung disease. Somewhat in contrast to patients with X-LA, disease of the GI tract occurs with almost equal frequency as disease of the respiratory tract in patients with CVID. As many as 30% to 60% of patients with CVID have chronic diarrhea. An infectious agent is identified in only about half of the patients; many of the others have idiopathic inflammatory bowel diseases. The most frequently documented GI pathogen is Giardia lamblia. Bacterial overgrowth of the small bowel is another recognized cause of chronic diarrhea in patients with CVID; enteroviruses are less of a problem.

Patients with CVID have a variety of associated disorders for which no infectious etiology has been established. These disorders may be the result of infections caused by unidentified pathogens, but many are believed to be autoimmune in origin, perhaps the result of the same disordered immunoregulation that is presumed to be responsible for the hypogammaglobulinemia in some CVID patients. GI and hematologic disorders predominate. Chronic idiopathic

diarrhea is the single biggest problem. Intestinal biopsy samples typically demonstrate nodular lymphoid hyperplasia as well as villous blunting and epithelial atrophy in the small bowel. Inflammatory bowel diseases, achlorhydria, and pernicious anemia occur with significant frequency. Hematologic abnormalities include the development of persistent splenomegaly, immune thrombocytopenia, leukopenia, and autoimmune hemolytic anemia. Curiously, a few patients have developed a clinical picture typical of sarcoidosis with granulomatous lesions and elevated angiotensin-converting enzyme levels, although without hypergammaglobulinemia. There appears to be an increased susceptibility to malignancy (particularly thymoma and lymphoma) in adults with CVID, but the risk in children is not known.

Treatment of these patients is the same as for those with X-LA: replacement with gamma globulin and aggressive management of infections.

■ SELECTIVE IgA DEFICIENCY

The diagnosis of selective IgA deficiency is established when a patient has a serum IgA level less than 5 mg/dL with normal levels of other immunoglobulin classes, normal serum antibody responses, and normal cell-mediated immunity. Selective IgA deficiency is the most prevalent primary immunodeficiency disease, occurring in approximately 1 of 600 individuals in the population. Usually, there is no recognized pattern of inheritance, although the incidence of selective IgA deficiency is higher in families with other lymphocyte disorders.

IgA has several unique biologic features. Although IgA makes up only 15% of serum immunoglobulins, it is the predominant immunoglobulin class on the mucosal surfaces of the GI and respiratory tracts. IgA is secreted onto mucosal surfaces as a macromolecular complex consisting of two IgA molecules joined to a J chain and a secretory component. The majority of patients with IgA deficiency lack both serum and secretory IgA, but there are rare cases in which there is a deficiency of secretory but not serum IgA. Unlike the other major serum immunoglobulin classes IgG and IgM, IgA is largely silent as a mediator of inflammatory responses. IgA is an antimicrobial defense that inhibits microbial adherence and neutralizes virus. It also has an important role in antigen clearance, thus excluding soluble antigens from penetrating the mucosa and entering the systemic circulation. The unique biologic features of IgA may help to explain the clinical associations of IgA deficiency with infection, atopic disease, and rheumatic disorders.

Some patients with selective IgA deficiency are more susceptible to infection, although there is disagreement about the relative risk of infection that IgA deficiency imposes on the host. Among patients referred to tertiary care centers for evaluation of recurrent sinopulmonary infections, the incidence of IgA deficiency is significantly higher compared to that of the general population. Apparently, asymptomatic individuals have been identified as IgA deficient by population-based screening. As might be expected by its role as the predominant secretory immunoglobulin, the most common infections in IgA-deficient patients occur on mucosal surfaces. Otitis media, sinusitis, bronchitis, pneumonia, and diarrhea are common; meningitis and bacterial sepsis are rare. In some series, as many as 50% of patients with selective IgA deficiency have chronic respiratory tract infections. A subgroup of IgA-deficient patients have additional deficiencies of the IgG subclasses IgG2 and IgG4. Studies suggest that these are the IgA-deficient patients who tend to experience the most severe and chronic sinopulmonary infections. Because IgG subclass deficiencies are treatable (see section below), IgG subclass determinations should be included in the workup of all IgA-deficient patients. The second major target for infections in IgA-deficient patients is the GI tract. Chronic diarrhea is often idiopathic. *Giardia* is the most frequently identified pathogen. Gluten-sensitive enteropathy, ulcerative colitis, and Crohn's disease have each been associated with selective IgA deficiency.

Atopic diseases such as allergic rhinitis, asthma, urticaria, eczema, and food allergy have been reported to occur in as many as 50% of patients with selective IgA deficiency. It has been postulated that lack of secretory IgA allows inhaled and ingested antigens to penetrate the mucosal epithelium and to elicit antibody responses in the bronchial and GI lymphoid tissues. A particularly hazardous allergic reaction in IgA-deficient patients is the development of anaphylactic reactions after the infusion of plasma or gamma globulin.

A variety of autoimmune and rheumatic diseases have been associated with selective IgA deficiency. These include juvenile rheumatoid arthritis, systemic lupus erythematosus, thyroiditis, and pernicious anemia. A unifying etiology to explain the association of these disorders with selective IgA deficiency has not been established. It has been hypothesized that penetration of environmental antigens may lead to production of antibodies with specificity for self, or that disordered immunoregulation underlies both IgA deficiency and autoimmune disease.

Children with low but not absent IgA (5 to 10 mg/dL) share many of the same disease manifestations, but they tend to be less severely affected. Furthermore, in longitudinal studies, it has been observed that serum IgA levels increase to within the normal range in more than half of these less severe cases, and, concomitantly, symptoms cease.

Immunoglobulin therapy is generally contraindicated in selective IgA deficiency. Commercial gamma globulin preparations contain trace amounts of IgA, which are insufficient to provide replacement therapy but are sufficient to sensitize the patient to IgA, thereby inducing an IgG or IgE anti-IgA antibody response. This is a relative and not an absolute contraindication to gamma globulin therapy. Patients with IgA deficiency and associated IgG subclass deficiencies who suffer from recurrent infections may benefit from immunoglobulin prophylaxis. In such cases, an intravenous gamma globulin preparation that contains less than 0.01 g/L of IgA can be used, but with caution.

■ IgG SUBCLASS DEFICIENCIES

The four subclasses of IgG differ somewhat in their biologic activities. IgG1, IgG2, and IgG3 fix complement, bind to Fc receptors on monocytes, and participate in antibody-dependent cellular cytotoxicity; IgG4 does not. The IgG response to protein antigens occurs predominantly within the IgG1 and IgG3 subclasses, whereas the IgG response to polysaccharide antigens generally is restricted to the IgG2 and IgG4 subclasses. Because antibodies to the polysaccharide capsules of bacteria such as *S pneumoniae* and *H influenzae* are important for host defense, deficiencies of IgG2 and IgG4 may predispose the host to infections caused by these and other encapsulated bacteria.

Deficiencies of IgG subclasses have been described in association with other primary immunodeficiency diseases such as selective IgA deficiency, ataxia-telangiectasia, and Wiskott-Aldrich syndrome. Isolated IgG subclass deficiencies have been only recently identified. The clue to the diagnosis is often the presence of borderline or low normal total serum IgG levels in a patient with recurrent sinopulmonary infec-

tions. In such individuals, further tests should include quantitation of IgG subclasses and measurement of antibody responses to protein (*eg,* diphtheria and tetanus toxoids) and polysaccharide (*eg,* pneumococcal) vaccines. Some patients with selective deficiency of IgG2 or deficiencies of IgG3 and IgG4 suffer from recurrent pyogenic infections of the respiratory tract. They may benefit from antibiotic prophylaxis or therapy with gamma globulin, but formal studies documenting efficacy are lacking. Only a small number of patients have been identified with isolated deficiencies of IgG3 or IgG4, and the biologic significance of these deficiencies is uncertain. Isolated IgG1 deficiency has not been reported.

(Abridged from Howard M. Lederman, Disorders of Humoral Immunity, in Oski, DeAngelis, Feigin, McMillan, Warshaw: *Principles and Practice of Pediatrics, Second Edition,* J.B. Lippincott, 1994.)

Oski's Essential Pediatrics,
edited by Kevin B. Johnson and Frank A. Oski.
Lippincott–Raven Publishers,
Philadelphia © 1997

189

Complement Deficiencies

The complement system is composed of a series of plasma proteins and cellular receptors, which, when functioning in an ordered and integrated fashion, serve as important mediators of host defense and inflammation. Although the complement system was first described at the turn of the century, it was not until 1960 that the first patient with a genetically determined complement deficiency was identified. Since then, deficiencies have been described for nearly all components of the complement system (Table 189–1).

■ CLINICAL PRESENTATION

Individuals with genetically determined complement deficiencies have a variety of clinical presentations. Most patients present with an increased susceptibility to infection, a variety of rheumatic diseases, or angioedema.

Increased Susceptibility to Infection

An increased susceptibility to infection is a prominent clinical finding in patients with complement deficiencies. The kinds of infections relate to the biologic functions of those components that are missing. The third component of complement (C3) is an important opsonic ligand. Therefore, patients with a deficiency of C3 or of a component in either of the two pathways that activate C3 are more susceptible to infections caused by encapsulated bacteria for which opsonization is the primary host defense (*eg, Streptococcus pneumoniae, Streptococcus pyogenes,* and *Haemophilus influenzae*). Similarly, C5–C9 form the membrane attack complex and are responsible for the bactericidal functions of complement. Patients with deficiencies of C5, C6, C7, C8, or C9 opsonize bacteria normally and are not unduly susceptible to gram-positive bacteria. They are, however, susceptible to gram-negative bacteria, notably *Neisseria* species, because

TABLE 189-1. Genetically Determined Complement Deficiencies

Deficiency	Inheritance	Major Clinical Manifestation
C1q	Autosomal recessive	Rheumatic disorders and pyogenic infections
C1r/s	Autosomal recessive	Rheumatic disorders
C4	Autosomal recessive	Rheumatic disorders and pyogenic infections
C2	Autosomal recessive	Rheumatic disorders and pyogenic infections
C3	Autosomal recessive	Pyogenic infections
C5	Autosomal recessive	Meningococcal sepsis and meningitis
C6	Autosomal recessive	Meningococcal sepsis and meningitis
C7	Autosomal recessive	Meningococcal sepsis and meningitis
C8	Autosomal recessive	Meningococcal sepsis and meningitis
C9	Autosomal recessive	Meningococcal sepsis and meningitis
Factor I	Autosomal recessive	Pyogenic infections
Factor H	Autosomal recessive	Hemolytic uremic syndrome
Properdin	X-linked recessive	Meningococcal sepsis and meningitis
C1 Inhibitor	Autosomal dominant	Angioedema

serum bactericidal activity is an important host defense against these organisms.

A number of studies have examined groups of patients with specific infectious diseases to determine the frequency of complement deficiencies and to evaluate the utility of screening for complement deficiencies. Between 5% and 15% of patients with systemic meningococcal infections have a genetically determined complement deficiency. The differing estimates may reflect differences in populations examined. In general, the prevalence is higher if the patient has had recurrent meningococcal disease, if the patient has a positive family history for meningococcal disease, or if the patient is infected with an uncommon meningococcal serotype. Therefore, it seems reasonable to screen children with systemic meningococcal infections for the presence of a complement deficiency. In contrast, many patients with complement deficiencies present with systemic pneumococcal or *H influenzae* infections, but the prevalence of complement deficiencies in patients with these specific infections appears low. Recommending screening for complement deficiencies in patients with bacteremia or meningitis caused by pneumococcus or *H influenzae* is more difficult to justify.

Rheumatic Diseases

Patients with complement deficiencies also have a variety of clinical conditions that best can be described as rheumatic diseases. These include a disorder that resembles systemic lupus erythematosus (SLE) as well as glomerulonephritis, dermatomyositis, anaphylactoid purpura, and vasculitis. The prevalence of these inflammatory disorders is highest in those patients with deficiencies of the classical

activating pathway (C1, C4, and C2) and of C3. The pathophysiologic basis for the occurrence of these diseases in complement-deficient patients is unclear but may relate, in part, to the physiologic role of the complement system in processing immune complexes or its role in the induction of a normal humoral immune response.

Some important differences between the rheumatic diseases are seen in complement-deficient patients and their counterparts in "normal" noncomplement-deficient individuals. For example, the SLE-like illness seen in complement-deficient individuals is often characterized by onset in childhood, skin lesions resembling discoid lupus, and relatively limited renal and pleuropericardial involvement. In addition, complement-deficient individuals with the lupuslike syndrome usually have absent or low titers of antinuclear antibodies and negative lupus preparations. In contrast, their incidence of anti-Ro antibodies is significantly higher than in noncomplement-deficient patients with lupus. Thus, clinical manifestations of and serologic findings for complement-deficient patients with the lupuslike syndrome resemble a subgroup of lupus patients who are "ANA-negative" or have subacute, cutaneous lupus.

■ SPECIFIC DISORDERS

C2 Deficiency

A deficiency of C2 is the most common of the inherited complement deficiencies. The frequency of the gene for C2 deficiency is estimated at 1 in 100 with homozygous-deficient individuals occurring as frequently as 1 in 10,000. Complement-mediated serum activities such as opsonization and chemotaxis are present in patients with C2 deficiency, presumably because their alternative pathway is intact, although they are not generated as quickly nor to the same degree as in individuals with an intact classical pathway. The clinical manifestations of C2 deficiency vary from individuals who are asymptomatic to individuals who are clinically affected with either an increased susceptibility to infection or rheumatic diseases or both. The infections are mostly bloodborne and systemic (*eg,* sepsis, meningitis, arthritis, and osteomyelitis) and caused by encapsulated bacteria. A variety of rheumatic diseases are associated with C2 deficiency. The most common are disorders that resemble systemic lupus erythematosus and discoid lupus. Glomerulonephritis, dermatomyositis, anaphylactoid purpura, and vasculitis have also been seen.

C3 Deficiency

Patients with C3 deficiency generally have less than 1% of the normal amount of C3 in their serum. Those serum activities that are either directly dependent on C3 (opsonization) or indirectly dependent on C3 because of its role in the activation of C5–C9 (chemotaxis and bactericidal activity) are also markedly reduced. The clinical manifestations of C3 deficiency in humans include increased susceptibility to infection and rheumatic disorders. Patients with C3 deficiency have a variety of infections, including pneumonia, bacteremia, meningitis, and osteomyelitis, caused by encapsulated pyogenic bacteria. A number of patients have presented with arthralgias and vasculitic skin rashes and a clinical picture consistent with systemic lupus erythematosus. Renal disease has also been seen in C3-deficient patients. Histologically, the lesions most closely resemble membranoproliferative glomerulonephritis.

C1 Inhibitor Deficiency

A genetically determined deficiency of C1 inhibitor (C1-INH) is responsible for the clinical disorder hereditary angioedema (HAE). C1 inhibitor deficiency is inherited in an autosomal dominant fashion. There are at least two forms of C1-INH deficiency. In the most common form (Type I), which accounts for about 85% of patients, the serum of affected individuals is deficient in both C1-INH protein (5% to 30% of normal) and C1-INH activity. In the less common form (Type II), a dysfunctional protein is present in normal or elevated concentrations, but its functional activity is markedly reduced. In either case, the level of C4 in serum is commonly reduced both during and between attacks, making it a useful diagnostic clue.

The pathophysiologic mechanisms by which the absence of C1-INH activity leads to the angioedema characteristic of the disorder are still incompletely understood. Neither the mediators responsible for producing the edema nor the mechanisms initiating their production have been clearly identified, although evidence implicates both the complement system and the kinin system in the pathogenesis of the edema.

The clinical symptoms of HAE are the result of submucosal or subcutaneous edema. The lesions are characterized by noninflammatory edema associated with capillary and venule dilation. The three most prominent areas of involvement are the skin, respiratory tract, and gastrointestinal tract.

Attacks involving the skin may involve an extremity, the face, or genitalia. The edema may vary in size from a few centimeters to involvement of a whole extremity. The lesions are pale rather than red, are usually not warm, and are characteristically nonpruritic. There may be a feeling of tightness in the skin caused by accumulation of subcutaneous fluid. Attacks usually progress for 1 to 2 days and resolve over an additional 2 to 3 days.

Attacks involving the upper respiratory tract represent a serious threat to the patient with HAE. Pharyngeal edema occurs at least once in nearly two thirds of the patients. The patients may initially experience a "tightness" in the throat, and swelling of the tongue, buccal mucosa, and oropharynx follow. In some instances, laryngeal edema, accompanied by hoarseness and stridor, progresses to respiratory obstruction and represents a life-threatening emergency.

The gastrointestinal tract can be affected by HAE. Symptoms are secondary to edema of the bowel wall and may include anorexia, dull aching of the abdomen, vomiting, and crampy abdominal pain. Abdominal symptoms can occur in the absence of concurrent cutaneous or pharyngeal involvement.

The onset of symptoms referable to HAE occurs in more than half the patients before adolescence, but, in some patients, symptoms do not occur until adulthood. Although trauma, anxiety, and stress are frequently cited as events that initiate attacks, more than half of patients cannot clearly identify an event that initiated an attack. Dental extractions and tonsillectomy can initiate edema of the upper airway, and cutaneous edema may follow trauma to an extremity.

Therapy of HAE is divided into two categories: prophylaxis of attacks and treatment of attacks. Long-term prevention of attacks may be indicated in those patients who have had laryngeal obstruction or have suffered frequent and debilitating attacks. Antifibrinolytic agents such as epsilon aminocaproic acid (EACA) or its cyclic analogue, tranexamic acid, have been used with some success in the long-term prevention of attacks. "Impeded" androgens such as danazol and stanozolol, which have attenuated androgenic potential, have been found to be useful in long-term prophylaxis of HAE. These agents have not been used extensively in children, however, because of their androgenic effects. Apparently, they act by stimulating the synthesis of functionally intact C1-INH by the normal gene. In some instances, patients may need short-term prophylactic therapy (eg, before oral surgery). In these circumstances, danazol therapy may be initiated 1 week before surgery or EACA the day before surgery.

A number of drugs have been used in an attempt to interrupt an attack of HAE once it has begun. Epinephrine, antihistamines, and corticosteroids are of no proven benefit. Recent trials with partially purified C1-INH are encouraging. Infusion of C1-INH has been accompanied by resolution of edema and symptoms within a few hours.

(Abridged from Jerry A. Winkelstein, Complement Deficiencies, in Oski, DeAngelis, Feigin, McMillan, Warshaw: *Principles and Practice of Pediatrics, Second Edition*, J.B. Lippincott, 1994.)

Oski's Essential Pediatrics, edited by Kevin B. Johnson and Frank A. Oski. Lippincott–Raven Publishers, Philadelphia © 1997

190

Functional Disorders of Granulocytes

Mobile blood granulocytes and monocytes and fixed phagocytic cells of reticuloendothelial tissues function as a first-line defense against invasion by bacterial or fungal microorganisms. Impaired granulocyte production as well as functional abnormalities of granulocytes or other professional phagocytes may significantly compromise host defense, thus increasing susceptibility to infection. Early animal studies demonstrated a critical 2- to 4-hour period after cutaneous invasion by pathogenic bacteria during which phagocytes must localize at a site of invasion to prevent or suppress an infectious process. Recurrent bacterial or fungal infections of the skin or mucous membranes are prominent in patients with quantitative deficiencies of blood granulocytes and in patients with functional deficits of granulocytic cells.

Two broad categories of functional disorders are those typified by impaired motility, recruitment, or localization of granulocytes at or to sites of infection; and those resulting from defective ingestion or intracellular killing of microorganisms by granulocytes and other phagocytic cells. In this latter group of patients, granulocytes accumulate normally in inflamed tissues but are unable to eradicate invading microorganisms. Laboratory studies of representative patients of both categories can be used to define abnormalities of one or more cellular functions (eg, directed migration or chemotaxis, adhesion, ingestion, degranulation, and oxidative intracellular killing) in vitro. In selected disorders, molecular deficits have been defined, which allows important new approaches to the diagnosis or clinical management of disease.

■ CHÉDIAK-HIGASHI SYNDROME

The Chédiak-Higashi syndrome is an autosomal recessive disorder of mink, cattle, beige mice, and humans. This condition is characterized clinically by partial oculocutaneous albinism, the presence of giant lysosomal granules in all granular cell types, susceptibility to bacterial infection, variable occurrence of neutropenia and thrombocytopenia, and an accelerated lymphomalike proliferative phase generally occurring in the first decade of life. Infectious complications are attributable to both neutropenia and functional deficits of neutrophils, monocytes, and natural killer (NK) cells. A comprehensive review in 1972 documented the significance of infectious morbidity and mortality in this syndrome. Among 56 cases reviewed, 33 individuals died before age 10 years; among 27 cases for which a cause of death was determined, infections was the sole cause in 17 and a contributing factor in 9 more cases. Pulmonary, cutaneous, subcutaneous, and upper respiratory infections were observed most. *Staphylococcus aureus* accounted for about 70% of all infections for which an etiologic agent was determined; group A *Streptococcus*, gram-negative enteric organisms (*Klebsiella, Pseudomonas, Proteus, Shigella* spp), *Aspergillus,* and species of *Candida* represented occasional etiologic agents.

Neutrophils, monocytes, and lymphocytes from these patients demonstrate large intracellular inclusions or granules, which represent the pathologic hallmark of the disease. Although they are most easily demonstrated in leukocytes, they also are present in renal tubular epithelium, gastric mucosa, pancreas, thyroid, neural tissue, and melanocytes. In neutrophils, inclusions contain azurophilic granule markers (myeloperoxidase and acid phosphatase) and are assumed to represent abnormal azurophilic granules. These abnormal granules, however, contain both azurophilic and specific granule markers. Normal-appearing specific granules are present, but normal azurophilic granules have not been seen. Analysis of bone marrow samples from patients with Chédiak-Higashi syndrome suggest that abnormal granules are formed during granulocyte maturation by the progressive aggregation and fusion of azurophilic and specific granules. Such findings are consistent with a proposed membrane abnormality.

Several functional abnormalities of neutrophils, monocytes, and natural killer cells of these patients have been identified. Defective neutrophil and monocyte chemotaxis has been consistently reported, but the molecular determinants of these abnormalities are undefined. Neutrophils demonstrate delayed and diminished intracellular killing of both gram-positive and gram-negative bacterial organisms, despite a normal capacity to ingest these organisms and a normal or elevated oxidative burst. Microbicidal abnormalities are attributed to impaired postphagocytic phagolysosomal fusion. A selective impairment of the functions of natural killer cells (as opposed to other lymphocyte functions) has been reported. Dysfunction of the natural killer cell system may account for the ultimate development of an aggressive lymphoproliferative syndrome in most patients.

A diagnosis of Chédiak-Higashi syndrome is made by identifying characteristic clinical features of the disorder in addition to characteristic large cytoplasmic inclusions in all granular cells, including peripheral blood granulocytes. Giant melanosomes can be demonstrated from hair of patients. Neutropenia and thrombocytopenia are most characteristic during the accelerated phase of disease. When bone marrow aspirates are examined, common abnormalities include hypercellularity with extensive vacuolization and inclusions in myeloid precursors. Elevated serum lysozyme levels probably reflect intramedullary granulocyte destruction. The accelerated phase of Chédiak-Higashi syndrome is characterized by widespread tissue infiltrates of lymphoid and histiocytic cells, usually without malignant histologic characteristics. Splenomegaly and associated hypersplenism contribute to anemia and thrombocytopenia

and may also contribute to neutropenia. Although viral agents and immunologic mechanisms may contribute to the pathogenesis of the accelerated phase, the precise mechanisms are undefined.

Most patients with Chédiak-Higashi syndrome succumb to infectious or infiltrative complications within the first decade of life. Successful bone marrow transplantation with reversal of the defect in natural killer activity has been reported in one case. The determination of definitive preventive or therapeutic strategies awaits definition of the disease's molecular pathogenesis.

■ SCHWACHMAN-DIAMOND SYNDROME

Clinical features of a syndrome first described by Schwachman and Diamond include exocrine pancreatic insufficiency, bone marrow hypoplasia with associated neutropenia, metaphyseal chondrodysplasia, growth retardation, and recurrent soft tissue infections. In a series of 21 patients, otitis media, bronchial pneumonia, osteomyelitis, dermatitis, and septicemia occurred in 17 (81%), from which 3 (14% of total series) died. Neutropenia was intermittent in most patients in this and other series. Bone marrow aspirations from patients with this disorder have demonstrated absent myeloid precursors or maturation arrest with variable degrees of hypoplasia. Normal bone marrow aspirates in neutropenic patients have also been described, suggesting that marrow hypoplasia is patchy in distribution. Diminished chemotaxis of neutrophils without other functional abnormalities was found in 12 of 14 patients with this syndrome. Nine of these patients were neutropenic, and 4 demonstrated low levels of serum IgA or IgM without other immunologic abnormalities. Intermediate abnormalities of neutrophil chemotaxis were recognized in parents of some of these individuals, suggesting that the individuals were heterozygous for the abnormality and that the abnormality is inherited as an autosomal recessive trait. A pathogenic basis for hematologic and other features of this multisystem disease has not been determined, and the relative contributions of impaired cellular motility, as opposed to neutropenia, to infectious susceptibility in affected patients remain uncertain.

■ CHRONIC GRANULOMATOSIS DISEASE

The chronic granulomatous diseases (CGD) are a genetically heterogeneous group of disorders of the oxidative metabolism of phagocytes. CGD result in impairment of intracellular killing of catalase-positive bacteria, fungi, or other microbes. CGD occur at a frequency of 1 in 1 million and are identified most often in males. Most patients with CGD develop recurrent soft tissue infections during the first year of life; a high proportion of these become clinically ill before age 3 months. Rarely, individuals may be clinically well until early adolescence or adulthood, possibly reflecting less deleterious genetic phenotypes. Disease-free intervals may increase in some patients with increasing age, but older individuals are still at high risk for life-threatening infections. Improved prophylactic or therapeutic regimens may diminish mortality rates in CGD. The routine use of prophylactic antibiotics and the introduction of interferon gamma in clinical management of CGD are likely to affect significantly the severity of this disease.

The basis for abnormal oxygen-dependent microbicidal activity in CGD cells is related directly to impaired generation of superoxide anion, H_2O_2, and other oxygen intermediates. This abnormality is expressed in a number of cell types including neutrophils, macrophages, eosinophils, and lymphocytes. Abnormal NADPH oxidase activity caused by one of several molecular defects recognized among CGD patients represents the fundamental basis for diminished microbicidal function.

Distinct forms of CGD are defined to involve deficits of each of the components of the NADPH oxidase complex, including the unique membrane associated cytochrome b and soluble cytosolic factors. Such definition is possible because of the availability of cDNAs or monoclonal antibodies reactive with patient mRNA or protein components. Historically, three genetic forms of CGD were described based on inheritance patterns and spectrophotometric detection of the cytochrome b in phagocytes of affected patients; X-chromosome linked (about 70%), autosomal recessive (about 30%), and autosomal dominant (rare cases).

Evidence suggests the following types of molecular defects in X-linked patients: subtle mutations in the 91kd cytochrome b gene, regulatory defects in mRNA transcription of cytochrome b components, structural mutations altering the stability of mRNA for these components, and abnormal assembly of the 91kd cytochrome protein with other components of NADPH oxidase.

The most common form of autosomal disease is a recessive trait in which cytochrome b levels are normal, implying defects of other components of the membrane oxidase complex. A study of 25 autosomal recessive CGD patients shows that 22 lacked a 47kd cytosolic protein and 3 lacked a 67kd cytosolic factor. Rare cases of autosomally transmitted CGD demonstrate deficient expression of cytochrome b, which appears to reflect mutations of the gene that encodes the 22kd subunit of this membrane protein. Genotypic heterogeneity appears to account for the considerable range of clinical severity among CGD kindreds. Precise definition of the molecular lesions in individual patients may even allow prognostic information or unique insights concerning novel therapeutic approaches (*eg*, somatic cell gene therapy).

Patients with CGD demonstrate a specific predilection for infection due to catalase-positive microorganisms that generally do not elaborate H_2O_2. *S aureus* represents the most common infecting agent, accounting for 30% to 56% of clinical isolates in reported series of patients. Catalase-positive, gram-negative bacteria including *Escherichia coli*, *Klebsiella*, and *Enterobacter* species, *Serratia marcescens*, *Salmonella*, and *Pseudomonas* species account for approximately 30% of infections overall. In specific geographic locations, *Chromobacterium violacium* infections have been recognized in several CGD patients. Fungal pathogens also represent frequent and important etiologic agents. Fungal infections occurred in 20% of 245 cases reviewed in one report. *Aspergillus* species accounted for 78% of these; *Candida albicans* and species of *Torulopsis* accounted for most of the remaining isolates. Other reports document the pathogenic importance of obligate intracellular pathogens such as *Pneumocystis carinii* and *Mycobacterium* species. Thus, patients with CGD are susceptible to infection by a variety of endogenous flora as well as ubiquitous organisms.

Clinical infections in CGD largely reflect an inability of circulating phagocytes to kill invading bacteria or fungi at sites of heavy colonization on or beneath skin or mucous membranes. Predictable clinical features in CGD are infections on body surfaces including inflammatory lesions of skin or subcutaneous tissues, ulcerative stomatitis, pneumonitis, perianal abscesses, and conjunctivitis. More widespread and deep-seated infections in CGD further reflect the persistence of invading organisms within circulating phagocytes, which allows localized or generalized seeding of tissue macrophages

throughout the reticuloendothelial system. As a result, typical granulomas, which constitute the histopathologic hallmark of this disorder, commonly develop in lymph nodes, lungs, liver, spleen, gastrointestinal tract, bone, and other tissues. Once established, these infections generally remain localized but may overwhelm the reticuloendothelial barriers leading to the development of septicemia or meningitis. Prolonged intracellular microbial residence in tissue abscesses or granulomas accounts for the indolent nature of observed clinical infections, considerable difficulties encountered in identifying specific infecting agents, and a delayed or refractory response to antimicrobial, surgical, or other therapeutic regimens in patients with CGD.

A diagnosis of CGD should be considered when a history of recurrent systemic infections or other clinical features beginning in infancy is elicited. Patients with CGD often are referred to tertiary care centers with histories of recurrent or chronic illness or inflammatory disease for which no etiology has been determined despite extensive diagnostic evaluations. They frequently present with fever of unknown origin or carry a presumptive diagnosis of rheumatoid disease, and they may be misdiagnosed as examples of other granulomatous inflammatory disorders such as Crohn's disease or tuberculosis. Particularly typical is a history of sterile tissue aspirates of superficial or deep-seated abscesses. The identification of unusual etiologic agents such as *Serratia marcescens* or *Pseudomonas maltophilia*, the occurrence of infections in unusual locations such as osteomyelitic involvement of small bones of hands or feet, and the occurrence of characteristic types of infections such as liver or other deep-seated abscesses should alert the clinician to the possibility of CGD.

Laboratory findings suggestive of CGD include leukocytosis, elevation of erythrocyte sedimentation rate, abnormal chest radiographs, and hypergammaglobulinemia. Serum levels of immunoglobulin G, A, and M generally are elevated, whereas IgE levels are variably increased or normal. Specific antibody synthesis and delayed hypersensitivity skin test responses generally are normal. Microscopic evaluations of postmortem or biopsy tissues almost uniformly reveal granulomas at sites of infection. Commonly, histiocytes contain pigmented (yellow or tan) lipid material that may result from persistent residence of microorganisms within macrophages.

A definitive diagnostic test for CGD is the demonstration of impaired intracellular bactericidal activity by neutrophils, eosinophils, or mononuclear phagocytes. Because bactericidal assays require special laboratory facilities and experience, other screening tests including the nitroblue tetrazolium (NBT) dye test are applicable for use in the general diagnostic laboratory. Oxidized NBT is colorless. When reduced by superoxide, it precipitates in the cytosol as blue formazan, which can be identified histochemically. Absence of superoxide evolution by CGD neutrophils or monocytes precludes their reduction of formazan in response to soluble oxidative stimulants or during phagocytosis. A modified qualitative NBT slide test employing the stimulant phorbol myristate acetate was originally developed by Newberger to allow a prenatal diagnosis of CGD using fetal blood. This rapid, inexpensive, and highly accurate assay is useful for both the identification of patients and family studies. Employing this technique, essentially no CGD leukocytes demonstrate a normal reduction of NBT, whereas essentially all of those of normal individuals are NBT positive. Heterozygous carriers of X-linked recessive CGD have nearly equal proportions of NBT-positive and NBT-negative cells.

Other laboratory techniques can be used to demonstrate impairment of the respiratory burst and thereby confirm a diagnosis of CGD. During phagocytosis, normal neutrophils or monocytes produce highly energized and unstable oxygen radicals, which return to more stable intermediates by emission of light energy or chemiluminescence. Chemiluminescence associated with phagocytosis or after stimulation by soluble stimulants can be conveniently measured in a scintillation counter. Leukocytes from patients with CGD generate no or markedly diminished chemiluminescence under most experimental conditions. The chemiluminescence assay may allow recognition of heterozygous CGD carriers in family studies, and it may be used to detect other heritable disorders of leukocyte oxidative metabolism including myeloperoxidase deficiency, G6PD deficiency, and abnormalities of glutathione metabolism, each of which can be confirmed by more specific biochemical assays. Because molecular heterogeneity has been increasingly recognized among identified patients with CGD and their kindreds, more detailed investigations to delineate a precise molecular lesion in selected cases should be performed in specialized laboratories.

The major clinical objectives in the management of CGD include prevention of infection, early identification of infection, and antimicrobial or surgical treatment. Superficial lesions such as furuncles, paronychia, and areas of cellulitis warrant concern, even with no fever or other systemic symptoms. Vigorous efforts should be made to isolate etiologic agents from involved tissues and to promptly initiate antimicrobial therapy. For recognized acute infections, appropriate antibiotics (based on susceptibility studies) should be administered for at least 10 to 14 days, even if the clinical response is prompt and favorable. Longer intervals of administration may be required when delayed defervescence is observed or when leukocytosis, an elevated sedimentation rate, or local inflammatory signs persist. Fever without an obvious site of infection is common. Noninvasive diagnostic procedures such as ultrasonography or radionucleotide scans should be considered early in the management of febrile episodes. The early administration of parenteral antibiotics is justified in febrile patients without localizing findings.

When possible, aggressive and early surgical intervention including incision and drainage of abscesses should be considered. Antibiotic administration should be continued for about 1 to 2 weeks after complete wound healing, even if a specific and highly sensitive etiologic agent is recovered. Administration of oral antibiotics may be justified for several weeks to several months longer even in the complete absence of clinical signs or laboratory abnormalities. The general rationale for this prolonged therapeutic interval is based on the knowledge that microorganisms are sequestered and not killed within phagocytes defective in microbicidal mechanisms and on the high incidence of relapsing infections in these patients.

The use of leukocyte transfusions in selected clinical settings should be considered. Although several investigators have reported beneficial effects in managing infectious complications, comparative evaluations of the efficacy or possible complications associated with leukocyte transfusions in these patients are lacking. Possible benefits of transfused leukocytes must be weighed against possible complications associated with their use. Foremost is the possibility of sensitization to granulocyte or monocyte antigens in patients who have the McLeod phenotype. Three clinical indications for leukocyte transfusions in CGD include failure of conventional medical and surgical therapy to control infection or inflammation, rapidly progressive or life-threatening infection, and failure to appropriately localize an infectious process or focus, thereby obviating the possibility of conventional medical or surgical approaches.

In addition to the therapeutic and supportive measures described above, the recent availability of recombinant interferon-gamma (INF-γ) provides a potentially important advantage in the clinical management of CGD. In vitro studies show that INF-γ enhances expression of cytochrome b 91kd mRNA and superoxide production in phagocytic cells from normal and some X-linked CGD patients. Administration of subcutaneous INF-γ resulted in enhanced superoxide production and staphylococcal killing (to near normal levels) in association with increased cytochrome b levels when studied in one series of CGD patients. In another report, the enhancement of the 47 kd cytosolic factor and its mRNA as well as increased production of superoxide and mRNA for the 91 kd cytochrome b subunit were evident in INF-γ treated normal macrophages. These findings suggest possible clinical applications of INF-γ in autosomal as well as X-linked phenotypes of CGD.

In addition to requiring management of infections, patients with CGD must be evaluated carefully with respect to their erythrocyte phenotype. Some individuals with CGD lack known antigens from the Kell series, a phenotype termed K_o, whereas others have the McLeod phenotype, characterized by erythrocytes that react weakly with antibodies defining some Kell antigens. Because both phenotypes are rare, these patients are at risk of forming antibodies to antigens on erythrocytes of most blood donors. Thus, transfusion should be avoided in patients who have these rare Kell-associated phenotypes, or their erythrocytes should be stored for possible future use. Additional management involves the identification of a carrier state among family members and the provision of appropriate genetic counseling.

(Abridged from Donald C. Anderson and C. Wayne Smith, Functional Disorders of Granulocytes, in Oski, DeAngelis, Feigin, McMillan, Warshaw: *Principles and Practice of Pediatrics, Second Edition*, J.B. Lippincott, 1994.)

Oski's Essential Pediatrics,
edited by Kevin B. Johnson and Frank A. Oski.
Lippincott–Raven Publishers,
Philadelphia © 1997

191

Combined Immunodeficiency Diseases

The first report of an immunodeficiency disease appeared in 1952 with the description of agammaglobulinemia. During the next dozen years, many other immunodeficiency disorders characterized by recurrent infections were reported. Confusion ensued because the types of infection that dominated the clinical picture in one group of patients appeared to cause few or no problems for patients with a different syndrome. In the 1960s, the immune system was shown to consist of two components with distinct but complementary roles in defense against infectious agents. Studies in rabbits, mice, and chickens established the presence of these two systems: the T cell, or cellular immune system, and the B cell, or humoral immune system.

Patients with defects in their B-cell system usually experience infections with high-grade encapsulated microorganisms such as *Haemophilus influenzae* and *Streptococcus pneumoniae*. These organisms cause infections ranging in severity from otitis media and pneumonia to septicemia and meningitis. In contrast, patients with abnormal T-cell function more frequently experience infections with opportunistic pathogens, resulting in infections such as disseminated fungal infections, *Pneumocystis carinii* pneumonia, mucocutaneous candidiasis, and overwhelming viral infections such as fatal chickenpox or cytomegalovirus infection.

Several of the unique genetic immunodeficiency disorders appeared to involve both groups of infectious agents, and patients with these disorders were shown to have defects in both the T-cell and the B-cell immune systems. These combined or dual system immunodeficiency disorders are the focus of this chapter.

SEVERE COMBINED IMMUNODEFICIENCY

Severe combined immunodeficiency (SCID) is the most extreme form of the inherited or primary immunodeficiency diseases. It is characterized by profound functional defects in both the humoral and the cell-mediated immune systems. A family history of similarly affected relatives occurs in about half the cases. Within the general classification of SCID are several distinct disorders with different modes of inheritance and different patterns of cellular deficiency. Both autosomal-recessive and X-linked inherited forms have been described in SCID. One type is associated with agranulocytosis as well as dual-system immunodeficiency. Other forms of SCID are characterized by an absence of all lymphocytes or by an absence of T cells but not B cells. Originally, SCID was seen only in infants because the immune deficit was so severe that patients usually died of infection within the first weeks or months of life. With earlier diagnosis and improved medical care, longevity is no longer so limited, and curative therapy for all patients is now available.

■ CLINICAL FEATURES

Infants with SCID often present with infections within the first months of life. Recurrent pneumonia, failure to thrive, chronic diarrhea, and persistent candidiasis of the mouth, esophagus, and skin of the face and diaper area are common. These infants may have infections with all types of microorganisms, but opportunistic pathogens tend to dominate the clinical picture. Death has occurred from generalized chickenpox, measles with Hecht's (giant cell) pneumonia, disseminated mycobacterial infection, and cytomegalovirus and adenovirus infections. When smallpox vaccination was used routinely, SCID infants regularly developed fatal generalized vaccinia infections. Live attenuated polio vaccine may cause paralytic poliomyelitis in infants with SCID, although it is often tolerated without symptoms in these patients. In addition to infections, many infants with SCID have developed graft-versus-host disease (GVHD) after transfusions of whole blood containing immunocompetent donor T lymphocytes. Maternal lymphocytes entering fetal circulation during labor and delivery or during gestation also have caused GVHD in infants with SCID.

■ IMMUNOLOGIC FINDINGS

SCID is classified as a profound dual-system immunodeficiency, meaning that SCID patients essentially have no normal function in either their T- or B-cell systems. Careful laboratory evaluation, however, reveals great heterogeneity within

this general diagnostic group with certain cellular components of the immune system preserved in some patients. Serum immunoglobulins vary from panhypogammaglobulinemia to variable partial immunoglobulin deficiency involving only one or two of the major isotypes. Antibody responses, however, almost always are profoundly impaired. B lymphocytes are absent in some SCID patients, whereas other patients have normal or even elevated B-cell numbers. Particularly in the X-linked variety, B cells may account for all of the circulating lymphocytes. Most tests of T-cell function are abnormal. The children are anergic to cutaneous delayed-hypersensitivity skin testing. Usually, the number of T cells in the blood is depressed to less than 10% of normal in more than 80% of SCID patients. In vitro tests show T-cell function is markedly impaired with defective proliferative, cytotoxic, and immunoregulatory activity. Patients occasionally retain some proliferative capacity to respond to allogeneic cells (lymphocytes from a nonidentical twin) or to one or more mitogens. In these patients, however, antigen proliferation is always nil.

■ PATHOGENESIS

SCID is a disease category that includes a heterogeneous group of disorders; no single pathogenic mechanism is common to all patients. Defects that lead to immunodeficiency include failure of differentiation into mature T or B cells, failure to transduce the antigen signal, poor cytokine secretion, and failure to recognize antigen. SCID is inherited as either an autosomal or X-linked recessive disease.

■ TREATMENT OF SCID

Development of effective treatment for these desperately ill children is a major challenge to clinical immunology. In 1968, bone marrow transplantation was introduced to clinical medicine when an infant with SCID was given a bone marrow transplant from a histocompatible sibling donor. The transplanted marrow completely reconstituted both the T- and the B-cell immune systems in this infant, and this reconstitution has persisted. Although the bone marrow is generally considered to provide a source of stem cells, at least some of the restoration is due to post-thymic T cells and mature B cells that apparently are long-lived and replicating. Overall, 50% to 60% of SCID patients treated by bone marrow transplantation are cured. The percentage would be higher if patients were all in good general health at the time of transplantation.

In many forms of combined immunodeficiency, conditioning of the patient with myeloablative or immunosuppressive drugs or x-ray is not necessary. Occasionally sufficient immunity to reject a marrow is present even in those children with profound deficiencies, and pretransplant conditioning is required. Laboratory tests to identify this variant of combined immunodeficiency precisely are not available.

Bone marrow transplantation may cause fatal GVHD because of the disparity of histocompatibility antigens. The donor and recipient must be matched appropriately to minimize this complication. When donors are matched, prophylaxis for GVHD is unnecessary, and only occasionally is GVHD severe enough to require therapy. The inheritance of the transplantation antigens is such that, except in rare circumstances, only siblings are a match. This event occurs about 25% of the time. With today's small families and the frequency with which first children are affected, the actual number of matched donors available for bone marrow transplantation is slightly less than 25%. Because GVHD primarily is caused by mature T cells, if they are eliminated, bone marrow can be transplanted even from a mismatched donor without fatal GVHD. This strategy enlarges the donor pool. In practice, a parent is used as the donor, because at least 50% of the antigens (haploidentical) including minor antigens that are not assessed by tissue-typing techniques, will match. A haploidentical sibling also is a suitable donor if age and size are not precluding factors.

More than 300 transplantations for SCID using haploidentical bone marrow donors have been performed. The long-term survival rate appears to be equal to that achieved with matched donors. Bone marrow transplantation using haploidentical partners, however, is significantly more complicated. Conditioning is more often necessary, implying that the mature T cells of the nondepleted marrows are actively involved in the engraftment process. Second and third transplants are necessary more often. The B-cell engraftment may be less complete, and the incidence of post-transplant B-cell lymphomas is higher. Nevertheless, haploidentical bone marrow transplantation is the preferred method of treatment if no fully matched sibling or close relative is available. Strides are being made in understanding and overcoming the problems of haploidentical bone marrow transplantation. Matched unrelated donors (MUD) have been used with success. In this strategy, a national or worldwide search for an individual with closely matched histocompatibility antigens is conducted. A major problem with unrelated transplants is the difficulty in finding donors for minority groups that are underrepresented in the available donor pools.

Alternative forms of treatment have included thymus transplantation, combined thymus and fetal liver transplantation, and intrauterine transplantation. Overall, the results of these transplantations are inferior to those of bone marrow transplantation. A few long-term survivors, however, have impressive degrees of reconstitution.

Bone marrow transplantation has been successful in both ADA(+) and ADA(-) SCID patients. As an alternative to transplantation, enzyme replacement has also been tried in ADA(-) SCID. Initially, exchange transfusions with irradiated whole blood were used because erythrocytes are a rich source of ADA. Red blood cell (RBC) transfusions have not proven to be effective treatment, although they have resulted in some improvement in lymphocyte function in vitro and in correction of the levels of deoxyadenosine in the blood and deoxyATP in the lymphocytes. Recently, bovine ADA has been conjugated with polyethylene glycol (PEG-ADA) and given as weekly intramuscular injections to ADA(-) SCID patients. The PEG conjugation renders the bovine enzyme less immunogenic and extends the serum half-life of the ADA from minutes to several hours. In the few patients treated with this material, there is a striking increase in lymphocyte numbers in the blood, an improvement in in vitro lymphocyte function tests, and some indication of clinical benefit. Antigen-specific immune responses, however, have not been consistent in treated patients, so PEG-ADA treatment may not result in sustained clinical correction.

ADA deficiency is the first immunodeficiency disease to be treated by gene therapy. Already, T-cell lines established from ADA(-) SCID patients have been "cured" in vitro after successful transfer of the human ADA gene into these cells using a recombinant retrovirus vector gene transfer system. A limited number of children have received monthly infusions of 1 billion transfected cells. After several months of treatment, one child's immunity improved enough to stop infusions; the length of persistent benefit is being assessed. This patient now attends a regular school. Successful transfection of stem cells is the next step.

ATAXIA-TELANGIECTASIA

Ataxia-telangiectasia (AT) is an autosomal-recessive multisystem disorder characterized by severe cerebellar ataxia, oculocutaneous telangiectasia, variable immunodeficiency, and high incidence of malignancy. The neurologic symptoms usually dominate the clinical picture with onset at about the time the child is learning to walk. The disorder frequently results in profound disability, and the patient becomes almost totally dependent on others for care and feeding.

■ CLINICAL FEATURES

The cerebellar dysfunction is manifested early as ataxia and is followed by choreoathetosis, severe involuntary myoclonic jerking movements, and oculomotor abnormalities. The telangiectasia usually appear first on the bulbar conjunctiva at between 2 and 5 years of age (Figure 191–1). They then begin to appear on the skin of exposed areas and on areas of trauma such as the nasal bridge, ears, and flexor folds on the neck and extremities. Other features involving the skin include café-au-lait spots, vitiligo, and prematurely gray hair. Multiple endocrine abnormalities are common, and half of patients have abnormal glucose tolerance tests. Hypoplasia or agenesis of the ovaries is common in females, but hypogonadism is less common in males. Cancer develops in as many as 15% of AT patients. Non-Hodgkin's lymphomas predominate in these patients as they do in many other primary immunodeficiency diseases, whereas carcinomas are more common in older patients. Adult males with AT who have IgA deficiency have a 70-fold increase in risk of developing carcinoma of the stomach.

Recurrent infections are a major feature in some patients, whereas other patients have relatively little trouble with infections until late in life. The degree of immune deficit correlates to the frequency of infectious episodes experienced by patients. Sinopulmonary infections are most common, and chronic bronchopulmonary disease is usually a contributing factor in a patient's demise.

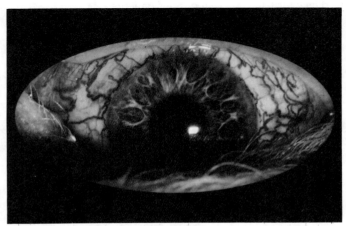

Figure 191-1. Striking telangiectasia on the bulbar conjunctiva of a 22-year-old patient with ataxia-telangiectasia. These dilated vessels typically appear between ages 2 and 5 years, first in the eye and later on cutaneous areas of chronic exposure or trauma.

■ IMMUNOLOGIC DEFECTS

Patients with AT, even within the same family, have varying degrees of immunodeficiency. Defects in both the T- and the B-cell immune systems have been reported. The most consistent defects in humoral immunity are IgA deficiency in 75% and IgE deficiency in 85% of cases. IgG_2 and IgG_4 deficiency are also common. Eighty percent of patients have serum IgM in a monomeric 7S form rather than the pentameric 19S molecule usually seen in the blood. The T-cell system also has a variety of abnormalities, including skin-test anergy in about half the patients and depressed lymphocyte proliferative responses in an equal proportion. An even higher percentage have depressed cytotoxic T-cell responses, and many have defects in immunoregulatory T-cell function as well.

■ PATHOGENESIS

The fundamental defect underlying the immune system and neurologic dysfunction in AT is unknown. One hypothesis arises from observations that patients are sensitive to ionizing radiation and radiomimetic drugs. Further, cultured fibroblasts from AT patients have a markedly reduced ability to form colonies and grow in vitro after being exposed to x-irradiation. There is presumed to be a major defect in one or more of the repair mechanisms for DNA in these patients, but the precise nature of the defect has not been elucidated. In more than half the cases, the sites of chromosomal breakage involve chromosomes 7 and 14 at the sites of the T-cell receptor genes and the immunoglobulin heavy-chain genes. These are chromosomal regions that regularly undergo DNA rearrangements, deletions, and repair during the course of the generation of the cellular antigen receptors and during heavy-chain class switch.

It has been suggested that normal levels of IgA and IgE and normal numbers of mature T cells with alpha/beta T-cell receptors require an immune system that differentiates efficiently and successfully over a protracted period of time, because more gene rearrangement events are required for their development. With the DNA repair defect in AT patients, the generation of these more "downstream" immune products is less efficient. Thus, the immune deficit is characterized by a lack of IgA, IgE, and alpha/beta T cells. The translocations also are associated with the high tendency for leukemia found in AT patients.

■ TREATMENT

No specific useful therapy corrects both the neurologic and the immunologic defects in this disease. Immunoglobulin replacement therapy and blood transfusions have been associated in some instances with fatal episodes of anaphylaxis in AT patients. These episodes occur because IgA-deficient AT patients may make IgG antibodies to IgA, which then react with IgA in the transfusion and cause a serious anaphylactic reaction. Administration of any blood product to an AT patient should be done with caution, and treatment for shock should be instituted as soon as any signs of a reaction appear.

WISKOTT-ALDRICH SYNDROME

Wiskott-Aldrich syndrome (WAS) is an X-linked disorder showing the triad of recurrent infection with all classes of microorganisms, hemorrhage secondary to thrombocytopenia, and eczema of the skin. Bleeding episodes or symptoms due to infection typically begin during the first 6 months of life.

■ CLINICAL FEATURES

WAS is characterized by recurrent infections and a variety of significant clinical abnormalities, which frequently overshadow the infections as management problems. Both high-grade and opportunistic pathogens cause infections. Patients frequently come to medical attention initially with otitis media or pneumonia caused by *S pneumoniae* or *H influenzae*. They also are prone to septicemia or meningitis with these organisms. *Candida albicans*, cytomegalovirus, and *P carinii* are also causes of significant infectious episodes in these children. WAS patients have died of generalized vaccinia after smallpox vaccination, and disseminated herpes simplex has also been reported. Chickenpox has also been lethal to WAS patients, particularly to those treated with corticosteroids (Figure 191–2).

The thrombocytopenia in WAS is unique because the platelets are very small in size and depressed in number, often in the 15,000 to 30,000 range. Small or microthrombocytes are not found regularly in any other thrombocytopenic disease, and their presence is perhaps the best single test to confirm the diagnosis of WAS. Bleeding accounts for about 30% of the mortality in WAS with intracranial hemorrhage being the greatest threat.

The third component of the clinical triad defining WAS is eczema of the skin. In addition, patients experience a high incidence of severe autoimmune disease. This autoaggressive disorder may take on many forms, including severe

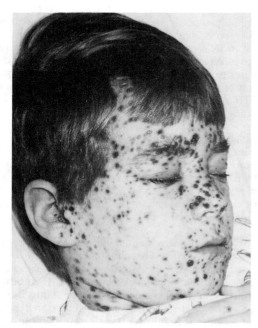

Figure 191-2. A Wiskott-Aldrich syndrome (WAS) patient with severe chickenpox covering every square inch of his skin. Patients with combined immunodeficiency are at particular risk for overwhelming varicella infection. This is especially true for WAS patients who are receiving corticosteroid treatment for the autoimmune disease that occasionally complicates management of their WAS disorder.

Coombs positive or negative hemolytic anemia, a JRA-like disorder with fevers and joint involvement, leukocytoclastic vasculitis usually involving the lower legs, and larger-vessel vasculitis affecting the coronary or cerebral arteries. In addition to their intrinsic thrombocytopenia, patients also develop an ITP-like thrombocytopenia, which is usually only appreciated after their original thrombocytopenia is corrected by splenectomy. This is often seen in association with high levels of circulating immune complexes and may be an ominous sign of clinical deterioration.

Another striking feature of WAS is a high incidence of malignancy. Patients with many of the primary immunodeficiency diseases show an increased frequency of cancer, and WAS patients have been estimated to have a cancer frequency 128 times that in the normal population. Most cancers are non-Hodgkin's lymphomas with the brain involved in more than half of cases. Despite this high incidence of lymphoma, the peripheral lymph nodes almost never contain cancer, although they often become markedly enlarged. Since the introduction of routine antibiotic prophylaxis and splenectomy, the incidence of cancer with this disease may be falling.

■ IMMUNOLOGIC DEFECTS

Wiskott-Aldrich syndrome is unique among the immunodeficiency diseases because it has selective defects involving each component of the host defense system, rather than having the more global defects seen in diseases like SCID. The patients have variable patterns of immunoglobulins in their serum, with the most typical profile consisting of normal levels of IgG, IgA elevated to about twice normal levels, and IgM at about half the normal level. Antibody responses to many antigens, such as tetanus, are normal, whereas responses to others are absent. WAS is the only disease that fails to produce antibodies to an entire class of antigens, the polysaccharides. Because of this unique defect, these patients have low or absent isohemagglutinins and do not produce antibody to the capsular polysaccharides of H influenzae or the pneumococci. This immune defect explains patients' susceptibility to infection with encapsulated organisms despite normal or elevated immunoglobulin levels, and their ability to make antibody to protein antigens like tetanus toxoid.

Another abnormality unique to WAS patients is that they hypercatabolize their serum immunoglobulins and albumin at a very rapid rate. The serum half-life of IgM, IgG, IgA, and albumin in WAS patients is only one third to one half of normal rates, so to keep serum levels normal, these proteins are synthesized at far greater than normal rates.

The cellular immune system also has selective defects in many functions. WAS patients are anergic and even have impaired rejection of skin allografts. They do have normal or near-normal numbers of T lymphocytes in their blood and a normal ratio of CD4+ to CD8+ T cells. The T cells can proliferate normally to mitogens and can produce IL-1, IL-2, gamma interferon, and other cytokines when stimulated appropriately. Nevertheless, cells usually respond poorly to antigens like tetanus and to allogeneic cells in mixed lymphocyte culture, and they do not develop self-restricted antigen-specific cytotoxic T cells, even to antigens to which they make antibodies, such as influenza.

The monocytes from WAS patients have defects in chemotaxis and cytotoxic function mediated by antibodies and by the endogenous mannosyl-fucosyl membrane receptor. Even the granulocytes from these patients are involved with defective chemotactic responsiveness, a common finding although their bactericidal capacity seems to be normal.

■ PATHOGENESIS

The fundamental defect in WAS that leads to all the diverse manifestations is not known. The selective defects in the function of T cells, B cells, platelets, granulocytes, and monocytes demonstrate that this disorder cannot be the result of a defect in the differentiation of a single cellular lineage such as is seen in X-linked agammaglobulinemia. Rather, some more general cellular defect must be present. A cell-membrane glycoprotein, sialophorin, has been shown to be defective on the lymphocytes of WAS patients, as well as on those from other immunodeficient subjects. A different glycoprotein is also abnormal on the platelets from WAS patients. A defect in an X-linked transacting factor involved in cell membrane structure or stability might be the site of the primary defect in this disease. There are at least seven distinct immunodeficiency diseases that are inherited as X-linked traits, and each of those studied has mapped to a different region of the X chromosome. The WAS maps to the short arm of X near the centromere.

As with most X-linked diseases, the female carriers of this genetic defect are immunologically and hematologically normal, displaying none of the abnormalities found in the affected males. Because females are mosaic for genes encoded on their X chromosomes (random X-inactivation—lyonization—occurs in the embryo), it is expected that some defect in immune or platelet function would be found in the carriers. This would be true unless those precursors whose X-chromosomes bore the defective WAS gene were at a selective disadvantage and not differentiating or developing. Normally, all cell lineages in a female have the same ratio of cells in which each of the parental X chromosomes is active. On the average, half of a female's cells use the paternally derived X chromosome and the other half use the maternally derived X. Skin biopsy samples from WAS carriers show this expected pattern of X inactivation, with roughly half the cells using either the maternally or the paternally derived X chromosome. All T cells, B cells, and granulocytes from these carriers, however, use only one of the two possible X chromosomes, the chromosome carrying the normal WAS gene. This striking unbalanced pattern of X-chromosome inactivation is not seen in normal females, and, therefore, its presence provides a convenient test to detect carriers of this X-linked disease.

■ TREATMENT

There are several approaches to the treatment of WAS. HLA-matched bone marrow transplantation is the treatment of choice if a matched sibling donor is available. After transplantation, all of the manifestations of this disease, including the eczema and autoimmune problems, are corrected.

Treatment for patients lacking an HLA-identical sibling donor presents a more difficult decision. T-cell-depleted, haploidentical bone marrow transplantation has been successful depending on the treatment center. There is a high incidence of failure of engraftment, GVHD, and B-cell proliferative disease complicating this form of treatment. There is increasing success with matched unrelated donors.

Splenectomy cures the thrombocytopenia in more than 90% of patients, has a major impact on the quality of life, and simplifies medical management. It is essential that prophylactic antibiotics or intravenous gamma globulin be used regularly, because these patients are more susceptible to overwhelming sepsis after removal of the spleen. The platelet size also becomes normal after splenectomy.

The autoaggressive syndrome recently recognized as a common complication of this disease may be very difficult to treat. The leukocytoclastic vasculitis usually responds to nonsteroidal anti-inflammatory drugs but may require systemic corticosteroids. The thrombocytopenia that sometimes occurs after splenectomy usually resolves without specific treatment, although some patients require aggressive treatment with intravenous gamma globulin, steroids, and even vincristine therapy to control this complication. As with all patients with severe T-cell immunodeficiency, all transfusions containing blood cells should be irradiated to prevent the development of GVHD.

Although these patients experience many different and sometimes serious medical problems, the overall prognosis is improving. Several patients treated by splenectomy have reached adulthood, married, and had children; patients treated successfully by bone marrow transplantation should have a nearly normal life expectancy.

DIGEORGE'S ANOMALY (THYMIC HYPOPLASIA, THIRD AND FOURTH PHARYNGEAL POUCH SYNDROME)

DiGeorge's anomaly (formerly DiGeorge's syndrome) is a congenital immunodeficiency disease caused by the maldevelopment of structures derived from the first through sixth branchial pouches during embryonic development. Structures derived from the branchial pouches include portions of the ear and certain facial features, portions of the aortic arch and heart, the parathyroids and thyroid, and the thymus.

■ CLINICAL FEATURES

Patients with DiGeorge's anomaly usually present in early infancy with symptoms unrelated to immunodeficiency. Congenital heart lesions, particularly conotruncal defects such as truncus arteriosus and interrupted aortic arch type B, are common presenting problems during the first 2 weeks of life. Abnormal calcium homeostasis because of hypoparathyroidism is seen in nearly all patients, and hypocalcemic tetany is the most common initial problem. Facial abnormalities include microstomia, hypertelorism,

upturned nose, posteriorly rotated and small, low-set ears with notched pinnae, and anti-Mongoloid slant of the eyes (Figure 191–3). Hypothyroidism, esophageal atresia, tracheoesophageal fistula, and a bifid uvula also have been described in these patients. If the patients survive the newborn period and they fall in the approximately 25% who have a significant immune deficit, then they will experience an increased susceptibility to infections, including recurrent pneumonia, diarrhea, and candidiasis of the mouth, oropharynx, esophagus, and skin of the diaper area.

■ IMMUNOLOGIC DEFECTS

DiGeorge's anomaly is extremely variable in extent of clinical manifestations and degree of immunodeficiency. Immunologic defects are the direct consequence of the failure of thymus development, and vary from severe deficiency to normal. Some patients may show a slight deficiency at birth but improved immune responses with time. About 25% of DiGeorge's anomaly patients have a persistent immune defect that is severe enough to require correction. They may be defined by measurement of the number of CD4+ T cells (less than 400/mm³) or their response to phytohemagglutinin stimulation (less than 10 times background). The total lymphocyte count is usually normal but consists mostly of B cells and non-T cells. The morphology of the spleen and lymph nodes reflects the T-lymphopenia with depletion seen in the usual "thymic-dependent areas." Immunoglobulin production is variable.

■ PATHOGENESIS

The structures affected in the DiGeorge's anomaly derive from the pharyngeal pouches. The third pouch gives rise to the parathyroids, the third and fourth produce the thymus, the first and second contribute to the lip and ear, and the sixth produces the pulmonary artery and the ultimobranchial body. These pouch derivatives all depend on a major contribution from the cephalic neural crest. If neural crest development is inhibited, multiple pouches are deprived. Multiple insults can affect the neural crest; in this way, the association of DiGeorge's anomaly with many apparently unrelated intrauterine insults is explained. These

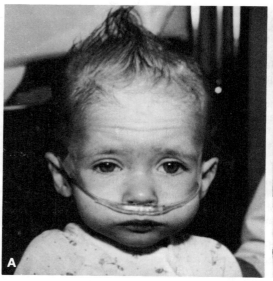
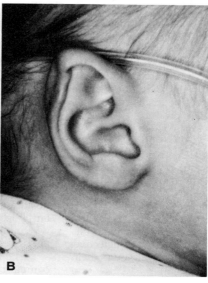

Figure 191-3. DiGeorge's anomaly is a congenital disorder involving maldevelopment of the structures derived from the first through the sixth pharyngeal pouches during embryonic life. As a consequence, these children often have facial abnormalities, as illustrated in this child by hypertelorism, defective low-set ears, hypoplastic mandible, and upward bowing of the upper lip (**A**). Closeup of the ears shows notched pinna and deficient helix formation (**B**).

causes range from teratogen exposure (retinoids, alcohol) to chromosomal abnormalities (monosomy 22) to midline developmental defects such as arrhinencephaly.

■ TREATMENT

The nonimmunologic features of DiGeorge's anomaly are often more life-threatening to newborns than is the immunodeficiency. Initial treatment should be directed at controlling the congenital heart disease and the metabolic abnormalities of these infants. Hypoparathyroidism and associated hypocalcemia are treated with vitamin D and calcium, and may require long-term replacement. The congenital heart disease frequently is severe and often requires immediate surgical intervention. Treatment of the heart lesion should not be deferred until after correction of the immune defect. Despite the immune system compromise, patients tolerate the surgical procedures very well. All blood products must be irradiated, however.

When a deficiency state is confirmed, immunologic reconstitution can be accomplished. Thymus transplantation using cultured glands obtained from small children has been successful. Bone marrow transplantation using a matched sibling has been successful.

(Abridged from Richard Hong, Combined Immunodeficiency Diseases, in Oski, DeAngelis, Feigin, McMillan, Warshaw: *Principles and Practice of Pediatrics, Second Edition*, J.B. Lippincott, 1994.)

Oski's Essential Pediatrics,
edited by Kevin B. Johnson and Frank A. Oski.
Lippincott–Raven Publishers,
Philadelphia © 1997

192

Pediatric AIDS

Pediatric acquired immunodeficiency syndrome (AIDS) is a severe clinical manifestation of infection with human immunodeficiency virus, type 1 (HIV-1). Most pediatric HIV-1 infections are transmitted perinatally from infected mothers; as such, pediatric AIDS resembles other sexually transmitted diseases with perinatal consequences, such as syphilis and hepatitis B. The etiologic agent of AIDS, HIV-1, infects and kills thymus-derived lymphocytes bearing the CD4 molecule. The loss of these cells results in immunodeficiency and the clinical consequences thereof. Thus, pediatric AIDS is a viral-associated secondary immunodeficiency.

■ ETIOLOGIC AGENT AND PATHOGENESIS

The virus etiologically associated with AIDS is a human retrovirus belonging to the subfamily Lentivirinae. Visna, a neurotropic "slow" virus of sheep, is the prototype of this viral subfamily. A closely related sheep virus, Maedi, is also known as progressive pneumonia virus (PPV); it produces a lymphocytic interstitial pneumonitis (LIP) in sheep. Histologically, the pulmonary lesions caused by PPV are similar to those noted in HIV-1 infected pediatric patients.

HIV-1 infects CD4-bearing lymphocytes by way of high-affinity binding of the viral envelope to the CD4 receptor molecule. Because the affinity of viral binding to the CD4 receptor is higher than for most HIV-1 neutralizing antibodies, HIV-1 infection is favored over neutralization. A second characteristic of HIV-1 is its ability to replicate in T lymphocytes. Retroviral replication depends on cellular DNA synthesis and cell division. Because lymphocytes generally undergo cell division in response to specific antigenic stimuli or differentiation signals, the virus has a number of accessory genes that regulate viral replication. Genetically, HIV-1 is one of the most complicated retroviruses. This complexity is associated with the unique life cycle of the virus—a combination of tropism for highly differentiated cells such as lymphocytes and the ability of the virus to be transmitted horizontally from person to person. As the virus replicates in the lymphocyte, the CD4+ cells are killed and immunologic dysfunction ensues. Exposure to any body fluid with HIV-1 infected lymphocytes carries a potential for transmission; however, blood has the highest titers. The immune system may control the infection within a host but cannot eliminate HIV-1 infected T lymphocytes from the body. The immunologic dysfunction associated with lymphocyte killing eventuates in dysgammaglobulinemia. This is manifest as hypergammaglobulinemia in most cases with about 10% of children having a panhypogammaglobulinemia. Also associated with significant dysfunction is the inability of the host to mount a normal primary immune response to new antigens. This, in turn, is associated with an increased susceptibility to pathogenic bacteria and fungi. Similarly, the virally mediated destruction of CD4+ lymphocytes results in lower numbers of absolute CD4+ lymphocytes, a relatively specific sign of immune dysfunction. The progressive loss of CD4+ lymphocytes is associated with the loss of the ability of the HIV-1 infected host to respond rapidly to primary infections or to regulate latent infections such as herpes viruses.

The host immune response to HIV-1 can be measured by both antigen-binding (serologic) and functional (neutralization of viral infectivity) antibody tests. Antibody responses in children are quantitatively similar to those in adults. In infants, however, particularly in the first 6 months of life, antibody levels may be low and are confounded by the presence of maternal antibody. As in adults, there is evidence that the host immune response partially inhibits replication of HIV-1. In certain clinical disease patterns such as LIP, there is a marked lymphocytic inflammatory component. In contrast to the process for most viral infections, the host's immune response does not eliminate virus-infected cells. Virus can usually be recovered from the blood of all infected children. Thus, HIV-1 infection is a chronic, persistent infection directed principally at CD4+ lymphocytes.

HIV-1 evades immune elimination by several mechanisms. Several potentially relevant characteristics of the persistence phenomenon include direct infection and elimination of subsets of T lymphocytes that are important in immune regulation. The external envelope glycoprotein coat of HIV-1 contains more carbohydrate than most human viruses; this may block recognition of immunogenic epitopes of the virus. Also, there is a high error rate of reverse transcription of the viral genome that results in enormous heterogeneity of the protein sequence of the HIV-1 envelope. This causes the immune response to be continually redirected as new B- and T-cell epitopes are generated, particularly in the external glycoprotein gp120. Finally, HIV-1 can infect macrophages. Because macrophages generally divide slowly and present antigen to lymphocytes, HIV-1 infection of macrophages offers an opportunity for the virus to remain latent and to be able to infect CD4+ lymphocytes without having to pass outside the cell and thereby risk destruction by the immune system.

■ EPIDEMIOLOGY

Pediatric AIDS and HIV-1 infections generally occur in three settings. First and most common, infection is transmitted perinatally from an infected mother. This may occur in utero, during delivery by exposure to the mother's infected blood, or postpartum, by ingestion of breast milk. There is no evidence of casual transmission of HIV-1 in households, day care settings, or schools. The perinatally infected child usually exhibits signs of HIV-1 infection in the first 2 years of life but may asymptomatically harbor virus for years before developing clinical manifestations. Perinatal transmission accounts for more than 80% of pediatric AIDS cases in the United States and nearly all new cases worldwide. The second setting involves blood or blood-product recipients. Pediatric patients who received blood products before March 1985, the time when HIV-1 donor screening began, have a higher risk of HIV-1 infection than do more recent recipients; however, the number of units received is an important variable. Finally, adolescents constitute the third setting in which HIV-1 infection is acquired. At least three factors contribute to adolescent risk. First, adolescent risk behavior in general is high, and exposure to drugs and higher-risk sexual behavior is increased. Second, sexually active adolescent women have a 1000-fold higher risk of acquiring any sexually transmitted disease, including HIV-1. Third, male homosexual behavior often begins in the adolescent period, and the opportunity for HIV-1 infection is particularly high in receptive anal intercourse. The incidence of AIDS in adolescents remains relatively low because of the latent period of disease, but the HIV-1 infection rate is likely to be increasing.

The Centers for Disease Control and Prevention (CDC) pediatric case definition for AIDS forms the basis for the pediatric AIDS surveillance system. This system includes pediatric patients younger than age 13 years and depends on local and state reporting. Approximately 1.7% of overall AIDS incidence in the United States is due to pediatric cases. This proportion is higher in parts of the world where heterosexual transmission of HIV-1 is more common. Pediatric AIDS incidence in the United States parallels the incidence of AIDS in women. The actual number of children with HIV infection in the United States is not known, but it is estimated that, in 1990, 6000 at-risk infants were born in the United States to mothers with HIV-1 infection. In addition, more cases are being identified in rural areas. Cases of AIDS in women and children continue to increase, whereas the incidence in other populations has stabilized.

Clinically asymptomatic women are the major source of perinatal HIV-1 infection. Immunologically, HIV-1 infected women have elevated IgG and lowered absolute levels of CD4+ lymphocytes. Generally, it is only through serologic screening for HIV-1 that women at risk of infecting newborn infants can be identified, because clinically they are often asymptomatic. The major risk factors for mothers appear to be either intravenous drug abuse or heterosexual contact with an HIV-1 infected male. A number of independent studies in different populations indicate that the risk that an infected mother will transmit HIV-1 and infect her infant is 13% to 39%.

The geographic distribution of HIV-1 infected women and children mirrors other aspects of the AIDS epidemic. In general, perinatal pediatric AIDS in the United States has been noted predominantly in East Coast urban areas and Puerto Rico. Worldwide, the urban pattern predominates, and areas with an increased incidence of sexually transmitted diseases and intravenous drug abuse (IVDA) are expected to be sources of pediatric AIDS cases. A more specific characteristic of perinatal AIDS in the United States is the preponderance of cases in lower socioeconomic classes and in racial and ethnic minorities. Seventy percent of perinatal AIDS cases are associated with IVDA. The CDC reports a doubling of pediatric AIDS incidence approximately every 16 months.

■ CLINICAL MANIFESTATIONS

HIV-1 infection is a chronic, multisystem infection. Thus, the presentation of clinical disease is varied. The CDC has devised a pediatric classification system that outlines the spectrum of clinical disease. A number of nonspecific findings may herald the onset of clinical disease. These include failure to thrive, generalized lymphadenopathy, hepatosplenomegaly, persistent oral candidiasis, recurrent or chronic diarrhea, and, rarely, parotitis. Similar findings occur in other congenital infections, primary immunodeficiencies, and other secondary immunodeficiencies, including malnutrition and cancer. Initially, the differential diagnosis is extensive. To shorten the time to diagnosis, consideration should be given to the epidemiologic setting in which such nonspecific findings exist. If the prevalence of HIV-1 infection is high, then appropriate testing should be done early, when clinical signs manifest. Testing should be done with parental consent, counseling, and confidentiality.

Pneumocystis carinii pneumonia (PCP) is the most common and serious opportunistic infection in children with AIDS. As a consequence of HIV-1 infection acquired perinatally, PCP usually occurs in the first year of life and is associated with high morbidity and mortality. Onset of the disease may be acute or subacute, with fever and tachypnea as common presenting signs. Bilateral interstitial perihilar infiltrates develop as the disease progresses. Diagnosis is made by demonstration of the organism in endotracheal aspirates, bronchial washings, or lung tissue. Because other pneumonias can present with a similar picture in immunocompromised hosts, aggressive diagnosis and treatment are necessary. *Candida* esophagitis is another common opportunistic infection. Children with poor oral intake, dysphagia, vomiting, and fever associated with oral candidiasis are candidates for diagnostic studies. A barium swallow suggests the diagnosis, which can be confirmed by endoscopy with biopsy and appropriate culture. Other opportunistic infections include disseminated cytomegalovirus infection, *Mycobacterium avium* intracellulare complex infection, cryptosporidiosis, recurrent herpes simplex infection, and, less commonly, cryptococcosis and toxoplasmosis.

LIP occurs in about 30% of HIV-1 infected children and is an AIDS-defining diagnosis. LIP is characterized by the presence of bilateral reticulonodular infiltrates with or without hilar lymphadenopathy. Diagnosis is confirmed by lung biopsy, although in most instances the diagnosis is made presumptively, based on the persistence of typical radiographic findings and a failure to demonstrate infectious agents. The onset of LIP is usually insidious; histologically, the lesions are characterized by the presence of lymphocytes, plasmacytes, and mononuclear cells in the interstitial and peribronchiolar areas. The disease may be static or progressive, resulting in chronic lung disease with the development of hypoxemia and pulmonary hypertension. The pathophysiology of LIP remains unclear, although regional immunity of bronchial associated lymphoid tissue is involved.

Recurrent bacterial infections in HIV-1 infected children have been seen with increasing frequency and include infections with *Streptococcus pneumoniae*, *Haemophilus influenzae* type b, *Salmonella* species, and *Staphylococcus aureus*. The spectrum of infections reported is broad and includes bacteremia, meningitis, septic arthritis, osteomyelitis, pneumonia, urinary tract infections, otitis media, and deep and superficial abscesses. Gram-negative enteric infections occur, particularly in the chronically ill host. The paradoxically high levels of immunoglobulin G, likely secondary to T-cell dysfunction, mask an associated inability to produce specific antibody to protein and polysaccharide antigens.

Central nervous system (CNS) abnormalities have been described in as many as 50% to 90% of HIV-infected children. Neurodevelopmental abnormalities range from mild developmental delay to progressive encephalopathy. The encephalopathy may be static or progressive, and is characterized by loss of developmental milestones, weakness usually beginning in the lower extremities with extension to the trunk and upper extremities, and secondary microcephaly. Seizures, ataxia, pseudobulbar palsy, myoclonus, and extrapyramidal rigidity are associated findings. The cerebrospinal fluid frequently is normal, but mild pleocytosis or elevated protein may be present. Computed tomography of the brain may show cortical atrophy or calcifications in the basal ganglia. There is increasing evidence that HIV-1 encephalopathy results from direct invasion of HIV-1 into the brain. HIV-1 nucleotide sequences have been demonstrated in the brains of both adults and children at autopsy. HIV-1 also has been cultured from spinal fluid, and intrathecal production of specific antibody has been demonstrated. The mechanism of CNS damage, however, is not clear because the virus does not directly infect neurons. Evidence suggests that some of these effects can be mediated by cytokines.

Nephropathy in children with HIV-1 infection is an important complication. Proteinuria is an early finding, and nephrotic syndrome with renal failure has been described. Pathologic lesions in the kidney include glomerulitis with focal segmental sclerosis or mesangial hyperplasia. Cardiomyopathy may occur as an acute or a subacute process. The clinical picture is similar to that in other cardiomyopathies, presenting with signs of heart failure along with cardiac enlargement and evidence of left ventricular hypertrophy with ST-T wave changes. It is not known if this is a direct effect of HIV-1, is secondary to another virus, or is an immune response to HIV-1.

Other associated clinical manifestations include anemia, leukopenia, and thrombocytopenia. Craniofacial dysmorphia has been described in HIV-infected children, but there is controversy whether this is related to HIV-1 or represents the influence of secondary factors such as maternal alcohol or drug abuse during pregnancy, the consequences of immunodeficiency, or other intercurrent processes. A number of cutaneous viral infections such as Herpes simplex stomatitis, herpes zoster, molluscum contagiosum, and condylomata may be presenting, persistent, or recurrent problems. Cutaneous Kaposi's sarcoma (KS) in children has been reported rarely; the limited number of KS cases in infants have been a diffuse lymphadenopathic form of the disease. Malignancies, most commonly B-cell lymphomas, have been reported in about 2% of children with AIDS.

What factors influence clinical expression of disease in children is not understood. In children reported with AIDS, the mortality ranges from 58% to 61%. Of those diagnosed before 1 year of age, there is a 50% mortality rate within 6 months after diagnosis. Survival varies, depending on clinical presentation. Progressive encephalopathy and PCP tend to be associated with a worse outcome than that for children with LIP. Thus, both age at onset of disease and type of clinical disease appear to influence prognosis. In addition, the effect of newer modalities of therapy such as antiretroviral drugs and PCP prophylaxis on survival has not yet been fully assessed. This illness, however, is among the 10 leading causes of death in children of all ages in the United States and has had a significant effect on infant and child mortality. In major urban areas (eg, New York City), AIDS is the leading cause of death in children 2 to 5 years of age.

■ DIAGNOSIS

The diagnosis of pediatric HIV infection remains a complicated algorithm. The primary and most successful diagnostic procedure objectively documents infection with HIV-1 by direct virus isolation. Studies indicate that virus isolation and polymerase chain reaction (PCR) detection of viral DNA in patient lymphocytes are of comparable sensitivity. Both are positive usually by 2 to 3 months of age if the infant is infected. Serologic tests that measure antibody to HIV-1 reliably indicate either exposure or infection. In the first year of life, serologic tests for HIV-1 remain positive because of the persistence of passively transferred maternal IgG; maternal antibody may persist through age 18 months in some cases. Diagnosis in this age group is most difficult and often rests on viral culture or a combination of clinical findings, documented exposure, or abnormal immunologic findings such as elevated IgG or lowered absolute numbers of CD4+ lymphocytes. HIV-1 core p24 antigen is noted in the serum of symptomatic patients in approximately 25% of cases and is a specific indicator of HIV-1 infection. More sensitive tests for detection of p24 antigen that dissociate antigen and antibody complexes may increase the usefulness of p24 antigen tests for primary diagnosis. A number of new laboratory tests developed for early diagnosis of HIV infection include polymerase chain reaction, detection of IgA antibody to HIV, use of an immune complex dissociation assay for p24, and in vitro methods detecting antibody production against HIV from lymphocytes isolated from the infant. None of these tests are licensed for use in neonatal diagnosis of HIV. In the research setting, a combination of the tests provides a diagnosis by age 3 to 6 months in most children. Infants born to HIV-1 infected mothers and who show no evidence of infection should be closely followed until at least age 18 months. Precision of detecting HIV-1 infection early continues to improve as new techniques become generally available. When perinatal exposure is suspected, the mother should be studied for evidence of infection. Identification of a maternal–child infection indicates the father and other siblings may be infected and necessitates family counseling.

■ TREATMENT

Treatment strategies for HIV-1 infected children have changed dramatically and continue to evolve. Available therapies include antiretroviral drugs and PCP prophylaxis. Selected patients receive intravenous gamma globulin. Supportive treatment and frequent medical monitoring are important. Source of fever and cause of infection should be diagnosed and treated promptly, just as for any severely immunocompromised patient. The immunization schedule for HIV-1 infected or exposed infants includes diphtheria-tetanus-pertussis (DPT), inactivated polio (IPV), measles, mumps, and rubella (MMR), H influenzae type b (HIB), and hepatitis B vaccines. Influenza vaccine and pneumococcal polyvalent vaccines are also recommended. Live attenuated oral poliovirus vaccine (OPV) and Bacille Calmette-Guérin (BCG) are not recommended, although the former has been inadvertently administered to hundreds of HIV-1 infected infants without evidence of problems.

Children with HIV-1 infection may have significant B-cell defects, with a resultant inability to form specific antibody. Such children may benefit from intravenous gamma globulin (IVIG) therapy monthly. A double-blind, placebo-controlled study showed that intravenous gamma globulin administered monthly delayed development of serious bacterial infections in children with CD4$^+$ lymphocyte counts more than 200/mm^3 but did not affect survival. Thus, children with recurrent serious bacterial infection, recurrent pneumonia, hypogammaglobulinemia, or poor antibody formation are candidates for IVIG therapy.

In 1991, a panel of experts convened to determine guidelines for beginning PCP prophylaxis in infants younger than 15 months at risk for HIV as well as for all children with known HIV infection. The basis for these recommendations included the age distribution of PCP among children, CD4$^+$ lymphocyte counts in children with PCP, the high mortality and normative data on CD4$^+$ lymphocyte counts in healthy children at various ages. The following age-adjusted CD4$^+$ lymphocyte counts are recommended thresholds for beginning PCP prophylaxis: 1 month to 11 months, less than 1500 cells/mm^3; 12 months to 23 months, 750 cells/mm^3; 24 months through 5 years, less than 500 cells/mm^3; 6 years and older, less than 200 cells/mm^3. In addition, any infected child with a CD4$^+$ lymphocyte percentage of 20% or less or with a prior episode of PCP should receive prophylaxis. Because of its proven efficacy in prevention of PCP in children with cancer and adults with AIDS, trimethoprim-sulfamethoxazole given three times weekly is the drug of choice for prophylaxis.

Two antiviral agents, zidovudine (ZDV) and dideoxyinosine (DDI), are licensed for use in children. Both are potent inhibitors of HIV-1 replication. ZDV is indicated for children with symptomatic disease. Anemia and neutropenia are the most common adverse effects. Didanosine (ddI) is licensed for use in children with advanced HIV disease who are intolerant to ZDV or who demonstrate significant immunologic or clinical deterioration while on ZDV. Adverse effects reported with ddI therapy include pancreatitis and neutropenia. The drugs are well tolerated in infants and children, and beneficial effects include weight gain, increased energy, an increase in CD4$^+$ lymphocyte count and a decrease in p24 antigen levels. The effect of combination therapy (ZDV plus ddI) and other antiviral agents, dideoxycytosine (ddc) and nevirapine, and immunomodulators such as alpha interferon are being systematically studied in children.

■ PREVENTION

Vaccination appears distant. Although as an adjunct to immune serum globulin and chemotherapy in newborns vaccines may have a future role, at present the most concrete means of preventing pediatric AIDS is to further reduce the risk of blood or blood-product transfusion by improved testing for HIV-1 in blood donors and voluntary donor deferral. To alter the incidence of perinatal pediatric AIDS, it is first necessary to identify HIV-1 infected women. Second, it is essential to counsel known HIV-1 positive women regarding the risk of perinatal transmission of HIV-1 and offer information regarding contraception and family planning. Breast-feeding by HIV-1 positive women is not recommended. These procedures may be only partially successful but are integral to any HIV-1 control program.

One important goal is the prevention of perinatal transmission. The timing and mechanism of perinatal transmission are not well understood. Infection of aborted fetal tissue with HIV has been reported as early as 12 weeks of gestation. Stud-

ies of twins born to HIV seropositive mothers indicate a higher incidence of infection in twin "A," suggesting perinatal exposure to infected secretions during the birth process. One study found that infection in the infant occurred with a subset of the maternal HIV-1 strain, suggesting that immune factors may be important. Other studies of maternal risk factors for perinatal transmission suggest that maternal stage of disease, maternal immune status, and lack of certain antibodies to specific viral epitopes might promote transmission.

Several approaches to the prevention of perinatal AIDS are being considered. One study uses chemotherapy with ZDV in second- and third-trimester pregnant women with CD4$^+$ lymphocyte counts more than 200 and randomizes them to treatment with ZDV or placebo. Their newborns will receive 6 weeks of therapy with the same drug the mother received. The purpose of this approach is to decrease the likelihood of HIV-1 transmission to the fetus. Other drugs such as hyperimmune globulin to HIV (HIVIG) and soluble CD4 linked to IgG are also candidates for drug trials in this population of HIV-1 infected women. To prevent pediatric AIDS, it is apparent that a combination of approaches by teams of health care workers throughout the world is necessary, and the focus must be the HIV-1 infected or at-risk woman.

(Abridged from Gwendolyn B. Scott and Wade P. Parks, Pediatric AIDS, in Oski, DeAngelis, Feigin, McMillan, Warshaw: *Principles and Practice of Pediatrics, Second Edition,* J.B. Lippincott, 1994.)

Oski's Essential Pediatrics,
edited by Kevin B. Johnson and Frank A. Oski.
Lippincott–Raven Publishers,
Philadelphia © 1997

193

General Considerations in Allergy

In the past 20 years, there has been a virtual explosion in our knowledge of the immunologic and biochemical mechanisms responsible for allergic disorders. Data support the pathogenic role of allergy in many cases of asthma, allergic rhinitis, atopic dermatitis, urticaria/angioedema, adverse food reactions, drug and biologic agent reactions, and stinging insect hypersensitivity. Information is available to approach the diagnosis and treatment of these disorders in a rational medical fashion. Much remains to be learned about allergic disorders, but allergy is firmly planted on a scientific base.

Allergy may be defined as any untoward physiologic event caused by an immunologically mediated response. This definition has several components that restrict its scope. First, there must be a demonstrable event or disease, which must be both symptomatic and pathologic. This disease must be related to an antigen or environmental factor, which could be airborne pollen, ingested foods, industrial chemicals, or a parenterally administered drug. Finally, the disease must have a demonstrable immunologic mechanism and must occur as a result of this immune mechanism.

Atopy, on the other hand, is a constellation of chronic diseases based on an IgE-mediated mechanism and that have a strong genetic predisposition. Coca and Cooke initially coined the term *atopy* in 1923 and later suggested that atopy was made up of asthma, allergic rhinitis, and atopic eczema (or atopic dermatitis). Not all asthma, rhinitis, or eczema is IgE-mediated, which results in considerable semantic confusion.

■ CLASSIFICATION OF ALLERGIC DISEASES

Allergic diseases were classified into four types by Gell and Coombs in 1963. The classification is simple and presumes that only one mechanism participates in the pathophysiology of immunologically mediated disease, when diseases usually are associated with diverse immunologic responses. Nevertheless, the classification is helpful and is still used. Although there are four types of allergic reactions, this chapter deals primarily with type I reactions.

Type I (Anaphylactic Reactions)

Type I reactions begin with a response to an antigen that includes IgE antibodies. This class of antibody can bind to the surface of mast cells or circulating basophilic granulocytes. Exposure of these IgE-coated cells to antigen results in cell activation and release of a variety of pharmacologically potent mediators. The interaction of these mediators with blood vessels, bronchi, or mucus-secreting glands causes disease. Examples of this type of allergy include anaphylactic reactions to insect stings, food-induced urticaria, or allergic rhinitis.

Type II (Cytotoxic Reactions)

In type II reactions, antibodies of the IgG or IgM class are formed by the patient to an environmental antigen or self-antigen (as in autoimmune disease). Upon subsequent exposure, the antigen may adsorb to the surface of a cell (because of certain chemical properties) and result in binding of antibody to the adsorbed antigen. Complement activation may ensue, whereupon the cell is damaged or destroyed by the membrane attack complex. Common clinical examples of this allergic reaction include drug-induced leukopenia, hemolytic anemia, and thrombocytopenia.

Type III (Arthus or Immune Complex Reactions)

In type III reactions, as in type II responses, IgG and IgM antibodies to an environmental antigen are produced. In this type of reaction, however, the antigen does not bind to cells but circulates in soluble form. The antigen–antibody complexes that are formed may be small, intermediate, or large. Small complexes may remain harmlessly in the circulation, whereas large complexes are rapidly cleared by the reticuloendothelial system. Intermediate size complexes, however, may become deposited in vessel walls and tissues. Vascular damage is then initiated by activation of complement, granulocytes, platelets, and probably basophils. The most common example of this reaction is classic serum sickness.

Type IV (Cell-Mediated Reactions)

Type IV reactions do not involve antibody but rather involve T-lymphocytes with specific receptors for an antigen. After primary exposure, these cells respond to subsequent exposure by proliferating, by differentiating into cells capable of causing cytolysis (natural killer cells), or by recruiting other cytolytic cells (macrophages). Classic examples of these reactions are contact dermatitis from poison ivy or other chemicals, graft-versus-host reactions, and tuberculin skin tests.

■ CLINICAL PRESENTATION OF THE ATOPIC SYNDROME

Atopy is a syndrome of various chronic disorders of the skin and respiratory tree associated with type I mechanisms. These disorders include atopic dermatitis, allergic rhinitis, and asthma. They constitute a syndrome because each has an identifiable IgE-dependent mechanism, and, therefore, each is frequently associated with one or more of the other disorders. For instance, asthma occurs in 20% to 50% of children with atopic dermatitis, and 80% to 90% of children with asthma have concomitant allergic rhinitis.

A number of allergic signs and symptoms are not included in the atopic syndrome, although some occur frequently in atopic individuals. These include food allergy, drug allergy, insect hypersensitivity, urticaria, angioedema, and contact dermatitis. Epidemiologic studies have not confirmed the suggestion that drug allergy, especially allergy to penicillin, occurs more frequently in atopic individuals. Similarly, anaphylactic allergy to stinging insects is not more common in atopic individuals.

Atopic disease has a strong familial tendency. In a study of college-age persons, the incidence of atopic disease was 15% when no first-degree relative had one of the diseases, 33% when one other relative was atopic, and 68% when two or more relatives were atopic. There is no clear pattern of inheritance, and it is felt to be polygenic. Exposure to several environmental factors such as cigarette smoke, air pollutants, allergens (foods, pollens, and molds), and viral infection have been associated with increased risk of atopic disease.

■ PREVALENCE AND NATURAL HISTORY

Allergic diseases affect 50 million people in the United States, or approximately 20% of the population. Epidemiologic data on the prevalence of atopic dermatitis, asthma, and allergic rhinitis are difficult to obtain because of considerable discrepancies in diagnostic criteria. The cumulative prevalence of asthma among preteenage children is considered 10% to 12% and in school-age children, 8.5% to 12.2%. In western societies, 50% of children with asthma have onset of their disease before age 3 years. Allergic rhinitis is more frequent in boys than girls at a young age; one study of 7 year olds found a prevalence of 6% in boys and 1.5% in girls. Similarly, a study of 5 to 15 year olds found a prevalence of 5% in boys and 3.6% in girls. Atopic dermatitis occurs in 8.3% to 10% of children, with more than 85% of cases presenting before age 5 years. These differences may be related to environmental factors. The incidence of atopic diseases is low (less than 1%) in West Indian populations but quickly rises to levels comparable to Western Europeans when West Indians emigrate. Several studies indicate that the incidence of atopic disease in Western Europe and the United States is increasing.

The natural history of atopic diseases is complex. Each disorder generally appears for the first time at a characteristic age, frequently becomes more severe over a period of months to years, then undergoes a period of prolonged remission. For example, asthma begins by age 4 years in the majority of children and may be "outgrown" by late adolescence, whereas allergic rhinitis more commonly appears in late adolescence and remits less frequently. Eczema and food allergy appear in the first few months of life and may resolve during the first several years of life.

■ PREDICTION AND PREVENTION

The development of atopic disease depends on sufficient contact between a genetically predisposed host and an allergen. Sensitization may take weeks or years and depends on host genetic factors, allergen dose and time of exposure, and adjuvant factors such as infection. Because external factors are important in the sensitization of a predisposed individual, appropriate identification of subjects at risk and modification of their environment may prevent atopic disease.

Several historical and laboratory parameters may be used to determine a child's likelihood of developing atopic disease. The incidence of atopy in a child when neither parent has atopic disease is 10%, approximately 40% when one parent is atopic, and 60% to 80% when both parents are atopic. Atopy tends to affect the same organ system within families (eg, lung, skin, nasal passages), but this is not consistent. A history of recurrent bronchitis or multiple episodes of croup during infancy is associated with an increased risk of asthma, although these episodes may actually be early manifestations of asthma. Infantile colic with proven food intolerance is associated with atopy in about 50% of infants.

Peripheral blood eosinophilia (more than 500 cells/mm^3) at the time of bronchitis is associated with the development of atopic disease in 75% of infants. In children undergoing adenoidectomy, two thirds of children with peripheral eosinophilia and elevated serum IgE concentrations developed atopic disease. Several studies have investigated the predictive value of cord blood serum IgE. In one large series, 70% of infants with cord blood IgE more than 1.3 IU/mL developed atopic symptoms by 1.5 years of age, and 82% by 4.5 years of age. In another series, approximately 50% of healthy infants and children with serum IgE concentrations greater than one standard deviation above age-matched controls developed atopic disease within 18 months. The presence of antigen-specific IgE, as determined by radioallergosorbent test (RAST) or skin testing, also may predict future allergic disease. In one study of wheezing infants, a positive RAST was found in 44% of infants who developed asthma or other allergic symptoms, and in only 3% who remained healthy on follow-up.

Although genetic constitution appears to be of primary importance in developing atopic disease, several environmental factors are major contributors. Because allergen exposure induces specific IgE, avoidance of allergen exposure early in life may reduce the incidence of atopic disease. In general, well-controlled prospective studies demonstrate that breast-feeding exclusively in the first year of life can affect the natural history of atopic disease. Allergic symptoms can be postponed until after the first or second year of life with exclusive breast-feeding for the first 6 months of life. More recent studies suggest that placing a lactating mother of a high-risk infant on a diet free of major allergens (egg, milk, peanut) may be even more protective, because food allergens are transmitted in maternal breast milk. The addition of solid foods to an infant's diet in the first 4 months of life has been directly correlated with increased risk of developing food allergy and atopic disease.

Exposure to inhalant allergens such as animal dander (especially cat dander), molds, and pollens in the first 6 months of life is associated with increased risk for developing atopic disorders. Consequently, measures to diminish exposure to animal products, dust mites, and molds seem justified in high-risk infants. Exposure to irritants or infection also may increase the risk of atopy. Several studies show that infants exposed to tobacco smoke develop higher serum IgE levels, have skin tests more positive to pollens, and develop respiratory disease at an earlier age than do infants in a nonsmoking environment. Furthermore, maternal smoking during pregnancy is associated with a twofold increased risk of atopy in offspring. A few studies suggest that certain viral infections (eg, respiratory synctial virus [RSV], parainfluenza) may act as adjuvants for increased IgE responses to environmental allergens. Further study is needed before strong recommendations can be made about avoiding likely settings of infectious exposures.

Multiple atopic disorders (asthma, allergic rhinitis, atopic dermatitis), one of which is severe, and markedly elevated serum IgE levels (more than 600 IU/mL) are bad prognostic indicators. If patients remove themselves from pertinent allergens by controlling their environment or moving to an area of country free of offending pollen or allergens, they often experience remission. Many will develop sensitivities to new local allergens, so moving is not frequently recommended.

■ DIAGNOSTIC EVALUATION

No single historical, physical, or laboratory finding is diagnostic of atopic disease. In fact, practically every symptom or sign of atopic disease can be seen in nonatopic disorders. Although clinical history provides the majority of information, a firm diagnosis must be based on accumulation of historical, physical, and laboratory data.

It is important to develop a clear understanding of the age of onset and progress of symptoms in terms of increasing or decreasing severity. A patient with relatively severe disease that is worsening warrants a more aggressive diagnostic approach than does someone with mild or remitting disease. Symptoms sometimes are related to allergen exposure, but more frequently overt symptoms do not follow contact with an isolated allergen. Recent studies suggest that immediate symptoms experienced by an allergic subject may go unrecognized, as distinct from the chronic disease state. Instead, a late-phase response, which is largely unresponsive to theophylline and beta-agonists, sets up a state of hyperirritability that causes the child to respond to a variety of nonspecific and often minor stimuli. For example, a pollen-sensitive asthmatic may respond to a histamine bronchoprovocation challenge for up to 4 weeks after a single allergen exposure.

A variety of allergens may affect the atopic patient. Pollen-sensitive subjects generally experience seasonal difficulty, so knowledge of local flora helps in making the appropriate diagnosis. In general, most tree pollens are released during early spring (February to March), and, in most parts of the country, grass pollens are released from late spring to midsummer. In the eastern and midwestern United States, ragweed is a major source of pollen in late summer and early fall. Whereas pollens are windborne during dry weather and are cleared from the air during rainy periods, mold spores are found in high counts in clouds and mist. High humidity provides favorable conditions for mold growth. House dust (composed of dust mites, animal danders, molds, pollens) is nonseasonal and may be increased to high concentrations when cleaning or when a child plays in a closet or under a bed. Domestic animals are common sources of potent allergens, but families often deny that their pet causes symptoms, suggesting that the problem is just pets in the neighborhood. Molds, especially in high concentrations frequently found in basements or around vegetation (hay, cut grass, barns, forests), can be a major source of difficulty. Foods, especially cow's milk, eggs, and peanuts, are frequent causes of allergic symptoms. A complete accounting of a patient's environment (indoors and outdoors), daily activities, and eating habits is necessary to assess potential allergen exposure.

Several features in the physical examination will suggest atopy. Characteristic features of specific atopic disorders are covered more thoroughly in subsequent chapters. Atopic children without overt atopic dermatitis may have dry skin with follicular prominence, mild scaling, and white dermographism. Children with nasal symptoms frequently have characteristic "allergic facies," with allergic shiners and Dennie-Morgan folds below the eyes due to venous congestion, a transverse crease across the bridge of the nose secondary to the "allergic salute," and persistent mouth breathing with "adenoid facies" characterized by deepened nasolabial folds, high arched palate, and some degree of malocclusion and overbite. Tonsils and adenoids frequently are enlarged in children with atopic disease, presumably in response to allergy and more frequent infection. Serous otitis media also is a common finding in atopic children. Chest deformities are uncommon except in severe, longstanding asthma.

Laboratory tests help substantiate clinical impressions formed from a careful history. Peripheral blood eosinophilia (more than 500 cells/mm^3) often occurs in atopic patients with asthma and atopic dermatitis but is seen less commonly in patients with allergic rhinitis. Eosinophilia in respiratory or gastrointestinal secretions highly suggests allergic disease. Secretions may be collected, dried on a microscope slide, and stained with Hansel stain, which stains eosinophils in a few minutes. Both circulating and secretory eosinophils are related directly to the severity of disease and may be absent when the disease is asymptomatic. A peripheral blood eosinophil count may be elevated with other illnesses such as malignancy, collagen vascular disease, and parasites, but secretory eosinophilia is seen in few other conditions.

Total serum IgE concentration is somewhat useful as a screening test for allergic disease, but levels may be elevated with so many other illnesses that they are even less specific than an eosinophil count. Normal values are age dependent, with highest levels normally found in late adolescence. Quantitation of IgE usually is performed by radioimmunoassay; values range from 0 to 100 IU/mL in childhood. An IgE concentration of greater than 100 IU/mL in the first year of life is correlated highly to future development of atopic disease.

Specific sensitivity may be confirmed with immediate wheal and flare skin tests. These are performed using various epicutaneous methods: prick, puncture, or scratch techniques. The skin is lightly abraded by "catching" the skin with the tip of a needle, pressing a needle onto the skin, or scratching the skin through a drop of allergen solution. An intracutaneous (intradermal) technique is a solution injected into the skin. The size of the resulting wheal using either method is determined at about 15 minutes and is compared to sizes of a positive and a negative control. The magnitude of the wheal and flare response correlates roughly with the severity of symptoms produced by natural exposure to the same allergens, although a positive skin test does not always reflect current clinical sensitivity. The intradermal test is more sensitive but less specific than the epicutaneous methods. Skin tests provide a rapid response and are relatively inexpensive. Disadvantages include moderate patient discomfort, minor risk of anaphylaxis, and suppression by antihistamines (for up to 1 week in some patients taking hydroxyzine).

As an alternative to the skin test, several serologic assays used to measure allergen-specific IgE are available. The RAST was developed first and is used most widely. Other methods are variations of the RAST: enzyme allergosorbent test (EAST), fluorescent allergosorbent test (FAST), multiple-thread allergosorbent test (MAST), and ventrex allergosorbent test (VAST). Although these assays measure circulating allergen-specific IgE antibodies that did not fix to mast cells, blood levels correlate with skin tests quite well. The tests are performed by incubating sera with solid materials to which allergen is chemically coupled. Nonspecific antibody is washed away, and adherent antibody is detected by incubation with a radiolabeled (enzyme-linked or fluorescein-linked) antihuman IgE antibody. The amount of radioactivity (enzyme activity or fluorescence) bound to the solid material directly correlates to the quantity of allergen-specific IgE. Serum can be drawn anywhere and sent to a competent technical facility, there is no risk of anaphylaxis, and patient medications do not interfere with the test. However, the tests are more expensive than skin tests and are somewhat less sensitive, and results are not available immediately.

■ TREATMENT

Treatment of allergic diseases falls into three categories: allergen avoidance, drug intervention, and allergen immunotherapy. Allergen avoidance is the treatment of choice and is the most effective. It is often impossible, however, to implement this mode of therapy effectively. Use of drug intervention and allergen immunotherapy depends on the disease state. Effective drug therapy usually is available and practical, but treatment merely provides symptomatic relief. Immunotherapy is time-consuming, expensive, and has risk, but it may abrogate specific hypersensitivities. In some allergic disorders (*eg*, life-threatening stinging insect allergy), immunotherapy is the preferred treatment.

Allergen avoidance not only reduces symptoms, it sometimes reverses allergic disease activity. Specific IgE antibody production frequently diminishes over time without continued allergen exposure (stimulation). When total avoidance is possible for long periods of time (penicillin allergy, food allergy), reexposure frequently is possible without risking recurrence of symptoms. For example, in a large series of patients with atopic dermatitis and food hypersensitivity, about one third of food allergies were "lost" after 1 to 2 years on a food allergen elimination diet.

Animal dander from household pets, such as cats and dogs, are potent allergens that frequently lead to allergic symptoms. Removal of the pet from the household is the most effective form of therapy, although it may take months for the allergen content to drop to insignificant levels. Dust mites, the major allergen in house dust, also are a major cause of allergic symptoms. To date, there are no measures known to eradicate dust mites completely, but exposure can be reduced. "Dust-proof" covers can be put on pillows and mattresses, throw rugs and nonwashable bedding can be removed, nonwashable stuffed animals and dolls ("mite farms") can be removed, and electrostatic filters can be used. Because mites thrive in humid environments, room humidifiers may aggravate the problem. These practices should be directed primarily at the child's bedroom, because children spend so much time there. When household molds are a problem, they are best dealt with by installing a dehumidifier, because most available fungicides are only partially effective. Exposure to outdoor allergens is difficult to avoid. Using air conditioning instead of leaving windows open during pollen season decreases exposure significantly.

Drug intervention is the second arm of allergy therapy. Certain drugs prevent IgE-mediated activation of mast cells and basophils. Corticosteroids inhibit mast cell activation and interleukin production and also interfere with the late-phase reaction through direct effects on granulocyte chemotaxis.

These drugs are especially important in treating chronic atopic diseases because topically active agents with minimal toxicity are available for use in the airway. Cromolyn interferes with allergen-induced immediate and late-phase reactions through mechanisms that are still poorly defined after 20 years of clinical use. Antihistamines are competitive antagonists that interfere with immediate reaction by blocking the effects of histamine released by mast cells and basophils. Theophylline, beta-adrenergic drugs, atropinic drugs, and decongestants largely attempt to reverse effects of mast cell and basophil mediators. These are discussed in more detail in sections on specific allergic disorders.

Immunotherapy is an attempt to modify immune mechanisms involved in allergic disease. Immunotherapy, or allergy-injection therapy, consists of repeated injections of allergenic material to increase the patient's tolerance of those allergens. Immunotherapy is indicated only for stinging insect hypersensitivity and for allergic rhinitis and asthma (where allergen-related symptoms are implicated by history and laboratory testing). Immunotherapy is begun with subcutaneous injections of very small doses of allergens. The treatment solutions may contain various extracts of windborne pollens, mold spores, or dust mites. There is no evidence to substantiate the effectiveness of use of food or bacterial proteins for immunotherapy. Although immunotherapy with animal dander extracts is effective, it is not generally recommended because removal of the pet from the household is the preferred treatment. Immunotherapy with any allergen extract begins with subcutaneous injection of very dilute solutions. The concentration is gradually increased at weekly intervals until doses approximately 10,000 times higher are tolerated. At these levels, the therapy is extremely effective for allergy to venom of stinging insects and has been shown to be efficacious in treating seasonal allergic rhinitis (hay fever), perennial allergic rhinitis, and extrinsic asthma. The mechanism of this beneficial effect is uncertain but may relate to the IgG-"blocking" antibodies produced, specific suppressor cell activation, and subsequent decreased IgE production or decreased releasability by mast cells and basophils. Immunotherapy carries a small (1% to 5%) risk of systemic anaphylaxis. Its effectiveness should be analyzed critically, because some individuals do not respond; ineffective treatment should be discontinued within 2 to 3 years.

■ UNPROVEN DISEASES AND THERAPY

A variety of disorders affecting every system of the body are attributed to allergy, although most allergists doubt their association. Examples include learning disorders, behavioral problems (especially hyperactivity), depression, schizophrenia, fatigue, insomnia, myalgia, inability to concentrate or think clearly, arthralgia and arthritis, assorted gastrointestinal complaints including obesity, pounding heart, and enuresis. A new subspecialty—Clinical Ecology—has emerged, proponents of which believe that the above symptoms are caused by an accumulation of low-dose exposures to chemicals in the environment and in our food supply. An evaluation includes a variety of unproven tests (eg, sublingual or subcutaneous provocation, leukocyte cytotoxic tests, tests for IgG antibodies or antigen–antibody complexes, and trace metal hair analysis). Although the concept that environmental exposure causing human disease is similar to the concept of allergy, there is no scientific basis for clinical ecology and the methods have never been validated by objective clinical trials.

The tension-fatigue syndrome has received considerable attention in pediatric literature. Proponents believe a large number of emotional symptoms (anxiety, inattention, fatigue, headaches, hyperactivity) are caused by exposure to food or food additives. Many children with severe atopic disorders become irritable, moody, fatigued, secondary to the physical discomfort or sleep deprivation caused by their disease. The concept of tension-fatigue, however, is that symptoms are a direct consequence of allergy. Attempts to validate this syndrome in controlled, blinded clinical trials have failed.

Several therapeutic methods are practiced under the guise of allergy therapy with either no adequate experimental support or clear experimental evidence that the method is not effective. These include administration of low doses of inhalant allergens to reduce allergic rhinitis (Rinkle therapy). Another example is the administration of small doses of food extracts (sublingual food drops or subcutaneous neutralization) to treat symptoms caused by food allergy.

Finally, several widely practiced therapeutic approaches are simply irrational. These include injection of the patient's urine to reduce symptoms, enzyme-potentiated transepidermal desensitization, extreme and arbitrary dietary manipulation including rotational diets, the use of nystatin to eliminate intestinal *Candida,* and confinement to aluminum foil lined rooms.

(Abridged from Hugh A. Sampson and Peyton A. Eggleston, General Considerations in Allergy, in Oski, DeAngelis, Feigin, McMillan, Warshaw: *Principles and Practice of Pediatrics, Second Edition,* J.B. Lippincott, 1994.)

Oski's Essential Pediatrics, edited by Kevin B. Johnson and Frank A. Oski. Lippincott–Raven Publishers, Philadelphia © 1997

194

Asthma

Asthma is a chronic disease characterized by increased responsiveness of the airways to various stimuli and manifested by widespread obstruction, which changes in severity either spontaneously or as a result of therapy.

A leading cause of morbidity among children throughout the world, asthma accounts for 2.2 million pediatrician visits per year and 28 million restricted activity days. Asthma is the most commonly cited reason for school absenteeism. In the United States, it accounts for one third of school days lost, and, in most urban hospitals, it is the most frequent cause for hospitalization of children. In most Western countries, between 2% and 10% of children younger than age 16 years are affected; the prevalence in Scandinavian countries is somewhat lower, 2% to 3%. In tropical and Third World countries, the prevalence is significantly lower.

For at least the past 15 years, asthma's prevalence in the United States has increased. In children aged 6 to 11 years, the prevalence in 1963 to 1965 was 5.3%; it rose to 7.6% in 1976 to 1980. The frequency of hospitalization also is increasing. The reason for this increase is not clear, but it has been seen throughout the Western world and is likely related to increasing urbanization in these populations, increasing pollution, and more accurate diagnosis of asthma.

Death from asthma is uncommon in children and represents a small fraction of the total causes of death in children of all ages in the United States. In 1985, for instance, the rate was 0.2 per 100,000 children 5 to 14 years of age, compared to 12.5 per 100,000 for accidents in the same age group, 3.5 per 100,000 for malignant neoplasm, and 1.2 per 100,000 for homicides. Death rates attributable to asthma have been increasing steadily in the last 20 years. In children in the United States, the rate has increased by approximately 6.2% per year. Again, this trend is worldwide, and mortality rates in the United States are generally small compared to other Western countries. For instance, general population mortality rates of 1.4 per 100,000 compare to 2.0 per 100,000 in Canada, 3.4 per 100,000 in Great Britain, 5.7 per 100,000 in Great Britain, and 6.5 per 100,000 in New Zealand.

Risk factors for general morbidity and mortality trends primarily relate to urbanization and poverty. When poverty is accounted for, hospitalization rate differences between black and white patients almost disappear. There are definite pockets of increased mortality in cities, especially among those in lower socioeconomic groups.

■ NATURAL HISTORY

The median age of onset of asthma is 4 years; more than 20% of children develop symptoms within the first year of life. Risk factors include atopy, especially multiple positive skin tests or radioallergosorbent test (RAST). This risk factor is genetic, in that the parental history is almost as strong a risk factor as is an elevated level of IgE in cord blood. The association with parental smoking is less clear, and most studies have shown a weak or insignificant association with either the onset or severity of asthma. Other obvious risk factors for early onset include neonatal lung disease, especially infants with reduced lung volumes, and respiratory infections, especially with the respiratory syncytial virus (RSV). Between 40% and 50% of children with RSV bronchiolitis develop chronic asthma.

In 60% of cases, asthma beginning in childhood resolves by young adult life. Fifty percent of those who undergo remission in adolescence become symptomatic again as young adults, and tests of airway hyperactivity show that even in asymptomatic young adults, the airways have not returned to normal. In general, those who resolve have less severe, intermittent asthma, usually do not have multiple positive skin tests to inhalant allergens, and do not have persistent wheezing or rhonchi. Studies demonstrate that heavy exposure to pollution, allergens, or cigarette smoke makes resolution less likely.

■ PATHOPHYSIOLOGY

Inflammation

As shown in the pathologic specimen in Figure 194–1, asthma is an inflammatory disease. The infiltrate in the airway wall and the surrounding parenchyma is characteristically rich in eosinophils, but neutrophils, basophils, and mononuclear cells are common, without organized lymphoid nodules or granulomata. Large areas of respiratory epithelium are desquamated, and collagen is deposited in the area of the basement membrane. Bronchial smooth muscle is hypertrophied. Respiratory epithelium and inflammatory cells frequently fill large mucus plugs in the airway lumen.

This inflammatory process is thought to be caused by mast cell activation. Mast cells are a fixed tissue cell that may increase in areas of intense inflammation either through

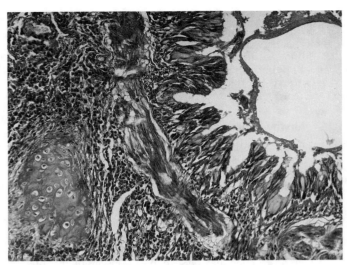

Figure 194-1. Pathology of asthma. Hematoxylin and eosin stained specimen of cross section of a small bronchus of an asthmatic patient.

migration or proliferation. The cell is activated by either lymphokines or IgE-dependent mechanisms to produce a variety of proinflammatory substances. IgE-dependent inflammation requires antigen-specific IgE antibody. IgE antibody participates with other immunoglobulins in the normal immune response. It is produced from plasma cells that derive from B lymphocytes influenced by T helper and suppressor cells. Characteristically, IgE binds with great avidity to mast cells and basophilic granulocytes and appears in the circulation in very small quantities. When it binds to mast cells, it confers on these cells the ability to respond to environmental allergens.

The nature of the antigen is an important component driving an IgE antibody response. Certain antigens such as penicillin, ovalbumin, ragweed pollen antigen, and parasitic proteins stimulate more IgE production than IgG. As a group, these allergens are 20,000- to 40,000-dalton molecular weight proteins that are constituent parts of such allergen vectors as plant pollens, foods, or animal dander. Although an IgE immune response occurs only after environmental exposure, modulation of IgE antibodies is genetically controlled. For example, certain inbred mouse strains preferentially produce IgE antibodies when immunized, whereas other strains produce IgG. The ability to respond to certain antigens has also been shown to be genetically controlled; for instance, the IgE response to certain pollen allergens is linked closely to the HLA-DW2 phenotype. Total serum IgE concentrations found in family and twin studies are inherited as a simple recessive trait.

On allergen exposure, the mast cell responds within seconds with an energy-dependent secretion of many pharmacologically active chemicals termed *mediators*. These mediators result in an "immediate response," within 15 to 30 minutes, which includes vasodilation, increased vascular permeability, smooth muscle constriction, and mucus secretion in the respiratory and gastrointestinal tracts. This immediate response evolves into a late-phase reaction (LPR) within 2 to 4 hours after antigen exposure. Eosinophils and neutrophils begin to infiltrate the area, but, by 48 hours, mononuclear cells predominate in the mixed cellular infiltrate. Symptoms associated with this LPR may include persistent tenderness or pain in the skin, persistent nasal congestion, or persistent asthma that responds poorly to beta-agonist treatment. Experimentally, it can be shown that the LPR is IgE-dependent. Recognizing LPR has been an important step in understanding asthma because it provides a mechanism for the chronic inflammation seen in asthma. In addition, an important physiologic element of asthma (ie, airway hyperresponsiveness) has been found to increase for days to weeks after LPR.

Airway Hyperresponsiveness

Highly variable levels of airway obstruction are characteristic of asthma and are called airway hyperresponsiveness. This hyperresponsiveness is best illustrated in Figure 194–2, which shows the record of daily peak expiratory flow rate (PEFR) measurements on two patients with asthma. The patient with milder asthma usually has normal PEFR values, but these measures vary by more than 20% daily. The person with severe asthma has more abnormal PEFR measures together with daily variations of more than 60%. These variations in obstruction may be seen in response to many "precipitants" of bronchospasm. Typically, any patient responds to multiple precipitants, and the more severe the degree of airway hyperactivity, the greater the response to a stimulus. These multiple stimuli include irritants (cigarette smoke, odors, pollution, sulfite preservatives), weather changes, and emotions. Common colds (RSV, influenza, rhinovirus, parainfluenza) typically precipitate prolonged severe attacks. Certain drugs (beta-adrenergic antagonists, aspirin, and all nonsteroidal anti-inflammatory agents, except acetaminophen) cause brief, severe obstruction. Exercise causes brief obstruction by forcing the airway to adapt to hyperventilation and exposure to large volumes of cold dry air. Allergens cause attacks when specific IgE antibody is present.

Airway inflammation and airway hyperresponsiveness recently have been linked. In persons with a late-phase allergic response, airway hyperresponsiveness increases within a few hours and remains increased for 2 to 3 weeks, long after the late-phase obstructive response has subsided. During this period, the airway response to many stimuli including cold air, exercise, and allergens is increased. It is hypothesized that chronic and persistent allergen exposure causes not only immediate obstruction that can be noticed by a child, but also airway inflammation and physiologic abnormality that gradually increases and becomes more chronic and severe. This process can be reversed by removal from an allergic stimulus. Both in children and adults who are allergic to house dust mite allergen, avoidance for weeks to months will decrease airway symptoms, medication requirements, and response to environmental stimuli.

■ PHARMACOTHERAPY FOR ASTHMA

Beta-Adrenergic Agonists

The beta-adrenergic agonist group of drugs is the most important symptomatic therapy for asthma available. Airway obstruction is reversed rapidly through their effects on the beta-2 receptor on bronchial smooth muscle. Available drugs and their doses are listed in Table 194–1. Because of its spectrum of effects and short duration, epinephrine is no longer the drug of choice for asthma, except as injectable preparations in infants when nebulized preparations cannot be given. The current drug of choice is either albuterol or terbutaline, which are beta-2 selective and longer acting. Newer drugs are being developed with much longer durations of action.

Whenever possible, beta-adrenergic agonists should be inhaled, because effective bronchodilation can be achieved with doses 10 to 20 times lower than with oral dosing. Toxicity includes tachycardia, palpitations, and central nervous system (CNS) excitement and muscular tremor. All these are dose-dependent and rarely are a problem with inhalation dosing. Nebulized drugs may be given with solutions from a nebulizer such as the DeVilbiss model 646 attached to a small compressor for home use or from a freon-powered inhaler. An inhaler is easier to administer when used with a reservoir device such as an Inspirease or Aerochamber; infants may be treated using an Aerochamber with a face mask. Adolescents must be cautioned against overuse of the inhaler and overreliance on its brief bronchodilatory effects.

In addition to being effective bronchodilators, beta-adrenergic agonists inhibit immediate asthmatic responses to allergens, exercise, and many inhaled irritants when given just before exposure. They have little effect on the LPR or on the resulting increase in reactivity.

Because beta-adrenergic agonists cannot inhibit inflammation, their use as primary chronic therapy is questionable. A double-blind, placebo-controlled study suggested that chronic therapy could be detrimental. During the 1-year

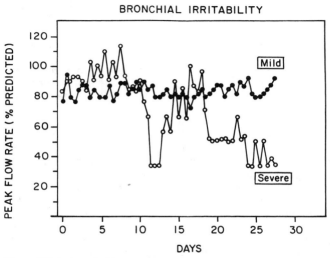

Figure 194-2. Daily PEFR measurement on two children with asthma.

TABLE 194-1. Available Drugs for Asthma

Preparations Available

BETA-ADRENERGIC AGONISTS	***CROMOLYN***
Oral	Metered-dose inhaler
Metaproterenol	Powder
Albuterol	Solution
Terbutaline	***CORTICOSTEROIDS***
Metered-Dose Inhaler	*Oral*
Metaproterenol	Prednisone
Albuterol	Prednisolone
Terbutaline	Methylprednisolone
Nebulized Solution	Dexamethasone
Metaproterenol	*Inhaled*
Albuterol	Beclomethasone
Terbutaline	Triamcinolone
THEOPHYLLINE	Flunisolide
Oral	*Injection*
Tablets	Prednisolone
Sustained-release tablets, capsules (except Theodur sprinkles)	Methylprednisolone
Aminophylline	
(About 80% theophylline 100, 200 mg/mL ampule)	

trial, asthmatic volunteers were treated regularly with inhalers containing beta-adrenergic agonists during one 6-month period and placebo during another 6 months. During the placebo period, the asthmatic volunteers had less acute medication requirements, fewer hospitalizations, more normal morning pulmonary function tests, and fewer chronic symptoms. The role of these drugs appears to be limited to controlling symptoms, and they should not be used as the only chronic therapy except in mild, episodic asthma.

Theophylline

Theophylline was the most popular drug for the treatment of asthma in the 1980s but is losing popularity to beta-adrenergic agonists because of toxicity and complex pharmacokinetics. The preparations available for clinical use are listed in Table 194–1. Toxic effects include both mild (nausea, vomiting, stomach pain, diarrhea, headache, irritability, distractibility) and severe and life-threatening (intractable convulsion, tachyarrhythmia) reactions. Both therapeutic and toxic effects are related directly to plasma levels, with a therapeutic range of peak levels suggested from 5 to 20 µg/mL. Distractibility, irritability, and poor school performance has been reported at all therapeutic levels; the consensus is that these effects are not significant when the effects of chronic illness are accounted for. Severe and life-threatening toxicity generally is not seen until plasma levels reach 30 µg/mL but has been reported to occur at these levels without milder toxicity warnings.

Plasma theophylline levels depend on the amount of drug absorbed and the amount cleared by hepatic metabolism. Of the two, hepatic clearance is the most variable, with a range of difference as great as fivefold among individuals. Clearance is affected by many other factors (Table 194–2). Absorption also is variable. Fatty meals delay absorption, and absorption rate is lowest between 2 AM and 4 AM. The absorp-

tion of certain time-released preparations (Theodur sprinkles) has been found to vary widely and unpredictably, although most are absorbed predictably. With the many variables described, it is imperative to measure serum theophylline concentrations when using the drug. In milder asthmatics treated with lower doses (10 mg/kg/day), a single level drawn at random may suffice. When the drug is used at higher doses, theophylline levels should be obtained whenever mild toxic symptoms occur, such as headache, stomachaches, or vomiting, or when the child is exposed to conditions that may affect clearance, such as viral infections or erythromycin therapy.

Theophylline is an effective bronchodilator, although not as effective as beta-agonists. In acute emergency room use, theophylline is definitely inferior to beta-agonists and does not add to therapeutic effects although it does add side effects. Studies with hospitalized acute asthmatic children suggest that theophylline does contribute significantly to improvement. Theophylline is a weak inhibitor of airway inflammation and of the LPR to allergens but is unable to prevent the increased airway reactivity after allergen LPR. On the other hand, chronic therapy with theophylline or cromolyn has comparable effects on pulmonary symptoms and airway reactivity.

Anticholinergics

Anticholinergic drugs are useful bronchodilators in acute asthma but are not effective when used chronically. These muscarinic antagonists inhibit vagal reflex at smooth muscle and glands but have no effect on CNS or neuromuscular transmission. Representative compounds in clinical use include atropine, ipratropium, and glycopyrrolate; only atropine is available for children younger than 12 years. Iprotropium bromide is a synthetic analogue of atropine. It is poorly absorbed and has less systemic toxicity. These drugs

TABLE 194-2. Factors Affecting Theophylline Clearance

Factor	Approximate Multiple of Dose Needed to Produce Therapeutic Level
INCREASED CLEARANCE	
Cigarette smoking	2.0
Phenytoin	1.9
Charcoal-broiled meats	1.3
DECREASED CLEARANCE	
Prematures, newborns	0.1
Cirrhosis	0.4
Congestive heart failure	0.4
Fever	0.5
Acute viral illness	0.5
Cimetidine	0.6
Erythromycin	0.8

are potent bronchodilators with peak effects that are delayed for 30 to 60 minutes. Treatment inhibits the response to irritants probably through interruption of vagal reflex, but exercise-induced and allergen-induced asthma is inhibited in only a fraction of patients. Toxic effects (xerostomia, mydriasis, tachycardia, and abdominal pain) are minor but are annoying enough that the drug is not well accepted.

Cromolyn

Cromolyn was the first drug shown to prevent allergen-induced asthma in humans without having bronchodilator properties. Initially, it was thought to function by inhibiting mast cell activation, but recent information suggests that its effects cannot be explained solely on mast cell activity. As shown in Table 194–1, it is available both as a solution for nebulization and as a metered-dose inhaler. In single doses, cromolyn inhibits bronchospasm due to allergen, exercise, and sulfur dioxide. It is the only drug available that effectively inhibits both early and late-phase asthma caused by allergen exposure. In chronic use, airway reactivity is improved slightly, and disease activity is decreased. This effect requires approximately 2 to 4 weeks of chronic therapy, and approximately 25% of patients do not benefit. In trials directly comparing theophylline and cromolyn for chronic use in mildly to moderately asthmatic children the two drugs are comparably effective, but theophylline is associated with a significantly higher rate of toxicity. Except for a rare allergic reaction, the cromolyn is nontoxic. A second drug, Nedocromil, has a very similar activity and has been approved for use in adults in the United States.

Corticosteroids

Corticosteroids are the most potent drugs available for asthma. The mechanism of their effectiveness in asthma may relate to inactivation of various inflammatory cells including macrophages, monocytes, lymphocytes, basophils, and eosinophils. Acutely, their effectiveness may relate to increased numbers of beta-adrenergic receptors on bronchial smooth muscle and increased responsiveness to beta-ago-nists. With pretreatment for several days, inhaled and systemic steroids inhibit the allergen-induced LPR but have little effect on immediate reaction. Chronically, airway hyperreactivity is significantly depressed.

Available preparations are listed in Table 194–1. For acute use, prednisone and methylprednisolone are equivalent. For chronic use, inhaled corticosteroids are an important new advance in asthmatic pharmacology. By modifying the glucocorticoid molecule, these compounds are about 100 times more potent than prednisone and methylprednisolone in anti-inflammatory activity. In addition, they are poorly absorbed from the respiratory tract and are rapidly cleared when absorbed from the gastrointestinal tract. This provides a wide therapeutic ratio and has led to recommendations for more widespread use in mild to moderate asthma. At the same time, studies show that signs of typical chronic toxicity may be seen with doses significantly higher than those shown in Table 194–1 and suggest the need for caution.

Corticosteroids have little serious acute toxicity except for hypokalemia. Eosinophil and mononuclear cells are reduced in peripheral blood, whereas neutrophils are increased and there is no demonstrable acute risk of infection. Chronic oral therapy with more than 5 mg/m^2/day of prednisone or equivalent other drug produces growth suppression, adrenal suppression, decreased cortical bone mass, decreased oscalcin, and posterior subcapsular cataracts. These toxic effects are minimized by alternate-day therapy or treatment with inhaled steroids.

■ CHRONIC MANAGEMENT

Management of asthma in children is best considered in separate phases: chronic management and management of acute episodes. The goals of chronic management are to establish the diagnosis of asthma, to determine the most appropriate treatment program, and to educate the child and family to foster independent management of the disease. The National Asthma Education Program of the National Institutes of Health (NIH) published a monograph entitled "Guidelines for the Diagnosis and Management of Asthma," which is a consensus of a number of experts in the field. This section relies heavily on its organization and recommendations.

In most cases, little medical evaluation is needed to confirm the diagnosis of asthma, especially when there is a history of acute reaction to appropriate stimuli and quick relief by appropriate therapy. Other useful supporting evidence includes eosinophilia (greater than 400 eos/mm^3 in blood; greater than 10% in secretions), a personal or family history of atopic disease, and an elevated serum level of total IgE. Another screening test, the Phadeotope assay, has been shown to be both more specific and sensitive than the total IgE. To provide a basis for specific allergen control advice, use of allergy skin testing or RAST (radioallergosorbent testing) to common inhalant and food allergens should be performed on all children with moderate and severe asthma. At the same time, it is important not to equate asthma and atopy because 20% to 40% of children with asthma have no evidence of allergic disease.

The differential diagnosis in childhood is limited and should be considered only when atypical features are present. These are discussed in subsequent paragraphs that discuss the wheezing infant, because most of the conditions that can be confused with asthma present first in infancy.

Allergic Aspects

Allergen avoidance is an essential first step in treating allergic asthma. The most common allergens associated with chronic asthma are house dust mites, cats, dogs, various molds, cockroaches, pollens, and various foods. House dust mite allergy is caused by pteroglyph mites that infest bedding, rugs, and other fabrics. The allergen is carried on fecal particles that are relatively large and settle quickly after disturbance; thus, close exposure (sleeping in an infested bed or lying on an infested rug) are important for sensitization and induction inflammation and symptoms. To avoid mite allergen, airtight covers must be installed to cover mattress and pillow completely. Bedding can be rendered mite-free by washing in hot water (55°C [131°C]) or by dry cleaning; infestation usually recurs within a few weeks. Wall-to-wall carpeting in the child's bedroom should be eliminated as should excessive numbers of fuzzy toys if they are closely associated with the bed.

Pets contribute potent allergens, and about one third of patients with asthma have positive skin tests to cat or dog.

The allergen originates in the animal's saliva. Pets should be eliminated from households with sensitized children. Because families often are unwilling to remove pets from the household, compromises may be employed. Keeping the pet out of the child's bedroom or in the yard is of questionable benefit. Washing the pet every 1 to 2 weeks does reduce concentrations in settled house dust, but cat antigen does not disappear from settled dust for more than 6 months after the animal has been removed. It is not clear whether compromise measures are adequate.

Mold antigens are ubiquitous in a home environment, and more than 25% of asthmatic children have positive skin tests. In general, the problem is worse in older houses or in moist environments. These sorts of environments are encountered with small room nebulizers, in basements, in homes in warm southern climates without air conditioning, or in rooms where vaporizers are used. The most effective way to remove mold and mildew is to remove contaminated materials and to reduce home moisture content.

Cockroaches recently have been found to contribute important allergens in urban environments, especially in the middle Atlantic and southeastern states. Elimination of the antigen usually requires pest control consultation and careful clean-up of the remaining insect parts and feces, which can be widespread and contain high concentrations of antigen.

Another approach to modifying the allergic response to environmental allergens is allergen immunotherapy, in which small amounts of aqueous extracts of source allergen vectors (pollens, dust mites, mold spores) are injected regularly over a period of months to years. Allergen immunotherapy reduces symptoms of allergic rhinitis but it is less useful for asthma.

Stepped Management of Medications

The first step in establishing stepped care is to establish the severity of asthma using a schema shown in Table 194-3. Symptoms of coughing and wheezing have the same significance in children. An episode occurs when an asthmatic child has more than two or three coughs or obvious wheezing. As asthma becomes more severe, intermittent episodes evolve to continuous symptoms.

In mild asthma, there are no symptoms or detectable signs of wheezing between episodes; they may, however,

TABLE 194-3. Assessment of Severity of Chronic Asthma

Symptom	Mild	Moderate	Severe
Episodes of cough or wheeze	Brief <2 per week	≥ 2 per week	Almost daily, continuous
Symptoms or signs between episodes	No	Occasional	Present
Exercise tolerance	EIA with strenuous exercise	EIA with most exercise	Activity limited even with medication
Nocturnal cough or wheeze	<2 per month	Weekly	Frequent
School loss	None	>7 days	>21 days
ER, office visits for acute asthma	None	≤3 per year	>3 per year
Hospitalization	None	None	1 per year
PEFR % reference	≥ 80%	60%–80%	<60%
PEFR variability	20%	20%–30%	>30% episodes while medicated
Response to optimal medication	Symptoms controlled with prn inhaler	Regular medication required to control	Symptoms even with regular medication

Adapted from NHILBI Expert Panel Report US Publication No. 91-3042.

occasionally be seen in moderate asthma. Mild asthma never requires an emergency room or office visit for an episode, whereas moderate asthma may require up to three a year. During exercise, mild asthma may produce symptoms that last a few minutes but do not interfere with activity. Nocturnal cough may be present but never more than two to three times a month in mild asthma.

Objective measurements of pulmonary functions are essential in managing asthma on a day-to-day basis. Symptoms and physical findings correlate poorly with objective measurements obtained in parallel. For chronic use, home peak expiratory flow meters should be used to educate patients about symptoms, to establish a baseline for measuring exacerbations, and to adjust medications. Acutely, peak flow meters should be used to establish the severity of obstruction. The PEFR is criticized as an inadequate measure of pulmonary function that provides little information compared to spirometry, but it is cheaper, more convenient, more easily performed by younger children, and correlates well with an FEV_1. Experience continues to confirm its usefulness. Equipment is inexpensive and includes the Assess and mini-Wright meters. Normal values are shown in Figure 194–3. Peak flows are within the normal range in mild asthma and never drop more than 20% during symptomatic episodes. Both figures escalate to more severe involvement in more severe asthma.

In general, children evolve from one stage of severity to another over long periods of time, usually months to years. Therefore, classification according to the categories described above can be used to plan therapy over extended periods of time.

■ TREATMENT OF ACUTE ASTHMA

The goal of treatment of acute asthma is to normalize pulmonary functions rapidly and to prevent progression of the attack. Essential to this process are early recognition of worsening lung function, prompt communication between patient and physician, removal from the allergen, irritant, or other trigger, and appropriate intensification of asthma medications.

A scheme to assess severity in acute asthma is shown in Table 194–4 and gives criteria for both home and hospital use. Generally, the most appropriate place to initiate treatment of an acute attack is in the home or at school. Certain patients are at risk for life-threatening severe attacks. These patients should be treated more aggressively than is outlined and sometimes cannot be treated at home at all. High-risk patients include those with prior intubation for asthma, two or more hospitalizations for asthma in the last year, three or more emergency room visits for asthma in the last year, hospitalization or emergency room use within the last month, a requirement for oral steroid therapy, a past history of syncope or hypoxic seizures during an asthma attack, and a history of serious psychiatric or psychosocial problems.

Home management is recommended whenever possible so treatment begins immediately and families gain some control of the disease. Always, a written, brief plan of assessment and treatment should be provided by the physician. The first step is to assess severity using Table 194–4. In mild to moderate attacks, albuterol should be given by nebulization or metered-dose inhaler. A good response is indicated by a return to evidence of mild obstruction. Routine medication should continue, albuterol should be given every 3 to 4 hours, and severity should be reassessed frequently. An incomplete response is indicated by persistent evidence of moderate obstruction. The physician should be contacted, oral prednisone should be given and inhaled, and beta-agonist treatment should continue. If severity subsides to mild over the next 4 hours, continued home treatment is appropriate. If moderate asthma continues, the patient should be seen in the physician's office or a hospital-based emergency room. If a patient has severe asthma according to Table 194–4, albuterol treatment should begin. The patient should then go immediately to a physician's office or to a hospital-based emergency room.

The decision to treat in a physician's office or a hospital-based emergency room depends on many factors, including accessibility of the emergency room, the ability and interest of the physician to manage severe asthma in the office, and the physician's previous relationship with the patient.

In the office, a reassessment should determine severity and rule out complications such as atelectasis, pneumomediastinum, and pneumothorax. Oxygen should be administered together with nebulized albuterol every 20 minutes for 1 hour. Prednisone should be given unless the patient responds imme-

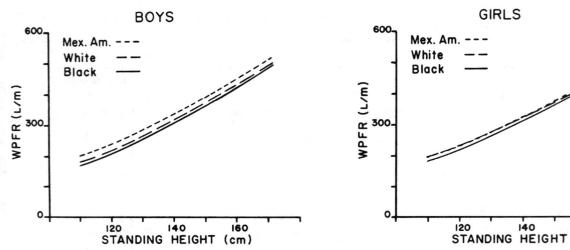

Figure 194-3. Prediction curves for PEFR measurements in children (Hsu KHK, Jenkins DE, Hsi BP, et al. Ventilatory functions of normal children and young adults–Mexican American, white and black: II wright peak flow meter. *J Pediatr.* 1979;95:192).

TABLE 194-4. Estimation of Severity of Acute Exacerbations of Asthma

Indication	Mild	Moderate	Severe
Alertness	Normal	Normal	May be decreased
Dyspnea	Absent, speaks complete sentences	Moderate, speaks phrases	Severe, speaks short phrases, words
Pulsus paradoxicus (mm Hg)	<10	10–20	20–40
Accessory muscle	None	Retractions sternocleidomastoid	Severe retractions, nasal flaring
Color	Good	Pale	Cyanotic
Auscultation	End-expiratory wheeze	Inspiratory, expiratory wheeze	Quiet breath sounds
O_2 saturation (%)	>95	90–95	<90
pCo_2 (mm Hg)	<35	<40	>40
PEFR predicted or % best	70–90	50–70	<50

Adapted from NHLBI Expert Panel Report US Publication No. 91-3042.

diately to a nebulized dose. Epinephrine, 0.01 mg/kg, should be given if the patient does not generate a peak flow, has decreased consciousness, or cannot cooperate for treatment with nebulized drugs. If treatment is required past 4 hours, hospitalization should be considered, and, if the response to treatment is poor, the patient should be admitted. Generally, a patient who has responded will be discharged on continued medication, which usually includes prednisone, and with a follow-up plan.

Hospital management offers little pharmacologically that cannot be provided as an outpatient. The major indication for hospitalization is to observe for continued deterioration so more intensive treatment can be given, in an intensive care unit if necessary.

■ THE WHEEZING INFANT

Because wheezy respiratory infections occur so commonly in infants and because chronic systemic illnesses present for the first time in infancy, the differential diagnosis of the wheezing infant is more extensive than that for older children. The most common cause of recurrent lower respiratory cough and wheeze in infants is simply recurrent colds, especially in day care settings. Asthma is the second most common cause, but congenital anomalies (vascular ring, TE fistulae, congenital heart disease), metabolic abnormalities (cystic fibrosis), foreign body aspiration, immunodeficiency syndromes, and gastroesophageal reflux must be considered. Any infant with significant steatorrhea, atypical wheezing with an inspiratory component or localization to one side, a history of aspiration or choking on food, or with failure to thrive or clubbing on physical examinations should receive further evaluation.

As a first step, any infant with recurrent wheezing should have a chest x-ray, a careful review of systems, and a careful physical examination. Laboratory evaluation and confirmation of an allergy history are more difficult because skin tests are generally smaller in infants and because RAST tests are more likely to be negative. In one study of 78 unselected asthmatic infants younger than 1 year of age, only 6 had positive skin tests. This contrasts with rates of 60% to 80% in older children and adults with asthma.

Treatment is more difficult in infants than in older children. Response to bronchodilator therapy is not striking, especially during an acute episode. Appropriate dosages for medication in infants are provided in Table 194–1. Specific problems with drug dosing include difficulty providing neb-

ulized medications, differences in theophylline clearance, and a general concern that the chronic toxicity of all drugs may differ in rapidly growing infants than in older children. Aerosol medication usually must be given with a portable nebulizer. Some infants tolerate a face mask, whereas others only allow the nebulizer outlet to be held close to the face while sitting on the parent's lap; support for the parent and imaginative methods for increasing acceptance by the infant are required. A spacer device, the Aerochamber, is available with a face mask, allowing some infants to be treated with metered-dose inhalers. Available drugs are not approved by the FDA for use in children younger than 6 years. Inhaled steroids, which have proven so important in the chronic therapy of older children, are not available for infants. In the United States, there is no available aerosol steroid preparation that can be used in a nebulizer; in Canada and Europe, however, budesonide has been used successfully.

(Abridged from Peyton A. Eggleston, Asthma, in Oski, DeAngelis, Feigin, McMillan, Warshaw: *Principles and Practice of Pediatrics, Second Edition*, J.B. Lippincott, 1994.)

Oski's Essential Pediatrics,
edited by Kevin B. Johnson and Frank A. Oski.
Lippincott–Raven Publishers,
Philadelphia © 1997

195

Urticaria and Angioedema

Urticaria (hives) is characterized by erythematous, edematous wheals of the superficial layers of the skin or mucous membranes. The lesions blanch with pressure, are often pruritic, and usually are distributed symmetrically. Individual urticarial lesions are usually evanescent, commonly lasting less than 4 hours, but occasionally persisting for 24 to 48 hours. If the lesions persist, there may be underlying vasculitis. Angioedema is a similar process occurring in deeper layers of the skin and subcutaneous tissues. Angioedema is characterized by well-demarcated areas of nonpitting, nondependent, and not-hot swelling. Whereas urticaria may occur on any part of the body, angioedema often involves the extremities, face (especially the perioral and periorbital areas), or genitalia.

Pruritus or a chronic itch does not equal chronic urticaria. Pruritus without visible lesions can be caused by a number of different diseases unrelated to urticaria, such as renal failure and azotemia. These patients have severe pruritus and no evidence of urticaria. Although urticarial lesions are often pruritic, the presence of pruritus without urticaria is cause to formulate a distinct list of differential diagnoses.

Traditionally, the duration of urticaria has defined whether the disease is acute or chronic. Chronic urticaria is a disease in which the patient has urticarial lesions that are either continuous or frequent for 6 weeks or longer. Acute urticaria is a disease in which the lesions are present for less than that period of time. However, one must also include in any classification scheme the physical urticarias. Physical urticarias may last for several years, but are manifested by recurrent episodes of acute lesions in relation to a physical stimulus such as cold, exercise, or pressure. In addition, chronic urticaria as opposed to acute and physical urticarias may be distinguished pathologically. Biopsy samples of chronic urticarial lesions tend to show a non-necrotizing perivascular infiltrate that is generally not noted during acute episodes of urticaria or physical urticarias. In most studies, an etiologic agent in chronic urticaria is found in only 5% to 20% of patients. Thus, most cases of chronic urticaria are labeled "idiopathic." The success rates for identifying specific causes of acute urticaria are higher.

The incidence of urticaria and angioedema is extremely high. It is estimated that 15% to 20% of the population experience an episode of urticaria or angioedema at some time in life. Acute urticaria may occur at any age and is the most common form seen in children. Chronic urticaria occurs more frequently in young adults (peak incidence in third and fourth decades) than in the pediatric population. Chronic urticaria may be persistent. In one long-term follow-up of pediatric and adult patients with chronic idiopathic urticaria or angioedema, the average duration of urticaria alone was 6 months, angioedema alone was 1 year, and urticaria with angioedema was 5 years.

Thus, it is readily apparent that all physicians can expect to see many patients with urticaria or angioedema. To facilitate the care of these patients, specific points about the pathophysiology, causes, diagnostic tests, and treatment of urticaria and angioedema are addressed in this chapter.

■ CAUSES

Because a number of mechanisms may lead to mast cell mediator release, a variety of etiologic factors have been found to cause urticaria and angioedema. The major etiologic factors producing acute and chronic forms of urticaria and angioedema are listed in Table 195–1. Acute urticaria is most frequently caused by a food or drug and usually dissipates within days to several weeks. As previously stated, the cause of chronic urticaria is usually not determined. The incidence of atopy in patients with chronic idiopathic urticaria does not appear to be higher than that found in the general population. The following paragraphs discuss many of the etiologic factors for urticaria and angioedema listed in Table 195–1.

Drug Reactions

Drug reactions are one of the most common causes of urticaria and angioedema. The reactions are mediated by type I or type III immune mechanisms or by direct nonimmunologic mast cell mediator release. Depending on the mecha-

TABLE 195-1. Major Causes of Urticaria and Angioedema

Drug reaction
Food
Infection
Inhalant
Systemic disease
   Collagen vascular diseases
   Malignancy
   Endocrine disorders
Urticaria pigmentosa and systemic mastocytosis
Hereditary disorder
   Familial cold urticaria
   Hereditary vibratory angioedema
   Urticaria with amyloidosis, deafness, and limb pain
   Hereditary angioedema (HAE)
Physical urticaria
   Dermatographism
   Cholinergic urticaria
   Exercise-induced anaphylactic syndrome
   Familial and acquired cold urticaria
   Localized heat urticaria
   Aquagenic urticaria
   Delayed pressure urticaria/angioedema
   Solar urticaria
   Familial and acquired vibratory angioedema
Chronic idiopathic

nisms involved, the urticaria may occur immediately or days to weeks after drug exposure (*eg*, serum sickness syndrome with urticaria). Many drugs are associated with urticaria. Antibiotics, especially penicillin and related compounds, remain the leading causes of drug-induced urticaria. Aspirin and other nonsteroidal anti-inflammatory agents are common causes of urticaria. There are no convincing data to indicate, however, that patients who are not allergic to these drugs have an exacerbation of their disease when taking aspirin or nonsteroidals. Some drugs such as the opioids can directly cause mast cell degranulation. Other classes of drugs frequently associated with urticaria include diuretics, radiocontrast dyes, muscle relaxants, and sedatives or barbiturates. All drugs taken by the patient must be determined because any drug can be a potential cause of urticaria. Vitamins, lotions, contraceptives, laxatives, and various over-the-counter drugs represent possible offenders. When a drug reaction is suspected, all unnecessary drugs should be eliminated, and an attempt should be made to switch to alternative, chemically distinct forms of necessary drugs.

Foods

Foods are a common cause of acute urticaria but may also cause chronic urticaria. Daily hives suggest foods eaten regularly, whereas sporadic, recurrent hives suggest foods eaten intermittently. The most common offenders include nuts, milk, eggs, chocolate, citrus fruits, tomatoes, and fish. Food dyes (tartrazine) and additives (benzoate derivatives, sulfates) may also infrequently cause urticaria. Patients with respiratory allergies to pollen may develop urticaria or angioedema after ingestion of certain foods with "cross-reactive" antigens. Reported examples include ragweed and banana and melons; birch and celery, nuts, and certain fruits; and grass and tomatoes.

Infection

Many types of infections have been associated with urticaria. Viral infections are common causes of acute urticaria in children and adolescents. Although undetected infections have been considered a cause of chronic urticaria, the incidence is probably low. The most common infections known to be associated with urticaria include infectious hepatitis, infectious mononucleosis, coxsackievirus infection, *Mycoplasma* infection, helminthic parasites, and acute beta-hemolytic streptococcal infection. The association of urticaria with *Candida* or tinea infections is probably coincidental. If an infection is found, it should be treated. However, extensive evaluation or empiric antimicrobial therapy for undetected infection is not warranted. Indeed, drugs used to treat suspected infections are more likely to cause hives.

Inhalants

Inhalant allergens including pollen, animal dander, and spores are infrequently associated with urticaria. Allergic respiratory symptoms to the inhalant generally occur concomitantly.

Insects

Children may get a hivelike reaction to biting insects such as fleas and mites, which is referred to as papular urticaria. These lesions are characterized by pruritic, papular lesions usually on exposed skin surfaces (especially the extremities). Acute urticaria and angioedema may also follow stings or bites from Hymenoptera in allergic individuals.

Systemic Diseases

A number of systemic diseases are associated with urticaria and angioedema. If the urticarial lesions are accompanied by fever, arthralgia, or elevated sedimentation rate, an underlying connective tissue disorder and cutaneous vasculitis should be considered. Systemic lupus erythematosus, rheumatic fever, and rheumatoid arthritis may be accompanied by urticarialike lesions. The rash associated with juvenile rheumatoid arthritis may appear before other signs of the disease. In patients with connective tissue disorders, lesional biopsy tests usually reveal vasculitis.

Urticaria also has been observed in adults and children with lymphoreticular malignancies, and in adults with carcinoma of the lung, rectum, or colon. Several studies suggest, however, there is not a higher incidence of malignancies in patients with chronic urticaria. Unless evidence suggests malignancy, an exhaustive search for cancer is not indicated.

Thyroid disease (especially Hashimoto's thyroiditis) and both hyperthyroidism and hypothyroidism are associated with urticaria. Exacerbations of chronic urticaria and cyclic urticaria have been noted during menses. These observations suggest a relationship among endocrine disorders, hormone levels, and urticaria.

■ URTICARIA DISORDERS

Urticaria Pigmentosa and Systemic Mastocytosis

Urticaria pigmentosa typically occurs during childhood and is characterized by persistent, pigmented, maculopapular lesions that urticate when stroked (Darier's sign). Biopsy of these lesions reveals mast cell infiltrations of the skin. Systemic mastocytosis is a generalized form of mast cell infiltration with involvement of the skin, bone marrow, long bones, liver, spleen, or lymph nodes.

Hereditary Disorders

Several rare inherited disorders are associated with urticaria and angioedema. Familial cold urticaria and hereditary vibratory angioedema are discussed in subsequent paragraphs. Familial urticaria has been seen in combination with amyloidosis, nerve deafness, and limb pain. This syndrome appears to be inherited as an autosomal dominant condition.

Hereditary angioedema (HAE) is an autosomal dominant disorder caused by the absence of functional C1 esterase inhibitor. HAE is clinically characterized by recurrent episodes of angioedema (without urticaria) precipitated spontaneously and variably after trauma. Multiple parts of the body may be involved including, and especially, the face, extremities, and gastrointestinal tract. Edema of the bowel wall may result in crampy abdominal pain, obstipation, vomiting, and abdominal rigidity. The most severe complication is laryngeal edema, which may result in asphyxiation and death. Most cases of HAE manifest in childhood but often worsen during adolescence. The severity and frequency of attacks vary greatly among patients. Only minor trauma is necessary to induce an attack with common triggers including contact sports and dental work. Sometimes an erythematous rash (erythema marginatum) may accompany attacks. The diagnosis of HAE is made by history and by evaluating complement levels (low C4, C2, and antigenic or functional C1 esterase inhibitor levels). Patients with HAE usually respond to androgen therapy.

Physical Urticarias

The physical urticarias are a unique subgroup of chronic urticarias in which wheals can be reproducibly induced by a physical stimulus. Cold, heat, pressure, vibration, light, water, exercise, and increases in core body temperature are all provoking stimuli. Physical urticarias make up as much as 17% of chronic urticarias and occur most frequently in young adults. The physical urticarias are distinguished by episodic lesions often limited to the areas of physical stimuli. In some patients, more than one type of physical urticaria may be present. The urticarial lesions are likely caused, in part, to mast cell activation and mediator release. Mast cell mediators, especially histamine, have been demonstrated in draining venous blood and in tissue fluids obtained from urticated areas in patients with various forms of physical urticarias. The mechanism by which a physical stimulus to the skin releases mast cell mediators is not fully understood but may involve neuropeptides. In some forms of physical urticaria, a passive transfer factor (usually IgE) in the serum has been reported. Only the more common physical urticarias are discussed here.

Symptomatic Dermatographism

Two percent to 5% of the general population may have dermatographism, but only a subgroup have symptomatic dermatographism. Dermatographism means "writing on the skin" and is manifest by transient wheal and erythematous responses occurring within minutes after stroking the skin with sufficient pressure ($3600 \ g/cm^2$). A transferable factor (probably IgE) has been identified in some patients. The disease usually can be treated with antihistamines.

Cholinergic Urticaria

Cholinergic urticaria is fairly common and occurs most frequently in teenagers and young adults. The skin lesions are often distinctive and appear as 2- to 4-mm pruritic wheals surrounded by extensive areas of macular erythema occurring most prominently on the upper trunk and arms. Systemic manifestations, including confluent urticaria, angioedema, hypotension, wheezing, and gastrointestinal complaints have been reported in patients with cholinergic urticaria after exercise. Furthermore, increases in blood histamine and neutrophil and eosinophil chemotactic factors have been demonstrated after provocative challenges. Cholinergic urticaria is a disease in which symptoms can be reproducibly induced by warming the body. It is postulated that the cholinergic nervous system effector mechanisms involved in the compensatory responses in thermoregulation may ultimately lead to mast cell degranulation. Elevation in core temperature induced by either exercise or passive heating (eg, hot bath), but not by endogenous pyrogen, has elicited symptoms in susceptible subjects. Attacks can be aborted sometimes by prompt cooling of the patient (eg, cold bath). Some patients have a refractory period after a severe attack. This effect can be used to develop a program to induce tolerance by subjecting the patient to carefully graded increasing stimuli.

Exercise-Induced Anaphylactic Syndrome

Exercise-induced anaphylactic syndrome (EIA) is clinically manifested by urticaria and the signs and symptoms of a classic anaphylactic reaction. Elevated plasma histamine levels have been demonstrated using provocative challenges. The disease appears to be more common among young adults. There have been reports of a family tendency in some subjects. Some subjects have symptoms only if exercise occurs postprandially. Celery, wheat, and shellfish are the foods most commonly implicated as precipitants, but any food may be associated with attacks. Subjects with postprandial EIA may avoid attacks by not eating for 4 to 6 hours before exercise. EIA and cholinergic urticaria are clinically similar in that both diseases may occur after exercise. EIA, however, is not related to core temperature and appears to be caused by either an abnormal release of a mast cell degranulating factor or an exaggerated response to a factor ordinarily released during exercise that is capable of inducing mast cell degranulation (eg, opioids). Because historical and clinical presentations of these two exercise-related syndromes are similar, diagnostic tests must be performed to distinguish those individuals having cholinergic urticaria/anaphylaxis from those with true exercise-induced anaphylaxis. Passive heat challenges are positive only in the subjects with cholinergic urticaria. A negative exercise challenge does not rule out the diagnosis of EIA because exercise does not always reproduce symptom development in these subjects.

Cold Urticaria

Familial urticarias are autosomal dominant disorders characterized by burning erythematous papules with inflammatory cell infiltrates occurring after cold exposure. There are two forms of familial cold urticaria, an immediate form with onset of symptoms at $1/2$ to 3 hours and a rare delayed form with onset of symptoms at 9 to 18 hours. The immediate familial form may be accompanied by a flulike syndrome. Essential (acquired) cold urticaria is more common than the familial forms. Essential cold urticaria appears within minutes of cold contact and rewarming and is manifested by pruritic wheals. Syncope and anaphylaxis may occur after intensive cold exposure in the essential form. Indeed, swimming has resulted in massive mediator release and drowning. Provocative testing for the familial forms involves cold air exposure. The essential form, but not the familial forms, may be elicited by placing a plastic-wrapped ice cube on the skin. Passive transfer has been accomplished only with the essential form. Connective tissue disorders, malignancies, or syphilis may be associated with acquired cold urticaria.

Delayed Pressure Urticaria/Angioedema

Delayed pressure urticaria/angioedema is manifested by deep tender swelling with or without urticaria. The lesions are localized and occur 3 to 12 hours after exposure to sustained pressure. Flulike symptoms may accompany these lesions. Common precipitating events include walking (foot swelling), clapping (hand swelling), sitting (buttock swelling), and swelling under belts or tight articles of clothing. This disease may respond to nonsteroidal anti-inflammatory drugs.

Solar Urticaria

Solar urticaria can occur at all ages but is more common in the fourth and fifth decades. The disease is characterized by pruritic wheals or morbilliform erythema occurring within minutes on sun-exposed areas. Anaphylactic symptoms may occur when large body areas are exposed. If patients react only to the 400- to 500-nm wavelength, erythropoietic protoporphyria, and porphyria cutanea tarda should be excluded.

Vibratory Angioedema

Vibratory angioedema is characterized by the rapid onset of localized angioedema proportional to the intensity and duration of the vibratory stimulus and body surface area involved. Common precipitators include vigorous towelling, lawn mowing, and motorcycling. A familial autosomal dominant form of this disease exists. Delayed pressure urticaria/angioedema and dermatographism should be excluded with appropriate tests.

■ DIAGNOSTIC EVALUATION

As with most diseases, the history and physical examination are key to the evaluation of patients with urticaria and angioedema. A detailed history of drug and new food exposure is essential. Drugs that have been taken for several months or drugs that have just been added can cause urticaria. A diary containing information about urticarial outbreaks in relation to time of day, food ingestion, activity, and exposure to possible precipitants can be extremely helpful. A thorough physical examination should be performed.

Signs and symptoms of systemic diseases and infections should be followed up with diagnostic tests. Provocative testing should be performed on patients thought to have a physical urticaria.

Because chronic urticaria in children is usually a benign disorder and most diagnostic tests are negative, extensive testing is indicated only when a systemic disease is suspected. Skin testing is generally not indicated for chronic urticaria and should be reserved for patients with histories suggestive of an allergen-induced disorder. If the cause is not obvious, I recommend a urinalysis, liver function tests, complete blood count, differential white blood cell count, and erythrocyte sedimentation rate or C-reactive protein to screen for hepatitis, infections, connective tissue diseases, eosinophilia, and leukemias. Stool for ova and parasites, complement assays, antinuclear antibodies, thyroid functions, and immunoglobulin levels are not routinely obtained unless a specific diagnosis is suspected.

Skin biopsy tests are generally not helpful. Skin biopsy tests should be performed, however, when individual urticarial lesions persist for more than 24 to 48 hours, or when the lesions are suggestive of cutaneous vasculitis or urticaria pigmentosa. Biopsy tests may be helpful if the lesions are hyperpigmented or leave a pigmented scar as they fade, or if the lesions have blisters. Another indication is refractoriness to therapy.

■ TREATMENT

The general principles of treatment of urticaria or angioedema are outlined in Table 195–2. When a causative agent is identified, the treatment of choice, if feasible, is avoidance. This generally applies when a specific allergen is identified, or when the patient has a physical urticaria. If an associated systemic disease is found, treatment of the underlying condition is necessary. Patients should also be advised to avoid potentiating factors such as alcohol, opioids, and heat. Induction of tolerance may be attempted for some forms of physical urticaria (cholinergic, solar, cold, and localized heat urticaria and vibratory angioedema). Immunotherapy (allergy shots) is not indicated for urticaria without accompanying respiratory symptoms.

Drug therapy to relieve symptoms should be instituted while the cause is investigated. Therapy should be aimed at relieving most symptoms while keeping side effects from the drugs to a minimum. The patient may have some lesions despite therapy. To minimize side effects, additional drug therapy is not indicated when remaining lesions are not physically or emotionally disturbing to the patient.

TABLE 195-2. Management of Chronic Urticaria or Angioedema

Avoidance or treatment of underlying cause

Avoidance of potentiating factors (*eg*, alcohol)

H_1 antihistamines

   Classic (*eg*, hydroxyzine)

   Nonsedating (terfenadine or astemizole)

   Tricyclic antidepressants

Combinations of H_1 antihistamines

Combinations of H_1 and H_2 antihistamines

Addition of sympathomimetics (*eg*, ephedrine)

Corticosteroids (rarely)

In acute severe urticaria or angioedema, subcutaneous epinephrine is the treatment of choice. Oral antihistamines of the H_1 class remain the drugs of choice for recurrent or chronic urticaria. Specific dosage recommendations are somewhat arbitrary. Therapy should begin with low doses and be titrated upward to relieve symptoms without causing significant adverse side effects (usually drowsiness). Terfenadine and astemizole are the only nonsedating antihistamines available, but neither is approved for children younger than age 12 years. If symptoms continue, the addition of a second, chemically distinct class of H_1 antihistamines, or the concomitant use of an H_2 antihistamine may be beneficial. Sympathomimetics such as ephedrine may also be useful adjuncts to H_1 antihistamine therapy. Tricyclic antidepressants such as doxepin and amitriptyline are potent antihistamines and are effective antiurticarial agents. For severe urticaria/angioedema unresponsive to these measures and disabling to the patient, corticosteroids may be tried. A short "burst" of corticosteroids usually relieves symptoms. Rarely, a patient requires low daily or alternate-day corticosteroids for a longer time. Prolonged treatment with large doses of corticosteroids should be avoided because of the potential side effects. Antihistamines should not be discontinued during corticosteroid treatment. Newer drugs capable of antagonizing mediators other than histamine or inhibiting mast cell degranulation may prove more effective than traditional antihistamines.

(Abridged from Thomas B. Casale, Urticaria and Angioedema, in Oski, DeAngelis, Feigin, McMillan, Warshaw: *Principles and Practice of Pediatrics, Second Edition,* J.B. Lippincott, 1994.)

Oski's Essential Pediatrics,
edited by Kevin B. Johnson and Frank A. Oski.
Lippincott–Raven Publishers,
Philadelphia © 1997

196

Food Allergies

■ FOOD ALLERGIES

Adverse food reactions are the result of food hypersensitivity (adverse immunologic responses) or food intolerance (adverse physiologic responses). Food intolerance makes up most adverse food reactions and is secondary to toxic or pharmacologic substances found in some foods, chemical or microbial contaminants, or metabolic disorders of the host (*eg*, lactose intolerance). Although an IgE-mediated mechanism is the most well-established form of hypersensitivity response, other less well-defined immunologic mechanisms are believed responsible for such disorders as celiac disease, milk- and soy-induced enterocolitis, and colitis syndromes.

■ PREVALENCE

The term *food allergy* is frequently used to denote any adverse food reaction, a misnomer that leads to considerable confusion in this field. In addition, the perceived prevalence of food allergy is far greater than actual prevalence. Household surveys suggest that one third of American families alter their eating patterns in the belief that at least one family member suffers from a food allergy. In one survey of a general pediatric practice involving 480 babies followed from birth until their third birthday, 28% of the infants were reported to have experienced adverse food reactions. Only 8%, however, had symptoms confirmed by oral food challenge. In three large studies of infants followed through their third birthday, the prevalence of cow's milk allergy was found to be 2.2% to 2.5%. The majority of food allergies present in the first year of life, but only a minority (25%) persist beyond a child's third birthday. Although comprehensive epidemiologic studies are not available, the prevalence of true food allergy is probably 3% to 4% in young children and 1% to 2% in adults.

■ PATHOGENESIS

The pathogenesis of food allergy involves three areas: the food or allergen, the gastrointestinal (GI) barrier and its handling of food, and the individual's genetic predisposition to develop an allergic response. Despite a widely varied Western diet, relatively few foods account for the majority of allergic responses. In children, egg, peanut, milk, soy, wheat, and fish account for about 90% of reactions. The allergenic fractions of these foods have several things in common: they are glycoproteins of about 20,000 to 60,000 daltons, they are largely heat and acid stable, and they are water soluble.

The GI tract uses both nonimmunologic and immunologic mechanisms to prevent intact foreign antigens from gaining access to the body while processing ingested food into forms that can be absorbed and used for energy and cell growth. IgA secreted into the gut lumen binds foreign antigens, such as food, and impedes their absorption. IgA–food antigen complexes become "hung up" in the glycocalyx, where enzymes in the mucosal cell brush border can break down these complex proteins. Food antigen-specific IgA and IgG in the blood may be involved in clearing antigens that enter the circulation. Although greater than 98% of ingested antigen is blocked by this GI barrier, minute amounts of intact food antigens are absorbed and transported throughout the body. Factors such as decreased stomach acidity or the ingestion of alcohol increase antigen absorption. Antigenically intact food proteins entering the circulation, however, generally do not cause adverse reactions because most individuals develop tolerance to ingested food antigens.

Studies in mice provide some insight into the development of oral tolerance. After "gut closure" at 4 days of life, a single antigen feeding suppresses antigen-specific IgM, IgG, and IgE antibody responses and cell-mediated immune responses. Gut processing of food antigens to a "tolerogenic" form is essential in developing this oral tolerance. Lymphoid cells in the GI tract are needed to generate the tolerogenic proteins; irradiation of mice abrogates their ability to form tolerogenic ovalbumin, whereas subsequent infusion of normal spleen cells restores their ability to form tolerogenic protein. Antigen-presenting cells also appear to play a critical role in the development of oral tolerance. Agents that enhance antigen-presenting cell activity interfere with generation of CD8$^+$ (suppressor) cells and the development of oral tolerance.

Young infants are at increased risk for developing food allergic reactions because of immunologic immaturity and, to some extent, immaturity of the gut. Consequently, genetically predisposed infants ingesting food antigens may generate excessive food-specific IgE antibodies or other abnormal immune responses. Several prospective studies suggest that exclusive breast-feeding may promote the development of oral tolerance and prevent some food allergy and atopic dermatitis in infants and young children. This protective effect is speculated to be the result of decreased exposure to foreign proteins, passive immunologic protection provided by breast milk s-IgA, and soluble factors in breast milk that induce earlier maturation of the GI barrier and the infant's immune response.

■ CLINICAL SYMPTOMS

A variety of food-allergic reactions have been confirmed by controlled trials. These reactions are outlined in Table 196–1.

Respiratory Reactions

Both upper and lower respiratory reactions have been provoked during double-blind, placebo-controlled oral food challenges (DBPCFC). Within minutes to 2 hours of ingestion, food allergens may induce typical signs and symptoms of rhinoconjunctivitis, although isolated upper airway symptoms are uncommon. These include periocular pruritus and erythema, and tearing; nasal congestion, pruritus, sneezing, and rhinorrhea. Nasal lavage fluid histamine levels rise significantly with the onset of nasal symptoms during DBPCFCs, strongly implicating a pathogenic role for nasal mast cell activation. Similarly, pulmonary function studies during DBPCFCs demonstrate significant drops in FVC, FEV$_1$, and maximal midexpiratory flow (MMEF) in patients experiencing a positive food challenge.

TABLE 196-1. Symptoms Substantiated by Controlled Food Challenges

GENERALIZED ANAPHYLAXIS WITH CARDIOVASCULAR COLLAPSE (SOMETIMES ASSOCIATED WITH EXERCISE)

RESPIRATORY

Upper airway—rhinoconjunctivitis, laryngeal edema

Lower airway—wheezing (asthma)

CUTANEOUS

Urticaria/angioedema

Atopic dermatitis

Urticaria associated with exercise

Dermatitis herpetiformis

GASTROINTESTINAL

IgE-mediated—lip swelling, palatal itching, tongue swelling, nausea, abdominal pain, cramps, emesis, and diarrhea

Coeliac disease and dermatitis herpetiformis

Protein gastroenteropathy, especially to soy and milk—diarrhea, gross or occult blood loss, malabsorption, and failure to thrive (FTT)

Milk-induced colitis—diarrhea and gross blood loss

Heiner's syndrome—pulmonary infiltrates, iron deficiency, anemia, emesis, diarrhea, and FTT

Colic—cow's milk-induced and allergen in breast milk

Eosinophilic gastroenteritis

NEUROLOGIC

Migraine

Consumption of food allergens rarely are the main aggravating factor in chronic rhinoconjunctivitis and asthma, and studies suggest that ingesting food allergens leads to bronchial hyperreactivity. Two large series of asthmatic patients followed in pulmonary clinics were evaluated for food allergy. In one survey, 300 patients of all ages were evaluated for food allergy by history, prick skin tests, or radioallergosorbent tests (RAST). Findings suggestive of food-induced symptoms were evaluated by blinded food challenges. Six patients (2%) had wheezing provoked by the food challenge. In the second series of 140 children with asthma, 8 patients (6%) had wheezing induced by oral food challenge. All asthmatic children with food-induced wheezing either had atopic dermatitis or a history of eczema.

Food-induced pulmonary hemosiderosis is a syndrome of chronic or recurrent pulmonary disease (with hemosiderosis), chronic rhinitis, GI blood loss, and iron deficiency anemia and failure to thrive secondary to milk ingestion; it was initially described by Heiner. Other foods rarely have been implicated.

Cutaneous Reactions

The skin is the most common target organ in IgE-mediated food hypersensitivity. Ingestion of food allergens may provoke rapid onset of cutaneous symptoms or aggravate more chronic conditions.

Urticaria/Angioedema

Acute urticaria and angioedema are among the most common symptoms of food allergic reactions. The exact prevalence of these reactions is unknown. In most cases, patients do not seek medical assistance (or even report the reaction) because the onset of hives or swelling occurs within minutes of ingesting the responsible food allergen, making the cause-and-effect nature of the reaction obvious to the patient. The foods most commonly incriminated include eggs, milk, peanuts, and nuts in children and fish, shellfish, nuts, and peanuts in adults. Food hypersensitivity is occasionally incriminated in chronic urticaria and angioedema (symptoms lasting longer than 6 weeks). In one series of 163 children with chronic or recurrent urticaria, food allergy was implicated in only 10% of patients.

■ DIAGNOSIS

Symptoms secondary to food hypersensitivity that have been confirmed by appropriate controlled studies are listed in Table 196–1. Other symptoms often attributed to "food allergy" have not been substantiated in controlled trials. Some of these symptoms may be due to pharmacologic properties of certain foods such as sleep disturbances in children who drink caffeinated beverages. The differential diagnosis of food sensitivity is broad (Table 196–2), but careful history often suggests the appropriate diagnostic category to pursue.

Although history can be verified in only 30% to 40% of cases, it is important to the evaluation. History should reveal types of symptoms, when symptoms occurred after ingestion, severity of symptoms, whether symptoms occurred more than once, and whether cofactors (eg, exercise) are necessary to elicit symptoms. In general, symptoms occurring soon after ingestion are more likely to be due to food hypersensitivity than are those that take hours or days to develop. Physical examination may exclude some disorders in the differential diagnosis, but there is nothing in the physical examination that is unique for individuals with food hypersensitivity.

TABLE 196-2. Differential Diagnosis of Adverse Food Reactions

GASTROINTESTINAL DISORDERS

Structural abnormalities—pyloric stenosis, hiatal hernia, tracheo-esophageal fistula

Enzyme deficiencies—(primary versus secondary) lactase deficiency, sucrase deficiency, etc.

Malignancy—lymphoma

Other—cystic fibrosis, gallbladder disease

PHARMACOLOGIC AGENTS

Caffeine (coffee, tea, soft drinks, cocoa)

Theobromine (chocolate, tea)

Tyramine (cheese, banana, tomato)

Tryptamine (tomato, blue plum)

Histamine (fish, beer, wine)

Phenylethylamine (chocolate)

CONTAMINANTS AND ADDITIVES

Flavorings and preservatives

Dyes

Toxins (bacterial, seafood-associated)

Infectious organisms

PSYCHOLOGICAL REACTIONS

Various diagnostic studies (eg, x-rays, breath hydrogen, biopsy tests) exclude many anatomic and metabolic abnormalities. Laboratory studies such as prick skin tests and IgE-specific food antibodies (eg, RAST, fluorescent allergosorbent test [FAST], multiple-thread allergosorbent test [MAST]) are of some value in discriminating among the foods responsible for immediate hypersensitivity reactions. There is no evidence to support the use of IgG-specific food antibodies or food antigen–antibody complexes in the diagnosis of food sensitivity.

To establish whether a patient has food hypersensitivity, a provocative oral food challenge is necessary. Food challenges may be performed openly, when both the patient and the physician know the contents of the challenge; single-blind, when only the physician is aware of the contents of the challenge; or double-blind, when neither the patient nor the physician knows the contents of the challenge. Placebo controls are necessary in the blinded challenges if they are to be truly blind. Only the double-blind procedure is free of psychological factors and inherent bias on the part of the patient and the physician. Several studies comparing results of single-blind and double-blind challenges in the same patient population have demonstrated the necessity of removing observer bias.

For research purposes, the DBPCFC should be the "gold standard" for diagnosing food allergy. In some cases, such as celiac disease, open challenge followed by intestinal biopsy is the diagnostic approach of choice. Although the DBPCFC provides a scientifically acceptable means of diagnosing food hypersensitivity, it is often not practical in the office practice setting. Table 196–3 outlines an approach that should be more useful to the pediatrician in the office setting. The initial evaluation consists of a careful history and physical examination, and laboratory studies suggested by the history or physical. If immediate hypersensitivity is suspected, results of prick skin testing to a battery of six to eight foods (egg, milk, peanut, fish, shellfish, nuts, soy, and wheat) or other foods suggested by history could be helpful. Nega-

TABLE 196-3. Evaluating Food Sensitivity

HISTORY AND PHYSICAL EXAMINATION

History—stress type of symptoms, timing, severity, and reproducibility

Physical examination—exclude many possibilities in differential

LABORATORY TEST

Studies suggested by history and physical examination (eg, x-rays, breath hydrogen, sweat test)

Skin tests—prick technique with commercial extract or fresh food

　If negative (wheal <3 mm), immediate hypersensitivity very unlikely, further workup probably unnecessary

　If positive (wheal >3 mm), proceed to allergen avoidance trial

STRICT ALLERGEN AVOIDANCE DIET FOR 2 WEEKS

Include foods suggested by history for most sensitivities, also foods suggested by prick skin tests for immediate hypersensitivity

If unequivocal improvement and only one major or one or two minor foods involved, continue restricted diet

If equivocal improvement or more than two foods involved, refer to allergist or gastroenterologist for evaluation

tive prick skin tests (ie, a wheal diameter less than 3 mm larger than the negative control wheal) make immediate hypersensitivity extremely unlikely and preclude the further evaluation, unless the history highly suggests otherwise. Such skin testing is valuable only when an IgE-mediated mechanism is suspected.

Foods suspected by history should be eliminated from the patient's diet for 2 weeks. If symptoms have unequivocally improved, the diet may be continued unless it requires the elimination of more than one major food (egg, milk, soy, wheat) or two or more minor foods (any food other than major food). If symptoms persist unabated and food sensitivity is still contemplated, a brief trial (no longer than 2 weeks) of a severely restricted diet may be warranted. The following diets may be used: for patients younger than 4 months old—milk substitute (Nutramigen, Pregestimil, or Vivonex); for patients aged 4 to 8 months—milk substitute, rice cereal (many infant cereals contain more than one grain), and pears; for patients aged 9 to 24 months—same as for 4- to 8-month-old patients plus rice, carrots, squash, and lamb; for patients older than 2 years—same as for 9- to 24-month-old patients plus fresh lettuce, potato, safflower oil, tea, and sugar.

If symptoms fail to improve, an adverse food reaction can be ruled out.

When improvement is not clear or several foods appear to be incriminated, a single-blind, or even an open, challenge should be performed in the office setting under observation. Because food challenges are time-consuming and may result in severe anaphylaxis, many pediatricians prefer to refer patients to a qualified allergist to perform these studies. When immediate hypersensitivity reactions are suspected, challenges should never be performed at home by parents. If challenges are performed in the office, appropriate equipment and personnel should be available in the office to deal with an emergency. If the office challenges reveal positive responses to only one major food or less than four foods in total, an appropriate elimination diet may be instituted. Such a diet would not be overly restrictive, and the results of such challenges would be acceptable.

Positive challenges to more than one major food or more than four foods in total should raise concern about the accuracy of the office challenges and suggest the need to refer the

patient for DBPCFC. Embarking on a diet restricted in a large number of foods without sound documentation subjects the patient to a diet that is extremely difficult to comply with and that may be nutritionally deficient.

If the clinician follows the protocol outlined in Table 196–3, it is likely that the DBPCFC is necessary in only a minority of patients. The need for sound documentation of food sensitivity by challenge procedures, however, cannot be overemphasized. Overly restricted diets in young children can lead to various eating disorders and create family conflict, especially around meal time. When various subjective complaints are ruled out (eg, vague abdominal complaints, behavioral problems), or when symptoms are reported to take several hours to days to develop, DBPCFC may be conducted at home. Extreme caution should be exercised, however, when recommending that parents administer a food at home. Only foods that are felt to be unlikely to elicit an immediate-type allergic reaction should be tested at home.

Other procedures advocated as useful in making the diagnosis of food hypersensitivity are leukocyte cytotoxicity tests, sublingual provocation with drops of antigen extracts, subcutaneous provocation with varying concentrations of food extracts, and measurement of IgG- or IgG4-specific antibody. None of these procedures has been demonstrated to be useful in controlled studies.

■ TREATMENT

Strict avoidance of the offending food allergen is the only proven therapy for food sensitivity. Drugs may modify symptoms in some cases, but such measures should only be considered palliative. Corticosteroids alleviate symptoms in some protein enteropathy syndromes and may be life-saving in some fulminant secretory diarrheas, but the side effects of long-term therapy generally are unacceptable. Antihistamines may modify symptoms of immediate hypersensitivity but rarely, if ever, block them completely. Oral cromolyn sodium has been advocated, but carefully controlled trials in patients with challenge-confirmed food sensitivity failed to demonstrate efficacy. Rotational diets, immunotherapy, and sublingual or subcutaneous neutralization has never been shown to be efficacious in controlled trials.

Young infants sensitive to cow's milk generally can be managed adequately with hypoallergenic formulas such as Alimentum or Nutramigen. Infants with cow's milk protein enteropathy syndrome develop sensitivity to soy in as many as 50% of cases. Many infants develop diarrhea and localized skin rashes after ingesting various fruits and fruit juices (citrus, apple, grapes, tomato). These reactions appear to represent "intolerance" and are generally short-lived. Most infants with food sensitivity can have their diets expanded appropriately (ie, addition of fruits, vegetables, and meats) without difficulty. Adding only one new food every 3 to 5 days, however, is probably a useful practice.

Children older than 2 years of age rarely, if ever, require an elemental diet for treatment of food sensitivity. Appropriate oral challenge studies generally reveal only one or two specific food sensitivities in more than 90% of cases. The most practical method for implementing strict allergen avoidance diets is to teach parents (and older patients) to read food labels. Long lists of foods that patients "may" or "may not" eat are difficult to follow and are readily outdated. Educating patients to recognize key words, ingredient listings that indicate the presence of a specific food, allows the least restrictive diet and results in good dietary compliance. For example, the presence of milk may be indicated by any of the following key words: milk, dried milk solids, whey, casein, lactalbumin, caseinates, cheese, butter, or curds. A dietitian's assistance in suggesting alternative food preparation techniques and ensuring a nutritionally sufficient diet is invaluable.

Strict allergen avoidance frequently leads to development of clinical tolerance to foods eliciting adverse responses. Virtually all young infants experiencing diarrhea in response to cow's milk or soy protein lose their sensitivity in 1 to 3 years. Several studies demonstrate the loss of immediate hypersensitivity reactions in about one third of patients after 1 year of antigen avoidance. Although young infants more consistently lose their food sensitivity, loss of hypersensitivity is not confined to the younger child. In addition, the clinical severity of the initial adverse reaction does not necessarily influence the longevity of the hypersensitivity. Infants younger than 2 years old with mild reactions may be rechallenged every 4 to 6 months to ascertain if symptoms persist. Older patients may be rechallenged every 1 to 2 years, depending on how difficult it is to avoid the food in question. Because loss of sensitivity varies with the antigen (eg, peanut, tree nuts, and fish appear to be persistent), rechallenging with some foods should be undertaken no sooner than every 4 to 5 years. In certain disorders, such as celiac disease or dermatitis herpetiformis, restricted diets should be continued indefinitely.

Clinical reactivity to a food appears to be highly specific, and rarely are children sensitive to more than one or two foods. Although results of skin tests and in vitro tests of specific IgE commonly demonstrate cross-reactivity among members of a botanical family or animal species, clinically relevant intrabotanical cross-reactivity and intraspecies cross-reactivity are rare. Consequently, it appears unwarranted to avoid all foods within a botanical family when one member is suspected of provoking allergic symptoms. By avoiding this practice, patient compliance with elimination diets is improved and a nutritionally deficient diet is less likely to be implemented.

Several contradictory reports discuss the role of breast-feeding in the prevention of food allergy. Several recent prospective studies suggest that exclusive breast-feeding for 6 months can reduce the infant's risk of developing food hypersensitivity and atopic dermatitis but may only postpone development of other atopic disorders. Avoidance of highly allergenic foods (peanut, egg, milk) by the lactating mother may be beneficial, but dietary manipulation in the third trimester of pregnancy appears to offer no advantage and may compromise the pregnant mother's nutritional status.

■ CONCLUSION

Food intolerance reactions probably represent the majority of food sensitivities in children, are more common in the young infant, and are short-lived. Both food intolerance and food hypersensitivity should be treated by strict avoidance of the inciting food. Repeated challenges should be conducted at varying intervals, depending on the age of the child, the type of reaction provoked, and the food involved to ascertain whether the sensitivity persists. Studies to document accurately the presence of food sensitivity will simplify the management of this disorder by reducing the number of foods that need to be eliminated from the patient's diet and the length of time they need to be avoided.

(Abridged from Hugh A. Sampson, Food Allergies, in Oski, DeAngelis, Feigin, McMillan, Warshaw: *Principles and Practice of Pediatrics, Second Edition*, J.B. Lippincott, 1994.)

Oski's Essential Pediatrics,
edited by Kevin B. Johnson and Frank A. Oski.
Lippincott–Raven Publishers,
Philadelphia © 1997

197

Atopic Dermatitis

Besnier, a French physician, presented the first comprehensive description of atopic dermatitis a century ago. He emphasized its hereditary nature, its chronically recurring course, and its association with hay fever and asthma. Wise and Sulzberger later coined the term *atopic dermatitis* to further emphasize the relationship between atopic eczema, hay fever, and asthma (the allergic triad). Like asthmatics, patients with atopic dermatitis may be divided into those with extrinsic and intrinsic forms of the disorder. Patients with extrinsic atopic dermatitis are generally younger than 20 years old, and flares of eczema are exacerbated by specific food or airborne allergens, whereas patients with intrinsic atopic dermatitis tend to be older and show no evidence of allergen-induced flares.

■ INCIDENCE

Epidemiologic studies suggest that atopic dermatitis affects between 10% and 12% of the pediatric population and has been increasing in prevalence over the past 20 years. More than 20% of pediatric dermatology visits and about 1% of pediatric visits are related to atopic dermatitis. Earlier reports that atopic dermatitis is primarily a disease of industrialized societies have been refuted by more recent epidemiologic studies.

■ DEFINITION AND CLINICAL FEATURES

Atopic dermatitis is a chronic cutaneous inflammatory disorder that generally begins in early infancy. About 60% of patients affected develop symptoms within the first year of life and 85% within the first 5 years. The skin symptoms generally present as an erythematous, papulovesicular eruption that progresses to a scaly, lichenified dermatitis over time. The distribution of the rash typically varies with age.

In infancy (3 to 6 months to 2 years), the cheeks, wrists, and extensor surfaces of the arms and legs typically develop papulovesicular, often weeping lesions that occasionally develop fine scaling or lichenification. The scalp and postauricular area frequently are affected with dermatitis. The eczematous dermatitis may involve the entire body, but generally the diaper area is spared. Frequent scratching results in obvious traumatic lesions and secondary infection.

Flexor surfaces, neck, wrists, and ankles generally are involved in the young child (2 to 12 years), with dry maculopapular lesions being a more prominent feature. Pruritus and scratching lead to excoriations, hyperpigmentation, and lichenification.

In the teenage patient and young adult, flexural surfaces, face (especially periorbital), hands, and feet frequently are involved. Extreme xerosis, marked papulation, and lichenification are characteristic of this stage. Older patients often have symptom-free periods that last for months, but even during remission, these patients retain a tendency toward dry, sensitive skin.

Unlike most dermatoses, atopic dermatitis has no primary skin lesion but is identified by a constellation of symptoms. The classification system described in Table 197-1 is the internationally accepted criterion for diagnosing atopic dermatitis. Modification of this criterion for the young infant is outlined in Table 197–2. Emphasis is placed on the extremely pruritic nature of the rash, its typical morphology and distribution, and its tendency toward a chronic or relapsing course. Some features, such as anterior subcapsular cataracts, nipple eczema, and upper lip cheilitis are uncommon but specific for diagnosing atopic dermatitis, whereas others such as orbital darkening, Dennie-Morgan infraorbital fold, and hyperlinearity of the palms are common but not specific.

There is no single, routine laboratory test that helps in diagnosing atopic dermatitis. Peripheral blood eosinophilia (5% to 20%) and elevated total serum IgE concentrations are present in as many as 80% of patients. Tests for specific IgE antibodies to foods and inhalants (eg, prick skin tests, radioallergosorbent tests [RAST]) are positive in at least 80% of pediatric patients. Intracutaneous injection of acetylcholine (0.1 mL of 1:1000) leads to increased sweating and

TABLE 197-1. Diagnostic Features of Atopic Dermatitis

MAJOR FEATURES*

Pruritus

Typical morphology and distribution
  Flexural lichenification or hyperlinearity in adults
  Facial and extensor involvement in infants and children

Chronic or chronically relapsing course

Personal or family history of atopy (asthma, allergic rhinitis, or atopic dermatitis)

MINOR FEATURES*

Xerosis

Ichthyosis/palmar hyperlinearity/keratosis pilaris

Immediate (type I) skin test reactivity

Elevated serum IgE

Early age of onset

Tendency toward cutaneous infections (especially S aureus and herpes simplex)/impaired cell-mediated immunity

Tendency toward nonspecific hand or foot dermatitis

Nipple eczema

Cheilitis

Recurrent conjunctivitis

Dennie-Morgan infraorbital fold

Keratoconus

Anterior subcapsular cataracts

Orbital darkening

Facial pallor/facial erythema

Pityriasis alba

Itch when sweating

Intolerance to wool and lipid solvents

Perifollicular accentuation

Food hypersensitivity

Course influenced by environmental/emotional factors

White dermographism/delayed blanch

Must have three or more.

TABLE 197-2. Diagnostic Features of Atopic Dermatitis for Infants

MAJOR FEATURES*

Family history of atopic disease

Typical facial or extensor eczematous or lichenified dermatitis

Evidence of pruritus

MINOR FEATURES*

Xerosis, icthyosis, hyperlinear palms

Perifollicular accentuation

Postauricular fissures

Chronic scalp scaling

Must have three or more.

delayed blanching at the injection site (normal response—erythema, sweating, and piloerection).

■ PHYSIOLOGIC ABNORMALITIES

Physiologic abnormalities described in patients with atopic dermatitis are decreased itch threshold, increased transepidermal water loss, abnormal cutaneous vascular responses, and abnormal pharmacologic responses including "beta-adrenergic blockade."

Itch is the dominant symptom in atopic dermatitis and the major cause of damaging excoriations, erosions, and lichenifications, which are characteristic of atopic dermatitis. The etiology of increased itching is unknown. Vasodilation precedes pruritus, suggesting that local release of mediators is responsible for increased pruritus. The increased number of mast cells and elevated tissue histamine in chronically involved areas support this hypothesis.

Increased transepidermal water loss is believed to be secondary to decreased sebum production. Sweating is abnormal in these patients. Studies evaluating amount of sweating are contradictory, but, in general, sweating is believed to be increased. A variety of abnormal vascular responses include exaggerated constrictor response of cutaneous vessels and poor adaptability (vascular hyperactivity), white dermographism, delayed blanch to cholinergic stimuli, and paradoxical response to application of nicotinic acid. None of these responses are specific for atopic dermatitis.

Atopic dermatitis patients have several features suggesting the presence of beta blockade. Their skin lacks the expected inhibition of DNA synthesis after treatment with beta-adrenergic agonists, and their leukocytes show functional responses that correlate with subnormal cellular cyclic-AMP levels after beta-adrenergic stimulation. Some studies show a consistent increase in cyclic-AMP phosphodiesterase activity in untreated mononuclear leukocytes from patients with atopic dermatitis, but not in patients with contact dermatitis. This increased phosphodiesterase activity could account for the reduced cyclic-AMP levels seen in patients with atopic dermatitis.

■ ETIOLOGY

The etiology of atopic dermatitis is unknown. Food and airborne allergens may reach cutaneous mast cells, lymphocytes, monocytes, and Langerhans cells by way of the circulation after entering at mucosal surfaces, or through breaks in the skin. The interaction of allergens with allergen-specific IgE on the surface of mast cells activates the cells to release histamine, LTC_4, platelet-activating factor, IL-4, and other cytokines that attract other cells (eg, eosinophils, lymphocytes, and monocytes) found in an IgE-mediated late-phase response. Release of IL-4 and IL-10 by infiltrating CD4 TH_2 lymphocytes inhibits local $CD4^+$ TH_1 cells and cell-mediated responses, and promotes up-regulation of IgE receptors on Langerhans cells and monocytes leading to allergen-induced IL-1 release and the efficient presentation of allergens to T cells. Studies demonstrate the presence of allergen-specific CD4 TH_2 cells in the skin of atopic dermatitis patients. Repeated allergen exposure provokes chronic inflammation secondary to IgE-mediated mast cell and lymphocytic responses and contributes to the pathogenesis of atopic dermatitis.

Skin biopsies from chronic eczematous lesions of patients with atopic dermatitis reveal large quantities of major basic protein (MBP), excreted almost exclusively by eosinophils, in the superficial dermis, indicating that eosinophils were in the area, whereas actual eosinophils may be seen in more acute lesions. MBP is not seen in uninvolved skin sites in these same patients or in lesions of patients with contact dermatitis. In one series, some subjects developed a pruritic, erythematous, macular, or morbilliform rash, and plasma histamine levels rose after double-blind, placebo-controlled food challenge. Skin biopsy specimens obtained 4 to 14 hours later revealed an infiltration of eosinophils and MBP deposition. This indicated that food allergen-induced mast cell activation triggered both an immediate and a late-phase response in the skin. Another eosinophil product, eosinophil-derived neurotoxin, may be responsible for the demyelination of nerves in the dermal layer seen in eczematous skin.

Inhalant allergens (pollens, molds, dust mites) may also play a role in IgE-induced pathology. Normal individuals passively sensitized to ragweed absorb sufficient pollen allergen by way of nasal challenge to produce a wheal and flare response at a distal skin site. In addition, eczematous skin changes are provoked by nasal challenge in some adult patients with *Alternaria* or ragweed allergy. Using a modified patch technique with dust mite antigen, eczematous changes and, later, increased mast cell numbers have been induced in patients with IgE antibodies to dust mite.

In addition to allergen-IgE initiated immediate and late-phase hypersensitivity responses, histamine-releasing factors (eg, lymphokines, monokines) have been discovered to bind surface-bound IgE molecules and activate mast cells and basophils to release various inflammatory mediators. IgE autoantibodies also have been found in 87% of patients with atopic disorders. Because low-affinity Fc ε receptors have been found on B cells, T cells, monocytes, macrophages, eosinophils, and platelets, histamine-releasing factors and IgE autoantibody immune complexes may affect a number of immunologic responses.

■ DIAGNOSIS

The diagnosis of atopic dermatitis is based on the presence of sufficient major and minor features (see Tables 197–1 and 197–2). Absence of pruritus, typical morphology or distribution, and history of chronic or relapsing course should raise serious question as to the accuracy of the diagnosis. Seborrheic dermatitis and allergic contact dermatitis are confused most frequently with atopic dermatitis. Seborrheic dermatitis may be indistinguishable from atopic dermatitis in some cases but often may be differentiated by its more frequent distribution in the axillae and diaper area, less prominent pruritus, and general absence of elevated serum total IgE and positive

skin tests to foods and inhalants. Other less common disorders may be mistaken for atopic dermatitis: hyper-IgE syndrome, Wiskott-Aldrich syndrome, and a variety of genetic disorders such as phenylketonuria, biotinidase deficiency, and erythrokeratoderma variabilis, and histiocytosis X.

There are no consistent and distinctive laboratory abnormalities associated with atopic dermatitis. Skin biopsies are not specific, except for IgE-bearing Langerhans cells. Consequently, there are no routine tests to evaluate atopic dermatitis.

■ THERAPY

Atopic dermatitis is characterized by intermittent inflammatory exacerbations superimposed on skin that is dry and easily irritated. The exacerbations may be infrequent with prompt resolution and healing, but, more commonly, exacerbations occur regularly. A variety of trigger factors are known to exacerbate flares. These vary in patients and must be delineated in each patient for successful management.

Atopic dermatitis patients have a decreased itch threshold and are more sensitive to a variety of cutaneous irritants. Bathing in hot water and scrubbing vigorously with soap is one of the most frequent sources of irritation. Patients should be encouraged to bathe in tepid water (especially for hydration), avoid soap, and pat dry with soft absorbent towels. Clothing should be rinsed carefully after washing to remove all residual detergent.

Most patients recognize early that sweating causes pruritus. Whether sweating is induced by thermal change, exercise, or anxiety, it generally leads to cutaneous pruritus, scratching, and subsequent skin changes characteristic of atopic dermatitis. Avoiding excessive room temperature, wearing light, nonocclusive clothing (eg, cotton instead of polyester), keeping the bedroom cool, and avoiding excessive bedclothing help reduce sweating.

Cutaneous infections are a frequent cause of acute flares in atopic dermatitis. *Staphylococcus aureus* is most frequently implicated, although streptococcal infections may be seen. Infection should be presumed in the presence of acute weeping or crusted lesions, small superficial pustules, or recalcitrant crusted patches. Staphylococcal organisms are generally resistant to penicillin (90% in the author's series of 120 patients), and many (31%) are resistant to erythromycin. Ideally, the physician is guided by results of culture and sensitivity tests. Antibiotic coverage generally can be started with erythromycin, but, if there is a slow clinical response, the presence of a resistant strain may be surmised. Oral dicloxicillin or cephalosporin may be substituted. Bactroban, a topical antibiotic effective for superficial *Staphylococcus* infections, may be used when infection is localized.

When lesions fail to respond to oral antibiotics, herpes simplex infection should be considered. A Giemsa-stained Tzanck smear or culture indicates the presence of the viral infection. Patients at risk for ocular involvement or serious dissemination and systemic involvement of herpes simplex should be treated with intravenous Acyclovir. Others may be treated with povidone–iodine compresses and ointment or topical Acyclovir. Occasionally, patients are flared from superimposed dermatophyte infections. These infections respond readily to either locally applied imidazole creams or oral Griseofulvin daily for 1 month.

Despite a longstanding debate on the significance of food allergens in the pathogenesis of atopic dermatitis, recent studies demonstrate a significant causative role in some patients. Eggs, milk, peanut, soy, and wheat are the most common offenders. Overall, about one third of children with atopic dermatitis have food hypersensitivity contributing to their symptoms. The role of inhalant allergens in the pathogenesis remains controversial. There is no evidence to support the use of immunotherapy in atopic dermatitis. In many cases, the dermatitis flares when allergy shots are initiated. Some attempt to reduce dust mite exposure appears warranted. Stuffed animals, stuffed furniture, and throw rugs may be removed, mattresses should be encased in plastic covers, and bedding should be laundered frequently.

Allergic contact dermatitis is uncommon in patients with atopic dermatitis. Occasionally, patients become sensitized, especially to topical medications or preservatives. Patch testing sometimes helps detect the offending contact allergen. Patients (or their parents) are generally aware that anxiety, anger, and frustration provoke pruritus and flares of atopic dermatitis. Patients should be encouraged to verbalize their emotional conflicts, and occasionally psychological counseling should be sought. In children, potential stressful situations in the home or school should be assessed and discussed.

Several general measures may be taken to reduce pruritus and consequent skin damage secondary to scratching. Fingernails should be trimmed short, and cotton gloves may be worn at night. Because dry skin is prone to itch, efforts to obtain maximal skin hydration are mandatory. Bathing for hydration, soaking in tepid water for 20 to 30 minutes, followed by immediate application of an emollient ointment or cream is the most effective form of therapy. Lubricant creams should be applied within 3 minutes of the child getting out of the tub so water absorbed into the stratum corneum does not evaporate. For patients with marked excoriation or weeping lesions, initial wet wraps with Burrow's solution (1:40) avoid the stinging or burning sensation sometimes seen with bathing. Adding oil to bath water is generally ineffective.

Topical corticosteroids are the mainstay of therapy for atopic dermatitis. For general management, midstrength corticosteroids such as 0.1% triamcinolone cream or ointment are optimal. Occasionally, more potent fluorinated steroids are required to suppress an acute flare. Use of these potent agents should be limited because of their accompanying side effects. In general, the least potent steroid that controls a patient's symptoms should be employed. Systemic corticosteroids should be avoided in this chronic dermatitis because many patients experience a rebound flare after a short course, which only leads to further requests for systemic therapy. A course of antibiotics or hospitalization should be considered before utilizing systemic corticosteroids.

Most patients experience some symptomatic relief with antihistamines; whether this relief is due to an antipruritic or soporific effect is debated. Patient response to antihistamines varies, but hydroxyzine or doxepin appears most effective. Antihistamines are competitive antagonists and are best used on a regular basis. Single large doses of hydroxyzine (2 mg/kg up to 75 to 100 mg before bedtime) or doxepin before bedtime generally circumvents daytime sedation and facilitates nighttime sleep.

Tar preparations provide a useful nonsteroidal approach to therapy. However, gel preparations frequently irritate dry skin, and the smell is unacceptable except to the most motivated patients. Ultraviolet light (UVA and UVB) therapy is beneficial in some recalcitrant cases but should be undertaken with extreme caution and careful professional supervision. PUVA (psoralen plus UVA) therapy has been beneficial in some severe cases. The dangers of squamous cell carcinomas and skin damage make these UV therapies unacceptable in most cases. Trials with immunomodulatory agents, thymopentin (TP-5) and interferon gamma are promising in severe cases of atopic dermatitis.

Hospitalization, or a simulated hospitalization at home, should be considered as a therapeutic modality. Whether removal from daily stresses or environmental factors, a brief period of bed rest often leads to considerable symptomatic improvement.

■ COURSE AND PROGNOSIS

The course of atopic dermatitis is capricious and marked by often unexplained exacerbations and remissions. A lack of distinct diagnostic criteria has interfered with epidemiologic studies of atopic dermatitis. Figures for persistent dermatitis vary from 10% to 83% of affected children, but studies indicate that the majority of patients retain some stigmata of the disorder throughout their lives. Less favorable prognostic signs include late onset and reverse pattern (involvement of extensor surfaces instead of flexors), severe widespread dermatitis in childhood, family history of atopic dermatitis, and associated allergic rhinitis or asthma. In general, the more severe the symptoms, the less likely is a permanent remission.

(Abridged from Hugh A. Sampson, Atopic Dermatitis, in Oski, DeAngelis, Feigin, McMillan, Warshaw: *Principles and Practice of Pediatrics, Second Edition*, J.B. Lippincott, 1994.)

Oski's Essential Pediatrics,
edited by Kevin B. Johnson and Frank A. Oski.
Lippincott–Raven Publishers,
Philadelphia © 1997

198

Allergic Rhinitis and Associated Disorders

Allergic rhinitis, or inflammation of the nasal mucosa, is the most common chronic disorder of the respiratory tract, occurring in 10% of children and 15% of adolescents. Some patients with allergic rhinitis have associated disorders such as allergic conjunctivitis, chronic sinusitis, or otitis media with effusion. In allergic rhinitis and allergic conjunctivitis, severity of symptoms is clearly related to allergen exposure. In contrast, in chronic sinusitis and in otitis media with effusion, the allergic basis for symptoms may be much more subtle and controversial.

ALLERGIC RHINITIS

■ ANATOMY

The nasal passages are separated by a cartilaginous and bony septum, which varies in thickness. The turbinates on the convoluted lateral wall of each nasal passage cause the incoming air stream to change direction and flow posteriorly and superiorly. The nasal cavities are lined anteriorly with nonkeratinizing squamous epithelium and posteriorly with ciliated pseudostratified columnar epithelium interspersed with goblet cells. The lamina propria is richly supplied with small seromucous glands, and there are large serous glands scattered anteriorly. Air passing through the nose is humidified by exudate from these glands. Nasal secretions consist of mucous from the goblet cells, watery materials from the serous and seromucous glands, condensed water from expired air, tears, and transudate from serum.

The vasculature of the nasal mucosa is erectile tissue containing abundant arterial-venous anastomoses and venous sinusoids capable of intermittent engorgement. The smooth muscle of this vasculature is primarily under sympathetic (adrenergic) nervous control. Parasympathetic or cholinergic fibers are numerous around the glands, and stimulation of these fibers results in secretion. In allergic rhinitis, there is autonomic imbalance in the nasal mucosa with relative overactivity of the parasympathetic nervous system and hyperresponsiveness to nonspecific physical and chemical stimuli including changes in air temperature and humidity, irritants (eg, cigarette smoke, paint, perfume), and changes in the emotional state. This results in sneezes that expel foreign particles and in rhinorrhea that dilutes foreign water-soluble material.

The physiologic functions of the nose include olfaction, humidification, warming and filtration of the inspired air, provision of vocal resonance for speech, and defense of the lower airways. All foreign particles larger than 10 microns in diameter, and even some particles as small as 2 microns, are filtered as they traverse the nasal cavities.

■ SYMPTOMS AND SIGNS

The cardinal symptoms of allergic rhinitis are nasal congestion (stuffy nose), paroxysmal sneezing, itching, and watery, profuse rhinorrhea. Other symptoms that may be reported include noisy breathing, oronasal breathing, snoring, hyposmia or anosmia, itching of the palate or pharynx, and repeated throat clearing or cough secondary to drainage of nasal mucus into the pharynx. Ocular symptoms such as redness, itching, or tearing may also be present.

Children with allergic rhinitis may have "allergic shiners," a term used to describe the dark discoloration of the infraorbital regions secondary to obstruction of venous drainage. If they are chronic oronasal breathers, they may have hypertrophied gingival mucosa and halitosis. In contrast to children who breathe through unobstructed nasal passages, they are more likely to have a gaping expression, a long, retrognathic facies with a high, narrow palate, and orthodontic anomalies such as posterior dental crossbite. Pharyngeal lymphoid tissue, adenoids, tonsils, and the lymphoid tissue of the anterior cervical region may be hypertrophied. If hypertrophy of the adenoids is severe, obstructive sleep apnea, alveolar hypoventilation, and cor pulmonale may develop.

Examination of the nose of the child with chronic allergic rhinitis may reveal a transverse external wrinkle, secondary to rubbing and dorsal manipulation of the nose, also known as the "allergic salute." The nasal mucosa is a variable color in health and disease. In patients with allergic rhinitis, it usually appears edematous, but it is not necessarily pale or violaceous. Watery, mucoid, or opaque material may be noted in the nasal cavity or the posterior pharyngeal wall. There may be evidence of recent epistaxis. Nasal polyps are rare in children, and, if they are observed, cystic fibrosis must be ruled out. Ideally, the nasal mucosa should be inspected before and after application of a topical vasoconstrictor such as oxymetazoline. Examination using an otoscope is not always adequate, and examination using

flexible fiberoptic rhinoscopy may be required for optimal diagnosis and management.

■ DIAGNOSTIC TESTS

Disorders that must be considered in the differential diagnosis of rhinitis are listed in Table 198–1. To confirm the diagnosis of allergic rhinitis, it is necessary to examine the nasal mucus or to obtain a specimen of nasal mucosa for cytologic examination using a disposable plastic Rhinoprobe scoop. The best method of collecting mucus is to have the child blow into a piece of nonporous paper, transfer the secretions to a glass slide, air-dry the specimen, and apply an eosin/methylene blue stain. In patients with allergic rhinitis, the percentage of eosinophils in specimens prepared in this manner will range from 10% to 100%. The total blood eosinophil count and the total serum IgE concentration may be elevated or normal in patients with allergic rhinitis.

Epicutaneous (prick) tests with common inhalant antigens may be helpful in patients with allergic rhinitis, especially those who have severe symptoms that do not respond to pharmacologic management and those who are curious about the etiology of their symptoms and are prepared to rid their environment of allergens to which they are sensitive. Skin tests cannot be interpreted accurately unless a positive control substance such as histamine and a negative control substance, preferably the antigen diluent, are tested concomitantly with the antigens. Measurement of allergen-specific IgE in serum by in vitro tests such as radioallergosorbent tests (RAST) or enzyme-linked immunosorbent assay (ELISA) is also useful in patients with allergic rhinitis, particularly in those who cannot tolerate withdrawal of H_1-receptor antagonists before skin testing, or who have, in addition to their rhinitis, severe widespread atopic dermatitis that precludes skin testing. Skin tests and allergen-specific IgE measurement should not be used in place of a history and physical examination to "screen" patients for allergic rhinitis. The correlation among skin tests, allergen-specific IgE measurements, and nasal challenge tests is excel-

TABLE 198-1. Differential Diagnosis of Rhinitis

Allergic rhinitis

Nonallergic eosinophilic rhinitis

Vasomotor rhinitis

Rhinitis medicamentosa from overuse of topical decongestants

Hormonal changes (pregnancy, oral contraceptives, hypothyroidism)

Infection: viral or bacterial

Acute or chronic sinusitis

Ciliary dyskinesia

Granulomatous disease (eg, Wegener's granulomatosis)

Foreign body

Trauma (nasal septal deviation, septal hematoma, fracture of nasal bones, synechiae)

Adenoid hypertrophy

Nasal polyps

Choanal atresia

Cerebrospinal fluid leak

Congenital intranasal lesions (dermoid cysts, meningomyelocele, nasal glioma)

Neoplasm

lent for allergens such as pollens. Intranasal challenges with antigen, although not necessary for clinical diagnosis, have become a useful research tool, facilitating study of the pathophysiology of allergic rhinitis.

■ MANAGEMENT OF ALLERGIC RHINITIS

The management of allergic rhinitis consists of avoidance of allergens, irritants, and other factors known to provoke symptoms; pharmacologic treatment to prevent or relieve symptoms; and, in selected patients, alteration of the immune response to allergens using immunotherapy (allergy shots).

The nasal mucosa of patients with allergic rhinitis is hyperreactive to many different environmental stimuli, including, in addition to allergens, irritants such as cigarette smoke or perfumes, and physical factors such as cold air or ingestion of hot liquids. The patient should avoid any environmental stimulus that is known to provoke symptoms. Well-maintained air conditioning units are effective in reducing indoor pollen and mold counts and associated symptoms in patients allergic to pollens and molds. Similar beneficial effects are claimed for high-efficiency particulate air (HEPA) filter units.

Major advances in the pharmacologic treatment of allergic rhinitis have occurred. Treatment must be highly individualized. A patient's medication requirements may vary from season to season, or from year to year, and may range from occasional use of one medication for a few days to year-round use of several medications. Some of the newer H_1-receptor antagonists (antihistamines) such as terfenadine, astemizole, loratadine, and cetirizine do not cross the blood–brain barrier readily, and are associated with a lower incidence of sedation and other central nervous system adverse effects than older H_1-receptor antagonists such as chlorpheniramine. The newer medications also lack anticholinergic effects. Neither the new nor the older H_1-receptor antagonists relieve the symptom of nasal congestion as well as they relieve itching, sneezing, or rhinorrhea. Most of the new H_1-receptor antagonists are no more effective than chlorpheniramine.

Topically applied sympathomimetic medications such as xylometazoline and oxymetazoline should be used only in patients with severe nasal blockage, and only for brief periods. These medications increase nasal patency and facilitate examination of the nasal mucosa. They can be used to advantage during initiation of intranasal glucocorticoid treatment; to decrease blockage of the eustachian tube orifices during air travel; or to decrease obstruction of the sinus ostia and facilitate mucociliary clearance of the sinuses in patients with allergic rhinitis complicated by sinusitis. They may cause rebound congestion and, with long-term use, rhinitis medicamentosa. In infants and young children, they may even cause systemic symptoms, including central nervous depression and coma. Orally administered sympathomimetics such as phenylpropanolamine and pseudoephedrine are also best used for short-term relief of nasal congestion, rather than for long-term therapy, because they may exacerbate hypertension, and cause visual hallucinations, insomnia, and agitation in some patients.

Disodium cromoglycate (cromolyn sodium) 2% solution sprayed into the nasal cavity prophylactically four to six times daily is an antiallergic medication that prevents sneezing, rhinorrhea, and nasal itching in some patients with allergic rhinitis. It is not very effective in preventing nasal congestion. The chief advantage of cromolyn is its lack of toxicity. Nedocromil, which in vitro is more potent and has a broader spectrum of antiallergic and anti-inflammatory effects than cromolyn, is being introduced.

Topically active, synthetic glucocorticoids such as beclomethasone, flunisolide, triamcinolone, or the newer agents budesonide and fluticasone, which are not yet available in the United States, are highly effective in the treatment of allergic rhinitis. In the nasal mucosa, these medications are rapidly degraded enzymatically to less active metabolites. Unchanged medication that is absorbed is metabolized in the first pass through the liver, and, therefore, the risk of hypothalamic–pituitary–adrenal axis suppression is small in patients receiving these medications intranasally in manufacturers' recommended doses. About 90% of patients with seasonal allergic rhinitis using an inhaled glucocorticoid regularly have excellent improvement of symptoms, and can reduce or eliminate the need for concomitant medications such as H_1-receptor antagonists and decongestants. Optimally, children should begin inhaling glucocorticoids 1 week before the pollen "season" begins. Regular monitoring of their technique of inhalation is essential. The spray should be directed away from the nasal septum.

Antibiotics are not required in the treatment of chronic rhinitis unless it is complicated by sinusitis or otitis media, or is associated with purulent nasal secretions, structural abnormalities of the upper respiratory tract, immunodeficiency disease, or ciliary dysfunction.

Immunotherapy for allergic rhinitis is time-consuming, inconvenient, and expensive, but it may reduce morbidity and medication requirements in patients whose symptoms are poorly controlled by optimal modification of the environment and by optimal pharmacologic management, including topical glucocorticoid treatment. Immunotherapy consists of a series of subcutaneous injections of increasing doses of specific antigens, identified on the basis of the patient's history, as well as on the basis of positive skin tests, RAST or ELISA performed and interpreted according to acceptable techniques. Placebo-controlled, double-blind studies in patients with pollen-induced allergic rhinitis have shown that the response to immunotherapy is clearly antigen-specific and dose-related. Immunotherapy results in immunologic changes such as increase in antigen-specific IgG-blocking antibody, eventual decline in specific IgE antibody, reduction in sensitivity of basophils to antigen (as measured by their ability to release histamine), and decreased lymphocyte proliferation and lymphokine production in response to antigen, also an increase in blocking IgG and IgA antibodies in secretions.

The most common adverse effect of immunotherapy is a large local reaction at the injection site. Generalized systemic reactions, such as anaphylaxis or serum sickness, occur rarely. Standardized antigens for immunotherapy are available.

DISORDERS ASSOCIATED WITH ALLERGIC RHINITIS

■ ALLERGIC CONJUNCTIVITIS

Allergic conjunctivitis is an IgE-mediated reaction to an airborne, antigenic stimulus. In temperate climates, it is usually a seasonal disorder. Symptoms include conjunctival erythema, tearing, lid edema, intense itching, and, occasionally, a mucopurulent discharge. Patients with allergic conjunctivitis often have associated allergic rhinitis, asthma, or eczema. Conjunctival scrapings show eosinophils, and skin tests with airborne antigens are positive.

Vernal conjunctivitis is a severe form of seasonal conjunctivitis in which patients have intense eyelid and conjunctival itching, as well as photophobia. In the palpebral form of vernal conjunctivitis, giant papillary reactions produce a cobblestone appearance in the everted tarsal conjunctivae, accompanied by a thick, white, ropey discharge. In the limbal form of vernal conjunctivitis, yellow-gray gelatinous limbal masses and white Trantas' dots are observed. In both forms of vernal conjunctivitis, eosinophils are present in conjunctival scrapings. The IgE level is usually elevated in tears. Skin tests with airborne antigens are positive in most patients with this disorder. Patients with severe vernal conjunctivitis may develop secondary bacterial conjunctivitis, or corneal complications such as superficial keratitis and ulceration.

In management of allergic conjunctivitis, avoidance of airborne allergens, although ideal, is often impossible. Topical vasoconstrictors such as phenylephrine or naphthazoline can be helpful. Topical or oral H_1-receptor antagonists may contribute greatly to relief of itching and other symptoms. Cromolyn sodium in a 2% solution may be instilled in the conjunctivae four to six times daily. Topical glucocorticoids combined with a vasoconstrictor should be reversed for only severely affected patients, and monitoring of intraocular pressure before the start of treatment and every few weeks thereafter, by an ophthalmologist, is an important aspect of such therapy.

■ CHRONIC SINUSITIS

In children with allergic rhinitis and asthma, chronic sinusitis is remarkably common, causes considerable morbidity, and is easily overlooked. In this disorder, inflammation of one or more of the maxillary, ethmoidal, sphenoidal, or frontal sinuses is caused by partial or complete obstruction of the osteomeatal complex with subsequent hypooxygenation of the involved sinus, disturbance of ciliary function, and diminished local host resistance factors. In addition to allergic rhinitis and asthma, other conditions are predisposing to or associated with sinusitis: recurrent viral upper-respiratory infections, nasal obstruction due to foreign body, polyps, adenoid hypertrophy or tumor, cystic fibrosis, immotile cilia syndrome, hypogammaglobulinemia or other immunodeficiency disorders, nasal fracture, barotrauma, deviated septum, hypersensitivity to aspirin or other nonsteroidal anti-inflammatory agents, or damage to nasal and ostial mucosa from chronic use of topically applied drugs such as cocaine, oxymetazoline, and xylometazoline.

Symptoms of chronic sinusitis include nasal discharge, postnasal drip, frequent cough, nasal obstruction, and loss of smell or taste. Pharyngitis, headache, sore neck, malaise, nausea, irritability, fatigue, and low-grade fever may be reported. Pain over the sinuses is infrequent. The nasal mucosa is usually red and swollen. Mucopurulent material may be present in the nose and on the posterior pharyngeal wall. Adenoids may be enlarged.

Sinus radiographs reveal opacification, air fluid levels, or thickening of the sinus mucosa of greater than 6 mm. Occipitomental (Waters) views facilitate visualization of the maxillary sinuses, which are especially prone to chronic disease. Occipitofrontal (Caldwell) views for maximum visualization of ethmoid sinuses and lateral and submental vertical views may also be useful. Transillumination and ultrasonography generally are not helpful. Definitive methods used to diagnose chronic sinusitis are coronal computed tomography or nasal endoscopy. Polymorphonuclear cells, with or without intracellular bacteria, predominate in nasal secretions. There is poor correlation between organisms found in the nose and those found in the sinuses. Pathogens recovered from the sinuses of children with chronic sinusitis include *Streptococcus pneumoniae*, nontypable *Haemophilus influenzae*, and *Moraxella (Branhamella) catarrhalis* as well as *Bacteroides* species, *Fusobacterium* species, and anaerobic gram-positive cocci.

In the management of chronic sinusitis in children, an antimicrobial such as amoxicillin or trimethoprim-sulfamethoxazole should be administered for 21 days. If beta-lactamase–producing *H influenzae* or *M catarrhalis* is implicated, amoxicillin-clavulanate or a second- or third-generation cephalosporin is recommended. Sometimes a second course of antibiotic treatment is required. Topical or oral decongestants administered for 5 to 7 days may improve drainage. For noninfectious chronic sinusitis, intranasal glucocorticoids may reduce mucosal inflammation around the osteomeatal complex and facilitate drainage. Occasionally, surgical intervention is required.

Patients with chronic sinusitis may also have refractory asthma, said to be caused by "seeding" of the lungs with bacteria in the mucopurulent discharge from the sinuses, reflex bronchospasm by way of the parasympathetic nervous system, or enhancement of beta-adrenergic blockade by infection. Although the association between sinusitis and asthma is not fully understood, relief of chronic sinusitis is often associated with marked improvement in asthma symptoms.

■ CONCLUSION

Allergic rhinitis and associated disorders such as allergic conjunctivitis, chronic sinusitis, and otitis media with effusion are common in childhood, and cause considerable morbidity. Physicians providing primary care for children should be careful not to overlook these disorders, and should be aware of the relief that aggressive, modern management can provide for young patients who suffer from them.

(Abridged from F. Estelle R. Simons, Allergic Rhinitis and Associated Disorders, in Oski, DeAngelis, Feigin, McMillan, Warshaw: *Principles and Practice of Pediatrics, Second Edition*, J.B. Lippincott, 1994.)

Oski's Essential Pediatrics,
edited by Kevin B. Johnson and Frank A. Oski.
Lippincott–Raven Publishers,
Philadelphia © 1997

199

Insect Sting Allergy

For most children, insect stings are common, painful, but not particularly hazardous. In about 1% of the general population, however, stings trigger systemic anaphylactic reactions that account for about 40 fatalities in the United States each year. Although the risk of a fatal reaction is lower in children than in adults, insect-allergic children cause anxiety in parents and pediatricians because children are more likely to be stung and young children cannot handle emergencies and provide self-treatment. During the past 15 years, major advances in understanding the biochemistry of insect venoms and the pathophysiology of the immune response have led to the development of safe and effective venom immunotherapy for highly allergic individuals. At the same time, long-term studies of the epidemiology and natural history of insect allergy have provided reassuring evidence that, for most children, the "allergic state" is a transient, self-limited process that may not require treatment.

■ THE INSECTS

True "stinging insects" that account for the majority of allergic reactions belong to the order Hymenoptera (Table 199–1). The females of each species have a modified ovipositor stinger through which an injection of venom is delivered. Biting insects, such as mosquitoes, flies, and bugs, only rarely produce systemic reactions and are not considered in this discussion.

Honeybees are the most common members of the apid family. They are small, fuzzy, relatively docile insects that usually live in domestic hives and often are seen pollinating clover and flowering plants. They usually sting only when sat on or caught under foot, and leave their barbed stinger embedded in the victim. Bumblebees are large, slow-flying, yellow- and black-striped bees that are usually solitary and only rarely sting. Honeybees and bumblebees survive the winter and are present throughout the summer.

The vespid family includes yellow jackets, hornets, and wasps. In most areas of the United States, these insects account for the majority of stings. Yellow jackets are common in the Northeast, whereas wasps are dominant in the South and Southwest. Yellow jackets are small, black- and yellow-striped insects that usually nest in the ground or in decaying logs. They scavenge for food, are often seen around picnics and garbage, and become particularly aggressive late in the summer when their nests are crowded. White-faced hornets are large black insects with white faces that build teardrop-shaped paper nests suspended in trees. The thin-bodied brown- and yellow-striped Polistes wasp typically creates open-faced nests under the eaves of buildings.

The imported fire ants are less common members of the order. They inhabit the coastal areas of the Southeast and live in large dirt mounds. They attach themselves to the skin and deliver multiple stings that result in sterile pustules. Although they are a cause of systemic reaction, their venom has been less well studied and is not commercially available for diagnosis and treatment.

■ REACTION TYPES

After a sting, 90% of children experience transient redness, swelling, and pain localized to the sting site, usually

TABLE 199-1. Classification of Common Stinging Insects (Order Hymenoptera)

Apid family
　Honeybee
　Bumblebee
Vespid family
　Yellow jacket
　White-faced hornet
　Yellow hornet
　Polistes wasp
Imported fire ant

TABLE 199-2. Classification of Reactions to Insect Stings

Reaction

NORMAL
Swelling <2 in in diameter
Duration <24 h

LARGE LOCAL
Swelling >2 in in diameter
Duration 1 to 7 d

SYSTEMIC
Non–life-threatening
　Immediate-type generalized reaction confined to the skin (urticaria, angioedema, erythema, pruritus)
Life-threatening
　Immediate-type generalized reaction that may include cutaneous symptoms but also has respiratory (laryngeal edema or asthma) or cardiovascular (hypotension/shock) symptoms

less than 2 inches in diameter and lasting for less than 24 hours (Table 199–2). Hymenoptera venoms contain a variety of enzymes (phospholipase A, hyaluronidase), cytotoxic proteins (apamine, mellitin), and vasoactive compounds (histamine and kinins) which, in the normal individual, induces local vasodilatation, edema, and tissue damage.

In 10% of children, the sting results in a large local reaction that is extensively swollen and tender, is larger than several inches in diameter, and peaks in 3 to 7 days. Although the exact mechanism of this reaction is unknown, 75% of these individuals demonstrate venom-specific IgE, suggesting that immediate hypersensitivity plays some role in this exaggerated sting response.

True systemic anaphylactic reactions are less common. Estimates of their incidence in the general population range from 0.5% to 5%. Anaphylaxis is caused by the activation of mast cells sensitized by venom-specific IgE, with the release of large quantities of vasoactive mediators including histamine and kallikreins, leading to vasodilatation and increased vascular permeability. Most of these reactions (70% to 80%) are non–life-threatening. They begin several minutes to several hours after the sting and consist of simple urticaria, erythema, pruritus, and angioedema. The more serious life-threatening reactions begin within 5 to 10 minutes. Airway obstruction may occur secondary to laryngeal edema (tickle in the throat, gagging, difficulty in swallowing, or voice change) or bronchospasm (chest tightness or wheezing). Hypotension (dizziness or fainting) and frank cardiovascular collapse are accompanied by metabolic acidosis, clotting abnormalities (decreased Factor V, Factor VII, and fibrinogen), and evidence of complement activation. Although approximately 40 deaths per year are attributed to insect allergy, almost all of these occur in adults, particularly the elderly. Fatal outcome in children is rare.

Several types of non–IgE-mediated reactions include serum sickness, renal disease, neurologic manifestation, and delayed hypersensitivity phenomenon. Their pathophysiology remains unknown. When a child is stung many times simultaneously, a "toxic," nonallergic reaction consisting of delayed fever, nausea, vomiting, and other systemic symptoms sometimes occurs. With an extremely large number of stings such as may occur with Africanized honeybees or "killer bees," this type of nonallergic reaction is occasionally fatal.

■ DIAGNOSIS

The initial step in managing insect-sting allergy is an attempt, by careful history taking, to identify the insect culprit and clearly define the reaction by category, extent, and time course. The critical distinction to make is that between local and systemic reactions. If the reaction is systemic, particularly if life-threatening, referral for skin-test evaluation is necessary.

■ VENOM SKIN TESTING

For children with a history of a prior systemic reaction, venom skin testing is the quickest and most sensitive way to determine the presence of venom-specific IgE and identify which insects are responsible. Testing may be done as soon as 1 week after the reaction and has been useful in children as young as 9 months old. A panel of purified processed venoms, including those of honeybee, yellow jacket, white-faced hornet, yellow hornet, and Polistes wasp, is available for intradermal testing at concentrations from 0.001 to 1.0 µg/mL. Although testing identifies the "sensitive state," there is no good correlation among the intensity of skin-test reactivity, the severity of the previous reaction, and the likelihood of reaction to subsequent stings. Positive skin tests must always be interpreted in light of clinical history. A negative skin test in a patient with a history of systemic reactions suggests non–IgE-mediated anaphylactoid mechanisms.

■ RAST TESTING

Venom radioallergosorbent testing (RAST) detects the presence of venom-specific IgE in serum. Because it is less sensitive (15% false-negative) and more expensive than skin testing, it is not used routinely as a screening test but may be helpful in situations in which skin testing is equivocal.

■ MANAGEMENT

Treatment of the Acute Episode

Systemic reactions of immediate onset should be treated promptly with subcutaneous aqueous epinephrine (Table 199–3). An injection of long-acting epinephrine (Sus-phrine) may be administered to prevent late recurrences. Oral and injectable antihistamines, such as diphenhydramine, are often administered, but their use should not delay the administration of epinephrine. Oral corticosteroids such as prednisone may be given, but the delayed onset of action limits their effectiveness in the early stages of treatment. In any case, patients

TABLE 199-3. Treatment of Acute Anaphylactic Reaction

Epinephrine
Diphenhydramine
Prednisone
In the event of a severe reaction:
Oxygen/respiratory support
Intravenous volume expanders and vasopressor infusion

who are experiencing systemic reactions should be observed until all symptoms of the reaction are resolved.

The more severe anaphylactic reactions consist of hypotension or airway obstruction. The hypotension is secondary to a combination of loss of vascular tone and extravascular leakage of fluid. Initial treatment consists of intravascular volume support with as much as 50 mL/kg of normal saline over the first hour, followed, if necessary, by albumin or 5% plasma protein (Plasmanate) infusion. In prolonged or unresponsive cases, intravenous vasopressors such as epinephrine 1:10,000 may be required. Respiratory obstruction is treated with supplemental oxygen in all cases. Upper-airway obstruction that does not respond to parenteral epinephrine should be treated with nebulized racemic epinephrine, and unresponsive bronchospasm may benefit from nebulized beta-agonists or cautious intravenous aminophylline.

Treatment of large local reactions consists of ice, elevation, antihistamines, and pain relievers. In persons with severe local reactions, a short course of corticosteroids has been advocated, but no controlled studies of their effectiveness have been performed.

Emergency Self-Treatment

Patients who have experienced systemic reactions should be given an epinephrine-containing self-treatment kit to be carried when they are at risk for sting and medical care is not immediately available. The Epi-Pen device is an automatic self-injector that is available in two sizes (0.15 mg and 0.3 mg epinephrine) and is particularly useful in children.

Avoidance Measures

Careful sanitation and extermination of vespid nests can significantly reduce the chance of yellow-jacket sting. For children especially, wearing shoes while walking in the grass eliminates the most common cause of honeybee sting. The usual insect repellents are not effective against Hymenoptera. In severely allergic children, wearing a Medic-Alert bracelet or necklace provides quick and useful information in case of accidental sting reaction.

Venom Immunotherapy

In 1979, the Food and Drug Administration (FDA) licensed the use of purified extracts of insect venoms to prevent future systemic reactions in children and adults. The five venoms used in immunotherapy correspond to those used in skin testing. The selection of venoms for therapy is based on the demonstration of venom-specific IgE, either by skin testing or by RAST. The regimen consists of rapid advancement to maintenance doses at every 4- to 6-week interval for as long as 5 years of treatment. Children tolerate this regimen extremely well, although almost all of them sometime experience local redness or swelling at the injection site. About one fourth of them sometime experience a large local reaction at the injection site, and there is about a 5% risk of a systemic reaction at some time during the immunotherapy regimen. These are similar to risks encountered with other high-dose immunotherapy regimens using pollens or other inhalants. There is no evidence of any long-term adverse effects. Studies using in-hospital challenge stings after 15 weeks of venom immunotherapy, and at yearly intervals thereafter, demonstrate a 97% to 98% nonreaction rate in various groups of adults and children.

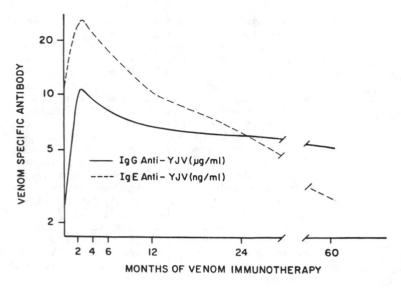

Figure 199-1. Antibody response to yellow-jacket venom immunotherapy.

During immunotherapy, a typical allergic patient responds initially by producing more venom-specific IgE at the same time that venom-specific IgG-blocking antibody increases. IgE peaks at about 8 weeks of therapy, then declines slowly over several years to a level lower than the initial baseline level (Figure 199–1). IgG antibody levels peak at about the same time and remain elevated for the duration of therapy. There is some correlation between the level of these antibodies and the certainty of protection conferred by immunotherapy so that, in very high-risk patients, it is useful to monitor IgG titers to ensure protection. After 3 years, venom sensitivity, as measured by positive skin tests or RAST, disappears in approximately 20% of patients. For these patients, immunotherapy can be safely discontinued. The remainder should complete 5 years of treatment, which confers long-term protection against stings regardless of skin test sensitivity at the time of discontinuation.

Patient Selection for Venom Immunotherapy

Only those patients who have experienced a significant systemic reaction and who have positive skin tests or RAST are candidates for venom immunotherapy. The more severe the prior reaction, the more likely it is that the subsequent reaction will be serious. Although positive skin tests identify sensitive individuals, they do not predict the risk of future reactions. As many as 40% to 60% of adults who have had a systemic reaction and are skin-test positive do not experience any systemic reaction if they are stung again. Children have an even lower risk, as evidenced by the high frequency of mild cutaneous systemic reactions and the extreme rarity of fatalities. For children who have had mild systemic reactions and are skin-test positive, the risk of systemic reaction on re-sting is less than 10% and the risk of progression to more serious reactions is much less than that. For these children, observation and emergency precautions, without venom immunotherapy, appear to be sufficient. For children with life-threatening systemic reactions and positive skin or RAST tests, venom immunotherapy is mandatory, as it is in all adults regardless of severity of prior systemic reaction. Although the guidelines for treatment listed in Table 199–4 are specific, the decision for or against venom immunotherapy must be made for each patient after careful discussion between physician and family of risks, benefits, and individual concerns.

TABLE 199-4. Indications for Venom Immunotherapy

Prior Reaction	Venom Skin Test	
	Positive	*Negative*
Life-threatening systemic	Yes	No
Non–life-threatening systemic	Yes	No
Adults		
Children	No	No
Large local	Not indicated	
Normal local	Not indicated	

(Abridged from Kenneth C. Schuberth, Insect Sting Allergy, in Oski, DeAngelis, Feigin, McMillan, Warshaw: *Principles and Practice of Pediatrics, Second Edition*, J.B. Lippincott, 1994.)

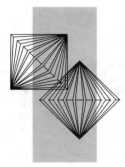

SECTION 14

Connective Tissue Diseases

Oski's Essential Pediatrics,
edited by Kevin B. Johnson and Frank A. Oski.
Lippincott–Raven Publishers,
Philadelphia © 1997

200

Connective Tissue Diseases

The connective tissue diseases are a group of heterogeneous afflictions that commonly inflame the connective tissues of the body. A frequent manifestation of these diseases is arthritis—objective inflammation of a joint. Etiologies of these disorders are mostly unknown. Many have an immunogenetic background and are characterized by prominent autoimmune phenomena: circulating autoantibodies such as rheumatoid factors and antinuclear antibodies and, in some cases, deposition of gammaglobulins in the affected tissues. There is also tissue accumulation of lymphocytes and plasma cells. The connective tissue diseases are often chronic and self-perpetuating, although many respond to glucocorticoid and anti-inflammatory drugs or immunosuppressive agents.

The combined prevalence of these disorders in the United States population in 1986 for children 15 years of age or younger would be about 70,000 for juvenile rheumatoid arthritis (JRA) and 17,500 for the other major connective tissue diseases. The total population of children with the various forms of juvenile arthritis would be about 175,000. Table 200–1 is a condensed diagnostic classification for juvenile arthritis.

JUVENILE RHEUMATOID ARTHRITIS

Juvenile rheumatoid arthritis is the most common pediatric connective tissue disease with arthritis as the principal manifestation. It is one of the more frequent chronic childhood illnesses and a leading cause of disability and blindness.

The etiology of JRA is unknown. It likely does not represent a single disorder but a spectrum of diseases of diverse pathogenesis.

■ CLINICAL MANIFESTATIONS

Although onset of JRA before 6 months of age is unusual, the mean age at onset is characteristically young— 1 to 3 years—with a substantial number of cases beginning throughout childhood and young adolescence. Girls are affected at least twice as frequently as boys.

Fatigue, low-grade fever, anorexia, weight loss, and failure to grow are common at onset of the disease in moderate to severely affected children. Morning stiffness, gelling after inactivity, and night pain are often encountered in uncontrolled disease. Children may not directly communicate these symptoms to their parents. The child may present, instead, with increased irritability, a posture of guarding the joints, or refusal to walk.

■ TYPES OF ONSET

The classification of JRA is strengthened by recognition of three distinct types of onset of the disease as listed in Table 200–2: polyarthritis, oligoarthritis (pauciarticular disease), and systemic disease. These types of onset are characterized by specific signs and symptoms at presentation and during the first 6 months of the illness.

Polyarthritis is disease that begins in five or more joints. This onset occurs in nearly half the children and may be acute or insidious. Systemic manifestations are usually not severe or persistent. The arthritis generally involves large joints such as the knees, wrists, elbows, and ankles. The smaller joints of the hands or feet may be affected early or late. The pattern of arthritis is usually symmetric. The child may not complain of pain even though the joints are tender and painful on motion. The cervical spine is often involved in this type of onset, although onset of JRA solely in the cervical spine is rare. The neck may be painful or stiff with an alarmingly rapid loss over time of extension and rotation. Atlantoaxial subluxation may occur early and place a child at risk to injury of the cervical cord in an accident or with attempted intubation before general anesthesia. Temporomandibular joint disease is relatively common in children with polyarthritis and leads to limitation or asymmetry of bite and micrognathia.

The onset of JRA in half of the children involves four or fewer joints. Oligoarthritis or pauciarticular disease often is confined to the knees or ankles or may involve a single joint at onset and throughout the course of the disease. The hips are usually spared at onset. Extra-articular systemic disease except for chronic uveitis is distinctly unusual.

A small number of children have onset of JRA with severe constitutional and systemic disease. This systemic onset may precede the appearance of overt arthritis by weeks, months, or years. A hallmark of this type of disease is a high spiking fever, often combined with a rheumatoid rash. Temperature elevations occur once or twice a day, often in late afternoon or evening, to a level of 39°C (102.2°F) or higher with a quick return to baseline temperature or lower. This quotidian pattern is highly suggestive of a diagnosis of JRA.

The rash of JRA develops with this fever and consists of 2- to 5-mm erythematous morbilliform macules (Figure 200–1). It is most commonly seen on the trunk and proximal

TABLE 200-1. Diagnostic Classification of Juvenile Arthritis

CONNECTIVE TISSUE DISEASES
Juvenile rheumatoid arthritis
Systemic lupus erythematosus
Dermatomyositis
Vasculitis
Scleroderma

SERONEGATIVE SPONDYLOARTHROPATHIES
Juvenile ankylosing spondylitis
Psoriatic spondyloarthritis
Reiter's disease
Inflammatory bowel disease

INFECTIOUS ARTHRITIS
Bacterial arthritis (including staphylococcal, gonorrhea, tuberculosis)
Viral arthritis
Fungal arthritis
Lyme disease

REACTIVE ARTHRITIS
Rheumatic fever
Post-*Yersinia* arthritis

RHEUMATIC DISEASES ASSOCIATED WITH IMMUNODEFICIENCY

CONGENITAL ANOMALIES AND GENETICALLY DETERMINED ABNORMALITIES OF THE MUSCULOSKELETAL SYSTEM
Constitutional diseases of bone
Lysosomal storage diseases
Heritable disorders of collagen and fibrous connective tissue
Amyloidosis

NONRHEUMATIC CONDITIONS OF BONES AND JOINTS
Traumatic arthritis
Reflex neurovascular dystrophy
Legg-Calvé-Perthes disease
Slipped capital femoral epiphysis
Toxic synovitis of the hip
Osteochondritis dissecans
Chondromalacia patellae
Plant-thorn synovitis

HEMATOLOGIC DISEASES
Sickle-cell anemia
Hemophilia
Thalassemia
Leukemia and lymphoma

NEOPLASTIC DISEASES
Neuroblastoma
Malignant and benign tumors of cartilage, bone, and synovium
Histiocytosis

ARTHROMYALGIA
Growing pains
Psychogenic rheumatism

onset but is never seen in children with oligoarthritis. The rash can sometimes be elicited in a child by rubbing or scratching the skin—the isomorphic response or Koebner phenomenon.

Children with systemic onset usually have hepatosplenomegaly and lymphadenopathy. Pericarditis, hepatitis, and other visceral disease may occur. Pulmonary involvement consists of a wide spectrum of abnormalities such as pleuritis and effusion, interstitial fibrosis, and hemosiderosis. The central nervous system (CNS) may be affected, but encephalopathy may be difficult to distinguish from drug toxicity, viral infection, or other complications of the systemic illness and fever.

Tenosynovitis and myositis are also accompaniments of active disease. A stenosing synovitis of the flexor tendon sheaths may lead to loss of extension of the fingers or a trigger finger. Rheumatoid nodules may occur on the tendons or subcutaneously over pressure points. They are particularly found in children with widespread polyarthritis who are older at onset and who have prominent small joint disease, an unrelenting course with erosions, and rheumatoid factor seropositivity.

■ CHRONIC UVEITIS

One of the most serious complications of JRA is the development of a chronic nongranulomatous uveitis involving the iris, ciliary body, and often the posterior choroid (Figure 200–2). This disease is usually bilateral and in 20% of children leads to blindness in the affected eye. Chronic uveitis characteristically has an insidious, asymptomatic onset and is only diagnosed by routine ophthalmologic and slit-lamp examinations at onset of the disease. These examinations should be repeated at frequent intervals during the first years after onset of JRA in all children. Chronic uveitis is confined to children with polyarthritis or oligoarthritis. It is particularly prone to occur in young girls of early age of onset with limited joint disease who are antinuclear antibody (ANA) seropositive. It is found in at least one fifth of these children.

■ GROWTH RETARDATION

Disturbances of growth and normal development are complications of a chronic disease such as JRA. Linear growth is retarded during periods of active disease and during use of glucocorticoid drugs. There is often delayed development of secondary sexual characteristics. Psychological stunting is a frequent and potentially severe complication. Localized growth retardation may also occur in selective areas such as the jaw (micrognathia). Unequal leg or arm lengths develop with monarticular disease involving a single limb.

■ LABORATORY EXAMINATION

Most children with active disease develop a normocytic, hypochromic anemia characteristic of the chronic anemia of inflammation. This is often moderately severe with the hemoglobin in the range of 7 to 10 g/dL. Leukocytosis and thrombocytosis are common with active disease. These findings are not seen or are much less pronounced in children with oligoarthritis.

The acute-phase reactants are often positive at onset of the disease and are moderately useful in following the

extremities, and over pressure areas, but may occur on the face, palms, or soles. The rash is not generally pruritic; the most characteristic feature is its transient nature. Any single lesion generally does not persist for more than an hour. This rash may also be seen in some children with polyarthritis at

TABLE 200-2. Classification of Types of Onset of Juvenile Rheumatoid Arthritis

Sign/Symptom of Onset	Polyarthritis	Oligoarthritis (Pauciarticular Disease)	Systemic Disease
Frequency of cases	40%–50%	40%–50%	10%–20%
Number of joints involved	≥ 5	≤ 4	Variable
Sex ratio (F:M)	3:1	5:1	1:1
Systemic involvement	Moderate involvement	Not present	Prominent
Occurrence of chronic uveitis	5%	20%	Rare
Frequency of seropositivity			
Rheumatoid factors	10% (increases with age)	Rare	Rare
Antinuclear antibodies	40%–50%	75%–85%*	10%
Course	Systemic disease is generally mild; articular involvement may be unremitting	Systemic disease is absent; major cause of morbidity is uveitis	Systemic disease is often self-limited; arthritis is chronic and destructive in 50%
Prognosis	Guarded to moderately good	Excellent except for eyesight	Moderate to poor

*In girls with uveitis.

course of the disease. The Westergren erythrocyte sedimentation rate, C-reactive protein level, and immunoglobulin concentrations reflect the inflammatory activity. Serum complement components usually are elevated at onset and with exacerbations. The serum amyloidlike protein is increased in concentration in children with JRA. Soluble immune complexes can be detected in the sera of some children, particularly those with systemic onset of the disease.

Tests for rheumatoid factors are positive in children with JRA less frequently than in adults with rheumatoid arthritis. Rheumatoid factors are IgM macroglobulins with antigenic specificity directed against the unfolded H-chains of IgG. About 20% of children with JRA eventually become seropositive, although few children at onset of JRA are seropositive and a positive latex fixation test is seldom observed in a child younger than 7 years of age. Rheumatoid factors tend to be present in a child of later age of onset or in the older child, and in one who has prominent symmetric polyarthritis with involvement of the small joints, subcutaneous rheumatoid nodules, articular erosions, and a poor functional outcome.

ANA seropositivity is present in at least 40% of children with JRA. The pattern of fluorescent staining is usually homogeneous or speckled; the titer is generally low to moderate. The presence of these antibodies is significantly correlated with development of chronic uveitis. They are less commonly found in older boys and in children with systemic disease. A positive ANA determination is a valuable diagnostic measure in a child suspected of JRA because ANA are not frequently positive in other childhood illnesses except for systemic lupus erythematosus (SLE), scleroderma, and transient acute viral disease.

The synovial fluid white cell count in JRA is usually moderately elevated in the range of 10,000/mm^3 to 20,000/mm^3. Synovial glucose concentration is low. Complement levels may be depressed, indicating intrasynovial complement activation.

Urinalysis generally is normal in children with JRA except for the few children who have a mild glomerulitis at onset. Proteinuria may occur with fever. Persistent proteinuria may be the first evidence of amyloidosis. Some children develop renal papillary necrosis during the course of the disease.

■ RADIOLOGIC EXAMINATION

A wide range of distinctive radiologic findings are present in children with JRA. Early changes consist of soft-tissue swelling, juxta-articular osteoporosis, and periosteal new bone apposition. Development of the ossification centers may be accelerated, or there may be premature epiphyseal closure leading to stunting of bone growth. In children with polyarthritis or systemic disease, especially late in the course, marginal erosions may develop along with narrowing of the cartilaginous spaces.

Cervical spine disease is characteristic of JRA. The upper cervical segments are principally affected with apophyseal joint fusion and atlantoaxial subluxation (Figure 200–3). The lower vertebrae may also be involved with failure to grow normally. Sacroiliac arthritis in children with JRA is not characterized by the degree of abnormality and reactive sclerosis that would be seen in ankylosing spondylitis. Fractures, particularly of the long bones and vertebrae, occur in children who develop generalized osteoporosis.

Routine radiographic studies generally are sufficient to delineate this progression of changes in evaluating a child's response to a management program. Newer methods of objectively evaluating joint disease can be employed, however, such as bone scans, computed tomography, and magnetic resonance imaging (MRI). MRI is more precise than routine x-ray examination in delineating soft tissue abnormalities in response to abnormal bone growth or fusion.

■ DIAGNOSIS

Classification criteria for JRA are listed in Table 200–3. JRA is defined as onset of idiopathic arthritis in a child younger than 16 years old. Arthritis is delimited objectively by the listed criteria. JRA is often a disease of exclusion, and, therefore, similar diseases must be considered (see Table 200–1). The differential diagnosis generally includes other rheumatic and connective tissue diseases, especially rheumatic fever, SLE, and ankylosing spondylitis. Other forms of arthropathy such as Reiter's syndrome and psori-

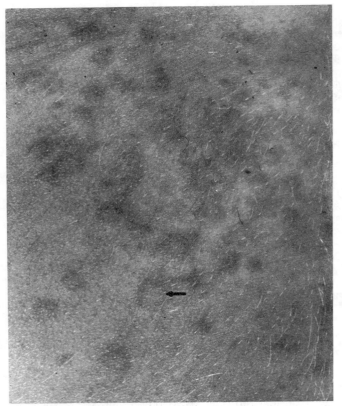

Figure 200-1. Rash of systemic onset JRA. This was a 4-year-old girl who presented with high spiking fever that occurred once a day accompanied by a transient nonpruritic rash. Shown is an area of active maculopapular rash on the back that was salmon pink in color. The arrow points to central clearing in a lesion. (Cassidy JT. Juvenile rheumatoid arthritis. In Kelley WN, Harris ED Jr, Ruddy S, Sledge CB, eds. *Textbook of rheumatology*. Philadelphia: WB Saunders;1993:1193.)

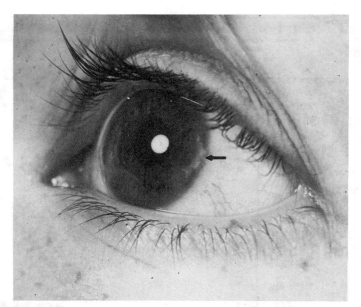

Figure 200-2. The arrow points to an area of band keratopathy just inside the limbus of the cornea in a girl who had ANA-positive oligoarticular JRA. Her chronic uveitis was bilateral and had resulted in a decrease in vision to 20/400 OD.

atic arthritis are uncommon in our experience. Particular attention must be accorded, however, to infectious arthritis, serum sickness, Henoch-Schönlein purpura, the enteropathies such as ulcerative colitis and regional enteritis, and the hematologic diseases such as leukemia, sickle-cell anemia, and hemophilia. The concurrence of arthritis and immunodeficiency has already been mentioned. Certain tumors may present as bone pain or arthritis in children, especially neuroblastoma in the young child. Onset of JRA in the hip is uncommon. In children with hip disease, transient synovitis, Legg-Calvé-Perthes disease, and slipped capital femoral epiphysis may mimic JRA, especially if the pain is referred to the knee.

■ MEDICAL TREATMENT

Conservative management of JRA attempts to control clinical manifestations of the disease and prevent or minimize deformity. This approach ideally involves a multidisciplinary team that follows the child throughout the course of the illness. Management should be family-centered, community-based, and coordinated. The long therapeutic program must be accepted by the child and family and must be judged to have a favorable risk/benefit ratio by the pediatric rheumatologist.

Prognosis is excellent for most children with JRA, so philosophy of management should stress the simplest,

safest, and most conservative measures. If this treatment proves inadequate, other therapeutic modalities should be chosen (Table 200-4).

Nonsteroidal anti-inflammatory drugs such as aspirin are effective in suppressing inflammation and fever. About 50% of children are treated satisfactorily with aspirin. The remainder should try another nonsteroidal anti-inflammatory drug.

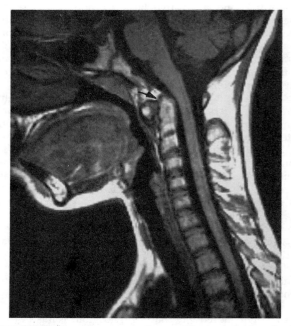

Figure 200-3. Magnetic resonance image of the cervical spine of a child with 7 mm of atlantoaxial subluxation. The arrow points to the odontoid, which is beginning to impinge on the upper cervical cord.

TABLE 200-3. Diagnostic Criteria for the Classification of Juvenile Rheumatoid Arthritis

Age of onset <16 years

Arthritis in ≥ 1 joints defined as *swelling or effusion*, or the presence of two or more of the following signs: *limitation of range of motion, tenderness or pain on motion, or increased heat*

Duration of disease ≥ 6 weeks

Type of onset of disease during the first 6 months

   Polyarthritis ≥ 5 joints

   Oligoarthritis or pauciarticular disease ≤ 4 joints

   Systemic disease: arthritis with intermittent fever

Exclusion of other forms of juvenile arthritis

Cassidy JT, Devenson JE, Bass JC, et al. A study of classification criteria for a diagnosis of juvenile rheumatoid arthritis. Arthritis Rheum. 1986; 29:274.

Hydroxychloroquine is a useful adjunctive agent for treatment of the child with more progressive disease. Gold salts either as intramuscular preparations or the oral compound are indicated in children whose polyarthritis is unresponsive to conservative management. Toxicities from these drug are primarily hematologic, renal, or hepatic, and those systems must be constantly monitored during treatment. D-penicillamine is not as widely employed as are gold salts. The expected response to treatment with D-penicillamine and its toxicities is similar to that for gold.

Glucocorticoid drugs should be reserved for treatment of the severely involved child who is recalcitrant to more conservative therapeutic regimens. Steroids have many toxicities associated with their use (*eg*, Cushing's syndrome) and severely retard normal growth and development. Steroids are indicated for resistant or life-threatening disease and its complications such as pericarditis. Ophthalmic administration is used for treatment of chronic uveitis. Occasionally intra-articular steroid is employed to achieve specific goals of a physical therapy program or for persistent monarticular involvement.

Methotrexate is the most successful and safe approach to advanced drug treatment of severe or resistant polyarthritis. This drug is attractive for pediatric use because it is taken only once a week orally as a pill or liquid, and has no proven oncogenic potential or untoward risk of sterility.

■ COURSE OF DISEASE AND PROGNOSIS

In general, 80% to 90% of children who develop JRA make a satisfactory recovery from their disease and enter adult life without serious functional disability. A small percentage of patients will have a recurrence of arthritis during the adult years. As many as 10% of children with JRA, however, enter adulthood with moderate to significant functional disability. The child most at risk is the one who has had polyarthritis of later age of onset, early symmetric involvement of the small joints of the hands or feet, the early appearance of erosions, unremitting activity of the joint disease, or prominent systemic manifestations, and the development of rheumatoid factor seropositivity and subcutaneous nodules. Progressive hip disease is also a major cause of long-term disability.

The prognosis for JRA is optimistic and in many children is excellent. It is important that both the child and parents understand the disease and share in its long-term management. The nature of JRA, the goals of therapy, and the course of the disease should be discussed in detail. A carefully selected program of coordinated care is initiated by the physician and needs constant reinforcement by the team nurse and social worker. Some families of children with JRA display psychiatrically important disruptions such as divorce, separation, death, and severe emotional disturbances. Thus, a priority in the management of a child with this chronic illness is to foster normal psychological and social development and peer group activities. Psychological regression to a more infantile pattern is present in most children who experience moderate to severe disease.

LYME DISEASE

Lyme disease has emerged in the last 15 years as a clinical entity of near-epidemic proportions in the summer and autumn in endemic areas of the United States. Initially, an unusually large number of cases of arthritis were diagnosed as JRA in children from Old Lyme, Connecticut. In subsequent epidemiologic investigations, it was ascertained to be a tickborne illness transmitted by *Ixodes dammini* and associated with widespread immune-complex disease. This arthropod vector multiplies in the white-footed deer mouse (adult ticks) and the white-tailed deer (larvae and nymphs). A spirochete, *Borrelia burgdorferi,* was isolated from adult ticks and proved to be a cause of this disease. The age of affected patients has been from 2 years to the ninth decade; the male-to-female ratio is equal. About half the patients are children. In endemic areas of the country, careful differentiation of Lyme disease from JRA (in particular the oligoarticular type) is essential.

A number of endemic areas are recognized within the United States: the Northeast, the upper Midwest, the West Coast, and Texas. The spirochete has worldwide distribu-

TABLE 200-4. Management of Children With Juvenile Rheumatoid Arthritis

MEDICATION PROGRAM—SUPPRESSION OF INFLAMMATION

Nonsteroidal anti-inflammatory drugs

Hydroxychloroquine

Gold (IM and oral)

Glucocorticoid drugs

Immunosuppressive drugs

PRESERVATION OF FUNCTION AND PREVENTION OF DEFORMITIES

Local and general rest

Physical therapy

Occupational therapy

Orthopedic surgery—preventive and reconstructive

PSYCHOSOCIAL DEVELOPMENT

Peer group relationships and schooling

Counseling of patient and family

Involvement of community agencies

MAINTENANCE OF ADEQUATE NUTRITION

Coordinated care

tion; a similar disease is described in Europe and other countries. In the infected patient, the spirochete has been identified in the cutaneous lesions, blood, synovial fluid, and the cerebrospinal fluid (CSF). Related ticks (*Ixodes pacificus, Amblyomma americanum*) or other vectors (birds or feral animals) may be involved in the expanding distribution of the disease. The *Borrelia* organisms can be transmitted to the fetus and result in congenital anomalies, prematurity, developmental delay, and intrauterine death.

■ CLINICAL MANIFESTATIONS

Constitutional symptoms including lethargy and fatigue are often prominent (Table 200–5). Most patients complain of intermittent headache, fever and chills, and musculoskeletal aching. Lymphadenopathy and hepatosplenomegaly are frequent. The sedimentation rate is elevated along with the serum muscle enzymes. Hematuria and proteinuria are often present.

The cutaneous hallmark of the acute illness, erythema chronicum migrans (ECM), is an annular lesion measuring 3 to 70 cm in diameter that follows the tick bite by 3 to 21 days and precedes the onset of arthritis by weeks or months. The early cutaneous lesions may resemble urticaria and are often located in groin or axillae. They do not involve the palms, soles, or mucous membranes. Although the cutaneous manifestations of the disease may progress through a number of recurrences, initial signs and symptoms generally resolve within 1 month. Only about one third of the children give a history of a tick bite at the site of the initial lesion. Multiple secondary and migratory lesions develop within the first week in about half the patients. Often, these are smaller than the initial ECM, are not associated with tick bites, and are less likely to become vesicular, indurated, or necrotic. Other mucocutaneous lesions including a malar rash and conjunctivitis may develop. A late manifestation is acrodermatitis chronica atrophicans, which has been primarily described in Europe.

The spectrum of Lyme disease includes carditis, neurologic disease, and arthritis. Cardiovascular abnormalities occur within the initial 4 to 6 weeks after onset and include atrioventricular block, pericarditis, cardiomegaly, and left ventricular dysfunction. Cardiac disease usually runs a brief course of up to 6 weeks and seldom recurs.

The initial neurologic abnormalities generally resolve within 3 months. These consist primarily of meningitis, cranial neuropathy, and peripheral radiculopathy. Other variable signs and symptoms of central or peripheral nervous system disease may be present. The CSF shows a mononuclear pleocytosis, slight elevation of the protein level, and a normal glucose concentration. The neurologic disease correlates with high antibody titers to the *Borrelia* spirochete. In 10% of patients, there is a late recurrence of CNS symptoms or peripheral neuritis including demyelinating disease or psychiatric illness years after onset.

Arthropathy follows the initial ECM by a few weeks to 2 years in about 80% of the children. Migratory arthralgia is characteristic initially. Recurrent attacks of asymmetric oligoarthritis occur months after onset of the illness and typically involve large joints such as the knees, although both large and small joints may be affected. A minority of children may have symmetric polyarthritis. The initial episodes of arthritis resolve in 2 to 4 weeks, but a child may experience exacerbations over several years. The synovial fluid white cell count is elevated to as high as 100,000/mm^3 with the polymorphonuclear leukocyte as the predominant cell. Synovial fluid protein concentration is increased, and the complement level is decreased. In a small percentage of children (10%), arthritis involving the large joints becomes chronic with subsequent appearance of radiologic erosions of cartilage and bone. The severity of the musculoskeletal disease and the risk of erosive arthritis appear to be immunogenetically related to HLA-DR2. CNS and cardiovascular symptoms also may be more severe in children with this alloantigen.

■ ANTIBODY TITERS

Specific IgM antibody titers against the spirochete reach a peak between the third and sixth week after the appearance of ECM. IgG antibody titers rise more slowly, are highest months after onset, and correspond to the time of the appearance of the arthropathy. The presence of an antibody titer in the diagnostic range is particularly important in differentiating Lyme disease from other rheumatic syndromes. Borderline results should be confirmed by Western blot analysis.

During the initial phases of illness, circulating immune complexes are present along with elevated IgM levels and IgM-containing cryoglobulins. There is a direct correlation between these observations and the severity and frequency of later CNS, cardiac, and joint involvement. The serum IgM concentration parallels disease activity in the neurologic and cardiac systems but may return to near normal levels at the onset of the arthritis. At that point, immune complexes are present in the synovial fluid but often are not detectable in the serum. Complement levels in the synovial fluid are depressed although serum complement concentrations often are elevated as acute-phase reactants. Tests for rheumatoid factors and antinuclear antibodies are usually negative.

■ TREATMENT

Oral tetracycline is the preferred treatment early in the illness for children older than 9 years. Doxycycline offers the

TABLE 200-5. Clinical Course of Lyme Disease

Time From Onset	Organ System	Clinical Manifestation
Early (1 day to 1 mo)	Cutaneous	ECM
		Lethargy/fatigue
		Fever/chills
		Headache
Intermediate (1/2 mo to 5 mo)	Cardiac	Syncope
		Pericarditis
		Congestive failure
	Neurologic	Meningoencephalitis
		Cranial neuritis
		Polyradiculitis
	Ophthalmologic	Uveitis
	Musculoskeletal	Arthalgia
		Myalgia
Late (5 mo to 1 y)	Cutaneous	Acrodermatitis chronica atrophicans
	Neurologic	Demyelinating and psychiatric illness
	Musculoskeletal	Oligoarthritis

advantage of twice-a-day administration and less concern over inactivation by food. In young children, phenoxymethyl penicillin or erythromycin are satisfactory alternatives. Established Lyme arthritis, a relapse, or major late complications such as meningitis or neuropathy may occur after early treatment. Intravenous penicillin-G, or ceftriaxone is the recommended therapy for those complications.

SYSTEMIC LUPUS ERYTHEMATOSUS

Systemic lupus erythematosus (SLE) is a multisystemic disease in which widespread inflammatory involvement of the connective tissues and immune-complex vasculitis occurs. It is a prototypic example of autoimmunity in humans that results from abnormal immunologic hyperreactivity and an immunogenetic predisposition to the disease.

■ CLINICAL MANIFESTATIONS

Although SLE can develop at any age, onset in children is usually after 5 years of age and becomes increasingly more common during the adolescent years. The female-to-male ratio is about 8 to 1 except in the youngest children, when relatively more boys are affected.

The manifestations of SLE are variable and present with any degree of severity from an acute, rapidly fatal illness to insidious, chronic disability with multisystemic exacerbations. In more than three fourths of the children, SLE is diagnosed within the first 6 months after onset because of the acute nature of the early illness, but diagnosis is often delayed by 4 to 5 years in the rest of the patients.

Fever, malaise, and weight loss are common (Table 200–6). Each exacerbation of the disease tends to mimic previous episodes. If serious renal disease develops, it does so within 2 years after onset. The major exception to the predictability of SLE is in the occurrence of CNS illness; CNS disease may intervene at any time in about one third of the children.

A malar erythematous rash in a butterfly distribution across the bridge of the nose and over each cheek is characteristic of an acute onset or exacerbation (Figure 200–4). Other forms of cutaneous and mucocutaneous involvement are common and varied in character and distribution. Raynaud phenomenon is frequent in SLE. It may result in digital ulceration and gangrene in a few children. Osteonecrosis, particularly of the femoral heads, is common in SLE and made worse by glucocorticoid therapy.

Arthritis affects the majority of children and commonly involves the small joints of the hands, wrists, elbows, shoulders, knees, and ankles. This arthritis is characteristically transient and may be migratory. Pain may be more severe than is suggested by objective changes. The arthritis of SLE is almost never erosive nor does it result in permanent deformity in 95% of instances.

Pericarditis is the most common manifestation of cardiac involvement. The child may also experience congestive heart failure, arrhythmias, or myocardial infarction. Valvular insufficiency develops in a few cases, and a sterile verrucous endocarditis (Libman-Sacks) is particularly characteristic of SLE. Although previously reported from necropsy examinations, echocardiography has become a sensitive premortem method of confirming its presence. Pleuritis is also common and may involve the diaphragmatic pleurae along with a

TABLE 200-6. Clinical Presentation and Course of SLE in Children

	At Onset (%)	During Course (%)
Nephritis	84	86
Hypertension	10	28
Arthritis	72	76
Dermatitis	69	76
Malar erythema	51	56
Photosensitivity	16	16
Alopecia	16	20
Oral or nasopharyngeal ulcerations	12	16
Pericarditis	40	47
Pleuritis	31	36
CNS disease	9	31
Raynaud's phenomenon	16	24
Hepatomegaly	43	47
Splenomegaly	20	20
Positive LE cells	86	100
Anemia	43	47
Leukopenia	60	71
Thrombocytopenia	22	24

Modified from Cassidy JT, Sullivan DB, Petty RE, et al. Lupus nephritis and encephalopathy: prognosis in 58 children. Arthritis Rheum. *1977; 20:316.*

basilar pneumonitis. Pulmonary hemorrhage is rare but can be fatal.

Abdominal pain often presents a diagnostic dilemma in a child with SLE, especially when under treatment with glucocorticoids. Mesenteric thrombosis and acute pancreatitis are life-threatening events. Hepatomegaly and splenomegaly are common, and splenic infarction may occur. Chronic active hepatitis is associated as an overlap syndrome with SLE.

Disease of the central and peripheral nervous systems are common causes of morbidity in these children. Pseudotumor cerebri may be a complication of SLE or the glucocorticoid therapy. Recurrent headaches, seizures, chorea, or frank psychosis are all encountered. Intracranial hemorrhage may result from hypertension, thrombocytopenia, or thrombosis associated with antiphospholipid antibodies. The so-called cytoid body of retinal vasculitis is often seen in disease involving the CNS or in lupus crisis. Systemic polyneuropathy, the Guillain-Barré syndrome, transverse myelopathy, and involvement of the cranial nerves have all been reported.

Some involvement of the kidneys is present in virtually all children with SLE. Even severe nephritis may not be detected early by the presence of an abnormal urinary sediment, proteinuria, or changes in the creatinine clearance. Evidence of active immune-complex disease such as increased levels of antinative DNA antibodies or hypocomplementemia correlate with active nephritis in most patients.

Lupus nephritis is categorized by the World Health Organization (WHO) classification of Type I–normal, Type II–mesangial, Type III–focal proliferative, Type IV–diffuse proliferative, and Type V–membranous disease. The relation

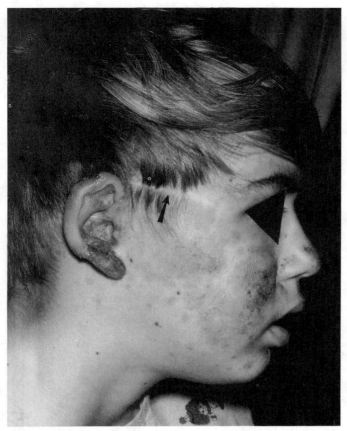

Figure 200-4. Excoriating erythematous facial rash of acute systemic lupus erythematosus in a 14-year-old boy. The crusting lesions are seen over the nose, malar areas, cheeks, and earlobes. The arrow points to a clear area corresponding to eyeglass frames, confirming the role of photosensitivity in the genesis of this lesion.

of these types of involvement to prognosis and eventual renal failure is shown in Table 200–7. Renal biopsy test is warranted in the majority of children with SLE unless there is no clinical evidence of significant involvement of the kidneys. The safest approach to long-term therapy is usually based on careful evaluation of the renal status. It is believed that serious renal lesions are more common in children with SLE than in adults, and prognosis for renal disease is more guarded.

■ LABORATORY FINDINGS

Otherwise unexplained leukopenia is particularly characteristic of SLE. The majority of children are leukopenic at onset with neutrophils predominating in the peripheral count. During the course of the illness, the white blood cell count often does not become elevated to an appropriate degree even with bacteremia. Thrombocytopenia and acute hemolytic anemia may also be present. Coombs' tests are often positive in these children. Other causes of anemia besides systemic disease include menorrhagia, septicemia, and gastrointestinal (GI) bleeding. SLE may present as thrombocytopenic purpura. The acute-phase indices are generally increased in active systemic disease.

Antinuclear antibodies are present in most children with SLE. They generally are found in high titer in a homogeneous pattern. A peripheral nuclear pattern is virtually synonomous with the presence of antinative DNA antibodies. Well-standardized assays for antinative DNA antibodies are critical to evaluating the degree of activity of the systemic immune-complex disease. Anti-Ro antibodies are characteristic of subacute cutaneous lupus and the neonatal lupus syndrome with congenital heart block. The LE-cell phenomenon is present in most children at onset of the disease and during acute exacerbations.

Rheumatoid factors and other antitissue antibodies such as antithyroglobulin are often positive in children with SLE. Cold agglutinins or cryoglobulins may result in peripheral anoxic phenomena. Antiphospholipid antibodies or circulating anticoagulants that cross-react with a phospholipid antigen of the Venereal Disease Research Laboratory (VDRL) test for syphilis predispose the child to repeated episodes of thrombosis. A young person with a biologic false-positive result for syphilis is at risk for development of SLE.

Components of both the classic and alternative complement pathways are consumed in the presence of active immune-complex vasculitis. The CH_{50} determination reflects the status of the total complement cascade; C3 concentration appears to be depressed less frequently, but a falling concentration of C4 is usually a reliable indicator of active disease. Occasionally, determination of circulating immune complexes, such as C1q binding or Raji cell assays, are useful in selected patients.

■ DIAGNOSIS

An early diagnostic suspicion that a child has SLE depends on recognizing an episodic, multisystemic constellation of clinical disease that is strongly associated with per-

TABLE 200-7. Classification of Lupus Nephritis

Type of Disease	Remission	Nephrotic Syndrome	Renal Failure	Uremic Deaths
Glomerular lesions				
Mesangial	+	−	−	−
Focal proliferative	++	+	+	+
Diffuse proliferative	+	++	++	+++
Membranous	+	+++	++	+
Extraglomerular lesions	+	+	++	++

−, absent; +, minimal; ++, moderate; +++, severe.

sistent ANA seropositivity. Eleven criteria have been tested by the American College of Rheumatology for the classification of SLE. These are listed in Table 200–8.

The differential diagnosis of SLE should consider JRA, other forms of acute glomerulonephritis, hemolytic anemia, leukemia, allergic or contact dermatitis, an idiopathic seizure disorder, mononucleosis, acute rheumatic fever with carditis, and septicemia. SLE remains today as the great masquerader!

■ TREATMENT

Long-term supportive care of the child with SLE should include adequate nutrition, fluid and electrolyte balance, early recognition and treatment of infections, and control of hypertension. Fevers and potential infection should be attended promptly. Pneumonitis, septicemia, and pyelonephritis are of particular concern.

Selected anti-inflammatory drugs are useful in treating minor manifestations of SLE such as arthralgia and myalgia. Hydroxychloroquine is an adjunctive medication that controls dermatitis or moderates glucocorticoid dosage. Glucocorticoid drugs are the mainstay of the basic regimen for children with this disease. Prednisone is the preferred analogue. A negative purified protein derivative (PPD) test for tuberculosis should be verified before a child is started on prednisone.

Immunosuppressive agents in addition to prednisone are necessary in some children. Although azathioprine has been employed extensively, recent data suggest that intravenous pulse cyclophosphamide is preferable, especially in children with severe nephritis. Dialysis and kidney transplantation have been successfully used in end-stage renal disease.

■ COURSE AND PROGNOSIS

Prognosis in children with SLE has improved substantially during the past 25 years. Therefore, there is a guardedly optimistic attitude toward this disease. It is estimated that 85% to 90% of children with SLE will survive over a 10-year period. The most recent data from Minnesota indicate an overall outcome in this range with a survivorship in children with diffuse proliferative glomerulonephritis of 70% at 10 years. Infection has replaced severe nephritis and CNS disease as the leading cause of death in children with SLE. Malignant hypertension, GI bleeding or perforation, acute pancreatitis, and pulmonary hemorrhage are also serious complications of the disease or its treatment.

SLE is characterized by repeated exacerbations and remissions; active disease is often prolonged over many years. Generalizations concerning prognosis for a specific child are especially unwise during the first 1 to 2 years after diagnosis. Later, a more reliable estimate can be offered the family based on the degree of systemic activity and its response to therapy and on the severity of nephritis, systemic vasculitis, and parenchymal organ involvement. Prognosis for life or function is poorest in diffuse proliferative nephritis or the organic brain syndrome and is best in minimal systemic disease, mesangial nephritis, and with a prompt sustained response to glucocorticoid therapy.

DERMATOMYOSITIS

A classification of idiopathic inflammatory myositis is presented in Table 200–9. Dermatomyositis in children is characterized by nonsuppurative inflammation of striated muscle and skin. These multisystemic findings are accompanied early in its course by an immune-complex vasculitis and late by development of calcinosis.

■ FREQUENCY AND AGE OF ONSET

Dermatomyositis occurs in about 5% of newly referred children to a pediatric rheumatology clinic. The disease is slightly more common in girls than boys at a ratio of about 1.6 to 1. The disease can present at any age, but onset is especially common from the 4th to 10th year.

■ ETIOLOGY

Investigations suggest that dermatomyositis is autoimmune in pathogenesis with both humoral and cell-mediated abnormalities. Immune-complex disease may be an initiat-

---

TABLE 200-8. Criteria for Classification of Systemic Lupus Erythematosus*

Malar (butterfly) rash

Discoid-lupus rash

Photosensitivity

Oral or nasal mucocutaneous ulcerations

Nonerosive arthritis

Nephritis
   Proteinuria > 0.5 g/day
   Cellular casts

Encephalopathy
   Seizures
   Psychosis

Pleuritis or pericarditis

Cytopenia

Positive immunoserology
   Antibodies to nDNA
   Antibodies to Sm nuclear antigen
   Positive LE-cell preparation
   Biologic false-positive test for syphilis

Positive antinuclear antibody test

Four of 11 criteria provide a sensitivity of 96% and a specificity of 96% for SLE.

Adapted from Tan EM, Cohen AS, Fries JF, et al. The 1982 revised criteria for the classification of systemic lupus erythematosus. Arthritis Rheum. 1982;25:1271.

TABLE 200-9. Classification of Inflammatory Myositis

Polymyositis

Dermatomyositis

Dermatomyositis or polymyositis with malignancy

Dermatomyositis with onset in childhood

Acute rhabdomyolysis

Polymyositis with Sjögren's or overlap syndrome

ing or perpetuating event. Immunoglobulins and complement are deposited in the walls of small blood vessels and in the skeletal muscles. There may be an immunogenetic predisposition to the development of dermatomyositis as HLA-B8 and DR3 may be increased in frequency in this disorder. Dermatomyositis has also occurred in patients with selective IgA deficiency and C2 complement component deficiency.

Dermatomyositis has developed after infections, vaccination, hypersensitivity reactions to drugs, and sunburn. A number of studies indicate that coxsackie B-virus or toxoplasmosis may play a role in onset. An acute transient inflammatory myositis has been observed in otherwise normal children after certain viral infections, especially influenza A and B. A similar myositis has been described in a few children with agammaglobulinemia in association with echovirus infection.

■ CLINICAL PRESENTATION AND COURSE

Table 200–10 lists characteristic clinical features of dermatomyositis in children. Most patients have prominent constitutional symptoms of fatigue, malaise, weight loss, anorexia, and low-grade fever. Unexplained fever may be the circumstance that prompts referral to a physician. The proximal limb-girdle muscles of the lower extremities are affected initially. The shoulder girdle and proximal arm muscles are next most frequently involved. The child may be unable to hold the head upright or maintain a sitting posture because of weakness of the anterior neck flexors and back muscles. The distal muscles of the extremities may be involved later in the disease or in children with an acute onset. The affected child may stop walking, may be unable to dress or climb stairs, or may complain of muscle pain. The affected muscles are occasionally edematous and indurated. There is usually a pronounced inability to get up off the floor unaided or out of bed.

Ten percent of children with dermatomyositis develop involvement of the pharyngeal, hypopharyngeal, and palatal muscles. Dysphonia and difficulty swallowing may be related to this involvement and also to esophageal hypomotility. Palatal speech and regurgitation of liquids through the nose are early signs of impending respiratory difficulty. These children are at risk for aspiration. Profound involvement of the thoracic and respiratory muscles is seen in a few children and leads to increasing dyspnea at rest, aspiration, or death.

The classic rash of dermatomyositis is seen in most of the children; in the remainder, it is less characteristic but suggests the diagnosis (Figure 200–5). The severity of cutaneous involvement is variable and may be the first sign of the disease. It is most distinctive over the upper eyelids, malar areas, and the dorsal surfaces of the knuckles, elbows, and knees. Often at onset of the disease, there is indurative edema of the skin and subcutaneous tissues. Later, there is thinning and atrophy of the accessory epidermal structures with loss of hair and development of telangiectases. Vasculitic ulcers at the corners of the eyes, around the axillae, and over stretch marks may become serious.

The course of dermatomyositis often is divided into four characteristic clinical phases (Table 200–11). About 75% of children with dermatomyositis pursue a uniphasic course that lasts from 8 months to 2 years. The remaining 25% continue to have acute exacerbations and remissions; about half of these patients eventually develop a clinical disease more typical of systemic vasculitis. A small number of children late in the course assume more of the characteristics of scleroderma with profound sclerodactyly and cutaneous atrophy. Other children, even years after onset, have persistent elevations of serum muscle enzymes and demonstrate characteristic histopathologic features of the disease if muscle biopsies are performed.

■ LABORATORY ABNORMALITIES

The acute-phase reactants such as the erythrocyte sedimentation rate (ESR) and C-reactive protein determination tend to correlate with the degree of clinical inflammation. Anemia is uncommon at onset except in the child with GI bleeding. Urinalysis is generally normal except in the few children with microscopic hematuria. Serum antinuclear antibodies are variably present in these children, and specific antibodies such as to the PM antigen have been described. Half the affected children at onset have positive tests for circulating immune complexes.

The three most important diagnostic laboratory abnormalities are elevated serum muscle enzyme levels, which are present in 98% of the children, abnormal electromyographic changes in 96%, and specific histopathologic abnormalities on muscle biopsy in 79%. The levels of the serum muscle enzymes are important for diagnosis and in monitoring effective therapy. Generally, a panel of the creatine kinase (CK), aspartate aminotransferase (AST), and aldolase is followed. The increase in serum concentrations ranges from 20 to 40 times normal for CK or AST. The appearance of MB bands on the isozyme pattern of serum creatine kinase in children with dermatomyositis is usually interpreted as evidence of regenerative striated muscle and not of cardiac damage.

Electromyography (EMG) helps confirm the diagnosis of dermatomyositis in some children and helps determine the best site for a muscle biopsy. EMG changes are those of myopathy and denervation. MRI is also abnormal in those children and distinguishes between unaffected and affected muscles.

TABLE 200-10. Clinical Features Associated With Dermatomyositis in Childhood

Muscle weakness
    Proximal pelvic girdle (95%)
    Proximal shoulder girdle (75%)
    Neck flexors (60%)
    Pharyngeal muscles (30%)
    Distal muscles of the extremities (30%)
    Facial and extraocular muscles (5%)
Muscle contractures and atrophy (60%)
Muscle pain and tenderness (50%)
Skin lesions (85%)
    Heliotrope rash of eyelids
    Malar rash
    Subcutaneous and periorbital edema
    Periungual and articular rash (Gottron papules)
Raynaud's phenomenon (20%)
Arthritis and arthralgia (25%)
Dysphagia, other GI symptoms (10%)
Calcinosis (40%)
Pulmonary fibrosis (5%)

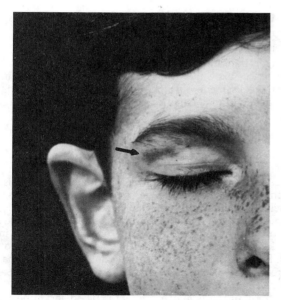

Figure 200-5. The arrow points to the violaceous suffusion of the upper eyelid in a boy with active juvenile dermatomyositis.

Although not often necessary for diagnosis, a muscle biopsy generally is indicated in the initial assessment of a child to support long-term glucocorticoid therapy or, eventually, immunosuppressive drugs. The muscle to be examined should be clinically involved but not atrophied. The best sites are generally a deltoid or quadriceps. The biopsy should be generous (2 cm) and usually is performed best by the open technique. Experience, however, is increasing with closed needle biopsy tests for diagnosis or at least for follow-up assessment.

■ TREATMENT

General supportive care and a coordinated team approach are necessary to manage this serious disease in children. Treatment should include a program of graduated rest and positioning along with physical therapy to minimize contractures. Generally, it is necessary to use prednisone for at least the first month after diagnosis. If clinical response is acceptable and the serum muscle enzyme concentrations decrease, then a lower dosage is instituted. Thereafter, the prednisone is slowly tapered by frequent monitoring of improvement in the clinical status of the child, the degree of muscle weakness documented by objective testing, and the serum muscle enzyme concentrations. Myositis is not controlled satisfactorily until serum muscle

enzymes return to normal (or nearly normal) levels and stay there while the steroid is tapered during an increase in the child's prescribed level of physical activity. Because long-term steroid administration is accompanied by significant toxicity in growing children, the glucocorticoid dose should be lowered as quickly as possible concomitant with continued improvement in indices of the disease.

Long-term survival in dermatomyositis approaches 90%. If death occurs, it is often within the first years after onset. This observation suggests that the major factors to be assessed in estimating prognosis are the basic nature of the inflammatory disease, its early treatment and response, and whether vasculopathy is present, or if there is involvement of organ systems such as the GI or pulmonary tracts.

The average child with dermatomyositis is expected to improve progressively to full functional recovery (Table 200–12). While the child heals, physical therapy is intensified to normalize function and minimize development of contractures secondary to muscle weakness or atrophy. Muscle-strengthening exercises should be added to the program only when acute inflammation subsides. Functional outcome appears best in children who have been seen early and treated vigorously. Most survivors function independently as adults, although some have residual atrophy of skin or muscle groups.

Late in the disease during the healing phase, about half the children develop calcinosis of the skin and subcutaneous tissues, about the joints, and within the interfascial planes of the muscles (Figure 200–6). The calcium salts have been identified as hydroxyapatite or fluorapatite. Many approaches to the therapy of calcinosis have been reported. None has been uniformly successful. Surgical excision of calcium tumors in areas of ulceration or pressure can be performed if necessary.

HENOCH-SCHÖNLEIN PURPURA

Henoch-Schönlein purpura (HSP) is the most common type of vasculitis of the small blood vessels that occurs in children and young adults and is an example of nonthrombocytopenic purpura. Table 200–13 lists the clinical characteristics of HSP. The classic purpuric rash consists of a maculopapular or purpuric eruption that affects the lower extremities and buttocks but may occur elsewhere.

■ EPIDEMIOLOGY

An upper respiratory tract infection or other illness, often in the spring, may precede the onset of HSP. In some cases, beta-hemolytic streptococcal pharyngitis has been diagnosed, and, in other instances, a recent vaccination, varicella, hepatitis B infection, insect bite, dietary allergy, malig-

TABLE 200-11. Clinical Phases of Dermatomyositis in Childhood

Prodromal period with nonspecific symptoms (weeks to months)

Progressive muscle weakness and rash (days to weeks)

Persistent weakness, rash, and active myositis (up to 2 y)

Recovery with residual muscle atrophy and contracture with or without calcinosis

Adapted from Hanson. Clin Rheum Dis. 1976;2:445.

TABLE 200-12. Prognosis for Dermatomyositis

Recovery with no disability	65%
Minimal atrophy or contractures	25%
Calcinosis*	20%
Wheelchair dependence	5%
Death	7%

Children with calcinosis are also included in the other categories.

nancy, or mycoplasmal disease has been cited. In rare cases, HSP appears to have familial predisposition, but no human leukocyte antigen (HLA) association has been identified. Hereditary C2 complement-component deficiency is a predisposing factor in some children with HSP.

■ CLINICAL MANIFESTATIONS

The extent of involvement of the necrotizing vasculitis determines the clinical manifestations of HSP in the skin, GI tract, joints, and kidneys. An isolated CNS vasculitis has been described in a few children. Onset of HSP is usually acute with sequential manifestations appearing during the next few days to weeks. Purpura over the lower extremities is the first manifestation of the disease in more than half of the children. The trunk is often spared. Purpuric lesions appear in crops; some may go on to develop hemorrhage or ulceration, and others mimic urticaria. The lesions may spread to form large areas of cutaneous involvement and may be interspersed with petechiae. Nonpitting edema occurs in 25% of the children and commonly affects the dorsal hands and feet, and, less commonly, the forehead, periorbital areas, scalp, perineum, and scrotum. Prominent edema is most common in the infant (younger than 2 years of age).

Involvement of the GI tract occurs in more than 85% of children. Colicky abdominal pain, melena, ileus, vomiting, or hematemesis may be the initial presentation. Severe hemorrhage or intussusception with obstruction or perforation occurs in less than 5% of cases. These complications are more common in the older child (more than 4 years of age). Arthritis occurs at onset or shortly thereafter in about 75% of the children. Knees and ankles are most commonly affected, but wrists, elbows, and the small joints of the hands may also be involved. Periarticular swelling and tenderness, usually without erythema or warmth, are most characteristic. Large effusions are unusual. This arthritis is transient, generally not migratory, and usually resolves within a few days.

Clinical Course

Most children with HSP have self-limited disease that consists of a single exacerbation lasting about 4 weeks. The younger the child, the shorter the course and the fewer recurrences expected. Most exacerbations occur within the first 6 weeks. Generally, the disease is over in 3 months. An unusual child may experience exacerbations for as long as 2 years after onset.

■ LABORATORY STUDIES

A moderate leukocytosis is seen in some children as is normochromic anemia, which may reflect GI blood loss. The platelet count is normal to elevated, and coagulation studies are normal. Although this is an immune-complex disease, the total hemolytic complement is generally normal during the initial attack of HSP. Hemolytic and C3 complement levels are normal, but the concentration of properdin and factor B may be decreased in half the children during the acute illness. Serum IgA and IgM concentrations are elevated in half the patients. Split fibrin products may be present in blood and urine.

■ DIAGNOSIS

Purpura and a normal platelet count must be present for a diagnosis of HSP. Abdominal pain, unexplained renal disease, and arthritis are additional diagnostic clues to the presence of HSP. This disease must be differentiated from a variety of other illnesses including acute poststreptococcal glomerulonephritis, rheumatic fever, SLE, septicemia, and disseminated intravascular coagulation. Other causes of an acute surgical abdomen or GI bleeding must be considered as must be intussusception or pancreatitis.

A skin biopsy may be useful to confirm a diagnosis in some children. Characteristic features are a leukocytoclastic vasculitis with intravascular deposition of IgA and C3. A kidney biopsy is generally not indicated except to clarify the

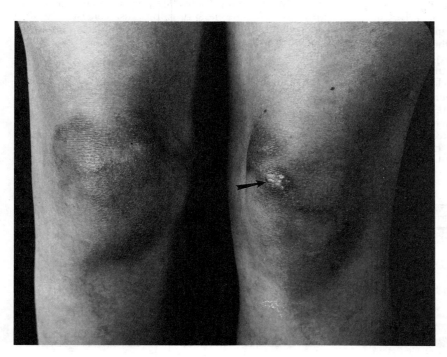

Figure 200-5. Knees of a girl with the erythematous prepatellar lesions of juvenile dermatomyositis. The arrow points to an area of calcinosis cutis.

TABLE 200-13. Clinical Characteristics of Henoch-Schönlein Purpura

Nonthrombocytopenic purpura
Arthritis
Abdominal pain
Nephritis

extent and nature of the renal disease in those children who are severely affected.

■ TREATMENT

General clinical support and meticulous observation for complications are critically important in the seriously ill child with HSP. Glucocorticoids are generally indicated only in GI hemorrhage. The response to the use of these drugs may be dramatic. Generally, prednisone is chosen, followed by a gradual reduction in the dose depending on response to therapy and extent of bleeding. Prednisone appears not to otherwise modify the extent of the disease, shorten its course, or affect the frequency or course of renal involve-

ment. Clinical studies have not thoroughly evaluated the efficacy of glucocorticoid therapy administered early to children with nephritis. In progressive renal disease, consideration should be given to glucocorticoids and cytotoxic agents. Antiplatelet drugs should also be evaluated. Renal transplants have been successfully performed in children with irreversible renal failure related to HSP. Nephritis has recurred in the allografts of some of these cases.

■ PROGNOSIS

Prognosis in HSP is generally excellent and depends on the extent of the disease and the age of the child; prognosis is better in the younger child. Morbidity and mortality are often related to the extent of involvement of the GI tract or kidneys. Less than 5% of children who develop HSP progressed to end-stage renal disease in early studies of its course. Recent estimates of long-term prognosis are more optimistic. In children admitted to a hospital during the initial illness, however, careful follow-up shows increased evidence of renal disease.

(Abridged from James T. Cassidy, Connective Tissue Diseases and Amyloidosis, in Oski, DeAngelis, Feigin, McMillan, Warshaw: *Principles and Practice of Pediatrics, Second Edition,* J.B. Lippincott, 1994.)

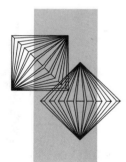

SECTION 15
Neurologic Disorders

Oski's Essential Pediatrics,
edited by Kevin B. Johnson and Frank A. Oski.
Lippincott–Raven Publishers,
Philadelphia © 1997

201

Evaluation of the Child With Neurologic Disease

■ PATIENT HISTORY AND NEUROLOGIC EXAMINATION

The most important parts of the evaluation of a child with neurologic symptoms are the history and physical examination. Principles used during the general portion of the evaluation are applicable to the child with a neurologic problem. Slight modification of the approach can increase the amount of information obtained. The purpose of the history is to obtain information that enables a tentative diagnosis to be made. With a tentative diagnosis in mind, the neurologic examination is performed to see if the findings are

consistent with the postulated diagnosis. For example, if a patient is thought to have idiopathic epilepsy but has an abnormal neurologic examination, the possibility of a structural lesion causing the seizures should be considered. In the case of the child with a complaint of weakness, cerebellar dysfunction should be considered, as well as disease of nerve or muscle, because unsteadiness may be interpreted as weakness. Tests of coordination, power of individual muscle groups, reflexes, and sensation can help differentiate the cause of the symptom.

Information obtained from the history should allow the tempo of the illness to be assessed and the findings to be interpreted in accord with neuroanatomic and neurophysiologic principles. The physician should determine if the disease process is acute or chronic and whether the onset was abrupt or insidious. Occasionally, an event such as intercurrent illness or trauma results in closer than usual observation of a child and discovery of a preexisting problem; a history dating the beginning of neurologic symptoms may not always be accurate. A decrease in the rate of acquisition of new developmental skills or loss of previously acquired skills suggests a degenerative process. Specific questions should be asked to help clarify the meaning of terms used by the historian. Dizziness may indicate vertigo or lightheadedness. Weakness may refer to loss of muscle power, fatigue, or unsteadiness. Blurred

TABLE 201-1. Normal Developmental Milestones

Newborn	8 Weeks	12 Weeks
In ventral suspension, head hangs down	In ventral suspension, head in same plane as rest of body	In ventral suspension, head held above rest of body
When prone, pelvis raised and knees under abdomen	When prone, chin lifts off couch	Head bobs when supported sitting
Complete head lag on traction	Hands held open part of the time	No grasp reflex
Walking reflex	Fixes and follows object through arc greater than 90 degrees	Turns head to sound, notices hands, follows object through 180-degree arc
Grasp reflex	Smiles and makes sounds	Recognizes mother

20 Weeks	28 Weeks	40 Weeks
When prone, chest off couch and weight on forearms	When prone, can support upper trunk with weight on hands and arms extended	Creeps on abdomen
No head lag on traction	Rolls prone to supine	Achieves sitting position independently
Can grasp objects and bring them to mouth	Sits on floor with support of hands	Pincer grasp
Smiles at mirror	Bears weight on legs in standing position	Waves bye-bye
Excites with feeding	Transfers objects	
Laughs aloud	Imitates sounds	
	Responds to name	
	Drinks from cup	
	States syllables	

52 Weeks	15 Months	18 Months
Walks like bear	Creeps upstairs	Pulls toys when walking
May walk independently	Can sit in chair	Takes off shoes and socks
Releases toys	Achieves standing position independently	Uses jargon and normal language
Plays simple games	Stacks 2 to 3 cubes	Imitates mother
Interest in picture books	Uses cup, rotates spoon	Follows simple request
Uses 2 to 3 words with meaning	Knows some body parts	Turns pages in groups
Understands simple phrases		

2 Years	2 ½ Years	3 Years
Walks up stairs placing both feet on each step	Jumps with both feet	Rides tricycle
Kicks ball	Holds crayon in hand	Draws circles and tries to imitate cross
Stacks more than 5 cubes	Toilet trained	Independent dressing skills except for buttons
Puts on socks	Knows name and sex	Normal speech
Some dressing skills	Follows instructions	Goes upstairs one foot at a time
Uses phrases	Identifies objects	May know nursery rhymes
Names common objects	May name a color	Beginning to understand prepositions
Turns pages singly		
Places objects in formboard puzzles		

4 Years	5 Years	6 Years
Walks downstairs with one foot on each step	Skips on both feet	Copies a diamond
Copies cross	Can tie shoelace	Repeats digits
Asks numerous questions	Copies square	Counts
Imaginative play	Knows age	Knows number of fingers
	Distinguishes morning from afternoon	
	Beginning to draw a man	

vision may indicate diplopia, decreased acuity, a visual field defect, or scotomata. Each of these would have different importance in terms of localizing the area of dysfunction. The physician has to decide if the symptoms can be explained by dysfunction of one part of the nervous system or if the process is diffuse or multifocal. Different physical findings correlate with each of these possibilities.

Information obtained during the history should include details of the mother's pregnancy, labor, and delivery. These are times when insults may affect the nervous system of the fetus or neonate and produce immediate or subsequent neurologic problems. Particular attention to the schedule of acquisition of motor and language developmental milestones yields information about the onset of the disease and whether the problem involves specific areas of function. A summary of normal developmental milestones is shown in Table 201–1.

Many neurologic illnesses are familial, and important clues to the child's illness may be obtained from careful review of the family history. Family members may not know the specific name of the disease being considered but may be familiar with symptoms and signs. This is particularly true with familial diseases involving the cerebellum, peripheral nerves, or muscle. Subtle manifestations of neurocutaneous syndromes may not have been appreciated previously, and the finding of tuberous sclerosis or neurofibromatosis in the child can result in identifying other affected relatives. Occasionally, diseases are diagnosed erroneously by family members. Any severe headache may be mistakenly referred to as migraine. It is important to elicit a detailed history in family members to see if the symptoms do suggest migraine.

The physical examination begins when the child enters the examining room; observations continue during the history taking. Significant information about the cranial nerves and cerebellar and motor function can be obtained by watching an infant crawl, walk, or play with toys. The general physical examination should include measurement of head size. Transillumination of the skull may be informative in children younger than 1 year of age and may help detect lesions such as chronic subdural hematomas, porencephalic cysts, and Dandy-Walker malformations. Dysmorphic features or cutaneous abnormalities may help establish a diagnosis. A Wood's lamp examination may be necessary to detect the depigmented ash-leaf lesion seen in tuberous sclerosis. Metabolic disorders resulting in the accumulation of excessive amounts of lipids or other materials may result in enlargement of the liver and spleen. Cardiac murmurs may predispose to neurologic complications such as embolic strokes and cerebral abscesses. A cranial bruit may suggest a large intracranial vascular malformation. Cutaneous abnormalities, dimples, vascular malformations, and tufts of hair over the lower back may be associated with occult spinal dysraphism. Limb growth asymmetry suggests a chronic hemiparesis.

The formal neurologic examination is used to confirm the information obtained by observation and to corroborate the suspected diagnosis based on the history. It is often easier to proceed with the infant seated in a parent's lap rather than seated or lying on an examining table. Beginning the examination with the legs and working upward results in better cooperation than if more unpleasant aspects of the examination, such as funduscopy, are performed first.

Cranial nerve testing is easy to perform. Cranial nerve I, the olfactory nerve, often is not tested unless there is a specific indication for doing so. Cranial nerve II, the optic nerve, can be inspected and tested. Vision can be assessed by several methods in children who are too young to cooperate for formal testing with visual charts. Various drums or tapes can be used to elicit opticokinetic nystagmus in young infants. With infants older than 6 months, various small objects, even a fleck of paper, can be placed in front of them, and their attempts to pick it up can be observed. Each eye can be tested separately. Cranial nerves III, IV, and VI are responsible for eye movements, pupillary responses, and lid opening. They can be tested by observing spontaneous eye movements and by having the child watch toys such as puppets. Facial sensation, governed by cranial nerve V, can be tested with a wisp of cotton. The motor branch of cranial nerve V supplies the muscles of mastication. These can be tested by having the child open his jaw against resistance and by palpating the masseter mus-

cles as the teeth are clenched. Facial movements, orchestrated by cranial nerve VII, can be assessed when the child smiles and laughs and with volitional movements. Asking the child to smile allows observations of the symmetry of the nasolabial folds; the symmetry of burying of eyelashes can be observed as the eyes are closed. The symmetry of the strength of the eyelids can be tested as attempts to open the upper lids are made when the child attempts to keep his eyes tightly closed. Auditory acuity, controlled by cranial nerve VIII, can be tested by using a tuning fork or watch or by giving whispered instructions out of sight of the child. Lower cranial nerves IX, X, XI, and XII can be tested by eliciting a gag reflex, watching the palate contract, and observing movements of the tongue.

The assessment of motor function in preschool children is made while watching the child play, crawl, climb, or walk. Activities can be designed to test upper or lower extremity function. Lifting a child with the examiner's hands placed in the patient's axillae tests shoulder girdle function. Lifting a child off the ground while he holds the examiner's thumbs tests hand strength. Tone is tested by passively moving the child's limbs.

Deep tendon reflexes are elicited in children by similar techniques used in adults. Infants have developmental reflexes in the newborn period that disappear with normal development. The more common developmental reflexes are listed in Table 201–2. The abnormal persistence of these reflexes usually is accompanied by other abnormalities of the neurologic examination or a lack of appropriate developmental skills. The isolated persistence of one of these reflexes should be interpreted cautiously because of the significant variation in normal age ranges during which they disappear.

Cerebellar function can be assessed in young infants and preschool children by watching them play. This is particularly useful for observing upper extremity function and balance. The skill with which young children perform fine motor tasks is age dependent, and the assessment of normalcy must take this into consideration. Infants often can be coaxed into reaching for small objects, and, during these maneuvers, fine motor coordination and hand function are observed. The presence of adventitial or associated movements can be evaluated at this time. Watching a child walk or run is helpful in determining cerebellar function and motor strength, peripheral nerve function, and abnormalities of tone.

The sensory examination often is difficult to perform and to interpret accurately in infants and preschool children. When performed near the end of a history taking and examination session, attention and cooperation may be lacking. Under these circumstances, completing the sensory examination at a later time may yield more useful information. Engag-

---

TABLE 201-2. Common Newborn Reflexes

Moro reflex—Present in normal newborns and disappears by 3 months of age

Grasp reflexes (palmar and plantar)—Present in normal newborns and disappear by 3 months of age

Lower extremity crossed extension reflex—Present at birth and disappears by 1 month of age

Extensor plantar response—Variably present in normal newborns and disappears by 8–12 months of age

Placing reflex—Present at birth and disappears by 1–2 months of age

Stepping reflex—Present at birth and disappears by 1–2 months of age

Asymmetric tonic neck reflex—Variably present in normal newborns and disappears by 3 months of age

ing the child to "play games" often enhances effort and interest. Testing of cortical or sensory modalities such as double simultaneous stimulation, stereognosis, or graphesthesia requires accurate reporting by the examinee. Reliable information often cannot be obtained until the child is of school age.

(Abridged from Marvin A. Fishman, Evaluation of the Child With Neurologic Disease, in Oski, DeAngelis, Feigin, McMillan, Warshaw: *Principles and Practice of Pediatrics, Second Edition*, J.B. Lippincott, 1994.)

Oski's Essential Pediatrics, edited by Kevin B. Johnson and Frank A. Oski. Lippincott–Raven Publishers, Philadelphia © 1997

202

Developmental Defects

HYDROCEPHALY

Hydrocephaly is a congenital or acquired disorder in which there is an excessive amount of cerebrospinal fluid (CSF) within the cerebral ventricles. More CSF is produced than can be reabsorbed. Increased pressure within the ventricular system may be transitory or persistent. Enlarged cerebral ventricles due to the loss of brain tissue (formerly called hydrocephalus ex vacuo) is excluded from consideration in this chapter, because it does not meet the definition of inadequate absorption of CSF and increased pressure. Noncommunicating hydrocephaly refers to conditions in which the ventricular fluid does not communicate with the fluid in the basal cisterns or spinal subarachnoid spaces. This implies a block of the CSF flow within the ventricular system. In communicating hydrocephaly, the block is outside the ventricular system or its exit foramina.

CSF is formed within the ventricular system, mainly by the choroid plexus through the processes of active secretion and diffusion. The fluid exits the ventricular system by way of foramina in the fourth ventricle and circulates into the lumbar and subarachnoid spaces. Most CSF absorption takes place at the arachnoid villi leading to venous channels of the sagittal sinus. In adults, the total CSF volume is approximately 150 mL, and only 25% is within the ventricular system. The rate of formation is approximately 20 mL/hour, and the CSF turns over three to four times per day.

■ PATHOGENESIS

Impaired absorption of CSF due to obstruction of flow or dysfunction of absorptive mechanisms is the most common mechanism for producing hydrocephalus. If flow is blocked within the ventricular system, there is a disproportionate dilatation of the ventricles proximal to the block. In aqueductal stenosis, the lateral and third ventricles are disproportionately dilated compared with the fourth ventricle. If the block is extraventricular, there is a relatively proportionate increase in size of all ventricles.

■ ETIOLOGY

Congenital hydrocephalus may result from congenital malformations of the nervous system, including isolated aqueductal stenosis, or may be associated with other malformations, including the Dandy-Walker malformation, which consists of a large cyst in the posterior fossa continuous with the fourth ventricle and partial or complete absence of the cerebellar vermis. A common associated malformation syndrome is that of meningomyelocele with Arnold-Chiari malformation. Other syndromes include a sex-linked form of aqueductal stenosis and chromosomal anomalies resulting in syndromes with additional multiple congenital malformations. Arachnoid cysts or congenital tumors may obstruct the ventricular system. Congenital hydrocephalus may be caused by intrauterine infections, which cause inflammation of the ependymal lining of the ventricular system or the meninges in the subarachnoid space, subsequently occluding the CSF pathways. Among the more common infections causing congenital hydrocephalus are rubella, cytomegalovirus, toxoplasmosis, and syphilis.

Hydrocephalus may be acquired postnatally secondary to infections of the nervous system (eg, bacterial meningitis), brain tumors, and arachnoiditis secondary to bleeding into the subarachnoid space from a ruptured arteriovenous malformation, aneurysm, or trauma. Premature infants may develop hydrocephalus secondary to intraventricular hemorrhage.

■ SYMPTOMS AND SIGNS

The primary process (eg, tumor, infection, bleeding) and the symptoms and signs caused by increased intracranial pressure secondary to the hydrocephalus may contribute to the clinical picture. The severity of the findings is influenced by the rate at which the hydrocephalus develops and the development of alternate pathways of CSF absorption. Nonspecific symptoms include headaches of various locations and intensities; they occasionally occur early in the morning and are associated with vomiting. Personality and behavior changes, including irritability or indifference, sometimes occur. Lethargy and drowsiness are relatively late symptoms. Nausea and vomiting are secondary to increased intracranial pressure, particularly in the posterior fossa. Nonspecific signs include third and sixth cranial nerve deficits, which result in paresis of extraocular muscles and may lead to diplopia. Papilledema may be a late finding if the intracranial pressure is not markedly elevated and the process is a slow, chronic one. Changes in vital signs occur relatively late and indicate distortion of the brain stem. In young children, the anterior fontanelle may become full or distended; this is accompanied by excessive head growth and dilatation of scalp veins. The setting sun sign is produced by paralysis of upward gaze and results in the sclera being visible above the iris. Spasticity develops first in the lower extremities and then in the arms and results from stretching of motor fibers around the bodies of the lateral ventricles. Dilatation of the third ventricle may cause pressure on the hypothalamus, resulting in disturbances in sexual development and in fluid and electrolyte imbalance.

■ DIAGNOSIS AND THERAPY

The advent of noninvasive neuroimaging techniques such as computed tomography (CT) or magnetic resonance imaging (MRI) has made the diagnosis of hydrocephalus relatively straightforward. The pattern of ventricular dilatation, the presence of interstitial edema (ie, CSF in the white matter surrounding the ventricles), and an underlying cause for obstruction of CSF flow are usually readily apparent (Figure 202–1). Examination of the CSF should be undertaken if there is suspicion of a relatively recent infection or if there is a clinical suspicion of subarachnoid bleeding but no evidence of such on neuroimaging studies. In infancy, chronic subdural hematomas may present in a similar fashion and can be detected by neuroimaging procedures.

Treatment includes specific therapy for any underlying condition associated with the hydrocephalus, such as brain tumor, abscess, and chronic meningitis. Surgery is the most effective means of treating progressive hydrocephalus, and a shunt system between the cerebral ventricles and the peritoneal cavity is the most commonly employed technique. The shunt, which allows diversion of the CSF into the peritoneal cavity where it is absorbed, is a palliative measure and not a cure. The complication rate is relatively high, and problems encountered include mechanical obstruction of the shunt system and infections within it, which may produce meningitis or ventriculitis. Shunt infections may be indolent and often are caused by organisms that usually are not considered pathogens, such as *Staphylococcus epidermidis*. Medical therapy designed to decrease CSF production may be used when the hydrocephalus is slowly progressive and perhaps transitory. This includes the ventricular enlargement that is sometimes seen after subarachnoid hemorrhage, meningitis, or intraventricular hemorrhage in premature infants. The therapeutic agents used include acetazolamide, furosemide, and glycerol. These agents also may be used in the interim period when an infected shunt system has to be removed and before a new system can be reinserted.

■ PROGNOSIS

Intellectual and motor function of the hydrocephalic child are determined by the problem causing the hydrocephalus rather than by the ventricular dilatation. The natural history of intrauterine infections, meningitis, brain tumors, or other disorders determines the prognosis. The disabilities produced by the hydrocephalus include motor problems related to spasticity or coordination deficits, visual impairment secondary to optic atrophy from longstanding increased intracranial pressure, and intellectual impairment. Intellectual ability is usually less significantly affected than motor performance, because the gray matter of the brain is less affected by the hydrocephalus than the white matter.

ARNOLD-CHIARI MALFORMATION

The Arnold-Chiari malformation involves the brain stem and lower portion of the cerebellum. These structures are displaced downward into the cervical canal. There are various degrees of the malformation. In type I, the medulla is displaced downward into the spinal canal with tonguelike processes of the cerebellum. In type II, in addition to the type I findings, the fourth ventricle is elongated and extends into the spinal canal. The downward displacement may be such that the cervical cord is kinked on itself and the foramen magnum and upper cervical canal may be packed tightly with the displaced tissue. In the rare type III malformation, there is an associated cervical spina bifida with herniation of brain tissue through the defect. As a result of the distal displacement, lower cranial nerves and cervical spinal nerve roots may be stretched. There often are associated nervous system abnormalities. Children with meningomyeloceles and hydrocephalus usually have an associated Arnold-Chiari malformation. It also may be associated with hydromyelia and syringomyelia. Other minor malformations include beaking of the tectal plate and large massa intermedia.

Arnold-Chiari malformations usually occur in children with spina bifida and hydrocephalus. The symptoms and signs are those caused by the malformations. With significant downward displacement of the hind brain, there may be stretching of the lower cranial nerves, which can produce facial paralysis, hoarseness or stridor, or difficulty with swallowing. If the upper segments of the spinal cord are involved, there may be motor deficits in the arms. Cerebellar

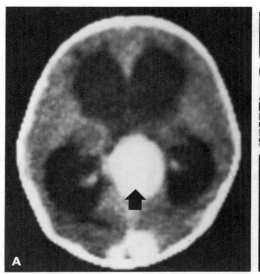
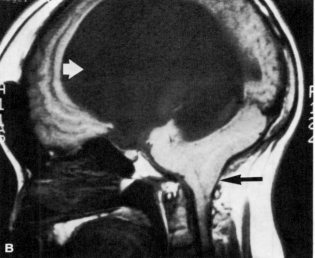

Figure 202-1. (A) CT scan with contrast enhancement demonstrating hydrocephalus secondary to an aneurysm of the vein of Galen (*arrow*). **(B)** MRI, sagittal plane, demonstrating hydrocephalus (*white arrow*) and an Arnold-Chiari type II malformation (*black arrow*) with downward displacement of the brain stem into the cervical canal. (Courtesy of Clark Carrol, MD, Texas Children's Hospital, Houston, TX.)

ataxia and vertical nystagmus also have been described in patients with Arnold-Chiari malformation.

The symptoms related to Chiari type I malformation include neck pain, back pain, scoliosis, torticollis, motor dysfunction, and apnea. The ages of the patients ranged from 1 month to 14 years. Several children had associated syringomyelia.

The downward displacement of the hind brain can be detected by neuroimaging procedures (see Fig 202–1*B*). In addition to CT or MRI of the posterior fossa, MRI of the spinal cord may be necessary to detect the associated malformations.

Shunting of an associated hydrocephalus would be the first procedure attempted in treating these patients. If this does not improve the symptoms attributable to hind brain or cervical cord dysfunction, occipital decompression and cervical laminectomy should be considered.

MACROCEPHALY AND MICROCEPHALY

■ MACROCEPHALY

Macrocephaly refers to a head size two standard deviations above the mean. There are many causes for large heads. Table 202–1 lists the more common conditions associated with large head size. In some children, a large brain (*ie,* megalencephaly) may be the underlying condition. This may be familial and not accompanied by any additional symptoms and signs, or there may be an associated mental deficiency and other neurologic abnormalities such as hypotonia.

Infants have been described who are macrocephalic and whose head growth parallels a normal growth pattern

---

TABLE 202-1. Large Head Syndromes

HYDROCEPHALY	**TOXIC-METABOLIC CAUSES**
Congenital	Benign increased intracranial hypertension associated with antibiotics, vitamins, endocrine disorders, "catch-up" growth after malnutrition, galactosemia, anemias
Aqueductal stenosis ⎫ with or without	
⎬ meningomyelocele	
Communicating ⎭ and Arnold-Chiari	
malformation	**CRANIOSKELETAL DYSPLASIAS**
Dandy-Walker syndrome	Anemias
Hydranencephaly	Achondroplasia
Porencephaly	Osteogenesis imperfecta
Holoprosencephaly	Osteopetrosis
Genetic:	Metaphyseal dysplasia
Chromosomal malformation	Platybasia
Sex-linked	Fibrous dysplasia (Albright's syndrome)
Cysts	
Infectious	**STORAGE AND DEGENERATIVE DISEASE**
Postinflammatory disease (meningitis)	Leukodystrophies
Viral (cytomegalovirus, mumps, other)	Canavan's spongy degenerative
Parasitic (toxoplasmosis)	Alexander's
Vascular	Lysosomal disease
Postsubarachnoid hemorrhage	Tay-Sachs
Arteriovenous malformation	Generalized gangliosidosis
Vein of Galen aneurysm	Mucopolysaccharidosis
Tumor	Metachromatic leukodystrophy
Choroid plexus papilloma	Peroxisomal disorders
Posterior fossa neoplasm	Neonatal adrenoleukodystrophy
Other	Amino acid disorders
	Maple syrup urine disease
SUBDURALS	
Effusion	**UNKNOWN CAUSES**
Hematoma	Cerebral gigantism
Hygroma	Megalencephaly
Empyema	Familial
	Dominant
NEUROCUTANEOUS DISORDERS	Wiedemann-Beckwith syndrome
Neurofibromatosis	
Tuberous sclerosis	
Multiple hemangiomatosis	
Incontinentia pigmenti	
Basal cell nevus syndrome	
Neurocutaneous melanosis	

but is above the 95th percentile. CT reveals slight ventricular dilation and increased width of the subarachnoid space over the convexities of the hemispheres. The development of most of these children is normal or only slightly delayed. If head growth continues parallel to the 95th percentile, no intervention is necessary. The exact cause of this condition is uncertain. It has been referred to as extraventricular obstructive hydrocephalus or external hydrocephalus. Another possibility is that the fluid over the convexities represents small subdural hematomas with secondary hydrocephalus. The diagnosis can be established by CT or MRI, and the children can be followed with serial head circumference measurements. Any deviation from the anticipated growth pattern warrants repeat neuroimaging studies. Usually by the preschool years, the head size deviates less from the 95th percentile, and the fluid collections remain stable or decrease.

■ MICROCEPHALY

Microcephaly indicates a head size less than two standard deviations below the mean. This indicates an accompanying small brain (ie, microencephaly). The causes are multiple. In primary microcephaly, there is no identifiable insult to the developing brain that subsequently inhibits its growth. The primary microcephalies include familial forms and the cases that seem to occur in isolation. Newborn infants often do not exhibit striking deficits, unlike the infants who have sustained a major insult in utero. Eventually, intellectual impairment becomes apparent, and some children develop motor deficits and epilepsy.

Other anomalies sometimes associated with microcephaly include agyria, lissencephaly, micropolygyri, schizencephaly, macrogyri, and heterotopia. These infants usually have severe deficits that are apparent in the neonatal period.

Microcephaly can be seen in a variety of chromosomal anomalies, intrauterine infections secondary to inherited metabolic disorders, intrauterine anoxia or vascular events, and insults in the perinatal period.

(Abridged from Marvin A. Fishman, Developmental Defects, in Oski, DeAngelis, Feigin, McMillan, Warshaw: *Principles and Practice of Pediatrics, Second Edition,* J.B. Lippincott, 1994.)

Oski's Essential Pediatrics,
edited by Kevin B. Johnson and Frank A. Oski.
Lippincott–Raven Publishers,
Philadelphia © 1997

203

Acute Encephalopathies

The term *encephalopathy* refers to a diffuse disturbance of brain function, resulting in behavioral changes, altered consciousness, or seizures. The term is usually reserved for noninfective causes of brain dysfunction. The term *encephalitis* refers to brain dysfunction resulting from an infectious process. Clinically, it may be difficult to differentiate the two, and an infectious process must always be considered in a patient with evidence of an acute disturbance of brain function.

Many conditions can cause acute brain dysfunction in children, resulting in progressive alterations of consciousness (Table 203–1). Many of these conditions are treatable and may have a favorable outcome if an accurate diagnosis is made and appropriate therapy instituted.

■ PATHOPHYSIOLOGY

To function normally, the brain must be adequately supplied with substrates and cofactors for energy production and for synthesis of structural components. There must be adequate blood flow to deliver the substrates and to remove waste products. Many encephalopathies are caused by cytotoxic injury, which occurs if energy production is disrupted by a lack of oxygen or glucose or by inadequate cerebral blood flow. Cytotoxic injury may also occur with direct poisoning of the neuron by exogenous toxins or drugs or by endogenous toxins arising from an error of metabolism or from inadequate removal of toxic wastes by the kidneys or liver. Cytotoxic injury is frequently accompanied by cerebral edema and increased intracranial pressure, amplifying cerebral ischemia.

Other encephalopathies may be caused by interference with neurotransmission rather than actual cytotoxic injury. Severe electrolyte disturbances may alter the electrical properties of cellular membranes. Various toxins and drugs may similarly interfere with membrane polarization or may alter neurotransmitters, interfering with neuronal activity.

■ CLINICAL PRESENTATION

The earliest signs of an acute encephalopathy may be subtle, including personality disturbances, a shortened attention span, and changes in mentation. Cognitive deficits, such as difficulty in processing new information and perceptual and memory deficits, are common in the initial stages. Abnormal movements, particularly fine tremors, asterixis, or myoclonus, may be present. Primitive reflexes, such as the grasp, snout, sucking, and rooting responses, may be elicited on examination. With increasing severity of brain dysfunction, alteration in the level of consciousness occurs, progressing from lethargy and obtundation to stupor and coma. Some patients retain their alert appearance but become increasingly disoriented and agitated. Other patients have alternating periods of hyperalertness and drowsiness, gradually progressing to longer periods of unresponsiveness. Seizures occur frequently and may be generalized or focal.

Diffuse symmetric abnormalities in motor tone and strength are common. Focal motor abnormalities are uncommon and, if present, tend to fluctuate in severity or change in location. The pupillary examination may be helpful in determining the cause of the encephalopathy. Preservation of the pupillary light reflexes in the presence of respiratory depression and deep coma suggests a metabolic coma. The absence of pupillary light reflexes suggests asphyxia, anticholinergic drug or glutethimide ingestion, or structural disease as the cause of coma. Alterations in the respiratory pattern are common in acute encephalopathies and may facilitate an accurate diagnosis if used in conjunction with direct determinations of the arterial blood pH, partial pressures of oxygen and carbon dioxide, and bicarbonate concentration (Table 203–2).

TABLE 203-1. Causes of Acute Encephalopathy in Childhood

OXYGEN, SUBSTRATE, OR COFACTOR DEPRIVATION	METABOLIC AND ENDOCRINOLOGIC DISTURBANCE	POSTINFECTIOUS DISORDERS
Hypoxia	Fluid/electrolyte imbalance	Acute disseminated encephalomyelitis
Pulmonary disease	Water intoxication	Reye's syndrome
Alveolar hypoventilation	Hypo- or hypernatremia	**EXOGENOUS TOXINS**
Carbon monoxide poisoning	Hypo- or hypermagnesemia	Drugs (sedatives, anticholinergics, psychotropics, salicylates)
Methemoglobinemia	Hypo- or hypercalcemia	Insecticides/pesticides
Anemia	Hypo- or hyperphosphatemia	Heavy metals, lead
ANOXIA OR ISCHEMIA	Acidosis or alkalosis	
"Near-miss" sudden infant death syndrome	Trace metal deficiency	**ABNORMAL TEMPERATURE REGULATION**
Cardiac arrest	"Scalds" encephalopathy	Hypothermia
Near-drowning	Endocrinologic disturbance	Heat stroke
Cardiac dysrhythmia	Diabetes mellitus	
Congestive heart failure	Hypo- or hyperthyroidism	
Hypotension	Hypo- or hyperparathyroidism	
Diffuse intravascular coagulation	Hypopituitarism	
Hypoglycemia	Organ failure	
Vitamin or cofactor deficiency	Hepatic	
Thiamine	Renal	
Niacin	Pancreatic	
Pyridoxin	Intussusception or volvulus	
B₁₂	Hypertensive encephalopathy	
Folate	Inborn errors of metabolism	
	Aminoacidurias (branched chain ketoacidosis)	
	Organic acidurias (propionic, methylmalonic, isovaleric acidemias, β- ketothiolase deficiency)	
	Urea cycle defects	
	Systemic carnitine deficiency	

Adapted from Plum F, Posner JB. The Diagnosis of Stupor and Coma. *3rd ed. Philadelphia: FA Davis; 1982.*

■ ETIOLOGY

Hypoxic-Ischemic Encephalopathy

Oxygen and glucose are the two major substrates needed for energy production in the brain. The supply of these two substrates and the cofactors necessary to allow usage of the substrates depends on an adequate cerebral blood flow. The brain is particularly vulnerable to even brief interruptions of blood flow or oxygen supply, because it possesses almost no reserves of nutrients and metabolizes at one of the highest rates of any organ in the body. If the brain's oxygen supply is insufficient, whether because of decreased availability or decreased delivery, consciousness is lost rapidly. If oxygenation is restored immediately, consciousness returns without sequelae. However, if oxygen deprivation lasts longer than 1 or 2 minutes, signs of an encephalopathy may persist for hours or permanently. Total ischemic anoxia lasting longer than about 4 minutes usually results in severe irreversible brain damage. In rare instances, especially near-drowning events, recovery of brain function occurs despite more prolonged periods of anoxia.

Major causes leading to hypoxic-ischemic encephalopathy include obstruction of the airway, as in drowning, choking, or suffocation, and a sudden decrease in cardiac output, as in cardiorespiratory arrest, severe dysrhythmias, severe hypotension, or massive systemic hemorrhage. Carbon monoxide poisoning may produce a hypoxic encephalopathy because carbon monoxide binds tightly to hemoglobin, diminishing its oxygen-carrying capacity. Subacute chronic hypoxia, as occurs in congestive heart failure, severe anemia, or pulmonary disease, may also cause an encephalopathy. However, severe neurologic changes usually occur only after a prolonged period of chronic hypoxia, and the cause of hypoxia is generally evident. Cerebral edema is a consistent feature in patients who have had an acute anoxic-ischemic event, and may be severe. Some patients may show a "lucent" interval of 12 to 24 hours before lapsing into coma with signs of cerebral edema. Occasionally, patients who have had oxygen deprivation or carbon monoxide intoxication develop a delayed postanoxic encephalopathy characterized by rapid neurologic deterioration several weeks after the initial insult.

The treatment of hypoxic-ischemic encephalopathy includes adequate oxygenation, rapid restoration of perfusion, and good fluid and electrolyte balance. Hyperosmolar agents and controlled hyperventilation may be necessary to reduce intracranial pressure. Anticonvulsants may also be necessary. The prognosis is difficult to determine early in the course, because patients may remain comatose for days, eventually recovering with few sequelae. Early evidence of brain stem dysfunction is a poor prognostic sign.

TABLE 203-2. Some Causes of Abnormal Ventilation in Unresponsive Patients

HYPERVENTILATION	HYPOVENTILATION
Metabolic Acidosis	*Respiratory Acidosis*
Anion gap	Acute (uncompensated)
Diabetic ketoacidosis*	Sedative drugs*
Diabetic hyperosmolar coma*	Brain stem injury
Lactic acidosis	Neuromuscular disorders
Uremia*	Chest injury
Alcoholic ketoacidosis	Acute pulmonary disease
Acidic poisons*	Chronic pulmonary disease*
Ethylene glycol	*Metabolic Alkalosis*
Methyl alcohol	Vomiting or gastric drainage
Paraldehyde	Diuretic therapy
Salicylism (primarily in children)	Adrenal steroid excess (Cushing's syndrome)
No anion gap	Primary aldosteronism
Diarrhea	Bartter's syndrome
Pancreatic drainage	
Carbonic anhydrase inhibitors	
NH_4Cl ingestion	
Renal tubular acidosis	
Ureteroenterostomy	
Respiratory Alkalosis	
Hepatic failure*	
Sepsis*	
Pneumonia	
Anxiety (hyperventilation syndrome)	
Mixed Acid–Base Disorders (Metabolic Acidosis and Respiratory Alkalosis)	
Salicylism	
Sepsis*	
Hepatic failure*	

*Common causes of stupor or coma.

Plum F, Posner JB. *The Diagnosis of Stupor and Coma. 3rd ed. Philadelphia: FA Davis; 1982: 186.*

Metabolic and Endocrinologic Disturbances

Hypoglycemia

Hypoglycemia is a serious, correctable cause of metabolic encephalopathy. The tolerance to hypoglycemia varies, but symptoms usually occur when blood glucose levels fall below 40 mg/dL. The severity of symptoms is determined by the availability of alternative substrates for cerebral metabolism. Patients with hypoglycemic encephalopathy may present with a variety of neurologic symptoms, including simple confusion, delirium, abrupt focal neurologic signs resembling a stroke, focal or generalized seizures, or coma. Because the spectrum of clinical presentations is so wide, hypoglycemia should be suspected in every patient with acute neurologic dysfunction. Blood should be drawn immediately for a glucose determination, and glucose should be administered. If treated promptly, neurologic symptoms are reversible. Persistent deficits may occur with prolonged or recurrent hypoglycemic attacks.

Diabetic Ketoacidosis

Diabetes mellitus is the most common endocrinologic disease presenting as an acute encephalopathy, although pituitary, adrenal, parathyroid, and thyroid disorders occasionally present with similar symptoms. Diabetic ketoacidosis typically occurs in patients with relatively severe diabetes who neglect to take their insulin or who have an associated acute infection. Polyuria, polydipsia, and fatigue lead to a dehydrated state with metabolic acidosis. Nausea, vomiting, and acute abdominal pain may be prominent early in the course. Hyperventilation is common and reflects the body's attempt to compensate for the metabolic acidosis. The neurologic examination is nonfocal, and brain stem function is usually intact.

The treatment of diabetic ketoacidosis may have serious neurologic consequences. Sudden lowering of serum osmolality may produce a shift of water into the brain, causing marked cerebral edema. This should be suspected when patients recovering from diabetic ketoacidosis complain of headache or become increasingly lethargic. Profound hypophosphatemia may occur as dehydration is corrected and the serum glucose level is lowered, causing further neurologic dysfunction. In addition to ketoacidosis, hypoglycemia, uremia, hypertension, and cerebral infarction should be considered in the diabetic presenting with an acute encephalopathy.

Disorders of Fluid and Electrolyte Balance

Disorders of electrolytes and serum osmolality are common causes of acute encephalopathy in childhood. Consciousness is altered if serum osmolality is less than 260 mOsm/kg or greater than 330 mOsm/kg. The total concentration of osmotically active materials in the interstitial and intracellular fluids is equal, because there is free diffusion of water across the cell membranes. A decrease in extracellular osmolality leads to cellular overhydration, and an increase in extracellular osmolality leads to cellular dehydration.

Hyponatremia

Hyponatremia or water intoxication may be caused by a sudden hypotonic water load, a disproportionate loss of sodium, or inappropriate retention of water. Numerous neurologic disorders stimulate antidiuretic hormone release in excess of the amount required to maintain a normal concentration of serum sodium. Meningitis, head trauma, brain neoplasms, and acute or subacute peripheral neuropathy have been associated with the syndrome of inappropriate antidiuretic hormone. A variety of endocrine disorders, pulmonary disorders, and drug ingestions increase antidiuretic hormone secretion and predispose the patient to hyponatremia. Chronic hyponatremia, which may occur in chronic renal disease, is better tolerated than acute changes in sodium balance. Clinical symptoms are caused by the accumulation of water within the cells, which is related in some way to altered excitability of the neural membrane. Moderately severe hyponatremia may cause confusion, delirium, and multifocal myoclonus. Seizures and coma are usually associated with severe hyponatremia and may be life threatening. Seizures may be multifocal or generalized and typically occur with serum sodium concentrations between 95 and 110 mEq/L.

The treatment of hyponatremia depends on the cause. Infants with hyponatremic dehydration are rehydrated with isotonic solutions. Patients with water intoxication due to antidiuretic hormone excess or a free-water load can often be treated with fluid restriction. Hypertonic saline solutions should be reserved for patients with severe hyponatremia manifested by seizures or coma.

Hypernatremia

Acute hypernatremia is most commonly caused by severe water depletion in children with diarrhea. It may also occur in patients receiving excessively concentrated solutions by tube feeding or in patients with diabetes insipidus. Symptoms of encephalopathy usually occur with serum sodium levels in excess of 160 mEq/L or total osmolalities of 340 or more mOsm/kg. Most of the dehydration in hypertonic states is intracellular. Because circulatory volume is relatively well maintained, clinical signs of dehydration such as tachycardia and poor skin turgor are less prominent than in

hyponatremic or isotonic dehydration. Brain shrinkage predisposes the child to petechial brain hemorrhages and to extra-axial hemorrhage. Venous sinus thrombosis and cerebral infarctions may also occur. There is a high mortality rate, and many of the survivors have permanent neurologic sequelae, including hemiparesis, seizure disorders, and mental retardation.

The treatment of hypernatremic dehydration involves the slow replacement of fluids. Rapid rehydration predisposes to cerebral edema with seizures and other manifestations of water intoxication.

Hypocalcemia

Hypocalcemia produces hyperexcitability of the peripheral and central nervous systems. Headaches and muscular cramping and twitching are early signs. Positive Chvostek's and Trousseau's signs are easily elicited, and carpopedal spasm may be prominent. Seizures are common and may be generalized, focal, or multifocal. Management consists of correction of the metabolic disturbance with intravenous administration of calcium gluconate. Chronic oral administration of calcium and vitamin D may be necessary, depending on the underlying cause.

Hypercalcemia

Neurologic manifestations of hypercalcemia include headaches, hallucinations, rigidity, tremor, and psychotic behavior. Some patients present with a slowly progressive dementia. Treatment depends on the cause. Severe hypercalcemia may require the use of a chelating agent.

Hypomagnesemia

Symptoms of hypomagnesemia, which occur when serum magnesium drops below 1 mEq/L, include confusion, irritability, hallucinations, and coma. Muscle twitching, myoclonic jerks, and tremors are common. Generalized seizures may occur. Examination shows increased muscle tone, carpopedal spasm, and positive Chvostek's and Trousseau's signs. Treatment consists of slow intravenous administration of magnesium sulfate.

Hypermagnesemia

Severe hypermagnesemia causes somnolence, lethargy, coma, and respiratory failure. There is a peripheral neuromuscular paralysis with loss of the deep tendon reflexes. Treatment is difficult. It may include the administration of calcium and neostigmine, and hemodialysis may be necessary in severe cases.

Other Causes

There are numerous other causes of encephalopathy, including hepatic failure, renal failure (uremic encephalopathy), hypertension, pancreatitis, inborn errors of metabolism, environmental toxins, and complications of medication overdoses. These causes are discussed elsewhere in this book.

(Abridged from Julie Thorne Parke, Acute Encephalopathies, in Oski, DeAngelis, Feigin, McMillan, Warshaw: *Principles and Practice of Pediatrics, Second Edition,* J.B. Lippincott, 1994.)

Oski's Essential Pediatrics,
edited by Kevin B. Johnson and Frank A. Oski.
Lippincott–Raven Publishers,
Philadelphia © 1997

204

Static Encephalopathy (Cerebral Palsy)

Static encephalopathy is a disorder of motor function against a background of a static or nonprogressive brain injury, usually as a result of a prenatal or perinatal event. The term encompasses a heterogeneous group of disorders whose causes are diverse and is synonymous with the term *cerebral palsy.* The motor dysfunction of the person with static encephalopathy clearly signifies to others the presence of a handicapping condition. In addition to the motor dysfunction, which may range from mild to severe, associated neurologic difficulties include mental retardation, seizures, communication dysfunction, and visual and hearing deficits. Individuals with static encephalopathy are, as a group, among the most handicapped in our society. In the United States, as many as 500,000 children may be affected and, thus, represent an important public health responsibility.

The classification of static encephalopathy has changed little from Freud's description of a century ago and represents the involvement, individually or in combination, of cerebral hemispheres, leading to upper motor neuron signs including spasticity; of basal ganglia, leading to extrapyramidal signs; and of the cerebellum, leading to hypotonia and ataxia. The resulting classification includes spastic forms (hemiplegia, tetraplegia, or diplegia); extrapyramidal forms (choreoathetosis or dystonia); and a cerebellar form (ataxia). Mixed forms also have been described. The comparative frequency of each form of static encephalopathy as determined from Swedish and American studies is shown in Table 204–1. The preponderance of spastic forms is evident. In general, males outnumber females at a ratio of 1.2:1. The increasing prominence of diplegic forms (symmetric lower extremity involvement greater than that in the upper extremities) is the result of increased survival of low-birth-weight infants with predominantly periventricular lesions.

The incidence of static encephalopathy has changed substantially over the last 30 years (Table 204–2). The declining incidence seen in the 1960s was attributed to improved prenatal and perinatal care. In particular, better treatment of Rh-incompatibility states, with a resulting decrease in damage to the basal ganglia from kernicterus, has led to a reduction in the extrapyramidal form. The increasing incidence noted in the past 2 decades also is related to better perinatal care, especially of low-birth-weight infants. Thus, the changing incidence pattern is felt to reflect improved survival yielding an apparent increase in incidence.

■ RISK FACTORS

Risk factors for static encephalopathy vary with the period or timing of the insult. More than a century ago, Little described cerebral palsy (static encephalopathy) and related it causally to difficulties in the birth process. Data from several large population-based studies confirmed the subsequent notion, first advanced by Freud, that static encephalopathy in the vast majority of children *cannot* be attributed to birth asphyxia, and that "difficult birth in itself is merely a symptom of deeper effects that influenced the development of the fetus." In fact, no specific cause can be identified for more than 50% of infants in whom the condition develops. Congenital disorders appear to account for 30% to 40% of the total and infections of the central nervous system (CNS) account for another 5% to 10%. In addition, multiple births (*ie,* twins) represent an increased risk for static encephalopathy. Neonatal events previously associated with asphyxia are at least as likely to occur with congenital disease. These include meconium in the amniotic fluid, low 10-minute Apgar scores, neonatal seizures, apnea, newborn neurologic abnormalities, and slow head growth. Furthermore, epilepsy and mental retardation alone do not follow birth asphyxia. Prematurity, low birth weight, and placental dysfunction are increasingly important factors in the genesis of static encephalopathy. The infant with low Apgar scores from a late asphyxial event, who does not show signs of newborn encephalopathy, will not have cerebral palsy.

Spastic diplegia most commonly is the result of prematurity and postnatal complications of premature birth. When seen in the full-term infant, it usually is the result of a complicated pregnancy and delivery. Spastic diplegia is not seen in the term infant whose only insult at birth is late asphyxia. That is, antenatal risk factors must have been present.

During the past 3 decades, infant mortality rates have fallen dramatically in the developed countries of the world. This has been attributed to improved prenatal and perinatal care. The fact that these improvements have not had a favorable impact on the incidence of static encephalopathy provides further support for causative factors other than the birth process in this disorder. Extensive evaluation of electronic fetal monitoring revealed that this technique did not improve the outcome in terms of neurologic development in either term or preterm infants. In addition, birth asphyxia that is significant enough to produce brain injury also damages the kidneys, liver, lungs, and heart. Finally, infants with neurologic sequelae that are secondary to a significant perinatal asphyxial event always have signs of newborn encephalopathy. Those infants injured sometime during the prenatal period may have had time to recover before parturition and may not have perinatal encephalopathy. Thus, their static problems can be assigned clearly to insults occurring at a time other than birth.

Static encephalopathy may result from postnatal events such as infection, trauma, or cardiac disease as well, although only 10% to 20% of cases have this origin. Less commonly, systemic disease (hematologic, immunologic, or metabolic), neoplasm, vascular malformation, or demyelinating disease are responsible. Postnatal events leading to static encephalopathy may occur throughout infancy and childhood. Of these, infection and trauma are the most significant.

■ ASSOCIATED ABNORMALITIES

Associated neurologic abnormalities may be seen in patients with each form of static encephalopathy. These include mental retardation, visual deficits, and seizures. About 50% of affected children have strabismus. Among the spastic forms of the disorder, those children with tetraplegia generally have profound retardation, cortical blindness, and seizures. In addition, they are likely to have swallowing difficulties as a manifestation of pseudobulbar palsy and to be at greater risk for aspiration and its attendant problems. The hemiplegic and diplegic forms of static encephalopathy are accompanied by retardation and seizures in one third of affected children. A hemianopia (visual field deficit) may

TABLE 204-1. Comparative Percentage Distribution of Static Encephalopathy

Type	Swedish Series*	Boston Children's Hospital†
Hemiplegia	37	41
Tetraplegia	7	19
Diplegia	41	5
Ataxia	5	—
Dyskinesia	10	22
Mixed	—	13

*1979–1982.
†1959.

occur in one third of all patients with hemiplegia. Children with choreoathetosis may have normal intellect and rarely have seizures. Their severe motor disorder limits meaningful interaction, however.

■ DIFFERENTIAL DIAGNOSIS

Static encephalopathy must be distinguished from progressive disorders and from familial disorders of similar appearance. A progressive static encephalopathy is a contradiction and should prompt careful review of the diagnosis. As an acquired disorder, static encephalopathy does not exhibit a familial pattern. It often presents with hypotonia and must be distinguished from other causes of hypotonia. In patients with static encephalopathy, the degree of hypotonia exceeds the degree of weakness, and the deep tendon reflexes usually are brisk. Injury to the spinal cord may produce weakness and hypotonia initially. Spinal muscular atrophy or anterior horn cell disease (Werdnig-Hoffmann disease) is characterized by weakness, hypotonia, and areflexia. Disorders of peripheral nerve and muscle cause

TABLE 204-2. Comparative Incidence Pattern of Static Encephalopathy

Rochester, Minnesota		Sweden	
Period	Incidence*	Period	Incidence*
1950–1958	2.3	1959–1962	1.9
		1963–1966	1.7
		1967–1970	1.3
1968–1976	1.6	1971–1974	1.6
		1975–1978	2.0
		1979–1982	2.2
		1983–1986†	2.5

*Incidence per 1000 live births.
†Preliminary.

weakness and hypotonia that are proportional and, in the case of peripheral nerve disease, hyporeflexia also is present.

The spastic forms of static encephalopathy must be differentiated from other neurologic disorders that are associated with upper motor neuron signs, including intracranial mass lesions such as a neoplasm, brain abscess, or subdural fluid collection; hydrocephalus; cerebrovascular disease such as vasculitis or arteriovenous malformation; and disorders of white matter such as multiple sclerosis or the various types of leukodystrophy. The clinical presentation of these disorders should be readily distinguishable from that of static encephalopathy.

The extrapyramidal forms of static encephalopathy must be differentiated from other extrapyramidal disorders of childhood, including the different forms of dystonia, benign familial chorea, and Huntington's disease.

■ TREATMENT AND PROGNOSIS

Treatment goals for patients with static encephalopathy include optimizing the motor and intellectual capabilities of each child and providing for realistic social interaction. Motor dysfunction requires an individualized physical and occupational therapy program and an appropriate educational curriculum. Physical therapy is essential to minimize contractures and orthopedic deformities from muscle imbalance. In some instances, surgical intervention may be required; in others, orthotic devices may be sufficient to treat these problems.

Regular reassessment is essential for the child with static encephalopathy to evaluate the status of the therapeutic and educational regimen and provide for appropriate modifications. In some instances, deterioration or apparent deterioration will occur and must be assessed carefully. Possible explanations for apparent deterioration are inaccurate initial assessment; inappropriate expectations of parents and therapists; an inadequate or inappropriate treatment program; depression; intoxication with anticonvulsant medications; medical-surgical problems such as excessive weight gain, dislocated hips, or fixed joint deformities; or unrecognized, slowly progressive disorders such as muscular dystrophy, spinal muscular atrophy, leukodystrophy, neuronal storage disease, or a neoplasm. The possible role of depression deserves emphasis. Children with static encephalopathy can be identified readily by their motor dysfunction. By preschool age, these children are capable of recognizing the fact that they are different, and appropriate attention must be given to their mental health as well.

The prognosis for a child with static encephalopathy depends on a number of factors, including the extent of the motor dysfunction, the extent of associated abnormalities, and the availability of appropriate educational and therapeutic programs. A child with spastic tetraplegia is least likely to demonstrate significant progress, whereas a child with mild spastic hemiplegia or diplegia has a very favorable prognosis. In either case, the role of the family and society will be a major determinant.

(Abridged from Alan K. Percy, Static Encephalopathy (Cerebral Palsy), in Oski, DeAngelis, Feigin, McMillan, Warshaw: *Principles and Practice of Pediatrics, Second Edition*, J.B. Lippincott, 1994.)

Oski's Essential Pediatrics,
edited by Kevin B. Johnson and Frank A. Oski.
Lippincott–Raven Publishers,
Philadelphia © 1997

205

Benign Intracranial Hypertension

Benign intracranial hypertension is a syndrome in which there is increased intracranial pressure in patients who have no history of an acute insult to the nervous system such as hypoxic ischemic disease, no acute encephalopathy such as Reye's syndrome, no focal or lateralizing neurologic signs, no evidence of intracranial tumor or obstruction to cerebrospinal fluid (CSF) flow, and normal results of CSF analyses except for increased pressure. This syndrome has occurred in children of all ages. There is no sex predilection as there is in adults, in whom there is a significant preponderance of females. The syndrome has been recognized for more than 80 years. Most of the earlier reported cases were associated with otitis media, mastoiditis, and lateral sinus thrombosis. The condition then was described as otitic hydrocephalus. Complications of otitis media have become less frequent precipitating factors, presumably related to the more aggressive use of antibiotics in the treatment of middle ear infections. A variety of conditions have been associated with this syndrome (Table 205–1). The most common cause now is "catch-up growth," which is confined to pediatric patients in some series. This may be seen in patients with a number of conditions, such as cystic fibrosis and nutritional deprivation syndromes, and after the correction of underlying chronic conditions such as patent ductus arteriosus and complications of prematurity. Rarely, a familial form of the syndrome has been reported.

■ PATHOGENESIS

The exact pathogenesis of increased intracranial pressure is not known. Different mechanisms may be operative in the various causes. Obstruction of the dural venous sinus system by thromboses resulting in increased intracranial venous pressure may cause decreased CSF absorption and intracranial hypertension. Alternatively, the increase in intracranial venous pressure may be transmitted directly to the CSF compartment. In other situations, the mechanism is less clear. Additional possibilities include an increased rate of CSF formation, a rise in brain volume secondary to an increase in interstitial fluid volume or cerebral blood volume, or a decreased rate of CSF absorption by arachnoid villi. Increased CSF production in the absence of a choroid plexus papilloma is highly unlikely. Studies using positron emission tomography have demonstrated that the intracerebral blood volume does not increase sufficiently to account for the rise in intracranial pressure. In addition, no evidence exists to support the presence of either vasogenic or cytotoxic brain edema to account for an increase in brain volume, which could produce intracranial hypertension. The most attractive hypothesis is that of altered absorption of CSF. Supporting evidence for this hypothesis has been derived from CSF perfusion studies in patients with benign intracranial hypertension, which have demonstrated reduced conductance to CSF outflow. Studies of the transport of intrathe-cal iodine 131 human serum albumin have revealed decreased plasma absorption of intrathecally injected isotope and abnormal transport of the material within the CSF pathways, thus indicating stasis and decreased absorption.

■ SYMPTOMS AND SIGNS

The onset of symptoms in patients with benign intracranial hypertension may be insidious or abrupt. The most common complaint is headache. Nausea, vomiting, and visual disturbances also are noted frequently. The visual complaints have included double vision, blurred vision, soreness of the eyes, and transient obscurations. Occasional complaints have included dizziness, vertiginous sensations, tinnitus, neck pain, paresthesias, radicular pain, and facial pain. The level of consciousness is relatively unimpaired.

The neurologic examination reveals no focal deficits. Occasionally, minor tremors and alterations in tone and reflexes have been noted. Abnormalities have been related primarily to the eyes and visual system. Papilledema has been noted in the vast majority of cases. Young infants whose fontanelles and cranial sutures are open may not have disc edema. Occasional cases have been reported in adults without papilledema, but they have met the diagnostic criteria and had documented increased intracranial pressure by lumbar puncture. The papilledema almost always is bilateral. Sometimes, unilateral or asymmetric involvement has been reported. In children old enough to cooperate for examination, visual field defects may be noted. The most common finding is an enlarged blind spot. Other findings include generally constricted visual fields, altitudinal defects, and nasal defects, often in the inferior quadrant. Decreased visual acuity is a late finding.

■ DIAGNOSIS

The diagnosis of benign intracranial hypertension has been facilitated by the development of noninvasive neuroimaging techniques, mainly computed tomography (CT) and magnetic resonance imaging (MRI). The diagnosis is one of exclusion. Clinically, the patient has a relatively normal neurologic examination, normal spinal fluid except for increased intracranial pressure, and an imaging procedure (CT or MRI) that shows no evidence of a mass lesion or obstruction to CSF flow. The majority of patients have one of the underlying conditions listed in Table 205–1. In some patients, however, no precipitating event can be identified. If all the diagnostic criteria are met, an overlooked cause of intracranial hypertension is unlikely. Before today's sophisticated imaging techniques were available, a midline neoplasm occasionally would go undiagnosed at the time of the initial evaluation. Other conditions that may be difficult to diagnose and may mimic benign intracranial hypertension include carcinomatous meningitis, fungal meningitis, and diffuse gliomatosis cerebri.

■ TREATMENT

Approaches to lowering intracranial pressure are applicable to all patients. In those children in whom a specific cause is identified (*eg,* iron deficiency anemia), treatment of the underlying disorder may result in resolution of the intracranial hypertension. Similarly, discontinuation of an antibiotic that is thought to precipitate the syndrome often will result in improvement. In those patients in whom no precipitating event or other identifying condition can be treated, symptomatic therapy is instituted. No reliable data are available regarding the effectiveness of any proposed method of therapy; in about 25% of patients, the problem resolves after the initial diagnostic lumbar puncture is performed.

Suggested treatment includes performing a lumbar puncture after obtaining a normal neuroimaging study. The lumbar puncture confirms the diagnosis of benign intracranial hypertension and is the first therapeutic intervention. Many patients experience relief of symptoms after the removal of CSF. A second lumbar puncture should be done several days later, even in an asymptomatic patient, to measure the CSF pressure again. If the pressure remains elevated after several additional examinations, pharmacologic intervention is indicated. Treatment with acetazolamide may help to decrease CSF formation and, thus, lower intracranial pressure. Raising the serum osmolality has been shown to decrease CSF production, and this may be the mechanism whereby these agents reduce increased intracranial pressure when they are administered on a long-term basis. If this approach does not result in resolution of the increased intracranial pressure, a course of steroids can be attempted. In children in whom the pressure remains elevated despite pharmacologic therapy, surgical intervention should be considered. CSF diversion procedures, optic nerve sheath decompression, and thecoperitoneal shunts have been used effectively.

The resolution of symptoms after the initiation of therapy does not necessarily indicate that the pressure has been relieved. Papilledema may take weeks to months to resolve and, therefore, is not a good parameter by which to judge the immediate effectiveness of therapy. Direct measurement of CSF pressure is necessary to monitor treatment. The goal of therapy is to relieve symptoms and avoid permanent visual disabilities. Therefore, whenever possible, visual fields and the blind spot should be assessed in patients who do not respond promptly to treatment. Dete-

---

TABLE 205-1. Causes of Benign Intracranial Hypertension

CIRCULATORY-HEMATOLOGIC	INFECTION
Gastrointestinal hemorrhage	Infectious mononucleosis
Polycythemia	Mastoiditis
Iron deficiency anemia	Lyme disease
Hemophilia	Postinfectious states
Dural sinus thrombosis	**NEUROLOGIC CONDITIONS**
Hypercoagulable state	Guillain-Barré syndrome
Pernicious anemia	Recurrent polyneuritis
Obstruction of superior vena cava	Head trauma
Sickle cell anemia	**SYSTEMIC CONDITIONS**
Cryofibrinogenemia	Lupus erythematosus
DRUGS	Sarcoidosis
Tetracycline	Paget's disease
Nalidixic acid	Chronic hypoxia
Steroid administration	Pulmonary hypoventilation
Steroid withdrawal	Serum sickness
Progestational agents	Cryoglobulinemia
Indomethacin	Catch-up growth
Sulfamethoxazole	Nephrotic syndrome
Oral contraceptives	Allergies
Lithium carbonate	Connective tissue syndromes
Thyroid hormone	Wiskott-Aldrich syndrome
Penicillin	Galactosemia
Minocycline	
Gentamicin	
ENDOCRINE	
Hyperparathyroidism	
Hypoparathyroidism	
Adrenal insufficiency	
Hyperadrenalism	
Menarche	
Obesity	
Menstrual abnormalities	
Pregnancy	
Hyperthyroidism	

rioration in the results of this examination is an indication for more aggressive therapy.

The main concern during treatment is the persistence of visual disabilities. The clinical findings early in the course of the disease do not differentiate those patients who are likely to have sequelae. Persistent impaired visual acuity is not related to the presence of transient visual obscurations or the degree of papilledema. Fortunately, only a minority of patients have persistent visual defects or diminished acuity. Loss of visual acuity and visual fields may be reversed with rapid, vigorous therapy, with good functional recovery. Therefore, close observation is extremely important.

A rare complication of benign intracranial hypertension is the development of the empty-sella syndrome. This is thought to occur in patients with congenital absence of the diaphragmatic sella. Continued pressure on the pituitary is thought to compress the gland and result in the eventual appearance of the sella being empty. There usually are no associated endocrine symptoms, but growth hormone deficiency may occur.

Recurrent episodes of benign intracranial hypertension have been noted. This is unusual and thought to occur in about 10% of all patients.

The papilledema usually resolves within 3 to 6 months. Symptoms in patients who have been treated effectively usually disappear before this time. Rarely, papilledema may persist for more than 12 months. Some patients have spontaneous resolution of the syndrome, and, in many others, the increased intracranial pressure remits as soon as any type of therapy is initiated.

(Abridged from Marvin A. Fishman, Benign Intracranial Hypertension, in Oski, DeAngelis, Feigin, McMillan, Warshaw: *Principles and Practice of Pediatrics, Second Edition*, J.B. Lippincott, 1994.)

Oski's Essential Pediatrics, edited by Kevin B. Johnson and Frank A. Oski. Lippincott–Raven Publishers, Philadelphia © 1997

206

Cerebrovascular Disease in Childhood

Cerebrovascular disease can be divided broadly into two primary pathophysiologic processes: occlusion and hemorrhage. In occlusive vascular disease , blood vessels are occluded by the formation of clot (thrombosis) or the migration of clotted material by way of other vessels from the heart, vessels, or other organs (embolism). In hemorrhagic vascular disease , there is rupture of blood vessels with bleeding into cerebral parenchyma and subarachnoid, subdural, and epidural spaces.

Both these broad processes have in common reduced blood flow to brain tissue and consequent ischemia of neural tissue. If the ischemia is severe enough, there is death of nerve cells and surrounding tissue, which is defined more properly as infarction or stroke. In addition, hemorrhage may cause pressure on parenchyma and consequent ischemia and infarction by further obstruction to blood flow locally and generally by the effects of pressure alone.

■ OCCLUSIVE CEREBROVASCULAR DISEASE

More than three fourths of all thrombotic events occur in the carotid artery or branches of the middle cerebral artery. A specific cause can be identified in about 50% to 60% of patients, and an arterial occlusion without a specific cause can be identified in a further 20% of patients. The cause of the event should be sought aggressively because treatment of the primary disorder may prevent recurrent episodes of stroke (Table 206–1).

Arteritis

The term *arteritis* refers to inflammatory changes in vessel walls. The arteritides affect vessels of many different sizes, with certain disorders typically affecting smaller vessels. The arteritides usually are associated with systemic symptoms such as fever, myalgia, arthralgia, and weight loss. Multiple organ systems, particularly the kidneys and lungs, often are involved. Significant laboratory findings include an elevated sedimentation rate, decreased serum complement levels, and increased antinuclear antibody titers. If the arteritis is limited to the central nervous system (CNS), however, these laboratory abnormalities may be absent. Treatment usually is with immunosuppressive agents such as corticosteroids.

Systemic lupus erythematosus (SLE) is one of the most common collagen vascular diseases in childhood. Between 13% and 30% of children with SLE have neurologic complications from their disease. In some series, cerebrovascular occlusive disease is reported to develop in 3% of children with SLE, with most of them having significant multisystem disease at the onset of complications.

Spasm or thrombosis of arteries at the base of the brain occurs in association with severe meningitic infections. This type of occlusive vascular disease is more common with chronic fungal and tuberculous meningitides but also can be seen with acute bacterial meningitis in children, particularly if treatment is delayed. The chances of a full recovery are poor. Major strokes rarely occur when bacterial meningitis is treated rapidly.

Trauma

Trauma probably is the single most common cause of occlusion of the extracranial portions of the carotid system in children. The pathophysiology associated with trauma initially is an intimal tear, then the formation of a dissecting aneurysm of the involved vessel, and subsequent occlusion of the vessel by thrombosis. The thrombus may extend distally, or an embolus can arise from the thrombus and occlude more distal vessels. The putative pathophysiology agrees well with the clinical syndromes seen with this type of injury. The neurologic deficit may be acute or associated with a delay in the onset of symptoms and a subsequent progressive stuttering course. Trauma may occur to the carotid artery externally in the neck or internally as a result of intraoral injury, such as results from a fall onto a pencil or stick. Vertebral artery dissections associated with twisting of the neck, such as can occur in chiropractic manipulations, have been described in adults and children.

Sickle-Cell Disease

Sickle-cell disease is a recessively inherited hemoglobinopathy in which hemoglobin S (HbS) comprises more

TABLE 206-1. Occlusive Cerebrovascular Diseases in Children and Adolescents

THROMBOSIS
Abnormalities of the arterial wall
  Atherosclerosis
    Lipid abnormalities
    Down's syndrome
    Progeria
  Arteritis
    Systemic lupus erythematosus
    Polyarteritis nodosa
    Takayasu disease
    Henoch-Schönlein purpura
    Radiation
    Infection
      Meningitis
      Mastoiditis
      Other
  Trauma
    External and internal trauma
    Dissection
  Congenital and hereditary disorders
    Kinking and tortuosity of vessels
    Fibromuscular dysplasia
    Neuroectodermal disorders
      Sturge-Weber syndrome
      Neurofibromatosis 1
      Tuberous sclerosis
    Sickle cell disease
    Metabolic disorders
      Homocystinuria
      MELAS syndrome (mitochondrial encephalomyopathy and stroke)
      Menke's disease
      Fabry's disease
      Other
  Moyamoya syndrome
  Moyamoya disease
  Migraine
Acute infantile hemiplegia
Hypercoagulable states
  Dehydration
  Hemolytic-uremic syndrome
  Nephrotic syndrome
  Cryoglobulinemia
  Polycythemia
  Leukemia and its treatment
  Thrombocytosis
  Antithrombin III deficiency
  Protein C deficiency
  Protein S deficiency

EMBOLISM
Cardiac disease
  Cyanotic heart disease
  Valvular disease
  Bacterial endocarditis
  Arrhythmias
  Tumor

PERIPHERAL THROMBOSIS AND EMBOLISM

than 50% of the hemoglobin in red cells. It is the most common hemoglobinopathy in the United States, and about 8% of the black population has the trait. The prevalence of stroke in individuals with sickle-cell disease ranges from 5% to 17% in different series. Most of these patients have the complications before they reach 15 years of age. Ischemic strokes tend to occur in younger individuals, whereas intracranial hemorrhage typically occurs in young adults.

HbS forms intracellular polymers, especially under conditions of low oxygen tension, and leads to a rigid, deformed red blood cell surface or membrane (the sickle cell). Initially, the sickling is reversible on reoxygenation, but with repeated episodes, the membrane is damaged and remains sickled. The abnormal shape of the red cell may impede movement though the microvasculature and cause regional hypoperfusion. Although this mechanism long has been presumed to be the cause of stroke, radiologic and pathologic studies have provided evidence that the mechanism actually is a large-vessel occlusive vasculopathy. The vessels primarily involved include the supraclinoid internal carotid artery and the proximal areas of the middle and anterior cerebral arteries. The stenosis or occlusion of large intracranial vessels at the base of the skull can lead to the angiographic appearance of moyamoya syndrome, and emboli from proximal vessels may cause distal hypoxia and further exacerbation of sickling and obstruction. The clinical features are similar to those that accompany other cerebrovascular events, but focal or generalized seizures commonly herald the onset of the stroke. The prognosis of a patient with an acute stroke in association with sickle-cell disease is poor. About 75% have permanent deficits, and seizures develop in 50% to 60%. Treatment involves providing adequate oxygenation and hydration, and instituting hypertransfusion therapy to maintain HbS levels less than 20%. The use of anticoagulation may be indicated in patients who have thrombotic events. Recurrent events are common, but a study showing the predictive value of transcranial ultrasonography in individuals with sickle-cell disease may enable hypertransfusion therapy to be used to prevent subsequent strokes in individuals who are at high risk.

Migraine

Migraine headaches occur in 10% to 25% of the population, with a significant percentage beginning in childhood or young adulthood. Complicated migraine (ie, migraine associated with neurologic deficits such as hemiplegia) has been estimated to occur in 1% of the population. Most migraine-related neurologic events are brief, last less than 1 hour, and are associated with a full recovery. Events of longer duration and permanent deficits are seen occasionally, however. Based on a review of 34 years of the literature, Featherstone defined individuals who are at risk of having a stroke associated with migraine as being more commonly female, with a history of classic or complicated migraine, and usually less than 40 years of age. Only about 15% of patients who have a stroke in connection with migraine are children. The prognosis for migraine-related stroke may be slightly better than for stroke of other causes. The diagnosis is based on other causes of stroke being excluded, the event occurring during a migraine attack, and the patient having a definite history consistent with migraine. Treatment is supportive, and vasodilators or anticoagulation given at the onset of a neurologic abnormality has not been shown to be of definite benefit. Prophylactic treatment of migraine reduces the frequency and severity of headache, and may decrease the risk of stroke.

TABLE 206-2. Causes of Hemorrhagic Vascular Disease

Abnormalities of the clotting mechanism
    Decreased clotting factors
    Thrombocytopenia
    Disseminated intravascular coagulation
Vascular malformation
    Arteriovenous malformation
    Cerebral aneurysm
        Congenital
        Acquired: mycotic, traumatic, embolic
Hypertensive cerebrovascular disease
Intracranial neoplasm
Trauma

■ INTRACRANIAL HEMORRHAGE

Abnormalities of the Clotting Mechanism

Deficiency of clotting factors, such as in hemophilia (Factor VIII deficiency), Factor IX deficiency (Christmas disease), von Willebrand's disease, thrombocytopenia (particularly idiopathic thrombocytopenic purpura), and disseminated intravascular coagulation, can be associated with spontaneous or post-traumatic intracerebral hemorrhage.

The presenting symptoms and signs of intracranial hemorrhage are seizures, focal neurologic signs, or evidence of increased intracranial pressure The underlying disease responsible for abnormalities in the clotting mechanism need to be corrected to ensure recovery and prevent recurrence. Occasionally, the clot may need to be evacuated surgically if control of the raised intracranial pressure cannot be achieved medically.

Vascular Malformations

Congenital abnormalities of cerebral blood vessels are the most common cause of intracranial bleeding (Table 206–2). These malformations include arteriovenous malformations (AVMs), angiomas, and aneurysms.

AVM is the most common abnormality and consists pathologically of normal and abnormal veins and arteries. These usually are found in the distribution of the internal carotid and middle cerebral arteries but also occur in the posterior circulation and posterior fossa. They may present clinically as an intracranial mass, a focal or generalized seizure disorder, or an acute hemorrhage. Presentation as a mass lesion is unusual, but symptoms of raised intracranial pressure and slowly progressive neurologic symptoms or signs typically occur. Between 50% and 70% of children with AVMs have intracranial hemorrhage, and about 25% to 40% have seizures. Of those who do have hemorrhage, the great majority have blood within the subarachnoid space. Some have blood within the brain substance, which produces acute focal signs.

At the time of acute rupture, blood mixed in the cerebrospinal fluid (CSF) may result in nuchal rigidity, severe headache, nausea, and vomiting. Excessive numbers of red blood cells or xanthochromia in the CSF may raise suspicion that a hemorrhage has occurred. Bruits can be heard over the cranial vault in about 25% of patients with symptomatic AVMs. The larger the malformation, the more likely it is that a bruit will be heard. Most AVMs are large enough to be iden-

tified by the radiographic scanning techniques now in use, but improvements in imaging techniques may improve diagnosis further. Occasionally, a small malformation will not be picked up by scanning if there is no surrounding hemorrhage or if the AVM is obliterated by the blood. If an AVM is suspected, arteriography is the most useful diagnostic procedure available. It also is needed to determine which vessels feed and drain the malformation, and to decide whether the lesion can be treated surgically. If the lesion is too extensive to be operated on, it may be possible to reduce its size by introducing artificial emboli to obstruct the arteries that feed it.

Telangiectasias are the second most common vascular malformation in children. They essentially are capillary angiomas. The vessels that make up the lesion look like widely dilated capillaries. These lesions occur anywhere in the brain but are seen frequently in the posterior fossa and in the bases pontis. Such malformations often are asymptomatic throughout life and can be inherited (Osler-Weber-Rendu disease). When they produce symptoms, it is almost always the result of intracerebral hemorrhage. Occasionally, these hemorrhages are large enough to produce elevated intracranial pressure, either by acting as a mass or by obstructing the flow of CSF and producing hydrocephalus. The most common presentation, however, is the acute onset of focal symptoms and signs without elevated intracranial pressure. The hemorrhage often can be seen on computed tomography (CT) scan. Usually, these hemorrhages are not large enough to require surgical evacuation. In many instances, the associated malformation is obliterated by the bleeding.

Other Causes of Intracranial Hemorrhage

A cerebral hemorrhage can be a manifestation of both leukemia and the drugs used to treat it.

Hypertension is a much less frequent cause of hemorrhage in children than in adults, but such catastrophes can occur because of elevated blood pressure levels in conjunction with renal, cardiovascular, or endocrine disorders.

Trauma certainly is the most common cause of subarachnoid hemorrhage in infants and young children, and is associated with accidental and nonaccidental injury.

Bleeding into a preexisting tumor may be responsible for an intracerebral accumulation of blood. An area of marked surrounding cerebral edema may indicate this diagnosis.

(Abridged from Andrew J. Kornberg and Arthur L. Prensky, Cerebrovascular Disease in Childhood, in Oski, DeAngelis, Feigin, McMillan, Warshaw: *Principles and Practice of Pediatrics, Second Edition*, J.B. Lippincott, 1994.)

Oski's Essential Pediatrics,
edited by Kevin B. Johnson and Frank A. Oski.
Lippincott–Raven Publishers,
Philadelphia © 1997

207

Acute Head Trauma

Pediatric head injuries are a very important cause of childhood morbidity and mortality. Each year in the United States, nearly 5 million children sustain a head injury; of these, about 200,000 are hospitalized. Such injuries, which are twice as frequent in boys as in girls, have many different causes: motor vehicle accidents, falls, bicycling and other recreational activities, competitive sports, and assaults (including child abuse). In 1986 in the United States, about 150,000 children suffered a traumatic brain injury. About 80% of these injuries were mild, 15% were moderate to severe, and 5% were fatal. Seven thousand of the children died from the direct effects of the trauma or from secondary complications or associated injuries, accounting for 30% of all childhood deaths from trauma that year. Each year in this country, almost 30,000 individuals 19 years of age and younger are left with permanent disabilities from moderate or severe head trauma, including posttraumatic epilepsy (PTE), motor handicaps, cognitive impairment, learning difficulties, and behavioral and emotional problems.

This chapter presents an approach to the diagnosis and treatment of acute head injuries in children, with consideration given to the clinical syndromes that are encountered most frequently. In addition, the prognosis of acute brain injuries in children is discussed. The scalp, skull, and brain all can suffer injury as a result of head trauma. Figure 207–1 depicts the brain, its surrounding structures, and the main associated pathologies that can complicate head trauma. The scalp, which is highly vascular, lies outermost, bounded on its inner surface by the galea aponeurotica, a tendinous sheath connecting the frontalis and occipitalis muscles. Beneath the galea is the subgaleal compartment. Immediately below this lies the skull, the outermost portion of which is the pericranium, or external periosteum. The outer and inner tables of the skull are separated by the diploic space, which is traversed by small veins. The dura, lying immediately below the inner table of the skull, contains few blood vessels (in contrast to the highly vascular leptomeninges, which are closely approximated to the brain). Small-caliber veins from the leptomeninges cross the subdural space to drain into dural sinuses. The brain is bathed in and protected by cerebrospinal fluid (CSF), which is located in the cerebral subarachnoid spaces, cisterns at the base of the brain, ventricular cavities, interconnecting channels, and foramina.

Intracranial pressure (ICP) is the sum total of pressures exerted by intracranial structures: brain tissue, the intracranial vascular tree, and the CSF. The skull of the newborn and infant is not a rigid box; rather, it consists of membranous bones, with fontanelles and unfused bony structures providing outlets for the increases in ICP that are seen so commonly in head-injured children. In older children, in whom the cranial sutures have fused, however, the foramen magnum provides the only major outlet through which increases in ICP can be accommodated.

■ MANAGEMENT

Patient History

It is essential that the specific circumstances of an episode of head trauma be determined and that predisposing factors be identified. Such information should be sought directly from the injured child whenever possible, and also from any observers. Attention should be paid to memory loss, perseverative questioning (persisting repetition of a question with no memory of having asked it before), confusion, visual disturbance, and symptoms of increased ICP such as irritability, altered consciousness, repeated vomiting, and severe headache.

General Physical Examination

The patient's vital signs demand immediate attention and, at times, emergency intervention. Alterations may indicate shock (decreased blood pressure, increased pulse rate) or intracranial hypertension (increased blood pressure, decreased or increased pulse rate, slowed or irregular respirations). Systemic hypotension in the head-injured child usually is caused by an injury outside the central nervous system (CNS), as with intra-abdominal bleeding (eg, from a ruptured spleen) or bleeding into soft tissues (eg, associated with a long-bone fracture or a major scalp laceration). Occasionally, however, systemic hypotension can be of intracranial origin (eg, from an epidural hematoma).

The child's entire body should be checked for signs of trauma. The neck should be examined with particular care because of possible injury that often is unsuspected. Neck injury is suggested by cervical abrasions, cervical spine tenderness, or meningism. The latter also can result from subarachnoid bleeding or cerebellar tonsillar herniation. Initial assessment may be limited because of immobilization of the neck by a collar or sandbags. The scalp should be inspected and all scalp lacerations examined. The skull should be palpated for areas of tenderness or loss of anatomic integrity. Tension of the anterior fontanelle should be assessed in the young child. Periorbital hemorrhage ("raccoon eyes" sign), ecchymosis behind the ear (Battle's sign) or behind the eardrum (hemotympanum), or bleeding from the ears or nose should be noted. These signs, along with CSF otorrhea or rhinorrhea, are indications of basal skull fracture.

Neurologic Examination

The neurologic examination should assess the child's alertness, orientation, and memory. The presence and extent of retrograde and anterograde (posttraumatic) amnesia should be determined. A child's repeated asking of the same question is reflective of a posttraumatic memory disturbance of anterograde type. The level of consciousness may range widely. The Glasgow Coma Scale (GCS; Table 207–1), with scores ranging from 3 (worst) to 15 (best), provides a useful and reproducible scoring system for quantifying the level of consciousness. Although most studies have reported a low GCS score to correlate with severe neurologic morbidity and substantial mor-

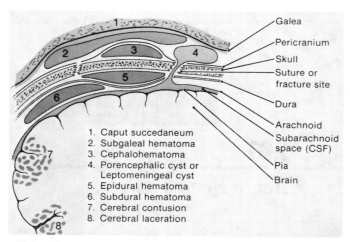

Figure 207-1. The brain, surrounding structures, and major types of pathology following acute head injury. (Rosman NP, Herskowitz J, Carter AP, et al. Acute head trauma in infancy and childhood. *Pediatr Clin North Am.* 1979;26:708.)

Galea
Pericranium
Skull
Suture or fracture site
Dura
Arachnoid
Subarachnoid space (CSF)
Pia
Brain

1. Caput succedaneum
2. Subgaleal hematoma
3. Cephalohematoma
4. Porencephalic cyst or Leptomeningeal cyst
5. Epidural hematoma
6. Subdural hematoma
7. Cerebral contusion
8. Cerebral laceration

TABLE 207-1. Glasgow Coma Scale

Response	Score
BEST MOTOR RESPONSE	
Obeys	6
Localizes pain	5
Withdraws	4
Flexion to pain	3
Extension to pain	2
Nil	1
BEST VERBAL RESPONSE	
Oriented	5
Confused conversation	4
Inappropriate words	3
Incomprehensible sounds	2
Nil	1
EYE OPENING	
Spontaneously	4
To speech	3
To pain	2
Nil	1

Rosman NP, Oppenheimer EY, O'Connor JF. Emergency management of pediatric head injuries. Emerg Med Clin North Am. 1983;1:144.

tality, it has been shown that many children with a GCS score of 3 to 5 can do surprisingly well if their head injury has not been complicated by a hypoxic-ischemic insult.

The neuro-ophthalmologic evaluation should include pupil size and reactivity. Small pupils are seen with diencephalic and pontine injuries; a unilateral dilated pupil suggests temporal lobe herniation on the same side. The fundi should be examined carefully, and evidence of retinal and preretinal (subhyaloid) hemorrhages and papilledema should be sought. Abnormalities of ocular gaze and position should be observed. If there is no neck injury, the oculocephalic ("doll's head") maneuver can be used to assess any apparent limitation of eye movements. With the child supine, the head is rotated to one side and then to the other. When the head is moved to the left, the eyes should deviate to the right (and vice versa) if brain stem pathways controlling eye movements are functioning normally. Lateral gaze also can be tested in the comatose patient by means of caloric stimulation. In this case, the child's head is elevated 30 degrees above the horizontal and one external auditory canal is irrigated with about 5 mL of ice water. If brain stem function is normal, the eyes should turn toward the ear being irrigated. It is important to be certain that the auditory canal is clear and the eardrum is intact before performing this test.

The extent to which the motor system can be examined depends on the child's alertness. Decorticate, decerebrate, and other abnormal posturing should be noted. Also, the distribution (hemiparetic or paraparetic) of any muscular flaccidity or spasticity should be observed. In the responsive child, more detailed motor, sensory, and coordinative testing is possible. Testing for abnormal reflexes (such as palmar grasp, suck, or rooting reflexes), eliciting deep tendon reflexes, and checking for plantar responses complete this portion of the examination.

Investigative Studies

Plain Radiographs

The need for radiologic examination of the child with a head injury is dictated by the severity of the head trauma, as reflected by the patient's state of consciousness and the presence or absence of focal neurologic signs. Severe head injury, with significant loss of consciousness and focal neurologic signs (GCS score 3 to 8), requires plain radiographs and further radiologic workup. The initial examination in a child with severe head trauma should include anteroposterior and lateral views of the cervical spine, as well as anteroposterior, inclined anteroposterior (Towne projection), and lateral views of the skull; the last is taken with a horizontal beam (cross table) to demonstrate any air–fluid levels in the cranial cavity or paranasal sinuses indicative of compound or basal fracture. With extensive head or facial trauma, radiographs should include a Waters projection of the facial bones and films of the orbits.

In a patient with moderate head trauma with localizing neurologic signs or a history of loss of consciousness (GCS score 9 to 12), routine skull radiographs alone usually suffice. If there is no history of neck injury, cervical spine films probably are unnecessary. In a child with mild head trauma without focal neurologic signs or loss of consciousness (GCS score 13 to 15), skull and spine films usually are not needed. If a depressed skull fracture is suspected, tangential views of the area should be obtained in addition to standard views.

Cranial Computed Tomography

In patients with severe head trauma or those with localizing neurologic signs regardless of the severity of the injury, the most helpful and least invasive imaging modality is the cranial computed tomography (CT) scan. Unilateral intracranial hemorrhage usually is readily evident on CT scan as a relatively dense mass in the immediate posttraumatic period, a time when the scan does not require the infusion of contrast medium. After several days, however, extravasated blood that is broken down incompletely may be of the same density as contiguous brain; thus, scans at that time should be done with and without contrast enhancement. In addition to disclosing blood within brain parenchyma (as in contusion) or outside the brain (as with subdural hematoma), cranial CT scanning can demonstrate brain edema, loss of brain tissue, hydrocephalus, midline displacements and other mass effects, and skull fractures. Some treatment centers have recommended that routine skull radiography be abandoned in favor of immediate cranial CT scanning with bone windows. Although it frequently is true that clinical decisions can be made on the basis of the findings on CT scanning alone, the scan may fail to demonstrate focal skull depressions, as well as stellate, facial, basal, and other fractures.

Ultrasonography

In the newborn or young infant with open fontanelles and sutures, real-time ultrasonography may be very helpful in demonstrating displacement or obstruction of the ventricular system and the presence of intraventricular, parenchymal, and subarachnoid blood. Thus, ultrasonography should be performed in all newborns who have suffered traumatic births, as well as in premature newborns (with or without a history of trauma), because the latter infants are at high risk for periventricular/intraventricular hemorrhage.

Magnetic Resonance Imaging

Magnetic resonance imaging (MRI), which provides a detailed demonstration of brain anatomy without exposing the patient to ionizing radiation, has become an increasingly valuable diagnostic tool. Advantages of MRI include safety (no known biologic hazards and no reported side effects), the ability to image in any plane, excellent depiction of normal and pathologic anatomy, the ability to identify vessels without contrast injections, and superiority to cranial CT in demonstrating the posterior fossa, where bone artifacts interfere with CT imaging. In cases of head trauma, however, MRI is of greatest assistance in evaluating injuries that are subacute or chronic, rather than ones that are acute.

Acute bleeding (ie, that occurring within the first 1 to 3 days after the injury), whether it is extra-axial (as with subdural and subarachnoid hemorrhage) or intra-axial (as with cerebral contusion), frequently is more difficult to recognize with MRI than with CT, because the deoxyhemoglobin in such lesions gives rise to a signal that is iso-intense with brain on T1-weighted images and of low or hypo-intensity on T2-weighted images. By contrast, edema surrounding areas of acute parenchymal hemorrhage is seen well with MRI, because T2-weighted images of edema have high signal intensity. Also, because of the ease with which sections can be obtained in multiple planes with MRI, and because no MRI signal is transmitted by bone, small collections of blood (eg, a thin convexity extra-axial hematoma) may be visualized more easily with MRI than with CT. It is because of this that MRI is more useful than CT in imaging the posterior fossa. MRI is especially useful for detecting lesions that are iso-dense on CT, such as subacute (3 to 14 days) and chronic (more than 14 days) extra-axial hematomas, which show high signal intensity on both T1- and T2-weighted images as a result of the formation of methemoglobin in subacute hematomas and increased protein content in chronic hematomas. Diffuse white matter shearing injuries are seen very well with MRI, because these lesions show increased signal intensity on T2-weighted images. A disadvantage of MRI compared to CT is the longer imaging time needed and its unsuitability for critically ill patients with life support systems that require continuous monitoring.

Lumbar Puncture

Lumbar puncture should not be performed in a child with a head injury unless complicating CNS infection is suspected. It usually is contraindicated in the presence of significantly elevated ICP and is absolutely contraindicated in the presence of an intracranial mass. Lumbar puncture may show evidence of CNS infection, recent or older subarachnoid bleeding, and elevated ICP.

Subdural Taps

Subdural taps may be indicated as a diagnostic measure, a therapeutic measure, or both. A maximum of 15 mL of fluid is removed from each subdural space, without aspiration; within a day or two, the taps can be repeated.

Other Studies

In moderately and severely injured children, and in those in whom the cause or circumstances of the injury are unknown, additional studies may be indicated. These include a complete blood count; determination of the serum amylase level; urinalysis; platelet and clotting studies; toxic screens on blood, urine, and gastric aspirate; and a skeletal survey for old and recent fractures.

■ TREATMENT

General Support

Treatment of the child with head injury is discussed in Chapter 20. In most children with severe head injuries

(GCS scores of 5 or less), the ICP should be monitored continuously (further discussion follows). If posttraumatic seizures occur, anticonvulsant drugs should be given, as described in the next section.

Posttraumatic Seizures

Early posttraumatic seizures (ie, those occurring within the first week after head injury) develop in about 5% of children who are hospitalized after sustaining head trauma. Of these children, about one in four has additional seizures after the first week.

The immediate treatment of posttraumatic seizures in children is essentially the same as the treatment of nontraumatic seizures. Phenytoin sodium (Dilantin) is the drug of choice because of its rapid entry into the brain and lack of prominent sedative effect. If seizure activity continues, intravenous diazepam (Valium) can be used. A benzodiazepine that is structurally similar to diazepam but has a much longer duration of action is lorazepam (Ativan). Phenobarbital is another drug that can be used.

In studies to date, the use of prophylactic anticonvulsant agents has not been shown to prevent the later development of epilepsy in the head-injured patient who has not had a seizure. A review of seven randomized, double-blind, controlled studies of head-injured adults and children given phenytoin, phenobarbital, or both to prevent posttraumatic seizures has shown phenytoin to reduce seizures in the first week after the head injury, but not beyond this point.

Raised Intracranial Pressure

ICP, the summation of pressures derived from structures within the cranium, is determined by pressures exerted by the brain, the cerebral blood vessels, and the CSF. ICP is elevated if it measures greater than 15 mm Hg in children, or greater than 7 mm Hg in newborns and infants. In patients with acute head trauma, causes of raised ICP include bleeding into the epidural, subdural, or subarachnoid spaces, or into the brain; brain hyperemia causing diffuse cerebral swelling (from days 1 to 3); brain edema accompanying brain contusion or hematoma (from days 2 to 10); acute hydrocephalus from subarachnoid bleeding; and pseudotumor cerebri.

The individual can adapt temporarily to increased ICP by displacing CSF through the foramen magnum into the distensible lumbar subarachnoid space; some adaptation also is accomplished by compression of the low-pressure intracranial venous system. The major adaptive mechanism, however, is an increase in the rate of CSF resorption, which can rise to as much as 2 mL/min, or six times its rate of formation. When these mechanisms no longer can compensate adequately for the rise in ICP, clinical signs of raised ICP become evident. The clinical symptoms and signs of acutely raised ICP are shown in Table 207–2. There is no single therapy for raised ICP. The therapeutic modalities employed include supportive measures and medical and surgical treatment.

Supportive Measures

When a patient's ICP is raised, respiratory and circulatory support must be provided. The head should be elevated to 30 degrees above the horizontal and stabilized in the midline. Fluids should be restricted to 1000 mL/m$_2$/day (two thirds of daily maintenance). Urine output should be maintained at 1 mL/kg/h. Elevated temperature should be reduced.

TABLE 207-2. Clinical Symptoms and Signs of Acutely Raised Intracranial Pressure

Infants	Children	Both
Full fontanelle	Headache	Altered mental state
Separated sutures	Papilledema	Vomiting
(Macrocrania)		Strabismus (CN VI, (III) palsies); "setting sun" sign
(Papilledemia)		Altered vital signs (increased blood pressure, decreased or increased pulse rate, decreased respirations)
		(Signs of herniation)

After Rosman NP, Oppenheimer EY, O'Connor JF. Emergency management of pediatric head injuries. Emerg Med Clin North Am. 1983;1:149.

Medical Management

A number of medical measures are useful in the treatment of patients with elevated ICP in association with acute head trauma. These treatments are outlined in Table 207–3.

Surgical Management

On occasion, elevations in ICP cannot be reversed adequately by specific interventions or by the empiric medical means just discussed. In such circumstances, surgical management may be indicated. Aspiration of the subdural spaces may be helpful therapeutically. When there is a marked elevation in ICP, with signs of impending or evolving brain herniation, a ventricular tap with slow withdrawal of CSF may be lifesaving. If the raised ICP continues in an unremitting fashion, decompression craniotomy may be needed.

Although no definite evidence exists that the control of ICP alters outcome in the head-injured child, anyone who has seen a substantial number of such patients can remember children in whom the control of intracranial hypertension was lifesaving.

CLINICAL SYNDROMES IN CHILDREN WITH ACUTE HEAD INJURIES

Skull Fractures

Six major kinds of skull fractures occur in childhood: (1) linear, (2) depressed, (3) compound, (4) basal, (5) diastatic, and (6) "growing." Linear fractures constitute about 75% of all skull fractures. They are especially frequent in children less than 2 years of age and occur most often in the temporoparietal region. Although these fractures need not be treated, they may overlie serious intracranial conditions, such as epidural hemorrhage, for which treatment is urgently required. Linear fracture in the infant or young child should raise the possibility of neglect or inflicted injury. Linear fractures heal within 1 to 2 months.

In depressed skull fractures, either continuity of the bony calvarium is disrupted or, particularly in the newborn, the skull simply may be indented, causing a so-called ping-pong ball or pond fracture, unaccompanied by a break in the cranial vault. Depressed skull fractures can be missed easily if tangential skull films, which usually demonstrate a double density (bone on bone) at the fracture site, are not obtained. Although depressed skull fractures are best seen with plain radiographs, many also can be seen on CT, particularly when a bone fragment is displaced. Depressed skull fractures are of particular concern because the underlying brain may be bruised or lacerated. Some clinicians advocate surgical elevation of depressed fractures if the depression is more than

TABLE 207-3. Medical Treatment of Acutely Elevated Intracranial Pressure in Patients With Head Trauma

Agent	Onset of Action	Peak Action	Advantages	Side Effects or Limitations
Passive hyperventilation	Seconds to minutes 20 mm Hg	2–30 min	Very prompt action	Effect may not be sustained; cerebral
Mannitol	5–30 min	15–90 min	Prompt action	Fluid/electrolyte imbalances; renal failure; intracranial bleeding; rebound
Glycerol	15–30 min	30 min (IV); 60–80 min (PO)	Prompt action PO or IV	Fluid/electrolyte imbalances; intracranial bleeding; possible rebound
Pentobarbital	1–2 min	Minutes	Prompt action; no rebound	Hypotension; renal failure; need for careful monitoring
Hypothermia	Approximately 1 h	2–3 h	No rebound	Cardiac arrhythmias; need for careful monitoring
Dexamethasone	18–24 h	12–24 h	No rebound	Slow onset of action; apparent lack of efficacy in head injury; gastrointestinal hemorrhage

IV, intravenously; PO, orally.

5 mm or if the depressed fragment extends below the inner table of the skull, but such elevation does not appear to reduce the risk of PTE, presumably because of brain injury sustained at impact.

Compound or open skull fractures, with laceration of the scalp extending to the fracture site, are of urgent concern because of the danger of complicating infection. Treatment involves meticulous debridement of the wound, search for a foreign body, copious irrigation with a sterile solution, and the administration of parenteral antibiotics and, if needed, tetanus prophylaxis. When a compound depressed fracture is found, the fracture should be elevated promptly to minimize the risk of complicating infection.

Only about 20% of basal skull fractures can be recognized on standard skull radiographs because of the anatomic complexity of the base of the skull. Although the addition of multiplanar tomography and thin-section cranial CT scanning appreciably increases the frequency with which such fractures can be seen on radiography, firm diagnosis frequently depends on the recognition of coexisting signs. These include hemorrhage in the nose, nasopharynx, middle ear, over the mastoid bone (Battle's sign), or about the eyes ("raccoon eyes" sign). Cranial nerve palsies sometimes occur, most frequently affecting cranial nerves I, VII, and VIII. CSF rhinorrhea and otorrhea, reflecting fractures of the cribriform plate or petrous temporal bone, respectively, are worrisome signs of basal skull fracture because of the risk of complicating bacterial meningitis, usually caused by *Streptococcus pneumoniae*. No clear evidence exists that prophylactic antibiotic therapy diminishes the frequency of this complication. Metrizamide CT cisternography can be very useful in identifying the location of a CSF leak complicating a fracture of the skull base. Hemorrhage into the cranial sinuses can cause an appearance on x-ray film simulating sinusitis. Skull films may show intracranial air (pneumocephalus), indicating continuity between a paranasal or mastoid sinus and the inside of the skull. Occipital fractures involving the foramen magnum may be accompanied by tachycardia, hypotension, and irregular respirations.

Diastatic skull fractures are traumatic separations of cranial bones at a suture site. They most frequently affect the lambdoid suture and are seen most often in the first 4 years of life. Diastatic fractures should be monitored closely in children younger than 3 years of age because they can become sites of "growing" fractures.

"Growing" skull fractures are caused by the herniation of tissue through torn dura and an associated fracture (linear or diastatic) into the overlying scalp. Such fractures occur most often in the parietal region (Figure 207–2). The herniating tissue either is solid brain or is cystic in nature, usually a porencephalic cyst (communicating with a lateral ventricle) or a leptomeningeal cyst. It is the pulsating, herniating tissue and associated scarring that prevent fusion of the fracture margins and cause the fracture to "grow." Although such fractures occasionally evolve immediately, they develop more often within weeks or months of the head injury. Only rarely do they occur in children older than 3 years of age.

Cerebral Concussion

Cerebral concussion is a clinical state characterized by a transient impairment of consciousness with loss of awareness and responsiveness immediately after a head injury and persisting for seconds, minutes, or, occasionally, hours. The force of injury needed to cause a concussion is somewhat less than that required to cause a skull fracture. The causative trauma usually is blunt. Concussion is much more likely to occur when the head moves freely after the impact

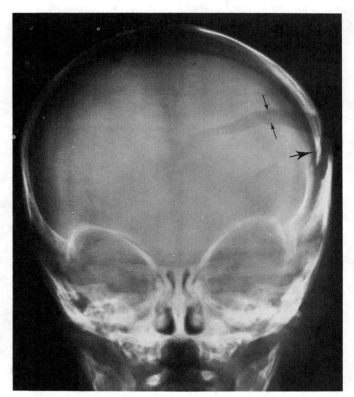

Figure 207-2. Posteroanterior radiograph of the skull shows a "growing" parietal skull fracture (*small arrows*) in a 9-week-old infant with an adjacent depressed parietal fracture; the depressed fragment (*large arrow*) lies beneath the squamous temporal bone.

(acceleration/deceleration) than when it is held firmly in place (compression). Concussive injuries cause an increase in ICP followed by a temporary shear strain on the upper brain stem, resulting in loss of consciousness. The concussed brain does not have any consistent morphologic abnormality. It seems likely that the clinical state is caused by suddenly increased and unmet energy demands of the brain.

Concussion is associated with three types of amnesia: a temporary retrograde amnesia that extends back to events predating the head injury by some years, a permanent retrograde amnesia that encompasses the few seconds or minutes that immediately preceded the injury, and a temporary posttraumatic (anterograde) amnesia characterized by an impaired ability to form new memories that usually lasts for some hours. In the absence of a history of definite loss of consciousness, demonstration of these types of amnesia is exceedingly useful in establishing the diagnosis of concussion. Also, the duration of the amnesia serves as a useful indicator of the severity of the head injury.

Children who have had a concussion should be observed closely for at least 24 hours; almost all recover uneventfully. A few, however, can be quite disabled by the development of a postconcussional syndrome, which is characterized by headache, dizziness, irritability, nervousness, inability to concentrate, and, occasionally, behavioral and cognitive impairment. The pathogenesis of the postconcussional syndrome is unsettled. Organic, environmental, and emotional factors have been cited, with evidence for an organic basis mounting.

A triad of symptoms that often follows minor head injury in young children includes lethargy, irritability, and vomiting, unaccompanied by loss of consciousness. These symptoms, which are attributed to torsion of the brain stem, usually subside within 48 to 72 hours.

Acute Epidural and Subdural Hematomas

The clinical points that aid in the diagnosis of and distinction between acute epidural and subdural hematoma are outlined in Table 207–4. Both types of hematoma are located much more frequently above the tentorium (supratentorial hemorrhage) than in the posterior fossa (infratentorial hemorrhage). Of the supratentorial hematomas, the subdural variety is 5 to 10 times more frequent than its epidural counterpart. An acute epidural hematoma most often is temporoparietal in location and is associated with a fracture of the squamous temporal bone in about 70% of cases. Although they usually are caused by laceration of the underlying middle meningeal artery, at least 25% of epidural hematomas in children are of venous origin (from dural sinuses, middle meningeal veins, emissary and diploic veins). Acute subdural hematomas characteristically are of venous origin, resulting from tearing of bridging meningeal veins; occasionally, they are arterial in origin. They usually are frontoparietal in location, with an accompanying skull fracture seen in only 30% of cases. Underlying brain contusion frequently is associated.

Acute subdural hemorrhages are seen most often in infancy, with a peak frequency at the age of 6 months, whereas acute epidural hematomas tend to occur in older children (when the dura is less firmly adherent to the inner table of the skull). In both types of hematomas, the degree of antecedent head trauma may be mild. Acute epidural hematomas usually are unilateral, whereas at least 75% of acute subdural hematomas are bilateral. Seizures occur in less than 25% of

children with acute epidural hematomas, but in 60% to 90% of those with acute subdural hematomas. Retinal and preretinal hemorrhages are found frequently in association with acute subdural hematomas but are uncommon with acute epidural hemorrhage. The "biphasic course" (impaired consciousness/alertness/impaired consciousness) said to be characteristic of acute epidural hematoma in adults is seen rarely in children.

The relatively large volumes of extravasated blood that are present in both types of hematoma produce symptoms and signs of intracranial hypertension. These include irritability or lethargy, vomiting, fullness of the anterior fontanelle, headache, papilledema, and elevation of the systolic blood pressure with a decreased or increased pulse rate and slowed, irregular respirations (see Table 207–2). With sufficient elevation of pressure in the supratentorial compartment, unilateral transtentorial herniation may occur.

The cranial CT scan is particularly valuable in differentiating acute epidural and subdural hematomas above the tentorium. The former tends to assume a lenticular configuration, whereas the latter characteristically is curvilinear or crescentic in appearance. The mortality rate in children with acute epidural hematoma has varied from 9% to 17%, but the survivors tend to be relatively free of neurologic sequelae. Although mortality with acute subdural hematoma often has been less than that with acute epidural hematoma, it has been as high as 17% to 20% in some series. Neurologic morbidity (motor deficits, seizures, cognitive impairment) is greater with acute subdural hematoma than with acute epidural hematoma because of the frequency with which the more deeply situated subdural hematoma is accompanied by injury to the underlying brain.

Epidural and subdural hemorrhages also can occur in the posterior fossa after head injury, but they are much less frequent in this infratentorial location than they are above

TABLE 207-4. Clinical Features of Acute Epidural and Subdural Hematomas

Clinical Feature	Epidural	Subdural
SUPRATENTORIAL		
Frequency	Less	5–10 times greater
Skull fracture	70%	30%
Source of hemorrhage	Arterial or venous	Almost always venous
Age	Usually older than 2 y	Usually younger than 1 y
Location	Usually temporoparietal	Usually frontoparietal
Laterality	Usually unilateral	75% bilateral
Seizures	Less than 25%	75%
Preretinal and retinal hemorrhages	Uncommon	Very frequent
Increased intracranial pressure	Present	Present
Computed cranial tomography (CCT) configuration	Usually lenticular	Curvilinear or crescentic
Mortality	Relatively high	Usually lower
Morbidity	Low	High
INFRATENTORIAL		
Frequency	2–3 times greater	Less
Skull fracture	Almost always	Frequent
Source of hemorrhage	Venous	Venous
Impaired consciousness	Frequent	Frequent
Acute hydrocephalus/medullary compression	Variable	Variable
Other posterior fossa signs	Variable	Variable

the tentorium. Here, in contrast to their relative frequencies above the tentorium, acute epidural hematomas are two to three times more frequent than are acute subdural hematomas. Occipital skull fractures are common with both types of infratentorial hematoma, particularly those that are epidural. In both types of infratentorial hematoma, the bleeding is venous. Clinical signs include impaired consciousness, headache, vomiting, and altered respirations. Only about half of the children have posterior fossa signs such as ataxia, nystagmus, and cranial nerve palsies. These posterior fossa hemorrhages may be complicated by upward herniation of the cerebellum through the tentorial notch or, more often, by downward displacement of the cerebellar tonsils through the foramen magnum.

If acute epidural hemorrhage is suspected clinically, the diagnosis should be confirmed promptly by a cranial CT scan; these hematomas sometimes enlarge so rapidly, with accompanying signs of acutely elevated ICP and progressive hemiparesis, that immediate neurosurgical treatment is usually required (craniotomy, surgical removal of blood clot, and attention to the bleeding source).

If acute subdural hemorrhage is suspected clinically, neurosurgical intervention rarely is needed before the diagnosis is confirmed by cranial CT scan. On occasion, however, with acutely elevated ICP in infants in whom a subdural hematoma is suspected, the subdural space should be tapped as a combined diagnostic and therapeutic measure.

■ PROGNOSIS

Most children who are hospitalized after head injury with loss of consciousness, skull fracture, or cerebral contusion recover completely, usually within 24 to 48 hours. A small number of these children have a postconcussional syndrome or posttraumatic seizures. A smaller group still has severe head injury resulting in prolonged coma, with persisting cognitive, behavioral, or motor deficits.

Severe Head Injuries and Neurologic Outcome

The GCS has proved useful in assisting in the prediction of mortality and neurologic morbidity after head injury. With this scale, head injuries can be classified as mild (GCS score 13 to 15), moderate (GCS score 9 to 12), or severe (GCS score 3 to 8). In the absence of accompanying systemic injury, children with a GCS score of 6, 7, or 8 rarely, if ever, die after head trauma, those with a GCS score of 4 or 5 are unlikely to die, but those with a GCS score of 3 face a mortality rate of 50% to 60% (usually within the first 2 to 3 days after injury). Children with a GCS score of 6 or more have an 80% to 90% chance of recovering with independent function and minimal neurologic deficit. With a GCS score of 4 or 5, cognitive, academic, and other neurologic deficits can be anticipated in 50% to 60% of cases. Children with a GCS score of 3 who survive their head injury have a high incidence of significant cognitive and other neurologic residua. In most such cases, cognitive deficits (attention, intelligence, memory, language), personality change, emotional upset, and social maladjustment are more disabling than is any residual motor handicap.

Age as a Factor in Neurologic Outcome

Of the many factors that influence outcome after head injury, the severity of the injury is the most significant. Next in importance is patient age. Numerous studies have shown that, after head injuries of comparable severity, children usually recover more fully than do adults. With regard to mortality in the head-injured child, the highest rates are seen in the first 2 years of life. After that point, mortality declines steadily throughout childhood, with the lowest rate seen at 12 years of age. Mortality then rises again, with the steepest increase occurring between the ages of 15 and 24 years (when motor vehicle accidents surpass both falls and bicycle accidents as the major cause of head injury).

(Abridged from N. Paul Rosman, Acute Head Trauma, in Oski, DeAngelis, Feigin, McMillan, Warshaw: *Principles and Practice of Pediatrics, Second Edition,* J.B. Lippincott, 1994.)

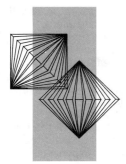

SECTION 16

Seizure Disorders

Oski's Essential Pediatrics,
edited by Kevin B. Johnson and Frank A. Oski.
Lippincott–Raven Publishers,
Philadelphia © 1997

208

Epilepsy

Epilepsy is the symptomatic expression of underlying brain pathology or disordered brain function, not a disease in the usual sense. The incidence of epilepsy has been reported to range from 0.8% to 1.1%. It is the most common neurologic disorder seen in children, and about 50% of all cases of epilepsy start in childhood. Epilepsy is defined as a randomly recurring symptom complex resulting from an episodic disturbance of central nervous system (CNS) function, associated with an excessive, self-limited, neuronal discharge. Variation in clinical manifestations is accounted for by variation in the portion of the brain involved.

Epilepsy is a clinical, not a laboratory, diagnosis, and errors in diagnosis, seizure classification, and subsequent treatment are most often the consequence of an inadequate history and physical examination. A number of relatively benign, episodic spells often are misdiagnosed and even treated as seizures. These include breath-holding spells, benign paroxysmal vertigo, syncope, tics, and even masturbation. The physician rarely has the opportunity actually to witness a clinical seizure and usually must rely on a description provided by the parents. A seizure often is a very frightening experience for parents, and it is understandable that their ability to recall details, time relationships, and the sequence of events can be limited. Frequently, the parents may not have witnessed the event and can report only what they were told by a teacher or other witness. It often is worthwhile to obtain a description by telephone from the actual witness. When the available clinical description is vague and unconvincing, it may be appropriate to delay definitive diagnosis and treatment and to instruct parents in what to look for should attacks recur.

The classification system for epileptic seizures (Table 208–1) is based on both clinical and electroencephogram (EEG) features. It divides seizures into two major categories, generalized and partial.

■ GENERALIZED SEIZURES

Generalized tonic-clonic seizures are characterized clinically by an abrupt arrest of activity and an immediate loss of consciousness. The tonic phase, consisting of sustained, generalized contraction of flexor or extensor muscles, usu-

ally lasts only a few seconds. The clonic phase that follows is characterized by symmetric, rhythmic, clonic activity consisting of alternating contraction and relaxation of major appendicular or axial muscle groups. The clonic phase is longer in duration than the tonic phase, but often terminates spontaneously in less than 5 minutes. Respiration may be irregular and stridulous, and sphincter incontinence may or may not be present. The clonic phase usually is followed by a variable period of confusion and lethargy, which may persist from minutes to hours, and sleep is common.

Clonic seizures are identical to the clonic phase of tonic-clonic seizures. Generalized tonic seizures are characterized by sustained contraction of flexor or extensor muscle groups, giving the child a stiff or rigid appearance. A coarse tremor may be superimposed, but it should not be confused with the rhythmic, alternating muscle contraction and relaxation of clonic activity. A distinction often can be made by asking the parents to supplement their verbal description with a demonstration of what they observed. Both clonic and tonic seizures also will be followed by postical signs and symptoms similar to those seen with generalized tonic-clonic seizures.

Atonic seizures are characterized by the abrupt loss of postural tone and limpness. In contrast to akinetic seizures, the loss of consciousness lasts for several minutes, and there usually is postictal confusion and lethargy or sleep.

Myoclonic seizures are characterized by very brief, random contractions of a muscle or group of muscles occurring unilaterally or bilaterally, and either singly or in clusters. Consciousness usually is preserved. Myoclonic seizures are seen most often with progressive or degenerative types of encephalopathy accompanied by intellectual deficits as well as other overt abnormalities on neurologic examination. Akinetic or "drop attacks" are a subclass of myoclonic seizures and are characterized by a precipitous loss of postural tone. The child abruptly becomes limp and drops to the floor. With nonambulatory infants, there may be precipitous loss of tone resulting in head nodding or slumping forward. The duration of myoclonic seizures is only a few seconds, and there is immediate resumption of normal activity with no postictal lethargy or confusion.

Absence seizures are characterized clinically by very brief episodes of altered awareness during which there is transient arrest of activity and the child appears to stare blankly. The duration of these episodes seldom is longer than 5 to 10 seconds, but they can recur many times a day. They rarely are seen in children less than 3 years of age, and most have their onset before 10 years of age. The child commonly is not aware that a seizure has occurred and frequently is assumed to be daydreaming. A child who is daydreaming, however, is aware of doing so and usually responds when his or her name is called or he or she is touched. In contrast, a child with absence seizures usually denies awareness of any lapse and does not respond to ver-

TABLE 208-1. Classification of Epileptic Seizures

GENERALIZED SEIZURES
Tonic-clonic
Clonic
Tonic
Atonic
Myoclonic
Absence

PARTIAL SEIZURES
Elementary symptomatology
    With motor symptoms
    With sensory symptoms
Complex symptomatology
    With impairment of consciousness only
    With cognitive symptomatology
    With affective symptomatology
    With psychosensory symptomatology
    Compound forms
Partial seizures secondarily generalized

Commission on Classification and Terminology of the International League Against Epilepsy. Proposal for revised clinical and electroencephalographic classification of epileptic seizures. Epilepsia. 1981;22:489.

bal or physical stimuli. Subtle motor activity such as rhythmic eye blinking, drooping of the head, or slight movements of the arms may accompany the staring episodes. The seizure is terminated by the immediate return of environmental awareness, and the child may resume an activity at the point where it was interrupted. A generalized, symmetric three-per-second spike and wave pattern is the EEG hallmark of absence seizures.

■ PARTIAL SEIZURES

The initial features of a partial seizure are especially important. Tonic deviation of the head and eyes to one side, or some other localized motor or sensory feature preceding a secondarily generalized tonic-clonic seizure may be a clue to focal cortical origin of the attack. In children, elementary partial seizures usually are focal motor or sensory. The initial feature may be focal twitching involving the distal portion of an extremity, which may remain localized or spread to become a hemiconvulsion. Similarly, focal sensory seizures may be initiated by the appearance of a sensation of numbness or tingling in an extremity, which may remain confined to that area or spread to involve the entire side of the body. Consciousness often is preserved, but will be lost if there is secondary generalization.

Complex partial seizures have a variety of clinical expressions and are subclassified on this basis. One form in which there is impairment of consciousness only is characterized by transient, blank staring or confusion. These episodes can be mistaken for absence seizures, but the attacks usually last 30 seconds or longer, whereas absence episodes commonly last less than 10 seconds. An EEG can be helpful in distinguishing between the two forms, because a three-per-second generalized spike and wave pattern is the hallmark of absence seizures, whereas focal discharge from temporal or frontal areas is antic-

ipated with complex partial seizures. Another form of partial complex seizure involves "cognitive symptomatology." This form is characterized clinically by an abrupt alteration in mental state that involves disruption of time relationships and memory. Older children sometimes describe feelings of unreality, remoteness, detachment, or depersonalization. Forced thinking, a deluge of thoughts, or perseveration of a thought also have been described. Déjà vu or jamais vu, the impression of an inappropriate familiarity or unfamiliarity with a place or situation, occasionally may be reported. Attacks characterized by "affective symptomatology" may be described as inexplicable feelings of fear or dread, or other emotional experiences that intrude abruptly on the patient's prevailing affective state. Attacks characterized by "somatosensory disturbances" are notable for distortions of perception or hallucinations. Some children report transient distortions of perception concerning the size of objects (micropsia or macropsia), and others describe hallucinations involving taste or smell as well as formed visual hallucinations.

Probably the most familiar complex partial seizure is the psychomotor attack that is characterized by semipurposeful motor automatisms. The stereotyped automatisms may be perseverative in nature, and the child will exhibit continuing repetition of the activity in which he was engaged before the onset of the seizure. For example, if the child was walking, he may continue to walk, but without purposeful direction. If the child was writing, he may continue to move the pencil across the page without producing decipherable script. The simplest type of automatisms are masticatory, sucking, and lip-pursing movements. Patting, scratching, or picking at clothing also may be seen. More complex behaviors such as fumbling with clothing as if to undress or turning about as if searching for something are less common. Finally, "compound forms" may be seen that incorporate various elements of the several varieties just described. In an individual child, the form taken usually is stereotyped from one attack to another.

■ EPILEPTIC SYNDROMES

Infantile spasms or infantile massive spasms are peculiar to infancy and early childhood, with a peak incidence of onset between 2 and 7 months of age. They have been described as occurring in three clinical forms. Flexor spasms consist of sudden flexion of the neck, trunk, and extremities, which may be so violent that the torso will "jackknife" at the waist. Extensor spasms consist of abrupt extension of the neck and trunk with adduction or abduction of the extremities. The predominant form is a mixed flexor-extensor spasm most commonly consisting of flexion of the neck, trunk, and arms, with extension of the legs and, less commonly, flexion of the legs and extension of the arms. Infantile spasms tend to occur in clusters, with each cluster consisting of 2 to 125 individual spasms. Each individual spasm lasts only a few seconds, although a cluster may extend over several minutes. Spasms rarely occur during actual sleep, but frequently occur on arousal. In most instances, the EEG shows the distinctive pattern of hypsarrhythmia.

Infantile spasms have occurred in association with numerous and seemingly unrelated pathologic states, and no one specific factor or circumscribed group of factors has been identified as a common etiologic abnormality. Etiologic associations provide the basis for division of these spasms into two broad groups. In the idiopathic or cryptogenic group, there is no demonstrable cause, the child's development usually has been normal until the onset of spasms, and the results of computed tomography (CT) scans of the brain are normal. In the symptomatic group, a specific etiologic factor can be identified, developmental or neurologic abnormalities have preceded the onset of spasms, and the results of CT scans of the brain often are abnormal. The cryptogenic group represents no more than 10% to 15% of the total, and they have a better prognosis than does the symptomatic group.

Causes associated with the symptomatic group of infantile spasms include cerebral dysgenesis, intrauterine infections, and genetic disorders. Two syndromes of cerebral dysgenesis that have been associated with infantile spasms are the Miller-Dieker syndrome (lissencephaly with or without a chromosome 17 abnormality) and Aicardi's syndrome (females with agenesis of the corpus callosum, distinctive chorioretinopathy, and mental retardation).

The Lennox-Gastaut syndrome is one type of symptomatic generalized epilepsy, and it is age-dependent. The Lennox-Gastaut syndrome is characterized by the onset in early childhood of mixed seizures (including tonic, tonic-clonic, atonic, akinetic or myoclonic, and absence), refractoriness to common antiepileptic drugs, an abnormal EEG (generalized, slow spike and slow wave activity), and a high incidence of developmental and mental retardation. This syndrome frequently is preceded by infantile spasms. Etiologic factors are similar to those outlined with infantile spasms. In 30% of the cases, the Lennox-Gastaut syndrome appears in children who have no antecedents, previous epilepsy, or clinical or neurologic evidence of brain damage, and who have had previously normal development.

■ ANCILLARY LABORATORY STUDIES

In approaching the laboratory evaluation, the physician must recall that epilepsy is primarily a clinical diagnosis. Some laboratory studies are necessary to establish a baseline for future comparison, and others can help with formulating medical treatment and prognosis. Indications for laboratory studies should be based on information extracted from the history and physical examination. If specific disease entities such as hypocalcemia, hypoglycemia, or other metabolic, toxic, or degenerative disorders are valid considerations, additional studies relevant to the particular entity are, of course, appropriate.

Electroencephalography

An EEG has value only when it is interpreted in the context of the child's age, the history, and the physical findings. The quality of information gained from an EEG is related directly to the standards of the laboratory and the training and experience of the personnel. A routine EEG always should be recorded during wakefulness and sleep, and, in older children, during hyperventilation and photic stimulation. Because normal organizational and frequency characteristics change rapidly with advancing age and cerebral maturation, it is particularly important that the interpretation of EEGs in infants and young children be done by an electroencephalographer who has had specific training and experience with this age group. EEGs in many laboratories are interpreted by adult neurologists with little or no experience with infants and young children.

Normal EEG results should not necessarily dissuade a physician from making a diagnosis of epilepsy in the face of a convincing clinical description. The initial EEG often does not contain epileptiform discharges. Investigators have found that the initial EEG in 25% to 58% of affected children may be normal or borderline without epileptiform abnormalities. Similarly, abnormal EEG results do not necessarily confirm a clinical suspicion of epilepsy. The type and location of an abnormality are expected to correlate with the clinical data. When available clinical and EEG data do not provide a basis for confident classification regarding seizure type, or in cases in which pseudoseizures are suspected, video-EEG monitoring may be justified. Protracted monitoring can be relatively expensive, however, and should be undertaken only when the frequency of the seizures suggests a reasonable probability that a clinical event will be captured during a 6- to 24-hour recording.

Neuroimaging

Routine skull radiographs seldom are indicated or helpful except when overt bony pathology is detected by physical examination. Neuroimaging studies may be indicated in cases of partial seizures or if the history and physical examination suggest structural lesions, degenerative diseases, or a congenital structural abnormality. There is no justification, however, for the routine use of these relatively expensive procedures.

■ MEDICAL TREATMENT

Successful treatment of a child with epilepsy demands more than just preventing recurrent seizures. The sensitive physician must adopt both an educational and an advocacy position, ensuring acceptance of the child's epilepsy by the family, by teachers and classmates, and by the community. Misconceptions about epilepsy still abound and often have an adverse impact on a child's self-esteem and psychosocial development. Time invested in providing a clear explanation, in lay language, of the nature of epilepsy, the objectives of treatment, and the simple fundamentals of pharmacokinetics can allay apprehensions, dispel misconceptions, and promote compliance with the prescribed drug regimen.

Population studies suggest that about 70% of patients in whom epilepsy is diagnosed ultimately will become seizure-free, and that the majority can expect to discontinue anticonvulsant medication. A higher likelihood of remission has been reported in children than in adults. Children with epilepsy in association with mental retardation or cerebral palsy, however, have very low rates of remission. The literature does not reflect universal agreement on the optimal duration of anticonvulsant therapy. In most instances, a seizure-free period of at least 2 to 3 consecutive years is a conservative objective before the gradual withdrawal of medication should be considered. Monitoring of serum drug levels at reasonable intervals can provide a guideline for the adjustment of drug dosages as the child grows. Complete seizure control is not possible in some children, and, in those instances, the occurrence of an occasional seizure is preferable to an increase in the dosage of anticonvulsants to levels that produce sedation and dysequilibrium, compromising both cognitive function and social interaction.

Treatment After the Nonfebrile First Seizure

The initiation of antiepileptic drug therapy after an initial, nonfebrile seizure in otherwise well children continues to be controversial. It may be argued that some children have a benign developmental disorder of seizure threshold that they will outgrow. These include children whose generalized tonic-clonic seizures begin between 1 and 10 years of age, and who have normal neurologic examinations and normal

TABLE 208-2. Commonly Used Antiepileptic Drugs

Drug	Side Effects
Carbamazepine (Tegretol)	Diplopia, vertigo, ataxia, sedation, nausea and vomiting, thrombocytopenia, leukopenia, and agranulocytosis
Ethosuximide (Zarontin)	Abdominal pain, anorexia; nausea, and vomiting, headache, dizziness, photophobia, aplastic anemia, leukopenia, agranulocytosis
Phenobarbital	Sedation, hyperkinesis, ataxia, nystagmus
Phenytoin (Dilantin)	Nystagmus, ataxia, sedation, hypertrichosis, gum hyperplasia, leukopenia, agranulocytosis
Primidone (Mysoline)	Sedation, hyperkinesis, ataxia, nystagmus
Valproic acid (Depakote, Depakene)	Nausea and vomiting, increased appetite with weight gain, anorexia with weight loss, transient alopecia, hepatic failure, anemia, leukopenia, thrombocytopenia, acute prancreatitis

or nonspecific abnormal EEG results, and children with benign epilepsy with rolandic spikes. Some physicians believe that the stigma attached to the diagnosis of epilepsy and the potential adverse side effects of antiepileptic drugs, especially on behavior and cognitive function, outweigh the risk of recurrent seizures. The risk for recurrence in children with a first, nonfebrile seizure has been addressed in only a few studies and has been reported to vary from 52% to 61%. Recurrence rates are much higher after a second seizure (79% to 90%), and most seizures recur within 6 months of the first (70% to 74%). Recurrence rates are highest in patients with abnormal results on neurologic examination, focal spikes in the EEG, and complex partial seizures. Recurrence rates in otherwise normal children, who have normal EEG results after the first, nonfebrile, generalized tonic-clonic seizure, range from 10% to 30%. As yet, there is no universally accepted consensus regarding withholding treatment after the occurrence of a first such seizure during childhood. A clinician who sees a child after a single seizure—especially a child who is neurologically and mentally normal, and who has normal EEG results—may consider, after discussion with the patient and parents, withholding therapy pending the occurrence of a second seizure.

Commonly Used Drugs

Eighteen drugs approved by the United States Food and Drug Administration (FDA) are available for the treatment of seizures. Six of these, either alone or in some combination, are used for seizure control in the majority of children who are responsive to medical therapy. These six are phenobarbital, phenytoin, carbamazepine, ethosuximide, valproic acid (VPA), and primidone (Tables 208–2 and 208–3). Evidence indicates that therapy with a single agent suffices for the majority of children, but a significant number require more than one drug.

■ COUNSELING PATIENTS AND PARENTS

Diagnosing the condition and initiating appropriate drug therapy are only the initial steps in caring for a child

with a seizure disorder. Parents and children often have many questions, misconceptions, and fears. They always want to know if the child will "outgrow" seizures, what to do during a seizure, and how seizures may influence participation in school and sports. Dispelling misconceptions and providing guidance are just as important as dispensing medication. Anxious and overprotective parents or overly solicitous teachers and peers can affect the child's psychosocial development adversely. Parents and older children should have a clear understanding that epilepsy is not a disease entity per se, but is the symptomatic expression of disordered cerebral function, and that the prognosis for seizure control depends on underlying etiologic factors and may vary significantly from one child to another. On the basis of specific etiologic factors, or the absence thereof, the physician can provide the family with an individualized understanding and prognosis.

TABLE 208-3. Commonly Used Antiepileptic Drugs

Drug	Half-life* (h)	Protein Bound (%)	Blood Levels (μg/mL)
Phenytoin (Dilantin)	N 30–60 C 20 ± 2 A 24 ± 12	90	10–20
Phenobarbital	N 70–100 C 55 ± 15 A 96 ± 12	50–60	15–40
Ethosuximide (Zarontin)	C 30 ± 6 A 55 ± 5	0	40–150
Valproic acid (Depakene)	12 ± 6	90	50–100
Primidone (Mysoline)	12 ± 6	3	5–15
Carbamazepine (Tegretol)	C 14 ± 5 A 17 ± 7	60–80	4–12

*N, *newborn;* C, *child;* A, *adult.*

Frequently, parents are very concerned that their child might die during a seizure. It should be emphasized that the objective of maintenance drug therapy is to prevent seizure recurrence and that a period of observation is required to optimize the medication dosage. If further seizures occur, they most likely will be brief in duration. Most seizures terminate spontaneously within 5 minutes, and death as a result of seizures is rare. Indeed, fatalities usually are the consequence of the patient being engaged in a potentially hazardous activity when a seizure occurs (swimming unattended, operating a motorized vehicle, or climbing to some high place).

Parents should be reassured that the brevity of most seizures obviates the necessity of making a dash for the emergency department. If a seizure persists beyond 10 to 15 minutes, it is appropriate to seek medical assistance. Teachers and school nurses also should be advised that it is not necessary to send a child home after a brief, uncomplicated seizure. Excessive zeal in this regard can only diminish self-esteem, raise anxiety levels, and alter social interaction with classmates. The family should be fully informed of the rationale for drug choice and use, and of the potential dose-related and non–dose-related side effects. Compliance can be enhanced by advising the use of an inexpensive pillbox that is compartmentalized to hold daily medications for 1 week.

Precautions

In general, the child with epilepsy should be treated as a normal child, with a few notable precautions. As with all children, swimming always should be supervised. Until seizures are well controlled, bicycle riding should be restricted to low-traffic residential areas, and climbing to rooftops should be discouraged. Sports and athletic activities often are extremely important to young people, and decisions regarding participation should involve the parents, patient, and physician in an open discussion. In most instances, epilepsy should not exclude a child from participation in sports activities. Situations in which a seizure could cause a dangerous fall, such as rope climbing, activities on parallel bars, and high diving, should be avoided. It is suggested that competitive underwater swimming also be avoided. Participation in contact or collision sports should be given individual consideration. Common sense suggests, however, that contact or collision sports might pose significant risks to a patient who is continuing to have several seizures per month.

(Abridged from Daniel G. Glaze, Epilepsy, in Oski, DeAngelis, Feigin, McMillan, Warshaw: *Principles and Practice of Pediatrics, Second Edition*, J.B. Lippincott, 1994.)

Oski's Essential Pediatrics,
edited by Kevin B. Johnson and Frank A. Oski.
Lippincott–Raven Publishers,
Philadelphia © 1997

209

Status Epilepticus

■ DEFINITION

Status epilepticus may be defined as seizure activity that lasts longer than 15 to 30 minutes or repeated seizures between which the child does not return to the baseline level of consciousness. In convulsive status, the child has a prolonged, generalized tonic-clonic seizure or the repetition of such seizures without a return to full consciousness between episodes. In nonconvulsive status, such as absence status and complex partial status, the clinical presentation is a prolonged "twilight" or semicoma state. In epilepsia partialis continua, consciousness is preserved in the face of continuous, focal motor activity.

About 12% of patients with newly diagnosed epilepsy will have a seizure lasting 30 minutes or longer. The greatest proportion of cases of status epilepticus occur in children, and less than 25% occur as an idiopathic event. The occurrence of status epilepticus should prompt a full diagnostic workup. Previously, overall mortality figures as high as 30% were reported, but more recent investigators have reported a mortality rate of 3% to 6% in children. This decrease in mortality is the result of more rapid diagnosis and support, combined with better medical treatment and improved intensive care. Death usually is attributable to the underlying cause of status epilepticus rather than to a prolonged seizure. When this information is considered, mortality related to prolonged seizures per se has been reported to be as low as 1% to 2%.

■ TREATMENT

Tonic-clonic status epilepticus is a life-threatening situation and represents a neurologic emergency. Prolonged seizures can lead to a series of metabolic derangements that potentially can cause neuronal damage. Tonic-clonic status epilepticus that progresses beyond 60 minutes may be associated with severe, permanent brain damage or death. The longer the seizure lasts, the more difficult it will be to stop. The therapeutic measures outlined here are appropriate in those cases in which a seizure or repeated seizures continue unabated for 15 to 30 minutes. Some clinicians consider almost any tonic-clonic seizure to be an episode of status epilepticus and intervene with both supportive and drug therapy. In children, infectious processes, toxic or metabolic disorders, and chronic forms of encephalopathy, as well as the sudden withdrawal of antiepileptic drugs may underlie or precipitate this condition.

Therapy must address the immediate problem of stopping the seizure, providing supportive measures (supplemental oxygen, a clear airway, an intravenous glucose source, and so forth), detecting and correcting any predisposing or precipitating factors, and incorporating a drug with a long half-life to prevent the recurrence of seizures once they have been arrested.

Supportive Measures

The preservation of vital functions takes precedence:

1. Blood pressure, respiration, and cardiac function are maintained to avoid hypoxic-ischemic damage to the brain. Resuscitation equipment should be available.

2. Blood samples are obtained for electrolyte, glucose, blood urea nitrogen, calcium, and magnesium measurements, and for antiepileptic drug level determinations if the patient has been treated previously for seizures.

3. An intravenous line is inserted for the infusion of a glucose solution to maintain the blood sugar level at about 150 mg/dL. Fluids should be limited initially to 1000 to 1200 mL/m².

4. Increased intracranial pressure is treated if evident.

Drug Therapy

Excluding infants who are less than 2 to 3 months of age, diazepam may be given. Because of its short half-life and characteristic distribution within body tissues, the effect of diazepam is very short. The duration of action of intravenous diazepam is less than 1 hour. Seizures may recur within 20 to 30 minutes. Therefore, if seizures are arrested, an antiepileptic drug with a longer duration of action must be given. Phenytoin is suggested. If seizures continue after about 20 to 30 minutes, phenobarbital may be used. If this regimen is unsuccessful, neurologic consultation is appropriate.

The use of lorazepam, a long-acting benzodiazepine, as the initial drug in the treatment of status epilepticus appears promising. Lorazepam has a rapid onset and a more prolonged duration of anticonvulsant action than does diazepam. Although its half-life of 10 to 15 hours is less than that of diazepam, lorazepam continues to achieve effective brain levels for 8 to 24 hours. Lorazepam has not been approved by the United States Food and Drug Administration (FDA) for use in children for this purpose. After additional clinical trials, it may be approved eventually and replace diazepam as the drug of choice for patients with status epilepticus.

(Abridged from Daniel G. Glaze, Status Epilepticus, in Oski, DeAngelis, Feigin, McMillan, Warshaw: *Principles and Practice of Pediatrics, Second Edition,* J.B. Lippincott, 1994.)

Oski's Essential Pediatrics,
edited by Kevin B. Johnson and Frank A. Oski.
Lippincott–Raven Publishers,
Philadelphia © 1997

210

Febrile Seizures

Febrile seizures are a worldwide problem and occur in 2% to 4% of children less than 5 years of age. A febrile seizure is defined as a convulsion associated with an elevated temperature greater than 38°C (100.4°F) occurring in a child who is less than 6 years of age. Exclusions to the diagnosis include a history of a previous afebrile seizure, central nervous system (CNS) infection or inflammation, or acute systemic metabolic abnormalities that may produce convulsions. Febrile seizures are classified into two groups based on their clinical features. Simple (benign) febrile seizures are those that last less than 15 minutes, do not have focal features, and, if they occur in a series, have a total duration of less than 30 minutes. Complex febrile seizures include those that last more than 15 minutes, have focal features or postictal paresis, and occur in series with a total duration greater than 30 minutes.

■ SIGNS AND SYMPTOMS

The vast majority of febrile seizures are simple. Prolonged convulsions occur in less than 10% of children with febrile seizures, and focal features are seen in less than 5%. Generalized seizures are mainly clonic, but both atonic and tonic episodes have been noted. Involvement of the facial and respiratory muscles is noted frequently. Children usually have a significantly elevated body temperature, but about 25% of febrile convulsions occur in children whose temperatures are between 38°C and 39°C (100.4°F and 102.2°F) The majority of febrile seizures are seen on the first day of illness, and, in some children, they are the first sign of the accompanying infection.

■ DIFFERENTIAL DIAGNOSIS

The main concern in evaluating an infant or child with a febrile convulsion is the possibility of underlying meningitis or encephalitis. Thorough evaluation by an experienced clinician almost always will detect the child with meningitis. If the only indication for performing a lumbar puncture is a febrile seizure, meningitis will be found in less than 1% of patients. Less than half of these will have bacterial meningitis. In children who have meningitis presenting with seizures, as many as 40% (particularly younger infants) may not have meningeal signs. They may have other symptoms and findings, however, that strongly suggest the presence of meningitis. Thus, it is rare for bacterial meningitis to be diagnosed solely on the basis of a "routine" evaluation of cerebrospinal fluid (CSF) after a febrile seizure.

■ DIAGNOSTIC TESTS

The routine performance of lumbar punctures in all children with febrile seizures does not seem warranted. Those children who might be considered candidates for examination of the CSF include young infants, children whose febrile seizure occurs after the second day of illness, cases in which the clinician is unsure of his or her judgment regarding the presence or absence of meningitis, and situations in which it is not possible to observe the patient. Other laboratory tests, such as complete blood counts, urine and blood cultures, should be obtained, as always, in young infants with no apparent source of their fever.

Prophylactic Treatment

Controversy exists regarding which children should be treated with continuous antiepileptic drug therapy to prevent recurrent febrile seizures. Although the incidence of recurrent febrile seizures can be reduced, no data prove that treatment decreases the incidence of sequelae associated with prolonged seizures or the development of epilepsy, which occurs at greater frequency in children who have febrile seizures than in the general population. Because febrile seizures have so few sequelae and such a good prognosis in the vast majority of children, the benefits of therapy must be considered carefully and compared to the side effects of the medication.

Because fever is the precipitating event in febrile seizures, attempts at reducing elevated temperature are a logical approach. Attempts at parent education have been made, however, including detailed written and oral instructions regarding the use of antipyretics, without success. The recurrence rate among patients whose parents were so instructed was 25%, which is similar to that of an untreated population.

■ PROGNOSIS

The prognosis for children with febrile seizures can be divided into three categories: recurrence rate for febrile seizures, development of neurologic sequelae, and development of epilepsy. The major factor influencing the recurrence of febrile seizures is the age of the infant at the time of the first seizure. The younger the child, the more likely it is that febrile convulsions will recur. If the first seizure occurs at less than 1 year of age, the recurrence rate is about 50% to 65%, in contrast to a rate of 28% if the first seizure occurs after that point. If the first seizure does not occur until at least 2½ years of age, the recurrence rate is reduced to about 20%. About 50% to 75% of recurrences take place within 1 year of the initial seizure, and about 90% occur within 2½ years. This recurrence rate can be influenced by the intermittent use of rapidly acting antiepileptic drugs or continuous prophylactic treatment.

Children who have febrile seizures are at increased risk for the development of epilepsy. In a normal child who has a simple febrile seizure, this risk may be twice that of the general population, or 1.0% versus 0.5%. Abnormal neurologic development in the presence of complex febrile seizures, particularly focal seizures, greatly increases the risk, by as much as 30- to 50-fold.

(Abridged from Marvin A. Fishman, Febrile Seizures, in Oski, DeAngelis, Feigin, McMillan, Warshaw: *Principles and Practice of Pediatrics, Second Edition,* J.B. Lippincott, 1994.)

Oski's Essential Pediatrics,
edited by Kevin B. Johnson and Frank A. Oski.
Lippincott–Raven Publishers,
Philadelphia © 1997

211

Reye's Syndrome

Reye's syndrome, first described in 1963, is an acute, life-threatening, postinfectious, metabolic encephalopathy that affects predominantly school-age children, occasionally infants, and rarely adults. Over the years, the disease and its clinical manifestations have received widespread recognition.

Characteristically, a prodromal illness—most often influenza or varicella infection—is followed in 3 to 5 days by the onset of persistent and intractable vomiting. Initially, patients are well oriented, but irritable and lethargic. Some patients have no change in consciousness and remain only lethargic with no progression to unconsciousness. The serum glutamic-oxaloacetic transaminase (SGOT) and serum glutamate pyruvate transaminase (SGPT) levels are 3 to 30 times normal. The serum bilirubin level rarely exceeds 1 mg/dL. Serum ammonia concentrations are variable at presentation. With encephalopathy worsening to a hyperexcitable state, the patient is intermittently out of contact with the environment. Further progression to a deeper comatose state is characterized by decerebrate and decorticate posturing, hyperventilation, and, finally, flaccid paralysis with loss of involuntary ventilatory control. The comatose patient uniformly has an elevated ammonia concentration ranging from 3 to 20 times normal. The encephalopathy typically persists for 24 to 96 hours, with gradual improvement in survivors. Recovery of consciousness in patients with permanent neurologic impairment may require weeks.

Criteria for the case definition of Reye's syndrome include the following: an acute, noninflammatory encephalopathy documented clinically by an alteration in consciousness and, if available, cerebrospinal fluid (CSF) containing less than eight leukocytes per cubic millimeter; hepatopathy documented by liver biopsy on autopsy or a threefold or greater rise in the SGOT, SGPT, or serum ammonia level; and no more reasonable explanation for the cerebral or hepatic abnormalities.

It is important to assess accurately the severity of the illness, because the therapies for severely affected children are aggressive, invasive, and dangerous. Several staging systems have been developed, culminating in the National Institutes of Health (NIH) Staging System. The most extensively used system includes electroencephalographic (EEG) information that previously was believed to have prognostic value. The EEG criteria have been replaced, and the resulting NIH Staging System consists of the following five stages:

Stage I: Lethargy; follows verbal commands; normal posture; purposeful response to pain; brisk pupillary light reflex; and normal oculocephalic reflex.

Stage II: Combative or stuporous; inappropriate verbalizing; normal posture; purposeful or nonpurposeful response to pain; sluggish pupillary reflexes; and conjugate deviation on doll's eyes maneuver.

Stage III: Comatose; decorticate posture; decorticate response to pain; sluggish pupillary reaction; and conjugate deviation on doll's eyes maneuver.

Stage IV: Comatose; decerebrate posture and decerebrate response to pain; sluggish pupillary reflexes; and inconsistent or absent oculocephalic reflex.

Stage V: Comatose; flaccid; no response to pain; no pupillary response; no oculocephalic reflex.

During the last 22 years, more than 3000 cases of Reye's syndrome have been reported to the United States Centers for Disease Control and Prevention (CDC), with a case fatality rate varying from 26% to 42%. From 1967 to 1973, between 11 and 83 cases were reported annually. Between 1974 and 1983, the reporting frequency increased to a peak of 555 cases in 1979–1980. Thereafter, there has been a steady decline in cases, such that Reye's syndrome now is a rare disease. In addition, there has been a trend in recent years toward diagnosis in earlier coma stages.

■ PATHOGENESIS

Despite intensive study, the pathogenesis of Reye's syndrome remains incompletely defined. It is unclear whether the pathogenesis can be explained by a primary injury to the mitochondria of multiple organs, including the brain, liver, and muscle, with its metabolic consequences, or whether a primary hepatic injury leads to metabolic consequences that produce the biochemical abnormalities and encephalopathy. Morphologic and biochemical studies have confirmed the presence of a characteristic injury. Pleomorphic, enlarged mitochondria with disrupted cristae, electron-lucent matrices, and reduced numbers of dense bodies are characteristic of the hepatic pathology of Reye's syndrome. Associated reductions in mitochondrial enzymes involved in ureagenesis and gluconeogenesis, and in enzymes associated with the citric acid cycle have been observed. Further evidence of mitochondrial injury is suggested by the finding of dicarboxylic acids in the urine and serum.

In 1982, the Committee on Infectious Disease of the American Academy of Pediatrics issued a statement warning against the use of salicylates in children with possible varicella or influenza infection, and a program of public education was initiated. Some authors have cited the reduction in aspirin use and the decrease in the occurrence of Reye's syndrome as an argument to support the association between aspirin administration and this disorder. Other authors dispute these conclusions, stating that even the prospective, controlled, epidemiologic study performed by the United States Public Health Service showed histologic support for the diagnosis of Reye's syndrome in only 27% of the patients, and no electron microscopic evidence was presented.

Based on available evidence, it appears that a primary mitochondrial injury stimulates multiple metabolic disturbances, and hyperammonemia, free fatty acidemia, lactic acidosis, and dicarboxylic acidemia are the results. Synergistically, the metabolic abnormalities and the underlying mitochondrial injury lead to the observed pathophysiology through incompletely understood mechanisms. Fatty acids, dicarboxylic acids, salicylates, and other factors may inhibit mitochondrial ureagenesis and potentiate their individual metabolic effects. Alternatively, they may inhibit adenosine triphosphate synthesis and lead to profound reductions in high-energy phosphate, which is required to catalyze an array of enzymatic reactions.

■ TREATMENT

The treatment of children with Reye's syndrome ranges from relatively simple provision of glucose to children with stage I findings to extremely complex neurologic intensive care for children with more severe stages of the disease. Therapy is significantly dependent on the stage of the disease in patients with Reye's syndrome.

Children who are in stage I require close neurologic evaluation, frequent glucose level determinations, and daily measurements of ammonia, transaminase, and electrolyte levels. Hypoglycemia is avoided by the provision of intravenous glucose, coupled with close monitoring of the glucose level. Children with stage I Reye's syndrome have an excellent prognosis if they undergo observation in the hospital and receive glucose and electrolyte intravenous therapy.

Children who have disease of stage II or higher require significantly more care and must be treated in the hospital's intensive care facility.

In all patients with stage III disease or stage II disease progressing toward stage III, aggressive therapy consisting of intubation, hemodynamic monitoring, intracranial pressure monitoring and control, and ammonia reduction therapies should be practiced.

Fluid and Electrolytes

Several types of electrolyte disturbances are seen in patients with Reye's syndrome, the most well recognized of which is hypoglycemia. There also may be abnormalities of potassium, calcium, and phosphorus. In the presence of inappropriate antidiuretic hormone secretion or diabetes insipidus, fluid balance is disordered.

Respiratory Support

Patients with stage I disease do not require respiratory support, but adequate oxygenation must be ensured. Those with more severe stages of Reye's syndrome need aggressive support to prevent hypoxia and hypercapnia. All children with stage III Reye's syndrome should undergo intubation and hyperventilation electively.

Hemodynamic Monitoring and Support

Arterial and central venous pressure lines are placed to monitor meticulously the fluid and cardiovascular status.

Coagulopathy

Most of these patients have a bleeding diathesis, which should be treated with the necessary blood products when clinical bleeding is noted.

Temperature Control

It is important to control the temperature in children with Reye's syndrome, because decreases may contribute to hemodynamic instability and increases will cause a rise in the cerebral metabolic rate.

Intracranial Pressure Management

The most significant advances in the care of children with this disease appear to be in the areas of supportive care and management of intracranial hypertension. Measures to decrease intracranial pressure include elevating the head of the bed, administering controlled mechanical hyperventilation, and using osmotic diuretics. The use of high doses of barbiturates in the treatment of elevated intracranial pressure in patients with Reye's syndrome is controversial. Although this pharmacologic treatment seems to be effective in reducing intracranial pressure, it also is associated with significant complications.

(Abridged from Penelope Terhune Louis, Reye Syndrome, in Oski, DeAngelis, Feigin, McMillan, Warshaw: *Principles and Practice of Pediatrics, Second Edition*, J.B. Lippincott, 1994.)

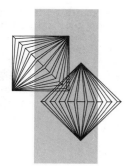

SECTION 17

Childhood Neuropathies

Oski's Essential Pediatrics,
edited by Kevin B. Johnson and Frank A. Oski.
Lippincott–Raven Publishers,
Philadelphia © 1997

212

Disorders of the Anterior Horn Cell

The anterior horn cells may be involved selectively in a number of acquired and inherited diseases. Certain viruses, particularly poliomyelitis, demonstrate a specific affinity for these nerve cells. Herpes zoster and coxsackievirus also occasionally affect anterior horn cells. Inherited conditions influencing the anterior horn cells include the spinal muscular atrophies (SMA) and a number of metabolic disorders. Damage to the anterior horn cells is characterized clinically by weakness, atrophy, and hyporeflexia. Fasciculations are common. Because the dorsal sensory root is not involved in these disorders, sensory abnormalities are not present. Motor nuclei in the brain stem are involved commonly, so bulbar involvement is seen frequently.

■ PROGRESSIVE SPINAL MUSCULAR ATROPHY

Progressive SMA is a degenerative disease affecting the anterior horn cells of the spinal cord and the motor cells of cranial nerve nuclei. It usually is inherited as an autosomal recessive trait, but autosomal dominant and X-linked recessive inheritance patterns also have been reported. Several classifications of the disease have been proposed based on patient age at the onset of symptoms, severity of the symptoms, and length of survival. Several distinct clinical presentations exist (Table 212–1). Within any individual family, there usually is a high level of concordance, so that affected siblings often have similar forms of the disease. A number of reports have described both mild and severe forms occurring within the same family, however, supporting the view that the different phenotypes are part of the same genotypic spectrum. In 1990, the genetic abnormality was localized to chromosome 5q11. The abnormality

TABLE 212-1. Progressive Spinal Muscular Atrophies (SMA)

Disorder	Inheritance	Age of Onset	Clinical Features
Acute infantile SMA (Werdnig-Hoffmann disease, SMA type 1)	Autosomal recessive	In utero to 6 months	Frog-leg posture
			Severe weakness with some movements of fingers and toes; most are unable to sit
			Areflexia
			Tongue atrophy and fasciculations
			Progressive swallowing and respiratory problems Survival less than 3 years
Intermediate SMA (chronic Werdnig-Hoffmann disease, SMA type 2)	Autosomal recessive; rarely autosomal dominant	3 months to 15 years	Proximal weakness; most sit, some walk until teens
			Decreased or absent reflexes
			Long periods of apparent arrest
			High incidence of scoliosis, contractures
			Unusual tremor (minipolymyoclonus)
			Survival varies several years to third decade
Kugelberg-Welander disease	Autosomal recessive; rarely autosomal dominant	5 years to 15 years	May be part of continuous disease spectrum of SMA type II
			Proximal weakness with hip and shoulder atrophy
			Calf hypertrophy
			Decreased or absent reflexes
			May remain ambulatory into fourth decade

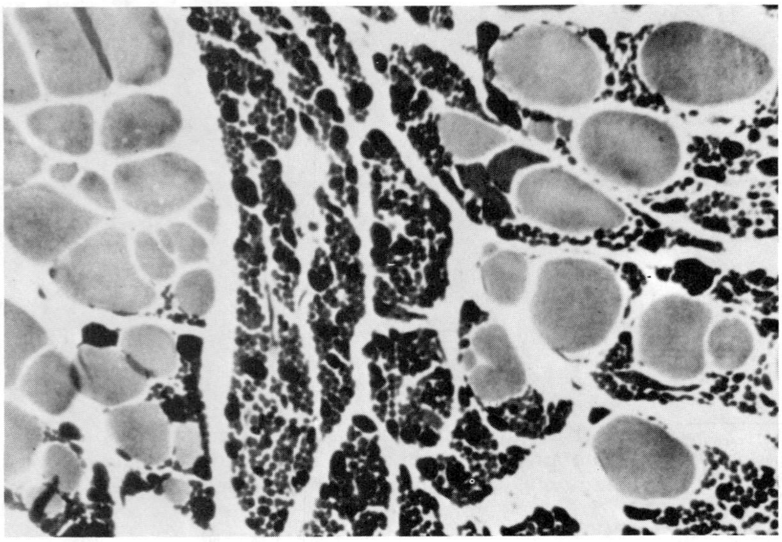

Figure 212-1. Muscle biopsy sample of a patient with Werdnig-Hoffman disease showing characteristic groups of rounded, atrophic type II (*dark*) muscle fibers adjacent to groups of normal-size or hypertrophic type I (*light*) muscle fibers.

appears to be the same in both the acute and the chronic form of the disease, indicating phenotypic heterogeneity with genetic homogeneity. Pathologically, there is a loss of anterior horn cells in the spinal cord. Surviving neurons show changes of chromatolysis and pyknosis. There is no sign of inflammation.

Acute Infantile Spinal Muscular Atrophy (Acute Werdnig-Hoffmann Disease, Spinal Muscular Atrophy Type 1)

Patients with the most severe form of SMA present a stereotypic picture, with the onset of symptoms occurring within the first 6 months of life. In one third of cases, the onset is in utero, with a notable decrease in fetal movements during the last months of pregnancy. These children are hypotonic and weak in the neonatal period, and they have significant feeding difficulties and respiratory distress. Other children may appear normal for the first few weeks of life while generalized weakness of the extremities, trunk, and bulbar muscles gradually develops. A typical "frog leg" posture, characterized by abduction of the arms with flexion at the elbows, and abduction of the legs with flexion at the knees, is seen in the early stages of the disease.

Physical examination reveals marked hypotonia and generalized and symmetric weakness. Movements may be limited to flickering of the fingers and toes. The tendon reflexes almost invariably are absent. The child is unable to support the head and cannot straighten the trunk when held in ventral suspension. Respirations are shallow, and chest movements may be paradoxic. Feeding difficulties occur early, and secretions pool in the mouth as swallowing becomes further impaired. There may be visible atrophy and fasciculations of the tongue. The extraocular muscles are not affected. The child appears alert and attentive, and development is normal with the exception of motor skills. Contractures are not common in the early stages of the disease, although a small percentage of patients have congenital contractures or dislocation of the hip. The natural course is one of gradually increasing weakness, with feeding difficulties and respiratory compromise. In most cases, death occurs from a pulmonary infection with respiratory failure before the patient reaches 3 years of age.

The two most useful diagnostic studies are electromyography and muscle biopsy. Serum creatine phosphokinase and aldolase levels may be increased slightly, but more often are normal. Electromyography typically reveals fibrillations at rest, suggestive of active denervation, and a marked reduction of motor unit potentials on voluntary effort. Regular, repetitive, involuntary firing of single motor units appears to be unique to the acute form of SMA. The large, complex, polyphasic motor unit potentials that are characteristic of chronic denervation are not seen in young infants with this disorder. The muscle biopsy findings in infantile SMA are diagnostic, revealing large numbers of round, atrophic fibers intermingled with clumps of hypertrophic fibers of uniform histochemical type (Figure 212–1).

The treatment of acute infantile SMA is limited to supportive care. Respiratory insufficiency frequently becomes a problem before 1 year of age, and survival beyond 2 years of age is rare. Because of the poor prognosis of these children, artificial ventilation rarely, if ever, is justifiable. Appropriate genetic counseling is mandatory.

(Abridged from Julie Thorne Parke, Disorders of the Anterior Horn Cell, in Oski, DeAngelis, Feigin, McMillan, Warshaw: *Principles and Practice of Pediatrics, Second Edition*, J.B. Lippincott, 1994.)

Oski's Essential Pediatrics, edited by Kevin B. Johnson and Frank A. Oski. Lippincott–Raven Publishers, Philadelphia © 1997

213

Peripheral Neuropathy

Involvement of the peripheral nerves may occur in a variety of different disorders, including systemic diseases, infections, and poisonings. In addition, there are a number of hereditary diseases in which degeneration of the peripheral nerves is a major feature. Diseases of the peripheral nerve have been classified in a number of different ways. They may be categorized according to type of functional impairment (motor, sensory, autonomic, or mixed), site of pathologic involvement (primary involvement of axon or myelin), clinical course and tempo (acute, subacute, or chronic), or presumed etiology. None of these systems of classification is entirely satisfactory, and combinations of clinical, electrophysiologic, and pathologic features usually are employed to determine the etiology. Despite a thorough diagnostic search, the cause of polyneuropathy remains obscure in more than half of all cases.

■ INFLAMMATORY POLYRADICULONEUROPATHY (GUILLAIN-BARRÉ SYNDROME)

The most common cause of acute weakness from peripheral nerve involvement is Guillain-Barré syndrome (GBS). This syndrome is characterized by the acute or subacute development of a polyradiculoneuropathy, usually after an upper respiratory tract infection or an episode of gastroenteritis. A number of infectious agents have been associated with the illness, including Epstein-Barr virus, coxsackievirus, influenza viruses, echoviruses, cytomegalovirus, and *Mycoplasma pneumoniae*. GBS also may follow immunization. Pathologically, the disorder is characterized by the presence of inflammatory lesions, with segmental demyelination scattered throughout the peripheral nervous system. The most severely involved segments are the rootlets and the proximal portions of the peripheral nerves.

Clinical symptoms typically follow an antecedent infection after a latent period that varies in length from several days to several weeks. The most common initial symptoms are numbness and paresthesias of the hands and feet, followed by progressive weakness involving all four extremities. Motor impairment usually begins in the lower extremities and progresses in an ascending pattern to involve the upper extremities, trunk, and cranial nerves. A descending pattern of weakness also has been observed. Occasionally, the onset is abrupt, with simultaneous involvement of all extremities. The weakness usually is symmetric, although minor differences between the sides may occur.

There is a spectrum of motor involvement, varying from mild weakness to a complete flaccid quadriplegia. Muscle stretch reflexes are markedly reduced or absent. Involvement of the cranial nerves is common, with facial diplegia occurring in 50% of patients. Lower cranial nerve dysfunction may give rise to dysarthria and difficulty in swallowing and coughing. Significant respiratory muscle weakness occurs in 20% of patients and may necessitate artificial ventilation. Sensory symptoms are much less prominent than is weakness, but distal sensory loss, particularly involving proprioception and vibratory sensation, may be present.

The autonomic nervous system is involved frequently, with episodes of paroxysmal hypertension or hypotension, tachycardia or bradycardia, and facial flushing, and sweating abnormalities. Bowel and bladder function may be impaired early in the course of the disease, but sphincter dysfunction usually is short-lived. The neurologic symptoms evolve fairly rapidly over the first few days, with maximum disability reached within 1 week in most cases. There is a stable period of 1 to 3 weeks, after which recovery begins. The recovery may be rapid, taking place in 6 to 8 weeks, or it may be slow, lasting many months.

Many patients with GBS have some variation in clinical presentation or laboratory test results. The accepted criteria for the diagnosis of this syndrome are listed in Table 213–1. Several variants of GBS are recognized. The most common of the variants occurring in childhood is a syndrome of acute external ophthalmoplegia, ataxia, and areflexia known as the Miller-Fisher syndrome. The ophthalmoplegia often is bilateral and may be complete with pupillary involvement. The

TABLE 213-1. Criteria for Diagnosis of Guillain-Barré Syndrome

REQUIRED

Progressive motor weakness in more than one extremity

Areflexia (or distal areflexia with hyporeflexia of biceps and knee jerks)

STRONGLY SUPPORTIVE

Clinical features (in order of importance):

    Progression up to 4 weeks into illness

    Relative symmetry

    Mild sensory symptoms or signs

    Cranial nerve involvement (facial weakness in 50%)

    Recovery beginning 2 to 4 weeks after progression ceases

    Autonomic dysfunction

    Absence of fever at onset of symptoms

Cerebrospinal fluid (CSF) features:

    Protein level elevated after first week of symptoms

    Ten or fewer mononuclear leukocytes per mm^3

Electrodiagnostic features:

    Nerve conduction slowing or block (80%)

    Prolongation of F-wave latencies

CASTING DOUBT

Marked, persistent asymmetry of weakness

Persistent bowel or bladder dysfunction

Bowel or bladder dysfunction at onset

More than 50 mononuclear leukocytes per mm^3 in CSF

Presence of polymorphonuclear leukocytes in CSF

Sharp sensory level

RULE OUT THE DIAGNOSIS

Current history of hexacarbon abuse

Abnormal porphyrin metabolism

Recent diphtheritic infection

Evidence of lead neuropathy or intoxication

Purely sensory syndrome

Definite diagnosis of poliomyelitis, botulism, hysterical paralysis, or toxic neuropathy

Adapted from Asbury AK. Diagnostic considerations in Guillain-Barré syndrome. Ann Neurol. 1981;9(Suppl):1.

course usually is benign, with recovery taking place within 3 to 6 months.

The most important laboratory finding in patients with GBS is an elevated cerebrospinal fluid (CSF) protein content without a pleocytosis (albuminocytologic disproportion). The total CSF protein level may be normal in the early stages of the illness but is elevated in almost all patients after an interval of several days. The protein content continues to increase after the disease stabilizes, reaching a peak 2 to 4 weeks after the onset of the disease and ranging from 45 to 800 mg/dL.

Electrophysiologic studies also are helpful in the diagnosis of GBS, with abnormalities of motor and sensory conduction occurring in 90% of patients. Characteristic electrodiagnostic features include marked slowing of conduction velocities, prolonged distal latencies, and dispersion of the evoked responses. Proximal nerve conduction is characteristically slow and can be measured by studying the latency of the F response. This may be the only abnormal electrophysiologic finding in the early stages of the disease. In later stages of the disease, electromyographic studies may show denervation potentials indicating axonal damage, which is associated with a poor prognosis for complete recovery.

The treatment of GBS is largely supportive. Careful monitoring of respiratory function is very important during the early stages of the illness to prevent death as a result of respiratory failure. Elective intubation and mechanical ventilation should be used aggressively in patients with any evidence of respiratory compromise, because respiratory failure may occur abruptly if they become fatigued. Good nursing care and physiotherapy are important in severely affected patients. Most children with GBS recover completely, although the convalescence may be prolonged. The value of corticosteroids in the treatment of GBS has been debated, but no convincing evidence exists to support their use. Plasmapheresis has been shown to be beneficial both in shortening the length of the illness and in lessening the associated long-term disability. Recent studies suggest that treatment with high-dose intravenous immunoglobulin is similar in efficacy to plasmapheresis, but has fewer adverse effects.

A number of entities may produce a clinical picture similar to that of GBS. The ascending form of acute transverse myelitis and early cord compression may be difficult to distinguish from GBS initially. The presence of pyramidal tract signs, a clear sensory level, and persistent sphincter disturbances support involvement of the spinal cord rather than the root and peripheral nerve. Acute paralytic poliomyelitis may present with weakness simulating GBS, but there generally are more systemic symptoms, more marked meningeal signs, and a cellular response in the CSF. Uncommon conditions that may cause acute symmetric weakness include porphyria, diphtheritic polyneuropathy, heavy metal intoxication, systemic lupus erythematosus, periodic paralysis, tick paralysis, rabies, and botulism.

■ POSTINFECTIOUS NEUROPATHIES

Bell's palsy, an acute paralysis of the face, is the most common postinfectious neuropathy. It frequently occurs after mild upper respiratory tract infections or episodes of otitis media. Patients often complain of pain localized in the ear, which is followed by the rapid development of weakness of the entire side of the face. The nasolabial fold on the affected side is flattened, and the child may be unable to close the eye. Taste sensation may be altered, and there may be hyperacusis as a result of involvement of the nerve to the stapedius muscle.

The prognosis for recovery is good, particularly if the paralysis is not complete. Convalescence begins within a few days to several weeks. Some evidence suggests that treatment with corticosteroids may be beneficial if it is started within 2 to 3 days of the onset of weakness. Therapy should include measures to protect the exposed cornea of the affected eye by taping and using artificial tears. The differential diagnosis of an acute facial palsy includes demyelinating disease, brain stem tumor, otitis media, and mastoiditis.

A painless abducens nerve paralysis also may occur after a nonspecific viral illness. The prognosis for this type of cranial nerve VI palsy is excellent, with improvement beginning in 3 to 6 weeks and total recovery seen in most children by 3 months. Isolated oculomotor, glossopharyngeal, and hypoglossal nerve palsies occur much less commonly.

■ BRACHIAL PLEXOPATHY

An acute brachial plexopathy may occur in children after acute febrile illnesses or immunizations. The disorder is characterized by the sudden onset of pain in the shoulder and upper arm, followed by the rapid development of flaccid weakness involving primarily the muscles that are innervated by the upper roots of the brachial plexus. The paralysis may be severe, and atrophy of the affected muscles occurs. Sensory loss is minimal or absent. Electrophysiologic studies reveal slowing of nerve conduction velocities, low-amplitude evoked responses, and evidence of denervation. Physiotherapy is required to prevent contractures, because recovery tends to be very slow, occurring over many months.

■ HEREDITARY MOTOR AND SENSORY NEUROPATHY TYPE I (HYPERTROPHIC PERONEAL MUSCULAR ATROPHY, CHARCOT-MARIE-TOOTH DISEASE)

Hereditary motor and sensory neuropathy (HMSN) type I is the most common of the hereditary neuropathies. This type of peroneal muscular atrophy usually is inherited in an autosomal dominant manner, but autosomal recessive

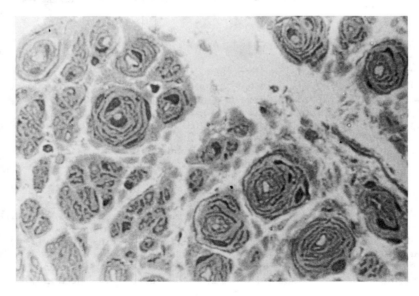

Figure 213-1. Sural nerve biopsy sample in a patient with hereditary motor and sensory neuropathy type 1 (Charcot-Marie-Tooth disease) shows multiple laminations of Schwann cells producing a characteristic "onion-bulb" formation.

and X-linked recessive modes of inheritance have been reported. The most common form of the disease is associated with a large, submicroscopic DNA duplication on the proximal 17p chromosome. There is marked variability in the clinical features among different family members. The onset is in childhood and the disorder is characterized by progressive weakness and atrophy beginning in the intrinsic foot muscles and the peroneal muscles. There often is a history of foot abnormalities such as pes cavus or hammer toe, and some family members with foot deformities do not have apparent weakness. The progressive footdrop causes the child to become progressively more clumsy and to trip frequently. The small muscles of the feet and the distal leg become atrophic, giving a "stork leg" or "inverted champagne bottle" appearance to the legs. As the disease progresses, intrinsic hand muscles and muscles of the proximal legs may become involved. Stretch reflexes are decreased or absent. Sensory function is normal or impaired only slightly. Peripheral nerves may be hypertrophic on palpation.

Reduced motor nerve conduction velocities are a hallmark of HMSN type I. Conduction velocities usually are less than one half of normal in the upper extremities and may be slowed profoundly in the lower extremities. Pathologically, there is a predominant loss of myelinated fibers in the peripheral nerves, with evidence of attempted remyelinization. Whorls of Schwann cells and multiple layers of poorly formed regenerating myelin cause a characteristic "onion bulb" appearance (Figure 213–1).

No specific treatment exists for HMSN type I, although ankle orthoses may help to alleviate the footdrop and improve the gait. Life expectancy is not reduced significantly, and patients usually remain ambulatory throughout life.

■ TOXIC NEUROPATHIES

Many pharmaceutical agents as well as toxic chemicals have been implicated as causes of peripheral neuropathy. The onset of these polyneuropathies usually is insidious after prolonged exposure to the toxin. A careful history of drug use and environmental exposure to toxins is of utmost importance in making a diagnosis. Some of the more common agents causing toxic neuropathies are listed in Table 213–2.

Lead poisoning in children typically produces symptoms similar to those of encephalopathy. On occasion, however, a peripheral neuropathy may precede the development of encephalopathic symptoms. Lead usually causes a motor neuropathy with only mild sensory impairment. The distribution of weakness is distal, with patients having either footdrop or wristdrop. The diagnosis is suggested by a history of pica and may be confirmed by an elevated lead concentration in the blood. Treatment consists of removal of the source of lead and administration of a chelating agent. Long-term arsenic intoxication may cause paresthesias and symmetric distal weakness, primarily in the feet and legs. Sensation is decreased in a glove and stocking distribution, and the tendon reflexes are depressed. Transverse white striae (Mees' lines) are seen in the fingernails 6 weeks after exposure. Cranial nerve involvement is unusual, and the CSF protein concentration is normal, helping to differentiate arsenic poisoning from GBS.

(Abridged from Julie Thorne Parke, Peripheral Neuropathy, in Oski, DeAngelis, Feigin, McMillan, Warshaw: *Principles and Practice of Pediatrics, Second Edition*, J.B. Lippincott, 1994.)

Oski's Essential Pediatrics,
edited by Kevin B. Johnson and Frank A. Oski.
Lippincott–Raven Publishers,
Philadelphia © 1997

214

Diseases of the Neuromuscular Junction

A number of different conditions may interfere with the transmission of the electrical impulse across the neuromuscular junction. The neuromuscular junction consists of the terminal portion of the motor nerve, the synaptic cleft, and the end plate region of the muscle. The nerve impulse originates in the anterior horn cell and is propagated down the axon of the motor nerve into the motor nerve terminals. Depolarization of the nerve terminals opens calcium channels, causing the release of acetylcholine into the synaptic cleft. Acetylcholine binds to receptors on the muscle end plate, altering the permeability to ions and causing localized depolarization of the end plate (the end plate potential). If the amplitude of the end plate potential reaches threshold, a muscle fiber action potential is generated. The muscle action potential is propagated along the muscle fiber and into the interior of the muscle fiber by the T tubules, initiating muscle fiber contraction. Acetylcholine acts at the postsynaptic membrane for only a brief period before it is broken down by an enzyme, cholinesterase, into two inactive components, choline and acetic acid. The choline is taken up by the presynaptic nerve terminal, where choline acetyltransferase catalyzes the resynthesis of acetylcholine.

TABLE 213-2. Toxic Neuropathies

INDUSTRIAL CHEMICALS AND INSECTICIDES
Acrylamide

Carbon disulfide

Cyanide

n-Hexane

Organophosphates (cholinergic symptoms with delayed-onset neuropathy)

Trichloroethylene (facial numbness)

Tri-orthocresylphosphate

METALS
Lead (especially neuropathy of radial nerve, causing wrist drop)

Arsenic (Mees' lines, sensory deficit)

Mercury

Thallium (ataxia, alopecia, seizures)

PHARMACEUTICAL AGENTS
Chloramphenicol

Cisplatin

Diphenylhydantoin

Disulfiram

Gold (may be acute)

Hydralazine

Isoniazid

Metronidazole

Vincristine

Neuromuscular transmission can fail if insufficient acetylcholine is released (presynaptic process) or if the number of acetylcholine receptors is insufficient to interact with the acetylcholine (postsynaptic disorder). Conditions interfering with the presynaptic events include some forms of congenital myasthenia gravis, botulism, hypocalcemia, hypermagnesemia, and neuromuscular blockade from antibiotics. Disorders affecting the postsynaptic events include autoimmune myasthenia gravis, some types of congenital myasthenia gravis, organophosphate poisoning, and iatrogenic neuromuscular blockade with curare (Table 214–1). Neuromuscular transmission failure also may occur if there is inhibition of or a deficiency in acetylcholinesterase, causing a depolarization block.

Disorders of neuromuscular transmission are manifested clinically by muscle weakness, which is exacerbated by exercise and improved by rest. Defects in neuromuscular transmission can be documented by pharmacologic tests and by electrophysiologic studies, including repetitive nerve stimulation and single-fiber electromyography.

JUVENILE MYASTHENIA GRAVIS

■ PATHOPHYSIOLOGY

The juvenile and adult forms of myasthenia gravis are autoimmune disorders characterized by an autoimmune attack on the acetylcholine receptor. Circulating antibodies to the acetylcholine receptor bind to the receptor on the muscle end plate, blocking its function. Morphologic studies show a simplified postsynaptic membrane with poorly developed folds and clefts, and a loss of functional acetylcholine receptor sites. Antibody can be demonstrated on the postsynaptic membrane, further implicating an immunologic process in its destruction. Circulating acetylcholine receptor antibodies can be measured, but the titer does not correlate well with the clinical condition of the patient. A lymphocyte-mediated immune response to acetylcholine receptors also has been identified. The thymus plays a role in the disease, possibly by sensitizing specific lymphocytes to produce acetylcholine receptor antibodies.

■ CLINICAL FEATURES

The onset of juvenile myasthenia gravis usually is after 10 years of age, although it can be much earlier. Girls are affected more commonly than are boys. The cardinal feature of the disease is easy fatigability. The onset usually is gradual, with symptoms most apparent in the afternoon or evening when the patient is tired. Occasionally, the onset is sudden and may appear to have been precipitated by an infectious illness. The weakness characteristically improves with rest and is made worse with sustained effort. In about one half of patients, weakness first appears in the ocular muscles, causing ptosis or diplopia (Figure 214–1). Ptosis frequently is asymmetric and may be unilateral. It tends to fluctuate during the day and to vary from day to day. Involvement of the ocular muscles is variable, but may be severe, causing a total ophthalmoplegia. About one fourth of patients have weakness of the bulbar musculature, resulting in difficulties speaking, swallowing, or chewing. The facial muscles are involved in most patients. Weakness of the palate and tongue may make speech unintelligible. The child's voice may be strong initially, becoming softer and less distinct during continued conversation. Difficulty chewing food is a common problem, and many patients support their jaw in one hand to assist with chewing. Swallowing difficulties and choking spells may occur. Weakness of the muscles of the neck, particularly the neck extensors, causes the head to fall forward. Patients with predominantly bulbar symptoms are at risk of the development of respiratory failure, particularly during an intercurrent infection.

TABLE 214-1. Disorders of Neuromuscular Transmission

PRESYNAPTIC
Botulism
Eaton-Lambert syndrome
Hypermagnesemia
Hypocalcemia
Snake bite
Antibiotics
Congenital myasthenia gravis
? Tick paralysis

INHIBITION OR DEFICIENCY OF ACETYLCHOLINESTERASE
Organophosphates
Congenital myasthenia gravis

POSTSYNAPTIC
Autoimmune myasthenia gravis
Curare (d-tubocurarine)
α-Bungarotoxin
Congenital myasthenia gravis

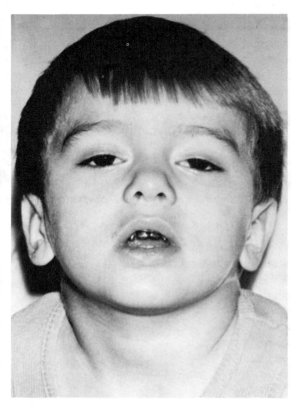

Figure 214-1. Four-year-old child with juvenile myasthenia gravis, exhibiting fluctuating ptosis and bilateral facial weakness.

A smaller number of children (about 20%) have generalized weakness of the extremities. Fatigability may be demonstrated in younger children by having them climb stairs or hold their arms outstretched for an interval. In older children, repetitive testing of deltoid strength or performance of multiple deep knee bends may help disclose the weakness. Regardless of the distribution of weakness, the principal features are a fluctuating quality to the weakness and susceptibility to fatigue. These features differ from those of other neuromuscular disorders, which produce relatively constant symptoms.

■ DIAGNOSTIC STUDIES

The diagnosis of myasthenia gravis usually can be made on the basis of the history and physical examination, and may be confirmed by pharmacologic tests. A small dose of an anticholinesterase drug produces a dramatic improvement in strength. Edrophonium chloride (Tensilon) is preferred because of its rapid onset and short duration of action. The availability of acetylcholine is increased by inhibiting the enzyme cholinesterase, thereby improving neuromuscular transmission. A marked but short-lived improvement in weakness usually is seen in patients with myasthenia. Neostigmine may be used if a longer effect is necessary to evaluate limb strength.

Electrophysiologic studies are helpful in documenting transmission failure at the neuromuscular junction. Repetitive nerve stimulation produces a characteristic fall in amplitude between the first and the fourth or fifth responses (decremental response). It may be necessary to test several muscles, because the abnormality may not be present in all muscles. Selective single-fiber electromyography is possible in some patients and may confirm the variability in synaptic transmission time in patients with rather mild disease. Antibodies to the human muscle acetylcholine receptor are found in the serum of as many as 90% of patients. Unfortunately, the patients with negative antibody test results typically are those with purely ocular weakness or mild generalized weakness in whom the diagnosis is uncertain. A negative test result does not exclude the diagnosis.

■ TREATMENT AND PROGNOSIS

A number of different therapeutic modalities are available for the treatment of myasthenia gravis. The approach selected should take into consideration the age of the patient, the severity of the disease, and the potential benefits and risks of each form of therapy. Cholinesterase inhibitors improve neuromuscular transmission by inhibiting the enzymatic degradation of acetylcholine, prolonging its effect on the muscle end plate. These agents result in symptomatic improvement in strength in most patients with myasthenia gravis and may be sufficient to produce normal or near-normal strength in some. Pyridostigmine bromide (Mestinon) and neostigmine bromide (Prostigmin) are the most commonly used agents (Table 214–2). Other treatment modalities, including thymectomy, corticosteroid therapy, and immunosuppressive agents, are aimed more directly at the basic immunologic mechanism of the disease.

The prognosis of patients with juvenile myasthenia gravis is relatively good, in that complete or partial remissions occur in 25% within 2 years of onset of the disease. The disease often is characterized by a fluctuating course of remissions and exacerbations, however. The severity of symptoms is variable, and some children have severe disease necessitating frequent hospitalizations and mechanical ventilatory support. About 80% of children improve after thymectomy.

CONGENITAL MYASTHENIA GRAVIS

There are several rare varieties of congenital myasthenia gravis with onset at birth or in early childhood and persistent symptoms. The disorders usually are familial, with autosomal recessive inheritance occurring most frequently. Similar to other disorders of neuromuscular transmission, the syndromes are characterized by fluctuating weakness. Recurrent episodes of apnea may occur. Severe ocular muscle weakness is characteristic of several of the syndromes. Congenital myasthenia gravis differs from acquired myasthenia gravis in that there is no evidence of an autoimmune etiology. Detailed physiologic and morphologic studies have identified specific abnormalities in the neuromuscular junction in patients with several of the syndromes (Table 214–3). Patients with these disorders do not respond to immunosuppressive therapy or to thymectomy. The response to cholinesterase inhibitors is variable.

BOTULISM

■ PATHOPHYSIOLOGY

The exotoxin of *Clostridium botulinum* is one of the most potent neurotoxins known. It is absorbed from the intestine or an infected wound and is distributed in a hematogenous manner to peripheral cholinergic nerve synapses, such as the neuromuscular junction. The toxin irreversibly blocks acetylcholine release from the presynaptic nerve terminals. Recovery occurs by sprouting of terminal motor neurons and the formation of new motor end plates.

In children and adults, poisoning may occur after ingestion of the toxin in inadequately cooked or improperly canned food. The anaerobic bacillus and the exotoxin it produces are destroyed by heat, so proper cooking of food should eliminate outbreaks. At high altitudes, water boils at a lower temperature and the exotoxin is not destroyed during boiling, accounting for the greater frequency of botulism in mountain locales. The majority of outbreaks of botulism can be traced to home-canned foods, particularly vegetables, fruits, fish, and condiments. Wound botulism results from infection of traumatized tissue by the organism, with subsequent toxin production. Most cases occur subsequent to wounds sustained in open fields or on farms, particularly compound extremity

---

TABLE 214-2. Cholinesterase Inhibitors in the Treatment of Myasthenia Gravis

Drug
Pyridostigmine bromide (Mestinon)
Neostigmine bromide (Prostigmin)
Neostigmine methylsulfate

*IM, *intramuscular;* IV, *intravenous.*

TABLE 214-3. Distinguishing Features of Congenital Myasthenic Syndromes

Features	Defect in ACh Synthesis or Mobilization	End-Plate AChE Deficiency	Slow-Channel Syndrome	End-Plate AChR Deficiency
Inheritance	Recessive	Recessive	Dominant	Recessive
Abnormal fatigability	+	+	+	+
Reduced muscle bulk	−	+	+	Occasionally +
Hyporeflexia	−	+	+, −	−
Age at onset of symptoms	At birth	At birth	Variable	At birth
Response to anticholinesterase drugs	+	−	+, −	+
Circulating AChR antibodies	−	−	−	−

AChR, *acetylcholine;* AChE, *acetylcholinesterase;* AChR, *acetylcholine receptor.*
After Engel A. Myasthenia gravis and myasthenic syndromes. Ann Neurol. *1984;16:519.*

fractures. A third type of botulism, infant botulism, differs from foodborne and wound botulism because it is caused by ingestion of the spores of *C botulinum* rather than the exotoxin. It occurs almost exclusively in children in the first year of life, usually in those between 5 and 12 weeks of age. The ingested spores colonize the intestinal tract and produce the *C botulinum* toxin. The source of the spores frequently is not found. Honey has been implicated as the source in about 20% of patients, however, and environmental sources, such as yard soil, have been implicated in other cases.

Seven antigenically distinct types of *C botulinum* toxin have been identified. Disease in humans is caused primarily by toxin types A, B, E, and F. Type E botulism almost always can be traced to fish and fish products. Almost all cases of infant botulism have been caused by toxin types A or B.

■ CLINICAL FEATURES

Clinical symptoms appear within 1 to 2 days after the consumption of contaminated food or within 1 to 2 weeks after wound inoculation. The initial symptoms of foodborne infection may resemble those of food poisoning: vomiting, diarrhea, and abdominal pain. Commonly, similar symptoms develop in several members of a family. Weakness of the extraocular muscles occurs, causing blurred vision and diplopia. Failure of convergence may be the first symptom. Visual problems often are accompanied by other bulbar symptoms, including dizziness, dysarthria, and dysphagia. Some patients have only bulbar symptoms; others have varying degrees of extremity weakness. Weakness may occur rapidly after the ingestion of large amounts of toxin, causing a flaccid paralysis and respiratory failure. In wound botulism, the toxin is released slowly into the circulation so that the onset of symptoms and the progression of weakness are slower. Examination reveals involvement of the extraocular muscles. Pupillary responses may or may not be affected. Tendon reflexes typically are absent, but may be present. Sensory abnormalities are not seen. In patients with milder disease, fatigability is not as prominent as in patients with myasthenia gravis.

The clinical appearance of infant botulism is different from that of foodborne or wound botulism. Constipation is the first sign of illness, although this symptom frequently may be overlooked. Infants gradually become listless and weak over a period of days to weeks. As the bulbar muscles become involved, there is difficulty feeding and the cry becomes weaker. Drooling and pooling of food and secretions in the posterior pharynx may occur. Ptosis, ophthalmoplegia, and diminished facial expression are present. Hypotonia and generalized muscle weakness most often are manifest initially as a loss of head control. Respiratory arrest may occur abruptly in patients with severe disease. Botulism may be responsible for some cases of unexpected sudden death in infancy.

■ DIAGNOSTIC STUDIES

Electrophysiologic studies are helpful in demonstrating a disturbance in neuromuscular transmission in patients with botulism. The compound muscle action potential elicited by a single stimulus to the nerve is small, and the amplitude declines with repetitive stimulation at a slow rate. Repetitive stimulation at fast rates produces an increase in the amplitude of muscle action potentials. Needle examination demonstrates a distinctive pattern of brief, small, abundant motor unit potentials that may be diagnostic of botulism in the context of the clinical syndrome. Confirmation of the diagnosis of botulism depends on detection of the toxin or the organism in the patient or the implicated food. In infant botulism, the organism may be isolated from stool culture.

■ DIFFERENTIAL DIAGNOSIS

Botulism in children must be distinguished from myasthenia gravis, Guillain-Barré syndrome, tick paralysis, and chemical intoxications. Patients with myasthenia gravis typically have preserved pupillary reactions and usually do not have areflexia. Fatigability is much more prominent in myasthenia gravis, and the edrophonium chloride (Tensilon) test result is dramatically positive. Clinical differentiation from Guillain-Barré syndrome may be difficult. Patients with Guillain-Barré syndrome usually have ascending weakness, with a later onset of cranial nerve involvement. Frequent paresthesias and elevated cerebrospinal fluid (CSF) protein content also help to distinguish this disorder. Electromyography is helpful in differentiating both Guillain-Barré syndrome and myasthenia gravis from botulism.

In addition to these disorders, the differential diagnosis of infant botulism includes Werdnig-Hoffmann disease, poliomyelitis, and diphtheria. The early extraocular muscle and pupillary involvement, the symmetry of weakness, and the absence of fever or pharyngitis, as well as the characteristic electrophysiologic findings, should increase the suspicion of botulism.

■ TREATMENT AND PROGNOSIS

The treatment of all forms of botulism is directed toward aggressive supportive care, with particular attention paid to respiratory support. The prognosis generally is good if the patient is supported adequately, although recovery may be very slow, taking weeks to many months in severely affected individuals. In cases of foodborne botulism, if the patient is seen early, emetics and gastric lavage should be used to reduce the amount of unabsorbed toxin. Antitoxin may be given, although evidence of its efficacy once neurologic manifestations have occurred is lacking. If foodborne botulism is suspected, state and federal health officials should be notified immediately. The treatment of wound botulism includes exploration and debridement of the site, in conjunction with antitoxin and antibiotic therapy. Guanidine may be of some value in improving muscle strength in mild or moderately severe cases of foodborne or wound botulism. Infant botulism is a self-limiting disease, generally lasting 2 to 6 weeks. The use of antitoxin and antibiotics has not been shown to influence its course. Antibiotics are not used because bacterial death may liberate *C botulinum* toxin, increasing the amount of toxin in the gastrointestinal tract. Aggressive supportive care is required throughout the period of hypotonia and weakness, and many infants require prolonged ventilator support. Constipation may persist for months and may improve with the use of stool softeners and adequate hydration. The mortality with botulism is 20% to 25% in cases of foodborne or wound botulism. The mortality of recognized cases of infant botulism is about 3%. Relapse of infant botulism after apparent resolution of clinical symptoms may occur, making close follow-up necessary.

TICK PARALYSIS

■ PATHOPHYSIOLOGY

A progressive, ascending flaccid paralysis may be caused by the attachment of certain species of ticks. In North America, the disease is caused most commonly by *Dermacentor andersoni* (wood tick) or *Dermacentor variabilis* (dog tick). *Ixodes holocyclus* (scrub tick) is the cause of the disease in Australia. Most cases of tick paralysis occur in the spring or summer and involve young children, especially girls with long hair. The tick frequently attaches near the hairline, where it remains unnoticed. Clinical symptoms begin within several days after the tick attaches. Tick paralysis is thought to be caused by a toxin released by the ticks, but the exact mechanism and site of the toxin's action are not known. It has been postulated that the toxin prevents depolarization in the terminal portions of the motor neurons.

■ CLINICAL FEATURES

Tick paralysis may begin with general symptoms such as irritability and diarrhea. Initial neurologic signs include gait ataxia and areflexia. Weakness of the legs then becomes apparent and advances in an ascending, symmetric pattern to involve the trunk and upper extremities. If the tick remains attached, the weakness may progress to involve the bulbar musculature, producing dysarthria, dysphagia, blurred vision, and facial weakness. Respiratory compromise may occur. Patients may complain of numbness and tingling of the extremities, but objective sensory abnormalities are rare.

■ DIAGNOSTIC STUDIES

Routine laboratory studies are not helpful in establishing the diagnosis of tick paralysis. The CSF protein level is normal, which helps to distinguish tick paralysis from Guillain-Barré syndrome. Electrophysiologic studies usually reveal a reduced amplitude of the compound muscle action potential, with no significant incremental or decremental response with repetitive stimulation. Motor and sensory nerve conduction velocities are decreased slightly in the distal segments.

■ TREATMENT AND PROGNOSIS

Recovery occurs within 1 to 5 days after removal of the tick. Intensive supportive care with assisted ventilation for respiratory failure may be required during this period. The tick must be removed for recovery to occur. Removal is achieved best by covering the tick with petrolatum to cause it to withdraw before removing it with forceps. Care should be taken to remove the entire tick so secondary infection does not occur.

NEUROMUSCULAR TOXINS

A number of pharmacologic and environmental agents may interfere with neuromuscular transmission (Table 214–4). Organophosphates, such as parathion, cause irreversible inhibition of acetylcholinesterase, resulting in an accumulation of acetylcholine in the synaptic cleft. These insecticides cause muscle paralysis with prominent autonomic symptoms. Common neuromuscular blocking agents used in anesthesia, such as succinylcholine, may cause prolonged paralysis in patients with clinical or subclinical myasthenia gravis. A number of antibiotics, such as neomycin,

TABLE 214-4. Drugs Affecting Neuromuscular Transmission

Antibiotics (tetracyclines, trimethoprim, polymyxins, aminoglycosides, lincomycin, clindamycin)

β-Adrenergic blockers (propranolol)

Phenytoin

Procainamide

Quinidine

Chloroquine

Lithium

Phenothiazines

Succinylcholine

Pancuronium bromide

Anticholinesterases

Adrenocorticotropic hormone

Corticosteroids

streptomycin, kanamycin, colistin, and tetracycline, interfere with the release of acetylcholine, aggravating preexisting neuromuscular transmission problems. Several other drugs, including propranolol, phenytoin, and corticosteroids, may have a similar effect on neuromuscular transmission. The treatment of drug-induced neuromuscular blockade consists of supportive care and the substitution of a different drug.

(Abridged from Julie Thorne Parke, Diseases of the Neuromuscular Junction, in Oski, DeAngelis, Feigin, McMillan, Warshaw: Principles and Practice of Pediatrics, Second Edition, J.B. Lippincott, 1994.)

Oski's Essential Pediatrics,
edited by Kevin B. Johnson and Frank A. Oski.
Lippincott–Raven Publishers,
Philadelphia © 1997

215

Hereditary and Acquired Types of Myopathy

■ DUCHENNE TYPE MUSCULAR DYSTROPHY

Duchenne type muscular dystrophy (DMD) is the most severe form of progressive primary muscular degeneration and is associated with a genetic abnormality in band 1 of region 2 of the short (p) arm of the X chromosome. This genetic locus is designated Xp2.1. About 1:3000 liveborn males has this condition, with one third of all cases representing new mutations. The dystrophy is manifest at birth, becomes clinically evident between 3 and 5 years of age, and progresses inexorably over the next 2 decades before culminating in the death of the patient. Most patients become wheelchair dependent between 10 and 12 years of age. Complications result from cardiac involvement, nervous system involvement, musculoskeletal deformities, and failing respiratory function. Levels of serum enzymes that originate from skeletal muscle are elevated, most notably creatine kinase (CK). The CK value is very high after birth and remains remarkably elevated during the presymptomatic phase, permitting early diagnosis of siblings at risk. Rarely, the infant is affected clinically. Infant macroglossia has been noted on occasion and motor milestones may be delayed. One third of patients with DMD are late walkers (*ie,* they do not walk independently until after 15 to 18 months of age). Parents retrospectively report developmental clumsiness and motor sluggishness in running, climbing stairs, rising from the ground after falling, and pedaling a tricycle. Abnormalities of gait and posture appear in middle childhood with the emergence of increasing lumbar lordosis, pelvic waddling, frequent falling, and Gowers' sign. Although it is distinctive in DMD, Gowers' sign may be seen in patients with any condition that causes pelvic girdle weakness. Enlargement of the musculature becomes evident, with characteristic involvement of calf, gluteal, lateral vastus, deltoid, and infraspinatus groups. Weakness is more evident in the proximal muscles, and tendon reflexes are diminished at the knees, biceps, and triceps. Only in the preterminal phase are the distal tendon reflexes noticeably affected. Contractures of the iliotibial bands, hip flexors, and heel cords develop before ambulation is lost. After ambulation is lost, the muscles decrease in size, contractures progress with loss of joint mobility, and kyphoscoliosis develops with further compromise of respiratory function.

Cardiac involvement is evident in all patients with DMD, but rarely is the cause of death. Similarly, cardiac abnormalities may be noted in female carriers of DMD, even when the serum CK values are normal. Degenerating muscle fibers and small foci of fibrosis are scattered throughout the myocardium and conduction systems. The posterobasal region and adjacent lateral wall of the left ventricle are involved commonly and prominently. The electrocardiographic (ECG) changes are distinctive: tall right precordial R waves and deep Q waves in the left precordial and limb leads.

Nervous system involvement has been recognized since the earliest descriptions of DMD. It is a nonprogressive process and may be associated with "atrophy" of the brain on computed tomography (CT). Some patients also have macrocephaly. The mean intelligence quotient (IQ) is about 80, and the individual IQ values correspond to a gaussian, bell-shaped distribution curve. It is not known whether the associated mental retardation is another example of a contiguous gene syndrome.

The electromyogram (EMG) is distinctively myopathic, with decreases in the amplitude and duration of the compound action potential and enrichment of the interference pattern. A large number of the motor units are polyphasic, and occasional sparse fibrillation potentials are observed consistently. Sensory and motor conduction velocities are normal.

The diagnosis of DMD can be made reliably in virtually every case with available information. The clinical presentation and course are constant in most instances. The CK value is very high in the preclinical phase and falls gradually as the muscle mass disappears in later years. The EMG and ECG findings are distinctive, and the morphologic findings on biopsy of the skeletal muscle are characteristic. Dystrophic immunoreactivity of muscle obtained on biopsy and analysis of blood DNA finalize the diagnosis. This constellation of clinical and laboratory findings permits the exclusion of those diseases that masquerade clinically as DMD in almost every case. The emerging molecular and biochemical advances should add measurably to our understanding of the phenotypic expressions of diseases associated with a genetic defect at the Xp2.1 locus, collectively referred to as dystrophinopathies.

■ BECKER'S MUSCULAR DYSTROPHY

Two other disorders share a genetic defect at or near the Xp2.1 locus: Becker's muscular dystrophy (BMD) and the McLeod syndrome. BMD represents a more benign version of DMD. Current information indicates that BMD and DMD are allelic gene abnormalities. BMD is similar to DMD, but the age of onset is later and the progression is slower (Table 215–1).

Pseudohypertrophy is striking and pes cavus deformities are present frequently in patients with BMD. Unlike in DMD, cardiac and nervous system involvement are unusual. Patients with BMD may have children, although infertility is higher in this population. All female progeny are obligate carriers, and all sons are unaffected.

■ LIMB-GIRDLE SYNDROMES

Walton and Nattrass, in 1954, introduced the term *limb-girdle muscular dystrophy* to describe a number of patients who did not fulfill the clinical criteria for DMD or facioscapulo-humeral (FSH) dystrophy. The patients were either male or

TABLE 215-1. Age (y) of Onset, Loss of Ambulation, and Death in BMD and DMD

Clinical Event	DMD	BMD
Onset	3–5	12
Loss of ambulation	9.0 ± 2.3	30.5 ± 12.0
Death	16.2 ± 3.7	42.0 ± 15.9

female, often were in middle to late childhood, and had serum enzyme, EMG, and skeletal muscle biopsy abnormalities of the type commonly encountered in patients with a muscular dystrophy. This large and ill-defined group of patients has been whittled down to a much smaller group as newer entities have been identified. We now recognize juvenile spinal muscular atrophy, congenital types of myopathy (*eg*, central core disease), and metabolic forms of myopathy, all of which previously were classified as limb-girdle muscular dystrophy. A small group of patients still exists who have a dystrophic process that is inherited as an autosomal recessive trait, however, justifying continued use of the term. Some of these patients will prove to have Xp2.1 locus genetic defects presenting in males or females. The availability of a biochemical probe for various types of dystrophy will help sort out these issues in the near future. For the moment, the term *limb-girdle* represents a convenient diagnostic pigeonhole when other diagnostic explanations fall short.

■ FACIOSCAPULOHUMERAL DYSTROPHY

The syndrome of FSH dystrophy and its variants are inherited as autosomal dominant traits, and their expression may be variable, even among family members. As the term implies, facial, periscapular, and humeral muscle groups are affected. Unlike most forms of dystrophy, involvement may be asymmetric and an isolated congenital absence of a muscle may occur. The condition generally is benign, presenting in adolescence and progressing slowly over decades, often with periods of clinical arrest. A few cases have started in infancy with a more malignant course. Initial presentation as Möbius' syndrome with congenital facial weakness also has been described. Early childhood onset may be associated with a sensorineural hearing loss or an exudative telangiectasia of the retina (Coats' disease). The clinical presentation in childhood, however, usually is more subtle. Patients may sleep with their eyes partially open and have difficulty whistling or sipping through a straw. One variant is known as the scapuloperoneal syndrome; scapular winging and footdrop are common signs. Subtle weakness of the facial muscles may coexist or develop later.

The pathogenesis of these syndromes is obscure. Some cases seem to have myopathic elements, and others are distinctly neurogenic. The biopsy samples also may have some prominent inflammatory features, raising the question of an inflammatory myopathy and justifying a clinical trial with corticosteroids. In some patients, surgical fixation of the scapulae to the posterior thoracic wall improves shoulder-girdle function.

■ MITOCHONDRIAL DISEASES

Defects of mitochondrial metabolism are being recognized with increasing frequency. Morphologic abnormalities of mitochondria have been observed in some patients. Mitochondria were either overly abundant, very large, or misshapen. A distinctive abnormality of mitochondria was evident at the light microscopic level with the modified Gomori trichrome stain, and fibers containing this abnormality were labeled "ragged-red." Ragged-red fibers are distinctive and usually represent the morphologic counterpart of suspected or proven biochemical defects that affect the inner mitochondrial membrane. Current information suggests that ragged-red fibers are seen in those mitochondrial diseases that are associated with a defect involving intramitochondrial protein synthesis. The muscle morphology may be normal in patients with other mitochondrial diseases, however, such as carnitine palmitoyl transferase (CPT) deficiency. This fact emphasizes the need for a classification scheme that is predicated on biochemical and molecular genetic criteria.

The classification of mitochondrial diseases is based on the principal metabolic pathways located in this organelle and on the dual genetic control of the respiratory chain (Figure 215–1). Organic acids, fatty acids, and amino acids are the principal sources of fuel, and each substrate is metabolized to acetylcoenzyme A (acetyl-CoA). Acetyl-CoA condenses with oxaloacetate to form citric acid. Citric acid is oxidized in the Krebs' cycle. The reducing equivalents that are generated during oxidation enter the respiratory chain and are reoxidized. The energy of oxidation is coupled to the phosphorylation of adenosine diphosphate, ultimately yielding adenosine triphosphate.

Primary mitochondrial DNA defects occur sporadically or are inherited as maternal, nonmendelian traits. Maternal inheritance resembles X-linked and autosomal-dominant inheritance patterns in that the maternally transmitted trait is passed from the mother to her children, and the disease appears in consecutive generations. The maternally inherited trait differs from the X-linked inherited trait because both male and female progeny inherit the condition from their mother. Similarly, the maternally inherited trait differs from the autosomal-dominant trait because a higher percentage (theoretically, 100%) of the progeny are affected. The phenotypic expression of a maternally inherited trait is modulated by replicative segregation and the threshold effect. These two concepts are predicated on the fact that there are multiple mitochondrial DNA copies in each mitochondrion, and there are hundreds or thousands of mitochondria in each cell. As a result, the distribution of wild-type mitochondrial DNA and mutated mitochondrial DNA drifts randomly in each successive cell division. As the percentage of mutated mitochondrial DNA copies approaches a theoretic threshold, the cellular phenotype reflects the genotype and displays energy failure.

Kearns-Sayre syndrome is characterized by three fundamental criteria: pigmentary degeneration of the retina, ophthalmoplegia, and clinical onset before 20 years of age. Other signs often occur, including heart block, cerebellar syndrome, and an elevated cerebrospinal fluid (CSF) protein concentration in excess of 100 mg/dL. Ragged-red fibers are present in skeletal muscle obtained at biopsy, and sensorineural hearing loss is frequent. Endocrine disturbances are associated with this syndrome, and short stature is the most common problem. Diabetes mellitus and hypoparathyroidism may develop, and may contribute to fatal episodes of coma or to seizures, respectively. A spongy degeneration is seen without exception in the brain of all patients examined at autopsy. Basal ganglia calcification is observed in all patients with hypoparathyroidism. Folic acid levels are reduced in the CSF, and coenzyme Q10 concentrations in serum and muscle are decreased. Replacement therapy has been proposed on the basis of these observations. A cardiac pacemaker is necessary as therapy for heart block.

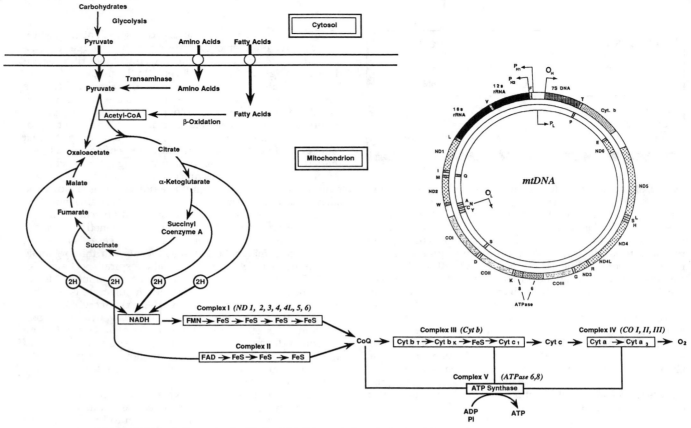

Figure 215-1. Pathways involved in the oxidative metabolism of mitochondrial fuels. The current classification of mitochondrial diseases is based on this scheme. Five events are important: (1) mitochondrial transport of substrates; (2) substrate utilization; (3) oxidation in the Krebs' cycle; (4) oxidation-phosphorylation; and (5) cellular respiration. The mitochondrial genome is inserted in the diagram to signify its role in the respiratory chain. The 13 mtDNA-encoded subunits of the respiratory chain are shown in parentheses above complexes I, III, IV, and V. *NADH*, the reduced form of nicotinamine-adenine dinucleotide; *ATPase*, adenosine triphosphatase; *ATP*, adenosine triphosphate; *ADP*, adenosine diphosphate; *FMN*, flavin mononucleotide; *FAD*, flavin adenine dinucleotide; *CoQ*, coenzyme Q; *PI*, inorganic phosphate.

Virtually all reported cases of Kearns-Sayre syndrome have been sporadic, and about 98% of affected patients have major deletions of the mitochondrial genome. Sporadic cases of progressive external ophthalmoplegia also have been associated with these deletions, suggesting that this abnormality of ocular motility is the minimal clinical expression of Kearns-Sayre syndrome. Large mitochondrial DNA deletions also have been observed in infants with Pearson syndrome, a frequently fatal sporadic disease of infancy manifested by pancytopenia and pancreatic exocrine dysfunction. In addition, large mitochondrial DNA deletions have been described in a family with maternally inherited diabetes mellitus and deafness.

Myoclonus epilepsy and ragged-red fibers (MERRF) is otherwise known as the Fukuhara syndrome. The clinical expression of this disease is dominated by myoclonus, ataxia, limb weakness, and generalized seizures. Most patients have symptoms in childhood or early adolescence. Associated signs often include dementia, optic atrophy, short stature, hearing loss, and proprioceptive sensory loss in the legs.

Spongy degeneration of the brain has been observed in all patients with MERRF who have been examined at autopsy. CT and magnetic resonance imaging scans reveal brain atrophy. The electroencephalogram characteristically shows paroxysmal epileptiform discharges that are either focal or generalized. The blood and CSF lactate values often are increased, but the CSF protein level usually is normal.

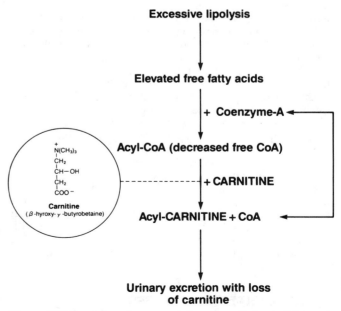

Figure 215-2. Schematic representation of carnitine esterification of activated fatty acids and urinary excretion resulting in secondary carnitine depletion.

Endocrine disturbances have been limited to one case of "hypothalamic disorder" and one case of isolated adrenocorticotropic hormone deficiency. Positron emission tomography revealed cerebral and cerebellar hypometabolism in one case. MERRF is inherited as a maternal trait. About 75% of affected patients have a mitochondrial DNA point mutation involving the transfer RNA^{lys} gene. No effective treatment is available for patients with MERRF aside from seizure control.

MELAS (mitochondrial myopathy, encephalopathy, lactic acidosis, and strokelike episodes) has been described in more than 70 patients. The original criteria included normal early development, short stature, seizures, and sudden onset of hemiparesis, hemianopsia, or cortical blindness. Dementia was prominent in several cases, as was episodic vomiting, headache, and hearing loss. CT scan revealed focal lucencies in several cases, and basal ganglia calcifications in some. Diffuse spongy degeneration of the brain and focal encephalomalacia were seen at autopsy. Acanthocytes were reported in one case. Marked deficiency of the reduced form of nicotinamide-adenine dinucleotide (NADH)–cytochrome c reductase (complex I) has been reported in about 35% of affected individuals. MELAS is inherited as a maternal trait, and

about 80% of patients fulfilling the clinical criteria for this condition have a mitochondrial DNA point mutation involving the transfer RNA $^{leu(UUR)}$ gene. Coenzyme Q10 is beneficial in treatment, and vigorous attempts should be made to control seizure activity.

Defects of Mitochondrial Transport

Carnitine deficiency represents an example of defective mitochondrial transport. Historically, two forms of carnitine deficiency have been discussed: one confined to muscle (myopathic) and the second involving a generalized defect in carnitine (systemic). The myopathic form involved a defect in the uptake of carnitine by muscle. Consequently, transport of long-chain fatty acids across the inner mitochondrial membrane is blocked, with resulting accumulation of neutral lipids in the cytoplasm. This lipid storage is associated with a progressive weakness that begins in childhood. The carnitine concentrations are decreased in muscle, but normal in blood and liver. A defect in the active transport of carnitine into muscle has been suspected, but never

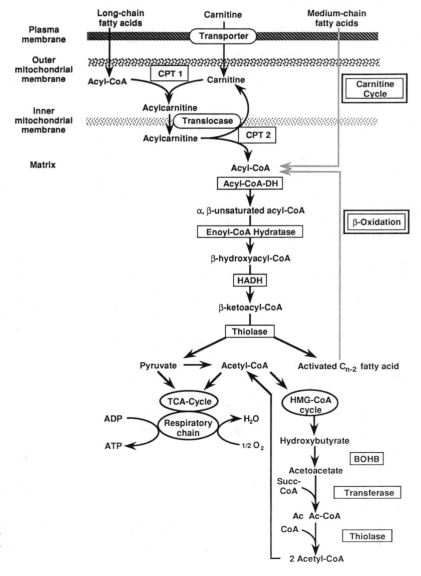

Figure 215-3. Schematic representation of fatty acid oxidation and ketone body synthesis. *ADP,* adenosine diphosphate; *ATP,* adenosine triphosphate.

proven. Patients with myopathic carnitine deficiency have been shown to have a skeletal muscle tissue–specific deficiency of short-chain acyl coenzyme A (acyl CoA) dehydrogenase. Some patients respond to carnitine supplementation or to prednisone. The mechanism of action of prednisone is unknown.

Systemic carnitine deficiency is manifested by recurrent encephalopathy that often is triggered by an intercurrent infection. This presentation is similar to that of Reye's syndrome. Carnitine concentrations are decreased in the serum and tissues, and there is excessive urinary excretion of carnitine. The legitimacy of systemic carnitine deficiency has been questioned since its first description in 1975. Most investigators believe that other biochemical mechanisms are at play to account for the reduced body stores of carnitine. Carnitine deficiency may result from excessive urinary loss, impaired hepatic synthesis, or associated genetic defects. Secondary carnitine deficiency is recognized with organic acidurias, respiratory chain defects, and defects of beta oxidation. Carnitine depletion results from the esterification of acyl CoA compounds that accumulate in these syndromes. The acyl-carnitine esters are water-soluble and are excreted in the urine, resulting in a net loss of carnitine (Figure 215–2). Several patients previously described as having systemic carnitine deficiency have been shown to have a deficiency of medium-chain acyl CoA dehydrogenase. Other patients have a genetically determined autosomal recessive carnitine-responsive cardiomyopathy resulting from a primary defect of the plasma membrane carnitine transporter system. Carnitine supplementation is lifesaving in these patients, and supplementation is recommended whenever carnitine deficiency is documented.

At least 13 defects of fatty acid and ketone body metabolism have been described, as shown in Figure 215–3. Some of the defects involving the carnitine cycle were discussed earlier in this section, including the membrane carnitine transporter defect and CPT II deficiency. A deficiency of CPT I has been described in about 10 patients. These patients have an illness similar to Reye's syndrome in infancy and may have associated renal tubular acidosis. This symptom responds to treatment with medium-chain triglycerides. Only one patient has been described with a defect of the carnitine-acylcarnitine translocase. This patient and the several patients described with the membrane carnitine transporter defect have very low tissue carnitine concentrations. Patients with CPT II deficiency have normal tissue and plasma carnitine concentrations. Patients with CPT I deficiency may have normal or high carnitine concentrations. Patients with defects involving the carnitine cycle demonstrate little, if any, dicarboxylic aciduria.

In contrast, patients with defects involving beta oxidation have remarkable dicarboxylic aciduria and carnitine deficiency. Five of these defects involve the first step in beta oxidation involving the conversion of acyl CoA to alpha-, beta-unsaturated acyl CoA. Three different acyl CoA dehydrogenases have been identified acting on either long-chain, medium-chain, or short-chain activated fatty acids. All three dehydrogenases use flavin adenine denucleotide (FAD) as a cofactor. Reoxidation of FAD is accomplished by two FAD-dependent electron carriers (electron transfer factor [ETF] and ETF-dehydrogenase). The electrons ultimately are transferred to coenzyme Q10, which is located centrally within the respiratory chain. Acetyl-CoA, resulting from the beta oxidation of fatty acids, enters the Krebs' cycle or the HMG-CoA cycle that is important in the biosynthesis of ketone bodies.

Severe hypoglycemic hypoketotic crises developing during prolonged fasting, physical exercise, or intercurrent infec-

tions characterize the clinical presentation of most patients with defects of beta oxidation. Medium-chain acyl CoA dehydrogenase deficiency is the most common of these defects. About 150 cases of medium-chain acyl CoA dehydrogenase deficiency have been described since 1983. The clinical description is reasonably uniform, with a history of recurrent metabolic crises in infancy or childhood, often triggered by infectious episodes and poor feeding. Hypoglycemia, with or without hyperammonemia, and inappropriately low urinary ketone body excretion are highly suggestive of a fatty acid oxidation defect. Liver biopsy may reveal fatty metamorphosis. Lipid accumulation in skeletal muscle is evident with long-chain acyl CoA dehydrogenase deficiency. Cardiac involvement also is prominent with the latter disorder.

(Abridged from Darryl C. De Vivo and Salvatore DiMauro, Hereditary and Acquired Types of Myopathy, in Oski, DeAngelis, Feigin, McMillan, Warshaw: *Principles and Practice of Pediatrics, Second Edition*, J.B. Lippincott, 1994.)

Oski's Essential Pediatrics, edited by Kevin B. Johnson and Frank A. Oski. Lippincott–Raven Publishers, Philadelphia © 1997

216

Adrenoleukodystrophy

Adrenoleukodystrophy, first described as an X-linked disorder, now is recognized as a multifaceted complex including adrenoleukodystrophy and adrenomyeloneuropathy, both of which are X-linked, and an autosomal recessive form that appears in infancy (Table 216–1).

■ FORMS OF THE DISEASE

Adrenoleukodystrophy, the most common of the three disease forms, is a progressive disorder of young males 3 to 16 years of age (mean age, 8 years) that generally begins with personality changes or altered school performance and motor deficit. Seizures occur in 20% of children and occasionally signal the onset of the disorder. Motor involvement may be unilateral at first. Progression generally is relentless and results in profound psychomotor retardation, spasticity, and extensor posturing. Death occurs within 10 years of diagnosis. Adrenal insufficiency is important clinically in about 40% of children, although an equal number may have inadequate cortisol response to adrenocorticotropic hormone challenge. An "Addison's disease only" phenotype of adrenoleukodystrophy is recognized and may account for 40% of males with Addison's disease.

Adrenomyeloneuropathy frequently is associated with adrenal insufficiency. This X-linked disorder usually appears in the third decade of life as a slowly progressive spastic paraparesis and a distal sensorimotor neuropathy. Bowel and bladder dysfunction accompany the motor disability.

TABLE 216-1. Adrenoleukodystrophy Complex

Characteristic	Adrenoleukodystrophy	Adrenomyeloneuropathy	Neonatal Adrenoleukodystrophy
Age at onset	3–16 y (mean age, 8 y)	20–40 y	Infancy
Prognosis	Death in 1–10 y	Prolonged survival	Death in 1–4 y
Mode of inheritance	XLR	XLR	AR
Neurologic signs	Behavior problems, poor school performance, quadriparesis, blindness	Spastic paraparesis, distal neuropathy, urinary retention, impotence	Hypotonia, seizures, rapid deterioration, mild dysmorphism, hepatomegaly
Systemic signs	Hypoadrenalism in 50%, diminished response to ACTH, skin hyperpigmentation	Hypoadrenalism, hypogonadism	Normal adrenal function, hypoplastic adrenal glands
Stored material	Very-long-chain fatty acids	Very-long-chain fatty acids	Very-long-chain fatty acids, phytanic acid, bile acids, reduced plasmalogens
Enzyme defect	Peroxisomal fatty acyl-CoA synthetase	Peroxisomal fatty acyl-CoA synthetase	Absent or deficient peroxisomes
Prenatal diagnosis feasible	Yes	Yes	Yes

AR, *autosomal recessive*; XLR, *X-linked recessive*; ACTH, *adrenocorticotropic hormone*; acyl-CoA, *acyl coenzyme A.*

Adrenoleukodystrophy and adrenomyeloneuropathy may occur in the same family.

Neonatal adrenoleukodystrophy is a somewhat different entity and is the least often seen of the three types of disease. Beginning in early infancy, this autosomal recessive disorder represents a fundamental abnormality of the subcellular organelle known as the peroxisome and is related thereby to Zellweger syndrome and neonatal Refsum's disease. Neonatal adrenoleukodystrophy is characterized by neonatal seizures, profound hypotonia, mild dysmorphic features, hepatomegaly with impaired function, and pigmentary abnormalities of the retina. Its progression is rapid, and death often occurs by the child's first birthday.

Neuropathologic evaluation of the adrenoleukodystrophy complex demonstrates a demyelinating process with a vigorous perivascular inflammatory response corresponding to the areas of clinical involvement. Adrenal atrophy is noted. The cortical cells are swollen, but the medullary cells are spared. In addition, birefringent laminar inclusions are present in patients with adrenoleukodystrophy and adrenomyeloneuropathy, but not in those with the neonatal form of the disease. The characteristic pathologic feature of neonatal leukodystrophy is the absence or marked reduction and morphologic alteration of peroxisomes. Definitive diagnosis of each of these disorders depends on the demonstration of elevated levels of very–long-chain fatty acids (26-carbon chain) or an elevated ratio of C26:0/C22:0 fatty acids. Thus, the metabolic defect is a failure of very–long-chain fatty acid beta oxidation, a function that is located in the peroxisome and is distinct from mitochondrial fatty acid beta oxidation, probably caused by defective long-chain fatty acid activation by the peroxisomal enzyme, fatty acyl coenzyme A synthetase.

■ DIAGNOSIS AND TREATMENT

The clinical diagnosis of adrenoleukodystrophy is based on results of the history and physical examination, charac-

teristic changes seen on computed tomography (CT; confluent hypodensities in parieto-occipital white matter with contrast enhancement at the margins suggesting active demyelination; Figure 216–1) or magnetic resonance imaging (MRI; symmetric periventricular signal increase) examination, normal nerve conduction velocities, abnormal brain stem auditory evoked responses (prolonged interpeak latency between waves I and V), and elevated cerebrospinal fluid (CSF) protein levels. Adrenomyeloneuropathy, in contrast, is characterized by normal CSF protein levels and normal results on CT of the brain (mild atrophy may be a late finding), but abnormal nerve conduction velocities and brain

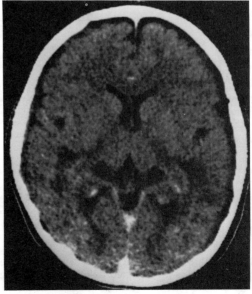

Figure 216-1. Enhanced brain CT scan of a child with adrenoleukodystrophy indicates symmetric low-density lesions located posteriorly in the parieto-occipital regions with areas of contrast enhancement.

stem auditory evoked responses. Children with neonatal adrenoleukodystrophy, in addition to having elevated very–long-chain fatty acid levels and altered peroxisomes, demonstrate reduced plasmalogens and elevated phytanic acid and pipecolic acid levels in plasma. Marked abnormalities of brain stem auditory evoked responses, visual evoked responses, and electroretinography results also may assist in the clinical diagnosis.

Heterozygote detection may be accomplished reliably for adrenoleukodystrophy by combining the measurement of very–long-chain fatty acid levels and ratios with brain stem auditory evoked responses. As many as 15% of possible heterozygotes for adrenoleukodystrophy still may escape detection, however. With regard to the neonatal form, heterozygote detection is not possible. Nevertheless, prenatal diagnosis is feasible for each disorder in families that are known to be at risk.

Fifteen percent or more of female heterozygotes for adrenoleukodystrophy may have a generally mild form of the disease that is characterized by a progressive spastic paraparesis, mild peripheral neuropathy, normal adrenal function, and elevated very–long-chain fatty acid levels in plasma or fibroblasts.

Effective therapy for the various forms of adrenoleukodystrophy is being sought actively. Bone marrow transplantation for enzyme replacement has not been helpful in neurologically impaired children with the disorder but may retard disease onset in normal or mildly affected patients. Dietary therapy aimed at restricting the intake of long-chain fatty acids and modifying their endogenous formation seems to function similarly by restricting disease onset in presymptomatic individuals. Nevertheless, the treatment of progressive disease is ineffective.

(Abridged from Alan K. Percy, The Leukodystrophies, in Oski, DeAngelis, Feigin, McMillan, Warshaw: *Principles and Practice of Pediatrics, Second Edition,* J.B. Lippincott, 1994.)

Oski's Essential Pediatrics,
edited by Kevin B. Johnson and Frank A. Oski.
Lippincott–Raven Publishers,
Philadelphia © 1997

217

The Metabolic Encephalopathies

DISEASES OF COPPER METABOLISM

■ MENKES' SYNDROME

Menkes' syndrome, also known as kinky hair disease or steely hair disease, is an X-linked disorder characterized by progressive neurologic deterioration beginning in the first 4 to 8 weeks of life, with apathy, somnolence, feeding difficulties, and myoclonic seizures. Many of these patients are born prematurely, fail to thrive, and have hypothermia. Patients also can be seen with acute sepsis. Their muscle tone varies

from hypotonia and flaccidity to hypertonia and spasticity. The descriptive names for this disorder derive from the macroscopic dull, hypopigmented, sparse, and kinky appearance of the hair resembling steel wool. Microscopically, there are pili torti and monilethrix with friable, short hair. The child's face typically is pale, with pudgy cheeks, a bow-shaped upper lip, and microcephaly. The arteries are tortuous, with defective, fragmented elastic fibers. Generalized or focal cerebral and cerebellar degeneration may be seen and may result from the vascular abnormalities. Low serum copper concentrations, low circulating ceruloplasmin levels, and decreased hepatic and brain copper content are observed. Copper absorption from the intestine is deficient, and elevated copper content in the intestinal mucosa, kidney, spleen, lung, muscle, pancreas, and placenta has suggested defective copper transport. The copper level is increased in cultured fibroblasts. Although progression followed by death in infancy or during the toddler years is typical, individuals with milder forms of this disorder have been described. Menkes' syndrome maps to chromosome xq13. Treatment with copper in the form of copper histidinate has been reported to prevent progression of the neurodegeneration, but this remains experimental, with considerable question regarding its general efficacy in patients with this disease.

■ WILSON'S DISEASE

Wilson's disease, or hepatolenticular degeneration, is a disorder with a variable clinical presentation, but typical features include neurologic manifestations, hepatocellular disease, Kayser-Fleischer rings of the cornea, a low serum ceruloplasmin level, and increased copper concentrations in the serum, urine, and liver. Two neurologic forms are recognized, although their signs and symptoms overlap. The dystonic form commonly is associated with liver disease in children, and symptoms include rigidity progressing to contractures. Choreiform or athetoid movements are manifestations of the lenticular degeneration. The pseudosclerotic form is typified by tremors and adult onset, with a more long-term progression than the dystonic form. The neurologic dysfunction associated with Wilson's disease is primarily motor, with no sensory component. Psychiatric manifestations may be seen and can be the primary complaint. Deterioration in school performance, alterations of mood, and acting out frequently are not recognized as manifestations of organic disease in these patients and are attributed to problems of preadolescent and adolescent socialization. The dementia caused by Wilson's disease may be severe, leading to the diagnosis of schizophrenia. Even if neurologic features are subtle or absent, the presence of Kayser-Fleischer rings by gross visual or slit lamp examination provides valuable clinical information. The corneal rings are present in virtually all patients with neurologic or psychiatric symptoms, but only in two thirds or less of those with hepatic abnormalities.

Additional features of Wilson's disease include acute or chronic hepatocellular disease, renal dysfunction, hemolytic anemia, neutropenia, thrombocytopenia, osteoporosis, osteomalacia, pathologic fractures, arthritis, cardiomyopathy, and hypoparathyroidism. Renal manifestations may range from generalized aminoaciduria to full renal Fanconi's syndrome, uricosuria with hypouricemia, renal lithiasis, nephrocalcinosis, and renal failure. In affected patients, the serum ceruloplasmin level generally is less than 20 mg/dL. Normal ceruloplasmin values are low in young infants (less than 3 months of age), however, and ceruloplasmin levels may be normal in as many as 5% of patients with Wilson's disease. An elevated copper content detected on liver biopsy is a particularly valuable measure. Although normal values vary among laboratories, the hepatic copper content of affected patients generally is at least $2^1/_2$- to 5-fold above the upper limit of normal and frequently is elevated 10-fold or more. The serum copper concentration may be low, but overlap with normal levels makes this a less useful diagnostic test. Urinary copper excretion is increased from less than 40 µg/24 h in normal individuals to 100 to 1000 µg/24 h in affected patients. A test dose of penicillamine at 10 mg/kg results in an increase in copper excretion to 1200 to 3000 µg/24 h in patients with Wilson's disease. It is important that all containers, solutions, and equipment (including biopsy needles) that are used to collect tissue and fluids for copper determination be free of contaminating copper, because this could interfere with accurate measurement. The incorporation of intravenously administered radioactive copper into ceruloplasmin also has been used in diagnosing this condition.

Wilson's disease is an autosomal-recessive disorder with linkage to retinoblastoma, esterase D, and other markers on chromosome 13 in the region of 13q14-21. Because the clinical features and age at onset of this disorder are so variable, physicians should subject siblings of affected patients to clinical and laboratory examination. Mildly symptomatic or presymptomatic individuals can be detected in this manner. Because of the variability in clinical expression of Wilson's disease, the differential diagnosis can be very broad, including acute viral hepatitis, chronic active hepatitis, α_1-antitrypsin deficiency, and other causes of liver disease that are associated with progressive neurologic deterioration or dementia, including the porphyrias. The presence of Kayser-Fleischer rings, however, is a definitive sign. Specific laboratory testing is required.

Treatment of Wilson's disease with D-penicillamine (Cuprimine) for copper chelation should be instituted as early as possible in the course of the disease, with the best results obtained in patients in whom treatment has been started before symptoms arise. It is an agent with a significant incidence of side effects, including allergic reactions, bone marrow suppression, and a variety of rashes. Restriction of copper intake should be considered, although strict restriction may be impractical. Zinc supplementation will prevent zinc deficiency from chelation and will decrease copper absorption by competition for uptake. Vitamin B_6 should be supplemented because penicillamine (particularly the L-isomer, but perhaps the D-isomer to a lesser extent) inhibits pyridoxine-dependent enzymes and can produce signs of pyridoxine deficiency.

The prognosis of patients with Wilson's disease and acute fulminant hepatitis is poor, but treatment should include peritoneal dialysis and possibly plasmapheresis. Aggressive and effective extraction of copper may not be successful in saving the life of such individuals. Liver transplantation has been effective in the treatment of patients with Wilson's disease, even those with acute disease, and should be considered in patients who do not respond to chelation, including those with acute, fulminant disease.

THE PORPHYRIAS

The porphyrias are inborn errors of the heme biosynthetic pathway. Not all the porphyrias are associated with encephalopathy, but all are described here for the purposes of differential diagnosis and completeness. Those porphyrias with neuropsychiatric features are readily identifiable, as outlined in Table 217–1.

Heme biosynthesis is diagrammed in Figure 217–1. Of the eight enzymatic steps in this pathway, four are mitochondrial: -aminolevulinic acid (ALA) synthase (step 1), coproporphyrinogen (coprogen) oxidase (step 6), protoporphyrinogen (protogen) oxidase (step 7), and ferrochelatase (step 8). Four enzymes are cytoplasmic: ALA dehydratase (step 2), porphobilinogen (PBG) deaminase (step 3), uroporphyrinogen III (urogen III) cosynthase (step 4), and urogen decarboxylase (step 5). Clinical disorders are associated with all eight steps: step 1 with X-linked sideroblastic anemia and steps 2 through 8 with porphyrias. ALA and coprogen III move between the mitochondrial and cytoplasmic compartments, but no defects in the transport of these intermediates have been noted. There are eight clinically distinct porphyrias associated with seven enzymes (steps 2 to 8): porphyria cutanea tarda (PCT) is caused by the heterozygous deficiency of step 5 (urogen decarboxylase), and hepatoerythropoietic porphyria (HEP) is caused by the homozygous deficiency of this same enzyme. Table 217–1 details the clinical

TABLE 217–1. The Human Porphyrias

Disease	Deficient Enzyme*	Genetics	Porphyria Classification	Major Symptoms		
				Neuropsychiatric	*Visceral*	*Photosensitivity*
ALAD porphyria	(2) ALA dehydratase	AR	Hepatic	+	+	−
Acute intermittent porphyria	(3) PBG deaminase	AD	Hepatic	+	+	−
Congenital erythropoietic porphyria	(4) Urogen III cosynthase	AR	Erythropoietic	−	−	+
Porphyria cutanea tarda	(5) Urogen decarboxylase	AD	Hepatic	−	−	+
Hepatoerythropoietic porphyria	(5) Urogen decarboxylase	AR	Hepatoerythropoietic	−	±	+
Hereditary coproporphyria	(6) Coprogen oxidase	AD	Hepatic	+	+	±
Variegate porphyria	(7) Protogen oxidase	AD	Hepatic	+	+	±
Erythropoietic protoporphyria	(8) Ferrochelatase	AD	Erythropoietic	−	±	+

*Number in parentheses is enzyme sequence in the heme synthetic pathway.

†Enzymatic diagnosis may be possible using other tissues, but has been well documented in those listed. Prenatal diagnosis at an enzymatic level is theoretically possible in all, but data are limited. In autosomal dominant disorders, family studies may be necessary to evaluate heterozygous levels of activity.

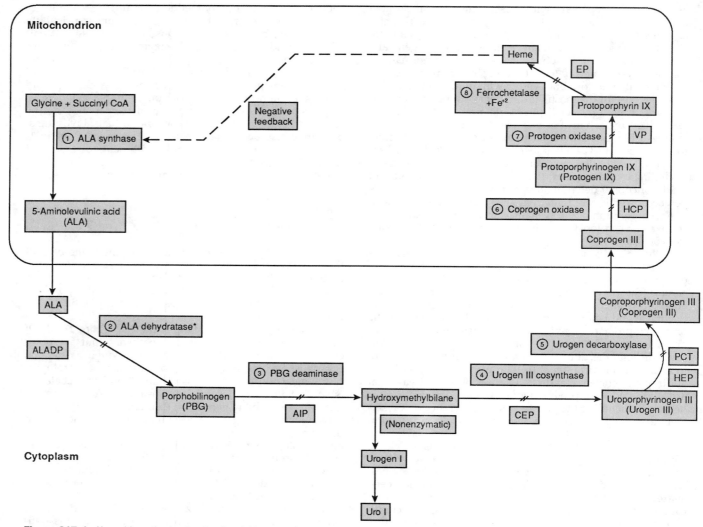

Figure 217-1. Heme biosynthesis, showing the eight enzymatic steps.

features of the porphyrias, listing them according to the enzyme sequence from step 2 through step 8. The disorders are discussed in the same sequence in the text.

ALA synthase is the initial and rate-limiting enzyme of heme biosynthesis, and it is regulated by negative feedback from the end product of the pathway heme. Two genes are recognized for this enzyme: ALAS1 encodes the housekeeping gene and maps to 3p21, and ALAS2 is the erythroid-specific gene and maps to Xp11. A defect in ALAS2 results in X-linked sideroblastic anemia, which is characterized by hypochromic microcytic anemia that frequently is detected in childhood, hemochromatosis that leads to death at a relatively young age, hyperferricemia, increased peripheral siderocytes after splenectomy, and reduced protoporphyrin levels in the microcytes.

■ ACUTE INTERMITTENT PORPHYRIA

Acute intermittent porphyria (AIP) is an autosomal-dominant deficiency of PBG deaminase, which maps to the long arm of chromosome 11 (11q23-Hq23-ter). It is considered the most common of the inborn errors of porphyrin metabolism, with an estimated incidence of 5 to 10 per 100,000 in the United States, although as many as 90% of individuals with PBG deaminase deficiency are asymptomatic.

The characteristic features of acute episodes are severe abdominal pain and port-wine urine. Associated vomiting, constipation, abdominal distention, and ileus may lead to the diagnosis of surgical abdomen, but surgery should be avoided whenever possible during these attacks. Diarrhea and urinary retention or incontinence may be seen. Tachycardia, hypertension or hypotension, fever, leukocytosis, and seizures may accompany attacks, in addition to psychiatric disturbances, including disorientation, hallucinations, paranoia, anxiety, and depression. Motor neuropathy is more common than is sensory neuropathy and is of extreme concern, because bulbar paralysis and respiratory insufficiency can occur and may be fatal.

Symptomatic AIP is rare before puberty but has been reported. Acute attacks are precipitated by a variety of drugs, most of which induce ALA synthase. Prominent among these agents are barbiturates, phenytoin (Dilantin), oral contraceptives, sulfonamides, and valproic acid. AIP attacks also may occur with menstrual periods, decreased food intake, and stress. Stress factors include infections, ethanol intoxication, and surgery.

PBG and ALA levels frequently are elevated in the urine but may be normal or minimally increased, especially in asymptomatic individuals with PBG deaminase deficiency. PBG deaminase activity in erythrocytes is reduced to about 50% of normal, but, as a result of wide variation in normal values leading to overlap of enzyme activity between patients with AIP and normal control individuals, enzyme activity should be measured in the parents of affected children and in other family members. Occasional patients have normal red cell PBG deaminase levels, and cultured fibroblasts may be used to measure enzyme activity. The enzyme deficiency also is expressed in amniotic fluid cells, liver, and lymphocytes. The PBG deaminase complementary DNA has been cloned and mutations analyzed.

The mainstay of treatment is prevention of attacks by avoidance of precipitating influences, including known exacerbating medications and stresses. Increased oral carbohydrate intake should be attempted early in an attack; if the patient does not respond to this treatment, then intravenous dextrose infusions should be used. These patients should be monitored for inappropriate antidiuretic hormone secretion. Propranolol has been used to control tachycardia and hypertension. The pain of an acute attack is severe but may be treated with a narcotic analgesic (*eg,* morphine) and a phenothiazine (*eg,* chlorpromazine), although the narcotic analgesic increases the tendency toward constipation and urinary retention. Intravenous hematin should be considered when an attack continues for longer than 2 days or when there is rapid neurologic progression. Phlebitis and thrombophlebitis are seen frequently with intravenous hematin.

■ PORPHYRIA CUTANEA TARDA

PCT is a common porphyria, which is subdivided into two types: type I, or sporadic, and type II, or familial. Urogen decarboxylase levels are decreased to 50% in both types, with the reduction found only in the liver in type I but generalized in the inherited type II. The sporadic form is seen in association with ethanol abuse, estrogen intake, or iron ingestion, as well as with other toxins or disorders. Type I PCT is seen more commonly in adults, whereas type II typically has its onset in childhood. Vesicles and bullae of the exposed skin, with crusting, scarring, and hyperpigmentation, are seen in both types, as is increased fragility of the skin. Hypertrichosis of the face may develop. Hepatic cirrhosis and siderosis are common findings, and there is an increased incidence of hepatocellular carcinoma.

Urogen decarboxylase deficiency may be documented in the liver in patients with types I and II PCT, and in the erythrocytes in patients with type II PCT. The urinary concentration of uroporphyrin exceeds that of coproporphyrin. The urogen decarboxylase locus maps to the short arm of chromosome 1 (1pter → p21). The urogen decarboxylase complementary DNA has been cloned and mutation analysis performed in familial PCT.

Treatment includes avoidance of precipitating exposures and protection from sunlight. Phlebotomy has been used and is presumed to work by decreasing total body iron levels. Chloroquine may be effective by forming a complex with porphyrins and improving their clearance, but its use has been associated with retinopathy.

■ ERYTHROPOIETIC PROTOPORPHYRIA

EP is the autosomal-dominant heterozygous deficiency of ferrochelatase, the final enzymatic step in heme synthesis that involves the insertion of iron into protoporphyrin. EP is the most common of the erythropoietic porphyrias. Cutaneous photosensitivity is relatively mild and is noted first in childhood, usually before 6 years of age, with exposure to the sun or other bright light causing burning, edema, itching, and erythema. Lesions generally resolve after a few hours, although petechiae, purpura, vesicles, and crusting may develop and last several days before clearing. Scarring and disfigurement are not typical features of this porphyria, although mild scarring and hyperkeratosis may be seen after chronic eczematoid lesions have resolved. Anemia is rare and, when present, is nonhemolytic. Gallstones are relatively common. Hepatocellular disease is rare, but may be severe, progressing rapidly to cirrhosis and death. The presence of protoporphyrin in the red cells, plasma, and stool is characteristic of patients with EP. Ferrochelatase activity can be assayed in erythrocytes and fibroblasts. The ferrochelatase complementary DNA has been cloned and mapped to chromosome 18g22, and mutations have been analyzed. The primary cause of clinical problems in patients with EP is sunlight or strong artificial light. If exposure cannot be avoided, topical sunscreens may be of some help if they have a high "sun protection factor" of 26 or 34. Oral high-dose β-carotene is considered useful but requires several weeks or months before tolerance to sunlight improves. In addition, the dosages necessary may lead to carotene discoloration of the skin. In the past, drugs and chemicals were not considered precipitating factors; with recognition of the potential severity of the associated liver disease, however, more attention is being paid to protecting patients from these agents. Iron, vitamin E, and cholestyramine have been recommended to prevent progression once hepatocellular disease is noted, but data on their efficacy are limited. There is a genetic animal model for EP, which is an autosomal-recessive deficiency of ferrochelatase in cattle.

(Abridged from Edward R.B. McCabe, The Metabolic Encephalopathies, in Oski, DeAngelis, Feigin, McMillan, Warshaw: *Principles and Practice of Pediatrics, Second Edition,* J.B. Lippincott, 1994.)

Oski's Essential Pediatrics,
edited by Kevin B. Johnson and Frank A. Oski.
Lippincott–Raven Publishers,
Philadelphia © 1997

218

Rett Syndrome

Rett syndrome is a pervasive developmental disorder affecting young females. After a period of apparently normal development, the patients reach a plateau and then experience a rapid decline in motor and cognitive function, usually beginning at 6 to 18 months of age. The principal clinical features consist of the loss of purposeful hand use; the development of stereotypic hand movements such as hand washing, hand wringing, or hand tapping (Figure 218–1); and the loss of communication skills. Generally, these children have developed the ability to speak a few words, but with the onset of the disorder, meaningful verbal communication is lost. In addition, affected individuals give very poor eye con-

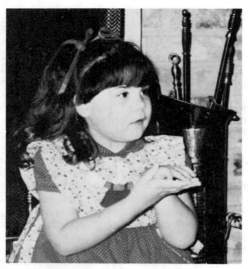

Figure 218-1. This photograph of a 5-year-old girl with Rett syndrome demonstrates the typical hand position associated with the disorder.

tact, which has led their behavior to be interpreted as autistic. An acquired-type deceleration of head growth is noted within the first 2 years of life; other features include periodic breathing while awake, with alternating periods of breath holding and hyperventilation. Seizures occur in many of these children and may consist of both staring spells and generalized tonic-clonic episodes. Growth failure is evident, with short stature and small hand and foot size. In addition, the hands and feet tend to be markedly cooler than the remainder of the extremities, and the children seem to have diminished responses to pain.

Although the behavioral mannerisms (hand stereotypies and periodic breathing) of children with Rett syndrome are confined to wakefulness, sleep often is interrupted and periods of uncontrollable screaming are reported frequently by parents during the first few years of life. After the early period of decline, there is a rather long, relatively stable phase during which the episodes of screaming and the behavioral mannerisms may become milder. Attentiveness and eye contact improve to the extent that communication may occur through eye gaze or eye pointing. In later childhood and early adolescence, scoliosis is common. Affected individuals may survive well into adulthood. Because this disorder has been recognized only for about 30 years and accurate diagnosis has been possible only within the last decade, however, the natural history of Rett syndrome has not been fully elucidated.

The occurrence of Rett syndrome exclusively in females has led to the suggestion that it is an X-linked disorder that is lethal in males. No affected males have been identified, and the precise genetic mechanism involved is unknown. It is possible, however, that nonrandom X-inactivation is occurring. The recurrence of Rett syndrome within individual families has been reported in less than 1% of cases. When recurrence has been described in more than one generation, the mode of transmission appears to be through the maternal side of the family. The prevalence rate of between 1:10,000 and 1:15,000 exceeds that of phenylketonuria in females.

No specific therapy is available for patients with Rett syndrome. The majority of children achieve independent walking but lose this capability in later stages and are susceptible to the complications of relative immobility, including orthopedic deformities, particularly progressive scoliosis. Anticonvulsant agents are indicated if seizures occur; carbamazepine has been particularly effective. Programs involving physical and occupational therapy as well as early childhood education should be tailored to the individual child.

(Abridged from Alan K. Percy, Rett Syndrome, in Oski, DeAngelis, Feigin, McMillan, Warshaw: *Principles and Practice of Pediatrics, Second Edition*, J.B. Lippincott, 1994.)

Oski's Essential Pediatrics,
edited by Kevin B. Johnson and Frank A. Oski.
Lippincott–Raven Publishers,
Philadelphia © 1997

219

Basal Ganglia and Neurotransmitter Disorders

Biochemical or structural pathology in the basal ganglia may be manifested by movement disorders, groups of neurologic diseases or syndromes that fall into one of two categories—those characterized by slowness, paucity, and "freezing" of voluntary movement (bradykinesia, akinesia), or those characterized by excess abnormal involuntary movement (hyperkinesia, dyskinesia).

The diagnosis of a particular movement disorder depends primarily on careful observation of the clinical phenomena. The bradykinetic movement disorders often are accompanied by rigidity, postural instability, and loss of automatic associated movements. The hyperkinetic involuntary movements are differentiated phenomenologically according to their characteristic clinical features, rapidity and duration of contractions, rhythmicity, pattern, and suppressibility (Table 219–1). In general, abnormal involuntary movements are exaggerated with stress and disappear during sleep; however, certain forms of myoclonus and tics may persist during all stages of sleep.

■ HUNTINGTON'S DISEASE

The usual onset of Huntington's disease (HD) is in the fourth and fifth decades of life, but about 10% of patients are seen during childhood or adolescence. Both juvenile and adult-onset HD are autosomal-dominant traits, with a defective gene mapped to a terminal band of the short arm of chromosome 4. The gene mutation was found to consist of an unstable enlargement of the CAG repeat sequence at 4p16.3. The majority of patients with juvenile HD have the akinetic-rigid syndrome termed the *Westphal variant.* Other features of juvenile HD include dementia, seizures, and ataxia. In addition, patients with juvenile HD are more likely to have inherited the abnormal gene from their father than from their mother, and they tend to segregate within families. Although the medium-sized spiny neurons (type I cells) usually are affected first in the adult form of HD, the large aspiny cells have been suggested to degenerate first in the juvenile form. In contrast to the caudate nucleus, which typically is involved in the adult form of HD, the putamen seems to be most damaged in the juvenile form of the disease.

There are no pathognomonic neurodiagnostic tests for HD, but the diagnosis can be established with at least 95% accuracy when the DNA marker is identified. The psychologic and social impact of such testing in identifying presymptomatic individuals is being investigated. The combination of DNA polymorphism and positron emission tomography may be used in the future to detect HD in the preclinical phase.

The most remarkable biochemical change observed in the brains of adults with HD is a reduction in the activity of glutamic acid decarboxylase, particularly in the corpus striatum, substantia nigra, and other basal ganglia. In contrast, thyrotropin-releasing hormone, neurotensin, somatostatin, and neuropeptide Y are increased in the corpus striatum. The depletion of τ-aminobutyric acid in the corpus striatum may result in disinhibition of the nigral-striatal pathway. Coupled with the accumulation of somatostatin, the net result may be the release of striatal dopamine, which results in chorea. Dopamine-blocking drugs, such as haloperidol, and dopamine-depleting agents, including tetrabenazine, often are useful in controlling chorea. In patients with childhood HD, which usually is manifested by parkinsonian features, levodopa may provide symptomatic relief.

■ HYPERKINETIC MOVEMENT DISORDERS

Tremor

Essential tremor (ET) probably is the most common cause of an oscillatory involuntary movement during childhood (Table 219–2, p 638). ET may start at any age, including infancy. One form of infantile ET is the hereditary chin tremor, which consists of rhythmic, three-per-second contractions of the chin that often are associated with deafness and are inherited in an autosomal-dominant pattern. Another form of ET that begins during infancy or early childhood is so-called shuddering attacks. Children may have more than 100 attacks a day, but symptom-free intervals may last as long as 2 weeks. The attacks are characterized by bursts of rapid trembling of the whole body, occasionally associated with head turning, involuntary sniffing, and throat clearing. During the course of the attacks, the child usually sinks to the floor; the attacks may even persist during sleep.

In addition to these forms of ET, the characteristic action-postural tremor also may be seen in children. The slower (about 6.5 Hz) tremor often involves the head and neck, whereas the more rapid tremor (8 to 12 Hz) tends to involve the hands. Many other variants of ET have been recognized, however. Although ET usually is "benign," it occasionally can progress to a very disabling movement disorder, interfering with writing, feeding, speaking, and other activities of daily living.

Although neurotransmitter abnormalities in the basal ganglia are suspected to underlie ET, no pathologic changes have been documented in the few brains that have been examined at autopsy. In addition to the beta blockers, essential tremor may improve with primidone, lorazepam, alprazolam, clonazepam, amantadine, clonidine, and ethanol.

Other oscillatory involuntary movements occasionally seen in infants and children are "head nodding," which often is associated with congenital nystagmus, including spasmus nutans; and the "bobble-headed doll's syndrome," which is seen with diencephalic lesions, including third-ventricle cysts or tumors, craniopharyngioma, hydrocephalus, and hypothalamic lesions.

Tics

About 25% of normal children have transient tics, making this the most frequent childhood-onset involuntary movement seen in a movement disorders clinic. One of the most common causes of pathologic tics in childhood is the

TABLE 219-1. Differential Diagnosis of Hyperkinetic Movement Disorders

| Clinical Features | Tremor | | | Chorea |
	At Rest	Postural	Kinetic	
Characteristics	3–7 Hz supination-pronation oscillatory ("pill rolling"): hands, legs, lips, jaw, (alternating contractions of antagonists)	4–12 Hz flexion-extension oscillatory movement with arms outstretched: hands arms, head, voice, legs (simultaneous contractions of antagonists)	3–5 Hz intention tremor on finger-to-nose and heel-to-shin test	Rapid, abrupt, flowing, unsustained, random, semipurposeful, non-patterned; *athetosis* is a slow chorea (writhing movement)
Associated features	Bradykinesia, rigidity (cogwheel), shuffling gait, postural instability, hypomimia, micrographia	Dystonia, parkinsonism, and hereditary peripheral neuropathy, torticollis, parkinsonism	Ataxia, titubation, dysdiadochokinesia, loss of check and other cerebellar or brain stem signs	"Milkmaid's grip," darting "darting tongue," orofacial dyskinesia, hypotonia, pendular or "hung-up" reflexes, dementia in Huntington's disease, carditis in Sydenham's chorea
Etiology	Parkinson's disease, secondary parkinsonism, heterogenous disorders with parkinsonian features	Physiologic, accentuated, physiologic, essential cerebellar outflow (midbrain rubral, wing beating)	Cerebellar disorders and tumor, multiple sclerosis brain stem and cerebellar strokes	Huntington's disease, rheumatic fever (Sydenham), drug-induced hyperthyroidism, static encephalopathy, pregnancy, vasculitis, electrolyte metabolic imbalance
Treatment	Anticholinergics, amantadine, levodopa/carbidopa, dopamine agonists	Propranolol and other beta-blockers, benzodiazepines, phenobarbital, pyrimidine, clonazepam, amantadine, alcohol	No effective treatment, wrist-arm weights, thalamotomy	Treat underlying disorder, dopamine blocking or depleting agents, cholinergic agents

Gilles de la Tourette's syndrome (TS). This motor-behavioral disorder is the expression of a genetic disturbance affecting the central nervous system. The onset of TS usually occurs between 2 and 15 years of age, and its expression is gender influenced; in boys, motor and vocal manifestations appears to dominate, whereas in girls, behavioral problems such as obsessive-compulsive disorder appear to be more common.

In addition to simple tics such as blinking, facial grimacing, shoulder shrugging, and head jerking, many patients with TS have complex sequences of coordinated movements, including bizarre gait, kicking, jumping, body gyrations, scratching, and seductive or obscene gestures. The waxing and waning nature of tics, the irresistible urge before a tic and relief after a tic, the temporary suppressibility of the tics, and the recurrence of tics during sleep often result in the disorder being misdiagnosed as having a psychogenic origin. The psychogenic nature of the condition also is suggested erroneously by the involuntary vocalizations that occur, which range from simple noises to coprolalia (obscene words), echolalia (repetition of words), and palilalia (repetition of a phrase or word with increasing rapidity). Coprolalia, although it is one of the most recognizable symptoms of TS, has been seen in only 40% of our patients thus far. Many patients also experience copropraxia, echopraxia, bizarre thoughts and ideas, thought fixation, compulsive ruminations, and perverse sexual fantasies. Sleep complaints, including restlessness, insomnia, enuresis, somnambulism, nightmares, and bruxism, have been noted in about half our patients, and about two thirds had evidence of motor tics recorded by polysomnography. If a broad spectrum of behavioral problems is included, then about 1% of all individuals manifest one or more aspects of the TS gene. Disturbance in the mesencephalic-mesolimbic system, which results in disinhibition of the limbic system, has been suggested as the pathogenetic mechanism underlying TS.

Although haloperidol is recommended most frequently for TS, we find fluphenazine, pimozide, and tetrabenazine to be more effective and better tolerated. Patients with predominant behavioral symptoms may benefit from clonidine and fluoxetine. When TS is associated with attention deficit disorder and hyperactivity, central nervous system stimulants such as methylphenidate may be needed, but should be used cautiously.

Myoclonus

In contrast to tics, myoclonus is a simple, jerklike movement that is not coordinated or suppressible, and often is activated by volitional movement (Table 219–3, p 639). Benign neonatal sleep myoclonus, which is seen in the first

| | | | Myoclonus | | |
Stereotypy	Dystonia	Ballism	*Generalized*	*Segmental*	Tics
Repetitive, purposeless movements esembling normal voluntary movements	Sustained, twisting, usually low but may be rapid and may progress to fixed contractures (dystonic postures)	Abrupt, random forceful, violent, flinging, usually proximal and unilateral, often spontaneously remits	Abrupt, irregular brief, jerklike contractions of one or more muscles occurring synchronously or asynchronously, may be stimulus-sensitive	Rhythmic contraction of agonists, not stimulus-sensitive, may persist during sleep	Rapid, sudden, unpredictable, coordinated jerks, preceded by inner urge, waxing and waning, temporarily suppressible
Often associated with *akathisia* sensory and motor restlessness)	Torticollis, writer's cramp, blepharospasm, spasmodic dysphonia, essential tremor, hypertrophy of contracted muscles	Initial hemiparesis, later choreoathetosis	Encephalopathy, seizures, dementia, periodic electroencephalogram, enhanced somatosensory evoked potentials	Palatal myoclonus may be associated with bulbar palsy; spinal myoclonus may be associated with myelopathy	Vocalizations, coprolalia, echolalia, copropraxia, echopraxia, obsessive-compulsive behavior, attention deficit disorder, sleep disturbance
Usually drug-induced (tardive dyskinesia) schizophrenia, autism, mental retardation, Rett syndrome	Dystonia musculorum deformans, adult-onset torsion dystonia drug-induced	Lesion of contralateral subthalamic nucleus (hemorrhage, infarction, rarely tumor)	Postanoxic, uremic and other encephalopathies, Creutzfeldt-Jakob disease, subacute sclerosing panencephalitis, myoclonic epilepsy, Ramsay Hunt syndrome	Brain stem or spinal cord infarction, hemorrhage, myelitis, demyelinating disease	Gilles de la Tourette's syndrome, transient tic of childhood
May improve with dopamine blockers or depletors, beta-blockers, opioid agonists or antagonists	Muscle relaxants, anticholinergics, tetrabenazine, baclofen, dopamine agonists, levodopa for diurnal dystonia, *C botulinum* toxin injections, thalamotomy	Dopamine blocking or depleting agents, thalamotomy	Clonazepam, 5-hydroxy-tryptophan, sodium valproate, piracetam, lisuride	Tetrabenzine, 5-hydroxy-tryptophan, clonazepam, anitcholinergics	Dopamine blocking or depleting agents

month of life, usually is stimulus sensitive and occurs in the early stages of sleep. It should be differentiated from neonatal seizures and infantile spasms. Essential myoclonus usually begins before 20 years of age. It is inherited in an autosomal-dominant pattern, and may be associated with essential tremor.

In patients with epileptic myoclonus, seizures often dominate the clinical presentation. Cortical reflex myoclonus is characterized by a time-locked electroencephalographic (EEG) event preceding the myoclonic movement and by enhanced amplitude of the somatosensory evoked potential. In contrast to the hyperexcitable sensorimotor cortex that underlies cortical myoclonus, reticular reflex myoclonus presumably is the result of hyperexcitable brain stem reticular formation, particularly the nucleus reticularis gigantocellularis. Progressive myoclonus epilepsy (PME) consists of myoclonus, seizures, and a progressive clinical course. One form of PME, Unverricht-Lundborg disease (also known as Baltic myoclonus), is characterized by stimulus-sensitive myoclonus that usually begins between 6 and 15 years of age. The patients also have dysarthria, ataxia, intention tremor, and mild intellectual decline, and most become bedridden within 5 years after

onset of the disease. Epileptiform EEG findings may be seen as long as 3 years before the onset of clinical symptoms. The disease is inherited in an autosomal-recessive pattern, and at least some cases may be associated with mitochondrial myopathy and encephalopathy. Another form of progressive myoclonus, Lafora's body disease, usually begins between 11 and 18 years of age, and is characterized by progressive dementia, apraxia, and cortical blindness, with total disability resulting within 5 to 8 years after onset. Biopsy of the skin (particularly the axillary skin), liver, muscle, or brain reveals typical inclusions (Lafora's bodies) that are positive on periodic acid–Schiff staining.

The idiopathic, generalized, or segmental forms of myoclonus may improve with treatment using clonazepam, sodium valproate, 5-hydroxytryptophan, tetrabenazine, reserpine, levodopa, and trihexyphenidyl. Two new drugs (lisuride and piracetam) have shown promise in the treatment of patients with myoclonus.

(Abridged from Joseph Jankovic, Basal Ganglia and Neurotransmitter Disorders, in Oski, DeAngelis, Feigin, McMillan, Warshaw: *Principles and Practice of Pediatrics, Second Edition*, J.B. Lippincott, 1994.)

TABLE 219-2. Classification of Tremors

REST TREMORS	ACTION TREMORS	
Parkinson Tremor	*Postural Tremors*	Factors that accentuate physiologic tremor also enhance or unmask essential tremor
Secondary parkinsonism	Physiologic tremor	Vitamin E deficiency
Postencephalic	Normal physiologic tremor	Action tremor of parkinsonism
Toxic: phenothiazines, butyrophenones, metoclopramide, reserpine, tetrabenazine, carbon monoxide, manganese, MPTP, carbon disulfide	Accentuated physiologic tremor	Neuropathic tremor
	Stress-induced: anxiety, fright, fatigue, fever	Peripheral neuropathies
Tumor	Endocrine: thyrotoxicosis, hypoglycemia, pheochromocytoma	Motor neuron disease
Trauma	Drugs, toxins: epinephrine, isoproterenol, caffeine, theophylline and other sympathomimetic agents, levodopa, amphetamines, lithium, tricyclic antidepressants, phenothiazines, butyrophenones, thyroxine, hypoglycemic agents, adrenocorticosteroids, alcohol withdrawal, mercury, lead, arsenic, bismuth, carbon monoxide, methylbromide, monosodium glutamate, sodium valproate, metrizamide, meperidine	Cerebellar postural hypotonic tremor (titubation)
Vascular		Midbrain ("rubral") tremor
Metabolic: hypoparathyroidism, chronic hepatocerebral degeneration		Dystonic (axial) tremor
Parkinsonism plus (heterogenous system degenerations)		*Kinetic (Intention) Tremor*
Olivopontocerebellar atrophy		Cerebellar outflow tremor (superior cerebellar peduncle lesion)
Progressive supranuclear palsy		Multiple sclerosis
Wilson's disease		Posterior circulation strokes
Huntington's disease	Essential tremor	Cerebellar degenerations
Spasmus Nutans	Autosomal dominant	Wilson's disease
Hereditary Chin Quivering	With peripheral neuropathy: Charcot-Marie-Tooth disease (Roussy-Lévy syndrome)	Drugs, toxins: phenytoin, barbiturates, lithium, meperidine, alcohol, mercury, 5-fluorouracil, vidarabine, amiodarone, cimetidine, tocainide
Other	With other movement disorders (parkinsonism, torsion dystonia, spasmodic torticollis, myoclonus)	Midbrain ("rubral") tremor
Midbrain (rubral) tremor		Primary handwriting tremor
Severe essential tremor		Dystonic (distal) tremor
Roussy-Lévy syndrome		

Familial benign chorea and tremor
Miscellaneous Tremors and Other Rhythmic Movements
Idiopathic
Hysterical
Involuntary rhythmic movements not classified as tremors
Cardiac and respiratory movements
Convulsions
Nystagmus
Segmental myoclonus
Oscillatory myoclonus
Asterixis
Fasciculations
Clonus
Minipolymyoclonus
Shivering
Shuddering
Head flopping or nodding movements

Modified from Jankovic J. Neurologic Consultant. New York: Lawrence Della Corte Publications; 1984:1.

TABLE 219-3. Classification of Myoclonus

PHYSIOLOGIC MYOCLONUS (NORMAL INDIVIDUALS)

Sleep jerks (hypnic jerks)
Anxiety-induced
Exercise-induced
Hiccough (singultus)
Benign infantile myoclonus with feeding

ESSENTIAL MYOCLONUS (NO KNOWN CAUSE AND NO OTHER GROSS NEUROLOGIC DEFICTS)

Hereditary (autosomal dominant)
Sporadic
Ballistic movement overflow myoclonus
Oscillatory myoclonus
Segmental myoclonus (rhythmic and nonrhythmic)
Nocturnal myoclonus
Restless leg syndrome

EPILEPTIC MYOCLONUS (SEIZURES DOMINANT AND NO ENCEPHALOPATHY, AT LEAST INITIALLY)

Isolated epileptic myoclonic jerks
Cortical reflex myoclonus
Reticular reflex myoclonus
Primary generalized epileptic myoclonus
Epilepsia partialis continua
Photoconvulsive response
Infantile spasms
Childhood epileptic encephalopathy with slow spike and slow waves (Lennox-Gastaut syndrome, myoclonic-ataxic epilepsy, cryptogenic myoclonic epilepsy)
Familial myoclonic epilepsy (Janz)
Familial myoclonic epilepsy (Rabot)
Progressive myoclonus epilepsy: Baltic myoclonus (Unverricht-Lundborg)

SYMPTOMATIC MYOCLONUS (PROGRESSIVE OR STATIC ENCEPHALOPATHY DOMINATES)

Progressive myoclonus epilepsy (PME)
Lafora's body disease
Neuronal ceroid lipofuscinosis
Sialidosis (types I, II)
Mitochondrial encephalopathy
Noninfantile neuronopathic Gaucher's disease
Biotin-responsive encephalopathy
Lipidoses (GM$_2$ gangliosidosis, Tay-Sachs, Krabbe's)
Spinocerebellar degeneration
Ramsay Hunt syndrome
Friedreich's ataxia
Ataxia-telangiectasia
Basal ganglia degenerations
Wilson's disease
Torsion dystonia
Hallervorden-Spatz disease
Progressive supranuclear palsy
Huntington's disease
Parkinson's disease
Dementias
Creutzfeldt-Jakob disease
Alzheimer's disease
Viral types of encephalopathy
Subacute sclerosing panencephalitis
Encephalitis lethargia
Arbovirus encephalitis
Herpes simplex encephalitis
Postinfection encephalitis

Metabolic
Hypoxic-ischemic encephalopathy
Hepatic failure
Renal failure
Dialysis syndrome
Hyponatremia
Hypoglycemia
Infantile myoclonic encephalopathy (polymyoclonus with or without neuroblastoma)
Nonketotic hyperglycemia
Toxic types of encephalopathy
Bismuth
Heavy metal poisons:
Methylbromide dichlorodiphenyltrichloroethane (DDT)
Drugs, including levodopa
Physical types of encephalopathy
Post-traumatic
Heat stroke
Electric shock
Decompression injury
Focal central nervous system damage
Post-stroke
Post-thalamotomy
Tumor
Trauma
Segmental myoclonus (branchial, spinal)

Modified from Patel V, Jankovic J. Myoclonus. In: Apel SH, ed. Current neurology. Vol 8. St. Louis: Mosby-Yearbook, 1988:77.

Oski's Essential Pediatrics,
edited by Kevin B. Johnson and Frank A. Oski.
Lippincott–Raven Publishers,
Philadelphia © 1997

220

The Phakomatoses and Other Neurocutaneous Syndromes

NEUROFIBROMATOSIS

Neurofibromatosis (NF) is more than one disorder. There are at least two specific types of NF, and perhaps as many as eight different forms of this disease. The most common type is von Recklinghausen's NF, or NF-1, which accounts for at least 85% of all patients with NF.

■ NF-1: VON RECKLINGHAUSEN'S NEUROFIBROMATOSIS

NF-1 occurs with a frequency of about 1 in 4000 persons. It is an autosomal-dominant trait, with about one half of the index cases representing new mutations, which means that a negative family history is common in the pediatric setting. The disorder is essentially the same whether it is inherited or results from a new mutation. NF-1 is highly variable in its expression, however, from one family to another, from one person to another within a family, and from one body part to another within a given person. On the other hand, its penetrance (*ie,* the likelihood tha the mutant gene will express itself at all if it is present) is virtually 100%.

The gene for NF-1 resides on the proximal long arm of chromosome 17, specifically in band 17q11.2.

■ FEATURES

A checklist of the features that are characteristic of all types of NF, with an emphasis on NF-1, is provided in Table 220–1.

Café au lait spots (CLS) are the hallmark of NF-1 and NF-6. In patients with NF-1, the hyperpigmented macules usually are larger than 15 mm in diameter and have sharply defined edges and a uniform intensity of coloration (Figure 220–1). CLS are different from freckling, which is most likely to occur in regions of skin apposition; other than axillary freckling, the onset of freckling is later in childhood or adulthood.

■ NATURAL HISTORY

Although some investigators and clinicians continue to claim that NF-1 is a generally benign disorder, NF of any type (except, perhaps, NF-6) always is a progressive disorder, with a significant likelihood of serious morbidity and premature death.

■ DIAGNOSIS

According to a 1987 National Institutes of Health Consensus Development Conference on NF, the diagnostic criteria for NF-1 are met in an individual if two or more of the following are found: six or more CLS greater than 5 mm in greatest diameter in prepubertal individuals and greater than 15 mm in greatest diameter in postpubertal individuals; two or more neurofibromas of any type, or one plexiform neurofibroma; freckling in the axillary or inguinal regions; optic pathway glioma; two or more iris Lisch nodules; a distinctive osseous lesion, such as sphenoid wing dysplasia or thinning of long-bone cortex, with or without pseudarthrosis; or a first-degree relative (parent, sibling, or offspring) with NF-1 diagnosed by the above criteria.

Establishing the diagnosis of NF-1 rarely is a problem in a child who is 1 year of age or older, because the requisite number of CLS usually are obvious by that age, one or more additional features are likely to be present, and alternative diagnoses are either rare or otherwise apparent by virtue of their own unique features. At any age, given the presence of six or more CLS that are 15 mm or greater in diameter, the likelihood of NF-1 is at or near 99%. Excluding the diagnosis of NF-1 in a child who is less than 1 year of age, however, may be difficult.

No laboratory tests are routinely available with which to confirm or exclude the diagnosis of NF-1. Although DNA-based genetic linkage data may be useful, clinical criteria usually suffice in patients older than 1 year of age. For cases of sporadic mutation, only 5% or so of the mutations are identifiable at the molecular level, making this test not feasible on a routine basis. Biopsies of CLS and neurofibromas (or other tumors) cannot establish the diagnosis of NF-1; they can only confirm the type of lesion.

Ordinarily, by 1 year of age, the diagnosis of NF-1 can be established using the criteria noted. If the diagnosis is suspected but cannot be established after that age, an alternative form of NF should not be discounted categorically. The assistance of an established NF referral center should be sought. Once the diagnosis of NF-1 is made, the presence of any of its features that are likely to cause serious problems should be noted, even if they currently are asymptomatic (*eg,* optic pathway glioma, sphenoid wing dysplasia, vertebral dysplasia, diffuse plexiform neurofibroma), and should serve as a basis for close follow-up.

■ TREATMENT

Medical therapy for NF-1 is similar to that used for the specific conditions seen in the absence of NF-1. Problems associated with NF-1 that are most likely to require medical treatment include constipation (*ie,* from colonic ganglioneuromatosis), seizures, headaches, hyperactivity and learning disabilities, anxiety, and renovascular hypertension. Pruritus in patients with NF is not treated effectively with histamine$_1$-blocking antihistamines, although some success has been obtained using the mast cell blocker, ketotifen. Mast cell blockers also may play a role in decreasing the rate of neurofibroma development. There is no absolute contraindication to the use of oral contraceptives in patients with NF-1, although evaluation on an individual basis obviously is appropriate. Antineoplastic chemotherapy has no role in the treatment of neurofibromas. Its role in the treatment of optic pathway gliomas still is investigational, and its utility in the treatment of neurofibrosarcomas is problematic. Radiotherapy for neurofibromas has no proven effect. It appears to be

TABLE 220-1. A Checklist of Anatomic-Structural and Functional Features of Neurofibromatosis Type 1

ANATOMIC-STRUCTURAL FEATURES

Skin Pigmentation

Café-au-lait spots; freckling: axillary, elsewhere; hyperpigmentation over a plexiform neurofibroma; other hyperpigmentation; hypopigmentation

Discrete Neurofibromas

Cutaneous; general, areola, nipple; subcutaneous; oral-pharynx-larynx; deep

Plexiform Neurofibromas

Craniofacial: orbital, other; chest wall; paraspinal: cervical, thoracic, lumbosacral; abdominal, retroperitoneal; limb; visceral

Central Nervous System (CNS)

Orbit: glioma, other; intracranial: chiasm, other; astrocytoma, schwannoma, meningioma, other; spinal

Other Tumors

Schwannoma (non-CNS); pheochromocytoma; carcinoid; other benign; malignancy

Ocular

Lisch nodules; hypertrophied corneal nerves; choroidal hamartomas; congenital glaucoma; eyelid ptosis; cataracts

Skeletal

Short stature; macrocephaly; craniofacial dysplasia; vertebral dysplasia; kyphoscoliosis/scoliosis; lumbar scalloping; pseudarthrosis: tibial, other; genu valgum/varum; pectus excavatum; other skeletal

Miscellaneous

Colon ganglioneuromatosis; xanthogranulomas (skin); vascular: angiomas, renal, cerebral, other; pulmonary fibrosis; cerebrospinal fluid: ventricle dilation, hydrocephalus, other abnormality; excess dental caries; electroencephalographic abnormality; other anatomic features

FUNCTIONAL FEATURES

Cosmetic disfigurement; hypertrophic impairment; weakness/paralysis; incoordination; pain; seizures; other neurologic features; strabismus; visual impairment; hearing impairment; speech impediment; developmental delay; learning disability; school performance problems; mental retardation; psychosocial burden; psychiatric; headache; puberty disturbance; pruritus; constipation; gastrointestinal bleeding; hypertension; surgery; other functional features

useful in the treatment of at least some optic pathway gliomas, although this is controversial.

Surgery is the mainstay of therapy for patients with NF-1, particularly for removing or debulking tumors (*eg*, neurofibromas, neurofibrosarcomas, pheochromocytomas), for treating skeletal dysplasia (*eg*, tibial pseudarthrosis, sphenoid wing dysplasia), for correcting scoliosis or kyphoscoliosis, and for treating at least some individuals with renovascular or other types of vascular compromise. In general, the surgical removal of neurofibromas is associated with suboptimal results; the tumors tend to recur and the possibility of a consequent neuropathy is significant. Surgical removal of a neurofibroma should be undertaken only if a specific major goal can be established beforehand.

Because 50% of the index cases of NF-1 represent new mutations, it is not surprising that the family history often fails to reveal another affected family member, especially if the index case (proband) is a child. For each offspring of a patient with NF-1, however, the recurrence risk is 50%. The severity of NF-1 in the offspring is unrelated to the severity of the disorder in the affected parent. Prenatal diagnosis is

available relatively routinely for families with at least two or more affected or at-risk members. Prenatal diagnosis is not yet available for a patient with a new mutation who has not borne at least one offspring. Rapid progress is being made, however, and in each instance, consultation with a geneticist or NF specialist is warranted.

TUBEROUS SCLEROSIS

Tuberous sclerosis (TS) is characterized by depigmented lesions of the skin, tumors of the central nervous system (CNS), ocular hamartomas, and an autosomal-dominant pattern of inheritance. It is the combination of developmental abnormalities of the skin, nervous system, and eyes that traditionally has led to this disorder being grouped with the phakomatoses.

■ NATURAL HISTORY

TS is a progressive disorder; the initial problems become worse and new lesions or complications appear with increasing patient age. There is marked variation in expression of the mutant gene. For a patient in whom the gene is expressed mildly, the natural history will be different than for a patient in whom the gene is expressed severely. The majority of patients have serious, compromising problems throughout their lives, most commonly mental retardation and seizures. Relatively few data are available to clarify the way in which patients with other problems (*eg*, renal angiomyolipomas, pulmonary interstitial fibrosis) fare over a lifetime. One exception may be the cardiac rhabdomyomas; these congenital cardiac tumors tend to regress at least to some degree with age. In any event, once the diagnosis of TS is made, the patient must be observed closely, and the appropriate clinical, laboratory, and radiologic techniques must be used to iden-

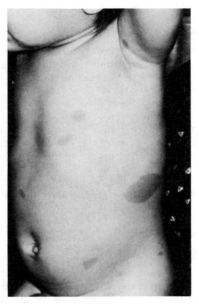

Figure 220-1. In patients with neurofibromatosis type 1, café au lait spots are usually larger than 15 mm in diameter, the edges are usually sharply defined, and the intensity of the coloration is uniform.

tify new lesions and monitor the progression of those already identified. The malignant degeneration of benign tumors (*eg*, astrocytomas, fibromas) is not a feature of TS.

In view of the fact that pertussis immunization rarely can lead to a severe neurologic syndrome, the use of vaccines with a pertussis component is contraindicated in patients with TS. The point is not that we know that pertussis vaccination actually aggravates TS, but that the vaccine is at least a confounding factor in understanding the contributing factors if the child's course deteriorates after the vaccine is administered.

■ DIAGNOSIS

When multiple features of TS are present, the diagnosis is relatively easy to make. When only one feature is present, the diagnosis is likely to be considered only tentatively, if not overlooked entirely. Establishing the diagnosis of TS depends on detecting the presence of two or more of the following features:

Skin: Hypopigmented macules, usually elliptic in shape (ash-leaf spots); fibroadenomas (adenoma sebaceum), typically involving the malar regions of the face; periungual fibromas; shagreen patches, seen most commonly over the lower trunk; and a distinctive brown patch on the forehead. The latter lesion is especially important, because it may be the first and most readily recognized feature of TS to be appreciated on physical examination of neonates and infants with the disorder.

Teeth: Characteristic pits of the enamel

Eye: Choroidal hamartomas; hypopigmented defects of the iris

CNS: Periventricular tubers; cerebral astrocytomas; sacrococcygeal chordomas; nonspecific electroencephalogram (EEG) abnormalities, including hypsarrhythmia

Cardiovascular: Cardiac rhabdomyomas; aortic and major artery constrictions

Kidney: Renal angiomyolipomas

Lungs: Diffuse interstitial fibrosis

Seizures of all types, but particularly myoclonic jerks associated with hypsarrhythmia, and mental retardation are the most common symptoms leading to the consideration of the diagnosis of TS. Magnetic resonance imaging (MRI) scans of the brain in patients with TS are virtually diagnostic and must be used in all individuals who are suspected of having the disorder. Heart failure or a cardiac murmur may indicate the presence of a cardiac rhabdomyoma, and deficient circulation or decreased pulses may indicate the presence of arterial tree involvement. Renal failure or an abdominal mass may lead to the recognition of hamartomatous kidney involvement. Dyspnea may indicate the presence of pulmonary involvement, but this anatomic feature of TS often is found coincidentally.

TS is the result of an autosomal-dominant mutant gene. Precisely because new mutations are relatively common, a previously negative family history does not exclude the diagnosis. Moreover, once the diagnosis of TS has been established in the proband, all first-degree relatives must be evaluated carefully for subtle signs of the disorder before a new mutation is presumed. Anyone who bears the mutant gene for TS carries a 50% risk that each of his or her offspring will have the disorder.

■ TREATMENT

No medical treatment is available for TS per se. The medical treatment used for seizures and other complications (*eg*, heart failure, renal failure) is the same as if TS were not present, unless surgery on the primary lesions is indicated. For example, surgical removal of a cardiac rhabdomyoma may be warranted, and some clinicians encourage an aggressive surgical approach to the renal angiomyolipomas, at least in advanced cases.

Because of the high frequency of new mutations and the variable expression of the disorder, counseling regarding recurrence among the siblings of an apparently sporadic case is difficult and is handled best by a center that specializes in TS. For an affected patient, the recurrence risk among offspring is 50%. Reliable prenatal diagnosis that relies on DNA genetic linkage data is not yet available. There is broad worldwide experience, however, in identifying several manifestations of TS in fetuses using high-resolution ultrasound techniques. Cervical cystic tumors, renal cystic abnormalities, and cardiac rhabdomyomas all have been used to identify TS prenatally. The manifestation of cardiac rhabdomyoma is particularly susceptible to this approach. Thus, it is reasonable to subject to prenatal diagnosis using ultrasound technology all pregnancies of a parent with TS.

STURGE-WEBER DISEASE

Sturge-Weber disease (SWD) also is referred to as encephalofacial angiomatosis and traditionally is known as the "fourth phakomatosis." It differs from the neurofibromatoses, TS, and VHLD by virtue of the absence of three features, however: cutaneous pigmentation defects, a clear excess of tumors, and heritability. In addition, the relatively large number of variant or atypical cases makes accurate comparisons difficult.

■ FEATURES

In addition to a facial port-wine stain and intracranial angiomatosis, primary involvement of the anterior chamber of the eye, specifically the trabecular network, and Schlemm's canal may lead to glaucoma (in either eye) in as many as 30% of patients with SWD. Macrocephaly and cutaneous xanthogranulomas also may be seen. No one feature is associated uniformly with any other, and histopathologic features cannot establish a diagnosis beyond confirming the type of lesion.

■ NATURAL HISTORY

The anatomic features of SWD may be associated with mental retardation, seizures, hemiparesis, and visual deficits, including homonymous hemianopsia. The disorder is progressive, with worsening associated with continued development of calcifications in the vascular defects.

■ DIAGNOSIS

The diagnosis of SWD depends on the presence of a port-wine stain (nevus flammeus) of the face, primarily in the first division of the trigeminal nerve; leptomeningeal angiomatosis (including angiomatous involvement of the choroid plexus or choroid of the eye); or both.

■ TREATMENT

No medical treatment is available for SWD, and the role of surgical treatment has yet to be defined. The use of lasers to treat the facial and ocular angioma lesions has been at least partially successful.

There is no precedent for SWD being recognized as a genetic or heritable disorder. Recurrence among siblings to the proband is unlikely. Caution is advised against prematurely discounting recurrence among offspring, however; the lack of precedence may reflect merely the lack of procreation of prior patients with SWD.

(Abridged from Vincent M. Riccardi, The Phakomatoses and Other Neurocutaneous Syndromes, in Oski, DeAngelis, Feigin, McMillan, Warshaw: *Principles and Practice of Pediatrics, Second Edition*, J.B. Lippincott, 1994.)

Oski's Essential Pediatrics,
edited by Kevin B. Johnson and Frank A. Oski.
Lippincott–Raven Publishers,
Philadelphia © 1997

221

Headache

Chronic and recurrent headaches are one of the most common neurologic complaints of children. Bille found that 2.5% of schoolchildren suffered from frequent headaches at 7 years of age and that 15.7% had similar complaints at 15 years of age. Other surveys indicate an even higher prevalence; in several Scandinavian countries, as many as 7% of all schoolchildren between 7 and 8 years of age have more than one headache each month. Ten percent to 20% of the adolescent population suffers from chronic headache syndromes.

■ MIGRAINE

The generally accepted criteria for the diagnosis of migraine in childhood is repeated episodes of headache accompanied by at least three of the following symptoms: recurrent abdominal pain (with or without headache) or nausea or vomiting; an aura, which usually is visual, but may be sensory, motor, or vertiginous; throbbing or pounding pain; pain that is restricted to one side of the head (although it may shift sides from one headache to the next); relief of pain by brief periods of sleep; and a family history of migraine in one or more immediate relatives. Most children who have migraine have nausea or some type of abdominal distress, are helped by sleep, and have a family history of migraine. Localized, throbbing pain, and an aura are seen more frequently during and after puberty.

Migraine headaches in children differ from those in adults in that about 60% of the affected patients are male (this drops to about 33% in the adult population); unilateral headaches are less common before puberty; and a visual aura is much less frequent. The incidence of epilepsy with migraine varies from 5.4% to 12.3% in various series, but is less than 3% in adults. Nausea and vomiting occur in about the same percentage of individuals in both groups, and about 70% of children and adults have a strong family history of migraine.

Childhood migraine is more likely to vary in frequency than in severity. Children who otherwise fit the criteria for the diagnosis of migraine may have one headache per month and then begin gradually or abruptly to have three to five headaches per week. If they are not treated, these headaches will last for a period of weeks or months and can interfere with school and other usual activities. Occasionally, these exacerbations can be related to changes in mood, particularly depression or stress. Much of the time, however, no predisposing factor can be found to explain the increased headache frequency.

Diagnosis

Migraine is a clinical diagnosis that is made by obtaining the patient's history. The physical examination generally is normal. Laboratory studies are not needed for confirmation unless there are physical signs or a doubtful history. In many published series of children with migraine headache, electroencephalogram (EEG) tracings often are abnormal and as many as 10% may be paroxysmal. Unless the abnormality seen on the EEG is focal, however, the tracing does not have any prognostic significance. Focal tracings do suggest the increased possibility of a lesion in the central nervous system (CNS) and make it necessary to perform a computed tomography (CT) or magnetic resonance imaging (MRI) scan to rule out a mass lesion or vascular disorder. Occasionally, certain aspects of the clinical history should alert the physician to study the child further. These include a strong family history of cerebrovascular disease early in life or of intracranial hemorrhage, headaches that localize persistently to one side of the cranium without shifting, the onset of motor or sensory symptoms well after the headache has started, the failure of motor or sensory symptoms to clear within 24 hours after the headache has ceased, and the association of focal headaches with partial seizures involving the same hemisphere. Focal physical findings or evidence of increased intracranial pressure on examination also indicate the need for further evaluation or even hospitalization.

Many children have symptoms that are said to be "migraine variants." These patients may not have a headache with each attack. The relationship of migraine variants to migraine is based on one of two pieces of information: a strong family history of migraine or the known tendency of more typical forms of migraine to develop in children with these disorders later in life.

The most common and easily related of these variants is basilar migraine, which is most prevalent in adolescent girls. The symptoms that occur lie within the territory of the basilar circulation. Vertigo, syncope, unilateral or bilateral numbness, and dysarthria can be seen at the onset of the attack. Some children feel weak and unsteady, but do not faint. On recovery, there may be visual loss for a brief period and there usually is a pounding occipital headache. Confusion and memory loss also can occur. A small subgroup has generalized seizures, which sometimes are difficult to control.

Motion sickness is common in patients who have migraine, but it is not clear that recurrent attacks of paroxysmal vertigo are a migraine variant. Patients with migraine may experience isolated attacks of confusion or memory loss. They may have recurrent attacks of delirium. These patients may not complain of headaches, and there may be only a strong family history to suggest migraine.

Some children with recurrent episodes of abdominal pain have typical migraine later in life. Certainly, paroxysmal abdominal pain is more likely to be a migrainous than an epileptic syndrome, although paroxysmal EEG tracings are common with the disorder. Most children with recurrent abdominal pain do not suffer from either disorder.

Patients who have a genetic predisposition to migraine seem to react more severely to relatively minor head injuries. Sometimes, a minor episode of trauma is followed by the onset of common or classic migraine. Transient blindness or motor or sensory loss may occur without significant headache. These episodes are short-lived and this, as well as the absence of any evidence of intracranial injury on CT scan, suggests that the symptoms and signs are the response of a migraineur and not the result of a contusion.

Treatment

Many migraine headaches can be relieved with simple analgesics such as aspirin or acetaminophen. Because aspirin may be associated with Reye's syndrome, acetaminophen is recommended for younger children. If these mild analgesics are not effective, commercial preparations such as Fiorinal (butalbital, aspirin, and caffeine) or Midrin (a combination of isometheptene mucate, acetaminophen, and dichloralphenazone) may be used in older children. Older children with more severe migraines that occur less frequently (no more than twice a month) may benefit from the use of ergotamine tartrate at the onset of a headache. Frequently, the long-term use of ergots is associated with vascular disease. Intractable migraine headaches often can be relieved by the use of a combination of intravenous metoclopramide followed by intravenous dihydroergotamine. In older patients, dihydroergotamine can be administered subcutaneously at home. This frequently relieves the pain sufficiently to permit the patient to resume normal activities.

A novel new drug called sumatriptan, a serotonin agonist, soon will be available for the treatment of patients with acute migraine headaches. This agent is a selective agonist of 5-hydroxytryptamine–like receptors in the CNS. It can be administered orally or subcutaneously.

Migraine also may be treated prophylactically. This is particularly beneficial for children who tend to get frequent headaches and otherwise would require a large amount of analgesic medication or ergot for relief. Average doses of prophylactic medications include propranolol cyproheptadine hydrochloride, phenobarbital or phenytoin, amitriptyline hydrochloride, or calcium channel blockers.

The most common forms of headache in children also have begun to be treated with biofeedback and relaxation therapy. Initial studies were poorly controlled and involved very few children. Evidence is increasing, however, that pediatric as well as adult patients with common migraine and tension headaches do respond to this type of treatment. Of all children who can complete successfully a course of training in either biofeedback or relaxation techniques, 60% to 80% have a positive response consisting of reduction in the frequency and severity of their headaches. This compares favorably with the response obtained with medication. Follow-up studies suggest that the benefits of this training last for at least 1 year. Problems associated with these forms of behavioral therapy include limited facilities,

cost, and failure of children to practice these learned techniques regularly.

■ TENSION HEADACHES

As noted earlier, it often is difficult to differentiate common migraine from tension headaches solely by the clinical description. No single factor in the history differentiates the two types. People who suffer from either type of headache tend to have a normal physical examination. A constellation of factors does help the physician to make a diagnosis, however. Tension headaches usually occur and are most severe during periods of obvious stress. This association is seen with migraine, but it is not as clear-cut. Migraine tends to involve the frontal and, to a lesser degree, temporal regions of the head, or to be localized retro-orbitally; tension headaches tend to involve the occipital or temporal regions bilaterally and often extend to the neck, or they are diffuse. Tension headaches often are continuous; they fluctuate throughout the day, but never disappear. Patients who have this constellation of features indicating a probable diagnosis of tension headaches are less likely to have immediate family members who have typical migraine. Nausea and vomiting occur with both types of headache when the pain is severe, but are much more common in children with migraine, as are isolated attacks of abdominal pain. The diagnosis is made by careful review of the history.

A subgroup of patients with tension headaches (as well as patients with migraine) suffer from an overt depression with a history of a clear-cut change in mood, self-image, interest in their usual day-to-day activities, appetite, and sleep habits. They often have multiple other somatic complaints. The headaches that these children have will not disappear until the underlying mood disorder is recognized and treated.

The pain resulting from tension headaches usually can be relieved with analgesics. Analgesics combined with codeine sometimes may be required, but the repeated use of codeine should be avoided. When tension headaches recur frequently, biofeedback and relaxation therapy is very useful. In that population of children whose headaches are related to depression, an anxiety neurosis, or a conversion reaction, however, referral to a psychiatrist is indicated.

■ SINUS HEADACHES

Chronic or recurrent headaches occur in about 15% of children who have chronic sinusitis. Frequently, there is no increase in temperature. The most common accompanying symptoms or signs are rhinorrhea, postnasal drip, persistent cough, and recurrent ear infections. There may be pain with pressure over the frontal or maxillary sinuses, and these cavities can fail to transilluminate. (The frontal sinuses form later in childhood and are not developed fully in most children until the end of puberty.) Most sinus headaches in children result from infection of the sphenoid or ethmoid sinuses. There usually is no tenderness to palpation when these sinuses are inflamed, and signs of nasal congestion frequently are minimal. Pain usually is referred to the frontotemporal region, but it can occur over any part of the cranial vault. Sinus headaches often occur at the same time each day, build slowly, frequently have a throbbing quality, and vary markedly with change in position (because positional change may promote sinus drainage). The only certain means of diagnosing headaches that result from disease of one or more of the paranasal sinuses is by roentgenography.

The diagnosis should be made only if the sinuses are clouded, exhibit a fluid level, or have a thickened mucosa.

Simple analgesics may help decrease the pain of sinus headaches, but sustained relief usually depends on long-term therapy with nasal decongestants and appropriate antibiotics. Surgical drainage is reserved for patients with intractable disease.

■ OTHER EXTRACRANIAL CAUSES OF HEADACHE

Temporomandibular joint disease usually presents with pain that is maximal at the joint and extends into the face and the temporal region. In some patients, however, the pain occurs predominantly in the form of a temporal or frontotemporal headache, which can be unilateral or bilateral and usually does not throb. The diagnosis can be suspected by the child's history. The physical examination is especially helpful if there is limited movement of the temporomandibular joint, or if a click is palpated when the patient makes chewing movements. There also may be a noise that either the child or the examiner can hear when the joint is moved.

Inflammation of the vessels of the scalp and periodontal infections are other rare causes of chronic headache syndromes in children.

■ INTRACRANIAL CAUSES OF HEADACHE

Headaches from intracranial lesions occur for one of two reasons: there is a localized or generalized increase in pressure within the skull, which stretches or distorts vessels at the surface of the brain or the arachnoid and dural membranes that cover the brain; or the pain-sensitive fibers in these brain coverings become irritated by infection or bleeding. Tumors or other masses such as abscess or hemorrhage usually are responsible for local distortion of the brain vessels or meninges. Nearly 80% of tumors in children, however, occur either in the posterior fossa or near the midline. Thus, they frequently obstruct the circulation of cerebrospinal fluid, with resulting hydrocephalus. When this occurs, the elevation in intracranial pressure is more diffuse and the headache often is bifrontal or generalized rather than localized over one part of the hemicranium.

It may not be possible to distinguish intracranial from extracranial causes of headache. Certain features, however, may suggest the likelihood of an intracranial mass, including severe occipital headache, headache that is made worse by straining or by sneezing or coughing, headache that awakens the patient from a deep sleep, headache that is exacerbated or improved markedly by a change in position, headache that is associated with projectile vomiting or vomiting without nausea, and headache with a history of focal seizures. If they are allowed to continue, these headaches usually increase in intensity and severity week after week. Patients who have headaches caused by intracranial mass lesions almost always have physical findings if the headaches have been present for several months. These findings include papilledema, unilateral or bilateral sixth nerve palsies, ataxia, and spasticity (particularly in the lower extremities), as well as more localized indications of brain dysfunction involving movement, vision, or language, depending on the site of the lesion.

Pseudotumor cerebri produces the same type of headache that is found in association with elevated intracranial pressure resulting from a mass lesion or hydrocephalus. Vomiting and blurred vision are frequent accompanying complaints, and papilledema, sixth nerve palsies, ataxia, and, less frequently, spasticity may be noted on physical examination. As the name implies, no mass is found with further laboratory studies. Pseudotumor cerebri probably is caused by the expansion of one or more intracranial fluid spaces, such as the vascular and extracellular fluid compartments.

Meningeal irritation usually results in an acute, diffuse, rapidly progressive headache that becomes so intense that it may be unbearable. If the cause is bleeding, then the onset may be explosive and the headache may become excruciating within only a minute or two. Such patients may have focal neurologic signs, but many do not. There frequently is a disturbance of orientation or consciousness. On physical examination, there may be nuchal rigidity caused by meningeal irritation. Occasionally, the examiner can see perivenous or subhyaloid hemorrhages in the eye, resulting from high intracranial pressure and the extravasation of subarachnoid blood.

It is the physician's first responsibility to rule out the possibility of an intracranial lesion. The association of any type of headache with a history of recent onset or progression of neurologic signs warrants the performance of a CT or MRI scan. Focal headaches that are becoming increasingly frequent, more severe, or intractable to therapy also demand further investigation. Other situations indicating the need for an outpatient CT scan include the onset of chronic headaches after an episode of head trauma and the individual characteristics of the headache, such as a sudden change in its intensity accompanying a change in position.

The treatment of headaches resulting from intracranial catastrophies is not within the scope of this chapter. If the diagnosis of pseudotumor cerebri is made, the patient frequently may obtain relief from a single lumbar puncture performed for diagnostic reasons. If, as often is the case, symptoms recur and intracranial pressure returns to high levels within 3 to 4 days, dexamethasone may be used for 3 to 5 days and then withdrawn rapidly. Alternatively, acetazolamide can be given in three divided doses. If this fails to relieve the patient's symptoms, then repeated lumbar punctures may be needed whenever symptoms recur, or glycerol can be used in gradually increasing dosages as tolerated. Obesity and chronic diarrhea are complications of oral glycerol therapy. Because long-term elevation of the intracranial pressure can affect the vision without causing other symptoms or signs, regular eye examinations should be performed in this group of children. Fenestration of the optic nerve sheath may preserve vision under these circumstances.

■ ACUTE HEADACHE

A headache may be so severe that it brings a child to a doctor's office or to the emergency department seeking both a diagnosis and immediate relief of pain. Under these circumstances, it is extremely important that the physician distinguish between intracranial and extracranial causes of the headache, decide if admission to the hospital is necessary, and provide some plan to relieve the child's pain as quickly as possible. The basis of diagnosis still remains the history and physical examination, but, in the face of an acute cephalgia, it often is crucial to decide whether the child requires an immediate head scan or lumbar puncture to assist in the diagnosis and planning of immediate care.

Common intracranial causes of acute, severe headache are a mass lesion, infection, or intracranial hemorrhage. Extracranial causes include migraine, tension headaches, and, rarely, sinusitis. The most decisive factor in the history is whether this is the first such headache this child has experienced or whether it is another headache in an already established pattern of headaches that has been evaluated in the past. It also is important to know whether this particular headache has been associated with unusual antecedent events such as a head injury, seizure, fever, or change in sensory or motor function. Critical physical findings include meningismus, focal neurologic signs, papilledema or split sutures, evidence of cranial trauma (including blood in or behind the ear), and a depressed level of consciousness.

If this is the first attack of severe cephalgia without a significant prior headache history, immediate neural imaging is recommended if any of the following are present: a history of recent trauma, the recent onset of seizures, unusual behaviors predating the headache, fever, meningismus, papilledema, focal neurologic signs, or a depressed level of consciousness. The determination that it will be necessary to use drugs that will depress consciousness significantly to relieve the child's pain also may lead to early neural imaging. In the presence of a prior headache history with a presumed diagnosis, a recent history of trauma, unusual premorbid behaviors, meningismus, papilledema, and significant depression of consciousness indicate the need for immediate neural imaging, as do focal signs, unless they have been present in the past as part of a typical migraine syndrome.

A lumbar puncture should be considered if there is a fever without a cause accompanying the headache, meningismus, and new neurologic signs or abnormal behaviors in the presence of normal results on CT or MRI scanning.

The presence of abnormal results on lumbar puncture or an acute or subacute abnormality on brain scanning dictates that the child be hospitalized. The patient should be admitted to the hospital in the presence of normal test results, however, if there is clinical evidence of elevated intracranial pressure, new neurologic signs, or meningismus. In the face of pernicious vomiting, children also may have to be admitted for rehydration. Children require hospitalization at times for the treatment of intractable pain and, rarely, for short-term psychiatric care.

If the child has no evidence of an intracranial lesion, excruciating pain can be relieved by the intramuscular administration of meperidine and hydroxyzine. An alternate approach, which is particularly useful if the child is agitated, is to sedate him or her with pentobarbital or chloral hydrate. This usually requires hospital admission for observation. If it is clear by the history that the child has migraine, the immediate intravenous administration of metoclopramide followed by dihydroergotamine (after a test dose), with the concomitant use of low-dose steroids may obviate hospitalization by relieving the headache rapidly in the emergency department. If this fails to relieve the pain over 2 to 3 hours, hospitalization for further parenteral therapy usually is indicated.

(Abridged from Arthur L. Prensky, Headache, in Oski, DeAngelis, Feigin, McMillan, Warshaw: *Principles and Practice of Pediatrics, Second Edition*, J.B. Lippincott, 1994.)

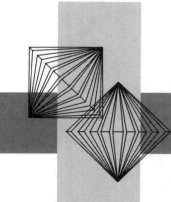

PART V

Pediatrician's Companion: Important Things to Remember

Oski's Essential Pediatrics,
edited by Kevin B. Johnson and Frank A. Oski.
Lippincott–Raven Publishers,
Philadelphia © 1997

222

Evaluation and Use of Laboratory Tests

More than 10% of all health care spending in the United States pays for clinical laboratory services, a percentage that continues to increase as new and more complex laboratory tests are developed and aggressively marketed. Increasing equally is the concern that not all of this spending is in the best interests of good medical care. Laboratory tests can be powerful aids in diagnosis and patient management, but evidence shows that many physicians know little about the tests they commonly order. The result is often extra expense and, at times, avoidable morbidity.

It is one thing to prescribe what a physician should know about a test and another to find that information and make it available in clinically useful form. As with many medical technologies, the common use of most laboratory tests has preceded study of how well they perform and in what settings they should be used. Thus, this chapter has four goals:

- To list the characteristics of laboratory tests and how the clinician can use these characteristics to select the proper test for a given task

- To describe how laboratory tests fit into the larger process of medical diagnosis and screening

- To suggest ways in which clinicians can find information about test characteristics when that information is not generally available in popular texts or laboratory manuals

- To provide information about some laboratory tests commonly used by clinicians caring for children.

In this chapter, the term *test* means a laboratory or clinical procedure such as a determination of serum sodium level or a urinalysis. The concepts discussed here apply equally to most other procedures used to gather clinical information. For example, questions in a medical history or maneuvers in a physical examination can be considered tests for which performance characteristics can be defined and measured.

■ PERFORMANCE CHARACTERISTICS OF TESTS

How well a test performs can be described by several parameters, each of which is important in determining when the test may be useful.

A test's precision reflects how much difference to expect if the same specimen was tested repeatedly. For example, it is important for a clinician to know whether a change from 20% to 30% of neutrophils on a patient's differential white blood-cell count (WBC) reflects a resolution of the patient's neutropenia or is likely to be a variation in test performance.

A test's precision is not always related to its accuracy (*ie*, the relationship of test result to true value of the measured

parameter). A machine may measure serum potassium with great precision, but values are meaningless if one does not recognize that hemolysis may render them inaccurate.

The "Two-by-Two" Table

The following paragraphs refer to Figure 222–1, the standard "two-by-two" cross-tabulation frequently used to describe basic test characteristics. Suppose test 1 is designed to detect disease X. The columns in Figure 222–1 represent two groups of individuals: those on the left (+) are known to have disease X; those on the right (–) are known to be free of the condition. The rows classify individuals based on results of test 1: the top row (+) counts all those whose test results were positive; the bottom row (–) counts all those whose test results were negative. Each cell (A, B, C, D) divides the group of tested individuals into four categories:

Cell	Have Disease X	Test Result	Label
A	yes	positive	true-positive
B	no	positive	false-positive
C	yes	negative	false-negative
D	no	negative	true-negative

If the test worked perfectly, there would be 100% agreement between test results and true presence of disease (individuals only in cells A and D). This almost never occurs, which is a reminder in interpreting test results: a positive (or negative) test result does not guarantee that a disease is (or is not) present. The test only tells how great a chance there is that the disease is present.

Sensitivity and Specificity

Test characteristics derived from sums and ratios of the four cell values (see Figure 222–1) determine how well a test performs a diagnostic task.

Sensitivity is the likelihood that a test will be positive in the presence of a targeted disease. Sensitivity is $A/(A + C)$, that is, the proportion of all individuals with disease X who have a positive result on test 1 (see Figure 222–1), or, sensitivity is the probability that test 1 will be positive in the presence of disease X. Test sensitivity is critical in screening for asymptomatic disease and ruling out specific diagnoses. When A is large compared to C (*eg*, when $A/(A + C)$ is greater than .99), there is relative confidence that if test 1 is negative, an individual does not have disease X. This does not make any claims for what a positive test result means.

Specificity is the likelihood of a test to be negative in individuals who do not have the disease. Specificity is defined as $D/(B + D)$ (see Figure 222–1), the probability of a negative test result in an individual without disease X. Very specific tests often are used to confirm or "rule in" a suspected diagnosis. When D is very large compared to B ($D/(B + D)$ is close to 1), a positive result is unlikely to occur in an individual who truly does not have disease X. Based on specificity alone, this does not make any claims for what a negative test result means.

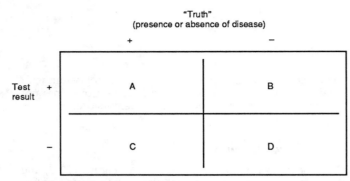

Figure 222-1. The "two-by two" cross-tabulation used to describe basic test characteristics.

Sensitivity and specificity are further diagrammed in Figure 222–2. The vertical axis corresponds to the columns of Figure 222–1. Counting up the axis represents persons from the (−) column, those without disease X, and counting down represents persons from the (+) column, persons with disease X. The horizontal axis corresponds to the rows of Figure 222–1. Test values considered to be positive are on the right, and test values considered to be negative are on the left. Areas beneath the two curves represent the number of individuals in each cell of Figure 222–1.

Predictive Value

Usually, it is not enough to know that a test is very sensitive or very specific. What the clinician wants to know is how much confidence there is that a positive test result really means that disease is present or that a negative result really means that disease is absent. The most basic way to express this confidence is with two quantities, the test's positive and negative predictive values. Positive predictive value is the proportion of persons who test positive on test 1 who actually have disease X, or $A/(A + B)$ (see Figure 222–1), or the

probability that disease X will be present, given a positive test. The negative predictive value is $D/(C + D)$ (see Figure 222–1), or the probability that disease is not present, given a negative test.

A test's positive and negative predictive values vary with the prevalence of the target disease in the studied population. This is illustrated by example—the use of enzyme-linked immunosorbent assays (ELISA) for human immunodeficiency virus (HIV). Although the characteristics of the HIV ELISA vary from manufacturer to manufacturer, in experienced hands, the test is felt to have a sensitivity that approaches 100% and a specificity of more than 99%. These are impressive statistics, and the tests yield impressive results when used in a high-prevalence population such as a group of hemophiliacs who received blood products before the use of treatments to inactivate HIV (Figure 222–3). With a prevalence of HIV antibodies approaching 50%, the positive and negative predictive values of the test are both nearly 100%. Figure 222–4 shows how the same test performs in a population of male Army recruits, in whom the prevalence of HIV positivity is reported to be 0.16%. The positive predictive value of the test is about 24%. In other words, for every true-positive result, there are about three that are false positive. Thus, HIV testing of low-prevalence populations requires sequential use of other tests, usually a repeat ELISA followed by a Western blot, to separate the true-positive from the false-positive results.

Even such a series of tests does not reduce the false-positive rate to zero; thus, many authorities question the utility and ethics of HIV and other testing in low-risk groups. In general, however, performing individual tests in series reduces the overall sensitivity and increases specificity. If all individuals who are positive on test 1 (true and false positives) are retested with test 2, there is no opportunity to learn more about individuals who were negative on test 1, but there is a chance to reduce the number of false positives.

The Likelihood Ratio

An increasingly popular way of summarizing a test's capabilities is to state its positive or negative likelihood ratio. The likelihood ratio is similar to the predictive value in that

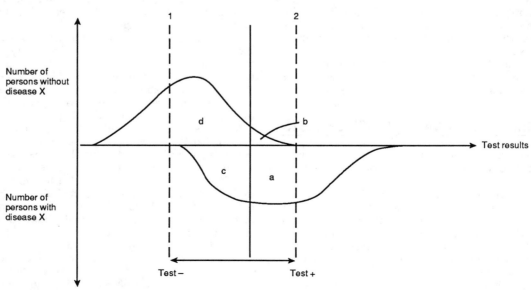

Figure 222-2. Sensitivity and specificity of tests (see Fig 222-1).

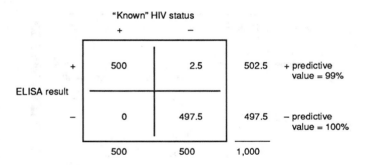

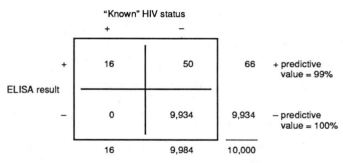

Total hypothetical population = 1,000
Prevalence = 50%
False-positive rate = 0.42%
False-negative rate = 0

Figure 222-3. Hypothetical data for use of a single ELISA test to detect antibodies to HIV in a high-prevalence population.

Total hypothetical population = 10,000
Prevalence = 0.16%
False-positive rate = 76%
False-negative rate = 0

Figure 222-4. Hypothetical data for use of a single ELISA test to detect antibodies to HIV in a low-prevalence population.

it helps in assessing the diagnostic benefit of a positive or negative test result. Unlike the predictive value, the likelihood ratio is independent of the prevalence of disease. The likelihood ratio, then, is useful in assessing how well a test will do in different populations or for individuals with higher or lower chances of having a certain disease.

The likelihood ratio is a ratio of probabilities—the probability that the test is positive in a person who really has the disease compared to the probability that the test is positive in a person who does not have the disease. For example, a person with disease X is so many times more likely to have a positive result on test 1 than is a person who does not have disease X. The chance that a person with disease X will have a positive test is the same as $A/(A + C)$ (see Figure 222–1), or the test's sensitivity. The chance that a person without disease X will have a positive test is $B/(B + D)$ (see Figure 222–1), or 1 minus the test's specificity.

Using a formula known as Bayes' theorem, the likelihood ratio can be used to calculate, for any level of disease prevalence or pre-test chance that a patient has disease, the revised, or post-test chance, given the test results that disease is present or absent.

For any test, there is usually a zone of pre-test probabilities within which the test offers maximum gain information. This zone can be used to define the threshold approach to making clinical decisions. At pre-test probabilities below the zone of usefulness, one would not test and, if this was a diagnostic test for a treatable condition, would not treat. At pretest probabilities above the zone, one would not test and would proceed as if the test was positive. Only for pre-test probabilities within the zone would one test first before going on to the next step in treatment or diagnosis. The test zone is determined by factors beyond sensitivity and specificity. For example, one would be more liberal with a test that was inexpensive and safe or more conservative with a test that had considerable risk or was less accurate.

Likelihood ratios may ultimately allow the elimination of single cut points for tests and, instead, provide information about the chances that disease is present at any point in the range of a test's possible results. This idea is appealing because many tested quantities do not lend themselves to "yes" or "no" dichotomies. For example, hyperglycemia may be defined as a blood-glucose level of greater than 130 mg/dL, but this definition falsely identifies some people with diabetes as normal. Table 222–1 shows hypothetical

post-test probabilities of diabetes for various blood-glucose levels and a range of pre-test probabilities of disease. It shows how a level of 130 mg/dL is more significant for a person with a 50–50 chance of having diabetes—someone giving a history of polyuria and polydypsia—than for a person with no symptoms and a low chance of having the disease. On the other hand, a level of 150 mg/dL has clinical significance for someone who is asymptomatic, and even a level of 100 mg/dL might be of concern in someone who had several clinical signs and symptoms and a high pre-test chance of illness.

■ ASSESSING INFORMATION ABOUT A TEST

Clinicians frequently must decide if a journal account of a new test warrants its use. The following questions may serve as guides to evaluating an account of a new or an old test.

What gold standard did the authors use in their study of the new test? In Figure 222–1, it was posited that the individuals in the left column really had the disease and those in the right column really did not. Usually, there is no such knowledge, and results of the new test are compared with results of another test that has its own degree of uncertainty. A variety of pitfalls can arise.

1. The old comparison test may not be performed properly. For example, an account of a new test that differentiates viral from streptococcal sore throats is compared with the gold-standard throat culture with its known susceptibility to false-negative results when improperly performed. Were throat swabs performed consistently and meticulously, carried promptly to the laboratory, and plated by a competent technician? Was identification of the organism carried out with an accepted method? This type of problem often surfaces when a new test is put into use while old diagnostic procedures are used, rather than being tested in the context of a deliberate research project. This sort of problem makes it difficult to establish how well the new test really works.

2. Even if performed properly, the old test may not be worthy of gold-standard status. Sometimes, there is no better alternative, but often there is. Using the

throat-swab example again, most research projects involving detection of streptococci in the pharynx use duplicate swabs as a gold standard because a single swab has been found to miss as many as 10% of true-positive cases.

3. Those performing the new test should be blind to how the patient is classified by the gold standard. Even relatively objective results can be swayed by biased observation.

What population was used to study the new test? As discussed, the population used to determine a test's characteristics can have profound influence on parameters such as positive and negative predictive values. Subtle problems also may arise related to the spectrum of disease among the studied patients.

1. All "disease-positive" patients may be individuals with advanced, unambiguous cases of the disease. It may be unknown how well the test will work in patients with earlier stages of illness or whose diagnosis is more debatable.

2. All control patients may be normal. The usual diagnostic task is not to differentiate persons with disease from those who are well but to choose who has a particular disease from among a group of people with similar symptoms. Thus, a test that separates children with rheumatoid arthritis from normal controls may not differentiate among those with collagen vascular disease, joint trauma secondary to overuse, and toxic synovitis.

How is "normal" defined, either for the new test or for the gold standard? Where a cut point divides normal and abnormal may influence greatly how a test performs and how it can be used. In most cases, the ideal way to define what is abnormal or normal is in terms of the target disease or body function being measured. For example, the best way to define an abnormally low hematocrit for diagnosing iron-deficiency anemia is to pick the point below which most individuals have a response to the administration of iron. Usually, however, cut points are calculated by performing a test on apparently normal individuals, then using statistical methods to define values of the test's results that are outside an expected normal range. In the hematocrit example, a large number of apparently healthy persons would be tested, and the lowest 5% of values would be declared too low. This method has a number of potential problems:

1. The population used to define normal may not be representative of all those on whom the test will be used. This is classically the case for tests developed in adult populations and for which normal values in children are not known. Similar problems can occur with race or sex differences.

2. The normal population may not be normal. It may contain persons who have the disease in question or other unrelated conditions that change the test's results.

TABLE 222-1. Table of Hypothetical Post-Test Probabilities of Diabetes, Given Varying Pre-Test Probabilities and Different Cut Points of Defining Hyperglycemia

	Cutoff Glucose Levels (mg/dL)		
	100	*130*	*150*
Pre-Test Probabilities			
0.1	.12	.35	.64
0.5	.56	.83	.94
0.9	.92	.98	.99
Hypothetical Likelihood Ratios			
100 mg/dL—1.3			
130 mg/dL—5.0			
150 mg/dL—16.0			

3. The use of statistical techniques to define normal and abnormal (*ie,* greater than two standard deviations from the mean; less than the fifth percentile) automatically labels a fixed proportion of the tested population as abnormal, regardless of whether this degree of deviation from the average has any physiologic significance. Failure to recognize this phenomenon can lead to unnecessary evaluations for problems that do not exist. If a healthy individual undergoes 12 tests, such as on a standard 12-test chemistry panel that uses the plus-or-minus-two-standard-deviations rule for normalcy, the chance that all 12 results will be normal is only 54%.

Is it clear how the new test is being used? Whether the new test is used alone or in conjunction with other diagnostic information must be clear. An x-ray film, for example, may be read as is or the radiologist may be given clinical data to aid in interpretation. Both methods may be valid depending on the setting in which the test is used, but the latter method may require additional study of the relative weights given to the film and to the clinical information.

Is the new test truly independent of the gold standard? The new test should not incorporate any element of the gold standard. This occurs most often when the proposed test is a symptom complex used to identify a high-risk group of patients. Problems arise, for example, if a new test for urinary tract infection (UTI) requires the presence of fever and dysuria, whereas the gold-standard diagnosis was defined as fever and a positive urine culture. The authors of the new test would then conclude that fever is a useful tool for identifying children at risk for UTI.

(Abridged from Lawrence S. Wissow, Evaluation and Use of Laboratory Tests, in Oski, DeAngelis, Feigin, McMillan, Warshaw: *Principles and Practice of Pediatrics, Second Edition,* J.B. Lippincott, 1994.)

Oski's Essential Pediatrics,
edited by Kevin B. Johnson and Frank A. Oski.
Lippincott–Raven Publishers,
Philadelphia © 1997

223
Laboratory Values

The following reference values for laboratory tests represent guidelines only, since the reference range from one institution to the next will vary, depending on the laboratory method used. To simplify the interpretation of laboratory results reported in International System (SI) units, conversion factors (from SI to conventional units) are provided. SI base units are the gram (g), the liter (L), and the mole (mol). Other abbreviations are listed below.

SI Prefixes

Factor	Prefix	Symbol
10^3	kilo	k
10^{-1}	deci	d
10^{-2}	centi	c
10^{-3}	milli	m
10^{-6}	micro	μ
10^{-9}	nano	n
10^{-12}	pico	p
10^{-15}	femto	f

Abbreviations

CI	confidence interval
d	day
F	female
h	hour
Hb	hemoglobin
M	male
MCHC	mean corpuscular hemoglobin concentration
MCV	mean corpuscular volume
mEq	milliequivalent
min	minute
RBC	red blood cell
s	second
SD	standard deviation
U	unit
WBC	white blood cell
yr	year

(Abridged from Peter C. Rowe, Laboratory Values, in Oski, DeAngelis, Feigin, McMillan, Warshaw: *Principles and Practice of Pediatrics, Second Edition*, J.B. Lippincott, 1994.)

Oski's Essential Pediatrics,
edited by Kevin B. Johnson and Frank A. Oski.
Lippincott–Raven Publishers,
Philadelphia © 1997

224
Common Syndromes With Morphologic Abnormalities

A *syndrome* is a running together of symptoms (usually), which, taken as a whole, presents a picture of a disease or disorder. Morphologic abnormalities often recur in patterns that create a recognizable picture. In this chapter, 50 syndromes with morphologic abnormalities are presented in abbreviated form, along with a list of common (and some less common) features, comments regarding key associations and prevalence, and information about performance and etiology. Distinctive phenotypic features of syndromes are shown in accompanying figures. Syndromes are listed alphabetically below.

Aarskog's
Achondroplasia
AIDS embryopathy
Anhidrotic (hypohidrotic) ectodermal dysplasia
Aniridia-Wilms' tumor
Apert's
Beckwith-Wiedemann
Bloom's
Camptomelic dysplasia
Carpenter's
Cerebral gigantism
Cerebrohepatorenal (Zellweger)
CHARGE
Cockayne's
Cornelia de Lange's
Cri du chat
Crouzon's
Down's
Fanconi's
Fetal alcohol
Fetal hydantoin
Hallermann-Streiff
Hurler's
Langer-Giedion
Larsen's
Leprechaunism
Marfan's
Menkes'
Morquio's
Mulibrey nanism
Noonan's
Oculoauriculovertebral
Oral-facial-digital

Prader-Willi
Progeria
Rothmund-Thomson
Rubinstein-Taybi
Russell-Silver
Saethre-Chotzen
Seckel's
Shprintzen's
Smith-Lemli-Opitz
Stickler's
TAR
Treacher Collins
Trisomy 13
Trisomy 18
Turner's
VATER
Williams

AARSKOG'S SYNDROME

Key Features (Figure 224-1)

Round face
Hypertelorism
Small, short, broad nose—anteverted nostrils
Long philtrum
Short stature
Shawl scrotum—scrotal fold encircles base of phallus

Other Findings

Ptosis of eyelids
Antimongoloid slant to eyes
Maxillary hypoplasia
Prominent metopic suture
Thin vermilion border of upper lip; pouting lower lip
Crease below lower lip
Widow's peak of hairline
Brachydactyly with clinodactyly of fifth fingers

Simian crease
Mild interdigital webbing
Mild pectus excavatum
Prominent umbilicus
Cryptorchidism
Low-set ears
Broad feet with bulbous toes
Proximal interphalangeal joint hyperextensibility with distal joint restriction

Comments. Short stature is usually not evident until 2 to 4 years of age. With age, the round face becomes triangular. The incidence of this syndrome is not known.

Performance. Mild mental retardation is common.

Etiology. X-linked recessive and autosomal-dominant inheritance have been reported.

ACHONDROPLASIA SYNDROME

Key Features (Figure 224-2)

Short stature
Macrocephaly
Low, broad nasal bridge
Frontal bossing
Midfacial hypoplasia
Short limbs

Other Findings

Brachycephaly
Narrow nasal passages
Prominent mandible
Dental malocclusion; crowding of teeth
Small, cuboid-shaped vertebral bodies
Lumbar lordosis
Elbows lacking full extension
Short, stubby hands
Bowed legs
Small foramen magnum; occipitalization of C-1

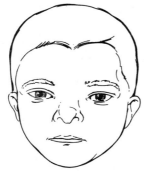

Figure 224-1. Aarskog's syndrome.

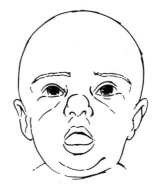

Figure 224-2. Achondroplasia syndrome.

Comments. These infants have an early delay in motor development, particularly in walking and in head control because of its relatively large size. A narrow spinal canal and instability of C-1 and C-2 predispose to spinal cord injuries. Hydrocephalus occurs with increased frequency. Disorders of respiration are common, especially those caused by thoracic cage restriction or upper airway obstruction.

The incidence is estimated at 1:10,000 to 1:20,000.

Performance. Normal mental development is the rule unless there are central nervous system (CNS) complications.

Etiology. Inheritance is autosomal dominant, although 80% to 90% of cases represent fresh mutations.

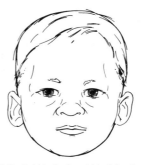

Figure 224-3. Anhidrotic (hypohidrotic) ectodermal dysplasia.

AIDS EMBRYOPATHY (FETAL AIDS SYNDROME)

Key Features

Microcephaly
Prominent boxlike appearance of forehead
Flat nasal bridge
Mild upward or downward obliquity of eyes
Prominent palpebral fissures with blue sclerae
Ocular hypertelorism
Short nose with flattened columella
Well-formed triangular philtrum
Full vermilion border of lip
Patulous lips
Growth failure

Comments. Whether maternal infection with human immunodeficiency virus (HIV) has distinct effects on the developing fetus is controversial.

ANHIDROTIC (HYPOHIDROTIC) ECTODERMAL DYSPLASIA

Key Features (Figure 224-3)

Small, saddle-shaped nose
Frontal bossing
Prominent supraorbital ridges
Midface hypoplasia
Prominent, pouting lips
Small, conical, or missing teeth
Hyperthermia from inadequate sweating
Fine, dry, sparse hair

Other Findings

Wide cheekbones
Small, pointed, low-set ears

Soft, thin skin
Dystrophic nails
Chronic rhinorrhea
Thin, wrinkled eyelid skin
Hoarse voice
Scaling skin in neonates

Comments. This disorder may be recognized first in infancy because of hyperthermia associated with the inability to sweat.

The incidence of this form of ectodermal dysplasia is about 1:100,000 male births.

Performance. Hyperthermia may result in mental and developmental delay.

Etiology. Inheritance is X-linked recessive; carrier females may express some features.

ANIRIDIA-WILMS' TUMOR ASSOCIATION

Key Features (Figure 224-4)

Prominent lips
Micrognathia
Poorly formed, low-set ears
Aniridia
Microcephaly

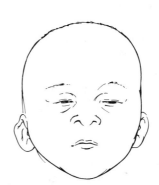

Figure 224-4. Aniridia-Wilms' tumor.

Other Findings

Poor growth

Ptosis of eyelids

Small palpebral fissures

Long, narrow face

High nasal bridge

Microcephaly

Cryptorchidism

Hypospadias

Kyphoscoliosis

Other ophthalmologic findings: congenital cataracts, nystagmus, blindness

Comments. Infants with aniridia have an increased incidence of development of Wilms' tumors. Infants who have aniridia and the chromosomal deletion (11p13) have a 50% incidence of Wilms' tumor before age 4 years.
The prevalence of this association is not known.

Performance. Moderate to severe mental retardation is usually present.

Etiology. An interstitial deletion of the short arm of chromosome 11p13 is present in infants and children with the above constellation of findings. Not all infants with aniridia and associated Wilms' tumors have the chromosomal defect. Almost all cases are sporadic in occurrence, although a familial occurrence has been recorded due to balanced translocation.

APERT'S SYNDROME (ACROCEPHALOSYNDACTYLY)

Key Features (Figure 224-5)

Craniosynostosis with flat occiput

Brachycephaly with high forehead

Midfacial hypoplasia—flat facies

Hypertelorism

Syndactyly, cutaneous or bony, of hands and feet

Other Findings

Shallow orbits with proptosis

Strabismus

Downslanting of palpebral fissures

Small nose, occasionally beaklike

Prominent mandible

High-arched palate; cleft soft palate in some cases

Ankylosis of elbow, shoulder, and hip

Hearing loss

Comments. Mortality is increased in the neonatal period. Despite the craniosynostosis, increased intracranial pressure is not common. Acne vulgaris with extension to the forearm is found in most adolescents with this syndrome.

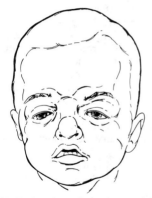

Figure 224-5. Apert's syndrome (acrocephalosyndactyly).

The incidence of this syndrome is estimated at 1:160,000.

Performance. Mental development varies, although many have decreased mental capacity.

Etiology. Apert's syndrome is autosomal dominant, with most cases representing fresh mutations.

BECKWITH-WIEDEMANN SYNDROME

Key Features (Figure 224-6)

Macrosomia—excessive postnatal growth

Macroglossia—large tongue

Prominent eyes

Capillary hemangioma (nevus flammeus) of the central forehead and eyelids

Abdominal wall defects: umbilical hernia, diastasis recti, omphalocele

Other Findings

Large fontanelle

Linear creases in ear lobule

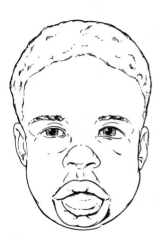

Figure 224-6. Beckwith-Wiedemann syndrome.

Prominent occiput
Visceromegaly: liver, kidneys, pancreas, uterus
Microcephaly
Midface hypoplasia
Large birth weight
Neonatal hypoglycemia
Advanced bone age

Occasional Findings

Hemihypertrophy
Absent gonads
Clitoral hypertrophy
Diaphragm abnormalities: eventration, hernia
Muscular hypertrophy

Comments. Although these infants are noted for their large size, they may not be abnormally large at birth. Phenotypic expression varies greatly. The neonatal hypoglycemia may be difficult to control. The enlarged tongue may result in significant feeding problems. An important association is the propensity to develop malignancies, particularly Wilms' tumor, adrenal carcinoma, and gonadoblastoma. Maternal hydramnios is common, and the incidence of prematurity is high.

The frequency of occurrence is estimated at 1:15,000 live births.

Performance. Mild to moderate mental retardation may occur, although some researchers think retardation may be the result of hypoglycemia.

Etiology. Most cases are sporadic in occurrence, but familial cases have been reported. Abnormalities of chromosome 11 have been reported in patients with features of this syndrome.

BLOOM'S SYNDROME

Key Features (Figure 224-7)

Short stature of prenatal onset
Small, narrow facies with protruding ears
Mild microcephaly
Malar hypoplasia
Small nose
Facial erythematous rash over malar area, sun-induced

Other Findings

High-pitched voice
Café-au-lait spots
Slender, delicate body build

Comments. Patients with Bloom's syndrome have a remarkable resemblance to one another. The photosensitive dermatitis combined with poor growth usually suggests the diagnosis. The rash usually occurs over the nose, lips, malar area, forearms, and dorsa of the hands. Children with this dis-

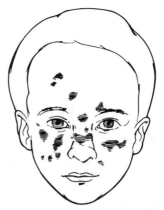

Figure 224-7. Bloom's syndrome.

order have a propensity for developing neoplasms, particularly lymphoreticular malignancies. Males may be sterile.

Slightly more than 100 cases have been described.

Performance. Mild mental retardation may be present.

Etiology. Almost half of the cases have been described in Ashkenazi Jews. Inheritance is autosomal recessive. On chromosomal analysis, a high incidence of sister chromatid exchange is found.

CAMPTOMELIC DYSPLASIA SYNDROME

Key Features

Anterior bowing of tibiae with pretibial skin dimple
Flat-appearing face
Low nasal bridge
Micrognathia
Short, narrow palpebral fissures
Dwarfism of prenatal onset
Small, bladeless scapulae

Other Findings

Dolichocephalic head
Long philtrum
Cleft palate
Small mouth
Hypertelorism
Dysplastic ears
Lower extremities appear short compared to upper extremities
Small thoracic cage
Dislocated hips
Talipes equinovarus
Mild brachydactyly and clinodactyly
Protuberant abdomen
Congenital heart disease

Renal anomalies (hydronephrosis)
Hypotonia
Dislocated joints
Pterygium colli
Unruly hair

Comments. The bowed tibiae and skin dimple should suggest this disorder, but they are not specific for this syndrome. These infants do poorly; most die soon after birth or in early infancy from respiratory problems. Tracheobronchial hypoplasia is common. Failure to thrive is a prominent feature. A sex reversal phenomenon, male karyotype with female phenotype, has been reported in a number of cases.
The incidence is unknown.

Performance. Infants with this disorder have significant retardation.

Etiology. The inheritance pattern is not established, although some seem to fit an autosomal-recessive pattern.

CARPENTER'S SYNDROME

Key Features

Obesity
Brachycephaly with variable synostosis of coronal, sagittal, and lambdoid sutures
Shallow supraorbital ridges
Flat nasal bridge
Lateral displacement of inner canthi
Short hands, stubby fingers
Partial syndactyly of third and fourth fingers
Preaxial polysyndactyly of the feet—duplication of first or second toe

Occasional Abnormalities

Downslanting palpebral fissures
Epicanthal folds
Cranial asymmetry
Short neck
Postaxial polydactyly
Low-set ears
Congenital heart defects: patent ductus arteriosus (PDA), ventricular septal defect (VSD), pulmonic stenosis
Hypogenitalism
Small stature

Comments. Obesity is generally mild.
The incidence of this uncommon syndrome is unknown.

Performance. Mental retardation is common and of variable degree.

Etiology. Inheritance is autosomal recessive.

CEREBRAL GIGANTISM (SOTOS SYNDROME)

Key Features (Figure 224-8)

Prenatal onset of excessive size
Large hands and feet
Macrocephaly
Prominent forehead
Downslanting palpebral fissures
Hypertelorism
Prognathism (prominent jaw); narrow anterior mandible
Coarse-looking facies

Other Findings

Advanced osseous maturation
High, narrow palate
Poor coordination; clumsiness
Premature eruption of teeth
Seizures
Strabismus
Kyphoscoliosis

Comments. Hypotonia is almost invariable during the first year of life. Rapid growth occurs in the first 2 to 3 years of life, then proceeds at a fairly normal rate. In the neonatal period, feeding and respiratory problems are common. Behavior may be aggressive. An abnormal glucose tolerance test is found in more than 10% of cases.
The incidence of this uncommon syndrome is unknown.

Performance. Most children with this syndrome would be categorized as having a mild or borderline mental handicap. The perceived developmental and behavioral problems, however, may seem more severe than real because of expectations based on size rather than age.

Etiology. Sporadic occurrence, although a few families have been reported with parent and child affected.

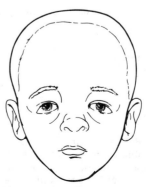

Figure 224-8. Cerebral gigantism (Sotos syndrome).

CEREBROHEPATORENAL (ZELLWEGER) SYNDROME

Key Features (Figure 224-9)

Hypotonia
High forehead
Shallow, flat supraorbital ridges
Long, flat face
Inner epicanthal folds
Large fontanelle with open metopic suture
Micrognathia
Abnormal external ears

Other Findings

Frontal bossing
Hepatomegaly; jaundice
Extra skin folds of the neck
Kidneys: albuminuria
Cardiac anomalies: patent ductus, septal defects
Simian crease
Contractures of joints, especially knee and fingers
Cryptorchidism
Corneal opacities, cataracts, glaucoma, Brushfield's spots
High-arched palate
Punctate epiphyseal calcifications of patellae, sternum, scapulae, and acetabulum
Talipes equinovarus

Comments. Infants with this syndrome do poorly from birth. Their suck is weak, failure to thrive occurs, and respiratory problems are common. Seizures occur in some infants. The generalized hypotonia is marked.

The incidence is estimated at 1:100,000, but identification of atypical cases and milder variants by biochemical means will result in a higher frequency. Early death is the rule.

Performance. Psychomotor development is retarded.

Etiology. Inheritance is autosomal recessive. In the classic syndrome, recognizable peroxisomes are missing from the liver and kidneys and are greatly reduced in skin fibroblasts. Elevated pipecolic acid concentrations in urine and plasma detected by routine amino acid chromatography are helpful but not diagnostic.

CHARGE ASSOCIATION

Key Features

Choanal atresia
Ear anomalies: small to cup-shaped lop ears
Deafness
Coloboma—retinal coloboma most common
Heart defects: tetralogy of Fallot, PDA, VSD, atrial septal defect (ASD)
Postnatal growth deficiency
Genital hypoplasia (males): microphallus, cryptorchidism

Occasional Other Findings

Microcephaly
Facial asymmetry, palsy
Malar flattening
Long philtrum
Cleft lip/palate
Small mouth
Swallowing difficulties
Polyhydramnios in 50% of cases

Comments. This is not a specific disorder or diagnosis. Patients who have choanal atresia or colobomas of the eyes should be examined for other anomalies. The acronym is derived from C, coloboma; H, heart anomalies; A, atresia of the choanae; R, retardation—mental and somatic; G, genital hypoplasia; E, ear anomalies. Feeding problems are common in infancy, and early death occurs in some infants. Hypocalcemia may reflect the presence of abnormalities of the parathyroid gland and indicate thymic and major vessel abnormalities as well.

The incidence of this association is not known.

Performance. Mental retardation is present in almost all cases. Significant CNS malformations may be present.

Etiology. The occurrence seems sporadic. An insult to the developing embryo during the second month of pregnancy is postulated.

COCKAYNE'S SYNDROME

Key Features (Figure 224-10)

Microcephaly
Loss of facial adipose tissue; prominent facial bones
Slender nose
Sunken eyes

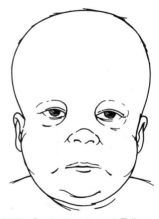

Figure 224-9. Cerebrohepatorenal (Zellweger) syndrome.

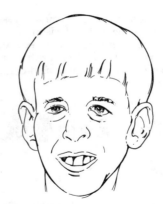

Figure 224-10. Cockayne's syndrome.

Large ears
Prominent chin
Growth deficiency, usually evident by age 2 years
Adipose tissue lost by mid-infancy to late infancy
Photosensitive, thin skin
Cool hands and feet—sometimes cyanotic

Other Findings

Unsteady gait
Tremor
Corneal opacity, cataract; pigmentary retinal degeneration; optic atrophy
Mild to moderate joint limitation of knees, elbows, ankles
Limbs seem long; hands and feet seem large
Congenital absence of some teeth; increased dental caries
Dorsal kyphosis
Sensorineural deafness
Blindness
Scalp hair and eyebrows may be sparse
Cryptorchidism and small testes in males
Lack of normal breast development in females

Comments. Infants with this disorder appear normal at birth, but develop the loss of adipose tissue and growth failure rapidly in the first years of life. Radiographs of the skull reveal thickening and often intracranial calcifications.

Children with Cockayne's syndrome usually are unable to care for themselves by the late teenage years. Earlier in life, they are affected adversely by heat. Death often occurs in early adulthood from inanition and respiratory infections.

The incidence of this uncommon disorder is unknown.

Performance. There is moderate to severe mental retardation.

Etiology. Inheritance is autosomal recessive.

CORNELIA DE LANGE'S SYNDROME

Key Features (Figure 224-11)

Microbrachycephaly (small, round head)

Bushy eyebrows and synophrys (eyebrows run together)
Long, curly eyelashes
Small nose, anteverted nostrils
Thin lips with small midline beak of the upper lip and a corresponding notch in the lower lip
Downward curving angle of the mouth
Micrognathia
Long philtrum
Generalized hirsutism
Hypoplastic nipples
Low-pitched, weak, growling cry in infancy
Short stature
Micromelia of feet
Failure to thrive

Other Common Findings

Abnormalities of the extremities: micromelia, phocomelia, oligodactyly, proximally placed thumbs, simian crease, flexion contractures of the elbows, syndactyly of the second and third toes
High-arched palate
Undescended tests; hypospadias; genital hypoplasia
Congenital heart defects—VSD most common
Gastrointestinal tract anomalies—duplication most common

Comments. The facial appearance of infants is quite characteristic. They are difficult infants, are irritable, feed poorly, and have recurrent respiratory infections and gastrointestinal upsets. As they become older, autistic and self-destructive behavior may appear. Seizures occur in one fourth of cases.

The frequency of occurrence is estimated at 1:10,000 to 1:20,000.

Performance. The IQ of these infants is generally less than 50, and less than 35 in the majority of cases.

Etiology. The cause of this syndrome is unknown. Most cases are sporadic, with few familial cases reported. A similar appearance to that in Cornelia de Lange's syndrome has been described with two chromosomal abnormalities, duplication of 3q and duplication of 4p.

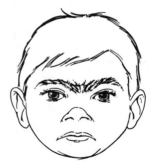

Figure 224-11. Cornelia de Lange's syndrome.

CRI DU CHAT SYNDROME (5p–)

Key Features (Figure 224-12)

Microcephaly

Hypertelorism

Epicanthal folds

Downward slanting of palpebral fissures

High-pitched, shrill cry similar to that of a cat—reflects abnormal laryngeal development

Marked poor growth

Other Common Features

Round face

Strabismus

Low-set or poorly formed ears; posteriorly rotated

Muscular hypotonia

Severe respiratory and feeding problems

Micrognathia

Prominent nasal bridge

Preauricular tags

Congenital heart defects of various types

Scoliosis

Transverse palmar creases

Low birth weight

Less Common Features

Short philtrum

Cleft lip/palate

Bifid uvula

Facial asymmetry

Premature graying of hair

Comments. The characteristic catlike cry is not present in all cases, and it disappears in the first few years of life in those who have this clue. Facial features of affected infants change with age. Older children have a thin rather than round face.

The incidence has been estimated at 1:20,000 to 1:50,000 live births.

Performance. Affected infants are severely retarded.

Etiology. A deletion of the short arm of chromosome 5 is responsible for 85% of cases, whereas the remaining 15% are the result of an unbalanced translocation from a parental carrier.

CROUZON'S SYNDROME (CRANIOFACIAL DYSOSTOSIS)

Key Features (Figure 224-13)

Prominent eyes due to shallow orbits

Strabismus

Hypertelorism

Midfacial hypoplasia

Prognathism

Craniosynostosis—especially coronal and lambdoid sutures

Brachycephaly

Other Findings

Flat nasal bridge

Nystagmus

Frontal bossing

Short upper lip

Drooping lower lip

High-arched palate

Crowded teeth, dental malocclusion

Bifid uvula, cleft palate

Atretic ear canals

Comments. Craniosynostosis occurs in the first year of life and may involve the sagittal as well as the coronal and lambdoidal sutures. Occasionally, increased intracranial pressure occurs. Headache and seizures may occur.

The incidence of this syndrome is not known.

Etiology. Inheritance is autosomal dominant, with 25% to 50% of cases representing new mutations.

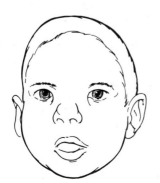

Figure 224-12. Cri du chat (5p-) syndrome.

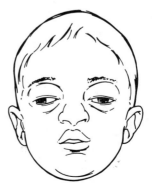

Figure 224-13. Crouzon's syndrome (craniofacial dysostosis).

DOWN SYNDROME

Key Features (Figure 224-14)

Short stature

Typical craniofacial composite:

>   Microcephaly-brachycephaly—small, round head; flat occiput
>
>   Upslanting of palpebral fissures (mongolian slant)
>
>   Inner epicanthal folds
>
>   Speckling of the iris (Brushfield's spots)
>
>   Small nose
>
>   Low nasal bridge
>
>   Small ears with small or absent ear lobes
>
>   Flat facial profile
>
>   Short neck
>
>   Mouth held open, often with tongue protruding

Hypotonia

Brachydactyly—short hands and fingers

Single flexion crease on fifth finger

Congenital heart disease in one third to one half of cases—endocardial cushion defect and VSD most common

Comments. This is the most common autosomal chromosomal abnormality in liveborn infants. The frequency of occurrence is estimated to be 1:700 to 1:1,000 live births.

In addition to the constellation of craniofacial findings, the newborn infant with Down's syndrome is hypotonic and has hyperextensible joints and excess skin on the back of the neck. Transverse palmar lines (simian creases) are present in about 50% of cases. Examination of dermatoglyphics reveals an increased number of ulnar loops.

There is significant morbidity and mortality in infancy and childhood due to congenital heart disease and an increased susceptibility to infection. One third of affected children die in the first year of life. Additional complications include an increased incidence of leukemia and, in newborns, a high incidence of duodenal atresia.

Performance. There is a wide range in IQ scores, but all are retarded in development.

Etiology. All children with this syndrome have an excess of chromosome 21 as either a trisomy or translocation. Mosaics may have a less severe phenotype. Trisomy 21 is the most common chromosomal abnormality, no matter what the maternal age. In infants with Down's syndrome born to mothers younger than 30 years of age, about 92% have trisomy 21 and 8% are the result of translocations. If the mother is older than 30 years, 98% of infants show trisomy 21 and 2% show translocations. In D/G 21 translocations, one third are inherited and two thirds are sporadic, whereas in G/G 21 translocations only 10% are inherited and 90% are sporadic. The risk of having another child with trisomy 21 is about 1%. As maternal age increases so does the chance of having a child with trisomy 21. In mothers younger than 20 years of age, the incidence of Down's syndrome is 1:2,500 live births, whereas in mothers 45 years of age, it is about 1:50.

FANCONI'S PANCYTOPENIA

Key Features

Short stature

Microcephaly

Hypoplasia to aplasia of the thumb

Hyperpigmentation of skin—uneven

Pancytopenia develops at about 8 years of age

Other Findings

Ptosis of the eyelid

Strabismus

Nystagmus

Microphthalmia

Aplasia of the radius

Clinodactyly

Syndactyly

Congenital hip dislocation

Rib and vertebral defects

Deafness—atresia of the auditory canal

Small penis, small testes, cryptorchidism

Urinary tract abnormalities: hydronephrosis, absent or ectopic kidneys

Comments. Some of these patients have no physical abnormalities. The first signs are those related to the pancytopenia—bleeding, pallor, and recurring infections. There is a higher incidence of leukemia and other cancers in these children. Most die late in the first decade of life.

A clue that helps separate this disorder from the TAR syndrome is that radial hypoplasia or aplasia occurs only with aplasia of the thumb in Fanconi's syndrome.

The incidence of this disorder is not known.

Performance. Patients occasionally are mentally retarded.

Etiology. Inheritance is autosomal recessive. Chromosomal fragility can be demonstrated on chromosomal examination.

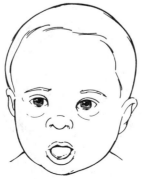

Figure 224-14. Down syndrome.

FETAL ALCOHOL SYNDROME

Key Features (Figure 224-15)

Mild to moderate microcephaly
Short palpebral fissures
Smooth philtrum
Thin vermilion border of upper lip

Other Findings

Maxillary hypoplasia
Short, upturned nose
Microphthalmia
Cleft lip or palate
Micrognathia
Short neck
Posteriorly rotated, prominent ears
Pectus excavatum
Clinodactyly
Small distal phalanges
Small fifth finger nails
Short stature
Hypotonia
Fine motor dysfunction
Cardiac murmurs: VSD, ASD usually gone by age 1 year

Comments. The features of this syndrome vary and, in part, are related to the amount of alcohol consumed by the mother during pregnancy. Two drinks per day may result in decreased birth weight, and four to six per day in subtle clinical findings. Hyperactivity in childhood is a common association. Affected infants are usually irritable and have a poor suck.

Performance. Borderline to moderate retardation is present, depending on the severity of the association.

Etiology. Ingestion of alcohol by the mother during pregnancy results in fetal alcohol syndrome.

FETAL HYDANTOIN SYNDROME

Key Features (Figure 224-16)

Broad, depressed nasal bridge
Short, anteverted nose
Wide mouth with bowed upper lip
Broad alveolar ridge
Cleft lip and palate
Short neck
Congenital heart defects: VSD, ASD, coarctation of the aorta, tetralogy of Fallot
Hypoplastic distal phalanges with small nails
Poor growth, usually of prenatal onset

Other Findings

Widely spaced small nipples
Coarse, profuse scalp hair
Hirsutism
Low-set hairline
Strabismus
Rib anomalies
Large anterior fontanelle; metopic suture ridging
Umbilical and inguinal hernias
Polydactyly; digitalized thumb
Microcephaly, brachycephaly
Coloboma, ptosis, glaucoma
Hypospadias

Comments. Features occur in varying prominence and combination in exposed infants. It is estimated that 10% of infants born to mothers taking hydantoin present a full picture of the syndrome, whereas 30% have some of the features.

Performance. Mild retardation occurs in many of these infants.

Etiology. Exposure to hydantoin in utero results in fetal hydantoin syndrome. It may be possible to identify fetuses at risk for this syndrome by measuring the activity of epoxide hydrolase in amniocytes.

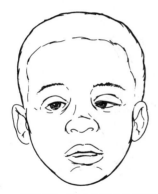

Figure 224-15. Fetal alcohol syndrome.

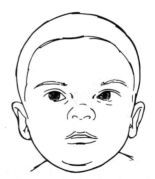

Figure 224-16. Fetal hydantoin syndrome.

HALLERMANN-STREIFF SYNDROME

Key Features (Figure 224-17)

Small stature
Brachycephaly
Frontal and parietal bossing
Malar hypoplasia
Micrognathia
Microphthalmia
Cataracts
Nose—thin, small, pointed, with hypoplastic cartilage
Microstomia—double chin

Other Findings

Hypoplastic and absent teeth, natal teeth, malocclusion
Atrophy of skin most prominent over nose and sutural areas of scalp
Thin, light hair with hypotrichosis; alopecia of frontal and occipital areas
Prominent scalp veins
Mild microcephaly
Delayed closure of fontanelles
High-arched, narrow palate
Cryptorchidism, hypogenitalism
Skeletal anomalies: syndactyly, spina bifida, lordosis, scoliosis
Cardiac defects—may have right-sided lesions

Comments. Feeding and respiratory problems often occur in the neonatal period. The temporomandibular joint has a characteristic forward displacement on radiographic examination.
The incidence of this uncommon syndrome is unknown.

Performance. Most children are developmentally normal, although 15% have mental retardation.

Etiology. The disorder seems to be sporadic in occurrence.

HURLER'S SYNDROME (MUCOPOLYSACCHARIDOSIS I)

Key Features (Figure 224-18)

Macrocephaly
Frontal prominence
Coarse facies
Wide, anteverted nostrils
Low, depressed nasal bridge
Hypertelorism
Corneal clouding
Enlarged lips
Claw hand
Hernias—umbilical, inguinal

Other Findings

Open mouth
Chronic nasal discharge
Enlarged tongue
Thickened gums
Abnormally spaced teeth
Inner epicanthal folds
Kyphosis
Short neck
Gibbus secondary to anterior vertebral wedging
Hirsutism
Hepatosplenomegaly
Pectus carinatum and excavatum
Growth failure after infancy

Comments. Infants with this syndrome appear normal at birth. During the first year of life, facial features become increasingly coarse and abnormalities become apparent. Recurrent respiratory infections are common. Death usually occurs before age 10 years from cardiorespiratory causes.
Radiographic changes that may help in the diagnosis include coarse bone trabeculation with sugarloafing of the

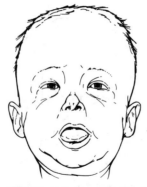

Figure 224-17. Hallermann-Streiff syndrome.

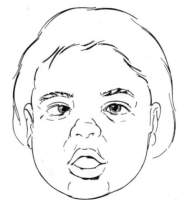

Figure 224-18. Hurler's syndrome (mucopolysaccharidosis I).

bones of the hand, abnormal vertebral bodies, and wide ribs.

The incidence of Hurler's syndrome is estimated at 1:100,000.

Performance. Increasingly severe developmental delay occurs with age. The children are markedly retarded.

Etiology. Inheritance is autosomal recessive. A deficiency of α-L-iduronidase allows for deposition of mucopolysaccharides in body tissues, leading to the typical picture. Dermatan sulfate and heparan sulfate are excreted in the urine.

LANGER-GIEDION TYPE OF THE TRICHORHINOPHALANGEAL SYNDROME

Key Features (Figure 224-19)

Large, bulbous, pear-shaped nose
Thickened alae nasi with tented nares
Sparse scalp hair
Mild micrognathia
Mild microcephaly
Large, laterally protruding ears
Multiple exostoses

Other Findings

Heavy eyebrows
Long, prominent philtrum
Thin upper lip
Mild postnatal onset of growth deficiency
Tendency toward fractures
Loose skin early in life
Multiple nevi
Asymmetric limb growth
Scoliosis

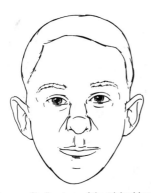

Figure 224-19. Langer-Giedion type of the trichorhinophalangeal syndrome.

Joint hypermobility
Winged scapulae
Exotropia
Hearing loss

Comments. Recurrent respiratory tract infections are common. Coning of phalangeal epiphyses, evident by 3 or 4 years of age, is a helpful radiologic finding in addition to the exostoses. A significant delay in speech development is common.

The Langer-Giedion type of trichorhinophalangeal syndrome differs from other types by the presence of multiple exostoses, loose skin, joint hypermobility, microcephaly, nevi, and delayed speech.

The incidence of this uncommon disorder is not known.

Performance. Mild to moderate mental retardation is found in many cases.

Etiology. The occurrence of this syndrome is sporadic, with a deletion at 8q24 found in most cases.

LARSEN'S SYNDROME

Key Features

Flat facies
Depressed, broad nasal bridge
Hypertelorism
Prominent forehead
Congenital dislocations of elbows, hips, and knees

Other Findings

Broad thumbs
Long, nontapering, cylindrical fingers
Short metacarpals
Talipes equinovarus
Short stature
Cleft palate
Congenital heart disease—various types, particularly septal defects
Kyphoscoliosis

Less Common Findings

Hydrocephalus
Hearing loss
Tracheomalacia and respiratory distress
Cervical spine instability

Comments. The dislocations often create major orthopedic problems. Acquired cardiac lesions similar to those found in Marfan's syndrome occur, including mitral valve prolapse, aortic dilatation, aortic insufficiency, and dissecting aneurysms.

The incidence of this disorder is not known.

Etiology. Inheritance is not known. Autosomal-dominant and autosomal-recessive cases have been reported.

LEPRECHAUNISM SYNDROME

Key Features (Figure 224-20)

Small face
Prominent eyes
Flat nasal bridge
Flared nostrils
Thick lips
Large, low-set ears
Body and facial hirsutism
Striking lack of subcutaneous tissue

Other Findings

Prenatal and postnatal growth deficiency
Gingival hypertrophy
Large mouth
Acanthosis nigracans
Large phallus
Breast hyperplasia
Clitoral and labia minora prominence
Hyperglycemia-hyperinsulinism
Microcephaly
Hypertelorism
Hernias—umbilical, inguinal
Hypotonia
Cryptorchidism
Large hands and feet

Comments. These infants demonstrate marked failure to thrive, and most die in the second half of the first year.
The incidence of this rare syndrome is unknown.

Performance. Mental and motor retardation is marked.

Etiology. Inheritance seems autosomal recessive.

MARFAN'S SYNDROME

Key Features (Figure 224-21)

Tendency toward tall stature
Long, slender limbs
Subluxation of lens—usually upward
Dilatation of the aortic root

Other Findings

Joint hyperextensibility
Scoliosis, kyphosis
Narrow face
Myopia, retinal detachment, glaucoma
Mitral valve prolapse
Hernias—inguinal, femoral
Large ears

Comments. There is no characteristic facies associated with Marfan's syndrome. The lower segment of the body, symphysis pubis to heel, is longer than the upper segment. The arm span is greater than the height. Lifespan is shortened secondary to cardiovascular complications, particularly dissection of the aorta. Spontaneous pneumothoraces are another common problem.
The incidence is estimated at between 1:16,000 and 1:60,000.

Performance. Mental retardation is not a characteristic of this disorder.

Etiology. Inheritance is autosomal dominant. The fundamental defect is caused by mutations of the fibrillin gene on chromosome 15.

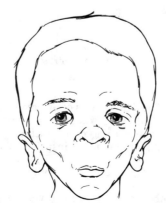

Figure 224-20. Leprechaunism syndrome.

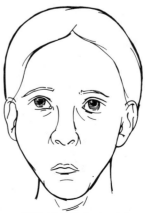

Figure 224-21. Marfan's syndrome.

MENKES' SYNDROME

Key Features (Figure 224-22)

Pudgy, full cheeks with lack of facial expression

Coarse, light-colored, wiry hair that breaks easily

Thick, dry, pale skin

Short, broad, upturned nose

Marked failure to thrive after birth

Severe and progressive neurologic deterioration in the first few months of life with hypothermia, irritability, feeding difficulties, and seizures

Other Findings

Micrognathia

Premature birth

Susceptibility to infection

Thickened periosteum, suggesting child abuse

Loss of vision

Spasticity, hyperreflexia

Comments. Infants with Menkes' syndrome appear normal at birth but rapidly deteriorate neurologically. The hair is normal at birth but becomes sparse, unruly, and light in color. Microscopically, the hair demonstrates a number of abnormalities, including twisting and beading.

The incidence is estimated at 1:50,000 to 1:100,000 births. Ninety percent of these infants die by age 2 years.

Performance. Severe retardation is progressive.

Etiology. Menkes' syndrome is inherited as an X-linked recessive trait. The defect is one of copper transport. Serum, urine, liver, brain, and hair copper levels are low, whereas other tissues demonstrate an increased amount of copper. The serum ceruloplasmin is low to absent. There is no effective treatment for this disorder.

MORQUIO'S SYNDROME (MUCOPOLYSACCHARIDOSIS IV)

Key Features (Figure 224-23)

Mild coarsening of facial features

Broad mouth

Short neck with restricted movement

Pectus carinatum

Short trunk

Short stature

Knocked knees

Other Findings

Short, anteverted nose

Cloudy corneas (late in first decade)

Abnormal teeth with pitting and enamel hypoplasia

Hepatomegaly

Short, stubby hands

Joint laxity

Scoliosis, lumbar lordosis

Comments. Not all of these children are coarse-featured. Generally, abnormalities begin to appear between ages 1 and 3 years. Neurologic complications occur secondary to spinal cord compression from C1/C2 dislocation. Aortic regurgitation is relatively common later in the course of the disorder. Progressive hearing loss is an additional feature.

The incidence is estimated at 1:40,000. Lifespan is shortened.

Performance. Affected children are normal mentally.

Etiology. Inheritance is autosomal recessive. A marked excretion of keratan sulfate and chondroitin sulfate A can be found in the urine.

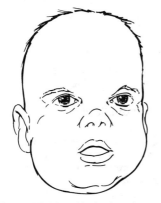

Figure 224-22. Menkes' syndrome.

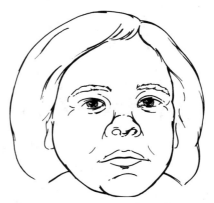

Figure 224-23. Morquio's syndrome (mucopolysaccharidosis IV).

MULIBREY NANISM

Key Features (Figure 224-24)

Triangular facies

Forehead prominent and high

Growth deficiency—prenatal onset

Development of a thick adherent pericardium

Hepatomegaly and distended neck veins develop because of the constrictive pericarditis

Other Findings

Hands and feet appear relatively large

High-pitched voice

Skull appears enlarged

Strabismus

Yellow spots on the retina

Variable fibrous dysplasia

Comments. This is an uncommon disorder, but it is important to diagnose early because of the constrictive pericarditis. True incidence is unknown.

Performance. The intelligence is normal to mildly retarded.

Etiology. Inheritance appears autosomal recessive.

NOONAN'S SYNDROME

Key Features (Figure 224-25)

Short stature in more than two thirds of cases

Broad forehead

Ptosis of eyelids

Low-set or malformed ears (fleshy folding of upper transverse portion of helix)

Low posterior hairline (webbed neck)

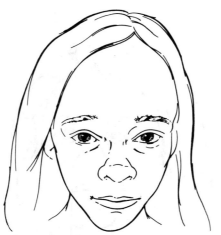

Figure 224-24. Mulibrey nanism.

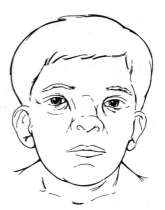

Figure 224-25. Noonan's syndrome.

Other Common Features

Cardiovascular abnormalities occur in almost half of cases. Right-sided defects are most common: valvular pulmonic stenosis, peripheral pulmonary artery stenosis, and PDA. ASDs and VSDs are less frequent. Coarctation of the aorta and Ebstein's anomaly occur occasionally.

Cryptorchidism

Epicanthal folds

Hypertelorism

Micrognathia

Flat nasal bridge—saddle nose

Deeply grooved philtrum

Mild antimongoloid slant to palpebral fissures

Dental malocclusion

High-arched palate

Bifid uvula

Shield chest

Pectus excavatum distally with proximal pectus carinatum

Lymphedema of lower extremities

Less Common Findings

Hypoplastic nails

Hirsutism

Hemangiomas

Sensorineural deafness

Hydrocephaly

Seizures

Autoimmune thyroiditis

Hernias—umbilical, inguinal

Skeletal abnormalities: cubitus valgus, osteoporosis, retarded bone age, clinodactyly, polydactyly, scoliosis, kyphosis

Hypospadias, renal duplication

Comments. Appearance of cases varies. Use of the term *male Turner's syndrome* is inappropriate and may lead to confusion. Although there is some resemblance to Turner's syndrome, a chromosomal abnormality has not been described in Noonan's syndrome.

If cardiac defects are not major, the prognosis for survival is generally good. Gonadal function may be compromised in some cases.

The prevalence of Noonan's syndrome is not established but may be as high as 1:1,000.

Performance. Mental retardation, usually mild, is present in almost half of cases.

Etiology. The basic defect resulting in Noonan's syndrome is unknown. Most cases are sporadic in occurrence, although several families with autosomal-dominant or autosomal-recessive inheritance have been reported.

OCULOAURICULOVERTEBRAL DYSPLASIA (GOLDENHAR'S SYNDROME)

Key Features (Figure 224-26)

Facial asymmetry with malar, maxillary, or mandibular hypoplasia

Macrostomia with cleftlike corner of mouth

Ear deformities: small, crumpled, complete absence, displaced

Preauricular tags or pits—most commonly in a line from the tragus to the corner of mouth

Other Findings

Vertebral anomalies: hemivertebra, occipitalization of the atlas

Epibulbar dermoid at lower lateral margin of the eye

Lipodermoid at upper lateral margin of the eye

Notched upper eyelid

Low-set eye on side of asymmetry

Hearing loss

Frontal bossing

Occasional Abnormalities

Coloboma of the iris or choroid

Rib anomalies

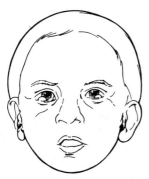

Figure 224-26. Oculoauriculovertebral dysplasia (Goldenhar's syndrome).

Talipes equinovarus

Cleft lip/palate

Ptosis

Congenital heart disease

Comments. The facial asymmetry is bilateral in 10% of cases.

The frequency of occurrence may be as high as 1:5,600 live births.

Performance. A minority of these children are mentally retarded.

Etiology. Sporadic in occurrence. It is thought to represent an anomalous development of the first and second branchial arches.

ORAL-FACIAL-DIGITAL SYNDROME (OFD)

Key Features

Thin nose with hypoplasia of the alar cartilage

Flat midfacial region

Lateral placement of the inner canthi

Partial clefts in mid-upper lip, tongue, and alveolar ridges

Cleft of soft palate

Anomalous teeth

Webbing between buccal mucous membranes and alveolar ridge

Asymmetric shortening of digits with clinodactyly, with or without syndactyly

Dry, rough, sparse hair

Other Findings

Hamartoma (lobules) of the tongue

Frontal bossing

Micrognathia

Flattened nasal tip

Dry skin

Polydactyly of the feet

Comments. This syndrome is often divided into two types, I and II. The description above best fits OFD I. In OFD II or Mohr syndrome, the tongue is cleft and polysyndactyly of the halluces, polydactyly of the hand, a broad nasal tip that may be bifid, ankyloglossia (bound-down tongue), and normal skin and hair are seen.

The incidence of OFD is estimated at 1:50,000. About one third of those with OFD I die in early infancy.

Performance. More than 50% of OFD I patients have mild mental retardation.

Etiology. OFD I is an X-linked dominant disorder, whereas OFD II has been described as both autosomal dominant and autosomal recessive.

PRADER-WILLI SYNDROME

Key Features (Figure 224-27)

Obesity—onset from infancy to 6 years (average 2 to 3 years)
Hypotonia—more severe in infancy
Hypogonadism—small penis and scrotum, cryptorchidism

Other Common Findings

Almond-shaped appearance of palpebral fissures
Narrow bifrontal diameter
Strabismus
Short stature
Small hands and feet
Fishlike mouth
Increased incidence of diabetes mellitus—nonketotic, insulin-resistant
Feeble fetal activity—often breech birth
Decreased oculocutaneous pigmentation

Less Common Findings

Congenital dislocated hips
Microcephaly
Clinodactyly
Syndactyly
Hyporeflexia, decreased Moro reflex
High-pitched voice
Primary amenorrhea or delayed menarche in females

Comments. Feeding problems and hypotonia are often the initial clues in infancy. Later, increased appetite and obesity become problematic. Speech development is retarded. Although these children are usually happy, they are irritable when food is denied.

The incidence of this relatively common disorder is 1:16,000 live births. Life expectancy is shortened as a result of the obesity and its effects on the cardiac and respiratory systems.

Performance. An IQ in the 40 to 60 range is most common.

Etiology. Most children with this syndrome lack paternal inheritance of a segment of chromosome 15 q11.2–q12 or maternal disomy of the entire chromosome 15.

PROGERIA (HUTCHINSON-GILFORD SYNDROME)

Key Features (Figure 224-28)

Alopecia—onset, birth to 18 months
Thin, warm, dry skin
Facial hypoplasia
Micrognathia (marked)
Thin nose—sculptured-appearing tip
Loss of subcutaneous fat (cheeks and pubic areas are last to be lost)
Head appears large for face
Fontanelles remain open
Stiff, partially flexed joints
Growth deceleration (between 6 and 18 months)
Slim bones

Other Findings

Delayed dentition
High-pitched voice
Prominent eyes
Thin lips
Dystrophic nails—thin, short, small
Skin develops increasing numbers of brownish spots and irregular pigmentation
Joints appear prominent

Comments. This syndrome is often referred to as one of premature aging. Affected children look remarkably similar to one another. Adult height rarely exceeds 110 cm and weight, 15 kg. Three early features are midfacial cyanosis, skin resembling scleroderma (thick, inelastic), and a glyphic (pointed or sculptured) nasal tip.

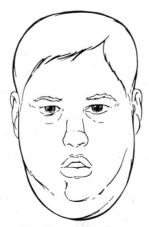

Figure 224-27. Prader-Willi syndrome.

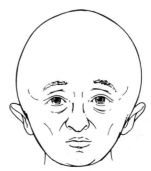

Figure 224-28. Progeria (Hutchinson-Gilford syndrome).

The incidence of this disorder is estimated at 1:250,000 to 1:4,000,000. Average age at death is 12 to 13 years, usually the result of complications of atherosclerosis, myocardial infarction, congestive heart failure, or stroke.

Etiology. The cause of this syndrome is not known.

ROTHMUND-THOMSON SYNDROME

Key Features (Figure 224-29)

Skin—marblelike or reticulated appearance due to erythema and telangiectasia, pigmentation, and hypopigmentation
Photosensitivity
Cataract (develops rapidly, usually after age 2 years)
Sparse or absent eyebrows and eyelashes

Other Findings

Short stature
Small hands and feet
Hypoplastic to absent thumbs; hypoplasia of radius, thumb, or ulna; absence of patella
Small saddle nose
Small dystrophic nails
Sparse hair—prematurely gray, occasional alopecia
Hyperkeratosis of palms and soles
Hypogonadism
Microcephaly
Frontal bossing
Defective dentition

Comments. Striking skin changes may be present at birth or develop later. Photosensitivity is common. Skin cancer may develop later in life.
The incidence of this uncommon disorder is unknown.

Performance. Mental retardation occurs in some children.

Etiology. Inheritance appears autosomal recessive.

RUBINSTEIN-TAYBI SYNDROME

Key Features (Figure 224-30)

Broad thumbs with radial angulation; broad great toes
Short stature
Microcephaly
Downslanting palpebral fissures
Hypoplastic maxilla with narrow palate
Beaked nose with nasal septum extending below alae nasi
Low-set or malformed auricles
Cryptorchidism

Other Common Findings

Epicanthal folds
Strabismus
Nevus flammeus of forehead
Other fingers broad
Prominent forehead
Large anterior fontanelle
Congenital heart defect

Less Common Findings

Long eyelashes, heavy eyebrows
Mild micrognathia
Ptosis of eyelids
Cataracts, colobomas
Hypertelorism, broad nasal bridge
High-arched palate
Dental malocclusion
Overlapping toes
Polydactyly
Pectus excavatum
Kyphoscoliosis
Hypospadias
Hirsutism
Stiff gait

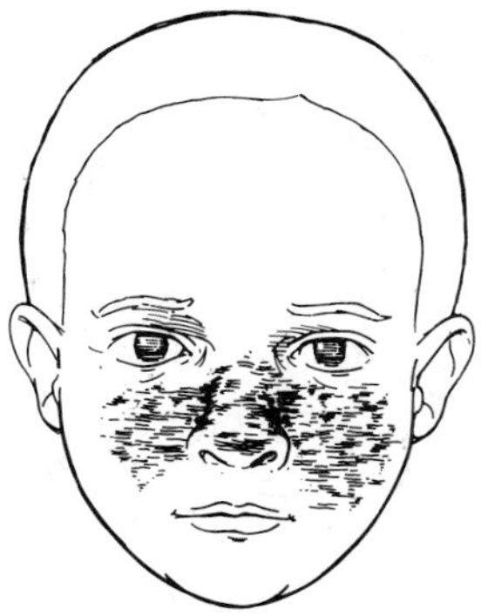

Figure 224-29. Rothmund-Thomson syndrome.

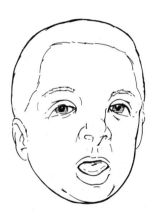

Figure 224-30. Rubinstein-Taybi syndrome.

Hyperextensible joints

Comments. The broad thumbs and toes are usually the features that focus attention on this diagnosis. Feeding and respiratory problems are common in infancy. Patients with Rubinstein-Taybi syndrome tend to form large keloids.

The frequency of occurrence of this syndrome is not known, but it is not uncommon.

Performance. All children affected with this disorder have mental, motor, and social retardation. In most, IQ is less than 50.

Etiology. Occurrence is sporadic in almost all cases.

RUSSELL-SILVER SYNDROME

Key Features (Figure 224-31)

Short stature—prenatal in onset

Small, triangular facies with downturning corners of the mouth

Clinodactyly—short, incurved fifth fingers

Asymmetry—most commonly of the limbs

Café-au-lait spots

Head appears disproportionately large

Other Features

Liability to fasting hypoglycemia

Prominent eyes

Frontal bossing and mandibular hypoplasia on profile

Long eyelashes

Thin lips

Palate high and narrow

Crowded teeth

Poor muscular development

Syndactyly of second and third toes

Delayed closure of anterior fontanelle

Precocious puberty

Urogenital abnormalities: hypospadias, ambiguous genitalia, small testes, cryptorchidism, posterior and anterior urethral valves, ureteropelvic stenosis, vesicoureteral reflux, horseshoe kidney.

Comments. Discussion continues whether there is one syndrome or two, Silver's and Russell's, the former with asymmetry.

Despite the short stature in infancy and childhood, Saal and colleagues reevaluated 15 patients later in life and found that 5 achieved normal adult height.

The incidence of this uncommon syndrome is not known.

Performance Mild developmental delay occurs in about one third of cases.

Etiology. The cause of this syndrome is not known. Hypopituitarism can closely mimic this disorder.

SAETHRE-CHOTZEN SYNDROME (ACROCEPHALOSYNDACTYLY TYPE III)

Key Features (Figure 224-32)

Short anterior-posterior diameter of skull

High forehead

Flat occiput

Flat facies

Shallow orbits

Hypertelorism

Strabismus

Downslanting of palpebral fissures

Small ears

Facial asymmetry

Other Findings

Small nose—often beaklike

Ptosis of eyelids

Large fontanelle

Microcephaly

Cutaneous syndactyly of second and third fingers, usually partial, and toes, usually third and fourth

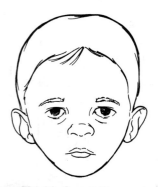

Figure 224-31. Russell-Silver syndrome.

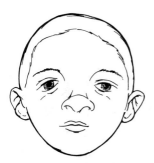

Figure 224-32. Saethre-Chotzen syndrome (acrocephalosyndactyly type III).

Short fingers
Broad thumbs and great toes
Fingerlike thumbs
Limited elbow extension
Short clavicles
Cleft palate
Cryptorchidism
Short stature

Comments. The abnormal head shape is felt to be the result of premature closure of the coronal suture. Some children develop increased intracranial pressure. Clinical expression varies.

The incidence of occurrence is not known, but this disorder may be the most common form of craniosynostosis.

Performance. Most affected individuals are normal in mental development.

Etiology. Inheritance is autosomal dominant.

SECKEL'S SYNDROME

Key Features (Figure 224-33)

Microcephaly—premature synostosis
Facial hypoplasia with prominent nose
Low-set, malformed ears—absent earlobes
Severe growth retardation

Other Findings

Micrognathia
Facial asymmetry
Eyes appear prominent
Clinodactyly of fifth fingers
Simian crease
Dislocated hips
Cryptorchidism

Occasional Findings

Strabismus
Partial adontia

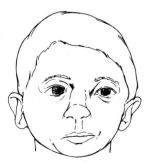

Figure 224-33. Seckel's syndrome.

Enamel hypoplasia
Sparse hair
Cleft lip
Scoliosis
Talipes equinovarus
Single flexion crease of fifth digit

Comments. This syndrome is also known as the "bird-headed dwarf syndrome" because of the phenotypic features. Affected children may have 11 pairs of ribs and hypoplasia of the proximal radius, resulting in inability to extend the forearm.

The incidence is unknown, but the syndrome is rare.

Performance. All affected children have mental retardation.

Etiology. Inheritance is probably autosomal recessive.

SHPRINTZEN'S (VELO-CARDIO-FACIAL) SYNDROME

Key Features (Figure 224-34)

Cleft of soft palate—overt or occult (submucous)
Long nose with a broad squared nasal root
Narrow alae nasi
Mandible set back slightly
Learning disabilities
Cardiac abnormalities: VSD, right aortic arch, tetralogy of Fallot

Other Findings

Narrow palpebral fissures
Long, myopathic facies
Malar flatness
Abundant scalp hair

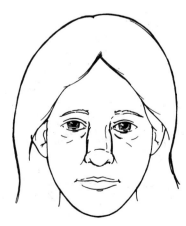

Figure 224-34. Shprintzen's (velo-cardio-facial) syndrome.

Conductive hearing loss
Slender limbs, hyperextensible fingers
Hypotonia in infancy
Microcephaly
Inguinal hernia
Malformed auricles
Laryngeal web
Cryptorchidism
Hypospadias
Scoliosis
Small stature
Hypocalcemia

Comments. Many of these children attend speech clinics because of cleft palate or hyponasal speech. Learning disabilities are present in almost all cases.

This diagnosis should be considered in any child with a conotruncal cardiac anomaly, particularly if associated with clefting.

The incidence of this disorder is not known.

Performance. Mental retardation occurs in fewer than half of cases.

Etiology. An autosomal-dominant or X-linked dominant inheritance is postulated.

SMITH-LEMLI-OPITZ SYNDROME

Key Features (Figure 224-35)

Ears—slanted or low-set
Ptosis of eyelids
Inner epicanthal folds
Broad nasal tip with anteverted nostrils
Micrognathia
Enlarged maxillary alveolar ridges
Syndactyly of the second and third toes
Cryptorchidism, hypospadias—mild to severe

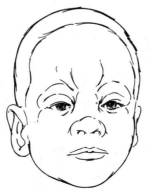

Figure 224-35. Smith-Lemli-Opitz syndrome.

Other Findings

Smallness for gestational age with failure to thrive postnatally
Microcephaly with narrow frontal area
Strabismus
Long philtrum
Simian crease
Congenital heart disease—various types
Variable muscle tone—hypotonia early and hypertonia later
Seizures
Cataract
Cleft palate
Skeletal defects: flexed fingers, polydactyly, vertical talus

Comments. Feeding difficulties and vomiting are especially common in early infancy. Infants with this syndrome are usually irritable. Early death is common, with one of five dying within the first year of life and half by 18 months of age.

The incidence of this uncommon syndrome is unknown.

Performance. There is moderate to severe mental retardation.

Etiology. Inheritance is autosomal recessive.

STICKLER'S SYNDROME (HEREDITARY ARTHRO-OPHTHALMOPATHY)

Key Features

Flat facies
Depressed nasal bridge
Epicanthal folds
Maxillary hypoplasia
Micrognathia
Myopia—before 10 years of age

Other Findings

Clefts of hard or soft palate
Long philtrum
Dental anomalies
Deafness—sensorineural, occurs in middle age
Hypotonia
Hyperextensible joints
Joint pains that may simulate juvenile rheumatoid arthritis
Marfanoid body build with slender body, long fingers, and increased arm span
Eye problems: retinal detachment, cataracts, strabismus, glaucoma, vitreous degeneration
Thoracic kyphosis or scoliosis
Pectus carinatum

Comments. Eye problems are frequently the reason that patients are referred. A family history of early-onset myopia should always suggest this disorder. A progressive multiple epiphyseal dysplasia results in bony enlargement of the ankles, knees, and wrists, and joint pains may simulate juvenile rheumatoid arthritis. In the newborn period, the micrognathia may be life threatening. The phenotypic findings are extremely variable, however.

The incidence of this disorder is not known.

Performance. Mental retardation is occasional.

Etiology. Inheritance is thought to be autosomal dominant.

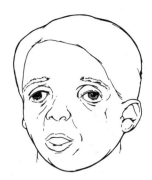

Figure 224-36. Treacher Collins syndrome.

TAR (RADIAL APLASIA-THROMBOCYTOPENIA)

Key Features

Aplasia or hypoplasia of radius—bilateral (thumbs are present, however)

Thrombocytopenia, present at birth

Leukemoid granulocytosis in the first year of life

Other Findings

Defects of the hands: club hand, syndactyly

Defects of the legs and feet: dislocated hips, coxa valga, small feet, hypoplasia or aplasia of lower limbs

Congenital heart defects: tetralogy of Fallot, ASD

Rib anomalies: cervical rib, asymmetric first rib

Fused cervical vertebrae

Micrognathia, maxillary hypoplasia

Low-set ears

Excessive perspiration

Pedal edema

Comments. Thrombocytopenia is most severe in early infancy. Anemia and eosinophilia are common. Death occurs in almost half of these infants in early infancy due to hemorrhage. Diarrhea is common in the first year of life.

Thumbs are present with the radial aplasia in this disorder, but are absent or hypoplastic with the radial aplasia in Fanconi's syndrome.

The incidence of this disorder is not known.

Performance. Mental retardation has occurred in some patients, but was felt to be secondary to intracranial hemorrhage.

Etiology. Inheritance is autosomal recessive.

TREACHER COLLINS SYNDROME

Key Features (Figure 224-36)

Antimongoloid slant of palpebral fissures

Malar hypoplasia

Micrognathia

Lower lid coloboma

Other Findings

Partial to total absence of lower eyelashes

Malformed auricles—microtia, crumpled, absent auditory canal

Projection of scalp hair onto cheek

Beaklike nose

Deafness

Extra ear tags, blind fistulas

High-arched palate

Dental malocclusion

Macrostomia—unilateral

Less Common Features

Cryptorchidism

Defects of cervical vertebrae

Congenital heart disease

Comments. Clinical expression varies. The incidence is 1:50,000 births.

Performance. Mental retardation is uncommon, and, if present, may be related to delayed detection of deafness.

Etiology. Inheritance is autosomal dominant, with as many as 50% of cases representing new mutations. The loci for the gene is thought to be in the region of 5q31–34.

TRISOMY 13

Key Features (Figure 224-37)

Microphthalmia (small eyes)

Cleft lip, cleft palate, or both

Moderate microcephaly with sloping forehead

Shallow supraorbital ridges

Localized scalp defects (cutis aplasia)

Broad, flat nose

Postaxial polydactyly of hands or feet

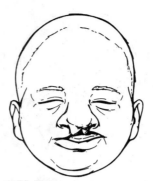

Figure 224-37. Trisomy 13.

Congenital heart defects: VSD, ASD, PDA, dextrocardia
Micrognathia

Less Common Findings

Head and Neck

Low-set, abnormally shaped ears
Loose skin of posterior neck
Short neck
Ocular hypotelorism or hypertelorism
Epicanthal folds
Capillary hemangioma of the glabella

Skeletal

Overlapping fingers
Short, dorsiflexed great toes
Rocker-bottom feet

Neurologic

Hypertonia or hypotonia, seizures, agenesis of corpus callosum

Ophthalmologic

Iris colobomas, cataracts, retinal detachment, retinal dysplasia

Other

Omphalocele, malrotation of intestines, Meckel's diverticulum, renal anomalies, cryptorchidism

Comments. About 5% of affected infants exhibit some form of holoprosencephaly. The prognosis is extremely poor: 65% die in the first 3 months of life and 95% by age 3 years. The incidence is estimated at 1:5,000 live births.

Performance. All of these infants are severely developmentally delayed.

Etiology. An older maternal age seems to be a factor for development of trisomy 13. Nondisjunction accounts for 75% of the cases. Young mothers with trisomy 13 infants should have their chromosomes analyzed to detect translocations. If one parent is a translocation carrier, the recurrence risk is about 10%, whereas if the parents are normal, the risk is less than 1%.

TRISOMY 18 (EDWARD'S SYNDROME)

Key Features

Low birth weight, generally less than 2,300 g
Common craniofacial findings:

Prominent occiput
Narrow bifrontal diameter of face-head
Low-set malformed ears—often posteriorly rotated and flattened
Short palpebral fissures
Microphthalmia
Small oral opening
Small mandible
Microcephaly

Congenital heart defects: VSD (90%), PDA (70%), ASD (20%)
Short sternum
Limited hip abduction
Short, dorsiflexed first toe
Clenched hand with overlapping fingers

Other Common Features

Inner epicanthal folds
Ptosis of the eyelids
Narrow nasal bridge
Narrow palate
Mild hirsutism of the forehead
Large fontanelles
Short neck
Hypotonia followed by hypertonia
Hypoplastic nails
Wide-spaced nipples
Rocker-bottom feet
Hypoplastic or absent thumbs
Cleft lip/palate
Cryptorchidism, hypoplastic labia, prominent clitoris

Comments. This is a relatively distinctive syndrome. More than 100 abnormalities have been described.

Trisomy-18 infants have feeble movements in utero. Polyhydramnios is present in more than half of the pregnancies. The placenta is small, and the umbilical cord has a single umbilical artery.

Affected infants have severe developmental retardation with failure to thrive. A poor suck leads to feeding difficulties. Seizures and hydrocephalus occur relatively frequently. Hernias, including umbilical, inguinal, and diaphragmatic hernias, occur in almost one fourth of these infants. Tracheoesophageal fistulas may be found as well.

The prognosis is poor, with one third dying in the first month of life and one half by 2 months of age. Less than 10% of cases survive the first year.

The frequency of occurrence is estimated at 1:3,500 to 1:7,000 live births.

Etiology. Eighty percent of cases are caused by nondisjunction. About 10% are due to translocations. The mean maternal age is elevated.

TURNER'S SYNDROME

CAUTION: Many patients with Turner's syndrome have minimal dysmorphic features.

Key Features (Figure 224-38)

Short stature—adult height usually less than 144 cm

Broad chest with widely spaced nipples

Webbed posterior neck (about 50%)

Low posterior hairline

Short neck

Increased carrying angle of arms (cubitus valgus)

Primary or secondary amenorrhea

Neonatal Clue

Lymphedema of the dorsa of the hands and feet

Other Phenotypic Clues

Abnormal ears—prominent

Epicanthal folds

Ptosis of the upper eyelids

Micrognathia

Downward and outward slant of palpebral fissures

Short fourth metacarpals

Toenails—hypoplastic, hyperconvex, deep set

Cutaneous nevi that increase with age

Sexual infantilism in postpubertal females

Comments. Congenital heart disease, particularly coarctation of the aorta, occurs in 15% to 30% of cases, and idiopathic hypertension in another 25%. Hearing loss occurs in 50% of cases, and various renal abnormalities in almost another 50%.

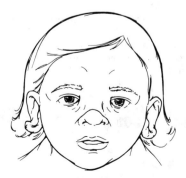

Figure 224-38. Turner's syndrome.

The prognosis is good for a normal lifespan if cardiovascular abnormalities and hypertension are absent.

The height of affected children is positively correlated with paternal height. Girls whose height is more than 2 STD below the mean for chronologic age should have a cytogenetic examination, even in the absence of dysmorphic features. Turner's syndrome should be considered in girls who develop lymphedema at any age.

The incidence of Turner's syndrome is estimated at 1:2,500 to 1:6,000 liveborn females, but about 20% of spontaneous abortions have a Turner karyotype.

Performance. Mental retardation is uncommon.

Etiology. The syndrome is the result of a partial or complete deletion of one X chromosome.

VATER ASSOCIATION

Key Features

No phenotypic facial abnormalities

Primary external abnormality is radial dysplasia

Anomalies that seem associated:

> Vertebral: hemivertebrae, sacral deformity
>
> Imperforate anus
>
> Esophageal atresia with tracheoesophageal fistula
>
> Radial dysplasia: thumb or radial hypoplasia, preaxial polydactyly, syndactyly
>
> Renal: aplasia, pelvic kidney, ureteropelvic obstruction
>
> Cardiac defects: VSD, ASD

Less Common Findings

Prenatal growth deficiency

Ear anomalies

Large fontanelles

Lower limb defects

Rib anomalies

Inguinal hernia

Malformation of the small intestine

Choanal atresia

Cleft lip/palate

Scoliosis/kyphosis

Comments. The acronym is derived from V, vertebral or vascular; A, anal malformation; TE, tracheoesophageal fistula; R, radial limb or renal defects. Usually, three of the major components are necessary to use this diagnostic association. The presence of one or two anomalies should always lead to close inspection for others.

The incidence of VATER association is not known, but it is not uncommon.

Etiology. Occurrence of this syndrome is sporadic. It seems to be related to an intrauterine event occurring between the fourth and seventh week of gestation.

WILLIAMS SYNDROME

Key Features (Figure 224-39)

Depressed nasal bridge

Epicanthal folds

Periorbital fullness of subcutaneous tissues

Blue eyes with stellate pattern of iris

Anteverted nares

Long philtrum

Prominent thick lips with open mouth; drooping lower lip

Short stature

Husky (hoarse) voice

Other Common Features

Mild microcephaly

Medial eyebrow flare

Full cheeks

Short palpebral fissures

Ocular hypotelorism

Strabismus

Mild antenatal growth deficiency

Friendly, loquacious personality

Hypoplastic nails (short, deep set, or brittle)

Cardiac defects: supravalvular aortic stenosis, valvular aortic stenosis, peripheral pulmonary artery stenosis, VSD, ASD, coarctation.

Renal artery stenosis (hypertension)

Pectus excavatum

Inguinal hernia

Partial adontia

Bladder diverticula

Nephrocalcinosis

Comments. The Williams syndrome was formerly called the syndrome of elfin facies, infantile hypercalcemia, supravalvular aortic stenosis, and failure to thrive. Evidence of infantile hypercalcemia is highly variable. In one series of patients, only 7 of 19 had supravalvular aortic stenosis, although murmurs were heard in 15 of 19. Children with this syndrome have a characteristic facial appearance. Their friendly, outgoing manner is often labeled as a cocktail-party personality.

As the children enter puberty, most attain heights above the fifth percentile. Normal sexual development occurs.

Renal or renovascular abnormalities occur in 50% of these patients.

The frequency of occurrence is not known, but this syndrome is not uncommon. The appearance is characteristic.

Performance. The average IQ is in the 50s. Testing reveals uneven developmental profiles compared to measured IQ, with reading abilities exceeding the expected level and visual motor skills lagging behind.

Etiology. The occurrence of this syndrome appears to be sporadic. There is some evidence of vitamin D sensitivity in many cases. Even patients who are normocalcemic and have

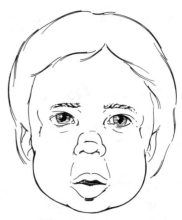

Figure 224-39. Williams syndrome.

no history of hypercalcemia have an abnormal response in levels of serum 25 OH vitamin D to pharmacologic doses of this vitamin.

(Abridged from Walter W. Tunnessen Jr, Common Syndromes With Morphologic Abnormalities, in Oski, DeAngelis, Feigin, McMillan, Warshaw: *Principles and Practice of Pediatrics, Second Edition*, J.B. Lippincott, 1994.)

Oski's Essential Pediatrics,
edited by Kevin B. Johnson and Frank A. Oski.
Lippincott–Raven Publishers,
Philadelphia © 1997

225

Presenting Signs and Symptoms

This chapter contains a group of common signs and symptoms. Each sign or symptom is followed by a list of possible causes, which are classified as common, uncommon, and rare. *Common causes* lists those diseases that, collectively, are responsible for the given sign or symptom in about 90% of patients who have it; the term is not meant to imply that the disease itself is necessarily common. *Uncommon causes* suggests that 1% to 10% of patients with the sign or symptom are found in that category. *Rare causes* lists the diseases that represent less than 1% of the causes of the symptom or sign under discussion. When confronted with a given symptom or sign, common causes should always be considered first.

ABDOMINAL MASSES

Common Causes

Appendiceal abscess

Bladder distention

Fecal collection
Hepatomegaly (any etiology)
Hydronephrosis
Multicystic dysplastic kidney
Neuroblastoma
Polycystic kidney disease (with or without liver involvement)
Pregnancy (with or without ectopic location)
Pyloric stenosis
Splenomegaly (any etiology)
Wilms' tumor

Uncommon Causes
Adrenal hemorrhage
Hernia (with or without incarceration)
Intestinal duplication
Intussusception
Leukemia
Lymphadenopathy
Ovarian cyst
Renal vein thrombosis

Rare Causes
Abscess
Anterior meningocele
Aortic aneurysm
Benign cystic causes
    Urachal cyst
    Mesenteric cyst
    Omental cyst
    Pancreatic cyst/pseudocyst
Bezoar
Hepatobiliary causes
    Cholecystitis/ascending cholangitis
    Choledochal cyst
    Hemangioendothelioma
    Hydrops of the gallbladder
Hydrometrocolpos
Intestinal causes
    Intestinal atresia (proximal dilatation)
    Malrotation with volvulus
    Meconium plug/ileus
    Regional enteritis
Retroperitoneal lymphangioma
Solid tumors
    Granulosa-theca cell tumor
    Hepatoblastoma
    Hepatocellular carcinoma
    Lymphoma
    Mesoblastic nephroma
    Nephroblastomatosis
    Rhabdomyosarcoma
    Teratoma (abdominal/ovarian)

ABDOMINAL PAIN

Acute

Common Causes
Appendicitis
Bacterial enterocolitis
    Campylobacter
    Salmonella
    Shigella
    Yersinia
Dietary indiscretion
Food poisoning
Mesenteric lymphadenitis
Pharyngitis
Pregnancy (with or without ectopic location)
Urinary tract infection
Viral gastroenteritis

Uncommon Causes
Cholecystitis/cholelithiasis
Diabetes mellitus
Hepatitis
Herpes zoster
Incarcerated hernia
Infectious mononucleosis
Intussusception
Meckel's diverticulum
Obstruction (adhesions)
Pelvic inflammatory disease
Peritonitis
    Post-trauma/instrumentation
    Spontaneous
Pneumonia
Sepsis
Trauma
    Bowel perforation
    Intramural hematoma
    Intraperitoneal blood
    Liver/spleen laceration or hematoma
    Musculocutaneous injury
    Pancreatic pseudocyst
Volvulus

Rare Causes
Abdominal abscess
Acute arrhythmia
Acute rheumatic fever
Adynamic ileus
    Drugs
    Metabolic
    Postsurgery/trauma
Ascites

Eosinophilic gastroenteritis
Glomerulonephritis
Hemolysis
Malignancy
> Leukemia/lymphoma
> Solid tumor (with or without rupture/hemorrhage)
> Mesenteric arterial insufficiency/occlusion
> Nephrolithiasis
> Nephrotic syndrome
> Obstructive nephropathy
> Pancreatitis
> Testicular torsion
> Vasculitis
> Henoch-Schönlein purpura
> Kawasaki disease
> Polyarteritis nodosa
> Systemic lupus erythematosus

Recurrent

Common Causes
"Psychophysiologic"
> Conversion hysteria
> Depression
> Idiopathic recurrent pain
> Reaction anxiety
> Secondary gain
> Task-induced phobia (*eg*, school, sports)

Uncommon Causes
Aerophagia
Constipation
Drugs
> Antibiotics
> Anticonvulsants
> Aspirin
> Bronchodilators
Dysmenorrhea
Enzymatic deficiency (*eg*, lactose intolerance)
Food allergy
Hepatosplenomegaly (any etiology)
Hiatal hernia
Inflammatory bowel disease
Irritable bowel syndrome
Mittelschmerz
Parisitic infection
> Ascariasis
> Giardiasis
> Strongyloidiasis
> Trichinelliasis
Peptic ulcerative disease
Sickle-cell anemia
Urinary tract infection

Rare Causes
Abdominal epilepsy
Abdominal masses/malignancies
> Lymphoma
> Neuroblastoma
> Ovarian lesions
> Wilms' tumor
Abdominal migraine equivalent
Acute intermittent porphyria
Addison's disease
Angioneurotic edema
Bowel anomaly with obstruction
> Duplication
> Malrotation
> Stenosis
> Web
Choledochal cyst
Collagen vascular disease
Cystic fibrosis (meconium plug/ileus equivalent)
Endometriosis
Familial Mediterranean fever
Heavy metal intoxication
Hematocolpos
Hirschsprung's disease
Hyperlipoproteinemia
Hyperthyroidism
Hypoperfusion states
> Coarctation of the aorta
> Familial dysautonomia
> Superior mesenteric artery syndrome
Mesenteric cyst
Neurologic
> Central nervous system (CNS) mass lesion
> Radiculopathy
> Spinal cord injury/tumor
Recurrent/chronic arrhythmia
Recurrent pancreatitis
Wegener's granulomatosis

ALOPECIA

Common Causes
Alopecia areata
Distal trichorrhexis nodosa
Physiologic (newborns)
> Temporal recession at puberty
Tinea capitis
Traction alopecia
Trichotillomania

Uncommon Causes

Acute bacterial infections
    Cellulitis
    Folliculitis decalvans
    Pyoderma
Burns
Cancer therapy
    Antimetabolites
    Radiation
Chemical injury
Kerion
Proximal trichorrhexis nodosa
Psoriasis
Seborrhea
Viral infections
    Herpes simplex
    Varicella

Rare Causes

Circumscribed alopecia
    Androgenic alopecia
    Aplasia cutis
    Conradi's disease
    Epidermal nevi—organoid
    Follicular aplasia
    Goltz's syndrome
    Hair follicle hamartoma
    Incontinentia pigmenti
    Infections
        Leprosy
        Tuberculosis
    Inflammatory etiologies
        Keratosis follicularis
        Lichen planus
        Morphea
        Porokeratosis of Mibelli
        Sarcoid
        Systemic lupus erythematosus
    Myotonic dystrophy
Diffuse alopecia
    Anagen effluvium
        Cytostatic agents in plants Mimosine Selemo-cystothionine
        Radium
        Thallium
    Anhidrotic ectodermal dysplasia
    Atrichia congenita
    Cartilage-hair hypoplasia
    Chondroectodermal dysplasia
    Crouston's syndrome
    Hair shaft deformities
        Monilethrix
        Pili torti

        Classic form
        Trichopoliodystrophy (Menkes' syndrome)
      Trichorrhexis invaginata
      Trichorrhexis nodosa
        Argininosuccinic aciduria
Hallermann-Streiff syndrome
Hidrotic ectodermal dysplasia
Langer-Giedion syndrome
Marinesco-Sjögren syndrome
Oculodentodigital dysplasia
Progeria
Rothmund-Thomson syndrome
Telogen effluvium
    Childbirth
    Chronic infection/illness
    Drugs
        Anticoagulants
        Anticonvulsants
        Antikeratinizing drugs
        Antithyroid drugs
        Heavy metals
        Hormones
    Excessive dieting
    High fever
    Hypothyroidism
    Stress
    Surgery

ANOREXIA

Common Causes

Acute infection
Apparent anorexia
    Dieting/fear of obesity
    Manipulative behavior
    Unrealistic expectations of caretakers

Uncommon Causes

Chronic infection
Drugs
    Aminophylline
    Amphetamines
    Anticonvulsants
    Antihistamines
    Antimetabolites
    Digitalis
    Narcotics
Esophagitis/gastroesophageal reflux
Food aversion in athletes
Iron deficiency
Irritable bowel syndrome

Pregnancy
Psychosocial deprivation (neglect/abuse)
Psychosocial factors
 Chronic mental/environmental stress
  Anxiety
  Fear
  Loneliness/boredom
 Depression
 Grief
 Mania

Rare Causes
Acquired immunodeficiency syndrome (AIDS)
Adrenogenital syndrome
Alcohol/drug abuse
Anorexia nervosa
Chronic disease
Collagen vascular disease
Congestive heart failure
Cyanotic heart disease
Electrolyte disturbances
 Hypercalcemia
 Hypochloremia
 Hypokalemia
Endocrine disease
 Addison's disease
 Diabetes insipidus
 Hyperparathyroidism
 Hypothyroidism
 Panhypopituitarism
Hypervitaminosis A
Inborn errors of metabolism
Kwashiorkor
Lead poisoning
Liver failure
Neurologic
 Congenital degenerative disease
 Diencephalic syndrome
 Hypothalamic lesions
 Increased intracranial pressure
 Mental retardation/cerebral palsy
Pain avoidance
 Appendicitis
 Constipation
 Gastrointestinal obstruction
 Inflammatory bowel disease
 Pancreatitis
 Superior mesenteric syndrome
Polycythemia
Postsurgery
Pulmonary insufficiency
Renal failure
Renal tubular acidosis

Schizophrenia
Zinc deficiency

APNEA

Common Causes
Breath-holding spells
Bronchiolitis
Extrinsic suffocation
Gastroesophageal reflux/aspiration
Idiopathic (? CNS immaturity)
Prematurity
Seizure

Uncommon Causes
Arrhythmia
Asthma
Bronchopulmonary dysplasia "spells"
CNS hypoperfusion
CNS trauma/bleed
Congenital airway anomaly
Hypoglycemia
Hypoxemia/hypercarbia (severe)
Infection
 Croup
 Meningitis/encephalitis
 Epiglottitis
 Pertussis
 Pneumonia
 Sepsis
Laryngospasm
Laryngotracheobronchomalacia
Obstructive sleep apnea
Sudden infant death syndrome (SIDS)
Toxins/drugs

Rare Causes
Anemia
Glossoptosis
Guillain-Barré syndrome
Hypocalcemia
Increased intracranial pressure
Infantile botulism
Intraventricular hemorrhage
Macroglossia
Metabolic disease
 Hyperammonemia
 Inborn errors
 Metabolic alkalosis
Micrognathia
Ondine's curse
Spinal cord injury

Cervical spine instability
>> Down's syndrome
>> Dwarfism
> Trauma
Tumor (CNS, airway)

BACK PAIN

Common Causes

Mechanical derangement (muscle strain or poor posture)
Scheuermann's kyphosis
Scoliosis
Spondylolysis/spondylolisthesis

Uncommon Causes

Disk space infection (diskitis)
Rheumatic disorders
Sacroiliac joint infections
Spina bifida occulta
Spinal cord tumors (lipomas, teratomas)
Vertebral osteomyelitis

Rare Causes

Aneurysmal bone cyst
Aseptic necrosis of vertebrae
Benign osteoblastoma
Eosinophilic granuloma of vertebrae
Hemangioma of bone
Hematocolpos
Herniated nucleus pulposus
Herpes zoster
Malignancy involving bone (neuroblastoma, leukemia metastatic)
Osteomalacia of the spine
Paraspinal tumor or infection
Secondary hyperparathyroidism
Tuberculosis of the spine
Vertebral osteoid osteoma

CHEST PAIN

Common Causes

Costochondritic
> Arthritis
> Infectious costochondritis
> Tietze's syndrome
Cough
Herpes zoster
Idiopathic
Indigestion (heartburn, esophagitis)

Mitral valve prolapse
Musculoskeletal (strain, occult trauma)
Pneumonitis
Psychogenic
Reactive airway disease
Sickle-cell disease
Trauma

Uncommon Causes

Arrhythmia
Congenital heart disease
Congestive heart failure
Esophageal (trauma associated with vomiting, foreign body)
Pleuritis/pleurisy
Pneumothorax
Precordial catch

Rare Causes

Cholecystitis
Diaphragmatic irritation
> Abscess
> FitzHugh-Curtis syndrome
> Peritonitis
> Ruptured viscus
> Tumor
Endocarditis
Juvenile rheumatoid arthritis
Myocardial ischemia (*eg,* anomalous coronary artery)
Myocarditis
Osteomyelitis (vertebrae, ribs)
Peptic ulcerative disease
Pericarditis
Pneumomediastinum
Pulmonary embolism
Rheumatic fever

COMA

Common Causes

CNS trauma
> Cerebral edema
> Concussion
> Hemorrhage
>> Epidural
>> Subarachnoid
>> Subdural
> Increased intracranial pressure
Drug intoxication
> Analgesics
> Anticonvulsants
> Antihistamines

Benzodiazepines
Digoxin
Ethanol
Heavy metals
Hydrocarbons
Hypnotics
    Barbiturates
Insulin
Lithium
Organophosphates
Phencyclidine
Phenothiazines
Salicylate
Tricyclic antidepressants

Uncommon Causes
Cardiorespiratory
    Cardiopulmonary arrest
    Hypercapnea
    Hypotension/shock
    Hypoxemia
Infection
    Abscess
    Encephalitis
    Meningitis
Metabolic
    Hypercalcemia/hypocalcemia
    Hypermagnesemia/hypomagnesemia
    Hypernatremia/hyponatremia
    Hypoglycemia
        Water intoxication
    Metabolic acidosis
    Metabolic alkalosis
Postictal state
Postoperative
    General anesthesia
    Hypotension/hypoxemia
Sepsis

Rare Causes
Cardiac
    Arrhythmia
    Hypertension
    Hypoperfusion
        Aortic stenosis
        Coarctation of the aorta
Cerebral tumors/metastases
Cerebrovascular
    Hemorrhage
    Thrombophlebitis
    Vasculitis
    Venous thrombosis
Dehydration

Diabetic ketoacidosis
Endocrine disorders
    Addison's disease
    Congenital adrenal hyperplasia
    Cushing's disease
Inborn errors of metabolism
    Hyperammonemia
    Hypoglycemia
Heat stroke
Hepatic failure
Hypothermia
Malignant hyperthermia
Porphyria
Postinfectious encephalomyelitis
    Measles
    Other viral infections
Psychiatric disturbances
    Fugue state
    Hysteria
Reye's syndrome
SIDS
Uremia

CONSTIPATION

Constipation is defined here as stools less frequent than expected by the caretaker.

Common Causes
Appendicitis
Breast-feeding (begins at about 6 weeks of age)
Cow's milk ingestion
Drugs
    Anticholinergics
    Antihistamines
    Narcotics
    Phenothiazines
Dysfunctional toilet training
Emotional disturbances
Functional ileus
Immobility
Inappropriate expectations of the caretaker
Intentional withholding
Intestinal abnormalities
    Atresia
    Hirschsprung's disease
    Microcolon
    Volvulus
    Web
Low dietary fiber
Meconium plug/ileus
Meningomyelocele

Mental retardation/cerebral palsy
Painful defecation (hemorrhoids, fissure, skin irritation)

Uncommon Causes
Diabetes mellitus
Electrolyte disturbances
      Hypercalcemia/hypocalcemia
      Hyperkalemia
Hypothyroidism
Imperforate anus/anal stenosis
Intestinal pseudo-obstruction
Lead poisoning
Salmonellosis
Spinal cord injury/tumor
Starvation

Rare Causes
Amyloidosis
Botulism
Dolichocolon
Multiple endocrine neoplasia
Myopathies/myotonias
Pheochromocytoma
Sacral malformations
Scleroderma
Tetanus
Tethered cord

COUGH

Common Causes
Allergic disease
Aspiration (direct or indirect)
Atelectasis
Bacterial infection
      Bronchiectasis
      Bronchitis
      Pneumonia
      Sinusitis
      Tracheitis
Congestive heart failure
Environmental pollution
Foreign body
Gastroesophageal reflux
Infections, other
      Chlamydia
      Mycoplasma
      Pertussis
Postnasal drip
Reactive airway disease
Smoking/passive smoking

Viral infection
      Bronchiolitis
      Croup
      Pneumonitis
      Upper respiratory infection

Uncommon Causes
Cystic fibrosis
Malformation of the airway
Malignancy (primary or metastatic)
Mediastinal adenopathy
Psychogenic
Tracheobronchomalacia
Tracheoesophageal fistula
Tuberculosis
Vascular ring

Rare Causes
Allergic bronchopulmonary aspergillosis
Auricular nerve stimulation
Bronchogenic cyst
Congenital lobar emphysema
Immotile cilia syndrome
Lymphocytic interstitial pneumonitis
Opportunistic infections (*Pneumocystis carinii* [PCP], cytomegalovirus [CMV], *Mycobacterium avium intracellulare* [MAI], fungal)
Parasitic infection
Pulmonary embolism
Pulmonary hemosiderosis
Pulmonary sequestration
Sarcoidosis

CYANOSIS

Common Causes
Acrocyanosis (especially cold stress)
Apnea of prematurity
Aspiration
      Direct (swallowing disorders, neuromuscular disease)
      Indirect (gastroesophageal reflux, emesis)
Atelectasis
Breath holding
Bronchiolitis
Congenital heart disease
      Decreased pulmonary blood flow (no pulmonary hypertension)
            Anomalous systemic venous return
            Ebstein's anomaly
            Hypoplastic right ventricle
            Pulmonary stenosis/atresia

Tetralogy of Fallot
Tricuspid stenosis/atresia/insufficiency
Eisenmenger's physiology
Increased pulmonary blood flow
Atrioventricular (AV) canal
Coarctation (preductal)
Hypoplastic left heart
Total anomalous pulmonary venous return (TAPVR)
Transposition
Truncus arteriosus
Ventricular septal defect (VSD) (large)
Pump failure
Aortic stenosis (severe)
Coarctation (postductal)
Patent ductus arteriosus
VSD
Croup
Crying
Drugs—respiratory depressants (*eg*, narcotics, benzodiazepines)
Hyaline membrane disease
Mucus plug
Nasal obstruction
Pneumonia
Pulmonary edema
Reactive airway disease
Seizures
Sepsis
Sleep apnea (tonsillar/adenoidal hypertrophy)

Uncommon Causes

Abdominal distention
Arterial thrombosis
Bronchopulmonary dysplasia
Chest wall abnormalities
Congenital bone/cartilage abnormalities
Pectus
Flail chest
Cystic fibrosis
Epiglottitis
Foreign body
Hypovolemia
Mediastinal mass
Persistent fetal circulation
Pickwickian syndrome
Pleural effusion
Pneumothorax
Polycythemia
Pulmonary hemorrhage
Retropharyngeal/peritonsillar abscess
Scoliosis
Tracheal compression

Abscess
Adenopathy
Hemorrhage
Tumor
Vascular ring
Tracheobronchomalacia/stenosis
Venous stasis

Rare Causes

Angioedema
Bronchogenic cyst
CNS disease
Edema
Hemorrhage
Infection
Trauma
Chylothorax
Diaphragmatic hernia
Factitious (blue paint/dyes/makeup)
Glossoptosis
Hemoglobinopathy (M, low oxygen affinity)
Hypoplastic lungs
Laryngeal web
Lobar emphysema
Methemoglobinemia
Methemoglobin reductase deficiency
Oxidant stress
Acetophenetidin
Antimalarials
Benzocaine
Crayons
Disinfectants
Ethylenediaminetetraacetic acid (EDTA)
Hydralazine
Marking dyes
Naphthalene
Nitrites
Amyl/butyl nitrate
Nitrate-contaminated well water
Nitrate food additives
Nitroglycerin
Plant nitrates (*eg*, carrots grown in contaminated soil)
Nitroprusside
Prilocaine
Pyridium
Sulfonamides
Vitamin K analogues
Ondine's curse
Primary pulmonary hypertension
Pulmonary AV malformation/fistula
Pulmonary embolism/thrombosis
Pulmonary hemosiderosis

Pulmonary sequestration
Pulmonary tumor (primary or metastatic)
Reflex sympathetic dystrophy
Respiratory muscle dysfunction
    Botulism
    Muscular dystrophy
    Myasthenia gravis
    Neuromuscular blockade
    Phrenic nerve damage
    Werdnig-Hoffmann disease
Superior vena cava (SVC) syndrome
Tracheoesophageal fistula
Tumor
Vocal cord paralysis

DIARRHEA, CHRONIC

Common Causes

Antibiotic-induced
Carbohydrate malabsorption, hereditary
    Lactose
Chemotherapy-induced
Cystic fibrosis
Dietary
    Allergy (milk, soy, other)
    Overfeeding
Infection
    Bacterial
    Human immunodeficiency virus (HIV)
    Parasitic
Postinfectious
    Carbohydrate malabsorption

Uncommon Causes

Anatomic lesions
    Hirschsprung's disease
    Malrotation
Celiac disease
Gastrointestinal bleeding
Irritable bowel syndrome
Malnutrition, starvation
Necrotizing enterocolitis
Parenteral infections
    Otitis media
    Urinary tract infections
Regional enteritis
Ulcerative colitis

Rare Causes

Abeta- and hypobetalipoproteinemia
Adrenal insufficiency
Biliary atresia

Blind loop syndrome
Carbohydrate malabsorption
    Sucrose, isomaltose, glucose, galactose
Chronic hepatitis
Enterokinase deficiency
Familial chloride diarrhea
Ganglioneuroma
Hyperthyroidism
Immunodeficiency
    Combined immunodeficiency
    Hypogammaglobulinemia
    IgA deficiency
Intestinal ischemia
Intestinal lymphangiectasia
Intestinal pseudo-obstruction
Liver abscess
Mesenteric artery insufficiency
Neuroblastoma
Pancreatic insufficiency and neutropenia (Schwachman-Diamond-Oski syndrome)
Pancreatic tumors
Radiation-induced
Short gut syndrome
Small bowel tumors; lymphosarcoma
Wolman's disease

DYSPHAGIA

Common Causes

Chemical mucositis
    Caustic ingestion
    Gastroesophageal reflux with esophagitis
    Radiation/chemotherapy
Immature sucking/swallowing mechanism
Oropharyngeal infections
    Cervical adenitis
    Epiglottitis
    Gingivitis
    Herpetic stomatitis
    Peritonsillar abscess
    Pharyngitis
    Retropharyngeal abscess
    Tooth abscess
Physiologic expulsion reflux

Uncommon Causes

Cerebral palsy
Cleft palate
Esophageal spasm
Esophageal stricture
External compression of the esophagus
    Esophageal diverticula

Esophageal duplication
Mediastinal masses/tumors
Vascular anomalies
Foreign body
Infectious esophagitis
Candida, herpes
Macroglossia (any cause)
Micrognathia
Pharyngeal diverticula
Physiologic (globus hystericus)
Submucosal cleft
Tracheoesophageal fistula

Rare Causes
Choanal atresia
Collagen vascular disease
Dermatomyositis
Scleroderma
Diphtheria
Esophageal atresia, web, cyst
Laryngeal cyst, cleft
Muscular hypertrophy of the esophagus
Neuromuscular causes
Botulism
Bulbar and suprabulbar palsy
Möbius' syndrome
Chalasia/achalasia of the esophagus
Congenital laryngeal stridor
Cranial nerve palsy
Demyelinating disease
Guillain-Barré syndrome
Hypotonias
Muscular dystrophy
Myasthenia gravis
Myotonic dystrophy
Pharyngeal or cricopharyngeal incoordination
Tetanus
Pharyngeal cyst, cleft
Rumination
Temporomandibular ankylosis/hypoplasia
Tumors (oropharynx, esophagus)

DYSRHYTHMIA

Common Causes
Acidemia
Congenital heart disease
Drugs
Antiarrhythmics
Beta blockers
Caffeine

Cocaine
Psychotropics
Sympathomimetics
Hypoxemia
Idiopathic
Postoperative (cardiac procedures)

Uncommon Causes
Cardiomyopathy (dilated, hypertrophic, infiltrative)
Electrolyte disturbances (especially K, Ca, Mg)
Myocarditis
Sickle-cell disease
Sick-sinus syndrome
Wolff-Parkinson-White syndrome (or other accessory bypass tracts)

Rare Causes
Anomalous coronary artery
CNS
Hemorrhage
Infection
Trauma
Collagen vascular disease
Complete congenital heart block
Endocrine (thyrotoxicosis, secondary electrolyte disturbance)
Kawasaki disease
Myocardial ischemia
Myocardial trauma
Myocardial tumors
Neonatal lupus
Prolonged QT syndrome
Rheumatic fever

DYSURIA

Common Causes
Candidal dermatitis/vaginitis
Chemical urethritis (bubble bath)
Contact dermatitis/vulvitis
Urethritis
Urinary tract infection
Viral cystitis

Uncommon Causes
Foreign body
Herpes simplex
Meatitis
Pinworms
Urethral trauma

Rare Causes
Appendicitis

Bladder diverticulum
Bladder outlet obstruction
      Posterior urethral valves
Bladder stones
Constipation
Drugs
      Amitriptyline
      Cytoxan
Hematospermia
Interstitial cystitis
Meatal stenosis
Posthitis
Prostatitis
Reiter's syndrome
Schistosomiasis
Stevens-Johnson syndrome
Tuberculosis
Urethral prolapse
Urethral stricture
Varicella

ENCOPRESIS

Common Causes
Chronic constipation
Diarrheal disorders
Emotional disturbance

Uncommon Causes
Hirschsprung's disease

Rare Causes
Diastematomyelia
Epidural abscess
Poliomyelitis
Post–anorectal surgery
Osteomyelitis of the vertebral body
Sacral agenesis
Spinal cord tumor
Syringomyelia
Transverse myelitis

ENURESIS

Common Causes
Developmental delay of bladder function and capacity
Psychological

Uncommon Causes
Diabetes

Food allergy
Obstructive abnormalities of the urinary tract
Urinary tract infection

Rare Causes
Compulsive water drinking
Diabetes inspidus, central or nephrogenic
Lumbosacral anomalies
Seizure disorder
Sickle-cell anemia
Spinal cord tumors

EPISTAXIS

Common Causes
Allergic rhinitis
Repeated sneezing
Secondary to dryness and crusting over anterior portion of nasal septum
Trauma
      External
            Self-inflicted (nose picking)
Upper respiratory infection

Uncommon Causes
Factor XI deficiency
Hypertension
Platelet dysfunction syndromes
Sickle-cell anemia
Thrombocytopenia (any cause)
Von Willebrand's disease

Rare Causes
Angiofibroma
Ataxia-telangiectasia
Congenital syphilis
Ehlers-Danlos syndrome
Foreign body
Malaria
Measles
Nasal angiomas
Nasal diphtheria
Nasal polyp
Oral contraceptives
Osler-Weber-Rendu disease
Pertussis
Rheumatic fever
Scarlet fever
Scurvy
Typhoid fever
Varicella
Wegener's granulomatosis

FAILURE TO THRIVE

Common Causes

Neglect
- Inadequate ingestion/metabolism of calories
  - Depression with anorexia
  - Manipulative behavior
  - Rumination as self-stimulation
  - Secondary malabsorption
    - Self-induced (vomiting, laxative abuse)
    - Specific deficiency (eg, zinc, biotin)
    - Starvation
  - Secondary neuroendocrine abnormalities
    - Abnormal cycling of growth hormone
    - Cortisol deficiency
- Physical neglect/abuse
- Psychosocial deprivation
- Withholding of food as neglect/abuse
  - Intentional withholding of food
  - "Unintentional" withholding of food
    - "Overwhelmed" caretaker
    - Lack of support systems (financial/social)
    - Primary personal needs (eg, drug/alcohol abuse)
    - Time constraints (eg, unsupervised eating, bottle propping)
  - Psychotic or depressed caretaker

Nonorganic failure to thrive
- Inadequate volume of feeds
  - Too few feeds per day
  - Too little per feed
    - Colic
    - "Difficult" feeder
    - Financial factors
    - Ignorance
    - Inexperienced/impatient caretaker with or without compounding child factors
- Inappropriate foods for age
  - Cultural factors
  - Fad diets
  - Financial factors
  - Ignorance
- Incorrect preparation of formula
  - Chronic dilution
  - Financial factors
  - Ignorance
  - Prolonged use after gastroenteritis
- Inappropriate additives

Normal variants
- Delayed growth spurt
- Early-onset growth retardation
- Genetic "slightness"

Organic failure to thrive
- CNS etiologies
  - Mental retardation/cerebral palsy
  - Neurodevelopmental retardation
- Gastrointestinal etiologies
  - Chronic gastroenteritis
  - Gastroesophageal reflux
  - Pyloric stenosis

Prematurity
Small for gestational age

Uncommon Causes

Defective utilization of calories
- Chronic hypoxemia
- Diabetes mellitus

Defects in absorption
- Cystic fibrosis
- Enzymatic deficiencies
- Food sensitivity/intolerance
- Hepatitis
- HIV infection
- Inflammatory bowel disease
- Milk allergy
- Starvation

Inadequacy of food intake
- Cleft lip/palate
- Dyspnea of any cause
  - Congenital heart disease
  - Respiratory disease/insufficiency
- Immature suck/swallow
- Pharyngeal incoordination

Increased metabolism
- Chronic anemias
- Chronic/recurrent infections
  - Otitis, sinusitis, pneumonia
  - Parasites
  - Tuberculosis
  - Urinary tract infection

Chronic respiratory insufficiency
Congenital heart disease
HIV infection
Malignancies

Rare Causes

Defective utilization of calories
- Adrenal insufficiency
- Chromosomal syndromes
- Diabetes insipidus
- Diencephalic syndrome
- Drugs/toxins
- Dysmorphogenic syndromes
- Fetal exposure syndromes
- Hypopituitarism

Hypothyroidism
Metabolic disorders
    Aminoacidopathies
    Galactosemia
    Organic acidurias
    Storage diseases
Parathyroid disorders
Renal tubular acidosis
Defects in absorption
    Acrodermatitis enteropathica
    Biliary atresia/cirrhosis
    Celiac disease
    Hirschsprung's disease
    Immunologic deficiency
    Necrotizing enterocolitis
    Pancreatic insufficiency
    Short gut syndrome
Inadequacy of food intake
    Choanal atresia
    CNS disorders
        Cerebral insults
        Degenerative diseases
        Drugs/toxins
        Subdural hematoma
    Diaphragmatic hernia/hiatal hernia
    Esophageal atresia
    Generalized muscle weakness
        Congenital hypotonia
        Myasthenia gravis
        Werdnig-Hoffmann disease
    Micrognathia/glossoptosis
    Tracheoesophageal fistula
Increased metabolism
    Acquired heart disease
    Adrenocortical excess
    Chronic inflammation (*eg,* juvenile rheumatoid arthritis, systemic lupus erythematosus)
    Chronic seizure disorder
    Drugs/toxins
    Hyperaldosteronism
    Hyperthyroidism

FATIGUE

Common Causes

Acute recovery from surgery, trauma, most illnesses
Anemia
Chronic atopy
Eating disorders
    Excessive dieting (with or without anorexia nervosa, bulimia)

Excessive physical exertion
Mononucleosis (and most viral infections)
Obesity
Pregnancy
Psychosocial
    Chronic boredom
    Chronic depression/anxiety
    Grief
    Stress (prolonged and severe)
Sedentary lifestyle
Sleep disorders
    Insomnia
    Sleep pattern disruption (lack of REM sleep)

Uncommon Causes

Acute bacterial infections
    Bacteremia
    Meningitis
Chronic hypoxemia
    Asthma
    Cardiomyopathy
    Chronic pulmonary disease
    Congenital heart disease
    Congestive heart failure
    Cystic fibrosis
    Heart disease
    Pericarditis
    Pulmonary hypertension
Chronic infections
    Brucellosis
    Cytomegalic inclusion disease
    Histoplasmosis
    Osteomyelitis
    Parasitic infestations
    Pyelonephritis
    Sinusitis
    Subacute bacterial endocarditis
    Toxoplasmosis
    Tuberculosis
    Urinary tract infection
Dehydration
Hepatitis
Upper airway obstruction (sleep apnea)
    Pickwickian syndrome
    Tonsillar-adenoidal hypertrophy

Rare Causes

AIDS
Allergic tension fatigue syndrome
Connective tissue diseases
    Dermatomyositis
    Juvenile rheumatoid arthritis
    Mixed connective tissue disease

Scleroderma
Systemic lupus erythematosus
Endocrine disorders
Diabetes insipidus
Diabetes mellitus
Hyperadrenalism/hypoadrenalism
Hyperparathyroidism
Hyperpituitarism/hypopituitarism
Hyperthyroidism/hypothyroidism
Hepatic insufficiency
Hypoglycemia
Inborn errors of metabolism
Inflammatory bowel disease
Intussusception
Malignancy
Leukemia
Lymphoma
Solid tumors
Metabolic disturbances
Hypermagnesemia/hypomagnesemia
Hypokalemia
Hyponatremia
Neurologic
Intracranial hematomas
Myasthenia gravis
Narcolepsy
Renal tubular acidosis
Toxins and drugs
Alcohol
Analgesics and salicylates
Anticonvulsants
Antihistamines
Barbiturates
Carbon monoxide
Corticosteroids
Digitalis
Heavy metals
Insulin
Nicotine
Pesticides
Progesterones
Sedatives
Tetracycline
Vitamin A
Vitamin D
Uremia

FEVER OF UNKNOWN ORIGIN

Fever is defined here as a temperature higher than 38.5°C for more than 2 weeks.

Common Causes

Collagen vascular disease
Juvenile rheumatoid arthritis
Lupus erythematosus
Periarteritis nodosa
Factitious
Infections
Atypical mycobacterial infections
Epstein-Barr virus infections
Osteomyelitis
Sinusitis, mastoiditis
Urinary tract infections
"Viral syndromes"
Inflammatory bowel disease
Regional enteritis
Ulcerative colitis
Malignancy
Acute lymphoblastic leukemia
Neuroblastoma
Hodgkin's disease
Non-Hodgkin's lymphoma

Uncommon Causes

Drug-induced
Infections
Cat-scratch disease
Cytomegalic inclusion disease
Lung abscess
Hepatitis
Histoplasmosis
Pelvic inflammatory disease
Salmonellosis
Kawasaki disease
Lyme disease

Rare Causes

Behçet's syndrome
Diabetes insipidus
Central
Nephrogenic
Diencephalic syndrome
Ectodermal dysplasia
Familial dysautonomia
Hepatoma
Infection
Blastomycosis
Brucellosis
HIV infection
Leptospirosis
Liver abscess
Lymphogranuloma venereum
Malaria
Perinephric abscess
Psittacosis

Q fever
Rocky Mountain spotted fever
Streptococcosis
Subdiaphragmatic abscess
Toxoplasmosis
Tuberculosis
Tularemia
Viral encephalitis
Visceral larva migrans
Myelogenous leukemia
Pancreatitis
Periodic disease (familial fever)
Reticulum-cell sarcoma
Sarcoidosis
Serum sickness
Thyrotoxicosis

GASTROINTESTINAL BLEEDING

In the Neonate

Common Causes
Esophagitis
Gastritis
Ingested maternal blood
Necrotizing enterocolitis
Stress ulcer (gastric)

Uncommon Causes
Acquired coagulopathy
Gastroenteritis (*Campylobacter* infections)
Hemophilia
Rectal trauma or gastrointestinal trauma
Thrombocytopenia
Vitamin K deficiency
Volvulus

Rare Causes
Acute ulcerative colitis
Gastric polyp
Gastrointestinal duplication cyst
Intussusception
Leiomyoma
Milk allergy
Nasal or pharyngeal bleeding
Severe cyanotic congenital heart disease
Vascular malformation of the gut (hemangioma, telangiecta-
sia, arteriovenous malformation)

In Infancy

Common Causes
Anal fissure

Cow's milk protein sensitivity
Esophagitis
Gastritis
Gastroenteritis

Uncommon Causes
Acute intestinal ischemia
Drug ingestion, such as aspirin or caustic
Hemophilia
Intussusception
Meckel's diverticulum
Peptic ulcer
Thrombocytopenia

Rare Causes
Duplication of the bowel
Gangrenous bowel
Hemangioma of the bowel
Henoch-Schönlein purpura
Polyps

In Childhood

Common Causes
Anal fissures
Esophagitis
Gastritis (possibly due to drug ingestion)
Gastroenteritis
Polyps

Uncommon Causes
Acquired coagulation disturbance
Hemophilia
Henoch-Schönlein purpura
Inflammatory bowel disease
Meckel's diverticulum
Parasitism
Peptic ulcer
Thrombocytopenia

Rare Causes
Chronic granulomatous disease
Diverticulitis
Ehlers-Danlos syndrome
Esophageal varices
Hemangiomas and telangectasia
Hemolytic-uremic syndrome
Hemorrhoids
Intestinal foreign body
Lymphosarcoma
Peutz-Jeghers syndrome
Pseudoxanthoma elasticum
Scurvy

HEADACHE

Common Causes

Extracranial infection
  Otitis/mastoiditis
  Pharyngitis
  Sinusitis
  Tooth abscess
Febrile illness
Migraine
Tension
  Anxiety
  Environmental stress

Uncommon Causes

Depression
Eye strain
Meningitis/encephalitis
Temporomandibular joint disease
Trauma
  Concussion
  Occipital neuralgia

Rare Causes

Allergy
Arnold-Chiari malformation
Cervical osteoarthritis
Chronic renal disease
Congenital erythropoietic porphyria
Cranial bone disease
Decreased intracranial pressure
  Post–lumbar puncture
Drugs
  Amphetamines
  Carbon monoxide
  Heavy metals
  Indomethacin
  Nalidixic acid
  Nitrates/nitrites
  Oral contraceptives
  Steroids
  Sulfa
  Tetracycline
  Vitamin A
Epilepsy
Hyperventilation
Increased intracranial pressure
  Hydrocephalus
  Mass/tumor/abscess
  Pseudotumor cerebri
Leukemia infiltration
Mastocytosis

Metabolic
  Hyperammonemia
  Hypercarbia
  Hypoglycemia
  Hyponatremia
  Hypoxia
  Metabolic acidosis
Myositis
Psychogenic
  Conversion reaction
  Mimicry
  Secondary gain
Orbit
  Glaucoma
  Orbital tumor
Pheochromocytoma
Vascular
  Anemia
  Aneurysm
  Arteritis
    Giant cell
    Periarteritis nodosa
    Subacute bacterial endocarditis
    Systemic lupus erythematosus
  AV malformation
  Cerebral infarct
    Embolus
    Thrombosis
  Cluster headache
  Hemorrhage
    Epidural
    Parenchymal
    Subdural
  Hypertension
  Phlebitis
  Venous sinus thrombosis

HEMATURIA

Common Causes

Benign causes
  Benign recurrent hematuria
  Familial hematuria
  Idiopathic recurrent gross hematuria
  Postural hematuria
Contamination
  Menstrual
  Munchausen's syndrome
  Munchausen's syndrome by proxy
  Pregnancy-related bleeding
Hemoglobinopathies

Hgb C
Hgb SC
Sickle-cell disease/trait (Hgb SS/SA)
Sickle-thalassemia trait
Hypercalciuria
Distal renal tubular acidosis
Diuretic therapy
Endocrine disorders
Diabetes mellitus
Hyperadrenocorticism
Hyperparathyroidism
Hypothyroidism
Hypercalcemia
Hyperphosphatemia
Hypertension
Immobilization
Juvenile rheumatoid arthritis
Medullary sponge kidney
Metabolic acidosis
Neoplasm
Renal tubular dysfunction
Sarcoidosis
Vitamin D excess
Hypoxia, asphyxia, and circulatory compromise
Acute tubular necrosis
Cortical and medullary necrosis
Infections
Cystitis (viral, bacterial)
Pyelonephritis
Urethritis
Meatal stenosis
Noninfectious cystitis
Cytoxan
Radiation
Perineal irritation
Phimosis
Post–infectious glomerulonephritis
Trauma
Fractured pelvis
Postcatheterization
Postcircumcision
Postsurgery
Renal contusion
Renal fracture
Urethral trauma
Urethral ulceration

Uncommon Causes

Bladder diverticula/polyps
Coagulopathies
Drug-induced
Analgesic nephropathy
Cephalosporins

Cytoxan
Penicillin
Sulfonamides
Exercise
Glomerular disorders
Mesangioproliferative
Minimal change disease
Hydronephrosis
Infections
Epididymitis
Prostatitis
Masturbation
Periureteritis (appendicitis, ileitis)
Polycystic disease
Reflux nephropathy
Renal calculi
Renal vein thrombosis
Thrombocytopenia
Ureteropelvic junction (UPJ) obstruction
Urethral foreign body
Wilms' tumor

Rare Causes

Allergy
"Apparent"
"Beeturia"
Betadine
Biliuria
Desferoxamine
Dyes
Analine
Congo red
Hemoglobinuria
Myoglobinuria
Phenothiazines
Porphyria
Diabetic nephropathy
Glomerular disorders
Amyloidosis
Crescentic glomerulonephritis (GN)
Familial nephritis (Alport's)
Focal segmental proliferative GN
Focal segmental sclerosis
Goodpasture's syndrome
IgA nephropathy
Membranous GN
Mesangiocapillary GN
Subacute bacterial endocarditis
Systemic lupus erythematosus
Wegener's granulomatosis
Hemangioma
Klippel-Trenaunay-Weber syndrome
Hematospermia

Immunologic
> Hemolytic-uremic syndrome
> Henoch-Schönlein purpura
> Polyarteritis nodosa
> Systemic lupus erythematosus

Infections
> Leptospirosis
> Malaria
> Schistosomiasis
> Toxoplasmosis
> Tuberculosis
> Varicella

Malignant hypertension
Medullary sponge kidney
Neoplasms
> Bladder cancer
> Prostatic cancer

Renal infarction
Retroperitoneal fibrosis
Vitamin deficiency
> Scurvy
> Vitamin K deficiency

HEMOPTYSIS

Common Causes

Aspiration
> Blood
>> Epistaxis
>> Gingivitis
>> Tonsillitis
>> Upper airway trauma (*eg,* intubation)
> Corrosives
> Foreign body
> Gastric contents
> Oral lesions

Cystic fibrosis
Pulmonary infection (bacterial)
> Bronchiectasis
> Bronchitis
> Pneumonia
> Tracheitis

Pulmonary infection (viral)
> Laryngitis
> Laryngotracheobronchitis
> Pneumonitis

Pulmonary trauma
> Contusion
> Penetrating injury

Uncommon Causes

Lung abscess

Pertussis
Pulmonary hemorrhage (barotrauma)
Pulmonary tuberculosis
Sickle-cell disease

Rare Causes

Arteriovenous malformation/fistula
> Rendu-Osler-Weber syndrome

Cardiac disease
> Endomyocardial fibrosis
> Mitral stenosis
> Pulmonary hypertension

Coagulopathy
Heiner's syndrome
Idiopathic pulmonary hemosiderosis
Munchhausen's syndrome
Munchhausen's syndrome by proxy
Pulmonary embolus
Pulmonary infection
> Aspergillosis
> Blastomycosis
> Coccidioidomycosis
> Hemorrhagic fevers
> Paragonimiasis

Pulmonary vasculitis
> Goodpasture's syndrome
> Polyarteritis nodosa
> Systemic lupus erythematosus
> Wegener's granulomatosis

Pulmonary venous thrombosis

HEPATOMEGALY

Common Causes

Benign cystic disease
Benign transient hepatomegaly (usually with gastrointestinal viral illness)
Biliary tract obstruction
> Alagille's disease
> Ascending cholangitis
> Biliary atresia
> Choledochal cyst

Congestive heart failure
Cystic fibrosis
Diabetes mellitus
Hyperalimentation
Iron-deficiency anemia
Leukemia, lymphoma
Malnutrition
Maternal diabetes
Neonatal hepatitis
Pulmonary hyperinflation ("apparent" hepatomegaly)

Septicemia

Sickle-cell anemia

Toxin/drug reactions (hepatitis, cholestasis, fatty infiltration)

        Acetaminophen

        Oral contraceptives

        Corticosteroids

        Hydantoins

        Phenobarbital

        Sulfonamides

        Tetracycline

Viral hepatitis

        Cytomegalovirus, Epstein-Barr virus, coxsackie virus

        Hepatitis A; hepatitis B; non-A, non-B hepatitis

Uncommon Causes

Chronic active hepatitis

Chronic anemias

Erythroblastosis fetalis

Hamartoma

Hemangioma

Klippel-Trenaunay-Weber syndrome

Hemolytic anemias

Hepatic abscess (pyogenic)

Hepatoblastoma

Inflammatory bowel disease

Liver hemorrhage

Metastatic tumors

Pericarditis

Reye's syndrome

Rocky Mountain spotted fever

Systemic inflammatory disease (*eg,* juvenile rheumatoid arthritis, systemic lupus erythematosus)

Visceral larva migrans

Rare Causes

α_1-Antitrypsin deficiency

Amyloidosis

Beckwith-Wiedemann syndrome

Brucellosis

Budd-Chiari syndrome

Candidiasis

Carnitine deficiency

Chédiak-Higashi syndrome

Crigler-Najjar syndrome

Farber's disease

Galactosemia

Gangliosidosis M_1

Gaucher's disease

Glycogen storage disease

Granulomatous hepatitis

        Chronic granulomatous disease

        Sarcoidosis

Tuberculosis

Hemochromatosis

Hemophagocytic syndrome

Hepatic porphyrias

Hepatocellular carcinoma

Hereditary fructose intolerance

Histiocytic syndromes

Histoplasmosis

Homocystinuria

Hyperlipoproteinemia 1

Hypervitaminosis A

Infantile pyknocytosis

Infantile sialidosis

Klippel-Trenaunay-Weber syndrome

Leptospirosis

Lipodystrophy

Malaria

Mannosidosis

Methylmalonic acidemia

Moore-Federmann syndrome

Mucolipidosis

Mucopolysaccharidoses

Mulibrey nanism

Niemann-Pick disease

Parasitic infections

        Amebiasis

        Flukes

        Schistosomiasis

Rendu-Osler-Weber syndrome

Rickets

Tangier's disease

Tyrosinemia

Urea cycle defects

Veno-occlusive disease

Wilson's disease

Wolman disease

Zellweger syndrome

HIRSUTISM

Common Causes

Familial or racial factors

Idiopathic hirsutism

Physiologic hirsutism

        Pregnancy

        Puberty

Uncommon Causes

CNS injury

Drugs

        Anabolic steroids

Oral contraceptives
Cyclosporine
Diazoxide
Dilantin
Minoxidil
Progesterones
Testosterone
Emotional stress (?)
Polycystic ovarian disease
Severe malnutrition

Rare Causes
Achard-Thiers syndrome
Acromegaly
Adrenal disorders
    Adrenal carcinoma
    Congenital adrenal hyperplasia
    Cushing's syndrome
    Virilizing adrenal adenoma
Congenital erythropoietic porphyria
Dysmorphogenic syndromes (many)
Hypothyroidism
Male pseudohermaphroditism
Ovarian disorders
    Pure gonadal dysgenesis
    Virilizing ovarian tumors
        Arrhenoblastoma
        Granulosa-theca cell tumors

HOARSENESS

Common Causes
Allergy
Caustic ingestion
Excessive use of the voice
Foreign body
Infectious mononucleosis
Instrumentation (naso/orogastric tube)
Laryngitis
Laryngotracheitis
Laryngotracheobronchitis
Postintubation hoarseness
Postnasal drip
Vocal cord nodules
Vocal cord paralysis (postsurgical trauma)

Uncommon Causes
Congenital vocal cord paralysis
Epiglottitis
Hypocalcemia (*eg*, hyperparathyroidism)
Hypothyroidism

Laryngeal trauma
Laryngomalacia
Sicca syndrome
Toxins (chemotherapy, lead, mercury, irradiation, smoke)
Tracheitis (bacterial)
Vocal cord polyps

Rare Causes
Amyloidosis
Angioneurotic edema
Chromosomal abnormalities
    Achondroplasia
    Bloom's syndrome
    Cockayne's syndrome
    Cri du chat syndrome
    De Lange's syndrome
    Diastrophic dwarfism
    Dubowitz's syndrome
    Dysautonomia
    Williams' syndrome
Congenital abnormalities
    Arytenoid cartilage displacement
    Clefts
    Cysts
    Webs
Cricoarytenoid arthritis (juvenile rheumatoid arthritis)
Diphtheria
Recurrent laryngeal nerve impingement
    Aberrant great vessels
    Cardiomegaly
    Hemorrhage
    Hilar adenopathy
    Neoplasm
Recurrent laryngeal nerve dysfunction
    CNS disease
        Arnold-Chiari malformation
        Chédiak-Higashi disease
        Encephalitis
        Hallervorden-Spatz disease
        Huntington's chorea
        Infection
        Ischemia
        Kernicterus
        Meningitis
        Metabolic disease
        Multiple sclerosis
        Polyneuritis
        Pseudobulbar palsy
        Ramsay Hunt syndrome
        Storage disease
        Syphilis
        Syringobulbia
        Toxin

Trauma
Tumor
Wilson's disease
Motor unit dysfunction
Botulism
Muscular dystrophy
Myasthenia gravis
Toxins
Werdnig-Hoffmann disease
Sarcoidosis
Storage diseases (*eg,* lysosomal)
Tetany
Tuberculosis
Tumors of the larynx
Adenoma
Carcinoma
Chondroma
Ectopic thyroid
Fibroangioma
Fibroma
Fibrosarcoma
Hamartoma
Hemangioma
Hygroma
Leukemia
Lymphoma
Myoma
Myxoma
Neuroblastoma
Neurofibroma
Papilloma
Rhabdomyosarcoma
Xanthoma
Vocal cord hemorrhage (nontraumatic)
Wegener's granulomatosis

HYPERHIDROSIS

Common Causes
Emotional stimuli
Exercise
Fever, recovery from fever
Increased environmental temperature
Ingestion of spicy foods

Uncommon Causes
Atopic predisposition
Chronic illness
Brucellosis
Pulmonary tuberculosis
Cluster headaches

Congestive heart failure
Drug withdrawal
Hypoglycemia
Respiratory failure
Salicylate intoxication

Rare Causes
Acrodynia
Acromegaly
Auriculotemporal syndrome
Carbon monoxide poisoning
Carcinoid syndrome
Citrullinemia
Diencephalic syndrome
Familial dysautonomia
Familial periodic paralysis
Hyperthyroidism
Insulin overdose
Ipecac ingestion
Myocardial infarction
Organophosphate poisoning
Phenylketonuria
Pheochromocytoma
Pyridoxine deficiency
Spinal cord injury
Thrombocytopenia-absent radius (TAR) syndrome
Vasoactive intestinal peptide-secreting tumor

HYPERKALEMIA

Hyperkalemia is defined here as a serum potassium level higher than 5.5 mEq/L.

Common Causes
Artifactual
Hemolysis during venipuncture
Acidosis
Renal failure
Severe dehydration

Uncommon Causes
Drugs
Spironolactone
Triamterene
Excessive potassium infusion
Shock

Rare Causes
Addison's disease (adrenal insufficiency)
Cell lysis syndromes
Crush injury
Malignant hyperthermia
Renal tubular acidosis

Theophylline intoxication

HYPERNATREMIA

Hypernatremia is defined here as a serum sodium level higher than 145 mEq/L.

Common Causes
Excessive loss of free water
    Diarrhea
    Diuretics
    High environmental temperature
    Hyperpnea
    Sweating
    Vomiting

Uncommon Causes
Nephrogenic diabetes insipidus
Post–obstructive diuresis
Salt poisoning
Sickle-cell nephropathy

Rare Causes
Cushing's disease
Diuretic phase of acute tubular necrosis (ATN)
Hypercalcemic nephropathy

HYPERTENSION

Common Causes
Agitation
Anxiety
Coarctation of the aorta
Essential hypertension
Immobilization
Obesity
Pain
Renal causes
    Acute tubular necrosis
    Congenital anomalies
        Hydronephrosis
        Nephrophthisis
        Polycystic kidneys
        Renal aplasia/hypoplasia/dysplasia
        Segmental hypoplasia
    Glomerulonephritis (acute and chronic)
        Membranoproliferative and so forth
        Postinfectious
    Liddle's syndrome
    Miscellaneous nephropathy
        Amyloidosis
        Diabetes mellitus

        Gout
        Nephrolithiasis
        Nephrotic syndrome
            Idiopathic
            Minimal change disease
    Obstructive uropathy
    Other nephritides
        Familial nephritis
        Hemolytic-uremic syndrome
        Henoch-Schönlein purpura
        Hypersensitivity/transfusion reaction
        Periarteritis nodosa
        Radiation
        Systemic lupus erythematosus
    Pyelonephritis
    Renal failure (acute and chronic)
    Renal transplantation
    Renal vascular disease
        Renal artery
            Aneurysm
            Arteritis
            Embolic disease
            External compression
        Fibromuscular dysplasia
        Fistula
        Stenosis
        Thrombosis
        Trauma
    Renal vein thrombosis
Retroperitoneal fibrosis
Trauma
Tumors
    Extrinsic tumors
        Adrenal carcinoma
        Neuroblastoma
    Renin-secreting tumors (J-G cell)
    Wilms' tumor
Small pressure-cuff size

Uncommon Causes
Cardiovascular etiologies
    Anemia
    Aortic aneurysm/thrombosis
    Arteriovenous fistula
        Aortic insufficiency
        Aorticopulmonary window
        Patent ductus arteriosus
    Bacterial endocarditis
    Iatrogenic hypervolemia
    Polycythemia
    Pseudoxanthoma elasticum
    Radiation aortitis
    Takayasu's arteritis

Drugs and chemicals
    Glucocorticoids
    Glycyrrhizic acid (licorice)
    Heavy metals (lead, cadmium, mercury)
    Methysergide
    Mineralocorticoids
    Monoamine-oxidase inhibitors
    Oral contraceptives
    Phencyclidine
    Sodium salts
    Sympathomimetics (decongestants)
    Tricyclic antidepressants

Rare Causes

Burns
CNS
    Dysautonomia (Riley-Day syndrome)
    Encephalitis
    Guillain-Barré syndrome
    Increased intracranial pressure
    Poliomyelitis
    Neurofibromatosis
Collagen vascular
    Dermatomyositis
    Scleroderma
Cystinosis
Endocrine
    Congenital adrenal hyperplasia
        11-β-hydroxylase deficiency
        17-hydroxylase deficiency
    Cushing's syndrome
    Hyperaldosteronism
        Primary
            Conn's syndrome
            Dexamethasone-suppressible
            Idiopathic nodular hyperplasia
        Secondary
    Hyperthyroidism
    Pheochromocytoma
Fabry's disease
Hypoxia
Malignant hyperthermia
Metabolic
    Hypercalcemia
    Hypernatremia
    Renal tubular acidosis (RTA) with nephrocalcinosis
Sickle-cell anemia
Stevens-Johnson syndrome

HYPOKALEMIA

Hypokalemia defined here as a serum potassium level lower than 3.5 mEq/L.

Common Causes

Chronic diarrhea
Diuretics
Malnutrition
Metabolic alkalosis
Vomiting/gastric suctioning

Uncommon Causes

Excessive corticoids
Renal tubular disorders

Rare Causes

Amphotericin B therapy
Bartter's syndrome
Colon cancer
Cushing's syndrome
Familial periodic paralysis
Laxative abuse
Primary aldosteronism
Pseudoaldosteronism
Ureterosigmoidostomy
Villous adenoma
Zollinger-Ellison syndrome

HYPONATREMIA

Hyponatremia is defined here as a sodium level lower than 130 mEq/L.

Common Causes

Diarrhea
Excessive salt-free infusions
Syndrome of inappropriate antidiuretic hormone (ADH) secretion
Water intoxication

Uncommon Causes

Acute renal failure
Chronic renal failure
Congestive heart failure
High environmental temperatures

Rare Causes

Adrenal insufficiency
Cirrhosis
Cystic fibrosis and excessive sweating
Spurious
Hyperlipidemia
Hyperglycemia

HYPOTONIA, NEONATAL

Common Causes

Asphyxia
Benign, congenital

Sepsis
Trauma

Uncommon Causes
Congenital joint laxity
Down's syndrome
"Hypermobility syndrome"
Hypothyroidism
Neonatal myasthenia
Spinal cord injury
Werdnig-Hoffmann disease

Rare Causes
Achondroplasia
Cerebrohepatorenal syndrome
Congenital lactic acidosis
Congenital myopathies
      Central core disease
      Myotubular myopathy
      Nemaline myopathy
Cri du chat syndrome
Ehlers-Danlos syndrome
Familial dysautonomia
Fetal warfarin syndrome
Generalized gangliosidosis
Glycogen storage disease (type II)
Hyperammonemia
Lidocaine toxicity
Mannosidosis
Maple-syrup urine disease
Marfan's syndrome
Myotonic dystrophy
Nonketotic hyperglycinemia
Osteogenesis imperfecta
Prader-Willi syndrome
Trisomy 13 syndrome
Williams' syndrome (idiopathic hypercalcemia)

JAUNDICE (BEYOND THE NEONATAL PERIOD)

Common Causes
Acute or chronic hemolytic anemias
Gilbert's disease
Hepatitis A; hepatitis B; non-A, non-B hepatitis; Epstein-Barr virus

Uncommon Causes
Cholelithiasis
Chronic active hepatitis
Cirrhosis

Cystic fibrosis
Drug-induced hepatitis
Total parenteral nutrition

Rare Causes
Alagille's syndrome
α_1-Antitrypsin deficiency
Benign recurrent cholestasis
Biliary atresia
Byler's disease
Chemical injury
Choledochal cyst
Dubin-Johnson syndrome
Fibrosing pancreatitis
Galactosemia
Glycogen storage disease
Hemophagocytic syndromes
Hereditary fructose intolerance
Niemann-Pick disease
Pheochromocytoma
Pyloric stenosis
Reye's syndrome
Rotor syndrome
Trisomy 18
Tyrosinemia
Wilson's disease

JOINT PAIN

Common Causes
Chondromalacia patellae
Growing pains
Osteomyelitis
Overuse
Septic arthritis
Sickle-cell disease
Sympathetic effusion
Tietze's syndrome
Transient synovitis
Trauma
      Contusion
      Fracture
      Hemarthrosis
      Sprain/strain
Viral arthritis
      Adenovirus
      Epstein-Barr virus
      Hepatitis
      Mumps
      Rubella
      Varicella

Uncommon Causes

Attention-seeking behavior
Child abuse
Foreign body
Legg-Calvé-Perthes disease
Mycoplasma
Osgood-Schlatter disease
Osteochondritis dissecans
Popliteal cyst
Psoriatic arthritis
Reactive arthritis
    Brucella
    Campylobacter
    Salmonella
    Shigella
    Yersinia
Referred pain (retroperitoneal/intraperitoneal inflammation)
Slipped-capital femoral epiphysis
Subluxation of the patella

Rare Causes

Bone tumors
Carpal-tarsal osteolysis
Congenital joint laxity
    Ehlers-Danlos syndrome
    Marfan's syndrome
    Stickler's syndrome
Cystic fibrosis
Fabry's disease
Gaucher's disease
Giardia
Gout
Hyperlipoproteinemia
Hyperparathyroidism
Idiopathic chondrolysis
Immunodeficiency
    Complement deficiency
    Hypogammaglobulinemia
Immunologic
    Acute rheumatic fever
    Ankylosing spondylitis
    Behçet's syndrome
    Dermatomyositis
    Giant-cell arteritis
    Henoch-Schönlein purpura
    Hepatitis
    Inflammatory bowel disease
    Juvenile rheumatoid arthritis
    Kawasaki disease
    Mixed connective tissue disease
    Polyarteritis nodosa
    Reiter's syndrome

    Scleroderma
    Serum sickness
    Sjögren's syndrome
    Systemic lupus erythematosus
Leukemia
Lipogranulomatosis
Lyme disease
Mucopolysaccharidosis
Mycobacterial disease
Psychogenic rheumatism
Reflex sympathetic dystrophy
Rickets
Sarcoidosis
Stevens-Johnson syndrome
Subacute bacterial endocarditis
Syphilis
    Charcot joint
    Infection
Thyroid disease
Villonodular synovitis
Whipple's disease

LIMB PAIN

Common Causes

Growing pains
Infection
    Cellulitis
    Osteitis
    Osteomyelitis
    Post–rubella vaccination
    Septic arthritis
    Soft-tissue abscess
    Toxic synovitis
    Viral myositis
Sickle-cell disease—vasoocclusive crisis
Trauma
    Chondromalacia patellae
    Compartment syndromes
    Dislocation and subluxation
    Fracture
    Hypermobility syndrome
    Joint strain, sprain, internal damage
    Myositis ossificans
    Pathologic fracture
    Postimmunization
    Shin splints
    Soft-tissue contusion or hemorrhage
    Stress fracture
    Tendonitis, fasciitis, bursitis
    Traumatic periostitis

Uncommon Causes

Accessory tarsal ossicle
Collagen vascular disease (dermatomyositis, lupus)
Conversion reactions
Henoch-Schönlein purpura
Juvenile rheumatoid arthritis
Legg-Calvé-Perthes disease
Osgood-Schlatter disease
Osteochondritis dissecans
Rheumatic fever
Tarsal coalition

Rare Causes

Bone tumors (osteogenic sarcoma, Ewing's sarcoma, chondrosarcoma)
Cushing's syndrome
Familial Mediterranean fever
Hemophilia
Histiocytosis X
Hyperparathyroidism
Hypervitaminosis A
Inflammatory bowel disease
Leukemia
Mucopolysaccharidosis
Myopathies
Neuroblastoma
Osteoporosis
Popliteal cyst
Rickets
Scurvy
Slipped-capital femoral epiphysis
Soft-tissue tumors (rhabdomyosarcoma, fibrosarcoma)
Sympathetic reflex dystrophy

LIMP

Common Causes

Attention-seeking behavior (usually after minor trauma)
Calluses/corns/ingrown toenails
Chondromalacia patellae
Contusion
Foreign body (especially plantar surface)
Fracture (may be occult)
Growing pains
Hemophilia (hemarthrosis, soft-tissue bleed)
Immunization (local reaction)
Leg length discrepancy
Mimicry
Myositis (acute viral)
Poorly fitting shoes (tight or loose)
Shin splints
Sickle-cell disease (painful crisis/infarction)

Soft-tissue/cutaneous infection
Sprain/strain
Tendonitis
Torsion deformities
Transient synovitis

Uncommon Causes

Arthritis (septic)
Baker's cyst
Blount's disease
Bone tumor (benign and malignant)
Calcaneal spurs
Child abuse
Congenital contractures
Coxa vera
Erythema nodosum
Legg-Calvé-Perthes disease
Leukemia
Neuromuscular disease
 Ataxia
 CNS bleed
 CNS infection
 Flaccid paralysis
 Migraine
 Muscular dystrophy
 Peripheral neuropathy
  Causalgia
  Diabetes mellitus
  Guillain-Barré syndrome
  Heavy metal intoxication
  Periodic paralysis
  Poliomyelitis
  Tick paralysis
 Radiculopathy
 Spastic paralysis
Osgood-Schlatter disease
Osteochondritis dissecans
Osteomyelitis
Phlebitis
Plantar wart
Referred pain
 Diskitis
 Epidural/paraspinal abscess
 Iliac adenitis
 Intraperitoneal infection/inflammation
 Pelvic inflammatory disease
 Retroperitoneal mass
Slipped-capital femoral epiphysis
Subluxation of the patella

Rare Causes

Arthritis/arthralgia
 Acute rheumatic fever
 Dermatomyositis

Henoch-Schönlein purpura
Inflammatory bowel disease
Juvenile rheumatoid arthritis
Kawasaki disease
Polyarteritis nodosa
Serum sickness
Systemic lupus erythematosus
Brucellosis
Caffey's disease
Congenital joint laxity (Ehlers-Danlos syndrome)
Erythromelalgia
Freiberg's disease
Hepatitis
Hypervitaminosis A
Hysteria
Intervertebral disk herniation
Köhler's disease
Larsen-Johansson disease
Neuroblastoma
Pott's disease
Psoas abscess
Pyomyositis
Rickets
Scurvy
Sever's disease
Sinding-Larsen disease
Trichinosis

LYMPHADENOPATHY (GENERALIZED)

Common Causes
Infection (viral, fungal, spirochetal)
Juvenile rheumatoid arthritis
Serum sickness

Uncommon Causes
Drug reactions
     Anticonvulsants, antithyroid, isoniazid
HIV infection
Hodgkin's disease
Infection, bacterial
Leukemia
Non-Hodgkin's disease
Systemic lupus erythematosus

Rare Causes
Angioimmunoblastic lymphadenopathy
Dysgammaglobulinemia
Gaucher's disease
Hemophagocytic syndromes
Histiocytic medullary reticulosis
Histiocytosis

Hyperthyroidism
Metastatic neuroblastoma
Niemann-Pick disease
Sarcoidosis

ODORS OF DISEASE

Common

Disease	Odor
Diabetes	Fruity; acetonelike
Uremia	Fishy (trimethylamine ammonia)

Uncommon

Disease	Odor
Intestinal obstruction	Feculent, foul
Intranasal foreign body	Fetid
Lung abscess	Foul, putrid
Vaginal foreign body	Foul

Rare

Disease	Odor
Glutaric acidemia (type III)	Sweaty feet
Hypermethioninemia	Fish, rancid butter, boiled cabbage
Isovaleric acidemia	Sweaty feet
Maple-syrup urine disease	Maple syrup, caramel-like
Oasthouse syndrome (methionine malabsorption)	Dried malt or hops
Phenylketonuria	Musty, wolflike, stale
Trimethylaminuria	Rotting fish
Tyrosinemia	Rancid butter, fish

POLYURIA

Common Causes
Diabetes mellitus
Diuretic abuse
     Alcohol
     Caffeine
     Medications
Iatrogenic
     Aggressive parenteral hydration
     Diuretic use
Psychogenic polydipsia
Renal failure
Sickle-cell anemia
Urinary tract infection

Uncommon Causes
Diabetes insipidus (central)
Interstitial nephritis

Analgesic abuse
Diphenylhydantoin
Mercury poisoning
Methicillin reaction
Sulfonamides
Renal calculi/hypercalcemia
Renal tubular acidosis

Rare Causes

Bartter's syndrome
Cystinosis
Medullary cystic disease of the kidney
Nephrogenic diabetes insipidus
Neuroblastoma/ganglioneuroblastoma
Pheochromocytoma

PROTEINURIA

Common Causes

Chronic pyelonephritis
Isolated transient/intermittent proteinuria
Cold exposure
Congestive heart failure
Exercise
Febrile illness
Idiopathic proteinuria
Orthostatic proteinuria
Pregnancy
Trauma
Urinary tract infection

Uncommon Causes

Nephritic sediment
Membranoproliferative glomerulonephritis
Postinfectious glomerulonephritis
Nephrotic sediment
Minimal change disease
Preeclampsia
Tubular proteinuria
Acute tubular necrosis
Obstructive uropathy
Polycystic kidney disease

Rare Causes

Drugs
Captopril
Fenoprofen
Gold
Penicillamine
Probenecid
Nephritic sediment
Hereditary nephritis

IgA nephropathy
Mixed cryoglobulinemia
Rapidly progressive glomerulonephritis
Subacute bacterial endocarditis
Systemic lupus erythematosus
Nephrotic sediment
Amyloidosis
Diabetes mellitus
Focal glomerulonephritis
Membranous nephropathy
Miscellaneous infections
Hepatitis B
Malaria
Syphilis
Overflow proteinuria
Bence Jones proteinuria
Lysozymuria (in leukemia)
Tubular proteinuria
Analgesic abuse
Chronic hypertension
Hypercalciuria
Hyperuricemia
Radiation nephritis

PRURITUS

Common Causes

Atopic dermatitis
Cholestasis of pregnancy
Contact allergens (plants, cosmetics, dyes, medications)
Contact irritants (soaps, chemicals, excrement, wool)
Drugs
Aminophylline
Aspirin
Barbiturates
Erythromycin
Gold
Griseofulvin
Isoniazid
Opiates
Phenothiazines
Vitamin A
Dry skin
Advanced age
Excess bathing/strong detergents
Low humidity
Foreign body
Hepatitis
High humidity
Insect bites/infestations

Fleas, mosquitoes, scabies mites, lice, mites, chiggers
Iron-deficiency anemia
Parasitic infection
  Pinworms
  Toxocara canis
Pityriasis rosea
Psoriasis
Seborrheic dermatitis
Skin infections (bacterial/viral/fungal)
Urticaria

Uncommon Causes

Biliary obstruction
  Drug-induced
  Extrahepatic biliary obstruction
  Primary biliary cirrhosis
Chronic renal failure
Hematopoietic malignancies
  Hodgkin's disease
  Leukemia
  Lymphoma
Neurodermatitis
Parasitic infection
  Cercaria
  Hookworms
  Trichinosis

Rare Causes

Autoimmune (sytemic lupus erythematosus, juvenile rheumatoid arthritis)
Congenital ectodermal disorders
Endocrine diseases
  Carcinoid syndrome
  Diabetes mellitus
  Hyperthyroidism/hypothyroidism
  Hypoparathyroidism
Erythropoietic protoporphyria
Hematopoietic malignancies
  Mastocytosis
  Multiple myeloma
  Polycythemia vera
Malignant solid tumors
Neurologic syndromes
Psychosis

PURPURA (PETECHIAL AND ECCHYMOSES)

Common Causes

Thrombocytopenia
Trauma
Viral infections

Uncommon Causes

Abnormal platelet function
Child abuse
Cupping and coin rubbing
Drug ingestion (aspirin)
Factitious
Henoch-Schönlein purpura
Hereditary coagulation disturbance
Infection
Septic emboli
Uremia
Vasculitis
Violent coughing

Rare Causes

Autoerythrocyte sensitization
Bernard-Soulier disease
Cushing's syndrome
Dysproteinemias
Exercise
Glanzmann's thrombasthenia
Hereditary hemorrhagic telangiectasia
Lyme disease
Macular cerulae
May-Hegglin anomaly
Osteogenesis imperfecta
Osteopetrosis
Platelet storage pool disease
Polyurethane exposure
Protein C deficiency
Protein S deficiency
Purpura fulminans
Schamberg's disease
Scurvy
Vitamin K deficiency

SCROTAL SWELLING

Common Causes

Hernia
Hydrocele
Orchitis
Torsion of the cord
Torsion of the testicular appendage
Varicocele

Uncommon Causes

Epididymitis
Henoch-Schönlein purpura
Idiopathic
Insect bites
Secondary to ascites

Rare Causes

Angiomas
Cysts
Healed meconium peritonitis
Hypertriglyceridemia
Leukemia
Sarcoidosis
Scrotal cellulitis
Tumors

SEIZURES

Common Causes

Febrile seizures
Idiopathic seizures

Uncommon Causes

CNS infections
    Aseptic meningitis
    Bacterial meningitis
    Viral encephalitis
CNS injury
    Anoxic encephalopathy
    Child abuse
    Concussion
    Hemorrhage
Hypoglycemia

Rare Causes

CNS infection
    Congenital infection
    Parasitic infection
    Syphilis
    Tetanus
    Tuberculosis
Congenital CNS malformation
    Agenesis/dysgenesis
        Holoprosencephaly
        Porencephaly
    Hydrocephalus
Drugs/toxins
    Aminophylline
    Amphetamines
    Antihistamines
    Atropine
    Camphor
    Carbon monoxide
    Drug withdrawal
    Heavy metals
    Hexachlorophine
    Hydrocarbons
    Local anesthetics

    Narcotics
    Organophosphates
    Penicillin
    Pertussis toxoid
    Phencyclidine
    Scabicides
    Steroids
    Tricyclic antidepressants
Inborn errors of metabolism
    Aminoacidopathy
    Galactosemia
    Organic aciduria
    Storage disease
Metabolic
    Hypernatremia
    Hypocalcemia
    Hypomagnesemia
    Hyponatremia
Miscellaneous
    Arrhythmia
    Dysmorphogenic syndromes (many)
    Kernicterus
    Metachromatic leukodystrophy
    Pyridoxine deficiency
    Rett syndrome
    Reye's syndrome
    Subacute sclerosing panencephalitis (SSPE)
Neurocutaneous syndromes
    Incontinentia pigmenti
    Linear sebaceous nevus
    Neurofibromatosis
    Sturge-Weber disease
    Tuberous sclerosis
Seizure mimics
    Breath-holding spells
    Hyperventilation
    Malingering
    Masturbation
    Migraine
    Myoclonus
    Narcolepsy
    Orthostatic hypotension
    Paroxysmal torticollis of infancy
    Pseudoseizures
    Sandifer's syndrome
    Shivering on urination
    Shuddering attacks
    Syncope
    Tics
    Vertigo
Systemic infection
    Roseola

Shigella
Tumors
Vascular
    Arteriovenous malformation
    Embolic phenomenon
    Hemorrhage
    Hypertension
    Sickle-cell disease
    Thrombosis
    Vasculitis

SPLENOMEGALY

Common Causes
Acute infections (bacterial, viral, rickettsial, protozoal, spirochetal, mycobacterial)
Congenital hemolytic anemias
    Hemoglobinopathies
    Hereditary spherocytosis
    Thalassemia major, thalassemia intermedia

Uncommon Causes
Congestive splenomegaly
Cyanotic congenital heart disease
Hodgkin's disease
Juvenile rheumatoid arthritis
Leukemia
Lupus erythematosus
Non-Hodgkin's disease
Severe iron-deficiency anemia

Rare Causes
Acquired autoimmune hemolytic anemia
Amyloidosis
Beckwith-Wiedemann syndrome
Brucellosis
Chronic granulomatous disease
Congenital erythropoietic porphyria
Dysgammaglobulinemia
Hemophagocytic syndromes
Histiocytosis
Hurler's syndrome and other mucopolysaccharide disorders
Malaria (in United States)
Metastatic neuroblastoma
Myelofibrosis
Osteopetrosis
Sarcoidosis
Serum sickness
Splenic cyst or hemangioma
Storage disease (*eg*, Gaucher's, Niemann-Pick)
Wolman's disease

STRIDOR

(Also see Hoarseness.)

Common Causes
Allergic reaction
Croup
Foreign-body aspiration
Hypertrophied tonsils/adenoids
Peritonsillar abscess
Postinstrumentation edema
Retropharyngeal abscess
Secretions
Spasmotic croup
Subglottic stenosis (congenital, postintubation)
Vocal cord nodules

Uncommon Causes
Corrosive ingestion
Epiglottitis
Granuloma (postintubation/tracheostomy)
Laryngeal trauma
Tracheitis (bacterial)
Vocal cord paralysis (congenital, postsurgical)
Vocal cord polyps

Rare Causes
Angioneurotic edema
Bronchogenic cyst
Congenital goiter
Cricoarytenoid arthritis (juvenile rheumatoid arthritis)
Diphtheria
Ectopic thyroid
Esophageal foreign body
External tracheal compression
    Hemorrhage
    Infection
    Tumors
Farber's disease
Glossoptosis
Hemangioma
Hypoplastic larynx
Internal laryngocele
Laryngeal papilloma
Laryngeal tumors
Laryngismus stridulus (rickets)
Macroglossia
Opitz-Frias syndrome
Pierre Robin syndrome
Post-tracheostomy stricture
Psychogenic stridor
Sarcoidosis
Tetany

Thyroglossal duct cyst
Tracheoesophageal fistula
Tracheolaryngoesophageal cleft
Vascular ring

TORTICOLLIS

Common Causes
Congenital, muscular, or vertebral anomalies

Uncommon Causes
Cervical adenopathy
Congenital nystagmus
Drug-induced (eg, phenothiazines, haloperidol, metoclopramide, trimethobenzamide)
Paroxysmal
Pharyngitis
Retropharyngeal abscess
Secondary to reflux esophagitis (Sandifer's syndrome)
Superior oblique muscle weakness

Rare Causes
Calcification of intervertebral disks
Dystonia musculorum deformans
Eosinophilic granuloma of cervical vertebrae
Fibromyositis
Focal myositis
Hepatolenticular degeneration
Juvenile rheumatoid arthritis
Kernicterus
Osteomyelitis of the cervical vertebrae
Pneumonia of an upper lobe
Posterior fossa tumor
Spasmus nutans
Spinal tumor
Subluxation or dislocation of cervical vertebrae

VERTIGO AND SYNCOPE

Vertigo (dizziness) and syncope (lightheadedness, fainting) may be difficult symptoms for a child to distinguish with certainty. Many entities that are traditionally thought to cause syncope may also cause vertigo. Syncope, therefore, is discussed as a subheading of causes of vertigo.

Common Causes
Benign paroxysmal vertigo
Drugs
    Alcohol
    Anticonvulsants
    Antihypertensives
    Aspirin

    Dilantin
    Gentamycin
    Narcotics
    Sedatives
    Streptomycin
Ear disease
    External canal impaction
        Cerumen
        Foreign body
    Inner ear disease
        Cholesteatoma (with extension)
        Fistula
        Mastoiditis (with extension)
        Suppurative labyrinthitis
        Vestibular neuronitis
        Viral (acute) labyrinthitis
    Middle ear disease
        Chronic suppurative otitis (with extension)
        Hemotympanum (basilar skull fracture)
        Otitis media (rare as isolated finding)
        Serous otitis media
        Tympanic membrane perforation
Headache
    Basilar artery migraine complex
    Migraine
Hyperventilation syndrome
Seizure
    Aura/recovery phase
    Reflex seizure
Visual impairment

Uncommon Causes
CNS infection
    Abscess
    Encephalitis
    Meningitis
    Hypotension
    Trauma
    Basilar skull fracture
    Cerebellar lesion/hemorrhage
    Labyrinthine trauma
    Postconcussion syndrome

Rare Causes
Adrenal insufficiency
Anemia
Arnold-Chiari malformation
Benign positional vertigo
Brain stem ischemia
Breath-holding spells
CNS tumors
    Acoustic neuroma
    Brain stem glioma

Cerebellar glioma
Ependymoma
Medulloblastoma
Demyelinating disease
Multiple sclerosis
Endocrine disorders
Adrenal insufficiency
Diabetes mellitus
Thyrotoxicosis
Hypertension
Hypoglycemia
Increased intracranial pressure
Meniere's syndrome
Pellagra
Psychosomatic illness
Ramsay Hunt syndrome
Syncope (many causes previously discussed)
Cardiovascular etiologies
Arrhythmia
Atrioventricular block
Cardioauditory syndrome
Emery-Dreifuss muscular dystrophy
Mitral valve prolapse
Paroxysmal atrial tachycardia
Paroxysmal ventricular tachycardia
Prolonged QT syndrome
Sick-sinus syndrome
Cardiac anomalies
Aortic stenosis
Pulmonary stenosis
Tetralogy of Fallot
Transposition truncus arteriosus
Carotid sinus syncope
Coronary artery spasm
Dysautonomia (Riley-Day syndrome)
Idiopathic hypertrophic subaortic stenosis
Left atrial myxoma
Myocardial infarction
Orthostatic hypotension
Pulmonary hypertension
Vasovagal stimulation
Vestibulocerebellar ataxia

WHEEZING

Common Causes

Aspiration
Direct (*eg,* defective swallow, neuromuscular disease)
Indirect (gastroesophageal reflux, emesis)
Asthma
Atopic disease
Bronchiectasis
Bronchiolitis
Bronchitis
Foreign-body aspiration
Pneumonitis

Uncommon Causes

Bronchopulmonary dysplasia
Congestive heart failure
Cystic fibrosis
Hypersensitivity pneumonitis
Allergic bronchopulmonary aspergillosis
Mediastinal mass/adenopathy
Pulmonary edema
Tracheobronchomalacia

Rare Causes

α_1-Antitrypsin deficiency
Angioneurotic edema
Carcinoid syndrome
Factitious wheezing
Lobar emphysema
Neoplasm/tumor
Psychogenic airway obstruction
Pulmonary hemosiderosis
Pulmonary sequestration
Pulmonary vasculitis
Sarcoidosis
Tracheobronchostenosis
Tracheoesophageal fistula
Vascular ring/sling
Visceral larva migrans

(Abridged from Harry C. Dietz and Frank A. Oski, Presenting Signs and Symptoms, in Oski, DeAngelis, Feigin, McMillan, Warshaw: *Principles and Practice of Pediatrics, Second Edition,* J.B. Lippincott, 1994.)

Oski's Essential Pediatrics,
edited by Kevin B. Johnson and Frank A. Oski.
Lippincott–Raven Publishers,
Philadelphia © 1997

226

Pediatric Pharmacotherapy

Contributed by Carlton K. K. Lee, Pharm. D., M.P.H.

■ PRESCRIPTION WRITING

Perhaps more than any other patient group, children require clinicians to practice good prescription writing techniques. The following is a list of medication order writing error prevention techniques that should be employed in both inpatient and ambulatory settings:

- Write all orders legibly with a ball point pen and include the following:
  - Inpatient Orders:

    Date & time of drug order, generic drug name, dosage in metric units, dosage form, route of administration, corresponding mg/kg calculation (when applicable), signature of prescriber, and professional designation with ID number
  - Ambulatory Prescriptions:

    Patient's full name, age, and weight (when applicable); date of prescription; drug name, dosage form and strength; number or amount to be dispensed; complete instructions for the patient; include applicable calculations so that dosage can be double-checked with weight; signature of prescriber with professional designation and DEA number for schedule II drugs
- Always express doses, when applicable, in mg, mcg, or units and avoid writing doses in ccs or mls when possible. Many drugs come in multiple concentrations.
- Write clear and concise orders and avoid ambiguity:
  - Do not abbreviate drug names; they can be misinterpreted.
  - Do not use the apothecary system or symbols.
  - Never use a tailing "0" after a decimal point (*ie*, 15.0); this can be mistaken for 150 should the decimal point not appear clearly on the medication order/prescription.
  - Always use a leading "0" before a point (*ie*, 0.15); this avoids ".15" being misinterpreted as 15.
  - Never use "μg" for expressing microgram because it can be mistaken for milligrams; use mcg.
  - Never use "U" for expressing units because it can be mistaken for micrograms or an additional zero; use UNT or UNIT.
  - Be aware of similar sounding drug names (*ie*, Xanax vs. Zantac).
- For inpatient medication orders, all changes or deletions should be rewritten out in their entirety. Changes written over a previous order may not be communicated to the pharmacist if the order copy has already been removed.

■ LIMITATIONS OF DRUG PRODUCTS

Certain commercially available drug products may not be in the most desirable form for a pediatric patient. Limitations of these products include:

- Lack of drug concentration that is adequate to deliver small pediatric specific doses accurately (especially for premature infants)
- Lack of a suitable dosage form for oral administration

These above limitations may be corrected by (1) properly diluting concentrated drug products; and (2) extemporaneously compounding a suitable oral dosage form such as a suspension. Such dosage form manipulations can be achieved by a pharmacist.

■ COMMONLY USED DRUGS LISTED BY GENERIC NAME

Note: all doses are for children, unless indicated. Routes of administration: PO = oral, IV = intravenous, IM = intramuscular, SC = subcutaneous, ETT = endotracheal tube, PR = rectal.

Acetaminophen: analgesic & antipyretic: 10-15 mg/kg/dose PO/PR prn q4h (**max dose: 4 gm/day, 5 doses/day**). *Comments:* caution with G6PD deficiency; acetylcysteine is the antidote for overdoses; many concentrations of the oral liquid product exist.

Acetazolamide: carbonic anhydrase inhibitor; *diuresis, child:* 5 mg/kg/dose PO/IV QD-QOD (**max dose: 1 gm/day**). *Comments:* **contraindicated** in hepatic failure; adjust dose in renal failure; may cause GI irritation, paresthesias, sedation, hypokalemia, acidosis; bicarbonate replacement therapy may be required for long-term use.

Acyclovir: antiviral; *mucocutaneous HSV:* IV: 15 mg/kg/day or 750 mg/m^2/day ÷ q8h X 7 days, PO: 1200 mg/day ÷ q8h X 7 days; *zoster:* IV: 30 mg/kg/day or 1500 mg/m^2/day ÷ q8h X 7-10 days, PO(> 12 yrs old): 4 gm/day ÷ 5X/day X 5-7 days; *varicella:* IV: zoster dose X 7 days, PO: 80 mg/kg/day ÷ QID X 5 days; *immunocompromised HSV:* IV: 750-1500 mg/m^2/day ÷ q8h X 7-14 days, PO: 1 gm/day ÷ 3-5X/day X 7-14 days. *Comments:* may cause renal impairment, headache, vertigo, insomnia, GI irritation; oral absorption is erratic; hydrating patient is essential to prevent renal tubule crystallization.

Albumin: blood product derivative; *hypoproteinemia & hypovolemia:* 1 gm/kg/dose IV (**max dose: 6 gm/kg/day**). *Comments:* available in 5% & 25% strengths each containing 130-160 mEq sodium /L; rapid infusion may cause fluid overload; **contraindicated** in CHF or severe anemia.

Albuterol: beta-2 agonist, bronchodilator; *inhalation use: aerosol:* 1-2 puffs Q4-6 hrs PRN; *nebulization:* age specific dose q4-6h (1-5 yr: 1.25 - 2.5 mg/dose; 5-12 yr: 2.5 mg/dose; > 12 yr: 2.5 - 5 mg/dose). *Comments:* the use of tube spacers may be useful for enhancing drug delivery of the aerosol dosage form; nebulized product is available in 2 concentrations (5mg/ml concentrate & 2.5mg/3ml pre-mixed solution); may cause tachycardia, palpitations, tremor, insomnia, and headache; monitor cardiac function & serum potassium when using high doses.

Alprostadil: prostaglandin E$_1$, vasodilator; *dilation of the ductus arteriosus:* start at 0.05-0.1 mcg/kg/min, increase to 0.2 mcg/kg/min if needed. *Comments:* provides palliative therapy prior to cardiac surgery; decrease dose to lowest effective dose when PaO_2 increases; may cause apnea, fever, seizures, flushing, bradycardia, hypotension, & diarrhea.

Amikacin: aminoglycoside antibiotic; *infant & child:* 15-22.5 mg/kg/day IV/IM ÷ q8h; *adult:* 15 mg/kg/day IV/IM ÷ q8h. *Comments:* monitor serum levels (peak: 20-30 mg/L; trough: 5-10 mg/L); may cause nephrotoxity & ototoxicity; adjust dose in renal failure; enhanced elimination of drug with burn, cystic fibrosis, & febrile neutropenic patients; risk for ototoxicity is increased with concomitant use of a loop diuretic.

Aminophylline: methylxanthine, bronchodilator; *IV loading dose:* 6 mg/kg (each 1.2 mg/kg increases serum theophylline level by 2 mg/L); *IV continuous infusion maintenance dose:* 1-9 yr: 1-1.2 mg/kg/hr, 9-12 yr & young adult smoker: 0.9 mg/kg/hr, 12-17 yr: 0.7 mg/kg/hr. *Comments:* monitor serum levels (asthma: 10-20 mg/L); aminophylline contains 80-85% theophylline, may cause arrhythmias, seizures, restlessness, & GI distress; see theophylline for drug interactions.

Amoxicillin: aminopenicillin; 20-50 mg/kg/day PO ÷ q8h (**max dose:** 2-3 gm/day). *Comments:* may cause diarrhea, rash, nausea, anemia & vomiting; renal elimination.

Amoxicillin/Clavulanic Acid: aminopenicillin with beta lactamase inhibitor; *based on amoxicillin:* 20-40 mg/kg/day PO ÷ q8h (**max dose:** 2 gm/day). *Comments:* covers beta-lactamase producing strains of *H influenzae, M cattarrhalis,* and some *S aureus;* causes significantly more diarrhea than amoxicillin.

Amphotericin B: antifungal; *test dose:* 0.1 mg/kg/dose IV up to **max** of 1 mg; *initial dose:* 0.25 mg/kg/day (including test dose); *increment:* increase as tolerated by 0.25-0.5 mg/kg/day QD or QOD; *maintenance:* 1 mg/kg/day QD or 1.5 mg/kg/day QOD (**max dose:** 1.5 mg/kg/day). *Comments:* may cause hypokalemia, renal failure, phlebitis, fever, chills, nausea and vomiting; meperidine useful for chills; acetaminophen & diphenhydramine premedication is commonly used.

Ampicillin: aminopenicillin; *mild infections:* 100-200 mg/kg/day IV/IM ÷ q6h; *severe infections:* 200-400 mg/kg/day IV/IM ÷ q6h (**max dose:** 12 gm/day). *Comments:* adjust dose in renal failure; may cause interstitial nephritis; similar side effect profile as penicillin.

Aspirin: analgesic & antipyretic: 10-15 mg/kg/dose PO q4h up to **max** of 80 mg/kg/day; *Kawasaki disease:* 80-100 mg/kg/day PO ÷ QID while febrile until patient defervesces then decrease dose to 3-5 mg/kg/day PO qam for 8 weeks or when platelet and ESR normalizes. *Comments:* **contraindicated** in children < 16 yr with chicken pox or flu symptoms because of Reye's syndrome; may cause liver toxicity, decrease platelet aggregation, tinnitus, & GI upset; interacts with drugs bound to albumin (*ie,* warfarin & sulfonamides); use with caution in bleeding disorders.

Azithromycin: macrolide antibiotic; *otitis media:* 10 mg/kg/dose (up to **max** of 500 mg) PO on day one followed by 5 mg/kg/dose PO QD on days 2-5 (**max dose:** 250 mg/day); *uncomplicated chlamydial urethritis or cervicitis:* 1 gm PO X 1. *Comments:* may cause increase in liver function tests, jaundice; take on an empty stomach and avoid antacids in order to assure adequate oral absorption.

Beclomethasone Diproprionate: corticosteroid; *oral inhaler:* 1-2 inhalations TID-QID (**max dose:** 6-12 yr. 10 inhalations/day, > 12 yr. 20 inhalations/day); *nasal inhaler:* 1 spray each nostril BID-TID; *aqueous nasal spray:* 1-2 sprays each nostril BID. *Comments:* not recommended for children < 6 yr; consider tube spacer device with oral inhaler; rinse mouth and gargle with water after oral inhalations to prevent thrush.

Bethanecol Chloride: cholinergic agent; *GE reflux:* 0.1-0.2 mg/kg/ dose PO 0.5 - 1 hr QAC and QHS (**max:** 4 doses/day). *Comments:* may cause hypotension (especially with ganglionic blockers), nausea, bronchospasm, salivation, flushing, abdominal cramps; **contraindicated** in asthma, GI or GU obstruction, peptic ulcer disease, seizures, & hyperthyroidism.

Bisacodyl: stimulant laxative; *oral:* 0.3 mg/kg/day or 5-10 mg; *rectal:* < 2yr: 5 mg, 2-11yr: 5-10 mg, > 11yr: 10 mg. *Comments:* effects seen within 6 hours with oral dosage form and 15 min with rectal; do not crush or chew tablets; may cause abdominal cramping, nausea, vomiting, & rectal irritation.

Calcitriol: active vitamin D; *renal failure:* 0.01-0.05 mcg/kg/day PO, dose may be titrated in 0.005-0.01 mcg/kg/day increments Q 4-8 weeks as needed. *Comments:* may cause weakness, headache, vomiting, constipation, hypotonia, polydipsia, polyuria & metastatic calcification; monitor serum calcium & phosphorus.

Calcium Carbonate: calcium supplement (40% elemental calcium); *hypocalcemia:* 50-162.5 mg/kg/day PO ÷ QID expressed as calcium carbonate. *Comments:* may cause constipation, hypercalcemia, hypophosphatemia, nausea, vomiting.

Calcium Gluceptate: calcium supplement (8.2% elemental calcium); *hypocalcemia:* 200-500 mg/kg/day IV ÷ q6h expressed as calcium gluceptate. *Comments:* may cause tissue necrosis due to extravasation, infusion related hypotension & bradycardia; **avoid** IM or SC administration.

Captopril: angiotensin converting enzyme inhibitor; *hypertension: infant/child:* 0.15-1 mg/kg/day PO ÷ q8h titrated to minimal effective dose (**max dose:** 6 mg/kg/day); *adolescents & adult:* 12.5-25 mg/dose PO TID increase weekly 25 mg/dose as needed up to **max** of 450 mg/day. *Comments:* may cause rash, proteinuria, neutropenia, cough, hypotension, and altered taste perception; adjust dosage in renal failure.

Carbamazepine: anticonvulsant; < *6 yr:* start with 5-10 mg/kg/day PO ÷ BID-QID, increase q 5-7 days up to 20 mg/kg/day PO; *6-12 yr:* start with 10 mg/kg/day PO ÷ BID up to **max dose** of 200 mg/day, increase 100 mg/day at 1 week intervals until desired response is obtained (÷ daily doses TID-QID), usual maintenance dose 20-30 mg/kg/day PO ÷ BID-QID (**max dose:** 1 gm/day); > *12 yr:* start with 200 mg PO BID, increase by 200 mg/day at 1 week intervals until desired response is obtained (÷ daily doses BID-QID), usual maintenance dose 600-1200 mg/day PO ÷ BID-QID (**max dose:** 12-15 yr: 1gm/day; adults: 1.6-2.4 gm/day). *Comments:* monitor levels (4-12 mg/L); may cause sedation, SIADH, dizziness, aplastic anemia, neutropenia, urinary retention, & Stevens-Johnson syndrome; **drug interactions:** erythromycin, verapamil, cimetidine, and INH may increase serum levels; carbamazepine may decrease effect of warfarin, doxycycline, oral contraceptives, theophylline, phenytoin, benzodiazepines, ethosuximide, & valproic acid.

Cefaclor: 2nd generation cephalosporin; 40 mg/kg/day PO ÷ Q8h (**max dose:** 2 gm/day). *Comments:* serum sickness has been reported in patients receiving multiple courses; adjust dose in renal impairment; use with **caution** in penicillin allergic patients; may cause false positive urine reducing substance.

Cefazolin: 1st generation cephalosporin; 50-100 mg/kg/day IV/IM ÷ q8h (**max dose:** 6 gm/day). *Comments:* provides gram-positive coverage; may cause phlebitis, leukopenia, thrombocytopenia, elevated liver enzymes, false positive urine reducing substance; adjust dose in renal impairment; use with **caution** in penicillin allergic patients.

Cefotaxime: 3rd generation cephalosporin; *infant & child:* 100-200 mg/kg/day IV/IM ÷ q6-8h; *meningitis:* 200 mg/kg/day

IV/IM ÷ q6h; *penicillin-resistant pneumococci:* 225-300 mg/kg/day IV/IM ÷ q6-8h. *Comments:* provides gram-negative coverage; similar side effects as with other cephalosporins; adjust dose in renal impairment; use with **caution** in penicillin allergic patients.

Cefoxitin: 2nd generation cephalosporin; 80-160 mg/kg/day IV/IM ÷ q4-6h (**max dose:** 12 gm/day). *Comments:* provides anaerobic coverage; similar side effects as with other cephalosporins; adjust dose in renal impairment; use with **caution** in penicillin allergic patients.

Ceftazidime: 3rd generation cephalosporin; *infant & child:* 90-150 mg/kg/day IV/IM ÷ q8h; *meningitis:* 225 mg/kg/day IV/IM ÷ q8h; *cystic fibrosis:* 150 mg/kg/day IV/IM ÷ q8h; (**max dose:** 6 gm/day). *Comments:* provides pseudomonas coverage; similar side effects as with other cephalosporins; adjust dose in renal impairment; use with **caution** in penicillin allergic patients.

Ceftriaxone: 3rd generation cephalosporin; *infant & child:* 50-75 mg/kg/day IV/IM ÷ q12-24h; *meningitis:* 100mg/kg/day IV/IM ÷ q12-24h (**max dose:** 4 gm/day). *Comments:* provides gram-negative coverage; causes significantly more diarrhea than other cephalosporins; may cause reversible cholelithiasis, sludging in gallbladder, and jaundice; use with **caution** in penicillin allergic & neonatal patients; does not require dosage adjustment in renal impairment.

Cefuroxime: 2nd generation cephalosporin; *IV/IM dosing:* 75-150 mg/kg/day ÷ q8h (**max dose:** 6 gm/day); *PO dosing for otitis media:* 30 mg/kg/day ÷ q12h with suspension **OR** 250 mg q12h with tablets (**max dose:** 1 gm/day). *Comments:* **not recommended** for meningitis; similar side effects as with other cephalosporins; adjust dose in renal impairment; use with **caution** in penicillin allergic patients.

Cephalexin: 2nd generation cephalosporin; 25-100 mg/kg/day PO ÷ q6-12h (**max dose:** 4 gm/day). *Comments:* use higher dose for severe infections & osteomyelitis; similar side effects as with other cephalosporins; adjust dose in renal impairment; use with **caution** in penicillin allergic patients.

Chloral Hydrate: sedative, hypnotic; *sedation:* 25-50 mg/kg/day PO/PR ÷ q6-8h (**max dose:** 500 mg/dose); *sedation for procedures:* 25-1000 mg/kg/dose PO/PR (**max dose:** 1 gm/dose for infant, 2 gm/dose for child). *Comments:* **does not** have analgesic effects; may cause GI irritation, excitation, hypotension, and respiratory depression; **contraindicated** in hepatic or renal disease.

Chloramphenicol: antibiotic; 50-100 mg/kg/day IV/PO ÷ q6h (**max dose:** 4 gm/day). *Comments:* monitor levels (Peaks: meningitis: 15-25 mg/L, other infections: 10-20 mg/L; Troughs: meningitis: 5-15 mg/L, other infections: 5-10 mg/L); may cause bone marrow suppression & aplastic anemia; **drug interactions:** phenobarbital & rifampin may lower chloramphenicol levels; chloramphenicol may increase phenytoin levels.

Chlorothiazide: thiazide diuretic; 20-40 mg/kg/day PO/IV ÷ q12h (**max dose:** 2 gm/day). *Comments:* **avoid** IM administration; may cause hypercalcemia, hypokalemia, alkalosis, pancreatitis, hyperglycemia, & hypomagnesemia; use with **caution** in liver and renal disease.

Ciprofloxacin: quinolone antibiotic; *IV dosing:* 10-20 mg/kg/day ÷ q12h (**max dose:** 800 mg/day); *PO dosing:* 20-30 mg/kg/day ÷ q12h (**max dose:** 1.5 gm/day). *Comments:* may cause GI upset, renal failure; do not administer with antacids or other divalent salts within 4 hours of ciprofloxacin dose; has caused arthropathy in beagle puppies; use with **caution** in children < 18 years old.

Cisapride: prokinetic agent; 0.2-0.3 mg/kg/dose PO TID-QID; *Comments:* may cause headaches & GI disturbances; use is highly discouraged in patient with underlying cardiac arrhythmias; **drug interactions:** fatal cardiac arrhythmias have been reported with concomitant use of ketoconazole, itraconazole, miconazole, fluconazole, erythromycin, clarithromycin, or troleandromycin.

Clarithromycin: macrolide antibiotic; 15 mg/kg/day PO ÷ q12h (**max dose:** 1 gm/day). *Comments:* may cause diarrhea, nausea, abnormal taste, dyspepsia, abdominal discomfort, & headache; **drug interactions:** may increase carbamazepine & theophylline levels; may cause cardiac arrhythmias when used with terfenadine or cisapride.

Clindamycin: antibiotic; *IV/IM dosing:* 25-40 mg/kg/day ÷ q6-8h (**max dose:** 4.8 gm/day); *PO dosing:* 20-30 mg/kg/day ÷ q6h; *topical use:* apply to affected area BID. *Comments:* may cause diarrhea, rash, Stevens-Johnson syndrome, granulocytopenia, thrombocytopenia & pseudomembranous colitis; **contraindicated** in meningitis.

Codeine: narcotic analgesic, antitussive; *analgesia:* 0.5-1 mg/kg/dose PO/IM/SC q4-6h (**max dose:** 60 mg/dose); *antitussive:* 1-1.5 mg/kg/day PO ÷ q4-6h PRN (**max dose:** child 2-6 yr: 30 mg/day; child 6-12 yr: 60 mg/day). *Comments:* **do not administer** via IV route due to risk for severe hypotension; may cause CNS and respiratory depression, constipation, cramping; used in combination with acetaminophen for analgesia; **do not use** as an antitussive for children < 2 years old.

Co-trimoxazole (Trimethoprim-Sulfamethoxazole): sulfonamide antibiotic; (**all doses based on trimethoprim**) *minor infections:* 8-10 mg/kg/day PO/IV ÷ q12h (**max dose:** 320 mg/day); *UTI prophylaxis:* 2-4 mg/kg/dose PO QD; *severe infections/pneumocystis carinii pneumonia:* 20 mg/kg/day PO/IV ÷ q6-8h; *pneumocystis prophylaxis:* 5-10 mg/kg/day or 150 mg/m²/day PO/IV ÷ q12h for 3 consecutive days per week (**max dose:** 320 mg/day). *Comments:* may cause kernicterus in newborns, blood dyscrasias, crystalluria, renal or hepatic injury, GI irritation, Stevens-Johnson syndrome; **avoid** in patients with G6PD deficiency; adjust dosage in renal compromise.

Cromolyn: anti-allergy agent; *nebulization:* 20 mg q6-8h; *aerosol inhaler:* 2 puffs TID-QID; *nasal:* 1 spray each nostril TID-QID; *comments:* may cause rash, cough, bronchospasm, nasal congestion; administer dose no longer than 1 hour for exercise induced asthma; requires at least 2-4 weeks of continuous use to assess efficacy.

Cyclosporine & Cyclosporine Microemulsion (Neoral): immunosuppressant; (**1:1 conversion with cyclosporine & Neoral is recommended**) *PO dosing:* 15 mg/kg/dose 4-12 hours prior to transplant followed by 15 mg/kg/day ÷ q12-24h for 1-2 week post-transplant then decrease dose by 5% per week to 5-10 mg/kg/day ÷ q12-24h; *IV dosing:* 5-6 mg/kg/dose 4-12 hours prior to transplant then 5-6 mg/kg/day post-transplant until converting to PO dosing. *Comments:* monitor serum trough levels (exact target serum concentration is based on specific transplant protocols); may cause nephrotoxicity, hypertension, hepatotoxicity, hirsutism, acne, hypomagnesemia, and leukopenia; **drug interactions:** fluconazole, ketoconazole, erythromycin, calcium channel blockers, and corticosteroids may elevate cyclosporine levels.

Dexamethasone: corticosteroid; *anti-inflammatory:* 0.08-0.3 mg/kg/ day PO/IV/IM ÷ q6-12h; *airway edema:* 0.5-2 mg/kg/day PO/IV/ IM ÷ q6h (start 24 hours before extubation and continue for 4-6 doses post-extubation); *croup:* 0.6 mg/kg/dose IM X 1; *cerebral edema:* 1-2 mg/kg/dose

PO/IV/IM X 1 followed by 1-1.5 mg/kg/day ÷ q4-6h. *Comments:* may cause hypertension, edema, headache, seizures, psychosis, pseudotumor cerebri, cataracts, peptic ulcers, & pituitary-adrenal axis suppression.

Diazepam: benzodiazepine; *anticonvulsant:* 0.2-0.5 mg/kg/dose IV q15-30 min (**max total dose:** < 5 yr: 5 mg, ≥ 5 yr: 10 mg); *muscle relaxant/sedative: IV/IM dosing:* 0.04-0.2 mg/kg/dose q2-4h (**max dose:** 0.6 mg/kg during an 8 hour period); *PO dosing:* 0.12-0.8 mg/kg/day ÷ q6-8h. *Comments:* may cause hypotension & respiratory depression (flumazenil is the antidote); do not administer faster than 2 mg/min & mix or dilute with IV fluids when using the IV dosage form; may be given rectally at 0.5 mg/kg/dose.

Didanosine (DDI): antiviral agent; 100-300 mg/m²/day PO ÷ q12h (check specific protocol for exact dosing). *Comments:* all doses must be administered on an empty stomach; may cause headaches, diarrhea, peripheral neuropathy, nausea, vomiting, rash, abdominal pain, & CNS depression; drug product contains significant amounts of sodium; reduces the absorption of drugs (ie, ketoconazole) requiring acidic GI environment.

Diphenhydramine: antihistamine; *children:* 5 mg/kg/day PO/IV/IM ÷ q6h (**max dose:** 300 mg/day); *anaphylaxis or phenothiazine overdose:* 1-2 mg/kg IV. *Comments:* may cause drowsiness, paradoxical CNS excitation in children; **contraindicated** with concurrent MAO inhibitor use and acute asthmatic attacks.

Divalproex sodium (Depakote): see Valproic Acid

Docusate Sodium: laxative, stool softener; *< 3 yr:* 10-40 mg/day ÷ QD-QID; *3-6 yr:* 20-60 mg/day ÷ QD-QID; *6-12 yr:* 40-150 mg/day ÷ QD-QID; *> 12 yr:* 50-500 mg/day ÷ QD-QID. *Comments:* onset of action may take up to 1-3 days of use; assure adequate hydration; relatively free of side effects; instilling a few drops of the 10 mg/ml liquid dosage form into the ear may be useful as a cerumenolyic.

Doxycycline: tetracycline antibiotic; *≤ 45 kg:* 5 mg/kg/day PO/IV ÷ BID (**max dose:** 200 mg/day) X 1 day then 2.5-5 mg/kg/day PO/IV ÷ BID; *> 45 kg:* 200 mg/day PO/IV ÷ BID X 1 day then 100-200 mg/day PO/IV ÷ BID. *Comments:* **contraindicated** in children < 9 yr; may cause photosensitivity, hemolytic anemia, GI disturbances; do not administer with dairy products or any divalent salts when using the oral dosing route.

EMLA (eutectic mixture of local anesthetics): transdermal anesthetic (**apply 60-90 minutes under occlusive dressings prior to intervention**); *weight of patient, maximum application area (cm²)):* < 10 kg: 100 cm²; 10-20 kg: 600 cm²; > 20 kg: 2000 cm². *Comments:* wipe cream off prior to intervention; use with **caution** in patients with G6PD deficiency, renal & hepatic failure; prilocaine (one of the drug's components) has been associated with methemoglobinemia.

Enalapril maleate (PO) & Enalapriat (IV): angiotensin converting enzyme inhibitor; *PO dosing:* start with 0.1 mg/kg/day ÷ QD-BID and increase as needed over 2 weeks up to a **maximum** of 0.5 mg/kg/day; *IV dosing:* 0.005-0.01 mg/kg/dose Q8-24h. *Comments:* enalapril maleate is a prodrug to the active form enalapriat; may cause nausea, diarrhea, headache, dizziness, hypotension, and cough; reduce dose in renal impairment.

Erythromycin Preparations: macrolide antibiotic; *PO dosing:* 30-50 mg/kg/day ÷ q6-8h (**max dose:** 2 gm/day); *pertussis:* 50 mg/kg/day PO (using estolate salt) ÷ q6h X 14 days; *IV dosing:* 20-50 mg/kg/day ÷ q6h (**max dose:** 4 gm/day); *preop bowel prep:* 20 mg/kg/dose PO (using erythromycin base)

X 3 doses with neomycin 1 day prior to surgery; *ophthalmic use:* apply 0.5 inch ribbon to the conjunctival sac of the affected eye BID-QID. *Comments:* various forms of the oral preparation exists (estolate salt is associated with cholestatic jaundice & hepatotoxicity); may cause nausea, vomiting, abdominal cramping & false positive urinary catecholamines; **drug interactions:** may increase effects of digoxin, theophylline, carbamazepine, cyclosporine, and induce cardiac arrhythmias with cisapride, astemizole, and terfenadine.

Erythromycin Ethylsuccinate & Acetyl Sulfisoxazole (Pediazole): macrolide antibiotic & sulfonamide combination product; *otitis media:* 50 mg/kg/day (erythromycin) and 150 mg/kg/day (sulfa) PO ÷ q6h (**max dose:** 2 gm erythromycin & 6 gm sulfisoxazole per day). *Comments:* see erythromycin preparations and sulfisoxazole.

Famotidine: histamine H₂ antagonist; *PO dosing:* start at 1-1.2 mg/kg/day ÷ q8-12h up to a **max** of 40 mg/day; *IV dosing:* start at 0/6-0/8 mg/kg/day ÷ q8-12h up to a **max** of 40 mg/day. *Comments:* may cause headaches, dizziness, constipation, diarrhea, and drowsiness; adjust dosage in severe renal failure; younger children may require q8h dosing interval due to enhanced elimination.

Fentanyl: narcotic analgesic; *intermittent IV/IM dosing:* 1-2 mcg/kg/dose q30-60 min prn; *continuous IV dosing:* 1-3 mcg/kg/hr; *PO sedation dosing:* 10-15 mcg/kg/dose up to **max** of 400 mcg/dose. *Comments:* drug in highly lipid soluble and distributes into fat tissue; may cause respiratory depression and chest wall rigidity (with rapid IV infusion); administer intermittent IV doses over 3-5 minutes; oralet is oral product.

Ferrous Sulfate: see iron preparations.

Flumazenil: benzodiazepine antagonist; start with 0.1 mg X 1, repeat dose of 0.1-0.2 mg if no response in 30-60 seconds after the initial dose, may repeat above doses to a **max** cumulative dose of 1 mg **or** 3 mg in 1 hour. *Comments:* onset of action is within 1-3 minutes; **does not** reverse effects of opiates; may cause seizures.

Fluoride: mineral; *fluoride supplementation:* (**all doses expressed as daily doses given QD**) *age 2 week - 2 years:* drinking water fluoride conc.: < 0.3 ppm give 0.25 mg; *age 2-3 years:* drinking water conc.: < 0.3 ppm give 0.5 mg, 0.3-0.7 ppm give 0.25 mg; *age 3-16 years:* drinking water conc.: < 0.3 ppm give 1 mg, 0.3-0.7 ppm give 0.5 mg. *Comments:* overdosages may cause GI distress, salivation, CNS irritability, tetany, seizures, hypocalcemia, hypoglycemia, & cardiorespiratory failure; chronic overdoses may result in mottled teeth.

Furosemide: loop diuretic; 0.5-2 mg/kg/dose PO/IV/IM q6-12h (**max dose:** 6 mg/kg/dose). *Comments:* may cause hypokalemia, alkalosis, dehydration, hyperuricemia, & increased calcium excretion; ototoxicity may occur when use is with an aminoglycoside.

Gentamicin: aminoglycoside antibiotic; *IV/IM dosing:* 6-7.5 mg/kg/day ÷ q8h; *ophthalmic drops:* 1-2 drops to affected eye q4h; *ophthalmic ointment:* apply to conjunctival sac of affected eye BID-TID. *Comments:* monitor serum levels (peak: 6-10 mg/L general, 8-10 mg/L for pulmonary infections, neutropenia, severe sepsis; trough: < 2 mg/L); may cause nephrotoxity & ototoxicity; adjust dose in renal failure; enhanced elimination of drug with burn, cystic fibrosis, & febrile neutropenic patients; risk for ototoxicity is increased with concomitant use of a loop diuretic.

Glucagon: antihypoglycemic agent; 0.03-0.1 mg/kg/dose IM/IV/SC q 20 min PRN (**max dose:** 1 mg/dose). *Comments:*

may cause cardiac stimulation at high doses; glucose infusion should also be administered.

Griseofulvin microcrystalline: antifungal agent; *microsize dosage form:* > 2yr: 10-15 mg/kg/dose PO QD to be administered with fatty foods (**max dose:** 1 gm/day); *ultramicrosize dosage form:* > 2 yr: 7 mg/kg/dose PO QD. *Comments:* **contraindicated** in porphyria & hepatic disease; may cause leukopenia & photosensitivity; **drug interactions:** phenobarbital may increase griseofulvin's clearance, griseofulvin may decrease the effects of warfarin, oral contraceptives, and cyclosporine.

Heparin: anticoagulant; *anticoagulation:* 50 units/kg IV bolus X 1 followed by 10-25 units/kg/hr IV or 50-100 unit/kg/dose IV q4h; *flushes: peripheral IV:* 1-2 ml of 10 unit/ml solution q4h, *central line IV:* 2-3 ml of 100 unit/ml solution q24h. *Comments:* adjust PTT to 1.5-2.5 times control value; may cause bleeding, allergic reactions, alopecia, & thrombocytopenia; protamine is the antidote.

Hydralazine: vasodilator, antihypertensive agent; *hypertensive crisis:* 0.1-0.2 mg/kg/dose IM/IV q4-6h PRN (**max dose:** 20 mg/kg/dose); *chronic hypertension:* 0.75-3 mg/kg/day PO ÷ q6-12 hr (**max dose:** 200 mg/day or 7.5 mg/kg/day). *Comments:* may cause reflex tachycardia and lupus-like syndrome (patients who are slow acetylators); maximum effects are seen in 3-4 days.

Hydrochlorothiazide: thiazide diuretic; 2-3 mg/kg/day PO ÷ BID (**max dose:** 200 mg/day). *Comments:* see chlorothiazide.

Hydrocortisone: corticosteroid; *status asthmaticus:* 4-8 mg/kg/dose IV (**max dose:** 250 mg) followed by 8 mg/kg/day IV ÷ q6h; *anti-inflammatory/immunosuppressive: PO dosing:* 2.5-10 mg/kg/day ÷ q6-8h; *IV dosing:* 1-5 mg/kg/day ÷ q6h. *Comments:* see dexamethasone for common side effects; various salt forms exist as their routes of administration differ (check each product for details).

Hydromorphone: narcotic analgesic; *IV dosing:* 0.015 mg/kg/dose q4-6h PRN; *PO dosing:* 0.03-0.08 mg/kg/dose q4-6h PRN. *Comments:* titrate dose to effect; similar side effects to morphine but causes less pruritus; naloxone is the antidote.

Ibuprofen: nonsteroidal anti-inflammatory agent; *analgesic/antipyretic:* 5-10 mg/kg/dose PO q6-8h (**max dose:** 40 mg/kg/day); *juvenile rheumatoid arthritis:* 30-50 mg/kg/day PO ÷ q6h (**max dose:** 2.4 gm/day). *Comments:* may cause GI discomfort, rashes, granulocytopenia, anemia, and platelet inhibition; use with **caution** in hepatic & renal insufficiency.

Intravenous Immune Globulin: blood product derivative; *antibody deficiency disorders:* 300-400 mg/kg/dose IV q monthly; *acute idiopathic thrombocytopenia:* 0.8-1 gm/kg in 1-2 doses X 1-5 days; *Kawasaki's disease:* 2 gm/kg/dose X 1, administered over 10-12 hours. *Comments:* **do not** exceed the product specific infusion rates, most adverse effects are related to rapid infusions; may cause flushing of face, hypotension, nausea, chills, fever, headaches, chest tightness, & diaphoresis; IgA containing products are **contraindicated** in IgA deficient patients.

Insulin, regular: pancreatic hormone; *diabetic ketoacidosis:* start at 0.1 unit/kg/hr and titrate to effect. *Comments:* **do not** rapidly decrease serum glucose because it may cause cerebral edema; be sure to flush the tubing with insulin infusion solution before beginning infusion, this will ensure proper drug delivery; may cause hypoglycemia, hypokalemia, & hypophosphatemia.

Ipecac: emetic agent; (**follow all doses with 10-20 ml/kg water**) *6-12 months:* 5-10 ml; *1-12 years old:* 15 ml. *Comments:* may cause GI irritation, cardiotoxicity, myopathy; **contraindi**cated in those who lack a gag reflex, have had seizures, or ingested strong acids, bases, volatile oils, or other corrosives.

Ipratropium: anticholinergic agent; *inhaler use:* < 12 yr: 1-2 puffs TID-QID, ≥ 12 yr: 2-4 puffs QID up to 12 puffs per day; *nebulized use:* < 2 yr: 250 mcg/dose TID-QID, ≥ 2 yr: 250-500 mcg/dose TID-QID. *Comments:* drug has fewer anticholinergic systemic effects than atropine; use with **caution** in narrow-angle glaucoma or bladder neck obstruction; may cause cardiac palpitations, tachycardia, rash, constipation, and dry mouth.

Iron Preparations: oral iron supplements; *iron deficiency anemia:* 3-6 mg elemental iron/kg/day PO ÷ QD-TID. *Comments:* two major oral salt forms used (ferrous sulfate: 20% elemental; ferrous gluconate: 12% elemental); may cause constipation, dark stools, nausea, GI discomfort; **drug interactions:** may decrease the absorption of tetracycline & ciprofloxacin; tetracycline & antacids may reduce iron's absorption.

Ketoconazole: antifungal agent; *PO dosing:* ≥ 2 yr: 5-10 mg/kg/day PO ÷ QD-BID (**max dose:** 800 mg/day); *topical use:* 1-2 applications per day; *shampoo use:* twice weekly for 4 weeks with at least 3 days between applications. *Comments:* requires acidic gastric medium for adequate absorption; may cause rash, vomiting, nausea, and fever; **drug interactions/ contraindications:** cardiac arrhythmias may occur when used with cisapride, terfenadine, astemizole.

Lactulose: laxative, ammonium detoxicant; *chronic constipation:* 7.5 ml/day PO after breakfast; *portal systemic encephalopathy:* 40-90 ml/day PO ÷ TID-QID. *Comments:* **contraindicated** in galactosemia; may cause GI discomfort, and diarrhea; therapeutic goal is to achieve 2-3 soft stools per day.

Lindane: scabicidal agent; *scabies:* apply thin layer of cream or lotion to skin, bathe and rinse off medication in 6-8 hours, may repeat once in 7 days PRN; *pediculosis capitis:* apply 15-30 ml of shampoo, lather for 4-5 minutes, rinse hair & comb with fine comb to remove nits, may repeat once in 7 days PRN. *Comments:* **contraindicated** in infants, young children, & during pregnancy (use permethrin); avoid contact with face and mucous membranes; may cause rash, seizures, & aplastic anemia; remember to change bedsheets and undergarments immediately after treatment.

Lorazepam: benzodiazepine; *anticonvulsant:* 0.05-0.1 mg/kg/dose IV over 2-5 minutes, may repeat 0.05 mg/kg X 1 in 10-15 minutes; *anxiolytic/sedative:* 0.05 mg/kg/dose PO/IV q4-8h. *Comments:* may cause respiratory depression, sedation, dizziness, ataxia, mood changes, & rash; onset of action for sedation: PO: 1 hr, IV: 15-30 minutes.

Magnesium Sulfate: magnesium salt; *hypomagnesemia or hypocalcemia: IV/IM dosing:* 25-50 mg/kg/dose q4-6h x 3-4 doses, repeat PRN (**max single dose:** 2 gm); *PO dosing:* 100-200 mg/kg/dose QID. *Comments:* use with **caution** in patients with renal insufficiency and receiving digoxin; may cause hypotension, respiratory depression, heart block with IV use.

Mebendazole: anthelmintic; *pinworms (children & adults):* 100 mg PO X 1, repeat in 2 weeks if not treated; *hookworms, round-worms, & whipworms:* 100 mg PO BID X 3 days, repeat in 3-4 weeks if not treated. *Comments:* may cause diarrhea & abdominal discomfort; entire family may need to be treated; concurrent phenytoin or carbamazepine use may decrease efficacy; administer all doses with food.

Methylphenidate: CNS stimulant; *attention deficit hyperactivity disorder:* ≥ 6 yr: start with 0.3 mg/kg/dose or 2.5-5 mg/dose PO given before breakfast and lunch, may increase by 0.1 mg/kg/dose or 5-10 mg/dose PO weekly until 0.6-1 mg/kg/day is reached (**max dose:** 2 mg/kg/day or 60 mg/day). *Comments:* **contraindicated** in glaucoma & anxiety disorders; may cause insomnia, weight loss, anorexia, rash, nausea, vomiting, tachycardia, hallucination, fever; use with **caution** in patients with hypertension & seizures.

Methylprednisolone: corticosteroid; *status asthmaticus:* 2 mg/kg IV/IM X 1 followed by 2 mg/kg/day IV/IM ÷ q6h; *anti-inflamatory/immunosuppressive:* 0.5-1.7 mg/kg/day PO/IV/IM ÷ q6-12h. *Comments:* see dexamethasone for common side effects; various salt forms exist as their routes of administration differ (check each product for details).

Metoclopramide: prokinetic agent, antiemetic; *GE reflux/GI dysmotility:* 0.1 mg/kg/dose PO/IV/IM 30 minutes QAC & QHS up to **max** of 0.8 mg/kg/day; *antiemetic:* 1-2 mg/kg/dose PO/IV/IM q2-6h (premedicate with diphenhydramine to reduce risk of EPS). *Comments:* extrapyramidal syndrome occurs at higher antiemetic doses; **contraindicated** in GI obstruction, seizures, pheochromocytoma, & patients receiving drugs with EPS potential.

Metronidazole: antiprotozoal antibiotic; *anaerobic infections:* 30 mg/kg/day PO/IV ÷ q6h (**max dose:** 4 gm/day); *C difficile infection:* 20-35 mg/kg/day PO ÷ q6h X 10 days; *amebiasis:* 35-50 mg/kg/day PO ÷ TID X 10 days; *trichomoniasis:* children: 15 mg/kg/day PO ÷ TID X 7 days, *adolescents & adults:* 2 gm PO X 1 or 250 mg PO TID X 7 days. *Comments:* may cause nausea, vomiting, urticaria, dry mouth, metallic taste, vertigo, discolored urine, & peripheral neuropathy; **contraindicated** in first trimester of pregnancy; **do not** consume alcohol for 24 hours after therapy because of disulfiram-like reaction; adjust dose in renal compromise.

Miconazole: antifungal agent; *vaginitis:* 1 applicator full of cream or 100 mg suppository QHS X 7 days **or** 200 mg suppository QHS X 3 days; *topical:* 1 application BID X 2-4 weeks. *Comments:* may cause pruritis & rash.

Morphine Sulfate: narcotic analgesic; *PO dosing:* 0.2-0.5 mg/kg/dose q4-6h PRN (immediate release product) **or** 0.3-0.6 mg/kg/dose q12h PRN (controlled release product); *IV/IM/SC dosing:* 0.1-0.2 mg/kg/dose q2-4h PRN; *continuous IV infusion:* 0.025-2.6 mg/kg/hr, titrate to effect. *Comments:* may cause CNS and respiratory depression, nausea, vomiting, urinary retention, constipation, dysphoria, biliary spasm, itching, bronchospasms and allergic reactions; naloxone is the antidote.

Mupirocin: topical antibiotic; *topical use:* apply to affected area TID X 5-14 days; *intranasal use:* apply small amount intranasally BID-QID for 5-14 days. *Comments:* intranasal use reduces *S aureus* carriage; may cause minor local irritation.

Naloxone: narcotic antagonist; *opiate intoxication (IM/IV/SC/ETT):* < 20 kg: 0.1 mg/kg/dose, ≥ 20 kg or > 5 yr: 2 mg/dose, all doses may be repeated q2-3 minutes PRN. *Comments:* use with **caution** in patients with chronic cardiac disease; abrupt reversal of narcotic depression may cause nausea, vomiting, diaphoresis, tachycardia, hypertension; naloxone has a short duration of action.

Nifedipine: calcium channel antagonist; *hypertension:* 0.25-0.5 mg/kg/dose of the immediate release product PO/SL p4-6h PRN (**max dose:** 10 mg/dose or 3 mg/kg/ day). *Comments:* may cause hypotension, peripheral edema, flushing, tachycardia, headaches, nausea, syncope, and palpitations; sublingual doses are administered by puncturing the capsule of the immediate release product (where 10mg capsules contain 0.34 ml & 20 mg capsules contain 0.45 ml); grapefruit juice may increase the bioavailability of the drug; **drug interactions:** may increase phenytoin, cyclosporine, and digoxin levels.

Nitrofurantoin: antibiotic; *general use:* 5-7 mg/kg/day PO ÷ q6h; *UTI prophylaxis:* 1-2 mg/kg/dose PO QHS, (**max dose** for both indications: 400 mg/day). *Comments:* may cause hypersensitivity, nausea, vomiting, diarrhea, & hemolytic anemia; **contraindicated** in severe renal disease, G6PD deficiency, infants < 1 month, and pregnancy at term; administer all doses with food or milk.

Nystatin: antifungal agent; *oral thrush: suspension:* 400,000-600,000 units (4-6 ml) swish & swallow QID, *troche:* 200,000-400,000 units 4-5 times a day. *Comments:* may cause diarrhea and GI discomfort; drug is not absorbed via the GI tract; **do not** swallow troches whole.

Omeprazole: gastric acid pump inhibitor; 0.7-3.3 mg/kg/dose PO QD. *Comments:* **do not** crush or chew capsules; enteric coated beads may be administered in acidic beverage (ie. apple juice); may decrease absorption of itraconazole, ketoconazole, & iron salts; may cause headache, diarrhea, nausea, vomiting.

Oxacillin: penicillinase resistant penicillin; 100-200 mg/kg/day IV/IM ÷ q6h (**max dose:** 12 gm/day). *Comments:* may cause diarrhea, nausea, vomiting, leukopenia, hepatoxicity, & acute interstitial nephritis.

Oxybutynin: anticholinergic agent, antispasmodic; ≤5 yr: 0.4-0.8 mg/kg/day PO ÷ BID-TID; > 5 yr: 10-15 mg/day PO ÷ BID-TID. *Comments:* **contraindicated** in glaucoma, GI obstruction, megacolon, myasthenia gravis, severe colitis, hypovolemia; may cause classical anticholinergic side effects.

Pemoline: CNS stimulant; > 6 yr: start with 37.5 mg PO qam, then increase at weekly intervals by 18.75 mg/day to a maintenance dose of 0.5-3 mg/kg/day PO qam (effective range: 56.25-75 mg/day) (**max dose:** 112 mg/day). *Comments:* effects may take up to 3-4 weeks; **do not** abruptly discontinue the drug; may cause insomnia, anorexia, hypersensitivity, depression, abdominal pain, hepatotoxicity, & growth inhibition.

Penicillin G Potassium & Sodium: penicillin antibiotic; 100,000- 400,00 units/kg/day IM/IV ÷ q4-6h (**max dose:** 24 million units/day). *Comments:* may cause anaphylaxis, hemolytic anemia, interstitial nephritis, & urticaria; use penicillin V potassium for oral use because of better absorption; adjust dose in renal compromise; use higher daily dose and shorter dosing interval for meningitis.

Penicillin V Potassium: penicillin antibiotic; 25-50 mg/kg/day PO ÷q6-8h (**max dose:** 3 gm/day). *Comments:* 250 mg is equivalent to 400,000 units; better GI absorption than penicillin G; administer doses 1 hour prior or 2 hours after meals; see penicillin G potassium & sodium for adverse effects.

Permethrin: scabicidal agent; *head lice:* after shampooing, rinsing & towel drying hair, use 1% cream rinse by saturating hair & scalp and leave on for 10 minutes, then rinse, dose may be repeated in 7 days; *scabies:* apply 5% cream from head to toe, leave on for 8-14 hours, then rinse off with water, dose may be repeated in 7 days. *Comments:* **avoid** contact with eyes; may cause pruritus, hypersensitivity, burning, stinging, erythema, and rash; patients **must** launder all clothing and bedding.

Phenobarbital: barbiturate; *status epilepticus: loading dose:* 15-20 mg/kg/dose IV X 1, may administer additional 5 mg/kg doses q15-30 minutes up to a **total maximum** of 30 mg/kg, *maintenance dose (PO/IV):* 1-5 yr: 6-8 mg/kg/day ÷ QD-BID, 6-12 yr: 4-6 mg/kg/day ÷ QD-BID, > 12 yr: 1-3 mg/kg/day ÷ QD-BID; *sedation:* 6 mg/kg/day PO ÷ TID; *pre-op sedation:* 1-3 mg/kg/dose PO/IV/IM X 1 given 60-90 minutes prior to procedure. *Comments:* monitor levels (therapeutic range: 15-40 mg/L); induces liver enzymes to enhance the elimination of hepatically metabolized drugs (ie, anticonvulsants);

may cause respiratory depression, hypotension, irritability, & insomnia.

Phenytoin: anticonvulsant; *status epilepticus: loading dose:* 15-20 mg/kg IV X 1, *maintenance dose:* (all doses divided q8-12h) *6 mon- 3 yr:* 8-10 mg/kg/day, *4-6 yr:* 7.5-9 mg/kg/day, *7-9 yr:* 7-8 mg/kg/day, *10-16 yr:* 6-7 mg/kg/day. *Comments:* monitor levels (therapeutic range: 10-20 mg/L of free & bound drug, 1-2 mg/L of free drug); need to asses serum albumin because drug is 90% bound to albumin, low albumin increases free fraction; **do not** administer IV dosage form at a rate > 1 mg/kg/min; may cause gingival hyperplasia, hirsutism, dermatitis, Stevens-Johnson syndrome, nystagmus, & liver toxicity; **contraindicated** in heart block or sinus bradycardia.

Phosphorus Supplements: phosphorus; *hypophosphatemia: acute IV dosing:* 5-10 mg/kg/dose over 6 hours; *maintenance therapy: IV dosing:* 15-45 mg/kg/day ÷ QD-BID, *PO dosing:* 30-90 mg/kg/day ÷ QD-BID. *Comments:* 31 mg is equivalent to 1 mM; **maximum** IV infusion rate is 0.2 mM/kg/hr; be aware of additional amounts of sodium and potassium (phosphorus products come in sodium and/or potassium salts); may cause tetany, hyperkalemia, & hypocalcemia; IV use may cause hypotension, renal failure, or myocardial infarction.

Piperacillin: extended spectrum penicillin; *general dose:* 200-300 mg/kg/day IV/IM ÷ q4-6h; *cystic fibrosis:* 350-600 mg/kg/day IV/IM ÷ q4-6h; (**max dose** for all use: 24 gm/day). *Comments:* good pseudomonal activity; see penicillin for adverse effects; reduce dosage in renal failure; may also cause fever, myoclonus, & seizures.

Piperacillin/Tazobactam: extended spectrum penicillin with beta-lactamase inhibitor; *general dose & cystic fibrosis:* see piperacillin (base all doses on piperacillin component). *Comments:* tazobactam extends the spectrum with good staph. activity; adjust dosage in renal failure; see piperacillin for adverse effects.

Potassium Supplements: potassium salts; *hypokalemia: PO dosing:* 1-4 mEq/kg/day ÷ BID-QID, *IV dosing:* 0.5-1 mEq/kg/dose administered at a rate of 0.5 mEq/kg/hr X 1-2 hours (**maximum IV infusion rate [only in critical situations]:** 1 mEq/kg/ hr). *Comments:* monitor serum potassium; oral administration may cause GI irritation and ulceration; IV administration may cause phlebitis, pain & irritation at injection site; patient receiving infusions at a rate > 0.5 mEq/kg/hr should be placed on a cardiac monitor.

Prednisolone: corticosteroid; *acute asthma:* 1-2 mg/kg/day PO ÷ QD-BID X 3-5 days (**max dose:** 80 mg/day); *anti-inflammatory/ immunosuppressive:* 0.5-2 mg/kg/day PO ÷ QD-QID. *Comments:* see dexamethasone for adverse effects; use methylprednisolone in the presence of hepatic disease.

Prednisone: corticosteroid; *acute asthma:* see prednisolone; *anti-inflammatory/ immunosuppressive:* see prednisolone. *Comments:* see prednisolone.

Prochlorperazine: phenothiazine, antiemetic; *antiemetic:* > 10 kg or > 2 yr: 0.4 mg/kg/day PO/PR ÷ TID-QID or 0.1-0.15 mg/kg/dose IM TID-QID (**max IM dose:** 40 mg/day). *Comments:* **do not** use IV route of administration; use **only** for vomiting of known etiology; may cause extrapyramidal reactions, orthostatic hypotension, & lower seizure threshold.

Prostaglandin E₁: see Alprostadil

Propranolol: beta adrenergic blocker; *hypertension:* start with 0.5-1 mg/kg/day PO ÷ q6-12h, increase dose q3-5 days PRN (**max dose:** 8 mg/kg/day); *migraine prophylaxis:* < 35 kg: 10-20 mg PO TID, ≥ 35 kg: 20-40 mg PO TID; *tetralogy spells: IV dosing:* 0.15-0.25 mg/kg/dose slow IV push, repeat X 1 PRN, *PO dosing:* 4-8 mg/kg/day ÷ q6h PRN. *Comments:* may cause

hypoglycemia, hypotension, nausea, vomiting, depression, impotence, bronchospasm, & heart block; **contraindicated** in asthma & heart block; use with **caution** in heart, liver, or renal failure; **drug interactions:** increased propranolol effect may occur with concomitant use of cimetidine, hydralazine, chlorpromazine, or verapamil.

Protamine Sulfate: heparin antidote; *IV dosing:* 1 mg will neutralize 115 units porcine intestinal or 90 units beef lung heparin, *if heparin administered immediately:* give 1-1.5 times above dose; *if heparin administered within 0.5-1 hr:* give 50% of above dose; *if heparin administered > 2 hours:* give 25% of above dose (**max dose:** 50 mg IV). *Comments:* may cause hypotension, bradycardia, dyspnea and anaphylaxis; monitor APTT or ACT.

Pyrethrins: pediculicide; *pediculosis:* apply to hair or affected area and leave in place for 10 minutes then wash thoroughly, may repeat dose in 7-10 days. *Comments:* **only** for topical use; **avoid** contact with eyes, face, or mouth; **do not** repeat administration in less than 24 hours.

Ranitidine: histamine H₂ antagonist; *PO dosing:* 4-5 mg/kg/day ÷ q8-12h; *IV/IM dosing:* 2-4 mg/kg/day ÷ q6-8h. *Comments:* may cause headache, malaise, insomnia, sedation, arthralgia, & hepatotoxicity.

Ribavirin: antiviral agent; *RSV infection:* administer 6 gm diluted in 300 ml preservative-free sterile water over a 12-18 hour period daily for 3-7 days. *Comments:* administer dose with a Viratek small particle aerosol generator (SPAG-2); may cause worsening of respiratory distress, bronchospasm, hypotension, anemia, and cardiac arrest.

Rifampin: antituberculosis agent, antibiotic; *tuberculosis:* 10-20 mg/kg/day PO/IV ÷ q12-24h **or** 10-20 mg/kg/day PO/IV as a single dose twice weekly (**max dose:** 600 mg/day); *prophylaxis for N meningitidis:* 0-1 mon: 10 mg/kg/day PO ÷ q12h X 2 days, > 1 mon: 20 mg/kg/day PO ÷ q12h X 2 days (**max dose for all ages:** 1200 mg/day). *Comments:* may cause GI irritation, allergic reactions, headache, fever, confusion, ataxia, hepatitis, blood dyscrasias, increased BUN & uric acid, and red discoloration of body secretions; **drug interactions:** may reduce effect of oral contraceptives, digoxin, corticosteroids, and theophylline.

Senna: stimulant laxative; *PO dosing:* 10-20 mg/kg/dose PO QHS (**max dose:** 1 mon - 1 yr: 218 mg/day; 1-5 yr: 436 mg/day; 5-15 yr: 872 mg/day); *PR dosing:* > 27 kg: 326 mg (0.5 suppository) QHS, adult: 652 mg QHS. *Comments:* onset of action within 6-24 hours after oral administration; may cause nausea, vomiting, diarrhea, & abdominal cramps.

Spironolactone: potassium-sparing diuretic; *diuretic:* 1-3.3 mg/kg/day PO ÷ BID-QID. *Comments:* may cause hyperkalemia, GI distress, rash, & gynecomastia; **contraindicated** in acute renal failure.

Succimer (DMSA): chelating agent; *lead chelation:* 10 mg/kg/dose **or** 350 mg/m²/dose PO q8h X 5-7 days, then 10 mg/kg/dose **or** 350 mg/m²/dose PO q12h X 14-21 days. *Comments:* monitor lead levels; GI distress, increased liver function tests, rash, headaches, dizziness, flu-like symptoms.

Sucralfate: anti-ulcer agent; 40-80 mg/kg/day PO ÷ q6h. *Comments:* may cause vertigo, constipation, dry mouth; contains aluminum and may accumulate in patients in renal failure; **drug interactions:** decreases absorption of phenytoin, digoxin, theophylline, cimetidine, ketoconazole, and oral anticoagulants.

Sulfacetamide Sodium: sulfonamide antibiotic; *ophthalmic ointment:* apply ribbon to conjunctival sac QID & QHS; *ophthalmic drops:* 1-2 drops to affected eye q2-3h. *Comments:* may cause stinging, local irritation, burning, & toxic necrolysis; 10% ophthalmic drops are most commonly used.

Sulfisoxazole: sulfonamide antibiotic; *> 2 months:* 75 mg/kg/dose PO X 1, followed by 150 mg/kg/day PO ÷ q4-6h (**max dose:** 6 gm/day). *Comments:* may cause photosensitivity, blood dyscrasias, CNS changes, nausea, vomiting, anorexia, diarrhea, and hemolysis in patients with G6PD deficiency; use with **caution** in infants < 2 months & renal or liver disease; **drug interactions:** enhances effects of oral anticoagulants.

Tetracycline: antibiotic; *> 9 yrs:* 25-50 mg/kg/day PO ÷ q6h (**max dose:** 2 gm/day). *Comments:* not recommended for children < 9 years old because of staining of teeth and decreased bone growth; may cause nausea, GI upset, hepatotoxicity, stomatitis, rash, photosensitivity, fever, & superinfection; **avoid** concomitant administration with dairy products or divalent cations.

Theophylline: methylxanthine derivative, bronchodilator; *bronchospasm: loading doses:* 1 mg/kg/dose for every 2 mg/L increase in serum theophylline level; *maintenance dose: < 45 kg:* start with 12-14 mg/kg/day PO ÷ q4-6h (immediate release products) **or** QD-TID (sustained release products, check specific product) up to **max** of 300 mg/day, if needed, gradually increase to 16-20 mg/kg/day PO (**max dose:** 600 mg/day); *≥ 45 kg:* start with 300 mg/day PO ÷ q6-8h (immediate release products) **or** QD-TID (sustained release products, check specific product), if needed gradually increase to 400-600 mg/day. *Comments:* monitor levels (bronchospasm: 10-20 mg/L); may cause nausea, vomiting, insomnia, abdominal pain, GE reflux, tachycardia, nervousness, seizures, & arrhythmias; **drug interactions:** allopurinol, alcohol, ciprofloxacin, cimetidine, clarithromycin, disulfiram, erythromycin, estrogen, propranolol, thiabendazole & verapamil can all increase theophylline levels; carbamazepine, isoproterenol, phenobarbital, phenytoin, & rifampin can all decrease theophylline levels.

Ticarcillin: extended spectrum penicillin; *general dose:* 200-300 mg/kg/day IV/IM ÷ q4-6h; *cystic fibrosis:* 300-600 mg/kg/day IV/IM ÷ q4-6h; (**max dose** for all use: 24 gm/day). *Comments:* provides good pseudomonal activity; reduce dosage in renal failure; may also cause decrease in platelet aggregation, bleeding diathesis, hypernatremia, hematuria, & hypokalemia.

Ticarcillin/Clavulante: extended spectrum penicillin with beta-lactamase inhibitor; *general dose & cystic fibrosis:* see ticarcillin (base all doses on ticarcillin component) (**max dose** for all use: 18-24 gm/day). *Comments:* clavulanate extends the spectrum with good *S aureus* & *H influenzae* activity; adjust dosage in renal failure; see ticarcillin for adverse effects.

Tobramycin: aminoglycoside antibiotic; *IV/IM dosing:* 6-7.5 mg/kg/day ÷ q8h; *ophthalmic drops:* 1-2 drops to affected eye q4h; *ophthalmic ointment:* apply to conjunctival sac of affected eye BID-TID. *Comments:* monitor serum levels (peak: 6-10 mg/L general, 8-10 mg/L for pulmonary infections, neutropenia, severe sepsis; trough: < 2 mg/L); may cause nephrotoxity & ototoxicity; adjust dose in renal failure; enhanced elimination of drug with burn, cystic fibrosis, & febrile neutropenic patients; risk for ototoxicity is increased with concomitant use of a loop diuretic.

Tolnaftate: antifungal agent; *tinea pedis, tinea cruris, tinea capitis & tinea manuum:* apply 1-2 drops of the solution or small amount of gel, liquid, or powder to affected area BID X 2-6 weeks. *Comments:* **do not** use for nail or scalp infections; may cause mild irritation & stinging.

Triamcinolone: corticosteroid; *PO inhalation: 6-12 yr:* 1-2 puffs TID-QID (**max dose:** 12 puffs/day), *> 12 yr:* 2 puffs TID-QID (**max dose:** 16 puffs/day); *intranasal use: ≥ 12 yr:* start with 2 sprays per nostril QD, may be increased to 4 sprays per nostril per day ÷ QD-QID; *topical use:* apply to affected areas QD-TID. *Comments:* gargle & rinse mouth with water after each use of oral inhaler dosage form; oral inhaler may cause oral candidiasis, dry throat & mouth; nasal dosage form may cause burning or stinging; topical use may cause dermal atrophy, telangiectasias, & hypopigmentation.

Ursodiol: gallstone solubilizing agent; *PO dosing:* 10-15 mg/kg/day ÷ TID. *Comments:* actual dissolution of gallstones may take several months; may cause GI disturbances, rash, arthralgias, & increase in liver enzymes; **drug interactions:** efficacy may be decreased with concomitant use of aluminum-containing antacids, cholestyramine, or oral contraceptives.

Valproic Acid: anticonvulsant: *PO dosing:* start with 10-15 mg/kg/day ÷ QD-TID then increase by 5-10 mg/kg/day at weekly intervals to a **maximum** of 60 mg/kg/day (usual maintenance dose is at 30-60 mg/kg/day, higher doses may be needed with concomitant use of other anticonvulsants); *PR dosing:* use the same oral dose by diluting the syrup dosage form with equal parts in volume (1:1) with water. *Comments:* monitor levels (therapeutic range: 50-100 mg/L); may cause GI, liver, & blood toxicities, weight gain, transient alopecia, vomiting, hyperammonemia, and rash; **drug interactions:** valproic acid increases the levels of phenytoin, diazepam, and phenobarbital; phenytoin, phenobarbital, and carbamazepine may decrease valproic levels.

Vancomycin: antibiotic; *general IV use:* 40 mg/kg/day IV ÷ q6h; *meningitis:* 60 mg/kg/day IV ÷ q6h; *C difficile colitis:* 40-50 mg/kg/day PO ÷ q6h X 7-10 days (**max PO dose:** 500 mg/day). *Comments:* may cause histamine mediated "Redman syndrome" especially if IV dose is rapidly infused (use diphenhydramine to reverse); recommended IV infusion rate is 1-2 hours; has been associated with ototoxcity & nephrotoxicity; monitor levels (peak: 25-40 mg/L, trough: 5-10 mg/L); consider alternative agents due to the prevalence of vancomycin resistant enterococcus (ie, consider metronidazole before vancomycin for *C difficile* colitis).

Warfarin: anticoagulant; *PO dosing:* start at 0.1 mg/kg/dose PO QD and adjust dose to achieve desired INR or PT (usual maintenance dose: 0.05-0.34 mg/kg/day). *Comments:* monitor INR after 5-7 days of new dosage; **recommended INR's:** DVT prophylaxis & treatment, pulmonary emboli, & prosthetic heart valves is at 2-3; mechanical prosthetic heart valves & prevention of recurrent systemic emboli is at 2.5-3.5; may cause fever, skin lesions, nausea, vomiting, hemorrhage, & diarrhea; **drug interactions:** chloramphenicol, cimetidine, fluconazole, metronidazole, indomethacin, aspirin, & sulfonamides may increase warfarin's effect; carbamazepine corticosteroids, chloral hydrate, griseofulvin, oral contraceptives, & vitamin K may decrease warfarin's effect; vitamin K and fresh frozen plasma is the antidote for toxicity.

Zidovudine (AZT): antiviral agent; *PO dosing: 3 mon - 12 yr:* 90-180 mg/m^2/day PO ÷ q6h (**max dose:** 200 mg/dose q6h), *> 12 yr (symptomatic):* 200 mg/dose q4h X 1 month then 100 mg/dose q4h, *> 12 yr (asymptomatic):* 100 mg/dose q4h while awake (500 mg/day); *IV dosing: 3 mon - 12 yr:* 100 mg/m^2/dose IV q6h, *> 12 yr:* 1-2 mg/kg/dose IV q4h; *Prevention vertical transmission: Gravid mother prior to labor during weeks 14-34 of pregnancy:* 100 mg PO 5 times per day. *Gravid mother during labor:* 2 mg/kg/dose IV over 1 hour followed by 1 mg/kg/hr IV until umbilical cord clamped. *Newborn infant:* 2 mg/kg/day PO ÷ q6h **or** 1.5 mg/kg/day IV over 1 hour ÷ q6h, start first dose within 12 hour after birth and continue for 6 weeks. *Comments:* may cause anemia, granulocytopenia, nausea, headache; use with **caution** in patients with renal or hepatic failure; **drug interactions:** drug associated with increased AZT toxicity include acyclovir, ganciclovir, and drugs that are glucurondated; **do not** administer via the IM route.

Index

Note: Page numbers followed by f indicate figures; those followed by t indicate tabular material.